Kaplan's Essentials of Cardiac Anesthesia for Cardiac Surgery

T0198044

Kaplan's Essentials of Cardiac Anesthesia for Cardiac Surgery

Second Edition

Editor

Joel A. Kaplan, MD, CPE, FACC

Professor of Anesthesiology
University of California, San Diego
La Jolla, California
Dean Emeritus
School of Medicine
Former Chancellor
Health Sciences Center
University of Louisville
Louisville, Kentucky

Associate Editors

Brett Cronin, MD

Assistant Clinical Professor
Department of Anesthesiology
University of California, San Diego
La Jolla, California

Timothy Maus, MD, FASE

Associate Clinical Professor
Director of Perioperative Echocardiography
Department of Anesthesiology
University of California, San Diego
La Jolla, California

ELSEVIER

ELSEVIER

1600 John F. Kennedy Blvd.
Ste 1800
Philadelphia, PA 19103-2899

KAPLAN'S ESSENTIALS OF CARDIAC ANESTHESIA FOR
CARDIAC SURGERY, SECOND EDITION

ISBN: 978-0-323-49798-5

Notices

Knowledge and best practice in this field are constantly changing. As new research and experience broaden our understanding, changes in research methods, professional practices, or medical treatment may become necessary.

Practitioners and researchers must always rely on their own experience and knowledge in evaluating and using any information, methods, compounds, or experiments described herein. In using such information or methods, they should be mindful of their own safety and the safety of others, including parties for whom they have a professional responsibility.

With respect to any drug or pharmaceutical products identified, readers are advised to check the most current information provided (i) on procedures featured or (ii) by the manufacturer of each product to be administered, to verify the recommended dose or formula, the method and duration of administration, and contraindications. It is the responsibility of practitioners, relying on their own experience and knowledge of their patients, to make diagnoses, to determine dosages and the best treatment for each individual patient, and to take all appropriate safety precautions.

To the fullest extent of the law, neither the Publisher nor the authors, contributors, or editors assume any liability for any injury and/or damage to persons or property as a matter of products liability, negligence, or otherwise or from any use or operation of any methods, products, instructions, or ideas contained in the material herein.

Previous edition copyrighted 2008

Library of Congress Cataloging-in-Publication Data

Names: Kaplan, Joel A., editor. | Cronin, Brett, editor. | Maus, Timothy, editor.
Title: Kaplan's essentials of cardiac anesthesia for cardiac surgery / editor,
   Joel A. Kaplan ; associate editors, Brett Cronin, Timothy Maus.
Other titles: Essentials of cardiac anesthesia. | Essentials of cardiac anesthesia
   for cardiac surgery
Description: Second edition. | Philadelphia, PA : Elsevier, [2018] | Preceded
   by Essentials of cardiac anesthesia / [edited by] Joel A. Kaplan. c2008. |
   Includes bibliographical references and index.
Identifiers: LCCN 2017042688 | ISBN 9780323497985 (pbk. : alk. paper)
Subjects: | MESH: Anesthesia | Cardiac Surgical Procedures | Heart–drug
   effects | Heart Diseases–surgery
Classification: LCC RD87.3.C37 | NLM WG 460 | DDC 617.9/6741–dc23
LC record available at https://lccn.loc.gov/2017042688

Executive Content Strategist: Dolores Meloni
Senior Content Development Specialist: Ann Anderson
Publishing Services Manager: Catherine Albright Jackson
Senior Project Manager: Doug Turner
Designer: Ryan Cook

Printed in India

Last digit is the print number: 9   8   7   6   5   4

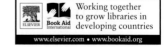

Dedication

To all of the residents and fellows in cardiac anesthesia with whom we have been fortunate to work over the past decades and to Norma, my loving wife of more than 50 years.

JAK

To my two girls, Hayley and Berkeley.

BC

To my wife, Molly, and my children, William, Owen, and Winston, for all of your love and support.

TM

Contributors

Shamsuddin Akhtar, MBBS

Associate Professor
Department of Anesthesiology and
Pharmacology
Yale University School of Medicine
New Haven, Connecticut

Sarah Armour, MD

Instructor
Anesthesiology
Mayo Clinic
Rochester, Minnesota

William R. Auger, MD

Professor of Clinical Medicine
Division of Pulmonary and Critical
Care Medicine
University of California, San Diego
La Jolla, California

John G.T. Augoustides, MD, FASE, FAHA

Professor of Anesthesiology and
Critical Care
Perelman School of Medicine
Hospital of the University of
Pennsylvania
Philadelphia, Pennsylvania

Gina C. Badescu, MD

Attending Anesthesiologist
Bridgeport Hospital
Stratford, Connecticut

James M. Bailey, MD

Medical Director
Critical Care
Northeast Georgia Health System
Gainesville, Georgia

Daniel Bainbridge, MD

Associate Professor
Department of Anesthesia and
Perioperative Medicine
Western University
London, Ontario, Canada

Dalia A. Banks, MD, FASE

Clinical Professor of Anesthesiology
Director, Cardiac Anesthesia
University of California, San Diego
La Jolla, California

Manish Bansal, MD, DNB CARDIOLOGY, FACC, FASE

Senior Consultant
Department of Cardiology
Medanta—The Medicity
Gurgaon, Haryana, India

Paul G. Barash, MD

Professor
Department of Anesthesiology
Yale University School of Medicine
New Haven, Connecticut

Victor C. Baum, MD

US Food and Drug Administration
Silver Spring, Maryland
Departments of Anesthesiology and
Critical Care Medicine and Pediatrics
George Washington University
Washington, District of Columbia

Elliott Bennett-Guerrero, MD

Professor and Vice Chair
Clinical Research and Innovation
Department of Anesthesiology
Stony Brook University School of
Medicine
Stony Brook, New York

Dan E. Berkowitz, MD

Professor
Anesthesiology and Critical Care
Medicine
Division of Cardiothoracic Anesthesia
Johns Hopkins University School of
Medicine
Baltimore, Maryland

Martin Birch, MD

Anesthesiologist and Critical Care
Physician
Hennepin County Medical Center
Minneapolis, Minnesota

Simon C. Body, MD

Associate Professor of Anesthesia
Harvard Medical School
Brigham and Women's Hospital
Boston, Massachusetts

T. Andrew Bowdle, MD, PhD, FASE

Professor of Anesthesiology and
Pharmaceutics
University of Washington
Seattle, Washington

Charles E. Chambers, MD

Professor of Medicine and Radiology
Heart and Vascular Institute
Penn State Hershey Medical Center
Hershey, Pennsylvania

Mark A. Chaney, MD

Professor and Director of Cardiac
Anesthesia
Anesthesia and Critical Care
The University of Chicago
Chicago, Illinois

Alan Cheng, MD

Adjunct Associate Professor
Johns Hopkins University School of
Medicine
Baltimore, Maryland

Davy C.H. Cheng, MD, MSC

Distinguished University Professor
and Chair
Department of Anesthesia and
Perioperative Medicine
Western University
London, Ontario, Canada

Albert T. Cheung, MD

Professor
Department of Anesthesiology
Stanford University School of
Medicine
Stanford, California

Joanna Chikwe, MD

Professor of Surgery
Co-Director, Heart Institute
Chief, Cardiothoracic Surgery Division
Stony Brook University School of
Medicine
Stony Brook, New York

David J. Cook, MD

Emeritus Professor of Anesthesiology
Mayo Clinic
Rochester, Minnesota
Chief Clinical and Operating Officer
Jiahui Health
Shanghai, China

Ryan C. Craner, MD

Senior Associate Consultant
Anesthesiology
Mayo Clinic
Phoenix, Arizona

Duncan G. de Souza, MD, FRCPC

Clinical Assistant Professor
Department of Anesthesiology
University of British Columbia
Vancouver, British Columbia, Canada
Director
Cardiac Anesthesia
Kelowna General Hospital
Kelowna, British Columbia, Canada

Patrick A. Devaleria, MD

Consultant
Cardiac Surgery
Mayo Clinic
Phoenix, Arizona

Marcel E. Durieux, MD, PhD

Professor
Departments of Anesthesiology and
Neurosurgery
University of Virginia
Charlottesville, Virginia

Harvey L. Edmonds, Jr., PhD

Professor Emeritus
Department of Anesthesia and
Perioperative Medicine
University of Louisville
Louisville, Kentucky

Joerg Karl Ender, MD

Director
Department of Anesthesiology
Intensive Care Medicine Heart Center
Leipzig, Germany

Daniel T. Engelman, MD

Inpatient Medical Director
Heart and Vascular Center
Baystate Medical Center
Springfield, Massachusetts
Assistant Professor
Department of Surgery
Tufts University School of Medicine
Boston, Massachusetts

Liza J. Enriquez, MD

Anesthesiology Attending
St. Joseph's Regional Medical Center
Paterson, New Jersey

Jared W. Feinman, MD

Assistant Professor
Department of Anesthesiology and
Critical Care
Hospital of the University of
Pennsylvania
Philadelphia, Pennsylvania

David Fitzgerald, MPH, CCP

Clinical Coordinator
Division of Cardiovascular Perfusion
College of Health Professions
Medical University of South Carolina
Charleston, South Carolina

Suzanne Flier, MD, MSC

Assistant Professor
Schulich School of Medicine
University of Western Ontario
London, Ontario, Canada

Amanda A. Fox, MD, MPH

Vice Chair of Clinical and
Translational Research
Associate Professor
Department of Anesthesiology and
Pain Management
Associate Professor
McDermott Center for Human
Growth and Development
University of Texas Southwestern
Medical Center
Dallas, Texas

Jonathan F. Fox, MD

Instructor
Anesthesiology
Mayo Clinic
Rochester, Minnesota

Julie K. Freed, MD, PhD

Assistant Professor of Anesthesiology
Medical College of Wisconsin
Milwaukee, Wisconsin

Leon Freudzon, MD

Assistant Professor
Department of Anesthesiology
Yale University School of Medicine
New Haven, Connecticut

Valentin Fuster, MD, PhD, MACC

Physician-in-Chief
The Mount Sinai Medical Center
Director
Zena and Michael A. Wiener
Cardiovascular Institute and Marie-Josee and Henry Kravis Center for
Cardiovascular Health
New York, New York
Director
Centro Nacional de Investigaciones
Cardiovasculare
Madrid, Spain

Theresa A. Gelzinis, MD

Associate Professor of Anesthesiology
Department of Anesthesiology
University of Pittsburgh
Pittsburgh, Pennsylvania

Kamrouz Ghadimi, MD

Assistant Professor
Cardiothoracic Anesthesiology and
Critical Care Medicine
Department of Anesthesiology
Duke University School of Medicine
Durham, North Carolina

Emily K. Gordon, MD

Assistant Professor
Department of Anesthesiology and
Critical Care
Perelman School of Medicine
Hospital of the University of
Pennsylvania
Philadelphia, Pennsylvania

Leanne Groban, MD

Professor
Director, Cardiac Aging Lab
Department of Anesthesiology
Wake Forest School of Medicine
Winston-Salem, North Carolina

Hilary P. Grocott, MD, FRCPC, FASE

Professor
Departments of Anesthesia and
Surgery
University of Manitoba
Winnipeg, Manitoba, Canada

Robert C. Groom, MS, CCP, FPP

Director of Cardiovascular Perfusion
Cardiovascular Services
Maine Medical Center
Portland, Maine

Jacob T. Gutsche, MD

Assistant Professor
Cardiothoracic and Vascular Section
Anesthesiology and Critical Care
Perelman School of Medicine
University of Pennsylvania
Philadelphia, Pennsylvania

Nadia Hensley, MD

Assistant Professor
Department of Anesthesiology and
Critical Care Medicine
Johns Hopkins University School of
Medicine
Baltimore, Maryland

Benjamin Hibbert, MD, PhD

Assistant Professor
CAPITAL Research Group
Department of Cardiology
University of Ottawa Heart Institute
Ottawa, Ontario, Canada

Thomas L. Higgins, MD, MBA

Chief Medical Officer
Baystate Franklin Medical Center
Greenfield, Massachusetts
Chief Medical Officer
Baystate Noble Hospital
Westfield, Massachusetts
Professor
Department of Medicine, Anesthesia,
and Surgery
Tufts University School of Medicine
Boston, Massachusetts

Joseph Hinchey, MD, PhD

Cardiac Anesthesia Fellow
Anesthesiology
The Mount Sinai Hospital
New York, New York

Charles W. Hogue, MD

James E. Eckenhoff Professor of
Anesthesiology
Northwestern University
Feinberg School of Medicine
Bluhm Cardiovascular Institute
Chicago, Illinois

Jay Horrow, MD, FAHA

Professor of Anesthesiology,
Physiology, and Pharmacology
Drexel University College of Medicine
Philadelphia, Pennsylvania

Philippe R. Housmans, MD, PhD

Professor
Anesthesiology
Mayo Clinic
Rochester, Minnesota

Ronald A. Kahn, MD

Professor
Department of Anesthesiology and
Surgery
Icahn School of Medicine at Mount
Sinai
New York, New York

Joel A. Kaplan, MD, CPE, FACC

Professor of Anesthesiology
University of California, San Diego
La Jolla, California
Dean Emeritus
School of Medicine
Former Chancellor
Health Sciences Center
University of Louisville
Louisville, Kentucky

Keyvan Karkouti, MD, FRCPC, MSC

Professor
Department of Anesthesia
Assistant Professor
Department of Health Policy,
Management, and Evaluation
University of Toronto
Scientist
Toronto General Research Institute
Deputy Anesthesiologist-in-Chief
Anesthesia
Toronto General Hospital
Toronto, Ontario, Canada

Colleen G. Koch, MD, MS, MBA

Mark C. Rogers Professor and Chair
Department of Anesthesiology and
Critical Care Medicine
Johns Hopkins University School of
Medicine
Baltimore, Maryland

Mark Kozak, MD

Associate Professor of Medicine
Heart and Vascular Institute
Penn State Hershey Medical Center
Hershey, Pennsylvania

Laeben Lester, MD

Assistant Professor
Anesthesiology and Critical Care
Medicine
Division of Cardiothoracic
Anesthesiology
Johns Hopkins University School of
Medicine
Baltimore, Maryland

Jerrold H. Levy, MD, FAHA, FCCM

Professor and Co-Director
Cardiothoracic Intensive Care Unit
Department of Anesthesiology,
Critical Care, and Surgery
Duke University School of Medicine
Durham, North Carolina

Warren J. Levy, MD

Associate Professor
Department of Anesthesiology and
Critical Care
Perelman School of Medicine
Hospital of the University of
Pennsylvania
Philadelphia, Pennsylvania

Adair Q. Locke, MD

Assistant Professor
Department of Anesthesiology
Wake Forest School of Medicine
Winston-Salem, North Carolina

Martin J. London, MD

Professor of Clinical Anesthesia
University of California, San Francisco
Veterans Affairs Medical Center
San Francisco, California

Monica I. Lupei, MD

Assistant Professor of Anesthesiology
and Critical Care Medicine
Department of Anesthesiology
University of Minnesota
Minneapolis, Minnesota

Michael M. Madani, MD

Professor of Cardiovascular and
Thoracic Surgery
University of California, San Diego
La Jolla, California

Timothy Maus, MD, FASE

Associate Clinical Professor
Director of Perioperative
Echocardiography
Department of Anesthesiology
University of California, San Diego
La Jolla, California

Nanhi Mitter, MD

Physician Specialist in Anesthesia
Clinical Anesthesiologist
Emory St. Joseph's Hospital of Atlanta
Atlanta, Georgia

Alexander J.C. Mittnacht, MD

Professor of Anesthesiology
Icahn School of Medicine at Mount
Sinai
Director, Pediatric Cardiac Anesthesia
Department of Anesthesiology
The Mount Sinai Medical Center
New York, New York

Christina T. Mora-Mangano, MD

Professor
Department of Anesthesiology,
Perioperative, and Pain Medicine
(Cardiac)
Stanford University Medical Center
Stanford, California

Benjamin N. Morris, MD

Assistant Professor
Department of Anesthesiology
Wake Forest School of Medicine
Winston-Salem, North Carolina

J. Paul Mounsey, BM BCH, PhD, FRCP, FACC

Sewell Family/McAllister Distinguished
Professor
Director, Electrophysiology
Department of Cardiology
University of North Carolina
Chapel Hill, North Carolina

John M. Murkin, MD, FRCPC

Professor of Anesthesiology (Senate)
Schulich School of Medicine
University of Western Ontario
London, Ontario, Canada

Andrew W. Murray, MBCHB

Assistant Professor
Anesthesiology and Perioperative
Medicine
Mayo Clinic
Phoenix, Arizona

Jagat Narula, MD, PhD, MACC

Philip J. and Harriet L. Goodhart
Chair in Cardiology
Chief of the Divisions of Cardiology
Mount Sinai West and St. Luke's
Hospitals
Associate Dean
Arnhold Institute for Global Health at
Mount Sinai
Professor of Medicine and Radiology
Icahn School of Medicine at Mount
Sinai
Director, Cardiovascular Imaging
Mount Sinai Health System
New York, New York

Howard J. Nathan, MD

Professor
Department of Anesthesiology
University of Ottawa
Ottawa, Ontario, Canada

Liem Nguyen, MD

Associate Clinic Professor
Department of Anesthesiology
UC San Diego Medical Center
La Jolla, California

Nancy A. Nussmeier, MD, FAHA

Physician
Department of Anesthesia, Critical
Care, and Pain Medicine
Massachusetts General Hospital
Boston, Massachusetts

Gregory A. Nuttall, MD

Professor
Anesthesiology
Mayo Clinic
Rochester, Minnesota

Daniel Nyhan, MD

Professor
Anesthesiology and Critical Care
Medicine
Division of Cardiothoracic Anesthesia
Johns Hopkins University School of
Medicine
Baltimore, Maryland

Edward R. O'Brien, MD

Professor
Department of Cardiology
Libin Cardiovascular Institute
University of Calgary
Calgary, Alberta, Canada

William C. Oliver, Jr., MD

Professor
Anesthesiology
Mayo Clinic
Rochester, Minnesota

Paul S. Pagel, MD, PhD

Professor of Anesthesiology
Medical College of Wisconsin
Clement J. Zablocki VA Medical
Center
Milwaukee, Wisconsin

Enrique J. Pantin, MD

Associate Professor
Department of Anesthesiology
Robert Wood Johnson University
Hospital
New Brunswick, New Jersey

Prakash A. Patel, MD

Assistant Professor
Department of Anesthesiology and
Critical Care
University of Pennsylvania
Philadelphia, Pennsylvania

John D. Puskas, MD

Professor of Cardiothoracic Surgery
Icahn School of Medicine at Mt. Sinai
New York, New York

Joseph J. Quinlan, MD

Professor
Department of Anesthesiology
University of Pittsburgh
Pittsburgh, Pennsylvania

CONTRIBUTORS

Harish Ramakrishna, MD, FASE, FACC

Professor of Anesthesiology
Vice Chair-Research and Chair
Division of Cardiovascular and
Thoracic Anesthesiology
Department of Anesthesiology
Mayo Clinic
Phoenix, Arizona

James G. Ramsay, MD, PhD

Professor of Anesthesiology
Medical Director
CT Surgery ICU
Department of Anesthesiology and
Perioperative Care
University of California, San Francisco
San Francisco, California

Kent H. Rehfeldt, MD, FASE

Associate Professor of Anesthesiology
Fellowship Director
Adult Cardiothoracic Anesthesiology
Mayo Clinic
Rochester, Minnesota

David L. Reich, MD

President and Chief Operating Officer
The Mount Sinai Hospital
Horace W. Goldsmith Professor of
Anesthesiology
Icahn School of Medicine at Mount
Sinai
New York, New York

Amanda J. Rhee, MD

Associate Professor
Department of Anesthesiology,
Perioperative and Pain Medicine
Medical Director of Patient Safety
Office for Excellence in Patient Care
Icahn School of Medicine at Mount
Sinai
New York, New York

David M. Roth, MD, PhD

Professor
Department of Anesthesiology
University of California, San Diego
San Diego, California

Roger L. Royster, MD

Professor and Executive Vice-Chair
Department of Anesthesiology
Wake Forest School of Medicine
Winston-Salem, North Carolina

Marc A. Rozner, PhD, MD

Professor
Anesthesiology and Perioperative
Medicine and Cardiology
University of Texas MD Anderson
Cancer Center
Houston, Texas

Ivan Salgo, MD, MBA

Senior Director
Global Cardiology
Philips Ultrasound
Andover, Massachusetts

Michael Sander, MD

Professor
Department of Anesthesiology
Director
Anesthesiology and Intensive Care
Medicine Clinic
Charite Campus Mitte
Universitätsmedizin Berlin
Berlin, Germany

Joseph S. Savino, MD

Professor
Department of Anesthesiology and
Critical Care
Hospital of the University of
Pennsylvania
Philadelphia, Pennsylvania

John Schindler, MD

Assistant Professor of Medicine
Cardiology
University of Pittsburgh Medical
Center
Pittsburgh, Pennsylvania

Partho P. Sengupta, MD, DM, FACC, FASE

Professor of Medicine
Director of Interventional
Echocardiography
Cardiac Ultrasound Research and
Core Lab
The Zena and Michael A. Weiner
Cardiovascular Institute
Icahn School of Medicine at
Mount Sinai
New York, New York

Ashish Shah, MD

Professor of Surgery
Department of Cardiac Surgery
Vanderbilt University Medical Center
Nashville, Tennessee

Jack S. Shanewise, MD

Professor
Department of Anesthesiology
Columbia University College of
Physicians and Surgeons
New York, New York

Sonal Sharma, MD

Attending Anesthesiologist
Department of Anesthesiology
St. Elizabeth Medical Center
Utica, New York

Benjamin Sherman, MD

Staff Cardiothoracic Anesthesiologist
TeamHealth Anesthesia
Portland, Oregon

Stanton K. Shernan, MD

Head, Cardiac Anesthesia
Brigham & Women's Hospital
Boston, Massachusetts

Linda Shore-Lesserson, MD

Professor
Department of Anesthesiology
Hofstra Northwell School of Medicine
Hempstead, New York

Trevor Simard, MD

Clinical Research Fellow
CAPITAL Research Group
Department of Cardiology
University of Ottawa Heart Institute
Ottawa, Ontario, Canada

Thomas F. Slaughter, MD

Professor and Section Head
Cardiothoracic Anesthesiology
Department of Anesthesiology
Wake Forest School of Medicine
Winston-Salem, North Carolina

Mark M. Smith, MD

Assistant Professor
Anesthesiology
Mayo Clinic
Rochester, Minnesota

Bruce D. Spiess, MD, FAHA

Professor and Associate Chair for
Research Anesthesiology
University of Florida College of
Medicine
Gainesville, Florida

Mark Stafford-Smith, MD, CM, FRCPC, FASE

Professor
Director of Fellowship Education and
Adult Cardiothoracic Anesthesia
Department of Anesthesiology
Duke University Medical Center
Durham, North Carolina

Marc E. Stone, MD

Professor and Program Director
Fellowship in Cardiothoracic
Anesthesiology
Department of Anesthesiology
Icahn School of Medicine at Mount
Sinai
New York, New York

Joyce A. Wahr, MD, FAHA

Professor of Anesthesiology
University of Minnesota
Minneapolis, Minnesota

Michael Wall, MD, FCCM

JJ Buckley Professor and Chair
Department of Anesthesiology
University of Minnesota
Minneapolis, Minnesota

Menachem M. Weiner, MD

Associate Professor
Department of Anesthesiology
Director of Cardiac Anesthesiology
Icahn School of Medicine at Mount
Sinai
New York, New York

Julia Weinkauf, MD

Assistant Professor
Department of Anesthesiology
University of Minnesota
Minneapolis, Minnesota

Stuart J. Weiss, MD, PhD

Associate Professor
Department of Anesthesiology and
Critical Care
Hospital of the University of
Pennsylvania
Philadelphia, Pennsylvania

Nathaen Weitzel, MD

Associate Professor
Department of Anesthesiology
University of Colorado School of
Medicine
Aurora, Colorado

Richard Whitlock, MD, PhD

Associate Professor
Department of Surgery
McMaster University/Population
Health Research Institute
Hamilton, Ontario, Canada

James R. Zaidan, MD, MBA

Associate Dean
Graduate Medical Education
Emory University School of Medicine
Atlanta, Georgia

Waseem Zakaria Aziz Zakhary, MD

Senior Consultant
Department of Anesthesiology and
Intensive Care Medicine
Heart Center
Leipzig, Germany

Preface

The second edition of *Kaplan's Essentials of Cardiac Anesthesia* has been written to further improve the anesthetic management of the patient with cardiac disease undergoing cardiac surgery. This book incorporates much of the clinically relevant material from the standard reference textbook in the field, *Kaplan's Cardiac Anesthesia,* seventh edition, published in 2017. *Kaplan's Essentials of Cardiac Anesthesia* is intended primarily for the use of residents, certified registered nurse anesthetists, and anesthesiologists participating in cardiac anesthesia on a limited basis, as opposed to the larger text that is designed for the practitioner, clinical fellow, teacher, and researcher in cardiac anesthesia.

The chapters in *Kaplan's Essentials* have been written by acknowledged experts in each specific area, and the material has been coordinated to maximize its clinical value. Recent information has been integrated from the fields of anesthesiology, cardiology, cardiac surgery, critical care medicine, and clinical pharmacology to present a complete clinical picture. This "essential" information will enable the clinician to understand the basic principles of each subject and facilitate their application in practice. Because of the large volume of material presented, several teaching aids have been included to help highlight the most important clinical information. Teaching boxes have been used, which include many of the "take home messages." In addition, the Key Points at the beginning of each chapter highlight the major areas covered in the chapter. Finally, the reference list for each chapter has been replaced by a small number of key articles, from which more information can be obtained. A complete list of references for each chapter can be obtained from the larger textbook, *Kaplan's Cardiac Anesthesia,* seventh edition, along with the basic experimental data and translational medicine underlying the clinical approaches covered in *Kaplan's Essentials.*

This book has been organized into six sections:

Section I: Preoperative Assessment and Management, including diagnostic procedures and therapeutic interventions in the cardiac catheterization and electrophysiology laboratories

Section II: Cardiovascular Physiology, Pharmacology, Molecular Biology, and Genetics, including the latest material on new cardiovascular drugs

Section III: Monitoring, with an emphasis on 2D transesophageal echocardiography (TEE)

Section IV: Anesthesia for Cardiac Surgical Procedures, which covers the care of most cardiac surgical patients

Section V: Extracorporeal Circulation, with an emphasis on organ protection

Section VI: Postoperative Care, which also addresses pain management in the postoperative cardiac patient

Kaplan's Essentials of Cardiac Anesthesia should further the care of the large number of cardiac patients undergoing noncardiac surgery. Much of the information learned in the cardiac surgical patient is applicable to similar patients undergoing major or even minor noncardiac surgical procedures. Some of the same monitoring and anesthetic techniques can be used in other high-risk surgical procedures. New modalities that start in cardiac surgery, such as TEE, will eventually have wider application during noncardiac surgery. Therefore the authors believe that *Kaplan's Essentials* should be read and used by all practitioners of perioperative care.

We gratefully acknowledge the contributions made by the authors of each of the chapters. They are the clinical experts who have brought the field of cardiac anesthesia to its highly respected place at the present time. In addition, they are the teachers of our residents and students, who will carry the subspecialty forward and further improve the care for our progressively older and sicker patients.

Joel A. Kaplan, MD, CPE, FACC
Brett Cronin, MD
Timothy Maus, MD, FASE

Contents

Section III
MONITORING

Section IV
ANESTHESIA FOR CARDIAC SURGICAL PROCEDURES

Section V
EXTRACORPOREAL CIRCULATION

Section VI
POSTOPERATIVE CARE

Section I
Preoperative Assessment and Management

Chapter 1

Cardiac Risk, Imaging, and the Cardiology Consultation

Manish Bansal, MD, DNB Cardiology, FACC, FASE •
Valentin Fuster, MD, PhD, MACC • Jagat Narula, MD, PhD,
MACC • Partho P. Sengupta, MD, DM, FACC, FASE

Key Points

1. Multivariate modeling has been used to develop risk indices that focus on preoperative variables, intraoperative variables, or both.
2. Key predictors of perioperative risk are dependent on the type of cardiac operation and the outcome of interest.
3. New risk models have become available for valvular heart surgery and for combined coronary and valvular cardiac procedures.
4. Perioperative cardiac morbidity is multifactorial, and understanding the predictive risk factors helps to define the risk for individual patients.
5. Assessment of myocardial injury is based on the integration of information from myocardial imaging (eg, echocardiography), electrocardiography (ECG), and serum biomarkers, with significant variability in the diagnosis depending on the criteria selected.
6. Echocardiography is the most widely used modality for cardiac imaging in almost any form of cardiac disease.
7. Stress echocardiography is helpful in the assessment of inducible myocardial ischemia, myocardial viability, and certain valve disorders.
8. Myocardial perfusion imaging can be performed using single-photon emission computed tomography (SPECT) or positron emission tomography (PET), and is useful in the evaluation of myocardial ischemia and viability.
9. Cardiac computed tomography and cardiac magnetic resonance are increasingly used when there are conflicting results or when further information is required in the preoperative phase of care.
10. Cardiac magnetic resonance is the gold standard for quantitative assessment of ventricular volumes, ejection fraction, and mass. It is also able to evaluate ventricular and valvular function, atherosclerosis, and plaque composition.
11. Computed tomographic aortography is the best modality for the evaluation of aortic aneurysms and dissections. Additionally, computed tomographic coronary angiography offers an alternative to invasive coronary angiography for excluding significant coronary artery disease in patients undergoing noncoronary surgery.

The first risk-scoring scheme for cardiac surgery was introduced by Paiement and colleagues at the Montreal Heart Institute in 1983. Since then, many preoperative cardiac surgery risk indices have been developed. The patient characteristics that affected the probability of specific adverse outcomes were identified and weighed, and the resultant risk indices have been used to adjust for case-mix differences among surgeons and centers where performance profiles have been compiled. In addition to comparisons among centers, the preoperative cardiac risk indices have been used to counsel patients and their families in resource planning, to identify high-risk groups for special care, to determine cost-effectiveness, to determine effectiveness of interventions, to improve provider practice, and to assess costs related to severity of disease.

CARDIAC RISK ASSESSMENT AND CARDIAC RISK STRATIFICATION MODELS IN PATIENTS UNDERGOING CARDIAC SURGERY

In defining important risk factors and developing risk indices, each of the studies has used different primary outcomes. Postoperative mortality remains the most definitive outcome that is reflective of patient injury in the perioperative period. Death can be cardiac and noncardiac related, and if cardiac related, it may be ischemic or nonischemic in origin. Postoperative mortality rate is reported as either the in-hospital rate or the 30-day rate. The latter represents a more standardized definition, although it is more difficult to capture because of the difficulty inherent in assessing death rates of discharged patients who may die at home or in another facility. Risk-adjusted postoperative mortality models permit assessment of the comparative efficacy of various techniques in preventing myocardial damage, but they do not provide information that is useful in preventing the injury in real time. The postoperative mortality rate is also used as a comparative measure of equality of cardiac surgical care.

Postoperative morbidity includes acute myocardial infarction (AMI), reversible events such as congestive heart failure (CHF), and need for inotropic support. Because resource utilization has become such an important financial consideration for hospitals, the length of stay in the intensive care unit (ICU) increasingly has been used as a factor in the development of risk indices.

Predictors of Perioperative and Postoperative Morbidity and Mortality

The original risk-scoring scheme for cardiac surgery (coronary artery bypass graft [CABG] and valve) identified eight risk factors: (1) poor left ventricular (LV) function, (2) CHF, (3) unstable angina or recent myocardial infarction (MI) (within 6 weeks), (4) age greater than 65 years, (5) severe obesity (body mass index >30 kg/m^2), (6) reoperation, (7) emergency surgery, and (8) other significant or uncontrolled systemic disturbances. The investigators identified three classes of patients: those with none of the listed factors (normal), those presenting with one factor (increased risk), and those with more than one factor (high risk). In a study of 500 consecutive patients undergoing cardiac surgery, it was found that operative mortality increased with increasing risk score (confirming the scoring system).

One of the most commonly used scoring systems for CABG was developed by Parsonnet and colleagues (Table 1.1). Fourteen risk factors were identified for in-hospital

1

3

Table 1.1 Components of the Additive Model

Risk Factor	Assigned Weight
Female sex	1
Morbid obesity (≥1.5 × ideal weight)	3
Diabetes (unspecified type)	3
Hypertension (systolic BP >140 mm Hg)	3
Ejection fraction (%):	
Good >50	0
Fair (30–49)	2
Poor (<30)	4
Age (y):	
70–74	7
75–79	12
≥80	20
Reoperation	
First	5
Second	10
Preoperative IABP	2
Left ventricular aneurysm	5
Emergency surgery after PTCA or catheterization complications	10
Dialysis dependency (PD or Hemo)	10
Catastrophic states (eg, acute structural defect, cardiogenic shock, acute renal failure)[a]	10–50[b]
Other rare circumstances (eg, paraplegia, pacemaker dependency, congenital HD in adult, severe asthma)[a]	2–10[b]
Valve surgery	
Mitral	5
PA pressure ≥60 mm Hg	8
Aortic	5
Pressure gradient >120 mm Hg	7
CABG at the time of valve surgery	2

[a]On the actual worksheet, these risk factors require justification.
[b]Values were predictive of increased risk for operative mortality in univariate analysis.
BP, Blood pressure; CABG, coronary artery bypass graft; HD, heart disease; Hemo, hemodialysis; IABP, intraaortic balloon pump; PA, pulmonary artery; PD, peritoneal dialysis; PTCA, percutaneous transluminal coronary angioplasty.
From Parsonnet V, Dean D, Bernstein A. A method of uniform stratification of risk for evaluating the results of surgery in acquired adult heart disease. Circulation. 1989;79:I3, by permission.

or 30-day mortality after univariate regression on analysis of 3500 consecutive operations. An additive model was constructed and prospectively evaluated in 1332 cardiac procedures. Five categories of risk were identified with increasing mortality rates, complication rates, and length of stay. The Parsonnet Index frequently is used as the benchmark for comparison among institutions. Since publication of the Parsonnet model, numerous technical advances now in routine use have diminished CABG mortality rates.

The Society of Thoracic Surgeons (STS) National Adult Cardiac Surgery Database (NCD) (Table 1.2) represents the most robust source of data for calculating risk-adjusted scoring systems. Established in 1989, the database included 892 participating hospitals in 2008 and has continued to grow. This provider-supported database, one of the largest in the world, allows participants to benchmark their risk-adjusted results against regional and national standards. New patient data are brought into the STS database on a semiannual basis.

Table 1.2 Risk Model Results

Variable	Odds Ratio
Age (in 10-year increments)	1.640
Female sex	1.157
Race other than white	1.249
Ejection fraction	0.988
Diabetes	1.188
Renal failure	1.533
Serum creatinine (if renal failure is present)	1.080
Dialysis dependence (if renal failure is present)	1.381
Pulmonary hypertension	1.185
Cerebrovascular accident timing	1.198
Chronic obstructive pulmonary disease	1.296
Peripheral vascular disease	1.487
Cerebrovascular disease	1.244
Acute evolving, extending myocardial infarction	1.282
Myocardial infarction timing	1.117
Cardiogenic shock	2.211
Use of diuretics	1.122
Hemodynamic instability	1.747
Triple-vessel disease	1.155
Left main disease >50%	1.119
Preoperative intraaortic balloon pump	1.480
Status	
Urgent or emergent	1.189
Emergent salvage	3.654
First reoperation	2.738
Multiple reoperations	4.282
Arrhythmias	1.099
Body surface area	0.488
Obesity	1.242
New York Heart Association class IV	1.098
Use of steroids	1.214
Congestive heart failure	1.191
PTCA within 6 h of surgery	1.332
Angiographic accident with hemodynamic instability	1.203
Use of digitalis	1.168
Use of intravenous nitrates	1.088

PTCA, Percutaneous transluminal coronary angioplasty.
From Shroyer AL, Plomondon ME, Grover FL, et al. The 1996 coronary artery bypass risk model: the Society of Thoracic Surgeons Adult Cardiac National Database. *Ann Thorac Surg.* 1999;67:1205, by permission of Society of Thoracic Surgeons.

There are currently three general STS risk models: CABG, valve (aortic or mitral), and valve plus CABG. These three models comprise seven specific, precisely defined procedures: the CABG model refers to an isolated CABG; the valve model includes isolated aortic or mitral valve replacement and mitral valve repair; and the valve plus CABG model includes aortic valve replacement with CABG, mitral valve replacement with CABG, and mitral valve repair with CABG. Besides operative mortality, these models were developed for eight additional end points: reoperation, permanent stroke, renal failure, deep sternal wound infection, prolonged (>24 hours) ventilation, major morbidity, operative death, and finally short (<6 days) and long (>14 days) postoperative length of stay. These models are updated every few years and are calibrated annually to provide an immediate and accurate tool for regional and national benchmarking, and they have been proposed for public reporting. The calibration of the risk factors is based on the ratio between observed and expected result (O/E ratio), and calibration factors are updated quarterly. The expected mortality (E) is calibrated to obtain a national O/E ratio.

The European System for Cardiac Operative Risk Evaluation (EuroSCORE) is another widely used model for cardiac operative risk evaluation. It was constructed from an analysis of 19,030 patients undergoing a diverse group of cardiac surgical procedures from 128 centers across Europe (Tables 1.3 and 1.4). The following risk

Table 1.3   Risk Factors, Definitions, and Weights (Score)

Risk Factors	Definition	Score
Patient-Related Factors		
Age	Per 5 years or part thereof over 60 years	1
Sex	Female	1
Chronic pulmonary disease	Long-term use of bronchodilators or steroids for lung disease	1
Extracardiac arteriopathy	One or more of the following: claudication; carotid occlusion or >50% stenosis; previous or planned intervention on the abdominal aorta, limb arteries, or carotids	2
Neurologic dysfunction	Disease severely affecting ambulation or day-to-day functioning	2
Previous cardiac surgery	Requiring opening of the pericardium	3
Serum creatinine	>200 µmol/L before surgery	2
Active endocarditis	Patient still under antibiotic treatment for endocarditis at the time of surgery	3
Critical preoperative state	One or more of the following: ventricular tachycardia or fibrillation or aborted sudden death, preoperative cardiac massage, preoperative ventilation before arrival in the anesthesia room, preoperative inotropic support, intraaortic balloon counterpulsation or preoperative acute renal failure (anuria or oliguria <10 mL/h)	3
Cardiac-Related Factors		
Unstable angina	Rest angina requiring IV nitrates until arrival in the anesthesia room	2
Left ventricular dysfunction	Moderate or LVEF 30–50%	1
	Poor or LVEF <30%	3
	Recent myocardial infarct (<90 days)	2
Pulmonary hypertension	Systolic pulmonary artery pressure >60 mm Hg	2
Surgery-Related Factors		
Emergency	Carried out on referral before the beginning of the next working day	2
Other than isolated CABG	Major cardiac procedure other than or in addition to CABG	2
Surgery on thoracic aorta	For disorder of the ascending aorta, arch, or descending aorta	3
Postinfarct septal rupture		4

CABG, Coronary artery bypass graft surgery; *LVEF,* left ventricular ejection fraction.
From Nashef SA, Roques F, Michel P, et al. European system for cardiac operative risk evaluation (EuroSCORE). *Eur J Cardiothorac Surg.* 1999;16:9.

Table 1.4 Application of EuroSCORE Scoring System

EuroSCORE	Patients (N)	Deaths (N)	95% Confidence Limits for Mortality	
			Observed	Expected
0–2 (low risk)	4529	36 (0.8%)	0.56–1.10	1.27–1.29
3–5 (medium risk)	5977	182 (3.0%)	2.62–3.51	2.90–2.94
≥6 (high risk)	4293	480 (11.2%)	10.25–12.16	10.93–11.54
Total	14,799	698 (4.7%)	4.37–5.06	4.72–4.95

EuroSCORE, European System for Cardiac Operative Risk Evaluation.
From Nashef SA, Roques F, Michel P, et al. European system for cardiac operative risk evaluation (EuroSCORE). *Eur J Cardiothorac Surg.* 1999;16:9, by permission.

BOX 1.1 *Common Variables Associated With Increased Risk for Cardiac Surgery*

Age	Reoperation
Female sex	Type of surgery
Left ventricular function	Urgency of surgery
Body habitus	

factors were associated with increased mortality: age, female sex, elevated serum creatinine level, extracardiac arteriopathy, chronic airway disease, severe neurologic dysfunction, previous cardiac surgery, recent MI, reduced left ventricular ejection fraction (LVEF), chronic CHF, pulmonary hypertension, active endocarditis, unstable angina, procedure urgency, critical preoperative condition, ventricular septal rupture, noncoronary surgery, and thoracic aortic surgery. For a given individual, each of these risk factors is assigned a score, and the sum total of these is used to predict surgical risk. In 2003 a more sophisticated logistic version of EuroSCORE was released to permit more accurate risk assessment in individuals deemed to be at very high risk.

In 2011 the EuroSCORE was recalibrated to keep up with the new evidence. The revised EuroSCORE, known as *EuroSCORE II*, permits more accurate risk estimation yet preserves the powerful discrimination of the original model. The EuroSCORE II is currently the recommended model for assessment of cardiac surgical risk. It can be accessed online (www.euroscore.org/calc.html) or downloaded as a smartphone application.

Consistency Among Risk Indices

Many different variables have been found to be associated with the increased risk during cardiac surgery, but only a few have consistently been found to be major risk factors across multiple and very diverse study settings. Age, female sex, LV function, body habitus, reoperation, type of surgery, and urgency of surgery were among the variables consistently present in most of the models (Box 1.1).

BOX 1.2 *Medical Conditions Associated With Increased Risk*

Renal dysfunction
Diabetes (inconsistent)
Recent acute coronary syndrome

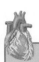

BOX 1.3 *Determinations of Perioperative Myocardial Injury*

Disruption of blood flow
Reperfusion of ischemic myocardium
Adverse systemic effects of cardiopulmonary bypass

Although a variety of investigators have found various comorbid diseases to be significant risk factors, no diseases have been shown to be consistent risk factors, with the possible exception of renal dysfunction and diabetes. These two comorbidities were shown to be important risk factors in a majority of the studies (Box 1.2).

SOURCES OF PERIOPERATIVE MYOCARDIAL INJURY IN CARDIAC SURGERY

Myocardial injury, manifested as transient cardiac contractile dysfunction ("stunning"), or AMI, or both, is the most frequent complication after cardiac surgery and the most important cause of hospital complications and death. Furthermore, patients who experience a perioperative MI have a poor long-term prognosis; only 51% of such patients remain free from adverse cardiac events after 2 years, compared with 96% of patients without perioperative MI.

Myocardial necrosis is the result of progressive pathologic ischemic changes that start to occur in the myocardium within minutes after interruption of its blood flow (eg, during cardiac surgery) (Box 1.3). The duration of the interruption of blood flow, either partial or complete, determines the extent of myocardial necrosis, and both the duration of the period of aortic cross-clamping (AXC) and the duration of cardiopulmonary bypass (CPB) have consistently been shown to be the main determinants of postoperative outcomes.

Reperfusion of Ischemic Myocardium

Surgical interventions requiring interruption of blood flow to the heart must be followed by restoration of perfusion. Reperfusion, although essential for tissue and organ survival, is not without risk because of the potential extension of cell damage as a result of reperfusion itself. Myocardial ischemia of limited duration (<20 minutes) that is followed by reperfusion leads to functional recovery without evidence of structural injury or biochemical evidence of tissue injury. However, reperfusion of cardiac tissue that has been subjected to an extended period of ischemia results in a phenomenon known as *myocardial reperfusion injury.*

Myocardial reperfusion injury is defined as the death of myocytes, which were alive at the time of reperfusion, as a direct result of one or more events initiated by reperfusion. Myocardial cell damage results from restoration of blood flow to the previously ischemic heart and extends the region of irreversible injury beyond that caused by the ischemic insult alone. The cellular damage that results from reperfusion can be reversible or irreversible, depending on the duration of the ischemic insult. If reperfusion is initiated within 20 minutes after the onset of ischemia, the resulting myocardial injury is reversible and is characterized functionally by depressed myocardial contractility, which eventually recovers completely. Myocardial tissue necrosis is not detectable in the previously ischemic region, although functional impairment of contractility may persist for a variable period, a phenomenon known as *myocardial stunning.* Initiation of reperfusion after longer than 20 minutes, however, results in escalating degrees of irreversible myocardial injury or cellular necrosis. The extent of tissue necrosis that develops during reperfusion is directly related to the duration of the ischemic event. Tissue necrosis originates in the subendocardial region of the ischemic myocardium and extends to the subepicardial region of the area at risk; this is often referred to as the *wavefront phenomenon.* The cell death that occurs during reperfusion can be characterized microscopically by explosive swelling, which includes disruption of the tissue lattice, contraction bands, mitochondrial swelling, and calcium phosphate deposition within mitochondria.

Adverse Systemic Effects of Cardiopulmonary Bypass

In addition to the effects of disruption and restoration of myocardial blood flow, cardiac morbidity may result from systemic insults due to CPB circuit–induced contact activation. Inflammation in cardiac surgical patients is produced by complex humoral and cellular interactions, including activation, generation, or expression of thrombin, complement, cytokines, neutrophils, adhesion molecules, mast cells, and multiple inflammatory mediators. Because of the redundancy of the inflammatory cascades, profound amplification occurs to produce multiorgan system dysfunction that can manifest as coagulopathy, respiratory failure, myocardial dysfunction, renal insufficiency, and neurocognitive defects. Coagulation and inflammation also are linked closely through networks of both humoral and cellular components, including tissue factor and proteases of the clotting and fibrinolytic cascades.

ASSESSMENT OF PERIOPERATIVE MYOCARDIAL INJURY IN CARDIAC SURGERY

There is a lack of consensus regarding how to measure myocardial injury in cardiac surgery because of the continuum of cardiac injury. Electrocardiographic changes, biomarker elevations, and measures of cardiac function have all been used (Box 1.4), but all assessment modalities are affected by the direct myocardial trauma of surgery. In 2000 the American College of Cardiology/European Society of Cardiology (ACC/ESC) published a definition of MI that included a characteristic rise and fall in blood concentrations of cardiac troponins or creatine kinase, myocardial bound (CKMB), or both, in the context of a coronary intervention; other modalities are less sensitive and specific (Fig. 1.1).

According to this most recent version, MI can be diagnosed based on detection of a rise and fall of cardiac biomarkers (preferably troponin) with at least one value above the 99th percentile of the upper reference limit, together with evidence of

1

BOX 1.4 *Assessment of Perioperative Myocardial Injury*

Assessment of cardiac function
Echocardiography
Nuclear imaging
Electrocardiography
Q waves
ST-T wave changes
Serum biomarkers
Myoglobin
Creatine kinase
Creatine kinase, myocardial bound isoenzyme
Troponin
Lactate dehydrogenase

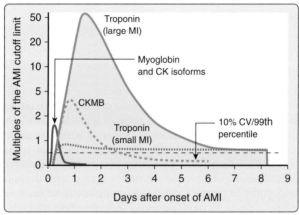

Fig. 1.1 Time course of the appearance of various markers in the blood after acute myocardial infarction *(AMI)*. Shown are the time concentrations/activity curves for myoglobin and creatine kinase *(CK)* isoforms, troponin after large and small infarctions, and CKMB. Note that with cardiac troponin, some patients have a second peak in addition. *CKMB,* Creatine kinase, myocardial bound; *CV,* coefficient of variation; *MI,* myocardial infarction. (From Jaffe AS, Babuin L, Apple FS: Biomarkers in acute cardiac disease: the present and the future. *J Am Coll Cardiol.* 2006;48:1–11.)

myocardial ischemia in the form of any of the following: symptoms of ischemia, electrocardiography (ECG) changes indicative of new ischemia (new ST-T changes or new left bundle branch block), development of pathologic Q waves on ECG, or imaging evidence of new loss of viable myocardium or new regional wall motion abnormality (RWMA). Because CABG itself is associated with cardiac trauma resulting in an increase in the serum levels of cardiac enzymes, an arbitrary cutoff level for elevation of cardiac biomarker values of more than 10 times the 99th percentile of the upper reference limit has been recommended for diagnosing MI during the immediate period after cardiac surgery. However, this threshold is more robust for diagnosing MI after an isolated on-pump CABG; cardiac biomarker release is typically considerably higher after combined valve replacement and CABG and considerably lower after an off-pump CABG.

CARDIOVASCULAR IMAGING

Imaging is fundamental to perioperative evaluation and management of patients undergoing cardiac surgery. For many years cardiac catheterization and nuclear imaging were the only modalities available for clinical use. The introduction of echocardiography in the early 1970s heralded a revolution in the field of cardiovascular imaging, and echocardiography soon surpassed all other modalities to become the cornerstone of cardiac imaging. Because of its noninvasive nature, safety, easy availability, portability, repeatability, and capacity to provide vast amounts of clinically relevant information, echocardiography has remained the most useful modality for cardiac imaging.

The last several decades have witnessed yet another explosion in imaging techniques with the evolution of cardiac computed tomography (CCT), cardiac magnetic resonance (CMR), and positron emission tomography (PET) as routine clinical evaluation tools. In the field of perioperative evaluation, these alternative imaging modalities have complemented more than supplemented traditional imaging.

ECHOCARDIOGRAPHY

Transthoracic echocardiography (TTE) is required in all patients scheduled for cardiac surgery and is often the basis for surgical decision making itself. In contrast to the nonsurgical setting, in which TTE is usually sufficient to provide most of the information needed to meet the clinical objectives, transesophageal echocardiography (TEE) is also frequently required for patients for whom surgery is being considered. Preoperatively, TEE helps provide information that is critical for surgical planning (eg, valve repair vs. valve replacement, coronary artery bypass surgery alone or with concomitant mitral valve repair). During the intraoperative period, TEE is the only modality available for cardiac imaging. In the immediate postoperative period, TEE is often called for because the presence of tissue edema, surgical dressings, and drains and the reduced ability to change the patient's position render transthoracic imaging extremely challenging.

Assessment of Left Ventricular Systolic Function

LV systolic function is one of the most important predictors of outcome in all cardiac conditions, and almost all therapeutic decisions in these patients are influenced by the status of LV systolic function. For cardiac anesthesiologists, preoperative knowledge of LV systolic dysfunction is crucial for anticipating and preparing for perioperative complications, whereas subsequent assessments are required for diagnosing and managing the cause of hemodynamic instability. Patients with LV systolic dysfunction who undergo CABG are known to require more inotropic support after CPB. Additionally, systolic dysfunction is a reliable prognosticator for surgical mortality.

LVEF is the simplest and the most widely used measure of global LV systolic function. A number of echocardiographic methods are currently available for estimation of LVEF, but the biplane modified Simpson method is the most accurate and is also the method recommended by the American Society of Echocardiography (ASE) (Fig. 1.2). In practice, however, LVEF is often estimated semiquantitatively by visual inspection alone, and this technique has been shown to have a reasonably high degree of accuracy when performed by an experienced echocardiographer.

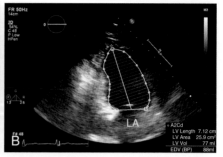

Fig. 1.2 Measurement of left ventricular volumes and ejection fraction using the Simpson summation-of-disks method. (A) Apical four-chamber view in end-diastole. (B) Same view in end-systole. *LA*, Left atrium; *RV*, right ventricle.

Regional Left Ventricular Systolic Function

In cardiac patients, assessment of regional LV systolic function has considerable clinical relevance. Coronary artery disease (CAD) is the prototype cardiac illness that affects the left ventricle regionally, and the presence of regional LV systolic dysfunction is virtually diagnostic of underlying CAD. The assessment of regional LV systolic function also provides an estimate of the overall extent of myocardial damage, permits recognition of the affected coronary arteries, and facilitates assessment of myocardial viability and inducible myocardial ischemia.

Assessment of Left Ventricular Diastolic Function

Abnormalities of LV diastolic function are common in patients undergoing cardiac surgery and have diagnostic and prognostic relevance. Diastolic dysfunction during and after CABG is associated with greater time on CPB and with greater inotropic support up to 12 hours postoperatively. This may be due to deterioration of diastolic function after CABG, which may persist for several hours. Diastolic dysfunction increases the risk of perioperative morbidity and mortality.

Echocardiography is currently the best modality for assessing LV diastolic function in clinical practice. Several echocardiographic measures of LV diastolic function are available. The examination usually begins with interrogation of the mitral inflow pattern. The specific mitral inflow measurements include the mitral inflow early diastolic (E) and late diastolic (A) velocities, the ratio of the two (E/A), and the deceleration time of the E wave (dtE).

Mitral annular early diastolic velocity (e′) is measured using tissue Doppler imaging. The ratio of mitral E to e′ (E/e′) provides an accurate and relatively load-independent measure of LV filling pressure (LVFP). Left atrial (LA) volume and tricuspid regurgitation (TR) jet velocity (a surrogate for pulmonary artery systolic pressure) are other useful measurements. Integrating all this information provides a quick assessment of LV diastolic function in most patients. When required, additional information can be obtained by evaluating pulmonary vein flow patterns, mitral inflow propagation velocity, isovolumic relaxation time, and pulmonary pressures. The ASE has recently published guidelines outlining a stepwise approach to assessment of LV diastolic function and estimation of LVFP or LA pressure in patients with and without LV systolic dysfunction. Using this algorithmic approach, LV diastolic dysfunction can be categorized as normal or abnormal and, when abnormal, can be grade 1 (impaired relaxation), grade 2 (pseudonormal pattern), or grade 3 (restrictive pattern) (Fig. 1.3).

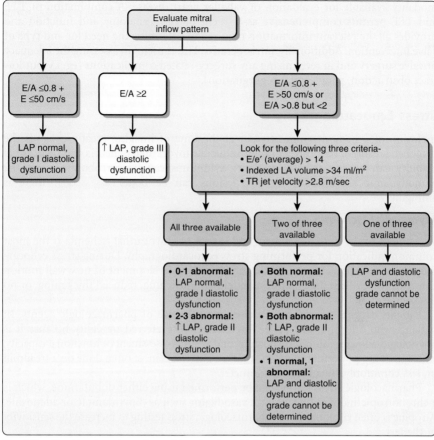

Fig. 1.3 Algorithm for echocardiographic estimation of left atrial pressure and grading left ventricular diastolic function in patients with myocardial disease but with or without left ventricular systolic dysfunction. *A,* Mitral inflow late diastolic velocity; *E,* mitral inflow early diastolic velocity; *e'* mitral annular early diastolic velocity; *LA,* left atrial; *LAP,* left atrial pressure; *TR,* tricuspid regurgitation. (Modified from: Nagueh SF, Smiseth OA, Appleton CP, et al. Recommendations for the evaluation of left ventricular diastolic function by echocardiography: an update from the American Society of Echocardiography and the European Association of Cardiovascular Imaging. *J Am Soc Echocardiogr.* 2016;29:277–314.)

Right Heart Evaluation

Dysfunction of the right side of the heart, in the absence of congenital heart disease, is most often secondary to left heart pathologies, especially mitral valve disease and severe LV systolic dysfunction. Additionally, obstructive airway disease and pulmonary thromboembolism are common in cardiac surgical patients. Primary right heart pathology is encountered less frequently and includes right ventricular (RV) MI and organic tricuspid valve disease.

Assessment of Valve Lesions

Valvular heart disease is the second most common primary indication, after CAD, for cardiac surgery. Valve lesions also frequently coexist in patients undergoing surgery for other cardiac and noncardiac indications. Echocardiography is currently the best modality available for evaluation of valvular heart disease. A combination of TTE and TEE permits comprehensive assessment of valve anatomy and function and provides all the relevant information required to determine the need for and type of valve intervention. Additionally, intraoperative TEE is useful in assessing the adequacy of valve surgery and in recognizing any surgery-related complications (eg, LV outflow tract obstruction, paravalvular regurgitation).

Stress Echocardiography

Inclusion of a hemodynamic stressor at the time of imaging greatly expands the diagnostic realm of echocardiography. Inducible myocardial ischemia and myocardial viability can be assessed, the patient's symptoms can be corroborated, and the hemodynamic significance of valve lesions can be better assessed if there is ambiguity.

Myocardial Ischemia

Assessment of the presence, extent, and severity of myocardial ischemia is the most common indication for performing stress echocardiography. During stress echocardiography, inducible ischemia is diagnosed by the development of new wall motion abnormalities, which may manifest as delayed thickening, reduced thickening, or no thickening at all.

Patients can be stressed by exercise or by the use of pharmacologic agents. In patients who are physically active, exercise is the preferred modality because it is physiologic, allows symptom correlation, and permits assessment of functional capacity, which itself is a powerful prognostic marker. Exercise is most often done on a treadmill or, less commonly, on a bicycle ergometer.

Pharmacologic stress testing can be performed using either dobutamine, which is a chronotropic/inotropic agent, or a vasodilator such as dipyridamole or adenosine. Atropine is often combined with pharmacologic stress testing to increase the sensitivity of the test.

The accuracy of stress echocardiography for detection of inducible ischemia has been examined in numerous studies. In a large metaanalysis, the average sensitivity and specificity of exercise echocardiography were found to be 83% and 84%, respectively. These values were 80% and 85%, respectively, for dobutamine echocardiography; 71% and 92% for dipyridamole echocardiography; and 68% and 81% for adenosine stress echocardiography.

MYOCARDIAL NUCLEAR SCINTIGRAPHY

Myocardial nuclear scintigraphy is the most widely used modality for assessment of myocardial ischemia and viability, at least in the preoperative setting. There are two main forms of myocardial nuclear imaging: single-photon emission computed tomography (SPECT) and PET. Both use the principles of radioactive decay to evaluate the myocardium and its blood supply. The radionuclides that are used in SPECT are technetium 99m (^{99m}Tc) and thallium 201 (^{201}Tl). Although PET also uses radioisotopes to produce images, the actual process of image formation is quite distinct from that of SPECT. The most common radioisotopes used for cardiac evaluation by PET imaging are rubidium 82, N-ammonia 13, and fluorine 18 (^{18}F).

Detection of myocardial ischemia is the most common indication for performing myocardial perfusion imaging. Either SPECT or PET can be used for this purpose, which is based on assessments of LV myocardial uptake of the radioisotope at rest and after stress. Myocardial uptake is reduced after stress in myocardial regions where significant coronary artery stenosis is present.

Nuclear scintigraphic methods, including both SPECT and PET myocardial perfusion imaging, can also be used to evaluate global and segmental LV systolic function. This is achieved by implementing ECG gating during data acquisition.

CARDIAC COMPUTED TOMOGRAPHY

CCT has grown significantly in clinical use since the advent, in the early 2000s, of multidetector CT (MDCT) scanners with submillimeter resolution that allow evaluation of the coronary anatomy. The x-ray tube produces beams that traverse the patient and are received by a detector array on the opposite side of the scanner. The tube and detector arrays are coupled to each other and rotate around the patient at a velocity of 250 to 500 microseconds per rotation. With today's advanced technology, 256-slice systems are standard, and 320-slice systems with 16 cm of coverage are able to capture the entire heart in one heartbeat and rotation.

CCT uses ionizing radiation for the production of images. Concern about excessive medical radiation exposure has been raised. Although several techniques, such as prospective ECG-gated acquisition, may be implemented to reduce the radiation dose, a risk-benefit assessment must be done for the selection of patients who have appropriate indications for CCT.

Coronary angiography is currently one of the most common indications for performing CCT. The patient's heart rate must be lowered to less than 65 beats/minute to achieve adequate results when imaging the coronary arteries. This usually requires the administration of oral or intravenous β-blockers. After the scan has been completed, images are reconstructed at various points of the cardiac cycle and analyzed on a computer workstation. Cardiac CT angiography (CCTA) has been well studied for the diagnosis of CAD in patients without known ischemic heart disease, demonstrating a sensitivity of 94% and a negative predictive value of 99%. It is being increasingly employed to exclude obstructive CAD before valve surgery in patients with low-to-intermediate pretest probability to avoid invasive testing.

CT aortography is the imaging modality of choice for evaluation of aortic pathologies such as aortic aneurysms and nonemergency dissections. Imaging protocols used for evaluation of the aorta are similar to those used for CCTA. It is important to have the scan gated to the patient's ECG because the ascending aorta moves significantly during the cardiac cycle. Nongated scans have inherent motion artifacts that can be confused with a dissection. Use of prospective ECG gating also minimizes radiation exposure. Visualization of the aortic root and coronary arteries is crucial because ascending aortic dissections can involve the ostia of the coronary arteries.

Although echocardiography is the gold standard for imaging valvular disease, advanced imaging with CCT or CMR may be required if TTE and TEE are technically difficult or if there are discrepancies in the findings. CMR offers more functional data than CCT, but CCT may be used if further anatomic information about a valve is required. For evaluating prosthetic valves, CCT is usually superior to CMR because of metallic artifact from the valve, which is visualized on CMR.

CCT, with its excellent spatial and temporal resolution, can also facilitate an accurate assessment of LV function. CCT uses actual 3D volumes to calculate LV systolic function. Retrospective scanning is used for functional analysis because the entire cardiac cycle (both systole and diastole) must be acquired. The raw data set is then reconstructed in cardiac phase intervals of 10%, from 0% (early systole) to 90% (late diastole), to derive functional information. Advanced computer workstations allow

1

cine images to be reconstructed and displayed in multiple planes. Segmental wall motion analysis can also be performed using the 17-segment model.

CARDIOVASCULAR MAGNETIC RESONANCE IMAGING

CMR is a robust and versatile imaging modality. It has the ability to evaluate multiple elements of cardiac status, including function, morphology, flow, tissue characteristics, perfusion, angiography, and metabolism. It can do this because of its unique ability to distinguish morphology without the use of any ionizing radiation by taking advantage of the influence of magnetic fields on the abundance of hydrogen atoms in the human body. Multicontrast CMR uses the intrinsic molecular properties of tissues and three types of contrast.

CMR is considered the gold standard for the quantitative assessment of biventricular volumes, ejection fraction, and mass while also offering excellent reproducibility. CMR has good spatial and temporal resolution, allowing for cine imaging.

CMR can also be used for perfusion imaging by evaluating the first pass of gadolinium contrast through the myocardium. ECG-gated images are acquired using three LV short-axis slices. As the contrast agent is injected, it is tracked through the right side of the heart and, subsequently, through the LV cavity and LV myocardium. The assessment of perfusion requires imaging over several consecutive heartbeats, during which time the contrast bolus completes its first pass through the myocardium. Imaging must be completed within a single breath-hold.

CMR has emerged as the gold standard for evaluation of myocardial scarring. Late gadolinium enhancement is used as the marker of myocardial scarring. Gadolinium contrast is injected intravenously, and imaging is performed 5 to 10 minutes later. Gadolinium tends to accumulate extracellularly; however, in normal myocardium, there is insufficient space for gadolinium deposition. In the setting of chronic scar, the volume of gadolinium distribution increases because of an enlarged interstitium in the presence of extensive fibrosis. Hence, normal or viable myocardium appears as nulled or dark, whereas scar appears bright. The advantage of delayed-enhancement imaging is that it allows for assessment of the transmural extent of the scar. The images are analyzed visually, and the thickness of scarring compared with wall thickness is quantified by percentage (ie, none, 1–25%, 26–50%, 51–75%, or 75–100%). A wall segment is considered to be viable and has a high probability of functional recovery if the scar thickness is no more than 50% of the wall thickness.

SUGGESTED READINGS

Allman KC, Shaw LJ, Hachamovitch R, et al. Myocardial viability testing and impact of revascularization of prognosis in patients with coronary artery disease and left ventricular dysfunction: a meta-analysis. *J Am Coll Cardiol.* 2002;39:1151–1158.

Bernard F, Denault A, Babin D, et al. Diastolic dysfunction is predictive of difficult weaning from cardio-pulmonary bypass. *Anesth Analg.* 2001;92:291–298.

Budoff MJ, Dowe D, Jollis JG, et al. Diagnostic performance of 64-multidetector row coronary computed tomographic angiography for evaluation of coronary artery stenosis in individuals without known coronary artery disease: results from the prospective multicenter ACCURACY (Assessment by Coronary Computed Tomographic Angiography of Individuals Undergoing Invasive Coronary Angiography) trial. *J Am Coll Cardiol.* 2008;52:1724–1732.

Fellahi JL, Gue X, Richomme X, et al. Short- and long-term prognostic value of postoperative cardiac troponin I concentration in patients undergoing coronary artery bypass grafting. *Anesthesiology.* 2003;99:270–274.

Gardner SC, Grunwald GK, Rumsfeld JS, et al. Comparison of short-term mortality risk factors for valve replacement versus coronary artery bypass graft surgery. *Ann Thorac Surg.* 2004;77:549–556.

Gibbons RJ, Balady GJ, Bricker JT, et al. ACC/AHA 2002 guideline update for exercise testing summary article. A report of the American College of Cardiology/American Heart Association Task Force on Practice Guidelines (Committee to Update the 1997 Exercise Testing Guidelines). *J Am Coll Cardiol.* 2002;40:1531–1540.

Greenson N, Macoviak J, Krishnaswamy P, et al. Usefulness of cardiac troponin I in patients undergoing open heart surgery. *Am Heart J.* 2001;141:447–455.

Gudmundsson P, Rydberg E, Winter R, et al. Visually estimated left ventricular ejection fraction by echocardiography is closely correlated with formal quantitative methods. *Int J Cardiol.* 2005;101:209–212.

Hillis LD, Smith PK, Anderson JL, et al. 2011 ACCF/AHA guideline for coronary artery bypass graft surgery: a report of the American College of Cardiology Foundation/American Heart Association Task Force on Practice Guidelines. Developed in collaboration with the American Association for Thoracic Surgery, Society of Cardiovascular Anesthesiologists, and Society of Thoracic Surgeons. *J Am Coll Cardiol.* 2011;58:e123–e210.

Khuri SF. Evidence, sources, and assessment of injury during and following cardiac surgery. *Ann Thorac Surg.* 2001;72:S2205–S2207, discussion S2267–S2270.

Lang RM, Badano LP, Mor-Avi V, et al. Recommendations for cardiac chamber quantification by echocardiography in adults: an update from the American Society of Echocardiography and the European Association of Cardiovascular Imaging. *J Am Soc Echocardiogr.* 2015;28:1–39 el 4.

Levy JH, Tanaka KA. Inflammatory response to cardiopulmonary bypass. *Ann Thorac Surg.* 2003;75:S715–S720.

Meijboom WB, Mollet NR, Van Mieghem CA, et al. Pre-operative computed tomography coronary angiography to detect significant coronary artery disease in patients referred for cardiac valve surgery. *J Am Coll Cardiol.* 2006;48:1658–1665.

Nashef SA, Roques F, Sharples LD, et al. EuroSCORE II. *Eur J Cardiothorac Surg.* 2012;41:734–744, discussion 744–745.

Nilsson J, Algotsson L, Hoglund P, et al. Early mortality in coronary bypass surgery: the EuroSCORE versus the Society of Thoracic Surgeons risk algorithm. *Ann Thorac Surg.* 2004;77:1235–1239, discussion 1239–1240.

Paiement B, Pelletier C, Dyrda I, et al. A simple classification of the risk in cardiac surgery. *Can Anaesth Soc J.* 1983;30:61–68.

Patel MR, Dehmer GJ, Hirshfeld JW, et al. ACCF/SCAI/STS/AATS/AHA/ASNC/HFSA/SCCT 2012 appropriate use criteria for coronary revascularization: focused update. A report of the American College of Cardiology Foundation Appropriate Use Criteria Task Force, Society for Cardiovascular Angiography and Interventions, Society of Thoracic Surgeons, American Association for Thoracic Surgery, American Heart Association, American Society of Nuclear Cardiology, and the Society of Cardiovascular Computed Tomography. *J Am Coll Cardiol.* 2012;59:857–881.

Rudski LG, Lai WW, Afilalo J, et al. Guidelines for the Echocardiography endorsed by the European Association of Echocardiography, a registered branch of the European Society of Cardiology, and the Canadian Society of Echocardiography. *J Am Soc Echocardiogr.* 2010;23:685–713 quiz 786–788.

Thygesen K, Alpert JS, Jaffe AS, et al. Third universal definition of myocardial infarction. *Eur Heart J.* 2012;33:2551–2567.

Vahanian A, Alfieri O, Andreotti F, et al. Guidelines on the management of valvular heart disease (version 2012). *Eur Heart J.* 2012;33:2451–2496.

1

17

Chapter 2

Cardiac Catheterization Laboratory: Diagnostic and Therapeutic Procedures in the Adult Patient

Theresa A. Gelzinis, MD • Mark Kozak, MD •
Charles E. Chambers, MD • John Schindler, MD

Key Points

1. The cardiac catheterization laboratory has evolved from a purely diagnostic facility to a therapeutic one in which many facets of cardiovascular disease can be effectively modified or treated.
2. Guidelines for diagnostic cardiac catheterization have established indications, contraindications, and criteria to identify high-risk patients.
3. Interventional cardiology began in the late 1970s as balloon angioplasty, with a success rate of 80% and emergent coronary artery bypass graft surgery (CABG) rates of 3% to 5%. Although current success rates exceed 95%, with CABG rates of less than 1%, failed percutaneous coronary intervention (PCI) presents a challenge for the anesthesiologist because of hemodynamic problems, concomitant medications, and the underlying cardiac disease.
4. Since the introduction of drug-eluting stents (DESs), acute closure owing to coronary dissection has diminished significantly, and restenosis rates have fallen precipitously.
5. The first-generation DESs were extremely effective at reducing in-stent restenosis when compared with bare metal stents (BMSs). However, DESs have demonstrated higher rates of late stent thrombosis (LST), especially in the setting of premature discontinuation of dual antiplatelet therapy. Second-generation DESs have LST rates comparable to those of BMSs and therefore are the preferred stent type.
6. In the United States, increasing numbers of diagnostic coronary angiograms and PCIs are performed from a transradial approach because of lower vascular complication rates and patient preference for this approach compared with the more traditional transfemoral approach.
7. In multivessel coronary artery disease, an angiographic synergy between percutaneous coronary intervention with taxus and an angiographic (SYNTAX) score should be calculated to assist with decision making regarding percutaneous versus surgical revascularization. A multidisciplinary heart team meeting (including a cardiologist, a cardiovascular surgeon, and, occasionally, an anesthesiologist) should then convene to discuss and optimize patient care by providing an individualized treatment recommendation.
8. Acute thrombotic PCI complications can usually be overcome with more aggressive antithrombotic and antiplatelet pharmacotherapy. These medications can complicate the management of a patient in an unstable condition who requires transfer for bailout CABG.

The cardiac catheterization laboratory (CCL) began as a diagnostic unit. In the 1980s percutaneous transluminal coronary angioplasty (PTCA) started the gradual shift to therapeutic procedures. Concomitantly, noninvasive modalities of echocardiography, computed tomography (CT), and magnetic resonance imaging (MRI) improved, and in some cases obviated, the need for diagnostic catheterization studies. The promise of PTCA led to various atherectomy and aspiration devices and stents, with or without drug elution. The evolution of the CCL has continued, with many laboratories commonly performing procedures for the diagnosis and treatment of peripheral and cerebral vascular disease. In addition, there has been an expansion of the treatment of noncoronary forms of cardiac disease in the CCL. Closure devices for patent foramen ovale (PFO), atrial septal defect (ASD), and ventricular septal defect (VSD) are emerging as alternatives to cardiac surgery. Many high-risk patients with valvular disease are now being treated with percutaneous valve repair and replacement, decreasing the incidence of balloon valvuloplasty.

This brief historical background serves as an introduction to the discussion of diagnostic and therapeutic procedures in the adult CCL. The reader must realize the dynamic nature of this field. In the past, up to 5% of percutaneous coronary interventions (PCIs) failed, but most centers now report procedural failure rates of less than 1%. Simultaneously, the impact on the anesthesiologist has changed. The high complication rates of years past required holding an operating room (OR) open for all PCIs, but complication rates are now so low that some procedures are performed at hospitals without on-site surgical backup. Despite the lower rate of adverse events, the anesthesiologist is occasionally confronted with a patient in need of emergent surgical revascularization. The anesthesiologist may find the information in this chapter useful in planning the preoperative management of these cardiac or noncardiac surgical procedures based on diagnostic information obtained in the CCL. When anesthesia is required for procedures in the hybrid laboratory or the CCL, this chapter will help the anesthesiologist, in collaboration with the cardiology and cardiac surgery team, to provide safe anesthesia care for these challenging patients.

▨ PATIENT SELECTION FOR CATHETERIZATION

Indications for Cardiac Catheterization in the Adult Patient

Box 2.1 lists indications for cardiac catheterization. The major indication is for the detection of coronary artery disease (CAD); the remaining indications are focused

BOX 2.1 *Indications for Diagnostic Catheterization in the Adult Patient*

Coronary Artery Disease

Symptoms

Unstable angina
Postinfarction angina
Angina refractory to medications

Continued

BOX 2.1 *Indications for Diagnostic Catheterization in the Adult Patient—cont'd*

Typical chest pain with negative diagnostic testing
Family history of sudden death

Diagnostic Testing

Strongly positive exercise tolerance test
Early positive, ischemia in ≥5 leads, hypotension, ischemia present for ≥6 min of recovery
Positive exercise testing after myocardial infarction
Strongly positive nuclear myocardial perfusion test
Increased lung uptake or ventricular dilation after stress
Large single or multiple areas of ischemic myocardium
Strongly positive stress echocardiographic study
Decrease in overall ejection fraction or ventricular dilation with stress
Large single area or multiple or large areas of new wall motion abnormalities

Valvular Disease

Symptoms

Aortic stenosis with syncope, chest pain, or congestive heart failure
Aortic insufficiency with progressive heart failure
Mitral insufficiency or stenosis with progressive congestive heart failure symptoms
Acute orthopnea/pulmonary edema after infarction with suspected acute mitral insufficiency

Diagnostic Testing

Progressive resting left ventricular dysfunction with regurgitant lesion
Decreasing left ventricular function and/or chamber dilation with exercise

Adult Congenital Heart Disease

Atrial Septal Defect

Age >50 years with evidence of coronary artery disease
Septum primum or sinus venosus defect

Ventricular Septal Defect

Catheterization for definition of coronary anatomy
Coarctation of the aorta
Detection of collaterals
Coronary arteriography if increased age and/or risk factors are present

Other

Acute myocardial infarction therapy—consider primary percutaneous coronary intervention
Mechanical complication after infarction
Malignant cardiac arrhythmias
Cardiac transplantation
Pretransplantation donor evaluation
Posttransplantation annual coronary artery graft rejection evaluation
Unexplained congestive heart failure
Research studies with institutional review board review and patient consent

on hemodynamic assessment to evaluate valvular heart disease, pulmonary hypertension, and cardiomyopathies. With respect to CAD, approximately 20% of the adult population studied will be found to have normal coronary arteries. Despite continued improvements in noninvasive assessment, coronary angiography is currently considered the gold standard for diagnosing and defining the extent of CAD. With advances in MRI and multislice CT scanning, the next decade may well see a further evolution of the CCL to an interventional suite with fewer diagnostic responsibilities.

Patient Evaluation Before Cardiac Catheterization

Diagnostic cardiac catheterization in the 21st century is universally considered an outpatient procedure except for the high-risk patient. Therefore the precatheterization evaluation is essential for quality patient care. Evaluation before cardiac catheterization includes diagnostic tests that are necessary to identify high-risk patients. An electrocardiogram (ECG) must be obtained for all patients shortly before catheterization. Necessary laboratory studies before catheterization include an appropriate coagulation profile (prothrombin time [PT], partial thromboplastin time [PTT], and platelet count), hemoglobin, and hematocrit. Electrolytes are obtained together with baseline blood urea nitrogen and creatinine (Cr) values to assess renal function. Recent guidelines express a preference for estimation of the glomerular filtration rate (GFR) using accepted formulas, and many clinical laboratories now report this value routinely. Urinalysis and chest radiography may provide useful information but are no longer routinely obtained by all operators. Prior catheterization reports should be available. If the patient had prior PCI or coronary artery bypass graft (CABG) surgery, anatomic information concerning stent or bypass placement also must be available.

Patient medications may need to be altered in preparation for a heart catheterization. On the morning of the catheterization, antianginal and antihypertensive medications are routinely continued, whereas diuretic therapy is withheld. Patients with diabetes are scheduled early, if possible, because the procedure requires nil per os (NPO) status. No short-acting insulin is given, and half of the long-acting insulin dose is usually administered. Patients on oral anticoagulation should stop warfarin (Coumadin) for 48 to 72 hours before catheterization to target an international normalized ratio (INR) of 1.8 or less if femoral artery access is used. Radial artery access is considered an option without discontinuation of warfarin. For patients who are managed with non–vitamin K antagonist novel oral anticoagulant (NOAC) therapy, the dose may need to be withheld for 24 to 48 hours depending on renal function and the bleeding risk of the procedure. In patients who are anticoagulated because of mechanical prosthetic valves, the best management may be intravenous (IV) heparin before and after the procedure, when the warfarin effect is not therapeutic. IV heparin is routinely discontinued 1 to 2 hours before catheterization, except in patients with unstable angina. Therapy with aspirin or P2Y12 platelet inhibitors or both is almost always continued for patients with angina or those with prior CABG.

■ CARDIAC CATHETERIZATION PROCEDURES

Whether the procedure is elective or emergent, diagnostic or interventional, coronary or peripheral, certain basic components are relatively constant in all circumstances.

Patient Monitoring and Sedation

Standard limb leads with one chest lead are used for ECG monitoring during cardiac catheterization. One inferior and one anterior ECG lead are monitored during diagnostic catheterization. During an interventional procedure, two ECG leads are monitored in the same coronary artery distribution as the vessel undergoing PCI. Radiolucent ECG leads permit monitoring without interfering with angiographic data.

Sedation in the CCL, from preprocedural administration or from IV administration during the procedure, may lead to hypoventilation and hypoxemia. The administration of midazolam, 1 to 5 mg intravenously, with fentanyl, 25 to 100 µg, is common practice. Institutional guidelines for conscious sedation typically govern these practices. Light to moderate sedation is beneficial to the patient, particularly for angiographic imaging and interventional procedures. Sedation is critical for patients who undergo a radial artery approach; conscious sedation has been shown to reduce the incidence of radial artery spasm, which, when severe, may force the operator to adopt a transfemoral approach to complete the procedure. Deep sedation, in addition to its widely recognized potential to cause respiratory difficulties, poses distinct problems in the CCL. Deep sedation often requires supplemental oxygen, which complicates the interpretation of oximetry data and may alter hemodynamics.

More complex interventions have resulted in longer procedures. Although hospitals require conscious sedation policies, individual variation in the type and degree of sedation is common. General anesthesia is rarely required for coronary procedures, but it is frequently used for percutaneous valve procedures. Advancements in intracardiac echocardiography have decreased the need for intubation and transesophageal echocardiography (TEE) in certain patients and procedures. Pediatric procedures require general anesthesia more commonly than those in adults. As the frequency of noncoronary procedures increases, the presence of an anesthesiologist in the CCL will be required more often.

Left-Sided Heart Catheterization

Catheterization Site and Anticoagulation

Left-sided heart catheterization (LHC) traditionally has been performed by means of a brachial or femoral artery approach. The femoral approach became almost universally accepted. The percutaneous radial artery approach was later developed to improve patient comfort and reduce vascular complications, but its use remained relatively stagnant for more than 10 years. Currently, only a small percentage of procedures are performed via the radial approach in the United States, but that number is increasing rapidly. Over the most recently reported 6-year time period, there was a 13-fold increase in radial artery PCI, with wide geographic variation.

Right-Sided Heart Catheterization

Indications

In the CCL, right-sided heart catheterization (RHC) is performed for diagnostic purposes. Routine RHC cannot be recommended. Box 2.2 outlines acceptable indications for RHC during LHC. Cardiac output (CO) measurements during RHC using the thermodilution technique allow for a further assessment of ventricular function.

> **BOX 2.2** *Indications for Diagnostic Right-Sided Heart Catheterization During Left-Sided Heart Catheterization*
>
> Significant valvular pathology
> Suspected intracardiac shunting
> Acute infarct—differentiation of free wall versus septal rupture
> Evaluation of right- and/or left-sided heart failure
> Evaluation of pulmonary hypertension
> Severe pulmonary disease
> Evaluation of pericardial disease
> Constrictive pericarditis
> Restrictive cardiomyopathy
> Pericardial effusion
> Pretransplantation assessment of pulmonary vascular resistance and response to vasodilators

Diagnostic Catheterization Complications

Complications are related to multiple factors, but severity of disease is important. Mortality rates are low. Complications are specific for RHC and LHC (Box 2.3). The registry reported incidences of major complications as follows: death, 0.1%; myocardial infarction (MI), 0.06%; cerebrovascular accident, 0.07%; arrhythmia, 0.47%; contrast reaction, 0.23%; and vascular complications, 0.46%. Infectious complications are infrequent, although they may be underreported.

VALVULAR PATHOLOGY

The number of patients presenting with valvular heart disease (VHD) in developed countries is growing, primarily because of the increasing age of the population. In 2014 the American College of Cardiology/American Heart Association (ACC/AHA) published updated practice guidelines for the management of VHD. These guidelines cover the invasive and noninvasive evaluation of valvular problems and the therapeutic approaches (see Chapter 15).

ANGIOGRAPHY

Ventriculography

Ejection Fraction Determination

Ventriculography routinely is performed in the single-plane 30-degree right anterior oblique (RAO) or biplane 60-degree left anterior oblique (LAO) and 30-degree RAO projections using 20 to 45 mL of contrast with injection rates of 10 to 15 mL/second (Box 2.4). Complete opacification of the ventricle without inducing ventricular extrasystoles is necessary for accurate assessment during ventriculography. Premature contractions not only alter the interpretation of mitral regurgitation (MR) but result in a false increase in the ejection fraction (EF).

2

BOX 2.3 *Complications of Diagnostic Catheterization*

Left-Sided Heart Catheterization

Cardiac Complications

Death
Myocardial infarction
Ventricular fibrillation
Ventricular tachycardia
Cardiac perforation

Noncardiac Complications

Stroke
Peripheral embolization
Air
Thrombus
Cholesterol
Vascular surgical repair
Pseudoaneurysm
Arteriovenous fistula
Embolectomy
Repair of brachial arteriotomy
Evacuation of hematomas
Contrast-related complications
Renal insufficiency
Anaphylaxis

Right-Sided Heart Catheterization

Cardiac Complications

Conduction abnormality
RBBB
Complete heart block (RBBB superimposed on LBBB)
Arrhythmias
Valvular damage
Perforation

Noncardiac Complications

Pulmonary artery rupture
Pulmonary infarction
Balloon rupture
Paradoxic (systemic) air embolus

LBBB, Left bundle branch block; *RBBB*, right bundle branch block.

The EF is a global assessment of ventricular function. It is calculated as follows:

$$EF = [EDV - ESV]/EDV = SV/EDV$$

where EDV is end-diastolic volume, ESV is end-systolic volume, and SV is stroke volume.

There are problems with the use of EF as a measure of ventricular function. EFs calculated by various techniques (eg, echocardiography, ventriculography, gated blood pool scanning) may not be identical because of the mathematical modeling involved.

BOX 2.4 *Angiography*

Coronary anatomy
- Left anterior descending coronary artery with diagonal and septal branches
- Circumflex artery with marginal branches
- Right coronary artery with conus, sinoatrial nodal, atrioventricular nodal, and right ventricular branches
- Dominant circulation (posterior descending): 10% circumflex; 90% right coronary artery

Coronary collaterals
Coronary anomaly
Ventriculography/aortography
Ejection fraction calculation
Valvular regurgitation

When single-plane ventriculography is used to calculate the EF, dysfunction of a nonvisualized segment (eg, the lateral wall in an RAO ventriculogram) and global function may be overestimated. Most important, the EF is a load–dependent measure of ventricular function. Changes in preload, afterload, and contractility can significantly alter the EF determination.

Abnormalities in Regional Wall Motion

Segmental wall motion abnormalities are defined in both RAO and LAO projections. A grading scale of 0 to 5 may be used to identify hypokinesis (decreased motion), akinesis (no motion), and dyskinesis (paradoxic or aneurysmal motion). The values are as follows: 0 = normal; 1 = mild hypokinesis; 2 = moderate hypokinesis; 3 = severe hypokinesis; 4 = akinesis; 5 = dyskinesis (aneurysmal).

Assessment of Mitral Regurgitation

A qualitative assessment of the degree of MR can be made with left ventricular (LV) angiography. The assessment is, by convention, done on a scale of 1+ to 4+, with 1+ being mild MR and 4+ being severe MR. As defined by ventriculography, 1+ regurgitation is that in which the contrast material clears from the left atrium (LA) with each beat, never causing complete opacification of the LA. Moderate or 2+ MR is present when the opacification does not clear with one beat, leading to complete opacification of the LA after several beats. In 3+ MR (moderately severe), the LA becomes completely opacified and equal in opacification to the left ventricle after several beats. In 4+ MR, the LA densely opacifies with one beat, and the contrast refluxes into the pulmonary veins.

By combining data from left ventriculography and RHC, a more quantitative assessment of MR can be made by calculating the regurgitant fraction (RF). The EDV and ESV are measured, and the difference between them is the total LV stroke volume. The total stroke volume calculated from angiography can be quite high, but in the setting of significant MR, a significant portion of this volume is ejected backward into the LA. The forward stroke volume (FSV) must be calculated from a measurement of forward CO by the Fick or thermodilution method:

$$FSV = CO/HR$$

where HR is heart rate. The regurgitant stroke volume (RSV) then can be calculated by subtracting the FSV from the total stroke volume (TSV):

$$RSV = TSV - FSV$$

The RF is the RSV divided by the TSV:

$$RF = RSV/TSV$$

An RF of less than 20% is considered mild, 20% to 40% is considered moderate, 40% to 60% is considered moderately severe, and greater than 60% is considered severe MR.

Aortography

The primary indication for aortography performed in the CCL is to delineate the extent of aortic regurgitation (AR). Similar to MR, AR is graded 1+ to 4+ based on the degree of contrast dye present in the LV chamber during aortography. In mild (1+) AR, there is transient filling of the LV cavity by contrast dye that clears after each systolic beat; in moderate (2+) AR, a small amount of contrast dye is regurgitated into the left ventricle and is present throughout the subsequent systolic beat; in moderately severe (3+) AR, a significant amount of contrast dye is present in the left ventricle throughout systole, but not at the intensity of that in the aorta; in severe (4+) AR, contrast dye is present in the left ventricle consistent with the intensity of that in the aorta, with rapid ventricular opacification and delayed clearance after aortic injection.

Coronary Arteriography

Description of Coronary Anatomy

The left main coronary artery (LM) bifurcates into the circumflex (Cx) and left anterior descending (LAD) arteries and is variable in length (Fig. 2.1). Occasionally, the Cx and LAD arise from separate ostia or the LM trifurcates, creating a middle branch, the ramus intermedius, which supplies the high lateral wall of the left ventricle. Both septal perforators and diagonal branch vessels arise from the LAD, which is described as having proximal, middle, and distal portions based on the location of these branch vessels. The proximal LAD is the portion located before the first septal and first diagonal branch; the middle LAD is between the first and second septal and diagonal branches; and the distal LAD is beyond the major septal and large diagonal vessels. The distal LAD provides the apical blood supply in two-thirds of patients, whereas the distal right coronary artery (RCA) supplies the apex in the remaining one-third.

The Cx artery is located in the atrioventricular (AV) groove and is angiographically identified by its location next to the coronary sinus. The latter is seen as a large structure that opacifies during delayed venous filling after left coronary injections. Marginal branches arise from the Cx artery and are the vessels in this coronary artery system usually bypassed. The Cx in the AV groove is often not surgically approachable.

The dominance of a coronary system is defined by the origin of the posterior descending artery (PDA), through which septal perforators supply the inferior one-third of the ventricular septum. The origin of the AV nodal artery often is near the origin of the PDA. In 85% to 90% of patients, the PDA originates from the RCA. In the

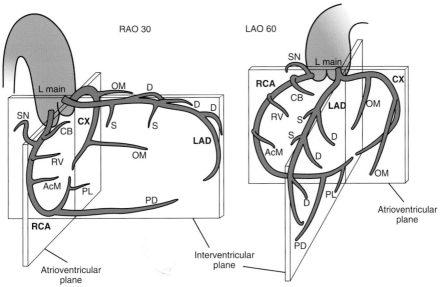

Fig. 2.1 Representation of coronary anatomy relative to the interventricular and atrioventricular valve planes. Coronary branches are indicated as follows: *AcM*, acute marginal; *CB*, conus branch; *CX*, circumflex; *D*, diagonal; *L main*, left main; *LAD*, left anterior descending; *OM*, obtuse marginal; *PD*, posterior descending; *PL*, posterolateral left ventricular; *RCA*, right coronary; *RV*, right ventricular; *S*, septal perforator; *SN*, sinus node branch. *LAO*, Left anterior oblique; *RAO*, right anterior oblique. (From Baim DS, Grossman W. Coronary angiography. In: Grossman W, Baim DS, eds. *Cardiac Catheterization, Angiography, and Intervention* [4th ed.]. Philadelphia: Lea & Febiger; 1991:200.)

remaining 10% to 15%, the PDA arises from the Cx artery. Codominance, or a contribution from both the Cx and the RCA, can occur and is defined when septal perforators from both vessels arise and supply the posteroinferior aspect of the left ventricle.

Assessing the Degree of Stenosis

By convention, the severity of a coronary stenosis is quantified as *percentage diameter reduction*. Multiple views of each vessel are recorded, and the worst narrowing is used to make clinical decisions. Diameter reductions can be used to estimate area reductions; for instance, if the narrowing were circumferential, 50% and 70% diameter reductions would result in 75% and 91% cross-sectional area reductions, respectively. Using the reduction in diameter as a measure of lesion severity is difficult if diffuse CAD creates difficulty in defining the "normal" coronary diameter. This is particularly true in patients with insulin-dependent diabetes mellitus (DM) and in individuals with severe lipid disorders. In addition, the use of percentage diameter reduction does not account for the length of the stenosis.

INTERVENTIONAL CARDIOLOGY: PERCUTANEOUS CORONARY INTERVENTION

A timeline of important events in the history of PCI is presented in Box 2.5. Catheter-based interventions were initially pioneered by Andreas Gruentzig in 1977 as PTCA, and they have expanded dramatically beyond the balloon to include a variety of PCIs. The use of PCI in the United States has grown considerably since the early 1980s;

BOX 2.5 *Interventional Cardiology Timeline*

1977 Percutaneous transluminal coronary angioplasty (PTCA)
1991 Directional atherectomy
1993 Rotational atherectomy
1994 Stents with extensive antithrombotic regimen
1995 Abciximab approved
1996 Simplified antiplatelet regimen after stenting
2001 Distal protection
2003 Drug-eluting stents (DES)
2008 Second-generation DES
2010 Percutaneous pulmonary valve approved
2011 Transcatheter aortic valve replacement (TAVR) approved
2012 MitraClip approved
2015 Impella approved

however, the annual volume of PCI procedures peaked in 2006 and has steadily declined since then.

General Topics for All Interventional Devices

Indications

Throughout the history of PCI, technology and operator expertise have continually advanced. The interventionalist now has the capability to approach places in the coronary tree that were previously inaccessible. This is reflected in the expanded role for PCI. Although PCI was first restricted to patients with single-vessel disease and normal ventricular function who had a discrete, noncalcified lesion in the proximal vessel, it now is performed as preferred therapy in many groups of patients, including selected patients with unprotected LM stenosis (ie, no bypass grafts). The most recently published guidelines state that LM PCI is a reasonable alternative to CABG in patients who have anatomic conditions associated with good procedural and longer-term outcomes and who are at increased risk for surgery. However, CABG remains the preferred therapy for many patients, particularly those with DM.

Box 2.6 provides a summary of current clinical indications for PCI. Primary PCI is the standard of care for patients with ST-elevation myocardial infarction (STEMI), with or without cardiogenic shock. Although PCI was initially reserved for patients who were considered suitable candidates for CABG, it is now routinely performed in patients who are not candidates for CABG in both emergent and nonemergent settings.

Equipment and Procedure

Although the femoral artery is still the most commonly used access site, the radial artery has seen increased adoption. Despite numerous advances, all PCIs still involve sequential placement of the following: a guiding catheter in the ostium of the vessel, a guiding wire across the lesion and into the distal vessel, and one or more devices of choice at the lesion site.

While a device is present in a coronary artery, blood flow is impeded to a varying degree. In vessels that supply large amounts of myocardium (eg, proximal LAD),

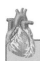

BOX 2.6 *Clinical Indications for Percutaneous Transluminal Coronary Interventional Procedures*

Cardiac Symptoms

- Unstable angina pectoris or non–ST-segment elevation myocardial infarction (NSTEMI)
- Angina refractory to antianginal medications
- Angina after myocardial infarction
- Sudden cardiac death

Diagnostic Testing

- Early positive exercise tolerance testing
- Positive exercise tolerance test despite maximal antianginal therapy
- Large areas of ischemic myocardium on perfusion or wall motion studies
- Positive preoperative dipyridamole or adenosine perfusion study
- Electrophysiologic studies suggestive of arrhythmia related to ischemia

Acute Myocardial Infarction

- Cardiogenic shock
- Unsuccessful thrombolytic therapy in unstable patient with large areas of myocardium at risk
- Contraindication to thrombolytic therapy
- Cerebral vascular event
- Intracranial neoplasm
- Uncontrollable hypertension
- Major surgery <14 days previously
- Potential for uncontrolled hemorrhage
- Probably preferred for all cases of ST-segment elevation acute myocardial infarction (STEMI)

prolonged obstruction of flow is poorly tolerated. However, when only smaller areas of myocardium are jeopardized or the distal vessel is well collateralized, longer occlusion times are possible.

Antiischemic medications may permit longer periods of vessel occlusion before signs and symptoms of ischemia become limiting. This additional time could permit the completion of a complex case or allow the use of distal protection devices. Most centers use either intracoronary or IV nitroglycerin (NTG) at some point during the procedure to treat or prevent coronary spasm. Intracoronary calcium channel blockers frequently are used to treat vasospasm and the "no-reflow" phenomenon. The latter term describes an absence of flow in a coronary vessel when there is no epicardial obstruction. No-reflow is associated with a variety of adverse outcomes; it is seen when acutely occluded vessels are opened during an MI or when PCI is performed in old saphenous vein grafts (SVGs). The cause is believed to be microvascular obstruction from embolic debris or microvascular spasm or both. Intracoronary calcium antagonists may help to restore normal flow, and nicardipine is preferred for its relative lack of hemodynamic and conduction effects. Continuous NTG infusions are rarely necessary after PCI unless symptoms or signs of ongoing ischemia are detected.

Restenosis

Once PTCA/PCI became an established therapeutic option for treatment of CAD, two major limitations were realized: acute closure and restenosis. The use of stents and antiplatelet therapy significantly decreased the incidence of acute closure. Before stents were available, restenosis occurred in 30% to 40% of PTCA procedures. With stent use, this figure decreased to about 20%. However, restenosis remained the Achilles heel of intracoronary intervention until the advent of the drug-eluting stent (DES).

Restenosis usually occurs within the first 6 months after an intervention and has three major mechanisms: vessel recoil, negative remodeling, and neointimal hyperplasia. Vessel recoil is caused by the elastic tissue in the vessel and occurs early after balloon dilation. It is no longer a significant contributor to restenosis because metal stents are almost 100% effective in preventing recoil. Negative remodeling refers to late narrowing of the external elastic lamina and adjacent tissue, which accounted for up to 75% of lumen loss in the past. This process also is prevented by metal stents and no longer contributes to restenosis. Neointimal hyperplasia is the major component of in-stent restenosis (ISR) in the current era. Neointimal hyperplasia is more pronounced in the patient with DM, which explains the increased incidence of restenosis in this population. DESs limit neointimal hyperplasia and have dramatically reduced the frequency of ISR.

The major gains in combating restenosis have been in the area of stenting. Intracoronary stents maximize the increase in lumen area during the PCI procedure and decrease late lumen loss by preventing recoil and negative remodeling. However, neointimal hyperplasia is enhanced because of a foreign body–like reaction to the stent. Different stent designs and strut thicknesses lead to different restenosis rates.

Anticoagulation

Thrombosis is a major component of acute coronary syndrome (ACS) and of acute complications during PCI; its management is continually evolving. Proper anticoagulation regimens are essential to limit bleeding complications and thrombotic complications, both of which negatively impact prognosis. This is most important with interventional procedures, in which the guiding catheter, wire, and device in the coronary artery serve as nidi for thrombus. In addition, catheter-based interventions disrupt the vessel wall, exposing thrombogenic substances to the blood. Table 2.1 summarizes current antiplatelet regimens in patients receiving stents.

The primary pathway for clot formation during PCI has proved to be platelet mediated. This has prompted a focus on aggressive antiplatelet therapy. Aspirin remains the foundation of antiplatelet therapy for patients with PCI.

Clopidogrel, prasugrel, ticagrelor, and cangrelor block the adenosine diphosphate (ADP) receptor P2Y12 on platelets. Cangrelor is an ADP inhibitor that is unique in its delivery form as an IV agent. Advantages of cangrelor, which might improve clinical outcomes over other antiplatelet agents, are its rapid onset of action and rapid return of platelet function after cessation.

Heparin has been used since the inception of PTCA, with the dose regimen undergoing significant evolution over time. Initially, high doses were used to prevent abrupt closure of the vessel. With experience and the introduction of stents, the dosing has evolved into a weight-based regimen (70–100 U/kg) that is routine and endorsed by the guidelines. The activated clotting time (ACT) is monitored to guide additional heparin therapy. Protamine is not routinely used, and the femoral sheaths are removed once the ACT is 150 seconds or less. If a transradial approach is used, the sheath is removed immediately after the procedure, and a transradial band is placed to apply hemostatic pressure while allowing for adequate perfusion to the

Table 2.1 Anticoagulation in the Catheterization Laboratory

Medication	Dose	Mechanism of Action	Half-Life	Monitoring
Antiplatelet Medications				
Aspirin	75–325 mg	Acetylates cyclooxygenase	3 h	Platelet function assays
Clopidogrel	300–600 mg loading dose	Irreversibly binds to P2Y12 platelet receptor	6 h	Platelet function assays
	75 mg daily			
Prasugrel	300 mg loading dose	Irreversibly binds to P2Y12 platelet receptor	7 h	Platelet function assays
	5–10 mg daily			
Ticagrelor	300 mg loading dose	Irreversibly binds to P2Y12 platelet receptor	7 h	Platelet function assays
	90 mg bid daily			
Glycoprotein (GP) IIb/IIIa Inhibitors				
Abciximab	0.25 mg/kg bolus	Monoclonal antibody GPIIb/IIIa platelet receptor inhibition	30 min	Platelet function assays
	0.125 µg/kg per min infusion			
Eptifibatide	180 µg/kg bolus	Cyclic heptapeptide GPIIb/IIIa platelet receptor inhibition	2.5 h	Platelet function assays
	2 µg/kg per min infusion			
Tirofiban	25 µg/kg bolus	Nonpeptide GPIIb/IIIa platelet receptor inhibition	2 h	Platelet function assays
	0.15 µg/kg per min infusion			
Anticoagulants				
Heparin	70–100 U/kg bolus	Indirect inhibitor of thrombin	Dose-dependent, ~1 h	Activated clotting time (ACT), partial thromboplastin time (PTT)
Enoxaparin	0.5–0.75 mg/kg bolus	Inhibitor of factor Xa	4 h	Anti-Xa levels
Bivalirudin	0.75 mg/kg bolus	Direct thrombin inhibitor	25 min	ACT
	1.75 mg/kg per h infusion			

affected hand (patent hemostasis). As an alternative to heparin, direct thrombin inhibitors have been investigated in the setting of PCI. The synthetic compound bivalirudin (Angiomax; The Medicines Company, Parsippany, NJ) is the best studied of these agents. The advantage of direct thrombin inhibitors is the direct dose response and the shorter half-life, which leads to a lower incidence of bleeding complications.

Operating Room Backup

When PTCA was introduced, all patients were considered candidates for CABG. The physician learning curve in the early 1980s was considered to be 25 to 50 cases; increased complications were seen during these initial cases. All PCI procedures had immediate OR availability, and often the anesthesiologist was present in the CCL. In the 1990s OR backup was necessary less often. Perfusion catheter technology had developed to allow for longer inflation times with less ischemia. Over time, the need for emergency surgery declined dramatically as a result of more experienced operators, improved techniques, better stents, and improved antiplatelet and anticoagulation regimens. Because the incidence of emergent CABG has been reduced to 0.2% of PCI procedures, more institutions are beginning to perform PCI despite lack of cardiac surgery facilities on-site. The main reasons are to provide timely access for primary PCI in patients with STEMI and to provide care to patients who do not want to travel. In 1911 the AHA, the American College of Cardiology Foundation (ACCF), and the Society for Cardiovascular Angiography and Interventions (SCAI) updated their recommendations for PCI without surgical backup (Table 2.2). Although many coronary lesions can be treated at stand-alone PCI centers, the 2014 SCAI/ACC/AHA guidelines state that intervention should be avoided in patients with specific coronary lesions (Box 2.7) and that transfer for emergency CABG must occur when there is high-grade LM or three-vessel disease with clinical or hemodynamic instability after a successful or unsuccessful PCI attempt in an occluded vessel, or if there is a failed or unstable PCI result and ongoing ischemia with intraaortic balloon pump (IABP) support. Transfer agreements with established oversight hospitals with on-site cardiac surgery capability are required; minimal requirements for operators and

Table 2.2 Recommendations for Percutaneous Coronary Intervention (PCI) Without Surgical Backup	
Primary PCI is reasonable in hospitals without on-site surgery provided that appropriate planning for program development has been accomplished.	Class IIa Level of Evidence B
Elective PCI might be considered in hospitals without on-site cardiac surgery provided that appropriate planning for program development has been accomplished and rigorous clinical and angiographic criteria are used for proper patient selection.	Class IIb Level of Evidence B
Primary or elective PCI should not be performed in hospitals without on-site cardiac surgery capabilities without a proven plan for rapid transport to a cardiac surgery operating room in a nearby hospital or without appropriate hemodynamic support capability for transfer.	Class III Level of Evidence C

From Levine GN, Piates ER, Blankenship JC, et al. ACCF/AHA/SCAI guideline for percutaneous coronary intervention. *J Am Coll Cardiol.* 2011;58:e44.

BOX 2.7   *Characteristics That Make Percutaneous Coronary Intervention Inappropriate in Stand-Alone Centers*

Avoid Treatment

- >50% Stenosis of the LM proximal to the infarct-related lesion, especially if the area in jeopardy is small and the overall LV function is not severely impaired
- Long, calcified, or severely angulated target lesions at high risk for PCI failure
- Lesions in areas other than the infarct artery unless they appear to be flow-limiting in patients with hemodynamic instability or ongoing symptoms
- Lesions with TIMI flow grade 3 in patients with LM or three-vessel disease if CABG is more likely to be a superior revascularization strategy
- Culprit lesions in more distal branches that jeopardize only a modest amount of myocardium if there is more proximal disease that could be worsened by attempted intervention
- Chronic total occlusion

Transfer for Emergency CABG

- High-grade LM or three-vessel disease with clinical or hemodynamic instability after successful or unsuccessful PCI attempt in an occluded vessel, preferably with IABP support
- Failed or unstable PCI result and ongoing ischemia, with IABP support

CABG, Coronary artery bypass graft surgery; *IABP*, intraaortic balloon pump; *LM*, left main coronary artery; *LV*, left ventricular; *PCI*, percutaneous coronary intervention; *TIMI*, Thrombolysis in Myocardial Infarction grading system.
Modified from Dehmer GJ, Blankenship JC, Cilingiroglu M, et al. SCAI/ACC/AHA expert consensus document: 2014 Update on percutaneous coronary intervention without on-site backup. *Catheter Cardiovasc Interv.* 2014;84:169.

institutions must be met, and a comprehensive quality assurance program must be in place.

Infrequently, high-risk interventional cases still may require a cardiac OR on immediate standby. This may occur in an emergent situation in which a patient with STEMI requires assistive support during primary PCI or, more electively, when a patient is identified as being at high risk but is not a candidate for a hybrid laboratory or no such facility is available. A preoperative anesthetic evaluation that allows for assessment of the overall medical condition, past anesthetic history, current drug therapy, and allergic history, as well as a physical examination concentrating on airway management considerations, is reserved for these high-risk cases.

Regardless of the location of the interventional procedure, when an emergency CABG is necessary, it is essential either to have an OR with a basic cardiac setup ready to go or to have the cardiology and surgery teams provide enough lead time to adequately prepare an OR. A basic cardiac setup includes the essential equipment to perform a CABG and an anesthesia setup with emergency medications such as heparin, epinephrine, vasopressin, and norepinephrine available to support the circulation until the patient is placed on cardiopulmonary bypass (CPB), as well as invasive monitors such as TEE and transducers to measure arterial blood pressure, central venous pressure, and pulmonary artery pressures, and resuscitative devices, including defibrillators and pacemakers. These patients are often critically ill, with ongoing

2

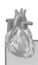

> ## BOX 2.8 *Preparation of the Patient for Surgery After Failed Intervention*
>
> Perform usual preoperative evaluation for an emergent procedure
> Inventory vascular access sites (eg, pulmonary artery catheter, intraarterial balloon pump)
> Defer removal of sheaths
> Review medicines administered:
> - Boluses may linger even if infusion is stopped (eg, abciximab)
> - Check medicines that have been administered before arrival at the catheterization laboratory (eg, enoxaparin, clopidogrel)
>
> Confirm availability of blood products

myocardial injury and circulatory collapse. Time is critical to limit the damage and prevent death. Therefore the sooner the anesthesiologist, staff, and OR personnel are aware of an arriving patient in this perilous condition, the better for all involved. In addition, because this situation occurs infrequently, cooperation among the interventionalist, the surgeon, and the anesthesiologist is essential for optimal patient care in this critically ill population.

In preparation for the OR, a perfusion catheter, pacemaker, and/or pulmonary artery catheter (PAC) may be inserted in the CCL, depending on patient stability, OR availability, and patient assessment by the cardiologist, cardiothoracic surgeon, and anesthesiologist. Although these procedures are intended to better stabilize the patient, this is achieved at the expense of ischemic time. An IABP or one of the newer support devices may be placed. Although these devices can reduce the myocardial oxygen requirements, myocardial necrosis still will occur in the absence of coronary or collateral blood flow. The anesthesiologist should examine the vascular sheaths that are in place and determine which are venous and which arterial. He or she should also review any inotropic, vasoactive, and anticoagulant medications that have been administered and determine whether blood products are available (Box 2.8).

In the OR, anesthetic management depends on the hemodynamic instability of the patient. Hemodynamically stable patients can have a controlled induction and intubation with placement of invasive monitors, including intraarterial and central venous catheters. If heart failure is anticipated after CPB, placement of a PAC with $S\bar{v}O_2$ and continuous CO measurements will be beneficial, especially if ventricular assist device placement is anticipated. A TEE is also beneficial in these patients. *Because these patients usually have received significant anticoagulation with heparin and antiplatelet drugs, attempts at catheter placement should not be undertaken when direct pressure cannot be applied to a vessel.* The most experienced individual should perform these procedures.

Patients who arrive in cardiogenic shock may require preinduction inotropic support to prevent cardiovascular collapse during induction and intubation. As with all patients with heart failure, it is important to remember that these patients have a slower circulatory time, and IV inductions will be slower; they also are more susceptible to the hemodynamic effects of the inhalation agents. For induction, medications that provide the most stable hemodynamics should be used.

The worst scenario is the patient who arrives in the OR in profound circulatory shock or in full cardiopulmonary arrest. In these patients, CPB should be established as quickly as possible, and it is important to have IV heparin prepared to anticoagulate the patient before bypass. No attempt to establish access for monitoring should be made if it would delay the start of surgery. The only real requirement to start a case such as this is to have good IV access, a five-lead ECG, airway control, a functioning blood pressure cuff, arterial access from the PCI procedure, and, if available, TEE. Preinduction inotropic support is required for these patients. If large doses of vasoactive medications were administered during the prebypass period, the patient may become severely hypertensive once on CPB, requiring the use of vasodilators.

In many cases of emergency surgery, the cardiologist has placed femoral artery sheaths for access during the PCI. *These should not be removed,* again because of heparin (or bivalirudin) and antiplatelet therapy during the PCI. A femoral artery sheath provides extremely accurate pressure measurements that closely reflect central aortic pressure. Also, a PAC may have been placed in the CCL, and this can be adapted for use in the OR.

Several surgical series have looked for associations with mortality in patients who present for emergency CABG after failed PCI. Complete occlusion, urgent PCI, and multivessel disease have all been associated with an increased mortality. In addition, long delays lead to increased morbidity and mortality. The paradigm shift in cardiovascular medicine toward PCI will be negatively impacted if significant numbers of serious complications occur because of prolonged delays in arranging emergent cardiac surgical care for the infrequent occurrence of failed PCI. As the frequency of PCI at institutions with no on-site cardiac surgery facility increases, cooperation among specialties and facilities will be required to ensure that timely transfer can be arranged after a failed PCI. Important time will be lost unless formal arrangements are in place ahead of time.

Support Devices for High-Risk Angioplasty

As devices and techniques in the CCL become more sophisticated, interventional cardiologists are expanding their practices to address more complex lesions and more high-risk patients who are deemed unsuitable candidates for surgical repair. Although there is no consensus on the definition of a high-risk PCI, a patient is considered to be at high risk when there is a combination of adverse clinical, anatomic, and hemodynamic factors that, when combined, will significantly increase the risk of periprocedural major adverse cardiac and cerebral events (MACCE) (Box 2.9). These patients are at higher risk for hemodynamic compromise from LV failure, arrhythmias, ischemia–reperfusion injury, or distal embolization of atherogenic material leading to cardiogenic shock or malignant arrhythmias.

Percutaneous mechanical circulatory systems (MCS) can provide a bridge by maintaining coronary perfusion pressure, supporting the right or left ventricle, and reducing myocardial workload, allowing the cardiologist time to complete the intervention. Another beneficial effect of MCS is to augment mean arterial pressure and CO, allowing vasopressor and inotropic support to be decreased or discontinued. The four mechanical circulatory devices that can be placed percutaneously in the CCL are the IABP, the Impella (Abiomed, Danvers, MA), the TandemHeart (CardiacAssist, Pittsburgh, PA), and extracorporeal membranous oxygenation (ECMO).

Controversies in Interventional Cardiology

Percutaneous Coronary Intervention Versus Surgical Revascularization in Complex Coronary Artery Disease

To address the changes in PCI and CABG therapy, four randomized trials were undertaken, and these are included in Fig. 2.2. The results of the newer studies were

> **BOX 2.9** *Clinical, Anatomic, and Hemodynamic Criteria Used to Identify High-Risk Percutaneous Coronary Interventions*
>
> 1. Clinical
>   a. Cardiogenic shock within 12 h or at the start of coronary intervention
>   b. Left ventricular systolic dysfunction on presentation with EF <30–40%
>   c. Killip class II–IV on presentation or congestive heart failure
>   d. Coronary intervention after resuscitated cardiac arrest within 24 h
>   e. STEMI
>   f. Acute coronary syndrome complicated by unstable hemodynamics, arrhythmia, or refractory angina
>   g. Mechanical complications of acute myocardial infarction
>   h. Age >70–80 y
>   i. History of cerebrovascular disease, diabetes, renal dysfunction, or chronic lung disease
> 2. Anatomic
>   a. Intervention in an unprotected left main coronary artery or left main equivalent
>   b. Multivessel disease
>   c. Distal left main bifurcation intervention
>   d. Previous CABG, including intervention in a graft, particularly a degenerated graft
>   e. Last remaining coronary conduit
>   f. Duke Myocardial Jeopardy score >8/12
>   g. Target vessel providing a collateral supply to an occluded second vessel that supplies >40% of the left ventricular myocardium
>   h. SYNTAX score >33
> 3. Hemodynamic
>   a. Cardiac index, <2.2 L/min per square meter
>   b. PCWP >15 mm Hg
>   c. Mean pulmonary artery pressure >50 mm Hg
>
> *CABG,* Coronary artery bypass graft surgery; *EF,* ejection fraction; *PCWP,* pulmonary capillary wedge pressure; *STEMI,* ST-segment elevation myocardial infarction.
> From Myat A, Patel N, Tehrani S, et al. Percutaneous circulatory assist devices for high-risk coronary intervention. *J Am Coll Cardiol Cardiovasc Interv.* 2015;8:229.

similar to the results of the earlier ones. In the Arterial Revascularization Therapy Study (ARTS), patients with DM had poorer outcomes with PCI, with rates of MACCE greater than 50% at 5 years. Overall, there was no difference in the rates of mortality, cerebrovascular accident, or MI between the groups at 5 years, but there was a higher MACCE rate in the stenting arm, which was driven by a higher rate of repeat revascularization because bare metal stents (BMSs) were utilized.

The well-known Synergy Between Percutaneous Coronary Intervention with Taxus and Cardiac Surgery (SYNTAX) trial randomized 1800 patients with three-vessel CAD and/or LM stenosis to either CABG or PCI with paclitaxel-eluting stents with the intention of obtaining complete revascularization. Patients were eligible regardless of clinical presentation on the condition that the angiograms were reviewed by both a cardiologist and a cardiac surgeon and complete revascularization was believed feasible by both techniques. After 1 year, 17.8% of the PCI patients and 12.4% of the CABG patients had experienced a MACCE (*P* = .002). Although this difference was driven primarily by a greater need for repeat revascularization in the PCI group, the

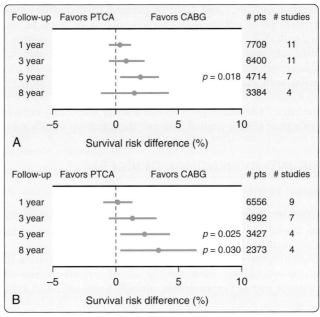

Fig. 2.2 Randomized trials of coronary artery bypass graft surgery *(CABG)* versus percutaneous coronary angioplasty *(PTCA)* in patients with multivessel coronary disease show risk differences for all-cause mortality in years 1, 3, 5, and 8 after initial revascularization. (A) All trials. (B) Multivessel trials. (Redrawn from Hoffman SN, TenBrook JA, Wolf MP, et al. A meta-analysis of randomized controlled trials comparing coronary artery bypass graft with percutaneous transluminal coronary angioplasty: one- to eight-year outcomes. *J Am Coll Cardiol.* 2003;41:1293. Copyright 2003, with permission from The American College of Cardiology Foundation.)

rate of death was not significantly greater in the PCI group, at 4.4%, compared with 3.5% in the CABG group. The rate of stroke was significantly greater in the CABG group, 2.2%, versus 0.6% in the PCI group ($P = .003$). The 5-year published data showed that outcomes were stratified based on the calculation of a SYNTAX score, which is an angiographically calculated score that takes into account the burden and location of CAD. For patients with low SYNTAX scores, including those with isolated LM disease, PCI appeared to be an acceptable alternative to CABG. However, in those with intermediate- to high-risk SYNTAX scores, CABG appeared superior mainly because of lower MACCE rates and lower repeat revascularization rates.

A metaanalysis of six major clinical trials that compared PCI with CABG for multivessel CAD revealed an unequivocal reduction in long-term mortality and MI in addition to reductions in repeat revascularizations favoring CABG. These findings were consistent in patients with and without DM.

Percutaneous Coronary Intervention Versus Coronary Artery Bypass Graft Surgery for Left Main Coronary Artery Disease

Of all patients undergoing coronary angiography, approximately 4% are found to have LM CAD. CABG has long been considered to be the gold standard revascularization method for patients with LM disease because it confers a survival benefit when compared with medical therapy. A metaanalysis of these trials demonstrated a 66% reduction in relative risk and mortality with CABG, with the benefit extending to 10 years.

More recently, in a significantly larger randomized controlled trial (RCT) using DESs, the composite end point of death, MI, or stroke at 2 years occurred in 4.4%

of patients treated with PCI and 4.7% of patients treated with CABG. However, ischemia-driven target-vessel revascularization was more often required in those patients treated with PCI (9.0% vs 4.2%). The publication of the results of the SYNTAX LM prespecified subgroup, which included 705 patients, contributed significantly to the data. This landmark study concluded that patients with LM disease who underwent revascularization with PCI had safety and efficacy outcomes comparable to those achieved with CABG at 1 year. The recently published 5-year outcomes from this study suggested that PCI-treated patients had a lower stroke rate but a higher revascularization rate than CABG-treated patients; there was no significant difference in mortality (12.8% vs 14.6% with PCI and CABG, respectively, $P = .53$).

▓ SPECIFIC INTERVENTIONAL DEVICES

Intracoronary Stents

The introduction of intracoronary stents has had a larger impact on the practice of interventional cardiology than any other development. The use of intracoronary stents exploded during the mid-1990s (Box 2.10).

Stent technology improved in incremental fashion. Modifications in coil geometry, alterations in the articulation sites, and the use of meshlike stents offered minor advantages. Various metals (eg, tantalum, nitinol) were used, and various coatings (eg, heparin, polymers, and even human cells) were applied. In addition, the delivery systems used to implant stents were decreased in size.

The early enthusiasm for first-generation DESs was tempered after widespread concerns about the increased risks of late stent thrombosis and very late stent thrombosis. In addition to the development of second-generation stents, research was also applied to produce a fully biodegradable scaffold. This new technology offers the possibility of transient scaffolding of the vessel to prevent acute vessel closure and recoil during elution of an antiproliferative drug to counteract constrictive remodeling and excessive neointimal hyperplasia. Currently, stents are placed at the time of most PCI procedures if the size and anatomy of the vessel permit. Multiple studies have been performed comparing BMSs with DESs in various clinical scenarios. There are several reasons not to use a DES in every procedure. First, DESs are not manufactured in sizes greater than

I

BOX 2.10   *Stents*

Antiplatelet therapy after stent placement: indefinite aspirin therapy plus:
- BMS: clopidogrel 4 wk for patients without ACS, 12 mo with ACS
- DES: clopidogrel 12 mo.

With BMS, thienopyridines reduce subacute thrombosis from 3% to <1%.
DES have never been tested without clopidogrel.
A concern with first-generation DES is delay in endothelial coverage of the stent.
With clopidogrel, subacute and late thrombosis rates for DES and BMS are identical.
Very late thrombosis rates are greater with first-generation DES.
Late stent thrombosis rates with second-generation DES are similar to those with BMS.

Options for elective surgery in patients with stents:
- Delay surgery until clopidogrel regimen is completed: recommended
- Perform surgery during clopidogrel therapy: accept bleeding risk.

ACS, Acute coronary syndromes; *BMS*, bare metal stents; *DES*, drug-eluting stents.

4.0 mm, making them useless in large vessels. Second, a longer course of thienopyridine is required, and this may not be desirable if a surgical procedure is urgently needed because it requires an uncomfortable choice between bleeding and increased risk for cardiac events. Stent thromboses, MIs, and deaths have been reported when antiplatelet therapy is interrupted. Third, there are cost considerations: DES is two to three times more expensive than a BMS. Finally, a DES may not be the ideal choice in a patient who requires long-term anticoagulation because bleeding rates are increased.

SUGGESTED READINGS

Baratke MS, Bannon PG, Hughes CF, et al. Emergency surgery after unsuccessful coronary angioplasty: a review of 15 years of experience. *Ann Thorac Surg*. 2003;75:1400.

Dehmer GJ, Blankenship JC, Cilingiroglu M, et al. SCAI/ACC/AHA expert consensus document: 2014 Update on percutaneous coronary intervention without on-site backup. *Catheter Cardiovasc Interv*. 2014;84:169.

Dehmer GJ, Blankenship JC, Cilingiroglu M, et al. Update on percutaneous coronary intervention without on-site surgical backup. *J Am Coll Cardiol*. 2014;63:2624.

Elli S, Tendera M, de Belder MA, et al. Facilitated PCI in patients with ST-elevation myocardial infarction. *N Engl J Med*. 2008;358:2205.

Feldman DN, Swamanathan RV, Kaltenback LA, et al. Adoption of radial access and comparison of outcomes to femoral access in percutaneous coronary intervention: an updated report from the National Cardiovascular Data Registry (2007–2012). *Circulation*. 2013;127:2295.

Hamid M. Anesthesia for cardiac catheterization procedures. *Heart Lung Vessel*. 2014;6:225.

Hanna EB, Rao SV, Manoukian SV, et al. The evolving role of glycoprotein IIb/IIIa inhibitors in the setting of percutaneous coronary intervention strategies to minimize bleeding risk and optimize outcomes. *JACC Cardiovasc Interv*. 2010;3:1209.

King S, Aversano T, Ballard W, et al. ACCF/AHA/SCAI 2007 update of the clinical competence statement on cardiac interventional procedures. *J Am Coll Cardiol*. 2007;50:82.

Kukreja N, Onuma Y, Garcia-Garcia HM, et al. The risk of stent thrombosis in patients with acute coronary syndromes treated with bare-metal and drug-eluting stents. *JACC Cardiovasc Interv*. 2009;2:533.

Mauri L, Kereiakes DJ, Yeh RW, et al. Twelve or 30 months of dual antiplatelet therapy after drug-eluting stents. *N Engl J Med*. 2014;371:2155.

Mohr FW, Morice MC, Kappetein AP, et al. Coronary artery bypass graft surgery versus percutaneous coronary intervention in patients with three-vessel disease and left main coronary disease: 5-year follow-up of the randomised, clinical SYNTAX trial. *Lancet*. 2013;381:629.

Morice MC, Serruys PW, Kappetein AP, et al. Outcomes in patients with de novo left main disease treated with either percutaneous coronary intervention using paclitaxel-eluting stents or coronary artery bypass graft treatment in the Synergy between Percutaneous Coronary Intervention with TAXUS and Cardiac Surgery (SYNTAX) trial. *Circulation*. 2010;121:2645.

Myat A, Patel N, Tehrani S, et al. Percutaneous circulatory assist devices for high-risk coronary intervention. *JACC Cardiovasc Interv*. 2015;8:229.

Nishimura RA, Otto CM, Bonow RO, et al. AHA/ACC guideline for the management of patients with valvular heart disease. *J Am Coll Cardiol*. 2014;63:e57.

Pursnani S, Korley F, Gopaul R, et al. Percutaneous coronary intervention versus optimal medical therapy in stable coronary artery disease. *Circ Cardiovasc Interv*. 2012;5:476.

Serruys PW, Chevalier B, Dudek D, et al. A bioresorbable everolimus-eluting scaffold versus a metallic everolimus-eluting stent for ischaemic heart disease caused by de-novo native coronary artery lesions (ABSORB II): an interim 1-year analysis of clinical and procedural secondary outcomes from a randomised controlled trial. *Lancet*. 2015;385:43.

Serruys P, Daemen J. Are drug-eluting stents associated with a higher rate of late thrombosis than bare metal stents? *Circulation*. 2007;115:1433.

Serruys PW, Ong AT, van Herwerden LA, et al. Five-year outcomes after coronary stenting versus bypass surgery for the treatment of multivessel disease: the final analysis of the Arterial Revascularization Therapies Study (ARTS) randomized trial. *J Am Coll Cardiol*. 2005;46:575.

Shahzad A, Kemp I, Mars C, et al. Unfractionated heparin versus bivalirudin in primary percutaneous coronary intervention (HEAT-PPCI): an open-label, single centre, randomised controlled trial. *Lancet*. 2014;384:1849.

Sipahi I, Hakan Akay M, Dagdelen S, et al. Coronary artery bypass grafting vs percutaneous coronary intervention and long-term mortality and morbidity in multivessel disease: meta-analysis of randomized clinical trials of the arterial grafting and stenting era. *JAMA Intern Med*. 2014;174:223.

Chapter 3

Cardiac Electrophysiology: Diagnosis and Treatment

Nadia Hensley, MD • Alan Cheng, MD • Ashish Shah, MD •
Charles W. Hogue, MD • Marc A. Rozner, PhD, MD

Key Points

1. Cardiac arrhythmias are common and result from an ectopic focus or a reentry circuit.
2. Surgical and catheter-based ablative therapies can abolish the origins of arrhythmias by interposition of scar tissue along the reentrant pathway or by isolating an ectopic area.
3. Supraventricular arrhythmias can be hemodynamically unstable, especially in the setting of structural heart disease. In some cases, persistent tachycardia can lead to tachycardia-induced cardiomyopathy.
4. Surgical treatment of atrial fibrillation (ie, maze procedure) has been employed with good success and has been modified to avoid the sinus node in an effort to minimize occurrences of chronotropic incompetence.
5. In adults, most episodes of sudden cardiac death are the result of ventricular tachyarrhythmias due to ischemic and nonischemic cardiomyopathy.
6. Preoperatively, identify the type of cardiac implantable electronic device (CIED) (eg, transvenous implantable pacemaker, intracardiac pacemaker, transvenous implantable cardioverter-defibrillator, subcutaneous implantable cardioverter-defibrillator) and the manufacturer of the generator.
7. Establish contact with the patient's CIED physician or clinic to obtain records and perioperative prescription (Heart Rhythm Society [HRS]). Have the CIED interrogated by a competent authority shortly before the procedure (American Society of Anesthesiologists [ASA]).
8. Determine the patient's underlying rate, rhythm, and pacing dependency to determine the need for asynchronous or external backup pacing support.
9. If magnet use is planned, then ensure that magnet behavior (pacing mode, rate, atrioventricular delay, shock therapy suspension) is appropriate for the patient.
10. If electromagnetic interference is likely or if a central venous catheter guidewire will be placed into the chest, then consider asynchronous pacing for the pacing-dependent patient and suspension of antitachycardia therapy for any implantable cardioverter-defibrillator (ICD) patient. Magnet application might be effective, although magnet use has been associated with inappropriate ICD discharge. Magnet application will never create asynchronous pacing in any type of ICD.
11. Monitor cardiac rhythm/peripheral pulse with pulse oximeter (plethysmography) or arterial waveform.
12. Ask the surgeon to avoid the use of the monopolar electrosurgical unit (ESU) or limit ESU bursts to less than 4 seconds separated by at least 2 seconds. Use the bipolar ESU if possible; if not possible, then pure cut (monopolar ESU) is better than "blend" or "coag."

13. Place the ESU dispersive electrode in such a way as to prevent electricity from crossing the generator-heart circuit, even if the electrode must be placed on the distal forearm and the wire covered with sterile drape.
14. Temporary pacing might be needed, and consideration should be given to the possibility of CIED failure.
15. Have the CIED interrogated by a competent authority postoperatively. Some rate enhancements can be reinitiated, and optimum heart rate and pacing parameters should be determined. The ICD patient must be monitored until the antitachycardia therapy is restored.

Cardiac rhythm disturbances are common and an important source of morbidity and mortality. Atrial fibrillation is the most common sustained cardiac arrhythmia in the general population. Prevalence is strongly associated with age, occurring in less than 1% of individuals younger than 55 years old but in almost 10% of those older than 80 years.

The treatment of cardiac arrhythmias has shifted over the past two decades to catheter-based and surgical ablation from pharmacologic therapy because of the drugs' limited efficacy and increased risk of death owing to their negative inotropic and proarrhythmic effects. Data from prospective, randomized trials showing improved survival for patients with implantable cardioverter-defibrillators (ICDs) compared with those given antiarrhythmic drugs bolstered the shift to nonpharmacologic treatments.

Current management options for cardiac arrhythmias include surgical and catheter ablative techniques using various energy sources. The principle in all cases is identification of the electrophysiologic mechanism of the arrhythmia followed by ablation of the involved myocardium using surgical incisions, cryothermy, or radiofrequency (RF) current. As the techniques have become more complex and time intensive, the need for anesthesia support has grown. Anesthesiologists caring for patients undergoing these procedures must be familiar with the anatomy of the normal cardiac conduction system, the electrophysiologic basis of common cardiac rhythm disorders, and the various approaches to ablative treatment.

3

▦ ELECTROPHYSIOLOGIC PRINCIPLES

Anatomy and Physiology of the Cardiac Pacemaker and Conduction Systems

Sinoatrial Node

The sinoatrial (SA) node (Fig. 3.1) is a spindle-shaped structure composed of highly specialized cells located in the right atrial sulcus terminalis, which is lateral to the junction of the superior vena cava (SVC) and the right atrium. Box 3.1 summarizes the anatomy of the cardiac pacemaker and conduction system.

Internodal Conduction

Despite previous controversy about the existence of specialized conduction pathways connecting the SA node to the atrioventricular (AV) node, electrophysiologists agree that preferential conduction unequivocally exists and that spread of activation from the SA node to the AV node follows distinct routes by necessity because of the peculiar

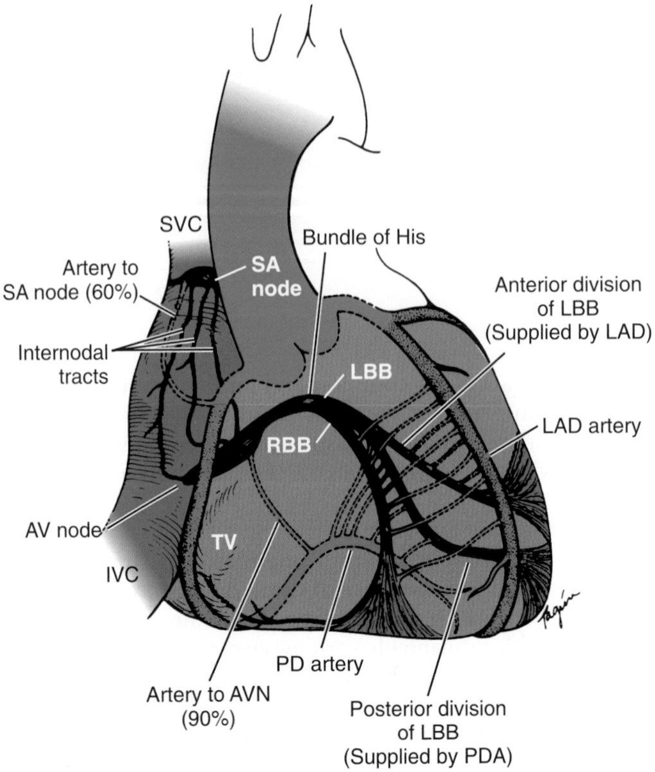

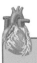

Fig. 3.1 Anatomy of the cardiac conduction system and arterial blood supply. In 60% of patients, the sinoatrial *(SA)* nodal artery is a branch of the right coronary artery, and in the remainder, it arises from the circumflex artery. The atrioventricular *(AV)* node is supplied by a branch from the right coronary artery or posterior descending artery *(PD artery)*. *IVC*, Inferior vena cava; *LAD*, left anterior descending coronary artery; *LBB*, left bundle branch; *RBB*, right bundle branch; *SVC*, superior vena cava; *TV*, tricuspid valve. (From Harthorne JW, Pohost GM. Electrical therapy of cardiac arrhythmias. In Levine HJ, ed. *Clinical Cardiovascular Physiology.* New York: Grune & Stratton; 1976:854.)

BOX 3.1   *Anatomy of the Cardiac Pacemaker and Conduction System*

Sinus node
Internodal conduction
Atrioventricular junction
Intraventricular conduction system
  • Left bundle branch
    • Anterior fascicle
    • Posterior fascicle
Right bundle branch
Purkinje fibers

geometry of the right atrium. The orifices of the superior and inferior cava, fossa ovalis, and ostium of the coronary sinus divide the right atrium into muscle bands, limiting the number of routes available for internodal conduction. These routes, however, do not represent discrete bundles of histologically specialized internodal tracts comparable to the ventricular bundle branches.

Atrioventricular Junction and Intraventricular Conduction System

The AV junction corresponds anatomically to a group of discrete, specialized cells that are morphologically distinct from working myocardium and divided into a transitional cell zone, compact portion, and penetrating AV bundle (ie, His bundle).

Basic Arrhythmia Mechanisms

The mechanisms of cardiac arrhythmias are broadly classified as focal mechanisms that include automatic or triggered arrhythmias or as reentrant arrhythmias (Box 3.2). Cells that display automaticity lack a true resting membrane potential and instead undergo slow depolarization during diastole. Diastolic depolarization results in the transmembrane potential becoming more positive between successive action potentials until the threshold potential is reached, producing cellular excitation. Cells possessing normal automaticity can be found in the SA node, subsidiary atrial foci, AV node, and His-Purkinje system.

Diagnostic Evaluation

Diagnosis of the underlying mechanisms of the arrhythmia may require invasive electrophysiologic testing. Studies involve percutaneous introduction of catheters that provide electrical stimulation and record electrograms from various intracardiac sites. Initial recording sites often include the high right atrium, bundle of His, coronary sinus, and the right ventricle. The catheters are most often introduced through the femoral vessels under local anesthesia. Systemic heparinization is required, particularly when catheters are introduced into the left atrium or left ventricle. The most common

BOX 3.2 *Arrhythmia Mechanisms*

Focal mechanisms
- Automatic
- Triggered

Reentrant arrhythmias

Normal automaticity
- Sinoatrial node
- Subsidiary atrial foci
- Atrioventricular node
- His–Purkinje system

Triggered mechanisms occur from repetitive delayed or early afterdepolarizations

Reentry
- Unidirectional block is necessary
- Slowed conduction in the alternate pathway exceeds the refractory period of cells at the site of unidirectional block

complications from electrophysiologic testing are those associated with vascular catheterization. Other complications include hypotension (1% of patients), hemorrhage, deep venous thrombosis (0.4%), embolic phenomena (0.4%), infection (0.2%), and cardiac perforation (0.1%). Proper application of adhesive cardioversion electrodes before the procedure facilitates rapid cardioversion-defibrillation in the event of persistent or hemodynamically unstable tachyarrhythmia resulting from stimulation protocols.

Anesthesia Considerations for Supraventricular Arrhythmia Surgery and Ablation Procedures

The approach to the care of patients undergoing percutaneous therapies for supraventricular arrhythmias involves similar principles (Box 3.3). Anesthesiologists must be familiar with preoperative electrophysiology study (EPS) results and the characteristics of associated supraventricular arrhythmias (eg, rate, associated hemodynamic disturbances, syncope), including treatments. Tachyarrhythmias may recur at any time during surgical and percutaneous treatments. Transcutaneous cardioversion-defibrillation adhesive pads are placed before anesthesia induction and connected to a defibrillator-cardioverter. Development of periprocedural tachyarrhythmias is unrelated to any single anesthetic or adjuvant drug.

Treatment of hemodynamically tolerated tachyarrhythmias is aimed at slowing conduction across the accessory pathway rather than the AV node. Therapy directed at slowing conduction across the AV node (eg, β-adrenergic–blocking drugs, verapamil, digoxin) may enhance conduction across accessory pathways and should be used only if proved safe by a prior EPS. Recommended drugs include amiodarone and procainamide. One consideration is that antiarrhythmic drugs may interfere with electrophysiologic mapping. Hemodynamically significant tachyarrhythmias developing before mapping are usually treated with cardioversion.

Accessory pathway ablation is typically performed under conscious sedation, and general anesthesia is reserved for selected patients such as those unable to tolerate the supine position.

Droperidol depresses accessory pathway conduction, but the clinical significance of small antiemetic doses is likely minimal. Opioids and barbiturates have no proven electrophysiologic effect on accessory pathways and are safe in patients with Wolff-Parkinson-White (WPW) syndrome. Normal AV conduction is depressed by halothane, isoflurane, and enflurane, and preliminary evidence suggests that these volatile anesthetics may also depress accessory pathway conduction. The major goal of managing

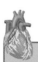

BOX 3.3   *Anesthesia Considerations for Supraventricular Arrhythmia Surgery and Ablation Procedures*

Familiarity with electrophysiologic study results and associated treatments
Transcutaneous cardioversion-defibrillation pads placed before induction
Hemodynamically tolerated tachyarrhythmias treated by slowing conduction across accessory pathway rather than the atrioventricular node
Hemodynamically significant tachyarrhythmias treated with cardioversion
Avoidance of sympathetic stimulation

supraventricular ablative procedures is to avoid sympathetic stimulation and the development of tachyarrhythmias. An opioid-based anesthetic technique with supplemental volatile anesthetics is typically used.

Anesthesiology teams are increasingly asked to care for patients undergoing catheter-based ablative procedures for atrial fibrillation. Monitored anesthesia care may be possible in some situations, but general anesthesia is typically chosen because of the duration of the procedure and the demand for no patient movement during critical lesion placement.

The choice of anesthesia depends on the patient's physical status, including comorbid conditions and ventricular dysfunction. General anesthesia with high-frequency jet ventilation (HFJV) can minimize thoracic excursion during respirations, which increases catheter-tissue contact. HFJV necessitates the use of intravenous anesthesia, which usually consists of a propofol infusion combined with a short-acting narcotic infusion such as remifentanil. HFJV risks include pneumothorax, barotrauma, inadequate ventilation or oxygenation, respiratory acidosis, pneumomediastinum, gastric distension, and aspiration.

Left atrial appendage (LAA) thrombus must be excluded with transesophageal echocardiography (TEE) before proceeding with catheter-based ablation. During catheter-based ablation of atrial fibrillation, patients undergo direct arterial pressure and esophageal temperature monitoring. Acute increases in esophageal temperature of only 0.1°C are communicated to the electrophysiologist. Immediately terminating RF energy and cooling the catheter tip with intraprobe saline at room temperature limit the spread of myocardial heating.

Because heparin is administered during the procedure, the activated clotting time is monitored. Constant vigilance is mandated for pericardial tamponade, and immediate transthoracic echocardiography should be performed when abrupt hypotension develops. Percutaneous pericardial drainage is emergently performed, which typically restores blood pressure. Continued collection of pericardial blood after protamine reversal of heparin anticoagulation may necessitate transfer of the patient to the operating room for a sternotomy and repair of the atrial defect.

VENTRICULAR ARRHYTHMIAS

As with supraventricular arrhythmias, the treatment of ventricular fibrillation (VF) and ventricular tachycardia (VT) is aimed at addressing underlying mechanisms (eg, myocardial ischemia; drug-induced, electrolyte, or metabolic abnormalities). In most patients with life-threatening ventricular arrhythmias and structural heart disease, ICD placement is the standard of care with or without concomitant antiarrhythmic drug therapy. In patients with significant structural heart disease, catheter ablation is considered as an adjuvant therapy for medically refractory monomorphic VT.

Rarely, VT occurs in the setting of a structurally normal heart. This syndrome of a primary electrical disorder usually is caused by a focal, triggered mechanism that occurs mostly in younger patients and originates from the right ventricular (RV) outflow tract or apical septum (Box 3.4).

Anesthesia Considerations

Anesthesia management of patients undergoing catheter-based procedures to ameliorate ventricular arrhythmias is primarily based on the patient's underlying cardiac disease and other comorbidities. Candidates often have coronary artery disease, severely impaired left ventricular function, and dysfunction of other organs (eg, liver, kidney).

BOX 3.4 *Ventricular Arrhythmias*

Most episodes of ventricular tachycardia or fibrillation result from coronary artery disease and dilated or hypertrophic cardiomyopathy.

Implantable cardioverter-defibrillator placement is the standard of care with or without medical treatment for life-threatening ventricular arrhythmias and structural heart disease.

Catheter ablation is adjuvant therapy for medically refractory monomorphic ventricular tachycardia.

Surgical therapy includes endocardial resection with cryoablation.

Anesthesia considerations focus on preoperative catheterization, echocardiography, and electrophysiologic testing.

Monitoring of surgical patients is dictated by the underlying cardiac disease.

Because they are receiving multiple medications that may interact with anesthetics (eg, vasodilation from angiotensin-converting enzyme inhibitors), a thorough review of the patient's underlying conditions and treatments is mandated. Special attention is given to cardiac catheterization results and preoperative echocardiogram findings. Information regarding characteristics of the patient's arrhythmia such as ventricular rate, hemodynamic tolerance, and method of arrhythmia termination should be sought.

Prior or current treatment with amiodarone is a particular concern. The long elimination half-life (about 60 days) of amiodarone requires that potential side effects such as hypothyroidism be considered perioperatively. The α-adrenergic and β-adrenergic properties of amiodarone may lead to hypotension during anesthesia. Much attention has been given to bradycardia associated with amiodarone during anesthesia that may be resistant to atropine. Methods for temporary cardiac pacing should be readily available to care for patients receiving amiodarone on a long-term basis. Retrospective reports suggest a greater need for inotropic support for patients receiving preoperative amiodarone therapy because low systemic vascular resistance has been observed.

Monitoring includes direct arterial pressure monitoring, and central venous access is necessary for administration of vasoactive drugs if needed. Means for rapid cardioversion-defibrillation should be readily available when inserting any central venous catheter. Self-adhesive electrode pads are used most often and connected to a cardioverter-defibrillator before anesthesia induction. Premature ventricular beats induced during these procedures can easily precipitate the patient's underlying ventricular arrhythmia, which may be difficult to convert to sinus rhythm. Selection of anesthetics for arrhythmia ablation is dictated mostly by the patient's physical status. General anesthesia with endotracheal intubation is typically chosen due to the duration of the procedures, but deep sedation is also employed.

Because anesthetics can influence cardiac conduction and arrhythmogenesis, there is concern about their ability to alter electrophysiologic mapping results. Effects of volatile anesthetics on ventricular arrhythmias vary according to the mechanism of the arrhythmia. Data showing proarrhythmic, antiarrhythmic, and no effects of volatile anesthetics on arrhythmias have been reported. Nonetheless, the small doses administered during ablative procedures may have minimal effects on electrophysiologic mapping. Opioids have had no effect on the inducibility of VT.

Battery-operated, implantable pacing devices (collectively, cardiac implantable electronic devices [CIEDs]) were first introduced in 1958, 4 years after the invention of the transistor. Although several generations of physicians have been trained since, these devices remain one of the most poorly understood aspects of medical care throughout the world. Often, these devices are ignored in the overall care of a patient with the erroneous (and possibly life-threatening) belief that mere application of a magnet will prevent any perioperative problem, as well as treat any situation that arises. Frequently, ICDs are labeled as a simple pacemaker, a situation during which the antitachycardia therapy or the inability to deliver magnet-driven asynchronous pacing in a pacing-dependent patient might be overlooked. Nevertheless, the presence of a CIED with therapeutic capability can significantly complicate a patient's life.

The natural progression of pacemaker developments led to the invention of the transvenous implantable cardioverter-defibrillator (TV-ICD) around 1980. As this technology has advanced, the lines between simple pacing generators and defibrillators have become less clear. For example, every TV-ICD currently implanted has robust antibradycardia pacing capability. The consequence of mistaking any TV-ICD for a conventional pacemaker can lead to patient harm, mostly attributable to electromagnetic interference (EMI) resulting in inappropriate ICD therapy. Fig. 3.2 shows a three-lead defibrillation system and identifies the RV shock coil, which differentiates a TV-ICD system from a conventional pacemaker system.

The development of the subcutaneous ICD (S-ICD) (Fig. 3.3), as well as the leadless transcatheter-deployed intracardiac pacemaker (IC-PM) (Fig. 3.4), further complicates this issue. S-ICDs are larger than their transvenous counterparts, cannot provide antitachycardia or sustained antibradycardia pacing, and generally have higher defibrillation thresholds (DFTs) than TV-ICDs. The IC-PMs likely behave differently from their transvenous-deployed cohorts, especially with respect to overall features and magnet placement.

The diversity and complexity of cardiac pulse generators, as well as the multitude of programmable parameters, limits the number of sweeping generalizations that can be made about the perioperative care of the patient with an implanted pulse generator. Population aging, continued enhancements in implantable technology, and new indications for implantation will lead to growing numbers of patients with these devices in the new millennium. Currently, four advisories or guidelines have been published in three countries endorsed by several societies regarding the care of the perioperative patient with a device. Table 3.1 compares and contrasts these statements. Work by the Association for the Advancement of Medical Instrumentation to standardize magnet responses has been ongoing since 2000 but without much success (see https://standards.aami.org/kws/public/projects/project/details?project _id=53).

PACEMAKERS

It is likely that well over 3 million patients in the United States have pacemakers today. Many factors lead to confusion regarding the behavior of a device and the perioperative care of a patient with a device.

No discussion of pacemakers can take place without an understanding of the generic pacemaker code (North American Society of Pacing and Electrophysiology [NASPE]/British Pacing and Electrophysiology Group [BPEG] generic [NBG] code),

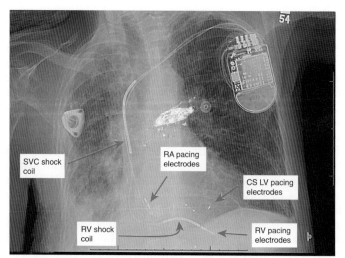

Fig. 3.2 Defibrillator system with biventricular (BiV) antibradycardia pacemaker capability. Note that three leads are placed: a conventional, bipolar lead to the right atrium; a true bipolar right ventricular (*RV*) lead with shock coils in the right ventricle and the superior vena cava (*SVC*), and a quadripolar lead to the coronary sinus (*CS*). This system is designed to provide "resynchronization (antibradycardia) therapy" in the setting of a dilated cardiomyopathy with a prolonged QRS complex (and frequently with a prolonged P-R interval as well). The bipolar lead in the right atrium will perform both sensing and pacing function. The true bipolar (discrete tip and ring) electrodes in the right ventricle provide pacing and sensing function. The presence of a "shock" conductor (termed *shock coil*) on the RV lead in the right ventricle distinguishes a defibrillation system from a conventional pacemaking system. The lead in the CS depolarizes the left ventricle, and this particular catheter has four electrodes in the CS to allow optimization of left ventricular (*LV*) pacing. Because of the typically wide native QRS complex in a left bundle branch pattern, failure to capture the left ventricle can lead to ventricular double-counting (and inappropriate antitachycardia therapy) in a BiV transvenous ICD system. Many defibrillation systems also have a shock coil in the SVC, which is most often electrically identical to the defibrillator case (called the *can*). When the defibrillation circuit includes the ICD case, it is called *active can configuration*. Incidental findings on this chest radiograph include the presence of a right-sided implanted central venous catheter, right pleural effusion, and scoliosis.

last updated in 2002. Shown in Table 3.2, the code describes the basic behavior of the pacing device.

Pacemaker Indications

Common indications for permanent pacing are shown in Box 3.5.

Pacemaker Magnets

Despite often-repeated folklore, most pacemaker manufacturers warn that magnets were never intended to treat pacemaker emergencies or to prevent EMI effects. Rather, magnet-activated switches were incorporated to produce pacing behavior that demonstrates remaining battery life and, sometimes, pacing threshold safety factors.

Placement of a magnet over a generator might produce no change in pacing because *not all pacemakers switch to a continuous asynchronous mode when a magnet is placed*. The Medtronic "Micra" leadless IC-PM has no magnet sensor. Pacemakers might also be nonresponsive to magnet placement owing to programming (including the default mode) or safety mode after an electrical reset from EMI or component

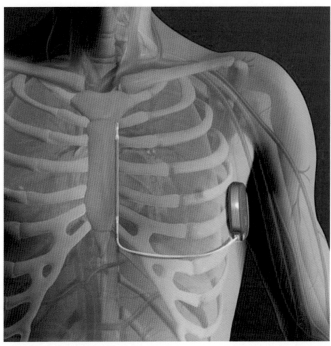

Fig. 3.3 The Boston Scientific subcutaneous implantable cardioverter-defibrillator (S-ICD). Illustration demonstrates an S-ICD (CE mark 2009; US Food and Drug Administration approval 2012), which consists of a generator implanted along the lateral chest wall with a subcutaneous lead tunneled into position over the heart. (From Hauser RG: The subcutaneous implantable cardioverter-defibrillator: should patients want one? *J Am Coll Cardiol*. 2013;61:20–22.)

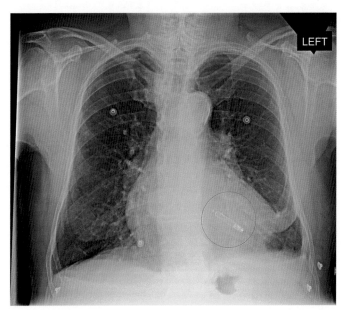

Fig. 3.4 The St. Jude Nanostim leadless intracardiac pacemaker. A leadless pacemaker is shown in the right ventricle *(circle)* on this posteroanterior chest film. Leadless pacemakers are currently approved for implant in several countries outside of the United States. (X-ray image courtesy of Vivek Reddy, MD, Icahn School of Medicine at Mount Sinai, New York, NY.)

Table 3.1 Comparisons of Perioperative Cardiac Implantable Electronic Device Advisories

	Preoperative Recommendation	Intraoperative Magnet Use	ESU Dispersive Electrode Placement	Postoperative Recommendation	Emergency Procedures PM	ICD
ASA Periop	"Timely interrogation" before elective surgery.	Shuns magnet use in favor of reprogramming.	Prevents presumed current path from crossing the chest and CIED system.	Interrogation is recommended. Footnotes added to 2011 revision suggest that CIED reinterrogation is not needed if no monopolar ESU is used.	(silent)	
HRS/ASA	PM interrogation within 12 months. ICD interrogation within 6 months. CRT interrogation within 3–6 months. CIED physician must provide prescription for perioperative care.	Magnet use is suggested for asynchronous pacing (when needed in PM patients) and disabling ICD high-energy therapy, provided that patient position does not interfere with magnet access or observation.	Prevents presumed current path from crossing the chest and CIED system.	For most cases involving EMI (especially those inferior to umbilicus and when no preoperative reprogramming was performed), interrogation can take place within 1 month as an ambulatory procedure. For reprogrammed CIEDs, hemodynamically challenging cases, cardiothoracic surgery, RFA, and external cardioversion, interrogation can take place before transfer from cardiac telemetry.	Use 12-lead ECG to identify pacing need, presume dependence if 100% pacing. Use magnet to mitigate pacing inhibition. Maintain cardiac monitoring until postoperative interrogation.	Use magnet to suspend ICD tachyarrhythmia therapy.

CAS-CCS	De-novo interrogation is not likely needed, but the CIED physician must provide a prescription for perioperative care.	Where reasonable, magnet use is suggested for asynchronous pacing (when needed in PM patients) and disabling ICD high-energy therapy.	No mention.	Clear plan for postoperative care is established before elective case.	Use 12-lead ECG to identify pacing need, presume dependence if 100% pacing; maintain careful monitoring to determine magnet action, >5-second pauses if ESU interferes with CIED.
MHRA[a]	Preoperative contact with the pacemaker ICD follow-up clinic for evaluation and perioperative recommendations.	Caution is advised since programming can affect magnet behavior.	"...ensure that the return electrode is anatomically positioned so that the current pathway between the diathermy electrode and return electrode is as far away from the pacemaker/ defibrillator (and leads) as possible."	Follow-up clinic prescribes postoperative follow-up.	Attempt to follow routine steps; postoperative interrogation is needed as soon as possible. Magnet might create asynchronous pacing. Magnet might prevent inappropriate discharge.

No recommendations have been published for the leadless intracardiac pacemaker or the subcutaneous ICD.
[a]Recommendations appear relevant only if EMI will be present.
ASA, American Society of Anesthesiologists; CAS, Canadian Anesthesiologists Society; CCS, Canadian Cardiovascular Society; CIED, cardiac implantable electronic device; CRT, cardiac resynchronization therapy (any CIED that has both right ventricular– and left ventricular–pacing capability); ECG, electrocardiography; EMI, electromagnetic interference; ESU, electrosurgical unit (Bovie); HRS, Heart Rhythm Society; ICD, implantable cardioverter-defibrillator; MHRA, Medicines and Healthcare Products Regulatory Agency; PM, pacemaker; RFA, radio frequency ablation.

3

Table 3.2 NASPE/BPEG Generic (NBG) Defibrillator Code

Position I: Pacing Chamber(s)	Position II: Sensing Chamber(s)	Position III: Response(s) to Sensing	Position IV: Programmability	Position V: Multisite Pacing
O = None	O = None	O = None	O = None	O = None
A = Atrium	A = Atrium	I = Inhibited	R = Rate	A = Atrium
V = Ventricle	V = Ventricle	T = Triggered	modulation	V = Ventricle
D = Dual (A+V)	D = Dual (A+V)	D = Dual (T+I)		D = Dual (A+V)

BPEG, British Pacing and Electrophysiology Group; *NASPE,* North American Society of Pacing and Electrophysiology,

BOX 3.5 *Pacemaker Indications*

Symptomatic bradycardia from sinus node disease
Symptomatic bradycardia from atrioventricular node disease
Long QT syndrome
Hypertrophic obstructive cardiomyopathy (HOCM)[a]
Dilated cardiomyopathy (DCM)[a]

[a]See text and Pacemaker Programming for special precautions.

failure. Although more than 90% of pacemakers have high-rate (85 to 100 bpm) asynchronous pacing with magnet application, some pacemakers respond with only a brief (10 to 100 bpm) asynchronous pacing event, reverting to the original pacing mode and rate thereafter. Box 3.6 provides common magnet behavior for conventional pacemakers.

Preanesthetic Evaluation and Pacemaker Reprogramming

For programmable devices, interrogation with a programmer remains the only reliable method for evaluating lead performance and obtaining current program information.

The timing of any preoperative interrogation depends on the local practice and selection of a pacemaker advisory. The American Society of Anesthesiologists (ASA) recommends interrogation within 3 months of the procedure. The Heart Rhythm Society (HRS)/ASA, Canadian Anesthesiologists Society (CAS)/Canadian Cardiovascular Society (CCS), and Medicines and Healthcare Products Regulatory Agency (MHRA) recommend review of CIED records and communication with the patient's CIED physician and clinic. For conventional pacemakers, HRS/ASA also recommends interrogation within 12 months of the procedure.

Important features of the preanesthetic device evaluation are shown in Box 3.7. Determining pacing dependency might require temporary reprogramming to a VVI mode with a low rate. In patients from countries where pacemakers might be reused,

BOX 3.6 *Pacemaker Magnet Behavior*[a]

Asynchronous pacing without rate responsiveness using parameters possibly not in the patient's best interest at 85–100 bpm. Asynchronous pacing is the most common behavior except for Biotronik pacemakers. All pacemakers manufactured by Biotronik, Boston Scientific, and St. Jude Medical have programmable magnet behavior.

Unexpected behavior (eg, VOO pacing in Medtronic or VDD pacing in Biotronik dual-chamber pacemaker), suggesting elective replacement has been reached and the pacemaker should be interrogated promptly.

No apparent rhythm or rate change.

Magnet mode permanently disabled by programming (possible with Biotronik, Boston Scientific, St. Jude Medical) or temporarily suspended (see Medtronic).

Program rate pacing in the patient who is already paced (many older pacemakers).

Improper monitor settings with pacing near the current heart rate (pace filter on).

No magnet sensor (Medtronic Micra leadless pacemaker, some pre-1985 Cordis, Telectronics models).

Brief (10–100 bpm) asynchronous pacing, then return to program values (most Biotronik and Intermedics pacemakers).

Continuous or transient loss of pacing.

Inadequate pacing output safety margin with failure to depolarize the myocardium.

Pacemaker enters diagnostic "Threshold Test Mode" (some Intermedics, Medtronic, St. Jude Medical devices, depending on model and programming).

Discharged battery (some pre-1990 devices).

Hypertrophic obstructive cardiomyopathy (HOCM).[a]

Dilated cardiomyopathy (DCM).[a]

[a]See text and Pacemaker Programming for special precautions.

BOX 3.7 *Preanesthetic Pulse Generator (Pacemaker, Implantable Cardioverter-Defibrillator) Evaluation*

Determining the indication for and the date of initial device placement

Identifying the number and types of leads

Determining the last generator test date and battery status

Obtaining a history of generator events (if any)

Obtaining the current program information (device interrogation)

Ensuring that generator discharges become mechanical systoles with adequate safety margins

Ensuring that magnet detection is enabled

Determining whether the pacing mode should be reprogrammed

battery performance might not be related to the length of implantation in the current patient.

Appropriate reprogramming (Box 3.8) might be the safest way to avoid intraoperative problems, especially if monopolar Bovie electrosurgery will be used. Whether CIED manufacturers stand ready to assist with this task or whether this task should be performed by industry-employed affiliated personnel remains controversial. Reprogramming a pacemaker to asynchronous pacing at a rate greater than the patient's underlying

> ### BOX 3.8 *Pacemaker Reprogramming Probably Needed*
>
> Any rate-responsive device (problems are well known, problems have been misinterpreted
>   with potential for patient injury, and the US Food and Drug Administration [FDA]
>   has issued an alert regarding devices with minute ventilation [MV] sensors)
> Special pacing indication (hypertrophic obstructive cardiomyopathy [HOCM], dilated
>   cardiomyopathy [DCM], pediatric patient)
> Pacing-dependent patient
> Major procedure in the chest or abdomen

rate usually ensures that EMI will not affect pacing. Reprogramming to asynchronous pacing will not protect it from internal damage or reset caused by EMI.

In general, rate responsiveness and other enhancements (eg, hysteresis, sleep rate, AV search) should be disabled by programming, since many of these can mimic pacing system malfunction.

Intraoperative (or Procedure) Management

No special monitoring or anesthetic technique is required for the patient with a pacemaker. However, monitoring of the patient must include the ability to detect mechanical systoles, since EMI, as well as devices such as a nerve stimulator, can interfere with QRS complex and pacemaker spikes on the ECG. To demonstrate pacing pulses, most ECG monitor filtering must be changed to eliminate or reduce high-frequency filtering. Mechanical systoles are best evaluated by pulse oximetry, plethysmography, or arterial waveform display; at least one of these monitoring modalities is recommended.

Monopolar Bovie electrosurgical unit (ESU) use remains the principal intraoperative issue for the patient with a pacemaker. Monopolar ESU is more likely to cause problems than bipolar ESU, and patients with unipolar electrode configuration are more sensitive to EMI than those with bipolar configurations. Coagulation ESU will likely cause more problems than nonblended "cutting" ESU. Additionally, the dispersive electrode should be placed such that the presumed current path from the hand tool to the electrode does not cross the chest.

The use of an ultrasonic cutting device, commonly called a *harmonic scalpel*, has been championed to prevent EMI while providing the surgeon with the ability to cut and to coagulate tissue. A number of case reports have demonstrated successful surgery without EMI issues in these patients.

Temporary Pacemakers

Several techniques are available to the anesthesiologist to establish reliable temporary pacing during the perioperative period or in the intensive care unit. Cardiovascular anesthesiologists are more likely than generalists to routinely use temporary transvenous or epicardial pacing in their practices. Temporary cardiac pacing can serve as definitive therapy for transient bradyarrhythmias or as a bridge to permanent generator placement. The various forms of temporary pacing include many transvenous catheter systems, transcutaneous pads, transthoracic wires, and esophageal pacing techniques.

Table 3.3 Temporary Pacing Indications

Patient Condition	Event Requiring Temporary Pacing
Acute myocardial infarction (AMI)	Symptomatic bradycardia, medically refractory
	New bundle branch block with transient complete heart block
	Complete heart block
	Postoperative complete heart block
	Symptomatic congenital heart block
	Mobitz II with AMI
	New bifascicular block
	Bilateral bundle branch block and first-degree AV block
	Symptomatic alternating Wenckebach block
	Symptomatic alternating bundle branch block
Tachycardia treatment or prevention	Bradycardia-dependent VT
	Torsade de pointes
	Long QT syndrome
	Treatment of recurrent supraventricular tachycardia or VT
Prophylactic	Pulmonary artery catheter placement with left bundle branch block (controversial)
	New AV block or bundle branch block in acute endocarditis
	Cardioversion with sick sinus syndrome
	Postdefibrillation bradycardia
	Counteract perioperative pharmacologic treatment causing hemodynamically significant bradycardia
	AF prophylaxis postcardiac surgery
	Postorthotopic heart transplantation

AF, Atrial fibrillation; *AV,* atrioventricular; *VT,* ventricular tachycardia.

Indications for Temporary Pacing

Temporary pacemakers are commonly used after cardiac surgery in the treatment of drug toxicity resulting in arrhythmias, with certain arrhythmias complicating myocardial infarction, and for intraoperative bradycardia attributable to β-blockade. On occasion, the placement of a temporary pacing system can assist in hemodynamic management in the perioperative period. Abnormal electrolytes, preoperative β-blocker use, and many of the intraoperative drugs have the potential to aggravate bradycardia and bradycardia-dependent arrhythmias. Because drugs used to treat bradyarrhythmias have a number of important disadvantages compared with temporary pacing, hemo-dynamically unstable perioperative bradyarrhythmias should be considered an indication for temporary pacing (Table 3.3). If the patient already has epicardial wires or a pacing catheter or wires, or transesophageal pacing is feasible, then pacing is preferred to pharmacologic therapy. However, transcutaneous and ventricular-only transvenous pacing, even if feasible, may exacerbate hemodynamic problems in patients with heart disease, because these pacing modalities do not preserve AV synchrony (ie, produce ventricular or global activation).

Transvenous Temporary Pacing

Transvenous cardiac pacing provides the most reliable means of temporary pacing. Temporary transvenous pacing is dependable and well tolerated by patients. With a device that can provide both atrial and ventricular pacing, transvenous pacing can maintain AV synchrony and improve cardiac output. Disadvantages include the need

3

for practitioner experience, time to place the wire(s) appropriately to provide capture, the potential complications of catheter placement and manipulation, and the need for fluoroscopy in many cases.

Rapid catheter position is most easily obtained by using the right internal jugular vein, even without fluoroscopy, although a prudent practitioner might want to document the final position(s) of the catheters clearly. The left subclavian vein is also easily used in emergent situations.

Once catheters are positioned, pacing is initiated using the distal electrode as the cathode (negative terminal) and the proximal electrode as the anode (positive terminal). Ideally, the capture thresholds should be less than 1 mA, and generator output should be maintained at three times threshold as a safety margin. In dual-chamber pacing, AV delays between 100 and 200 ms are used. Many patients are sensitive to this parameter. Cardiac output optimization with echocardiography and/or mixed venous oxygen saturation can be used to maximize hemodynamics when adjusting AV delay. AV sequential pacing is clearly beneficial in many patients, but starting emergency pacing with *ventricular* capture alone should be remembered.

Pacing Pulmonary Artery Catheters

The pulmonary artery AV-pacing thermodilution catheter allows for AV-sequential pacing via electrodes attached to the outside of the catheter, as well as routine pulmonary artery catheter (PAC) functions. The combination of the two functions into one catheter eliminates the need for separate insertion of temporary transvenous pacing electrodes. However, several potential disadvantages exist with this catheter, including: (1) varying success in initiating and maintaining capture; (2) external electrode displacement from the catheter; and (3) relatively high cost as compared with standard PACs. The Paceport PAC provides ventricular pacing with a separate bipolar pacing lead (Chandler probe), which allows for more stable ventricular pacing and hemo-dynamic measurements. This catheter has been used for successful resuscitation after cardiac arrest during closed chest cardiac massage when attempts to capture with transcutaneous or transvenous flow-directed bipolar pacing catheters have failed. However, this unit does not provide the potential advantages associated with atrial pacing capability. The pulmonary artery AV Paceport adds a sixth lumen to allow for the placement of an atrial J-wire, flexible-tip bipolar pacing lead. Both of these Paceport catheters are placed by transducing the RV port to ensure correct positioning of the port 1 to 2 cm distal to the tricuspid valve. This position usually guides the ventricular wire (Chandler probe) to the apex, where adequate capture should occur with minimal current requirements. Although ventricular capture is easily obtained, atrial capture can be more difficult and less reliable. This catheter has been successfully used after cardiac surgery.

Transcutaneous Pacing

Transcutaneous pacing is readily available and can be rapidly implemented in emergency situations. Capture rate is variable, and the technique may cause pain in awake patients, but it is usually tolerated until temporary transvenous pacing can be instituted. It may be effective even when endocardial pacing fails. Transcutaneous pacing continues to be the method of choice for prophylactic and emergent applications.

Typically, the large patches are placed anteriorly (negative electrode or cathode) over the palpable cardiac apex (or V_3 lead location) and posteriorly (positive electrode or anode) at the inferior aspect of the scapula. Typical thresholds are 20 to 120 mA, but pacing may require up to 200 mA at long pulse durations of 20 to 40 ms.

Transcutaneous pacing appears to capture the right ventricle, followed by near simultaneous activation of the entire left ventricle. The hemodynamic response is similar to that of RV endocardial pacing. Both methods can cause a reduction in left ventricular systolic pressure, a decrease in stroke volume, and an increase in right-sided pressures attributable to AV dyssynchrony. Palpation or display of a peripheral pulse should confirm capture. Maintenance current should be set at least 5 to 10 mA above threshold. Success rates appear to be highest when the system is used prophylactically or early after arrest—upward of 90%. When used in emergent situations, successful capture rates are usually lower but range from 10% to 93%. The technique poses no electrical threat to medical personnel, and complications are rare. There have been no reports of significant damage to myocardium, skeletal muscle, skin, or lungs in humans, despite continuous pacing up to 108 hours and intermittent pacing up to 17 days. Several commercially available defibrillators include transcutaneous pacing generators as standard equipment.

Postanesthesia Pacemaker Evaluation

Any pacemaker that has been reprogrammed for the perioperative period should be reevaluated and programmed appropriately. For nonreprogrammed devices, most manufacturers recommend interrogation to ensure proper functioning and remaining battery life if any monopolar ESU was used. The ASA advisory recommends interrogation before discharging the patient from monitored care, whereas the HRS/ASA statement suggests that immediate postoperative interrogation is needed only for hemodynamically challenging cases or when significant EMI occurs superior to the umbilicus while operating.

IMPLANTABLE CARDIOVERTER-DEFIBRILLATORS

The development of an implantable, battery-powered device able to deliver sufficient energy to terminate VT or VF has represented a major medical breakthrough for patients with a history of ventricular tachyarrhythmias. These devices prevent death in the setting of malignant ventricular tachyarrhythmias, and they clearly remain superior to antiarrhythmic drug therapy. Initially approved by the FDA in 1985, the implantation rate currently exceeds 12,000 TV-ICDs per month in the United States. Industry sources report that more than 300,000 patients have these devices today.

Similar to pacemakers, ICDs have a generic code to indicate lead placement and function, which is shown in Table 3.4.

Table 3.4 NASPE/BPEG Generic (NBG) Defibrillator Code

Position I: Shock Chamber(s)	Position II: Antitachycardia Pacing Chamber(s)	Position III: Tachycardia Detection	Position IV: Antibradycardia Pacing Chamber(s)
O = None	O = None	E = Electrogram	O = None
A = Atrium	A = Atrium	H = Hemodynamic	A = Atrium
V = Ventricle	V = Ventricle		V = Ventricle
D = Dual (A+V)	D = Dual (A+V)		D = Dual (A+V)

BPEG, British Pacing and Electrophysiology Group; NASPE, North American Society of Pacing and Electrophysiology

BOX 3.9 *Implantable Cardioverter-Defibrillator Indications*

Prophylactic use for patients with:
- Ischemic cardiomyopathy surviving 40 days and longer with EF of 30% or less and NYHA Class I or EF of 35% or less and NYHA Class II/III
- Nonischemic cardiomyopathy with an EF of 35% or less and NYHA Class II/III

Ventricular fibrillation or ventricular tachycardia from nonreversible cause
Ischemic cardiomyopathy, EF 40% or less, NSVT, inducible at electrophysiologic study
Brugada syndrome (right bundle branch block, S-T elevation V_1–V_3)[a]
Arrhythmogenic right ventricular dysplasia[a]
Long QT syndrome
Hypertrophic cardiomyopathy[a]
Infiltrative cardiomyopathy

[a]Requires one or more risk factors for sudden cardiac arrest.
EF, Ejection fraction; *NSVT,* nonsustained ventricular tachycardia; *NYHA,* New York Heart Association.

Implantable Cardioverter-Defibrillator Indications

Initially, ICDs were placed for hemodynamically significant VT or VF. Newer indications associated with sudden death include: long QT syndrome, Brugada syndrome (right bundle branch block, S-T segment elevation in leads V_1–V_3), and arrhythmogenic RV dysplasia. Recent studies suggest that ICDs can be used for primary prevention of sudden death (ie, before the first episode of VT or VF) in young patients with hypertrophic cardiomyopathy, and data from the second Multicenter Automatic Defibrillator Intervention Trial (MADIT II) suggest that any post-MI patient with ejection fraction (EF) less than 30% should undergo prophylactic implantation of an ICD. At the present time, however, the Centers for Medicare and Medicaid require a prolonged QRS interval (greater than 120 ms) to qualify for ICD placement in this group. A review of 318,000 implants in patients over 65 years of age for the period 2006 to 2010 demonstrated improvements in 6-month all-cause mortality, 6-month rehospitalization rate, and device complications when compared with matched control subjects (Box 3.9).

Implantable Cardioverter-Defibrillator and Magnets

Similar to pacemakers, magnet behavior in some ICDs can be altered by programming. Most devices will suspend tachyarrhythmia detection (and therefore therapy) when a magnet is appropriately placed to activate the magnet sensor. Some devices can be programmed to ignore magnet placement. If the magnet mode is off, then intraoperative EMI is likely to produce repeated shocks. In general, magnet application will not affect antibradycardia pacing rate or pacing mode. Interrogating the device and calling the manufacturer remain the most reliable method for determining magnet response.

Preanesthetic Evaluation and Implantable Cardioverter-Defibrillator Reprogramming

In general, *all* patients with an ICD should be evaluated for the need to disable high-voltage therapy before the commencement of any procedure, although such action might be unnecessary in a setting without EMI or placement of a metal guidewire into the chest. The comments in the pacing section apply here for any ICD with antibradycardia pacing. Guidelines from HRS/NASPE suggest that every patient with an ICD have an in-office comprehensive evaluation every 3 to 6 months.

Intraoperative (or Procedure) Management

At this time, no special monitoring (attributable to the ICD) is required for the patient with any ICD. ECG monitoring and the ability to deliver external cardioversion or defibrillation must be present during the time of ICD disablement.

Postanesthesia Implantable Cardioverter-Defibrillator Evaluation

Any ICD that underwent suspension of high-voltage therapy must be reinterrogated and reenabled. All stored events should be reviewed and counters should be cleared, since the next device evaluator might not receive information about the EMI experience of the patient and make erroneous conclusions regarding the patient's arrhythmia events.

SUGGESTED READINGS

Atlee JL, Bernstein AD. Cardiac rhythm management devices (part I): indications, device selection, and function. *Anesthesiology.* 2001;95:1265–1280.

Blomstrom-Lundqvist C, Scheinman MM, Aliot EM, et al. ACC/AHA/ESC guidelines for the management of patients with supraventricular arrhythmias—executive summary. A report of the American College of Cardiology/American Heart Association Task Force on practice guidelines and the European Society of Cardiology Committee for practice guidelines (writing committee to develop guidelines for the management of patients with supraventricular arrhythmias) developed in collaboration with NASPE-Heart Rhythm Society. *J Am Coll Cardiol.* 2003;42:1493–1531.

Connolly SJ, Gent M, Roberts RS, et al. Canadian implantable defibrillator study (CIDS): a randomized trial of the implantable cardioverter defibrillator against amiodarone. *Circulation.* 2000;101:1297–1302.

Crossley GH, Poole JE, Rozner MA, et al. The Heart Rhythm Society Expert Consensus Statement on the perioperative management of patients with implantable defibrillators, pacemakers and arrhythmia monitors: Facilities and patient management. *Heart Rhythm.* 2011. Available at: http://www.hrsonline.org/content/download/1432/20125/file/2011-HRS_ASA. Published.

Di Biase L, Conti S, Mohanty P, et al. General anesthesia reduces the prevalence of pulmonary vein reconnection during repeat ablation when compared with conscious sedation: results from a randomized study. *Heart Rhythm.* 2011;8:368–372.

Doll N, Borger MA, Fabricius A, et al. Esophageal perforation during left atrial radiofrequency ablation: is the risk too high? *J Thorac Cardiovasc Surg.* 2003;125:836–842.

Epstein AE. An update on implantable cardioverter-defibrillator guidelines. *Curr Opin Cardiol.* 2004;19:23–25.

Epstein AE, DiMarco JP, Ellenbogen KA, et al. 2012 ACCF/AHA/HRS focused update incorporated into the ACCF/AHA/HRS 2008 Guidelines for device-based therapy of cardiac rhythm abnormalities: a report of the American College of Cardiology Foundation/American Heart Association Task Force on Practice Guidelines and the Heart Rhythm Society. *J Am Coll Cardiol.* 2013;61:e6–e75.

Goode JS Jr, Taylor RL, Buffington CW, et al. High-frequency jet ventilation: utility in posterior left atrial catheter ablation. *Heart Rhythm.* 2006;3:13–19.

Guidelines for the perioperative management of patients with implantable pacemakers or implantable cardioverter defibrillators, where the use of surgical diathermy/electrocautery is anticipated. Medicines and Health Care products Regulatory Agency. Available at: http://heartrhythmuk.org.uk/files/file/Docs/Guidelines/MHRA; Published 2006.

3

Natale A, Newby KH, Pisano E, et al. Prospective randomized comparison of antiarrhythmic therapy versus first-line radiofrequency ablation in patients with atrial flutter. *J Am Coll Cardiol.* 2000;35:1898–1904.

Practice advisory for the perioperative management of patients with cardiac implantable electronic devices: pacemakers and implantable cardioverter-defibrillators: an updated report by the American Society of Anesthesiologists task force on perioperative management of patients with cardiac implantable electronic devices. *Anesthesiology.* 2011;114:247–261.

Preliminary report: effect of encainide and flecainide on mortality in a randomized trial of arrhythmia suppression after myocardial infarction. *N Engl J Med.* 1989;321:406–412.

Rozner MA, Roberson JC, Nguyen AD. Unexpected high incidence of serious pacemaker problems detected by pre-and postoperative interrogations: a two-year experience. *J Am Coll Cardiol.* 2004;43:113A.

Squara F, Chik WW, Benhayon D, et al. Development and validation of a novel algorithm based on the ECG magnet response for rapid identification of any unknown pacemaker. *Heart Rhythm.* 2014;11:1367–1376.

The Antiarrhythmics versus Implantable Defibrillators (AVID) investigators. A comparison of antiarrhythmic-drug therapy with implantable defibrillators in patients resuscitated from near-fatal ventricular arrhythmias. *N Engl J Med.* 1997;337:1576–1583.

The CAST investigators, Wyse DG, Waldo AL, et al. A comparison of rate control and rhythm control in patients with atrial fibrillation. *N Engl J Med.* 2002;347:1825–1833.

Zipes DP. Implantable cardioverter-defibrillator: a Volkswagen or a Rolls Royce: how much will we pay to save a life? *Circulation.* 2001;103:1372–1374.

Section II

Cardiovascular Physiology, Pharmacology, Molecular Biology, and Genetics

Chapter 4

Cardiac Physiology

Paul S. Pagel, MD, PhD • Julie K. Freed, MD, PhD

Key Points

1. The cartilaginous skeleton, myocardial fiber orientation, valves, blood supply, and conduction system of the heart determine its mechanical capabilities and limitations.
2. The cardiac myocyte is engineered for contraction and relaxation, not protein synthesis.
3. The cardiac cycle is a highly coordinated, temporally related series of electrical, mechanical, and valvular events.
4. A time-dependent, two-dimensional projection of continuous pressure and volume during the cardiac cycle creates a phase space diagram that is useful for the analysis of systolic and diastolic function of each cardiac chamber in vivo.
5. Each cardiac chamber is constrained to operate within its end-systolic and end-diastolic pressure-volume relationships when contractile state and compliance are constant.
6. Heart rate, preload, afterload, and myocardial contractility are the main determinants of pump performance.
7. Preload is the quantity of blood that a cardiac chamber contains immediately before contraction begins, and afterload is the external resistance to emptying with which the chamber is confronted after the onset of contraction.
8. Myocardial contractility is quantified using indices derived from pressure-volume relationships, isovolumic contraction, and the ejection phase.
9. Diastolic function is the ability of a cardiac chamber to effectively collect blood at a normal filling pressure.
10. Left ventricular diastole is a complicated sequence of temporally related, heterogeneous events; no single index of diastolic function completely describes this period of the cardiac cycle.
11. Left ventricular diastolic dysfunction is a primary cause of heart failure in as many as 50% of patients.
12. The pericardium exerts important restraining forces on chamber filling and is a major determinant of ventricular interdependence.

The heart is an electrically self-actuated, phasic, variable-speed hydraulic pump composed of two dual-component, elastic, muscular chambers, each consisting of an atrium and a ventricle connected in series that simultaneously provide an equal quantity of blood to the pulmonary and systemic circulations. All four chambers of the heart are responsive to the stimulation rate, muscle stretch immediately before contraction (ie, preload), and the forces resisting further muscle shortening after contraction has begun (ie, afterload). The heart efficiently provides its own energy supply through an extensive coronary circulation.

The heart rapidly adapts to changing physiologic conditions by altering its inherent mechanical properties (ie, Frank-Starling mechanism) and by responding to neuro-hormonal and reflex-mediated signaling. Overall performance is determined by the contractile characteristics of the atria and ventricles (ie, systolic function) and by the ability of its chambers to effectively collect blood at normal filling pressures before the subsequent ejection (ie, diastolic function). This innate duality implies that heart failure may occur as a consequence of abnormalities in systolic or diastolic function.

▣ FUNCTIONAL IMPLICATIONS OF GROSS ANATOMY

Structure

The heart's anatomy determines many of its major mechanical capabilities and limitations. The annuli of the valves, the aortic and pulmonary arterial roots, the central fibrous body, and the left and right fibrous trigones form the heart's skeletal foundation. This flexible, strong, cartilaginous structure is located at the superior aspect (ie, base) of the heart. It provides support for the translucent, macroscopically avascular valves, resists the forces of developed pressure and blood flow within the chambers, and provides a site of insertion for superficial subepicardial muscle.

The left atrium (LA) and right atrium (RA) are composed of two relatively thin, orthogonally oriented layers of myocardium. The walls of the right ventricle (RV) and left ventricle (LV) are thicker (approximately 5 and 10 mm, respectively) than those of the atria and consist of three muscle layers: interdigitating deep sinospiral, superficial sinospiral, and superficial bulbospiral.

The RV is located in a more right-sided, anterior position than the LV within the mediastinum. Unlike the thicker-walled, ellipsoidal LV that propels oxygenated blood from the pulmonary venous circulation into the high-pressure systemic arterial vasculature, the thinner-walled, crescentic RV pumps deoxygenated venous blood into a substantially lower-pressure, more compliant pulmonary arterial tree.

Valves

Two pairs of valves ensure unidirectional blood flow through the right and left sides of the heart. The pulmonic and aortic valves are trileaflet structures located at the RV and LV outlets, respectively, and they operate passively with changes in hydraulic pressure. The pulmonic valve leaflets are identified by their anatomic positions (ie, right, left, and anterior), whereas the name of each aortic valve leaflet is derived from the presence or absence of an adjacent coronary ostium. The pulmonic and aortic valves open as a consequence of RV and LV ejection, respectively.

The thin, flexible, and very strong mitral valve separates the LA from the LV. The mitral valve is an oval, hyperbolic paraboloid (ie, saddle-shaped structure) containing two leaflets, identified as anterior and posterior on the basis of their anatomic locations. The valve leaflets coapt in a central curve, with the anterior mitral leaflet forming the convex border.

The functional integrity of the mitral valve apparatus is crucial to overall cardiac performance. The apparatus ensures unidirectional blood flow from the LA to the LV by preventing regurgitant flow into the LA and proximal pulmonary venous circulation.

Blood Supply

Blood flow to the heart is supplied by the left anterior descending coronary artery (LAD), the left circumflex coronary artery (LCCA), and right coronary artery (RCA).

Most blood flow to the LV occurs during diastole, when aortic blood pressure exceeds the LV pressure, establishing a positive pressure gradient in the coronary arteries, all three of which contribute to the LV's blood supply. Acute myocardial ischemia resulting from a critical coronary artery stenosis or abrupt occlusion causes a predictable pattern of LV injury based on the known distribution of blood supply. The LAD and its branches (including septal perforators and diagonals) supply the medial one-half of the LV anterior wall, the apex, and the anterior two-thirds of the interventricular septum. The LCCA and its obtuse marginal branches supply the anterior and posterior aspects of the lateral wall, whereas the RCA and its distal branches supply the medial portions of the posterior wall and the posterior one-third of the interventricular septum.

The coronary artery that supplies blood to the posterior descending artery (PDA) defines the right or left dominance of the coronary circulation. Right dominance (ie, PDA supplied by the RCA) is observed in approximately 80% of patients, whereas left dominance (ie, PDA supplied by the LCCA) occurs in the remainder.

In contrast to the LV, coronary blood flow to the RA, LA, and RV occurs throughout the cardiac cycle because systolic and diastolic aortic blood pressures exceed the pressures within these chambers. The RCA and its branches supply most of the RV, but the RV anterior wall also may receive blood from branches of the LAD. RV dysfunction may occur because of RCA or LAD ischemia.

Conduction

The mechanism by which the heart is electrically activated plays a crucial role in its mechanical performance. The sinoatrial (SA) node is the primary cardiac pacemaker if marked decreases in firing rate, conduction delays or blockade, or accelerated firing of secondary pacemakers (eg, atrioventricular (AV) node, bundle of His) do not occur. The anterior, middle, and posterior internodal pathways transmit the initial SA node depolarization rapidly through the RA myocardium to the AV node (Table 4.1). A branch (ie, Bachmann bundle) of the anterior internodal pathway also transmits the SA node depolarization from the RA to the LA across the atrial septum.

The bundle of His pierces the connective tissue insulator of the cartilaginous cardiac skeleton and transmits the AV depolarization signal through the right and left bundle branches to the RV and LV myocardium, respectively, by an extensive Purkinje network located within the inner one-third of the ventricular walls. The

Table 4.1 **Cardiac Electrical Activation Sequence**		
Structure	Conduction Velocity (m/s)	Pacemaker Rate (beats/min)
SA node	<0.01	60–100
Atrial myocardium	1.0–1.2	None
AV node	0.02–0.05	40–55
Bundle of His	1.2–2.0	25–40
Bundle branches	2.0–4.0	25–40
Purkinje network	2.0–4.0	25–40
Ventricular myocardium	0.3–1.0	None

AV, Atrioventricular; SA, sinoatrial.
From Katz AM. *Physiology of the Heart.* 3rd ed. Philadelphia: Lippincott Williams & Wilkins; 2001.

bundle of His, the bundle branches, and the Purkinje network are composed of His-Purkinje fibers that ensure rapid, coordinated distribution of depolarization. This electrical configuration facilitates synchronous ventricular contraction and coordinated ejection.

Artificial cardiac pacing (eg, epicardial RV pacing) bypasses the normal conduction system and produces dyssynchronous LV activation. This dyssynchrony causes uncoordinated contraction that may reduce global LV systolic function, and it is a frequent cause of a new regional wall motion abnormality after cardiopulmonary bypass in cardiac surgical patients. This type of contractile dyssynchrony is also associated with chronic RV apical pacing (eg, for treatment of sick-sinus syndrome or an AV conduction disorder) and is known to cause detrimental effects on LV chamber geometry and function. Recognition of the key relationship between a normal electrical activation sequence and LV contractile synchrony forms the basis for the successful use of cardiac resynchronization therapy in some patients with heart failure.

◼ CARDIAC MYOCYTE ANATOMY AND FUNCTION

Ultrastructure

The myocyte contains large numbers of mitochondria that are responsible for the generation of high-energy phosphates (eg, adenosine triphosphate [ATP], creatine phosphate) required for contraction and relaxation (Fig. 4.1). The sarcomere is the contractile unit of the cardiac myocyte. Its myofilaments are arranged in parallel, cross-striated bundles of thin fibers that contain actin, tropomyosin, and the troponin complex, and thick fibers that are primarily composed of myosin and its supporting proteins. Sarcomeres are connected in series, and the long and short axes of each myocyte simultaneously shorten and thicken, respectively, during contraction.

Each cardiac myocyte contains a dense sarcoplasmic reticulum (SR) network that surrounds the contractile proteins. The SR is the primary calcium ion (Ca^{2+}) reservoir

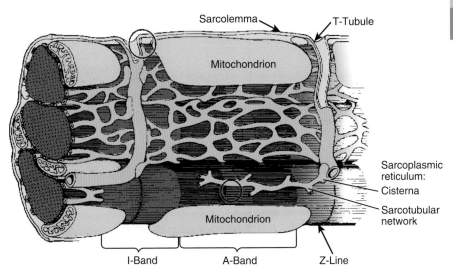

Fig. 4.1 Arnold Katz's schematic depiction of the ultrastructure of the cardiac myocyte. (From Katz AM. *Physiology of the Heart*. 3rd ed. Philadelphia: Lippincott Williams & Wilkins, 2001.)

of the cardiac myocyte, and its extensive distribution ensures an almost homogenous dispersal and reaccumulation of activator Ca^{2+} throughout the myofilaments during contraction and relaxation, respectively.

Proteins of the Contractile Apparatus

The contractile apparatus has six major components: myosin, actin, tropomyosin, and the three-protein troponin complex. Binding of the myosin head to the actin molecule stimulates a cascade of events initiated by activation of a myosin ATPase that mediates hinge rotation and actin release during contraction and relaxation, respectively. Actin is the major component of the thin filament. Tropomyosin is a major inhibitor of the interaction between actin and myosin in the myocyte sarcomere. The troponin complex consists of three proteins that regulate the contractile apparatus.

Calcium-Myofilament Interaction

Binding of Ca^{2+} and troponin C produces a sequence of conformational changes in the troponin-tropomyosin complex that exposes the specific myosin-binding site on actin (Fig. 4.2). Small amounts of Ca^{2+} are bound to troponin C when the intracellular Ca^{2+} concentration is low during diastole (10^{-7} M). Under these conditions, the troponin complex confines each tropomyosin molecule to the outer region of the groove between F-actin filaments and prevents the myosin-actin interaction by inhibiting the formation of cross-bridges between these proteins. The resting inhibitory state is rapidly transformed by the 100-fold increase in intracellular Ca^{2+} concentration (to 10^{-5} M) occurring as a consequence of sarcolemmal depolarization that opens L- and T-type Ca^{2+} channels, allows Ca^{2+} influx from the extracellular space, and stimulates Ca^{2+} release from the SR.

Binding of Ca^{2+} to troponin C stimulates several changes in the chemical conformation of the regulatory proteins that result in the exposure of the myosin-binding site on the actin molecule. Opening of the myosin-binding site allows cross-bridge formation and contraction to occur.

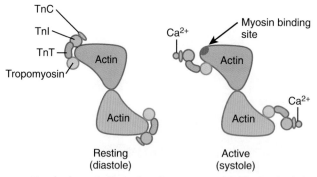

Fig. 4.2 Cross-sectional schematic illustration demonstrates the structural relationship between the troponin-tropomyosin complex and the actin filament under resting conditions (ie, diastole) and after Ca^{2+} binding (ie, systole). Ca^{2+} binding produces a conformational shift in the troponin-tropomyosin complex toward the groove between the actin molecules, exposing the myosin binding site on actin. *TnC*, Troponin C; *TnI*, troponin I; *TnT*, troponin T. (From Katz AM. *Physiology of the Heart*. 3rd ed. Philadelphia: Lippincott Williams & Wilkins, 2001.)

THE CARDIAC CYCLE

A schematic illustration of the cardiac cycle is useful for demonstrating the highly coordinated, temporally related series of electrical, mechanical, and valvular events that occur with contraction and relaxation of the cardiac chambers (Fig. 4.3). A single cardiac cycle occurs in 0.8 s at a heart rate of 75 beats/minute. Synchronous depolarization of RV and LV myocardium (as indicated by the electrocardiogram QRS complex) initiates contraction of and produces a rapid increase in pressure within these chambers (ie, systole). Closure of the tricuspid and mitral valves occurs when RV and LV pressures exceed the corresponding atrial pressures and causes the first heart sound (S_1).

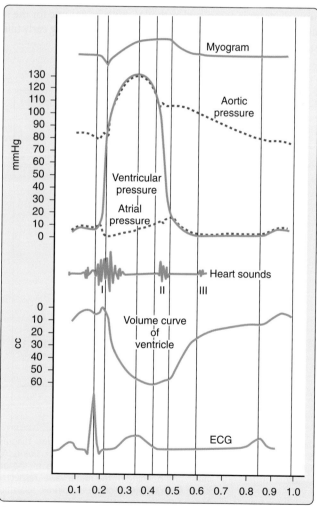

Fig. 4.3 Carl Wiggers' original illustration depicting the electrical, mechanical, and audible events of the cardiac cycle, including the electrocardiogram; aortic, left ventricular, and left atrial pressure waveforms; left ventricular volume waveform; and heart tones associated with mitral and aortic valve closure. (From Wiggers CJ: The Henry Jackson Memorial Lecture. Dynamics of ventricular contraction under abnormal conditions. *Circulation*. 1952;5:321–348.)

Pressure-Volume Diagrams

A time-dependent, two-dimensional plot of continuous LV pressure and volume throughout a single cardiac cycle creates a phase space diagram, which is useful for analysis of LV systolic and diastolic function in the ejecting heart (Fig. 4.4).

The cardiac cycle begins at end-diastole (see Fig. 4.4, point A). An abrupt increase in LV pressure at constant LV volume occurs during isovolumic contraction. Opening of the aortic valve occurs when LV pressure exceeds aorta pressure (see Fig. 4.4, point B) and ejection begins. LV volume decreases rapidly as blood is ejected from the LV into the aorta and proximal great vessels. When LV pressure declines below aortic pressure at the end of ejection, the aortic valve closes (see Fig. 4.4, point C). This event is immediately followed by a rapid decline in LV pressure in the absence of changes in LV volume (ie, isovolumic relaxation). The mitral valve opens when LV pressure falls below LA pressure (see Fig. 4.4, point D), initiating LV filling. The LV pressure-volume diagram is completed as the LV refills its volume for the next contraction concomitant with relatively small increases in pressure during early filling, diastasis, and LA systole.

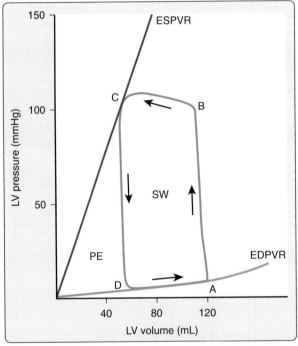

Fig. 4.4 As shown in the steady-state left ventricular (LV) pressure-volume diagram, the cardiac cycle proceeds in a time-dependent, counterclockwise direction (arrows). Points A, B, C, and D correspond to LV end-diastole (ie, closure of the mitral valve), opening of the aortic valve, LV end-systole (ie, closure of the aortic valve), and opening of the mitral valve, respectively. Segments AB, BC, CD, and DA represent isovolumic contraction, ejection, isovolumic relaxation, and filling, respectively. The left ventricle is constrained to operate within the boundaries of the end-systolic and end-diastolic pressure-volume relationships (ESPVR and EDPVR, respectively). The area inscribed by the LV pressure-volume diagram represents the stroke work (SW) (ie, kinetic energy) performed during the cardiac cycle. The area to the left of the LV pressure-volume diagram between ESPVR and EDPVR is the remaining potential energy (PE) of the system. The sum of SW and PE is the pressure-volume area.

The steady-state LV pressure-volume diagram provides advantages over temporal plots of individual LV pressure and volume waveforms when identifying major cardiac events without electrocardiographic correlation (eg, aortic or mitral valve opening or closing) or evaluating acute alterations in LV loading conditions. For example, end-diastolic and end-systolic volumes may immediately be recognized as the lower right (point A) and upper left (point C) corners of the diagram, respectively, allowing rapid calculation of stroke volume (SV) and ejection fraction (EF). Movement of the right side of the pressure-volume diagram to the right is characteristic of an increase in preload concomitant with a larger SV, whereas an increase in afterload causes the pressure-volume diagram to become taller (ie, greater LV pressure) and narrower (ie, decreased SV). The area of the diagram precisely defines the LV pressure-volume (stroke) work (ie, kinetic energy) for a single cardiac cycle.

As illustrative as a single LV pressure-volume diagram may be for obtaining basic physiologic information, the dynamic changes of a series of these LV pressure-volume diagrams occurring during an acute alteration in LV load over several consecutive cardiac cycles provide unique insights into LV systolic and diastolic function.

Pressure-volume analysis provides a useful illustration of the pathophysiology of LV systolic or diastolic dysfunction as underlying causes for heart failure. For example; a decrease in the end-systolic pressure-volume relationship (ESPVR) slope indicates that a reduction in myocardial contractility has occurred. This observation is consistent with pure LV systolic dysfunction. The event is often accompanied by a compensatory LV dilation (ie, movement of the pressure-volume diagram to the right) along a normal end-diastolic pressure-volume relationship (EDPVR) (Fig. 4.5). The increase in preload may preserve SV and cardiac output (CO), but occurs at the cost of higher LV filling and pulmonary venous pressures. In contrast, an increase in the EDPVR denotes a reduction in LV compliance such that LV diastolic pressure is higher at each LV volume. Under these circumstances, myocardial contractility may remain

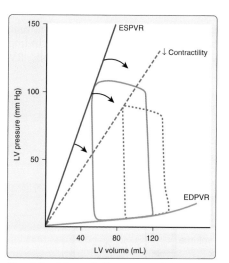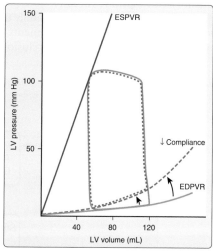

Fig. 4.5 Schematic illustrations of the alterations in the steady-state LV pressure-volume diagram produced by a reduction in myocardial contractility, as indicated by a decrease in the slope of the ESPVR (*left*), and a decrease in LV compliance as indicated by an increase in the position of the EDPVR (*right*). The diagrams emphasize that heart failure may result from LV systolic or diastolic dysfunction independently. *EDPVR,* End-diastolic pressure-volume relationship; *ESPVR,* end-systolic pressure-volume relationship; *LV,* left ventricular.

relatively normal (ie, ESPVR does not change), but LV filling pressures are elevated, producing pulmonary venous congestion and clinical symptoms (Fig. 4.5). Simultaneous depression of the ESPVR and elevation of the EDPVR indicate LV systolic and diastolic dysfunction.

▦ DETERMINANTS OF PUMP PERFORMANCE

From a clinical perspective, LV systolic function is most often quantified using CO (ie, product of heart rate and SV) and EF. These variables depend on the intrinsic contractile properties of the LV myocardium, the quantity of blood the chamber contains immediately before contraction commences (ie, preload), and the external resistance to emptying with which it is confronted (ie, afterload). The interactions among preload, afterload, and myocardial contractility establish the SV generated during each cardiac cycle (Fig. 4.6). When combined with heart rate and rhythm, preload, afterload, and myocardial contractility determine the volume of blood that the LV can pump per minute (ie, CO), assuming adequate venous return.

Preload

Preload is most often defined as the volume of blood contained within each chamber at its end-diastole. This blood volume effectively establishes the length of each myocyte immediately before isovolumic contraction and is related to LV end-diastolic wall stress.

LV preload may be estimated using a variety of other methods, each of which has inherent limitations (Fig. 4.7). LV end-diastolic pressure may be measured invasively in the cardiac catheterization laboratory or during surgery by advancing a fluid-filled or pressure transducer–tipped catheter from the aorta across the aortic valve or through the LA and across the mitral valve into the LV chamber. LV end-diastolic pressure is related to end-diastolic volume based on the nonlinear EDPVR and may not accurately quantify end-diastolic volume.

Cardiac anesthesiologists commonly use several other estimates of LV end-diastolic volume that depend on measurements obtained upstream from the LV, including mean LA, pulmonary capillary occlusion (wedge), pulmonary arterial diastolic, RV

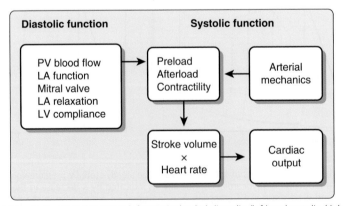

Fig. 4.6 Major factors that determine left ventricular *(LV)* diastolic *(left)* and systolic *(right)* function. Pulmonary venous *(PV)* blood flow, left atrial *(LA)* function, mitral valve integrity, LA relaxation, and LV compliance combine to determine LV preload.

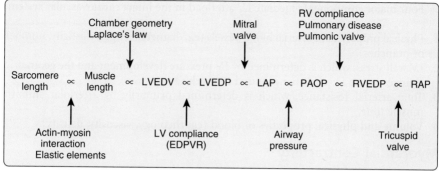

Fig. 4.7 Several factors influence experimental and clinical estimates of sarcomere length as a pure index of the preload of the contracting left ventricular *(LV)* myocyte. *EDPVR*, End-diastolic pressure-volume relationship; *LAP*, left atrial pressure; *LVEDP*, left ventricular end-diastolic pressure; *LVEDV*, left ventricular end-diastolic volume; *PAOP*, pulmonary artery occlusion pressure; *RAP*, right atrial pressure; *RV*, right ventricular; *RVEDP*, right ventricular end-diastolic pressure.

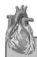

BOX 4.1 *Indices of Left Ventricular Afterload*

Aortic input impedance (magnitude and phase spectra)
Windkessel parameters
 Characteristic aortic impedance (Z_c)
 Total arterial compliance (C)
 Total arterial resistance (R)
End-systolic pressure
End-systolic wall stress
Effective arterial elastance (E_a)
Systemic vascular resistance

4

end-diastolic, and RA (central venous) pressures. These estimates of LV end-diastolic volume are affected by functional integrity of the structures that separate each measurement location from the LV.

Correlation among LV end-diastolic volume, pulmonary artery occlusion pressure, and RA pressure is notoriously poor in patients with compromised LV systolic function, and measurement of pressures upstream from the LV may be of limited clinical utility in the assessment of LV preload under these circumstances.

Afterload

Afterload is the additional load to which cardiac muscle is subjected immediately after the onset of a contraction (Box 4.1). Impedance to LV or RV ejection by the mechanical properties of the systemic or pulmonary arterial vasculature provides the basis for the definition of afterload in vivo.

The mechanical forces to which the LV is subjected during ejection may be used to define LV afterload. Increases in LV pressure and wall thickness occur during isovolumic contraction and are accompanied by a large reduction in LV volume (ie, radius) after the aortic valve opens.

Four major components mediate LV afterload in the intact cardiovascular system:

1. Physical properties of arterial blood vessels (eg, diameter, length, elasticity, number of branches).
2. LV wall stress, which is determined by LV pressure development and the geometric changes in the LV chamber required to produce it.
3. Total arterial resistance, which is determined primarily by arteriolar smooth muscle tone.
4. Volume and physical properties of blood (eg, rheology, viscosity, density).

Myocardial Contractility

Quantifying myocardial contractility in the intact heart is a challenging problem. Quantification of LV contractility would allow cardiac anesthesiologists to reliably evaluate the effects of pharmacologic interventions or pathologic processes on LV systolic function.

End-Systolic Pressure-Volume Relationships

Because the LV is an elastic chamber, the relationship between its pressure and volume may be described in terms of time-varying elastance (ie, ratio of pressure to volume) during the cardiac cycle (Box 4.2). LV elastance increases during systole as LV pressure

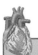

BOX 4.2 *Indices of Left Ventricular Contractility*

Pressure-Volume Analysis

End-systolic pressure-volume relation (E_{es})
Stroke work–end-diastolic volume relation (M_{sw})

Isovolumic Contraction

dP/dt_{max}
$dP/dt_{max}/50$
$dP/dt_{max}/P$
dP/dt_{max}-end-diastolic volume relation (dE/dt_{max})

Ejection Phase

Stroke volume
Cardiac output
Ejection fraction
Fractional area change
Fractional shortening
Wall thickening
Velocity of shortening

Ventricular Power

PWR_{max}
PWR_{max}/EDV^2

dE/dt_{max}, Slope of the dP/dt_{max}-end-diastolic volume relationship; *dP/dt_{max}*, maximum rate of increase of left ventricular pressure; *EDV*, end-diastolic volume; *E_{es}*, end-systolic elastance; *M_{sw}*, slope of the stroke work–end-diastolic volume relationship; *P*, peak left ventricular pressure; *PWR_{max}*, maximum left ventricular power (product of aortic pressure and blood flow).

rises and LV volume declines. Maximal LV elastance (E_{max}) occurs at or very near end-systole, most often corresponding to the left upper corner of the steady-state LV pressure-volume diagram. Analogously, minimal LV elastance is observed at end-diastole (Fig. 4.4).

The slope (ie, E_{es}) of the ESPVR is a quantitative index of LV contractile state that incorporates afterload because the analysis is conducted at end-systole (Fig. 4.8). An increase or decrease in the magnitude of E_{es} produced by a positive or negative inotropic

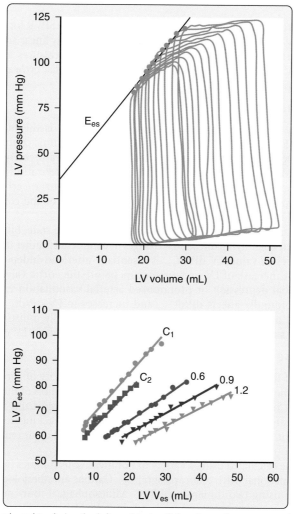

Fig. 4.8 Method used to derive the left ventricular *(LV)* end-systolic pressure-volume relationship (ESPVR) from a series of differentially loaded LV pressure-volume diagrams generated by abrupt occlusion of the inferior vena cava in a canine heart in vivo. *Top panel*: The pressure-volume ratio or maximal elastance (E_{max}) for each pressure-volume diagram is identified *(left upper corner)*, and a linear regression analysis is used to define the slope or end-systolic elastance (E_{es}) and volume intercept of the ESPVR. *Bottom panel*: The effects of isoflurane (0.6, 0.9, and 1.2 minimum alveolar concentrations) on the ESPVR are shown. C_1, Control 1 (before isoflurane); C_2, control 2 (after isoflurane); P_{es}, LV end-systolic pressure; V_{es}, LV end-systolic volume. (Modified from Hettrick DA, Pagel PS, Warltier DC. Desflurane, sevoflurane, and isoflurane impair canine left ventricular-arterial coupling and mechanical efficiency, *Anesthesiology*. 1996;85:403–413.)

drug (eg, dobutamine or esmolol), respectively, quantifies the corresponding change in LV contractility that has occurred.

Stroke Work–End-Diastolic Volume Relationships

Early studies defined a fundamental relationship between LV pump performance (eg, CO) and preload determined using indirect indices of LV filling (eg, central venous pressure). In this familiar framework, movement of an LV function curve upward or to the left indicated that an increase in the contractile state had occurred because the LV was able to generate more stroke work (SW) at an equivalent preload.

The SW-V_{ed} relationship offers several advantages over the ESPVR for the determination of LV or RV contractility. The SW-V_{ed} relationship is highly linear and reproducible over a wide variety of loading conditions, arterial blood pressures, and contractile states because LV pressure and volume data from the entire cardiac cycle are incorporated into its calculation.

Isovolumic Indices of Contractility

The maximum rate of increase of LV pressure (dP/dt_{max}) is the most commonly derived index of the global LV contractile state during isovolumic contraction. Precise determination of LV dP/dt_{max} requires high-fidelity, invasive measurement of continuous LV pressure and usually is performed in the cardiac catheterization laboratory. LV dP/dt_{max} also may be noninvasively estimated using transesophageal echocardiography (TEE) in patients undergoing cardiac surgery by analysis of the continuous-wave Doppler mitral regurgitation waveform.

LV dP/dt_{max} is sensitive to acute alterations in contractile state, but it is probably most useful when quantifying directional changes in contractility rather than establishing an absolute baseline value. LV dP/dt_{max} is essentially afterload-independent because the peak rate of increase of LV pressure occurs before the aortic valve opens unless severe myocardial depression or pronounced arterial vasodilation exists. However, LV preload profoundly affects dP/dt_{max}, and increases in LV dP/dt_{max} produced by greater preload or an enhanced contractile state are virtually indistinguishable. LV mass, chamber size, and mitral or aortic valve disease also affect LV dP/dt_{max}.

Ejection-Phase Indices of Contractility

Examination of the degree (eg, EF, SV) or the rate (eg, velocity of shortening) of LV ejection forms the basis of all currently used ejection-phase indices of the LV contractile state, including newer echocardiographic parameters derived from tissue Doppler imaging, myocardial stress-strain relationships, speckle tracking technology, and endocardial color kinesis. From a clinical perspective, the most common ejection-phase index of LV contractility is EF, for which $EF = V_{ed} - V_{es}/V_{ed}$.

LV EF may be calculated using a variety of noninvasive techniques (eg, radionuclide angiography, functional MRI, echocardiography). Cardiac anesthesiologists most often measure LV EF using two-dimensional TEE. Midesophageal four- or two-chamber images are obtained at LV end-systole and end-diastole. They are subsequently analyzed by applying Simpson's rule of disks, which defines the volume as the sum of a finite series of cylinders of various diameters and thicknesses (Fig. 4.9).

Two closely related parameters, fractional shortening (FS) and fractional area of change (FAC), are often calculated as surrogate measures of LV EF in the midpapillary short-axis plane using images obtained at end-systole and end-diastole. FS is calculated from endocardial measurements of anteroposterior (or septolateral) wall diameter as $FS = D_{ed} - D_{es}/D_{ed}$, in which D_{ed} and D_{es} are the endocardial end-diastolic and end-systolic diameters, respectively (Fig. 4.10).

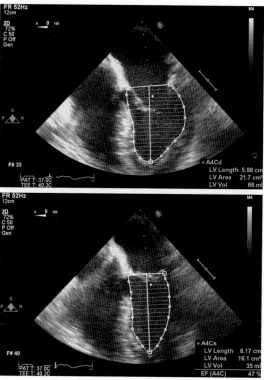

Fig. 4.9 Calculation of ejection fraction from midesophageal four-chamber images obtained at left ventricular (LV) end-diastole *(left)* and end-systole *(right)* using Simpson's rule. After the LV endocardial border is identified in each image, the software generates a series of thin cylindrical disks *(parallel white lines)* and determines the volume based on their sum. LV ejection fraction is then calculated using the standard formula. In this example, the LV ejection fraction is 47%.

FAC may be determined using the same midpapillary short-axis images by manually tracing the endocardial borders (with the papillary muscles most often excluded) at end-systole and end-diastole. Computer software automatically integrates the end-systolic and end-diastolic areas and FAC is calculated.

▣ EVALUATION OF DIASTOLIC FUNCTION

LV diastole encompasses a complicated sequence of temporally related, heterogeneous events (see Fig. 4.6), and no single index of LV diastolic function can comprehensively describe this period of the cardiac cycle or selectively identify patients at highest risk for developing clinical signs and symptoms of heart failure resulting from filling abnormalities. Most indices of LV diastolic function depend on heart rate, loading conditions, and myocardial contractility.

Despite inherent difficulties, the crucial nature of LV diastolic function is emphasized by the striking observation that as many as 50% of patients with heart failure do not have a substantial reduction in LV EF. This *heart failure with normal ejection fraction* (HF$_n$EF), previously called *diastolic heart failure*, occurs most frequently in elderly women with poorly controlled essential hypertension, obesity, renal insufficiency, anemia, general deconditioning, or atrial fibrillation. Many of these risk factors

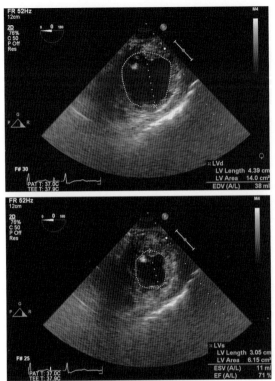

Fig. 4.10 Calculation of fractional area change (FAC) and fractional shortening (FS) from the left ventricular (LV) midpapillary short-axis images obtained at end-diastole *(left)* and end-systole *(right)*. The LV endocardial border is manually traced (excluding the papillary muscles). The software integrates the area inscribed and determines the diameter of the LV chamber. In this example, FAC is 69%, and FS is 59%.

contribute to the progressive development of LV hypertrophy and fibrosis that adversely affect LV filling characteristics, and increase the risk of heart failure.

The pathophysiology of HF_nEF appears to be multifactorial and involves delayed LV relaxation, reduced compliance, and abnormal ventricular-arterial stiffening. Regardless of the underlying cause (Box 4.3), diastolic dysfunction is a ubiquitous feature of HF_nEF. Diastolic dysfunction is uniformly identified in all patients with heart failure resulting from LV systolic dysfunction. The severity of LV diastolic dysfunction and its response to medical therapy are important determinants of exercise tolerance and mortality in patients with heart failure independent of concomitant LV systolic dysfunction.

From the perspective of the cardiac anesthesiologist, LV diastolic dysfunction has significant implications in determining the LV response to acute alterations in loading conditions that occur during and after surgery. For example, cardiopulmonary bypass temporally exacerbates preexisting LV diastolic dysfunction in cardiac surgical patients. Volatile and intravenous anesthetics alter LV relaxation and filling properties in the normal and failing heart. Assessing the existence and severity of LV diastolic dysfunction remains an important objective in the management of patients undergoing cardiac surgery.

BOX 4.3 *Common Causes of Left Ventricular Diastolic Dysfunction*

Age >60 years
Acute myocardial ischemia (supply or demand)
Myocardial stunning, hibernation, or infarction
Ventricular remodeling after infarction
Pressure-overload hypertrophy (eg, aortic stenosis, hypertension)
Volume-overload hypertrophy (eg, aortic or mitral regurgitation)
Hypertrophic obstructive cardiomyopathy
Dilated cardiomyopathy
Restrictive cardiomyopathy (eg, amyloidosis, hemochromatosis)
Pericardial diseases (eg, tamponade, constrictive pericarditis)

PERICARDIAL FORCES

The pericardium is a sac that encloses the heart, proximal great vessels, distal vena cavae, and pulmonary veins. The smooth surface of the visceral pericardium combined with the lubrication provided by 15 to 35 mL of pericardial fluid (ie, plasma ultrafiltrate, myocardial interstitial fluid, and a small quantity of lymph) and surfactant phospholipids reduce friction and facilitate normal cardiac movement during systole and diastole.

The pericardium also acts as a mechanical barrier that separates the heart from other mediastinal structures and limits abnormal displacement of the heart through its inferior (ie, diaphragmatic) and superior (ie, great vessels) attachments. The fibrous layer of the parietal pericardium determines the J-shaped pericardial pressure-volume relationship (Fig. 4.11),which indicates that the pericardium is substantially less compliant than LV myocardium. As a result of this lack of elasticity, the pericardium has very limited volume reserve and is capable of accommodating only a small increase in volume before a large increase in pressure occurs.

Pericardial pressure is usually subatmospheric (range, −5 to 0 mm Hg), varies with changes in intrathoracic pressure, and produces little or no mechanical effect in a normal heart under euvolemic conditions. Instead, the pericardium exerts a critical restraining force on the filling of all four cardiac chambers, and the effect is exaggerated during pericardial compression (eg, tamponade, constrictive pericarditis) or acute increases in chamber dimension (eg, volume loading).

Pericardial restraint is most apparent in the thinner-walled atria and RV, and it is the primary determinant of the diastolic pressure and volume of these chambers. The pericardium resists further increases in atrial and RV chamber size during volume loading, and pressure within these chambers rises more rapidly than predicted on the basis of myocardial elasticity alone.

The pericardium plays an essential role in ventricular interdependence (ie, influence of the pressure and volume of one ventricle on the mechanical behavior of the other). The pericardium restrains the LV and RV equally despite the inherent differences in compliance between the chambers. An increase in RV size (eg, ischemia, volume overload) causes pericardial pressure to increase, reducing LV compliance and restricting LV filling. Similarly, acute LV distension (eg, application of an aortic cross-clamp) encroaches on the RV, and limits RV filling.

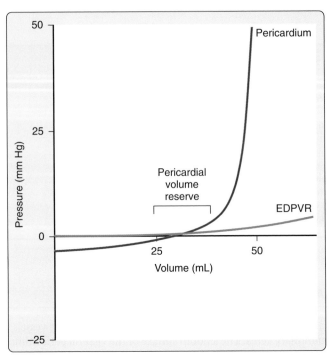

Fig. 4.11 Pressure-volume relationship of the pericardium compared with the left ventricular end-diastolic pressure-volume relationship *(EDPVR)*. Large increases in pericardial pressure occur after the reserve volume is exceeded.

Evidence for diastolic ventricular interaction is readily apparent using pulsed-wave echocardiography to determine changes in RV and LV filling during spontaneous ventilation. Inspiration decreases intrathoracic pressure, enhances venous return, and causes modest RV distension. These effects mildly reduce LV filling by decreasing compliance of the chamber, resulting in small declines in mean arterial pressure and CO. During expiration, RV filling is attenuated, and LV filling is augmented. Compression of the ventricular chambers during pericardial tamponade or constrictive pericarditis markedly exaggerates these respiratory changes in RV and LV filling. Maintenance of spontaneous ventilation is crucial under these circumstances because negative intrathoracic pressure preserves venous return to some degree, whereas institution of positive-pressure ventilation may rapidly cause cardiovascular collapse by profoundly limiting venous return.

SUGGESTED READINGS

Borlaug BA, Kass DA. Ventricular-vascular interaction in heart failure. *Heart Fail Clin.* 2008;4:23–26.

Burkhoff D, Mirsky I, Suga H. Assessment of systolic and diastolic ventricular properties via pressure-volume analysis: a guide for clinical, translational, and basic researchers. *Am J Physiol Heart Circ Physiol.* 2005;289:H501–H512.

Cowie B, Kluger R, Kalpokas M. Left ventricular volume and ejection fraction assessment with transoesphageal echocardiography: 2D vs 3D imaging. *Br J Anaesth.* 2013;110:201–206.

Dorosz JL, Lezotte DC, Weitzenkamp DA, et al. Performance of 3-dimensional echocardiography in measuring left ventricular volumes and ejection fraction: a systematic review and meta-analysis. *J Am Coll Cardiol.* 2012;59:1799–1808.

Gaasch WH, Zile MR. Left ventricular diastolic dysfunction and diastolic heart failure. *Annu Rev Med.* 2004;55:373–394.

Grossman W. Diastolic dysfunction and congestive heart failure. *Circulation.* 1990;81(2 suppl):III1–III7.

Katz AM. Influence of altered inotropy and lusitropy on ventricular pressure-volume loops. *J Am Coll Cardiol.* 1988;11:438–445.

Kitzman DW, Little WC, Brubaker PH, et al. Pathophysiological characterization of isolated diastolic heart failure in comparison to systolic heart failure. *JAMA.* 2002;288:2144–2150.

Little WC, Downes TR. Clinical evaluation of left ventricular diastolic performance. *Prog Cardiovasc Dis.* 1990;32:273–290.

Maeder MT, Kaye DM. Heart failure with normal left ventricular ejection fraction. *J Am Coll Cardiol.* 2009;53:905–918.

Meris A, Santambrogio L, Casso G, et al. Intraoperative three-dimensional versus two-dimensional echocardiography for left ventricular assessment. *Anesth Analg.* 2014;118:711–720.

Sagawa K. The end-systolic pressure-volume relation of the ventricle: definition, modifications and clinical use. *Circulation.* 1981;63:1223–1227.

Sidebotham DA, Allen SJ, Gerber IL, et al. Intraoperative transesophageal echocardiography for surgical repair of mitral regurgitation. *J Am Soc Echocardiogr.* 2014;27:345–366.

Solaro RJ, Rarick HM. Troponin and tropomyosin. Proteins that switch on and tune in the activity of cardiac myofilaments. *Circ Res.* 1998;83:471–480.

Pagel PS, Kehl F, Gare M, et al. Mechanical function of the left atrium: new insights based on analysis of pressure-volume relations and Doppler echocardiography. *Anesthesiology.* 2003;98:975–994.

Pagel PS, Nijhawan N, Warltier DC. Quantitation of volatile anesthetic-induced depression of myocardial contractility using a single beat index derived from maximal ventricular power. *J Cardiothorac Vasc Anesth.* 1993;7:688–695.

Paulus WJ, Tschope C, Sanderson JE, et al. How to diagnose diastolic heart failure: a consensus statement on the diagnosis of heart failure with normal left ventricular ejection fraction by the Heart Failure and Echocardiography Associations of the European Society of Cardiology. *Eur Heart J.* 2007;28:2539–2550.

Rakowski H, Appleton C, Chan KL, et al. Canadian consensus recommendations for the measurement and reporting of diastolic dysfunction by echocardiography: from the Investigators of Consensus on Diastolic Dysfunction by Echocardiography. *J Am Soc Echocardiogr.* 1996;9:736–760.

Rayment I, Holden HM, Whittaker M. Structure of the actin-myosin complex and its implications for muscle contraction. *Science.* 1993;261:58–65.

Zile MR, Baicu CF, Gaasch WH. Diastolic heart failure—abnormalities in active relaxation and passive stiffness of the left ventricle. *N Engl J Med.* 2004;350:1953–1959.

4

Chapter 5

Coronary Physiology and Atherosclerosis

Benjamin Hibbert, MD, PhD • Howard J. Nathan, MD •
Trevor Simard, MD • Edward R. O'Brien, MD

Key Points

1. To care for patients with coronary artery disease in the perioperative period safely, the clinician must understand how the coronary circulation functions in health and disease.
2. Coronary endothelium modulates myocardial blood flow by producing factors that relax or contract the underlying vascular smooth muscle.
3. Vascular endothelial cells help maintain the fluidity of blood by elaborating anticoagulant, fibrinolytic, and antiplatelet substances.
4. One of the earliest changes in coronary artery disease, preceding the appearance of stenoses, is the loss of the vasoregulatory and antithrombotic functions of the endothelium.
5. Although sympathetic activation increases myocardial oxygen demand, activation of α-adrenergic receptors causes coronary vasoconstriction.
6. It is unlikely that one substance alone (eg, adenosine) provides the link between myocardial metabolism and myocardial blood flow under a variety of conditions.
7. As coronary perfusion pressure decreases, the inner layers of myocardium nearest the left ventricular cavity are the first to become ischemic and display impaired relaxation and contraction.
8. The progression of an atherosclerotic lesion is similar to the process of wound healing.
9. Lipid-lowering therapy can help restore endothelial function and prevent coronary events.

When caring for patients with coronary artery disease (CAD), the anesthesiologist must prevent or minimize myocardial ischemia by maintaining optimal conditions for perfusion of the heart. This goal can be achieved only with an understanding of the many factors that determine myocardial blood flow in both health and disease.

ANATOMY AND PHYSIOLOGY OF BLOOD VESSELS

The coronary vasculature has been traditionally divided into three functional groups: (1) large conductance vessels visible on coronary angiography, which offer little resistance to blood flow; (2) small resistance vessels ranging in size from approximately 250 nm to 10 μm in diameter; and (3) veins. Although it has been taught that arterioles (precapillary vessels <50 μm in size) account for most coronary resistance, studies indicate that, under resting conditions, 45% to 50% of total coronary vascular resistance resides in vessels larger than 100 μm in diameter. The reason may be, in part, the relatively great length of the small arteries.

Normal Artery Wall

The arterial lumen is lined by a monolayer of endothelial cells that overlies smooth muscle cells). The inner layer of smooth muscle cells, known as the intima, is circumscribed by the internal elastic lamina. Between the internal elastic lamina and external elastic lamina is another layer of smooth muscle cells, the media. Outside the external elastic lamina is an adventitia that is sparsely populated by cells but consists of complex extracellular matrix (primarily collagen and elastin fibers) and the microvessels that comprise the vasa vasorum.

Endothelium

Although the vascular endothelium was once thought of as an inert lining for blood vessels, it is more accurately characterized as a very active, distributed organ with many biologic functions. It has synthetic and metabolic capabilities and contains receptors for a variety of vasoactive substances.

Endothelium-Derived Relaxing Factors

The first vasoactive endothelial substance to be discovered was prostacyclin (PGI_2), a product of the cyclooxygenase pathway of arachidonic acid metabolism (Fig. 5.1 and Box 5.1). The production of PGI_2 is activated by shear stress, pulsatility of flow, hypoxia, and a variety of vasoactive mediators. On production it leaves the endothelial cell and acts in the local environment to cause relaxation of the underlying smooth muscle or to inhibit platelet aggregation. Both actions are mediated by the stimulation of adenylyl cyclase in the target cell to produce cyclic adenosine monophosphate (cAMP).

It has been shown that many physiologic stimuli cause vasodilation by stimulating the release of a labile, diffusible, nonprostanoid molecule termed *endothelium-derived relaxing factor* (EDRF), now known to be nitric oxide (NO). NO is a very small lipophilic molecule that can readily diffuse across biologic membranes and into the cytosol of nearby cells. The half-life of the molecule is less than 5 seconds so that only the local environment can be affected. NO is synthesized from the amino acid L-arginine by NO synthase (NOS). When NO diffuses into the cytosol of the target cell, it binds with the heme group of soluble guanylate cyclase; the result is a 50- to 200-fold increase in production of cyclic guanosine monophosphate (cGMP), its secondary messenger. If the target cells are vascular smooth muscle cells, vasodilation occurs; if the target cells are platelets, adhesion and aggregation are inhibited. NO is probably the final common effector molecule of nitrovasodilators. The cardiovascular system is in a constant state of active vasodilation that depends on the generation of NO. The molecule is more important in controlling vascular tone in veins and arteries compared with arterioles. Abnormalities in the ability of the endothelium to produce NO likely play a role in diseases such as diabetes, atherosclerosis, and hypertension. The venous circulation of humans seems to have a lower basal release of NO and an increased sensitivity to nitrovasodilators compared with the arterial side of the circulation.

Endothelium-Derived Contracting Factors

Contracting factors produced by the endothelium include prostaglandin H_2, thromboxane A_2 (generated by cyclooxygenase), and the peptide endothelin. Endothelin is a potent vasoconstrictor peptide (100-fold more potent than norepinephrine). In vascular smooth muscle cells, endothelin 1 (ET-1) binds to specific membrane receptors

5

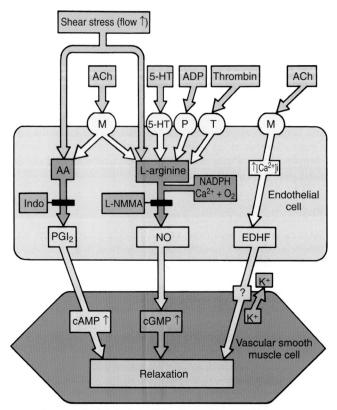

Fig. 5.1 The production of endothelium-derived vasodilator substances. Prostacyclin *(PGI₂)* is produced by the cyclooxygenase pathway of arachidonic acid *(AA)* metabolism, which can be blocked by indomethacin *(Indo)* and aspirin. PGI₂ stimulates smooth muscle adenylyl cyclase and increases cyclic adenosine monophosphate *(cAMP)* production, actions that cause relaxation. Endothelium-derived relaxing factor *(EDRF)*, now known to be nitric oxide *(NO)*, is produced by the action of NO synthase on L-arginine in the presence of reduced nicotinamide adenine dinucleotide phosphate *(NADPH)*, oxygen *(O₂)*, and calcium *(Ca²⁺)* and calmodulin. This process can be blocked by arginine analogs such as Nᴳ-monomethyl-L-arginine *(LNMMA)*. NO combines with guanylate cyclase in the smooth muscle cell to stimulate production of cyclic guanosine monophosphate *(cGMP)*, which results in relaxation. Less well characterized is an endothelium-derived hyperpolarizing factor *(EDHF)*, which hyperpolarizes the smooth muscle membrane and probably acts by activation of potassium *(K⁺)* channels. *ACh,* Acetylcholine; *ADP,* adenosine diphosphate; *[Ca²⁺]ᵢ,* intracellular calcium; *5-HT,* serotonin; *M,* muscarinic receptor; *P,* purinergic receptor; *T,* thrombin receptor. (From Rubanyi GM. Endothelium, platelets, and coronary vasospasm. *Coron Artery Dis.* 1990;1:645.)

(ETₐ) and, through phospholipase C, induces an increase in intracellular calcium resulting in long-lasting contractions. It is also linked by a guanosine triphosphate (GTP)-binding protein (Gᵢ) to voltage-operated calcium channels. This peptide has greater vasoconstricting potency than any other cardiovascular hormone, and in pharmacologic doses it can abolish coronary flow, thereby leading to ventricular fibrillation and death.

Endothelial Inhibition of Platelets

A primary function of endothelium is to maintain the fluidity of blood. This is achieved by the synthesis and release of anticoagulant (eg, thrombomodulin, protein C), fibrinolytic (eg, tissue-type plasminogen activator), and platelet inhibitory

> ## BOX 5.1 *Endothelium-Derived Relaxing and Contracting Factors*
>
> Healthy endothelial cells have an important role in modulating coronary tone by producing:
> - vascular muscle-relaxing factors
>   - prostacyclin
>   - nitric oxide
>   - hyperpolarizing factor
> - vascular muscle-contracting factors
>   - prostaglandin H_2
>   - thromboxane A_2
>   - endothelin

> ## BOX 5.2 *Endothelial Inhibition of Platelets*
>
> Healthy endothelial cells have a role in maintaining the fluidity of blood by producing:
> - anticoagulant factors: protein C and thrombomodulin
> - fibrinolytic factor: tissue-type plasminogen activator
> - platelet inhibitory substances: prostacyclin and nitric oxide

(eg, PGI_2, NO) substances (Box 5.2). Mediators released from aggregating platelets stimulate the release from intact endothelium of NO and PGI_2, which act together to increase blood flow and decrease platelet adhesion and aggregation (Fig. 5.2).

■ DETERMINANTS OF CORONARY BLOOD FLOW

Under normal conditions, coronary blood flow has four major determinants: (1) perfusion pressure; (2) myocardial extravascular compression; (3) myocardial metabolism; and (4) neurohumoral control.

Perfusion Pressure and Myocardial Compression

Coronary blood flow is proportional to the pressure gradient across the coronary circulation (Box 5.3). This gradient is calculated by subtracting downstream coronary pressure from the pressure in the root of the aorta.

During systole, the heart throttles its own blood supply. The force of systolic myocardial compression is greatest in the subendocardial layers, where it approximates intraventricular pressure. Resistance resulting from extravascular compression increases with blood pressure, heart rate, contractility, and preload.

The most appropriate measure of the driving pressure for flow is the average pressure in the aortic root during diastole. This value can be approximated by aortic diastolic or mean pressure.

5

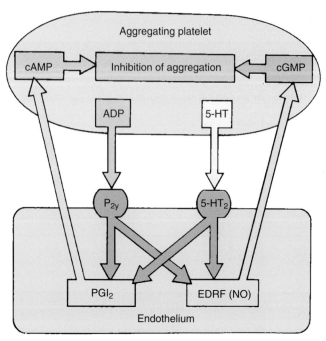

Fig. 5.2 Inhibition of platelet adhesion and aggregation by intact endothelium. Aggregating platelets release adenosine diphosphate (*ADP*) and serotonin (*5-HT*), which stimulate the synthesis and release of prostacyclin (*PGI₂*) and endothelium-derived relaxing factor (*EDRF;* nitric oxide *[NO]*), which diffuse back to the platelets and inhibit further adhesion and aggregation and can cause disaggregation. PGI_2 and EDRF act synergistically by increasing platelet cyclic adenosine monophosphate (*cAMP*) and cyclic guanosine monophosphate (*cGMP*), respectively. By inhibiting platelets and also increasing blood flow by causing vasodilation, PGI_2 and EDRF can flush away microthrombi and prevent thrombosis of intact vessels. P_{2y}, Purinergic receptor. (From Rubanyi GM. Endothelium, platelets, and coronary vasospasm. *Coron Artery Dis.* 1990;1:645.)

BOX 5.3 *Determinants of Coronary Blood Flow*

The primary determinants of coronary blood flow are:
- perfusion pressure
- myocardial extravascular compression
- myocardial metabolism
- neurohumoral control

Although the true downstream pressure of the coronary circulation is likely close to the coronary sinus pressure, other choices may be more appropriate in clinical circumstances. The true downstream pressure of the left ventricular subendocardium is the left ventricular end-diastolic pressure, which can be estimated by pulmonary artery occlusion pressure. When the right ventricle is at risk of ischemia (eg, severe pulmonary hypertension), right ventricular diastolic pressure or central venous pressure may be a more appropriate choice for measuring downstream pressure.

Myocardial Metabolism

Myocardial blood flow is primarily under metabolic control. Even when the heart is cut off from external control mechanisms (neural and humoral factors), its ability to match blood flow to its metabolic requirements is almost unaffected. Because coronary venous oxygen tension is normally 15 to 20 mm Hg, only a small amount of oxygen is available through increased extraction. A major increase in myocardial oxygen consumption ($M\dot{v}O_2$), beyond the normal resting value of 80 to 100 mL O_2/100 g of myocardium, can occur only if oxygen delivery is increased by augmentation of coronary blood flow. Normally, flow and metabolism are closely matched, so that over a wide range of oxygen consumption coronary sinus oxygen saturation changes little. Flow and metabolism could be coupled either through feedback or feedforward control or a combination of both. Feedback control requires myocardial oxygen tension to fall and provide a signal that can then increase flow. That would require vascular tone to be linked either to a substrate that is depleted, such as oxygen or adenosine triphosphate (ATP), or to the accumulation of a metabolite such as carbon dioxide or hydrogen ion. The mediator or mediators linking myocardial metabolism so effectively to myocardial blood flow are still unknown (Box 5.4).

Neural and Humoral Control

Coronary Innervation

The heart is supplied with branches of the sympathetic and parasympathetic divisions of the autonomic nervous system. Large and small coronary arteries and veins are richly innervated. The sympathetic nerves to the heart and coronary vessels arise from the superior, middle, and inferior cervical sympathetic ganglia and the first four thoracic ganglia. The stellate ganglion (formed when the inferior cervical and first thoracic ganglia merge) is a major source of cardiac sympathetic innervation. The vagus nerve supplies the heart with efferent cholinergic nerves.

Parasympathetic Control

Vagal stimulation causes bradycardia, decreased contractility, and lower blood pressure. The resultant fall in $M\dot{v}O_2$ causes metabolically mediated coronary vasoconstriction. These effects can be abolished by atropine.

5

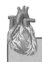

BOX 5.4 *Myocardial Metabolism*

Several molecules have been proposed as the link between myocardial metabolism and myocardial blood flow, including:
- oxygen
- reactive oxygen species
- carbon dioxide
- adenosine

Current evidence suggests that a combination of local factors, each with differing importance during rest, exercise, and ischemia, acts together to match myocardial oxygen delivery to demand.

β-Adrenergic Coronary Dilation

β-Receptor activation causes dilation of both large and small coronary vessels, even in the absence of changes in blood flow.

α-Adrenergic Coronary Constriction

Activation of the sympathetic nerves to the heart results in increases in heart rate, contractility, and blood pressure that lead to a marked, metabolically mediated increase in coronary blood flow. The direct effect of sympathetic stimulation is coronary vasoconstriction, which is in competition with the metabolically mediated dilation of exercise or excitement. Whether adrenergic coronary constriction is powerful enough to diminish blood flow in ischemic myocardium further or whether it can have some beneficial effect in the distribution of myocardial blood flow is controversial.

CORONARY PRESSURE-FLOW RELATIONS

Autoregulation

Autoregulation is the tendency for organ blood flow to remain constant despite changes in arterial perfusion pressure. Autoregulation can maintain flow to myocardium served by stenotic coronary arteries despite low perfusion pressure distal to the obstruction. This is a local mechanism of control and can be observed in isolated, denervated hearts. If $M\dot{v}o_2$ is fixed, coronary blood flow remains relatively constant between mean arterial pressures of 60 and 140 mm Hg.

Coronary Reserve

Myocardial ischemia causes intense coronary vasodilation. After a 10- to 30-second coronary occlusion, restoration of perfusion pressure is accompanied by a marked increase in coronary flow. This large increase in flow, which can be five or six times resting flow, is termed *reactive hyperemia*. The repayment volume is greater than the debt volume. However, no overpayment of the oxygen debt occurs because oxygen extraction falls during the hyperemia. The presence of high coronary flows when coronary venous oxygen content is high suggests that mediators other than oxygen are responsible for this metabolically induced vasodilation. The difference between resting coronary blood flow and peak flow during reactive hyperemia represents the autoregulatory coronary flow reserve—the further capacity of the arteriolar bed to dilate in response to ischemia.

Transmural Blood Flow

When coronary perfusion pressure is inadequate, the inner one-third to one-fourth of the left ventricular wall is the first region to become ischemic or necrotic. This increased vulnerability of the subendocardium may reflect an increased demand for perfusion or a decreased supply, compared with the outer layers.

If coronary artery pressure is gradually reduced, autoregulation is exhausted, and flow decreases in the inner layers of the left ventricle before it begins to decrease in the outer layers (Fig. 5.3). This finding indicates less flow reserve in the subendocardium than in the subepicardium. Three mechanisms have been proposed to explain the decreased coronary reserve in the subendocardium: (1) differential systolic intramyocardial pressure; (2) differential diastolic intramyocardial pressure; and (3) interactions between systole and diastole.

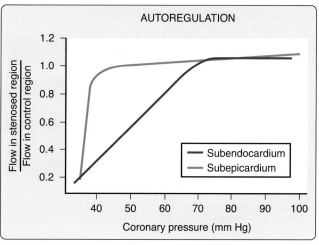

Fig. 5.3 Pressure-flow relationships of the subepicardial and subendocardial thirds of the left ventricle in anesthetized dogs. In the subendocardium, autoregulation is exhausted and flow becomes pressure-dependent when pressure distal to a stenosis falls to less than 70 mm Hg. In the subepicardium, autoregulation persists until perfusion pressure falls to less than 40 mm Hg. Autoregulatory coronary reserve is less in the subendocardium. (Redrawn from Guyton RA, McClenathan JH, Newman GE, Michaelis LL. Significance of subendocardial ST segment elevation caused by coronary stenosis in the dog. *Am J Cardiol.* 1977;40:373.)

BOX 5.5 *Atherosclerosis*

- The atherosclerotic process begins in childhood and adolescence.
- The progression of an atherosclerotic lesion resembles the process of wound healing.
- Inflammation, lipid infiltration, and smooth muscle proliferation have important roles in atherogenesis.
- Impairment of endothelial function is an early consequence of atherosclerosis.
- Statin therapy has been shown to improve endothelial function, impede development of atherosclerosis, and, in some cases, reverse established disease.

ATHEROSCLEROSIS

The atherosclerotic lesion consists of an excessive accumulation of smooth muscle cells in the intima, with quantitative and qualitative changes in the noncellular connective tissue components of the artery wall and intracellular and extracellular deposition of lipoproteins and mineral components (eg, calcium) (Box 5.5). By definition, *atherosclerosis* is a combination of "atherosis" and "sclerosis." The term *sclerosis* refers to the hard, collagenous material that accumulates in lesions and is usually more voluminous than the pultaceous "gruel" of the atheroma (Fig. 5.4).

The earliest detectable change in the evolution of coronary atherosclerosis is the accumulation of intracellular lipid in the subendothelial region that gives rise to lipid-filled macrophages or "foam cells." Grossly, a collection of foam cells may give the artery wall the appearance of a "fatty streak." In general, fatty streaks are covered by a layer of intact endothelium and are not characterized by excessive smooth muscle cell accumulation. At later stages of atherogenesis, extracellular lipoproteins accumulate

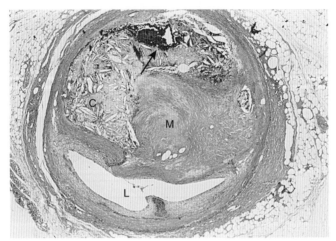

Fig. 5.4 Atherosclerotic human coronary artery of an 80-year-old man. He has severe narrowing of the central arterial lumen *(L)*. The intima consists of a complex collection of cells, extracellular matrix *(M)*, and a necrotic core with cholesterol *(C)* deposits. Rupture of plaque microvessels has resulted in intraplaque hemorrhage *(arrow)* at the base of the necrotic core (Movat's pentachrome–stained slide; original magnification ×40).

in the musculoelastic layer of the intima and eventually form an avascular core of lipid-rich debris that is separated from the central arterial lumen by a fibrous cap of collagenous material. Foam cells are not usually seen deep within the atheromatous core but are frequently found at the periphery of the lipid core.

Arterial Wall Inflammation

Monocytes or macrophages and T lymphocytes are found in arteries not only with advanced lesions but also in arteries with early atherosclerotic lesions in young adults. Leukocyte infiltration into the vascular wall is known to precede smooth muscle cell hyperplasia. Once inside the artery wall, mononuclear cells may play several important roles in lesion development. For example, monocytes may transform into macrophages and become involved in the local oxidation of low-density lipoproteins (LDLs) and accumulation of oxidized LDLs. Alternatively, macrophages in the artery wall may act as a rich source of factors that promote cell proliferation, migration, or the breakdown of local tissue barriers. The process of local tissue degradation may be important for the initiation of acute coronary artery syndromes because loss of arterial wall integrity may lead to plaque fissuring or rupture.

Role of Lipoproteins in Lesion Formation

The clinical and experimental evidence linking dyslipidemias with atherogenesis is well established. However, the exact mechanisms by which lipid moieties contribute to the pathogenesis of atherosclerosis remain elusive. Although the simple concept of cholesterol accumulating in artery walls until flow is obstructed may be correct in certain animal models, this theory is not correct for human arteries.

One of the major consequences of cholesterol accumulation in the artery wall is thought to be impairment of endothelial function. The endothelium is more than a physical barrier between the bloodstream and the artery wall. Under normal conditions, the endothelium is capable of modulating vascular tone (eg, through NO), thrombogenicity, fibrinolysis, platelet function, and inflammation. In the presence of traditional risk factors, particularly dyslipidemias, these protective endothelial functions are reduced or lost. The loss of these endothelium-derived functions may occur in the presence or absence of an underlying atherosclerotic plaque and may simply imply that atherogenesis has begun. Aggressive attempts to normalize atherosclerotic risk factors (eg, diet and lipid-lowering therapies) may markedly attenuate endothelial dysfunction, even in the presence of extensive atherosclerosis. Some clinical studies demonstrated dramatic improvements in endothelial function, as well as in cardiovascular morbidity and mortality, with the use of inhibitors of 3-hydroxy-3-methylglutaryl coenzyme A (HMG-CoA) reductase, or "statins."

■ PATHOPHYSIOLOGY OF CORONARY BLOOD FLOW

Coronary Artery Stenoses and Plaque Rupture

Coronary atherosclerosis is a chronic disease that develops over decades and remains clinically silent for prolonged periods (Box 5.6). Clinical manifestations of CAD occur when the atherosclerotic plaque mass encroaches on the vessel lumen and obstructs coronary blood flow to cause angina. Alternatively, cracks or fissures may develop in the atherosclerotic lesions and result in acute thromboses that cause unstable angina or myocardial infarction.

Patients with stable angina typically have lesions with smooth borders on angiography. Only a few coronary lesions are concentric; most have complex geometry varying in shape over their length. Eccentric stenoses, with a remaining pliable, musculoelastic arc of normal wall, can vary in diameter and resistance in response to changes in vasomotor tone or intraluminal pressure. Most human coronary artery stenoses are compliant. The intima of the normal portion of the vessel wall is often thickened, thus making endothelial dysfunction probable. In contrast, patients with unstable angina usually have lesions characterized by overhanging edges, scalloped or irregular borders, or multiple irregularities. These complicated stenoses likely represent ruptured plaque or partially occlusive thrombus, or both. On angiography these lesions may appear segmental, confined to a short segment of an otherwise normal proximal coronary artery. At autopsy, however, the most common pathologic finding is *diffuse* vessel involvement with superimposed segmental obstruction of greater severity. In a diffusely narrowed vessel, even modest progression of luminal narrowing can be significant. In such an artery, rating the significance of the obstruction by the percentage of diameter reduction relative to adjacent vessel segments

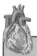

BOX 5.6   *Pathophysiology of Coronary Blood Flow*

- In most patients experiencing a myocardial infarction, the coronary occlusion occurs at the site of less than 50% stenosis.
- Plaque rupture leads to incremental growth of coronary stenoses and can cause coronary events.
- Plaque rupture occurs at the shoulder of the plaque where inflammatory cells are found.

underestimates its physiologic importance. Therefore understanding the characteristics of atherosclerotic plaques is of central importance to the management of acute coronary artery syndromes.

The intuitive notion that the severity of coronary artery stenoses should correlate with the risk of complications from CAD was disproved. The coronary angiograms of 38 patients who had had Q-wave myocardial infarction in the interval between serial studies were reviewed. On the preinfarct angiograms, the mean percentage of stenosis at the coronary segment that was later responsible for infarction was only 34%. Therefore, although the revascularization of arteries with critical stenoses in target lesions is appropriately indicated to reduce symptoms and myocardial ischemia, a risk of further cardiac events remains because atherosclerosis is a diffuse process, and mild or modest angiographic stenoses are more likely to result in subsequent myocardial infarction than are severe stenoses.

With this background comes the problem of predicting which arterial segments with minimal angiographic disease will later develop new critical stenoses. Superficial intimal injury (plaque erosions) and intimal tears of variable depth (plaque fissures) with overlying microscopic mural thrombosis are commonly found in atherosclerotic plaques. In the absence of obstructive luminal thrombosis, these intimal injuries do not cause clinical events. However, disruption of the fibrous cap, or plaque rupture, is a more serious event that typically results in the formation of clinically significant arterial thromboses. From autopsy studies it is known that rupture-prone plaques tend to have a thin, friable fibrous cap. The site of plaque rupture is thought to be the shoulder of the plaque, in which substantial numbers of mononuclear inflammatory cells are commonly found. The mechanisms responsible for the local accumulation of these cells at this location in the plaque are unknown; presumably, monocyte chemotactic factors, the expression of leukocyte cell adhesion molecules, and specific cytokines are involved. Currently, no effective strategies have been designed to limit the possibility of plaque rupture; however, aggressive lipid-lowering therapy may be a helpful preventive measure.

Hemodynamics

If accurate angiographic assessment of the geometry of a coronary stenosis is made, hydrodynamic principles can be used to estimate the physiologic significance of the obstruction.

Resting flow remains constant as lumen diameter decreases because the coronary arterioles progressively dilate, thereby reducing the resistance of the distal coronary bed sufficiently to compensate for the resistance of the stenosis. As the severity of the stenosis increases further, the arteriolar bed can no longer compensate, and flow begins to fall. As stenosis severity increases, distal perfusion pressure falls, arterioles dilate to maintain flow until autoregulation is exhausted (in the subendocardium first), and flow becomes pressure-dependent.

The frequently used term *critical stenosis* is usually defined as coronary constriction sufficient to prevent an increase in flow over resting values in response to increased myocardial oxygen demands. This is a greater degree of obstruction than angiographically significant stenosis, which is usually defined as a reduction in cross-sectional area of 75%, equivalent to a 50% decrease in the diameter of a concentric stenosis.

Coronary Collaterals

Coronary collaterals are anastomotic connections, without an intervening capillary bed, between different coronary arteries or between branches of the same artery. In the normal human heart, these vessels are small and have little or no functional role. In patients with CAD, well-developed coronary collateral vessels may play a critical role in preventing death and myocardial infarction. Individual differences in the capability of developing a sufficient collateral circulation are determinants of the vulnerability of the myocardium to coronary occlusive disease.

In humans, perfusion through collaterals can equal perfusion through a vessel with a 90% diameter obstruction. Although coronary collateral flow can be sufficient to preserve structure and resting myocardial function, muscle dependent on collateral flow usually becomes ischemic when oxygen demand rises to more than resting levels. Among patients with stable CAD, the presence of "high collateralization" is associated with a reduction in mortality rates of greater than 30% compared with patients with low collateralization. It is possible that evidence from patients with angina underestimates collateral function of the population of all patients with CAD. Perhaps persons with coronary obstructions but excellent collateralization remain asymptomatic and are not studied.

PATHOGENESIS OF MYOCARDIAL ISCHEMIA

Ischemia is the condition of oxygen deprivation accompanied by inadequate removal of metabolites consequent to reduced perfusion. Clinically, myocardial ischemia is a decrease in the blood flow supply-to-demand ratio that results in impaired function. No universally accepted gold standard exists for the presence of myocardial ischemia. In practice, symptoms, ECG changes, anatomic findings, and evidence of myocardial dysfunction must be combined before concluding that myocardial ischemia is present.

Determinants of Ratio of Myocardial Oxygen Supply to Demand

An increase in myocardial oxygen requirement beyond the capacity of the coronary circulation to deliver oxygen results in myocardial ischemia (Box 5.7). This is the most common mechanism leading to ischemic episodes in chronic stable angina and during exercise testing. Intraoperatively, the anesthesiologist must measure and control the determinants of $M\dot{v}_{O_2}$ and protect the patient from "demand" ischemia. The major determinants of $M\dot{v}_{O_2}$ are heart rate, myocardial contractility, and wall stress (chamber pressure × radius/wall thickness).

An increase in heart rate can reduce subendocardial perfusion by shortening diastole. Coronary perfusion pressure may fall in response to reduced systemic pressure or increased left ventricular end-diastolic pressure (LVEDP). With the onset of ischemia, perfusion may be further compromised by delayed ventricular relaxation (decreased

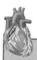

BOX 5.7 *Determinants of Myocardial Oxygen Supply-to-Demand Ratio*

The major determinants of myocardial oxygen consumption are:
- heart rate
- myocardial contractility
- wall stress (chamber pressure × radius/wall thickness)

subendocardial perfusion time) and decreased diastolic compliance (increased LVEDP). Anemia and hypoxia can also compromise delivery of oxygen to the myocardium.

Dynamic Stenosis

Patients with CAD can have variable exercise tolerance during the day and between days. Ambulatory monitoring of the electrocardiogram has demonstrated that ST-segment changes indicative of myocardial ischemia, in the absence of changes in oxygen demand, are common. These findings are explained by variations over time in the severity of the obstruction to blood flow imposed by coronary stenoses.

Although the term *hardening of the arteries* suggests rigid, narrowed vessels, in fact most stenoses are eccentric and have a remaining arc of compliant tissue. A modest amount (10%) of shortening of the muscle in the compliant region of the vessel can cause dramatic changes in lumen caliber. The term *spasm* is reserved for "situations where coronary constriction is both focal, sufficiently profound to cause transient coronary occlusion, and is responsible for reversible attacks of angina at rest" (ie, variant angina). Although this syndrome is rare, lesser degrees of obstruction in response to vasoconstrictor stimuli are common among patients with CAD.

Coronary Steal

Steal occurs when the perfusion pressure for a vasodilated vascular bed (in which flow is pressure-dependent) is lowered by vasodilation in a parallel vascular bed, with both beds usually distal to a stenosis. Two kinds of coronary steal are illustrated: collateral and transmural (Fig. 5.5).

Fig. 5.5A shows collateral steal in which one vascular bed (R_3), distal to an occluded vessel, is dependent on collateral flow from a vascular bed (R_2) supplied by a stenotic artery. Because collateral resistance is high, the R_3 arterioles are dilated to maintain flow in the resting condition (autoregulation). Dilation of the R_2 arterioles increases flow across the stenosis R_1 and decreases pressure P_2. If R_3 resistance cannot further decrease sufficiently, flow there decreases, thus producing or worsening ischemia in the collateral-dependent bed.

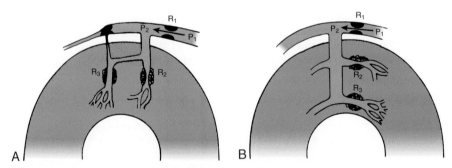

Fig. 5.5 Conditions for coronary steal in different areas of the heart and between the subendocardial and subepicardial layers of the left ventricle. (A) Collateral steal. (B) Transmural steal. See text for details. P_1, Aortic pressure; P_2, pressure distal to the stenosis; R_1, stenosis resistance; R_2 and R_3, resistance of autoregulating and pressure-dependent vascular beds, respectively. (From Epstein SE, Cannon RO, Talbot TL. Hemodynamic principles in the control of coronary blood flow. *Am J Cardiol.* 1985;56:4E.)

Transmural steal is illustrated in Fig. 5.5B. Normally, vasodilator reserve is less in the subendocardium. In the presence of stenosis, flow may become pressure-dependent in the subendocardium, whereas autoregulation is maintained in the subepicardium.

SUGGESTED READINGS

Ambrose JA. In search of the "vulnerable plaque": can it be localized and will focal regional therapy ever be an option for cardiac prevention? *J Am Coll Cardiol.* 2008;51:1539–1542.

Aude YW, Garza L. How to prevent unnecessary coronary interventions: identifying lesions responsible for ischemia in the cath lab. *Curr Opin Cardiol.* 2003;18:394–399.

de Bruyne B, Pijls NHJ, Kalesan B, et al. Fractional flow reserve-guided PCI versus medical therapy in stable coronary disease. *N Engl J Med.* 2012;367:991–1001.

Deussen A, Ohanyan V, Jannasch A, et al. Mechanisms of metabolic coronary flow regulation. *J Mol Cell Cardiol.* 2012;52:794–801.

Dole WP. Autoregulation of the coronary circulation. *Prog Cardiovasc Dis.* 1987;29:293–323.

Duncker DJ, Bache RJ. Regulation of coronary vasomotor tone under normal conditions and during acute myocardial hypoperfusion. *Pharmacol Ther.* 2000;86:87–110.

Fujita M, Tambara K. Recent insights into human coronary collateral development. *Heart.* 2004;90:246–250.

Goodwin AT, Yacoub MH. Role of endogenous endothelin on coronary flow in health and disease. *Coron Artery Dis.* 2001;12:517–525.

Harrison DG, Cai H. Endothelial control of vasomotion and nitric oxide production. *Cardiol Clin.* 2003;21:289–302.

Heusch G. Reprint of: the paradox of alpha-adrenergic coronary vasoconstriction revisited. *J Mol Cell Cardiol.* 2012;52:832–839.

Hoffman JIE, Spaan JAE. Pressure-flow relations in coronary circulation. *Physiol Rev.* 1990;70:331–390.

Koerselman J, Van der Graaf Y, De Jaegere PPT, et al. Coronary collaterals: an important and underexposed aspect of coronary artery disease. *Circulation.* 2003;107:2507–2511.

Konidala S, Gutterman DD. Coronary vasospasm and the regulation of coronary blood flow. *Prog Cardiovasc Dis.* 2004;46:349–373.

Maiellaro K, Taylor WR. The role of the adventitia in vascular inflammation. *Cardiovasc Res.* 2007;75:640–648.

Meier P, Hemingway H, Lansky AJ, et al. The impact of the coronary collateral circulation on mortality: a meta-analysis. *Eur Heart J.* 2012;33:614–621.

Pasterkamp G, de Kleijn D, Borst C. Arterial remodeling in atherosclerosis, restenosis and after alteration of blood flow: potential mechanisms and clinical implications. *Cardiovasc Res.* 2000;45:843–852.

Tonino PA, De BB, Pijls NH, et al. Fractional flow reserve versus angiography for guiding percutaneous coronary intervention. *N Engl J Med.* 2009;360:213–224.

Treasure CB, Klein JL, Weintraub WS. Beneficial effects of cholesterol-lowering therapy on the coronary endothelium in patients with coronary artery disease. *N Engl J Med.* 1995;332:481–487.

Zaugg M, Lucchinetti E, Uecker M, et al. Anaesthetics and cardiac preconditioning, part I: signalling and cytoprotective mechanisms. *Br J Anaesth.* 2003;91:551–565.

Zimarino M, D'Andreamatteo M, Waksman R, et al. The dynamics of the coronary collateral circulation. *Nat Rev Cardiol.* 2014;11:191–197.

5

Chapter 6

Molecular and Genetic Cardiovascular Medicine and Systemic Inflammation

Amanda A. Fox, MD, MPH • Sonal Sharma, MD •
J. Paul Mounsey, BM BCh, PhD, FRCP, FACC •
Marcel E. Durieux, MD, PhD • Richard Whitlock, MD, PhD •
Elliott Bennett-Guerrero, MD

Key Points

1. The rapid development of molecular biologic and genetic techniques has greatly expanded the understanding of cardiac functioning, and these techniques are beginning to be applied clinically.
2. Cardiac ion channels form the machinery behind the cardiac rhythm; cardiac membrane receptors regulate cardiac function.
3. Sodium, potassium, and calcium channels are the main ion channel types involved in the cardiac action potential. Many subtypes exist, and their molecular structure is known in some detail, thus allowing a molecular explanation for phenomena such as voltage sensing, ion selectivity, and inactivation.
4. Muscarinic and adrenergic receptors, both of the G-protein–coupled receptor class, are the main regulators of cardiac function.
5. Volatile anesthetic agents significantly affect calcium channels and muscarinic receptors.
6. Powerful genetic analysis techniques are being used to better understand adverse cardiovascular events through molecular approaches. Research using these techniques has begun to explore links between genomics and perioperative adverse cardiovascular events.
7. Treatment through gene therapy is evolving in cardiovascular medicine, although it currently does not have a prominent role in the perioperative setting.
8. Excessive systemic inflammation is proposed to be a cause of postoperative organ dysfunction.
9. No interventions that attenuate systemic inflammation have been proved in large, randomized clinical trials to protect patients from morbidity and mortality.

The past decades have witnessed what may be termed a revolution in the biomedical sciences, as molecular and genetic methodologies suddenly jumped onto the clinical scene. The birth of molecular biology is commonly identified with the description of the structure of deoxyribonucleic acid (DNA) by Watson and Crick in the 1950s. Now, the human genome has been sequenced completely. The development of the polymerase chain reaction, a technique of remarkable simplicity and flexibility, has dramatically increased the speed with which many molecular biology procedures can be performed, and it has allowed the invention of many new techniques. More recent years have seen the development of approaches allowing screening of large amounts of genetic material for changes associated with disease states.

Cardiovascular medicine has benefited from these advances. Not only have the electrophysiologic and pumping functions of the heart been placed on a firm molecular footing, but also the underlying molecular mechanisms have been determined for numerous pathologic cardiac states, thereby allowing progress in therapeutic development. Nothing indicates that the pace of progress in molecular biology is slowing down. If anything, the opposite is the case, and more dramatic advances may be expected in the years to come. Thus techniques such as gene therapy may become effective therapeutic options in cardiac disease.

MACHINERY BEHIND THE CARDIAC RHYTHM: ION CHANNELS

The cardiac action potential results from the flow of ions through ion channels, which are the membrane-bound proteins that form the structural machinery behind cardiac electrical excitability. In response to changes in electrical potential across the cell membrane, ion channels open and allow the passive flux of ions into or out of the cell along their electrochemical gradients. This flow of charged ions results in a current, which alters the cell membrane potential toward the equilibrium potential (E) for the ion, which is the potential at which the electrochemical gradient for the ion is zero. Depolarization of the cell could, in principle, result from an inward cation current or an outward anion current; for repolarization, the reverse is true. In excitable cells, action potentials are mainly caused by the flow of cation currents. Membrane depolarization results principally from the flow of sodium (Na^+) down its electrochemical gradient (E_{Na} is approximately +50 mV), whereas repolarization results from the outward flux of potassium (K^+) down its electrochemical gradient (E_K is approximately −90 mV). Opening and closing of ion channels selective for a single ion result in an individual ionic current. The integrated activity of many different ionic currents, each activated over precisely regulated potential ranges and at different times in the cardiac cycle, results in the cardiac action potential. Ion channels are usually highly (but not uniquely) selective for a single ion, hence the terms K^+ channels, Na^+ channels, and so forth. Channels may rectify; that is, pass current in one direction across the membrane more easily than the other. Electrical and chemical stimuli, which lead to opening and closing of the channel, cause a conformational change in the channel molecule (gating) (Box 6.1).

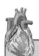

BOX 6.1   *Properties of Ion Channels*

Ion selectivity
Rectification (passing current more easily in one direction than the other)
Gating (mechanism for opening and closing the channel):
- activation (opening)
- inactivation (closing)

BOX 6.2   *Cardiac Action Potential*

Phase 0 (rapid upstroke): primarily Na$^+$ channel opening
Phase 1 (early rapid repolarization): inactivation of Na$^+$ current, opening of K$^+$ channels
Phase 2 (plateau phase): balance between K$^+$ and Ca^{2+} currents
Phase 3 (final rapid repolarizations): activation of Ca^{2+} channels
Phase 4 (diastolic depolarization): balance between Na$^+$ and K$^+$ currents

Ca^{2+}, Calcium; *K$^+$*, potassium; *Na$^+$*, sodium.

Phase 0: Rapid Upstroke of the Cardiac Action Potential

The rapid upstroke of the cardiac action potential (phase 0) is caused by the flow of a large inward Na$^+$ current (I_{Na}) (Box 6.2). I_{Na} is activated by depolarization of the sarcolemma to a threshold potential of −65 to −70 mV. I_{Na} activation, and hence the action potential, is an all-or-nothing response. Subthreshold depolarizations have only local effects on the membrane. After the threshold for activation of fast Na$^+$ channels is exceeded, Na$^+$ channels open (ie, I_{Na} activates), and Na$^+$ ions enter the cell down their electrochemical gradient. This action results in displacement of the membrane potential toward the equilibrium potential for Na$^+$ ions, approximately +50 mV. I_{Na} activation is transient, lasting at most 1 to 2 ms because, simultaneous with activation, a second, slightly slower conformational change in the channel molecule occurs: inactivation, which closes the ion pore in the face of continued membrane depolarization. The channel cannot open again until it has recovered from inactivation (ie, regained its resting conformation), a process that requires repolarization to the resting potential for a defined period. Thus the channels cycle through three states: (1) resting (and available for activation), (2) open, and (3) inactivated. While the channel is inactivated, it is absolutely refractory to repeated stimulation.

Phase 1: Early Rapid Repolarization

The early rapid repolarization phase of the action potential, which follows immediately after phase 0, results both from rapid inactivation of the majority of the Na$^+$ current and from activation of a transient outward current (ITO), carried mainly by K$^+$ ions.

Phases 2 and 3: Plateau Phase and Final Rapid Repolarization

The action potential plateau and final rapid repolarization are mediated by a balance between the slow inward current and outward, predominantly K$^+$, current. During the plateau phase, membrane conductance to all ions falls, and very little current flows. Phase 3, regenerative rapid repolarization, results from time-dependent inactivation of L-type Ca^{2+} current and increasing outward current through delayed rectifier K$^+$ channels. The net membrane current becomes outward, and the cell repolarizes.

Phase 4: Diastolic Depolarization and Pacemaker Current

Phase 4 diastolic depolarization, or normal automaticity, is a normal feature of cardiac cells in the sinus and atrioventricular nodes (AVN), but subsidiary pacemaker activity is also observed in the His-Purkinje system and in some specialized atrial and ventricular myocardial cells. Pacemaker discharge from the sinus node normally predominates because the rate of diastolic depolarization in the sinoatrial node is faster than in other pacemaker tissues.

Molecular Biology of Ion Channels

The preceding sections focus on the electrical events that underlie cardiac electrical excitability and on the identification of cardiac ionic currents on the basis of their biophysical properties. This section reviews the molecular structures behind these electrical phenomena. The first step in understanding the molecular physiology of cardiac electrical excitability is to identify the ion channel proteins responsible for the ionic currents.

Ion Channel Pore and Selectivity Filter

The presence of four homologous domains in voltage-gated Na^+ and Ca^{2+} channels suggests that basic ion channel architecture consists of a transmembrane pore surrounded by the four homologous domains arranged symmetrically (see Fig. 6.1).

Clinical Correlates

Ion Channels and Antiarrhythmic Drugs

Drug therapy of cardiac arrhythmias would ideally be targeted at an individual ionic current, thereby tailoring the cardiac action potential in such a way that abnormal excitability is reduced but normal rhythmicity is unaffected. This goal remains unrealized. The prototype antiarrhythmic agents (eg, disopyramide and quinidine) have diverse effects on cardiac excitability and, similar to agents introduced more recently, frequently exhibit significant proarrhythmic activity with potentially fatal consequences. In the Cardiac Arrhythmia Suppression Trial (CAST), the mortality rate among asymptomatic patients after myocardial infarction (MI) was approximately doubled by treatment with the potent Na^+ channel-blocking agents encainide and flecainide, an effect likely attributable to slowing of conduction velocity with a consequent increase in fatal reentrant arrhythmias. Drugs that prolong action potential duration all block I_{Kr}, and it is not clear that this therapeutic goal will result in arrhythmia control without induction of clinically significant proarrhythmia. The only drugs currently available that definitely prolong life by reducing fatal arrhythmias are β-blockers, and these agents have no channel-blocking effects.

Ion Channels in Disease

Elucidation of the molecular mechanisms of the cardiac action potential is beginning to have a direct impact on patient management. This is most obvious in patients with inherited genetic abnormalities of ion channels that lead to cardiac sudden death. Two groups of diseases illustrate this point: long QT syndrome (LQTS) and Brugada syndrome. An understanding of the molecular mechanism of cardiac electrical excitability is also starting to lead to the emergence of gene therapies and stem cell therapies that may in the future allow manipulation of cardiac rhythm and function.

6

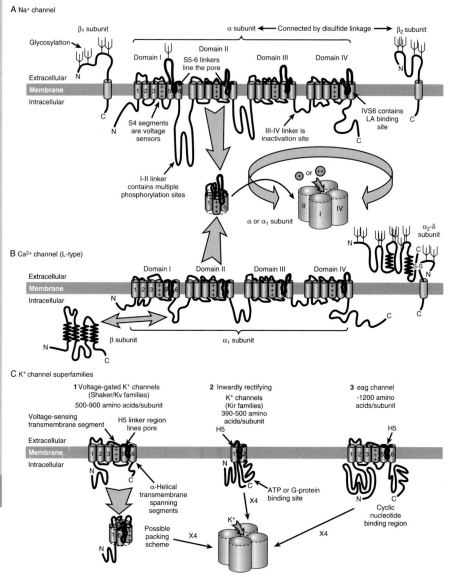

Fig. 6.1 Diagrams of ion channel molecular structure. (A) Sodium *(Na⁺)* channel. (B) Calcium *(Ca²⁺)* channel. (C) Potassium *(K⁺)* channels. *ATP,* Adenosine triphosphate; *LA,* local anesthetic.

CONTROLLING CARDIAC FUNCTIONING: RECEPTORS

Receptors are membrane proteins that transduce signals from the outside to the inside of the cell. When a *ligand*—a hormone carried in blood, a neurotransmitter released from a nerve ending, or a local messenger released from neighboring cells—binds to the receptor, it induces a conformational change in the receptor molecule. This process changes the configuration of the intracellular segment of the receptor and results in activation of intracellular systems, with various potential effects ranging from enhanced phosphorylation and changes in intracellular (second) messenger concentrations to activation of ion channels.

Receptor Classes

Receptors are grouped in several broad classes, and the most important are the *protein tyrosine kinase receptors* and the *G-protein–coupled receptors* (GPCRs). The protein tyrosine kinase receptors are large molecular complexes that incorporate phosphorylating enzyme activity in the intracellular segment. Ligand binding induces activation of this enzyme activity. Because phosphorylation is one of the major mechanisms of cellular regulation, such receptors can have numerous cellular effects. GPCRs are much smaller than protein tyrosine kinase receptors. Ligand binding results in activation of an associated protein *(G-protein)* that subsequently influences cellular processes (Box 6.3).

The heart and blood vessels express various GPCRs. The β-adrenergic and muscarinic acetylcholine (ACh) receptors are those most important for regulation of cardiac functioning, but several others play relevant modulatory roles. These include the α-adrenergic, adenosine A_1, adenosine triphosphate (ATP), histamine H_2, vasoactive intestinal peptide (VIP), and angiotensin II receptors (Fig. 6.2).

Adrenergic Receptors and Signaling Pathways

Adrenergic Receptors

Main control over cardiac contractility is provided by the β-adrenergic signaling pathways, which can be activated by circulating catecholamines (derived from the adrenal glands) or those released locally from adrenergic nerve endings on the myocardium.

The two main subtypes of β-adrenergic receptors are the β_1 and β_2 subclasses. A β_3 subtype also exists, but its role in the cardiovascular system is unclear; its most important role is in fat cells. Both β_1- and β_2-receptors are present in the heart, and both contribute to the increased contractility induced by catecholamine stimulation (this is different from the situation in vascular muscle, where β_2-adrenergic stimulation induces relaxation). Under normal conditions, the relative ratio of β_1- to β_2-receptors in heart is approximately 70 : 30, but this ratio can be changed dramatically by cardiac disease.

6

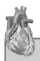

BOX 6.3 *G-Protein–Coupled Receptors*

β-Adrenergic receptors
α-Adrenergic receptors
Muscarinic acetylcholine receptors
Adenosine A_1 receptors
Adenosine triphosphate receptors
Histamine H_2 receptors
Vasoactive intestinal peptide receptors
Angiotensin II receptors

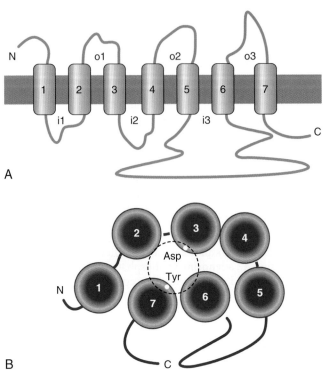

Fig. 6.2 Model of G-protein–coupled receptor. (A) Linear model. Seven hydrophobic stretches of approximately 20 amino acids are present, presumably forming α-helices that pass through the cell membrane, thus forming seven transmembrane domains (*t1* through *t7*). Extracellularly, the amino terminus *(N)* and three outside loops (*o1* through *o3*) are found; intracellularly there are similarly three loops (*i1* through *i3*) and the carboxy terminus *(C)*. (B) *Top-down view.* Although in (A), the molecule is pictured as a linear complex, the transmembrane domains are thought to be in close proximity, forming an ellipse with a central ligand-binding cavity *(dashed circle)*. Asp and Tyr refer to two amino acids important for ligand interaction. G-protein binding takes place at the i3 loop and the carboxy terminus.

The β-adrenergic receptors are closely related structurally as well as functionally. Both the β_1- and β_2-adrenergic receptors couple to G_s (a guanosine triphosphate (GTP)–binding protein) and thereby activate adenylate cyclase, thus leading to increased intracellular levels of cyclic adenosine monophosphate (cAMP). In addition to their effect on cAMP signaling, β-receptors may couple to myocardial Ca^{2+} channels.

The inotropic and electrophysiologic effects of β-adrenergic signaling are indirect results of increases in intracellular cAMP levels. cAMP activates a specific protein kinase (PKA) that, in turn, is able to phosphorylate several important cardiac ion channels (including L-type Ca^{2+} channels, Na^+ channels, voltage-dependent K^+ channels, and Cl^- channels). Phosphorylation alters channel functioning, and the resulting changes in membrane electrophysiology modify myocardial behavior.

The α-adrenergic receptors, like their β-receptor counterparts, can be divided into two groups: α_1- and α_2-receptors. Both groups consist of several closely related subtypes. In general, α_1-receptors couple to G_q proteins and thereby activate phospholipase C (PLC), a process that results in increases in intracellular Ca^{2+} concentrations. α_2-Receptors couple to G_i proteins, which inhibit adenylate cyclase and consequently reduce intracellular cAMP concentrations. In the heart, the primary subtype present is α_1. Activation of these receptors leads to a modest increase in cardiac contractility.

The primary role of α-receptors is in the vasculature, where α_1-receptors on vascular smooth muscle are the main mediators of neuronally mediated vasoconstriction. α_2-Receptors on the neurons themselves function in a negative feedback loop to control α-adrenergic vasoconstriction.

Regulation of β-Receptor Functioning

β-Receptor stimulation allows the dramatic increases in cardiac output of which the human heart is capable, but this β-receptor effect is clearly intended to be a temporary measure. Prolonged adrenergic stimulation has significant detrimental effects on the myocardium, with pronounced increases in cAMP levels resulting in increased intracellular Ca^{2+} concentrations, reduced ribonucleic acid (RNA) and protein synthesis, and finally cell death. Thus β-receptor modulation is best viewed as part of the "fight-or-flight" response: beneficial in the short term, but detrimental if depended on for too long. Cardiac failure, in particular, has been shown to be associated with prolonged increases in adrenergic stimulation, even to the extent that norepinephrine "spillover" from cardiac nerve endings can be detected in the blood of patients in heart failure.

One mechanism for decreasing β-receptor functioning is the *downregulation* (ie, decrease in density) of receptors. In cardiac failure, receptor levels are reduced up to 50%. β_1-Receptors downregulate more than β_2-receptors do, thus resulting in a change in the β_1/β_2 ratio; in the failing heart, this ratio is approximately 3:2. Various molecular mechanisms exist for this downregulation. In the long term, β_1-receptors are degraded and permanently removed from the myocyte cell surface. In the short term, receptors can be temporarily removed from the cell membrane and "stored" in intracellular vesicles, where they are not accessible by an agonist. These receptors are, however, fully functional and can be recycled to the membrane when adrenergic overstimulation has ceased.

Muscarinic Receptors and Signaling Pathways

Muscarinic Acetylcholine Receptors

The second major receptor type in cardiac regulation is the muscarinic receptor. Although five subtypes of muscarinic receptors exist, only one of these (M_2) is present in cardiac tissue. Most of these muscarinic receptors are present on the atria. Indeed, it was formerly thought that the ventricles had no vagal innervation, but this view turns out to be incorrect. The ventricles are innervated by the vagus nerve, and muscarinic receptors are in fact present in the ventricles, albeit at lower concentrations than in the atria. The amount of muscarinic receptor protein in atrium is approximately twofold greater than in ventricle. Thus, although the primary function of cardiac muscarinic signaling is heart rate control through actions at the atrial level, vagal stimulation can directly influence ventricular functioning.

Clinical Correlates

Understanding of the role of adenosine in cardiac regulation has expanded significantly over the past decades. Its established use as an antiarrhythmic compound and its probable role in cardiac preconditioning are two examples of clinical advances resulting from this increase in understanding. Adenosine acts through a GPCR by activating several intracellular signaling systems.

6

Adenosine Signaling

Although adenosine can be generated by several pathways, in the heart it is usually found as a dephosphorylation product of AMP. Because AMP accumulation is a sign of a low cellular energy charge, an increased adenosine concentration is a marker of unbalanced energy demand and supply; thus ischemia, hypoxemia, and increased catecholamine concentrations are all associated with increased adenosine release. Adenosine is rapidly degraded by various pathways, both intracellularly and extracellularly. As a result, its half-life is extremely short, of the order of 1 second. Therefore, not only is it a marker of a cardiac "energy crisis," but also its concentrations fluctuate virtually instantly with the energy balance of the heart; it provides a real-time indication of the cellular energy situation.

Adenosine signals through GPCR of the purinergic receptor family. Two subclasses of purinoceptors exist: P_1 (high affinity for adenosine and AMP) and P_2 (high affinity for ATP and adenosine diphosphate [ADP]). The P_1 receptor class can be divided into two main receptor subtypes: A_1 and A_2. A_1 receptors are present mostly in the heart and, when activated, inhibit adenylate cyclase; A_2 receptors are present in the vasculature and, when activated, stimulate adenylate cyclase. The A_2 receptors mediate the vasodilatory actions of adenosine. The A_1 receptors mediate its complex cardiac effects.

Antiarrhythmic Actions of Adenosine

The antiarrhythmic actions are largely a result of its activation of K_{ACh}. Recalling the tissue distribution of K_{ACh}, it could be anticipated that adenosine would be much more effective in the treatment of supraventricular arrhythmias than ventricular arrhythmias, and such is indeed the case. Because of its negative chronotropic effects on the atrial conduction system, the compound is most effective in treating supraventricular tachycardias that contain a reentrant pathway involving the AVN. The efficacy of adenosine in terminating such tachycardias has been reported as greater than 90%. In contrast, it is consistently ineffective in tachycardias not involving the AVN.

▨ ANESTHETIC ACTIONS

Interactions With Channels: Calcium Channels

Of the various ion channels present in the heart, those most likely to be significantly affected by anesthetic agents in the clinical setting are the voltage-gated Ca^{2+} channels. Almost all volatile anesthetic agents inhibit L-type Ca^{2+} channels. Inhibition is modest, approximately 25% to 30% at 1 monitored anesthesia care (MAC) anesthetic, but certainly sufficient to account for the physiologic changes induced by the anesthetic agents. Volatile anesthetic agents decrease peak current and also tend to increase the rate of inactivation. Maximal Ca^{2+} current is therefore depressed, and duration of Ca^{2+} current is shortened. Together, these actions significantly limit the Ca^{2+} influx into the cardiac myocyte.

▨ GENETIC CARDIOVASCULAR MEDICINE

Considerable progress has been made in the identification and understanding of the genetic basis of cardiovascular disease. These disorders, spanning all aspects of cardiovascular disease and affecting all parts of the heart, can be divided into two groups (Box 6.4). *Monogenic disorders* are Mendelian disorders for which changes in a

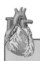

> ### BOX 6.4 *Examples of Important Cardiovascular Disorders With a Genetic Basis*
>
> Monogenic disorders
> - Familial hypercholesterolemia
> - Hypertrophic cardiomyopathy
> - Dilated cardiomyopathy
> - Long QT syndrome
>
> Multigenic disorders
> - Coronary artery disease
> - Hypertension
> - Atherosclerosis

single gene are implicated in the disease process and that usually exhibit characteristic inheritance patterns (ie, additive, dominant, or recessive genetic models). More than 40 cardiovascular disorders are known to be caused directly by single gene defects. Examples include familial hypercholesterolemia and hypertrophic cardiomy-opathies (HCMs).

More commonly, however, multiple genes influence the disease process by enhancing disease susceptibility or by augmenting the impact of environmental risk factors. The genetic component in those *multigenic disorders* comprises a collection of gene variants such as single nucleotide mutations, referred to as *single nucleotide polymorphisms* (SNPs). Each individual SNP may have a modest effect on the quantity or function of a translated protein product. However, when individual SNPs aggregate and interact with environmental risk factors, they may have a major impact on disease biology. Common complex diseases that appear to follow this paradigm include coronary artery disease (CAD), atherosclerosis, hypertension, and atrial fibrillation.

Clinical Applications

The ability to identify diseases before they become clinically manifest allows preventive treatment. For example, implantable cardioverter-defibrillators (ICDs) can prevent sudden cardiac death in patients with certain genetic cardiomyopathies and arrhythmias (Fig. 6.3). Medical therapy may ameliorate the progression of genetic dilated cardiomyopathy (DCM). Prospective identification of those patients who are asymp-tomatic but at greater risk for development of the disease enables closer surveillance and early intervention.

Common Complex Multigenic Cardiovascular Disorders

Identifying the gene variants associated with the development and progression of multigenic common complex cardiovascular diseases provides the potential for these variants to be used to better predict who will develop certain cardiovascular disorders, as well as to target preventive and treatment strategies more accurately and to develop novel treatments. The obvious challenges are to identify the genes and gene variants that collectively contribute to a cardiovascular disease such as CAD and to understand

6

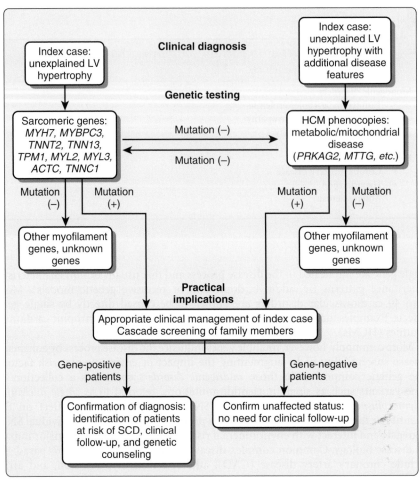

Fig. 6.3 Proposed sequence of genetic testing for patients with hypertrophic cardiomyopathy (*HCM*). *LV,* Left ventricular; *SCD,* sudden cardiac death. (*From Keren A, Syrris P, McKenna WJ. Hypertrophic cardiomyopathy: the genetic determinants of clinical disease expression.* Nat Clin Pract Cardiovasc Med. *2008;5:158–168.*)

how these genetic variants interface with environmental insults to perpetuate cardiovascular disease.

Clinical Applications

One way to translate genetic information into practice of clinical cardiovascular medicine is through a better understanding of genetic responsiveness of patients to medications prescribed to address cardiovascular diseases and their sequelae. This concept that drug selection can be personalized to a person's genetic susceptibility is a straightforward idea.

Knowledge of genetic variation has led to pharmacogenomic personalization of treatment in cardiovascular medications. The pharmacogenomics of warfarin is an example. Warfarin also has a narrow therapeutic window, is metabolized by cytochrome P450, and shows large variations in dose requirements between patients. Patients with CYP2C9*2 and CYP2C9*3 allele variants (cytochrome P450 2C9 enzyme) and patients with the A haplotype of the *VKORC1* gene (vitamin K epoxide reductase complex subunit 1) seem to require lower doses of warfarin to achieve an optimal state of anticoagulation. In 2005, the US Food and Drug Administration changed the label of warfarin to point out the potential relevance of genetic information to prescribing decisions. However, randomized trials of pharmacogenetic algorithms that have used *CYP2C9* and *VKORC1* genotyping to guide warfarin dosing have had mixed results, and further studies are needed to determine how these genotypes may effectively guide initial dosing of warfarin as well as long-term monitoring of international normalized ratio.

Perioperative Genomics in Cardiac Surgery

Despite advances in surgical, anesthetic, and cardioprotective strategies, the incidence of perioperative adverse events in cardiac surgical procedures continues to be significant and is associated with reduced short- and long-term survival. Because all surgical patients are exposed to perturbations that potentially activate inflammation, coagulation, and other stress-related pathways, but only a subset of patients experience adverse perioperative events, a genetic component is likely (Fig. 6.4).

Gene Therapy

Although molecular diagnostic techniques have advanced rapidly, gene therapy is still just tantalizingly out of the scope of routine clinical practice for treating

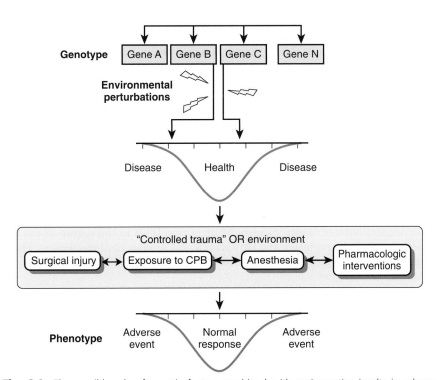

Fig. 6.4 The possible role of genetic factors combined with perioperative insults in adverse postoperative outcomes. *CPB,* Cardiopulmonary bypass; *OR,* operating room.

cardiovascular disorders. One overriding concept of gene therapy is to correct a faulty genetic sequence by using an affected cell's molecular workings. Another gene therapy objective is the targeting of drug delivery to specific organs by using molecular techniques. Gene therapies are designed to modify expression of genetic material. Although myriad approaches have been suggested, these all fall into three basic strategies: (1) gene transfer to restore or increase gene expression; (2) gene silencing to inhibit gene expression selectively; and (3) gene editing to "correct" DNA.

SYSTEMIC INFLAMMATION

An exaggerated systemic proinflammatory response to surgical trauma is a proposed cause of many postoperative complications, ranging from organ dysfunction to death. However, the cause and clinical relevance of systemic inflammation after cardiac operations are poorly understood. Systemic inflammation is a multifactorial process and has profound secondary effects on both injured and normal tissues. Proinflammatory mediators can have beneficial as well as deleterious effects on multiple organ systems. According to most theories, tissue injury, endotoxemia, and contact of blood with the foreign surface of the cardiopulmonary bypass (CPB) circuit are some of the major factors postulated to initiate a systemic inflammatory response.

SYSTEMIC INFLAMMATION AND CARDIAC SURGICAL PROCEDURES

The systemic inflammatory response after cardiac operations is multifactorial. A schematic of the inflammatory process is depicted in Fig. 6.5. Clinicians generally agree that all these processes may happen and may be associated with complications in cardiac surgical patients. Tissue injury, endotoxemia, and contact of blood with the foreign surface of the CPB circuit are thought to initiate a systemic inflammatory response after cardiac surgical procedures. What is least understood and most controversial is the issue of which of these many processes is the most clinically relevant.

Mechanisms of Inflammation-Mediated Injury

It is not entirely clear how inflammation ultimately damages cells and organ systems. Activation of neutrophils and other leukocytes is central to most theories of inflammation-induced injury. Neutrophil activation leads to the release of oxygen radicals, intracellular proteases, and fatty acid (ie, arachidonic acid) metabolites. These products, as well as those from activated macrophages and platelets, can cause or exacerbate tissue injury.

Another mechanism of inflammation-mediated injury involves microvascular occlusion. Activation of neutrophils leads to adhesion of leukocytes to endothelium and formation of clumps of inflammatory cells (ie, microaggregates). Activated leukocytes have less deformable cell membranes, and this affects their ability to pass through capillaries. Microaggregates can cause organ dysfunction through microvascular occlusion and reductions in blood flow and oxygen at the local level. After the disappearance of these microaggregates and restoration of microvascular flow, reperfusion injury may occur.

106

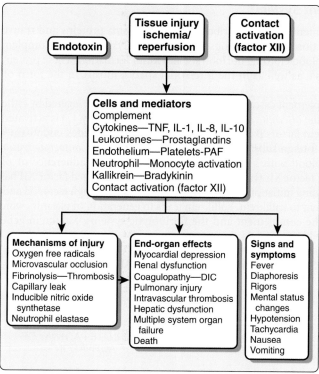

Fig. 6.5 Overview of inflammation. *DIC,* Disseminated intravascular coagulation; *IL,* interleukin; *PAF,* platelet-activating factor; *TNF,* tumor necrosis factor.

Physiologic Mediators of Inflammation

Cytokines

Cytokines are believed to play a pivotal role in the pathophysiology of acute inflammation associated with cardiac surgical procedures. Cytokines are proteins released from activated macrophages, monocytes, fibroblasts, and endothelial cells that have far-reaching regulatory effects on cells. They are small proteins that exert their effects by binding to specific cell-surface receptors. Many of these proteins are called *interleukins* because they aid in the communication between white blood cells (leukocytes).

Cytokines mediate this attraction of immune system cells to local areas of injury or infection. They also help the host through activation of the immune system, thus providing for an improved defense against pathogens. For example, cytokines enhance the function of both B and T lymphocytes, therefore improving both humoral and cell-mediated immunity. Most cytokines are proinflammatory, whereas others appear to exert an antiinflammatory effect, suggesting a complex feedback system designed to limit the amount of inflammation. Excessive levels of cytokines, however, may result in an exaggerated degree of systemic inflammation that may lead to greater secondary injury. Numerous cytokines (tumor necrosis factor [TNF], interleukin-1 [IL-1] to IL-16), as well as other protein mediators (eg, transforming growth factors, macrophage inflammatory proteins), have been described and may play an important role in the pathogenesis of postoperative systemic inflammation.

Complement System

The complement system describes at least 20 plasma proteins and is involved in the chemoattraction, activation, opsonization, and lysis of cells. Complement also is involved in blood clotting, fibrinolysis, and kinin formation. These proteins are found in the plasma, as well as in the interstitial spaces, mostly in the form of enzymatic precursors.

The complement cascade illustrated in Fig. 6.6 can be triggered by either the *classic pathway* or the *alternate pathway.* In the alternate pathway, C3 is activated by contact of complement factors B and D with complex polysaccharides, endotoxin, or exposure of blood to foreign substances such as the CPB circuit. *Contact activation* describes contact of blood with a foreign surface with resulting adherence of platelets and activation of factor XII (Hageman factor) (Fig. 6.7). Activated factor XII has numerous effects, including initiation of the coagulation cascade through factor XI and conversion of prekallikrein to kallikrein. Kallikrein leads to generation of plasmin, which is known to activate the complement and the fibrinolytic systems. Kallikrein generation also activates the kinin-bradykinin system.

The classic pathway involves the activation of C1 by antibody-antigen complexes. In the case of cardiac surgery, two mechanisms for the activation of the classic pathway

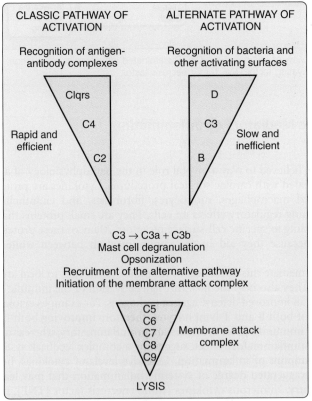

Fig. 6.6 Simplified components of the complement system. (*From Bennett-Guerrero E: Systemic inflammation. In: Kaplan J, Reich D, Savino J, eds.* Kaplan's Cardiac Anesthesia: The Echo Era. *6th ed. Philadelphia: Saunders, 2011.*)

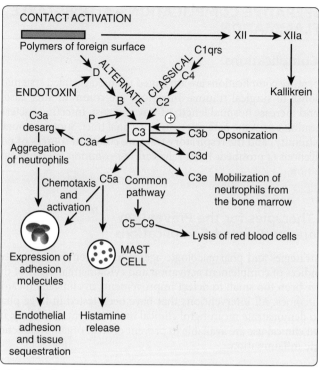

Fig. 6.7 Contact activation of the complement cascade during cardiopulmonary bypass. Activation of complement occurs primarily through the alternate pathway. (*From Ohri SK. The effects of cardiopulmonary bypass on the immune system.* Perfusion. *1993;8:121.*)

are likely. Endotoxin can be detected in the serum of almost all patients undergoing cardiac surgical procedures. Endotoxin forms an antigen-antibody complex with antiendotoxin antibodies normally found in serum that can then activate C1. The administration of protamine after separation from CPB has been reported to result in heparin-protamine complexes, which also can activate the classic pathway.

Activated C3 and other complement factors downstream in the cascade have several actions. The effects of activated complement fragments on mast cells and their circulating counterparts, the basophil cells, may be relevant to the development of postoperative complications potentially attributable to complement activation. Fragments C3a and C5a (also called *anaphylatoxins*) lead to the release of numerous mediators, including histamine, leukotriene B_4, platelet-activating factor, prostaglandins, thromboxanes, and TNF. These mediators, when released from mast cells, result in endothelial leak, interstitial edema, and increased tissue blood flow. Complement factors such as C5a and C3b complexed to microbes stimulate macrophages to secrete inflammatory mediators such as TNF. C3b activates neutrophils and macrophages and enhances their ability to phagocytose bacteria. The lytic complex, composed of complement factors C5b, C6, C7, C8, and C9, is capable of directly lysing cells. Activated complement factors make invading cells "sticky," such that they bind to one another (ie, agglutinate). The complement-mediated process of capillary dilation, leakage of plasma proteins and fluid, and accumulation and activation of neutrophils makes up part of the acute inflammatory response.

▣ POSTOPERATIVE COMPLICATIONS ATTRIBUTABLE TO INFLAMMATION

Types of Complications

Many postoperative complications are attributed to an exaggerated systemic proinflammatory response to surgical trauma. Infections are common after cardiac surgical procedures and increase hospital length of stay and cost. Infecting bacteria may arise from translocation across the patient's gastrointestinal tract. Surgical wounds (sternum and lower extremity) and the respiratory tract are common sources of postoperative infection. Infections of prosthetic heart valves are less common but represent a devastating complication.

Potential Therapies for the Prevention of Inflammation-Related Complications

Numerous strategies and pharmacologic agents have been demonstrated to reduce laboratory indices of complement activation and cytokinemia. Many of these studies, however, have been too small to detect improvements in clinically meaningful postoperative outcomes. All interventions that have been tested in large phase III trials have failed to demonstrate meaningful clinical improvement. Currently, no therapies in widespread clinical use are available to prevent or treat organ dysfunction resulting from systemic inflammation.

SUGGESTED READINGS

Benito B, Brugada R, Brugada J, et al. Brugada syndrome. *Prog Cardiovasc Dis.* 2008;51:1–22.

Dandona S. Cardiovascular drugs and the genetic response. *Methodist Debakey Cardiovasc J.* 2014;10: 13–17.

Dieleman JM, Nierich AP, Rosseel PM, et al. Intraoperative high-dose dexamethasone for cardiac surgery: a randomized controlled trial. *JAMA.* 2012;308:1761–1767.

DiFrancesco D. The onset and autonomic regulation of cardiac pacemaker activity: relevance of the f current. *Cardiovasc Res.* 1995;29:449–456.

Echt DS, Liebson PR, Mitchell LB, et al. Mortality and morbidity in patients receiving encainide, flecainide, or placebo: the Cardiac Arrhythmia Suppression Trial. *N Engl J Med.* 1991;324:781–788.

Fox AA, Shernan SK, Body SC. Predictive genomics of adverse events after cardiac surgery. *Semin Cardiothorac Vasc Anesth.* 2004;8:297–315.

Grocott HP, White WD, Morris RW, et al. Genetic polymorphisms and the risk of stroke after cardiac surgery. *Stroke.* 2005;36:1854–1858.

Ho CY, Seidman CE. A contemporary approach to hypertrophic cardiomyopathy. *Circulation.* 2006;113:e858–e862.

Huneke R, Fassl J, Rossaint R, et al. Effects of volatile anesthetics on cardiac ion channels. *Acta Anaesthesiol Scand.* 2004;48:547–561.

Korn SJ, Trapani JG. Potassium channels. *IEEE Trans Nanobioscience.* 2005;4:21–33.

Miller BE, Levy JH. The inflammatory response to cardiopulmonary bypass. *J Cardiothorac Vasc Anesth.* 1997;11:355–366.

Mythen MG, Purdy G, Mackie IJ, et al. Postoperative multiple organ dysfunction syndrome associated with gut mucosal hypoperfusion, increased neutrophil degranulation and C1-esterase inhibitor depletion. *Br J Anaesth.* 1993;71:858–863.

Nishimura RA, Holmes DR Jr. Clinical practice: hypertrophic obstructive cardiomyopathy. *N Engl J Med.* 2004;350:1320–1327.

Ragazzi E, Wu SN, Shryock J, et al. Electrophysiological and receptor binding studies to assess activation of the cardiac adenosine receptor by adenine nucleotides. *Circ Res.* 1991;68:1035–1044.

Robin NH, Tabereaux PB, Benza R, et al. Genetic testing in cardiovascular disease. *J Am Coll Cardiol.* 2007;50:727–737.

II

Rothenburger M, Soeparwata R, Deng MC, et al. Prediction of clinical outcome after cardiac surgery: the role of cytokines, endotoxin, and anti-endotoxin core antibodies. *Shock*. 2001;16(suppl 1):44–50.

Schwarz UI, Ritchie MD, Bradford Y, et al. Genetic determinants of response to warfarin during initial anticoagulation. *N Engl J Med*. 2008;358:999–1008.

Sigurdsson MI, Muehlschlegel JD, Fox AA, et al. Genetic variants associated with atrial fibrillation and PR interval following cardiac surgery. *J Cardiothorac Vasc Anesth*. 2015;29:605–610.

Verrier ED, Shernan SK, Taylor KM, et al. Terminal complement blockade with pexelizumab during coronary artery bypass graft surgery requiring cardiopulmonary bypass: a randomized trial. *JAMA*. 2004;291:2319–2327.

Welsby IJ, Podgoreanu MV, Phillips-Bute B, et al. Genetic factors contribute to bleeding after cardiac surgery. *J Thromb Haemost*. 2005;3:1206–1212.

6

Chapter 7

Pharmacology of Anesthetic Drugs

Laeben Lester, MD • Nanhi Mitter, MD •
Dan E. Berkowitz, MD • Daniel Nyhan, MD

Key Points

1. In patients, the observed acute effect of a specific anesthetic agent on the cardiovascular system represents the net effect on the myocardium, coronary blood flow (CBF), and vasculature; electrophysiologic behavior; and neurohormonal reflex function. Anesthetic agents within the same class may differ from one another quantitatively and qualitatively. The acute response to an anesthetic agent may be modulated by the patient's underlying pathology or pharmacologic treatment, or both.

2. Volatile agents cause dose-dependent decreases in systemic blood pressure. For halothane and enflurane, this mainly results from depression of contractile function, and, for isoflurane, desflurane, and sevoflurane, pressure changes result from decreases in systemic vascular responses. Volatile anesthetics cause dose-dependent depression of contractile function that is mediated at a cellular level by attenuating calcium currents and decreasing calcium sensitivity. Decreases in systemic vascular responses reflect various effects on endothelium-dependent and endothelium-independent mechanisms.

3. Volatile agents determine CBF by their effect on systemic hemodynamics, myocardial metabolism, and coronary vasculature. When these variables were controlled in studies, the anesthetics exerted only mild direct vasodilatory effects on the coronary vasculature.

4. In addition to causing acute coronary syndromes, myocardial ischemia can manifest as myocardial stunning, preconditioning, or hibernating myocardium. Volatile anesthetics can attenuate myocardial ischemia development through mechanisms that are independent of myocardial oxygen supply and demand and can facilitate functional recovery of stunned myocardium. Volatile agents also can simulate ischemic preconditioning, a phenomenon described as anesthetic preconditioning, the mechanisms of which are similar but not identical.

5. Intravenous induction agents (ie, hypnotics) belong to various drug classes, including barbiturates, benzodiazepines, N-methyl-D-aspartate receptor antagonists, and α_2-adrenergic receptor agonists. Although they all induce hypnosis, their sites of action and molecular targets are different, and their cardiovascular effects partially depend on the class to which they belong.

6. Studies of isolated cardiac myocytes, cardiac muscle tissue, and vascular tissue have demonstrated that induction agents inhibit cardiac contractility and relax vascular tone by inhibiting the mechanisms that increase intracellular calcium ion (Ca^{2+}) concentration. This may be offset by mechanisms that increase myofilament Ca^{2+} sensitivity in the cardiac myocyte and vascular smooth muscle, which can modulate cardiovascular changes. However, the cumulative effects of induction agents on contractility, vascular resistance, and vascular capacitance are mediated predominantly by their sympatholytic effects. Induction agents should be used judiciously and with extreme caution in patients with shock, heart failure, or other pathophysiologic circumstances in which the sympathetic nervous system is paramount in maintaining myocardial contractility and arterial and venous tone.

7. Opioids have diverse chemical structures, but all retain an essential T-shaped component necessary stereochemically for the activation of the μ-, κ-, and δ-opioid receptors. These receptors are not confined to the nervous system and have been identified in the myocardium and blood vessels where endogenous opioid proteins can be synthesized.
8. Acute exogenous opioid administration modulates many determinants of central and peripheral cardiovascular regulation. However, the predominant clinical effect is mediated by attenuation of central sympathetic outflow.
9. Activation of the δ-opioid receptor can elicit preconditioning, which is mediated by signaling pathways that involve G-protein–coupled protein kinases, caspases, nitric oxide, and other chemicals. In contrast with ischemia in homeotherms, hibernation is well tolerated in certain species. This phenomenon may partially depend on mechanisms that are activated by opioids or opioid-like molecules.

An enormous body of literature has described the effects of different anesthetic agents on the heart and the pulmonary and systemic regional vascular beds. More publications have been spawned by the great interest in anesthesia-induced preconditioning (APC). In this chapter, volatile agents, intravenous anesthetics, and opioids are discussed in terms of their acute and delayed effects on the cardiovascular system (CVS). The acute effects on myocardial function, electrophysiology, coronary vasoregulation, systemic and pulmonary vasoregulation, and the baroreceptor reflex are described. Discussion of the delayed effects focuses on APC.

▓ VOLATILE AGENTS

Acute Effects

Myocardial Function

The influence of volatile anesthetics on contractile function has been investigated extensively in several animal species and in humans using various in vitro and in vivo models. It is widely agreed that volatile agents cause dose-dependent depression of contractile function (Box 7.1). Different volatile agents are not identical in this regard, and the preponderance of information indicates that halothane and enflurane exert equal but more potent myocardial depression than isoflurane, desflurane, or sevoflurane, in part because of reflex sympathetic activation with the latter agents. In the setting of preexisting myocardial depression, volatile agents have a greater effect than in normal myocardium. At the cellular level, volatile anesthetics exert their negative inotropic effects mainly by modulating sarcolemmal L-type Ca^{2+} channels, the sarcoplasmic reticulum (SR), and contractile proteins. However, the mechanisms by which anesthetic agents modify ion channels are not completely understood.

Cardiac Electrophysiology

Volatile anesthetics reduce the arrhythmogenic threshold for epinephrine. For volatile agents, the order of sensitization is halothane > enflurane > sevoflurane > isoflurane = desflurane. The molecular mechanisms underlying the effect of volatile anesthetics are poorly understood.

Coronary Vasoregulation

Volatile anesthetics modulate several determinants of myocardial oxygen supply and demand. They also directly modulate the myocyte's response to ischemia.

7

BOX 7.1 *Volatile Anesthetic Agents*

All volatile anesthetic agents cause dose-dependent decreases in systemic blood pressure, which for halothane and enflurane predominantly result from attenuation of myocardial contractile function; and which for isoflurane, desflurane, and sevoflurane predominantly result from decreases in systemic vascular resistance.

Volatile agents obtund all components of the baroreceptor reflex arc.

The effects of volatile agents on myocardial diastolic function are not well characterized and await the application of emerging technologies that have the sensitivity to quantitate indices of diastolic function.

Volatile anesthetics lower the arrhythmogenic threshold to catecholamines. However, the underlying molecular mechanisms are not well understood.

When confounding variables are controlled (eg, systemic blood pressure), isoflurane does not cause coronary steal by a direct effect on coronary vasculature.

The effects of volatile agents on systemic regional vascular beds and on the pulmonary vasculature are complex and depend on many variables, including the specific anesthetic, precise vascular bed, and vessel size, and whether endothelial-dependent or endothelial-independent mechanisms are being investigated.

The effect of isoflurane on coronary vessels was controversial and dominated much of the relevant literature in the 1980s and early 1990s. Several reports indicated that it caused direct coronary arteriolar vasodilatation in vessels with diameters of 100 μm or less and that isoflurane could cause coronary steal in patients with steal-prone coronary anatomy. Several studies in which potential confounding variables were controlled found that isoflurane did not cause coronary steal. Studies of sevoflurane and desflurane showed similar results that were consistent with a mild direct coronary vasodilator effect of these agents.

Systemic Vascular Effects

All volatile anesthetics decrease systemic blood pressure (BP) in a dose-dependent manner. With halothane and enflurane, the decrease in systemic BP primarily results from decreases in stroke volume (SV) and cardiac output (CO), whereas isoflurane, sevoflurane, and desflurane decrease overall systemic vascular resistance (SVR) while maintaining CO.

Baroreceptor Reflex

All volatile agents attenuate the baroreceptor reflex. Baroreceptor reflex inhibition by halothane and enflurane is more potent than that observed with isoflurane, desflurane, or sevoflurane, each of which has a similar effect. Each component of the baroreceptor reflex arc (eg, afferent nerve activity, central processing, efferent nerve activity) is inhibited by volatile agents.

Delayed Effects

Reversible Myocardial Ischemia

Prolonged ischemia results in irreversible myocardial damage and necrosis (Box 7.2). Depending on the duration and sequence of ischemic insults, shorter durations of myocardial ischemia can lead to preconditioning or myocardial stunning (Fig. 7.1). Stunning, first described in 1975, occurs after brief ischemia and is characterized by

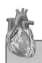

BOX 7.2 *Volatile Agents and Myocardial Ischemia*

Volatile anesthetic agents can attenuate the effects of myocardial ischemia (ie, acute coronary syndromes).

Nonacute manifestations of myocardial ischemia include hibernating myocardium, stunning, and preconditioning.

Halothane and isoflurane facilitate the recovery of stunned myocardium.

Preconditioning, an important adaptive and protective mechanism in biologic tissues, can be provoked by protean nonlethal stresses, including ischemia.

Volatile anesthetic agents can mimic preconditioning (ie, anesthetic preconditioning), which can have important clinical implications and provide insight into the cellular mechanisms of action of these volatile agents.

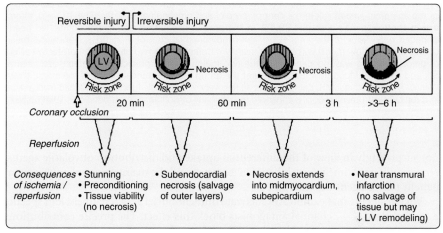

Fig. 7.1 Effects of ischemia and reperfusion on the heart based on studies using an anesthetized canine model of proximal coronary artery occlusion. Periods of ischemia of less than 20 minutes followed by reperfusion are not associated with development of necrosis (ie, reversible injury). Brief ischemia and reperfusion results in stunning and preconditioning. If the duration of coronary occlusion is extended beyond 20 minutes, necrosis develops from the subendocardium to subepicardium over time. Reperfusion before 3 hours of ischemia salvages ischemic but viable tissue. Salvaged tissue may demonstrate stunning. Reperfusion beyond 3 to 6 hours in this model does not reduce myocardial infarct size. Late reperfusion may still have a beneficial effect on reducing or preventing myocardial infarct expansion and left ventricular *(LV)* remodeling. (From Kloner RA, Jennings RB. Consequences of brief ischemia: stunning, preconditioning, and their clinical implications, part I. *Circulation.* 2001;104:2981.)

myocardial dysfunction in the setting of normal restored blood flow and by an absence of myocardial necrosis. Ischemic preconditioning (IPC) was first described in 1986 and is characterized by an attenuation of infarct size after sustained ischemia if the period of sustained ischemia is preceded by a period of brief ischemia (Fig. 7.2). This effect is independent of collateral flow. Short periods of ischemia followed by reperfusion can lead to stunning or preconditioning with a reduction in infarct size.

Anesthetic Preconditioning

Volatile agents can elicit delayed (ie, late) and classic (ie, early) preconditioning. APC is dose dependent, exhibits synergy with ischemia in affording protection, and perhaps

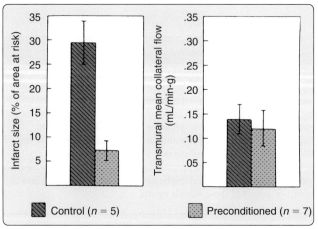

Fig. 7.2 Infarct size and collateral blood flow in a 40-minute study. Infarct size as a percentage of the anatomic area at risk in the control *(purple)* and preconditioned *(green)* hearts *(left)*. Infarct size in control animals averaged 29.4% of the area at risk. Infarct size in preconditioned hearts averaged only 7.3% of the area at risk (preconditioned vs control, $P < .001$). Transmural mean collateral blood flow *(right)* was not significantly different in the two groups. The protective effect of preconditioning was independent of the two major baseline predictors of infarct size: area at risk and collateral blood flow. Bars represent the group mean ± standard error of the mean. (From Warltier DC, al-Wathiqui MH, Kampine JP, et al. Recovery of contractile function of stunned myocardium in chronically instrumented dogs is enhanced by halothane or isoflurane. *Anesthesiology.* 1988;69:552.)

not surprisingly in view of the differential uptake and distribution of volatile agents, requires different time intervals between exposure and the maintenance of a subsequent benefit that is agent dependent.

Volatile agents that exhibit APC activate mitochondrial K^+_{ATP} channels, and specific mitochondrial K^+_{ATP} channel antagonists block this effect. The precise contributions of sarcolemmal versus mitochondrial K^+_{ATP} channel activation to APC remain to be elucidated (Fig. 7.3).

INTRAVENOUS INDUCTION AGENTS

The drugs discussed in this section are induction agents and hypnotics. The drugs belong to different classes (ie, barbiturates, benzodiazepines, *N*-methyl-D-aspartate [NMDA] receptor antagonists, and α_2-adrenergic receptor agonists). Their effects on the CVS depend on the class to which they belong.

Acute Cardiac Effects

Myocardial Contractility

With regard to propofol, the studies remain controversial about whether there is a direct effect on myocardial contractile function at clinically relevant concentrations. The weight of evidence, however, suggests that the drug has a modest negative inotropic effect, which may be mediated by inhibition of L-type Ca^{2+} channels or modulation of Ca^{2+} release from the SR.

In one of the few human studies using isolated atrial muscle tissue, no inhibition of myocardial contractility was found in the clinical concentration ranges of propofol,

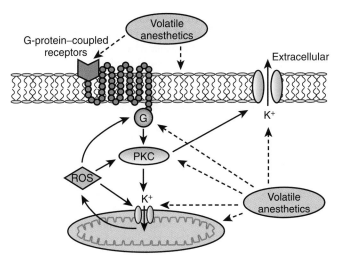

Fig. 7.3 Multiple endogenous signaling pathways mediate volatile anesthetic-induced myocardial activation of an end-effector that promotes resistance against ischemic injury. Mitochondrial K^+_{ATP} channels have been implicated as the end-effector in this protective scheme, but sarcolemmal K^+_{ATP} channels may also be involved. A trigger initiates a cascade of signal transduction events, resulting in protection. Volatile anesthetics signal through adenosine and opioid receptors, modulate G proteins *(G)*, stimulate protein kinase C *(PKC)* and other intracellular kinases, or directly stimulate mitochondria to generate reactive oxygen species *(ROS)* that ultimately enhance K^+_{ATP} channel activity. Volatile anesthetics may also directly facilitate K^+_{ATP} channel opening. *Dotted arrows* delineate the intracellular targets that may be regulated by volatile anesthetics; *solid arrows* represent potential signaling cascades. (From Tanaka K, Ludwig LM, Kersten JR, et al. Mechanisms of cardioprotection by volatile anesthetics. *Anesthesiology.* 2004;100:707.)

midazolam, and etomidate. Thiopental showed strong negative inotropic properties, whereas ketamine showed slight negative inotropic properties. Negative inotropic effects may partially explain the cardiovascular depression on induction of anesthesia with thiopental but not with propofol, midazolam, and etomidate. Improvement of hemodynamics after induction of anesthesia with ketamine cannot therefore be explained by intrinsic cardiac stimulation but is a function of sympathoexcitation.

The effect of drugs such as propofol may be affected by the underlying myocardial pathology. For instance, one study evaluated the direct effects of propofol on the contractility of human nonfailing atrial and failing atrial and ventricular muscles obtained from the failing human hearts of transplant recipients or from nonfailing hearts of patients undergoing coronary artery bypass graft (CABG). They concluded that propofol exerted a direct negative inotropic effect in nonfailing and failing human myocardium, but only at concentrations larger than typical clinical concentrations. Negative inotropic effects are reversible with β-adrenergic stimulation, suggesting that propofol does not alter the contractile reserve but may shift the dose responsiveness to adrenergic stimulation.

Vasculature

As with the heart, the physiologic actions of anesthetics in the vasculature represent a summation of their effects on the central autonomic nervous system (ANS), direct effects on the vascular smooth muscle, and modulating effects on the underlying endothelium.

Propofol decreases SVR in humans. This was demonstrated in a patient with an artificial heart in whom the CO remained fixed. The effect is predominantly mediated by alterations in sympathetic tone, but in isolated arteries, propofol decreases vascular tone and agonist-induced contraction. Propofol mediates these effects by inhibition of Ca^{2+} influx through voltage- or receptor-gated Ca^{2+} channels and inhibition of Ca^{2+} release from the intracellular Ca^{2+} stores.

The effects of induction agents on pulmonary vasoregulation may have important implications for the management of patients whose primary pathologies involve the pulmonary circulation when they undergo cardiothoracic surgery (ie, primary pulmonary hypertension for lung transplantation and chronic thromboembolic disease for pulmonary endarterectomy). The effects may be important for patients with right ventricular failure. In modulating hypoxic pulmonary vasoconstriction, induction agents may affect intraoperative alveolar-arterial (A-a) gradients, particularly during one-lung ventilation.

Propofol attenuates endothelium-dependent vasodilatation through a mechanism involving nitric oxide (NO) and endothelium-dependent hyperpolarizing factor.

INDIVIDUAL AGENTS

Thiopental

General Characteristics

Thiopental has survived the test of time as an intravenous anesthetic drug (Box 7.3). Since Lundy introduced it in 1934, thiopental has remained the most widely used induction agent for decades because of the rapid hypnotic effect (ie, one arm-to-brain circulation time), highly predictable effect, lack of vascular irritation, and general overall safety. The induction dose of thiopental is less for older than for younger healthy patients. Pharmacokinetic analyses confirm the awakening from thiopental is due to rapid redistribution. Thiopental has a distribution half-life ($t_{1/2}\alpha$) of 2.5 to 8.5 minutes, and the total body clearance varies according to sampling times and techniques from 0.15 to 0.26 L/kg per hour. The elimination half-life ($t_{1/2}\beta$) varies from 5 to 12 hours. Barbiturates and drugs such as propofol have increased volumes of distribution (V_d) when used during cardiopulmonary bypass (CPB).

Cardiovascular Effects

The hemodynamic changes produced by thiopental have been studied in healthy patients and in patients with cardiac disease (Table 7.1). The principal effect is a decrease in contractility, which results from reduced availability of calcium to the myofibrils. There is also an increase in heart rate (HR). The cardiac index (CI) is unchanged or reduced, and the mean arterial pressure (MAP) is maintained or slightly reduced. In the dose range studied, no relationship between plasma thiopental and hemodynamic effect was found.

Mechanisms for the decrease in CO include direct negative inotropic action; decreased ventricular filling, resulting from increased venous capacitance; and transiently decreased sympathetic outflow from the central nervous system (CNS). The 10% to 36% increase in HR that accompanies thiopental administration probably results from the baroreceptor-mediated sympathetic reflex stimulation of the heart. Thiopental produces dose-related negative inotropic effects that appear to result from a decrease in calcium influx into the cells and a resultant diminished amount of calcium at sarcolemma sites. Patients who had compensated heart disease and received 4 mg/ kg of thiopental had a greater (18%) BP decline than did other patients without heart

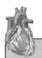

BOX 7.3 *Intravenous Anesthetics*

Thiopental

- Thiopental decreases cardiac output by:
    - A direct negative inotropic action
    - Decreased ventricular filling resulting from increased venous capacitance
    - Transiently decreasing sympathetic outflow from the central nervous system.
- Because of these effects, caution should be used when thiopental is given to patients who have left or right ventricular failure, cardiac tamponade, or hypovolemia.

Midazolam

- Small hemodynamic changes occur after the intravenous administration of midazolam.

Etomidate

- Etomidate is the drug that changes hemodynamic variables the least. Studies in noncardiac patients and those who have heart disease document remarkable hemodynamic stability after administration of etomidate.
- Patients who have hypovolemia, cardiac tamponade, or low cardiac output probably represent the population for whom etomidate is better than other induction drugs, with the possible exception of ketamine.

Ketamine

- A unique feature of ketamine is stimulation of the cardiovascular system, with the most prominent hemodynamic changes, including significant increases in heart rate, cardiac index, systemic vascular resistance, pulmonary artery pressure, and systemic artery pressure. These circulatory changes increase myocardial oxygen consumption with an appropriate increase in coronary blood flow.
- Studies have demonstrated the safety and efficacy of induction with ketamine in hemodynamically unstable patients, and it is the induction drug of choice for patients with cardiac tamponade physiology.

Dexmedetomidine

- Dexmedetomidine is a highly selective, specific, and potent adrenoreceptor agonist.
- α_2-Adrenergic agonists can safely reduce anesthetic requirements and improve hemodynamic stability. They can enhance sedation and analgesia without producing respiratory depression or prolonging the recovery period.

disease. The 11% to 36% increase in HR encountered in patients with coronary artery disease (CAD) who were anesthetized with thiopental (1 to 4 mg/kg) is potentially deleterious because of the obligatory increase in myocardial oxygen consumption ($M\dot{V}O_2$).

Despite the well-known potential for cardiovascular depression when thiopental is given rapidly in large doses, the drug has minimal hemodynamic effects in healthy patients and in those who have heart disease when it is given slowly or by infusion. Significant reductions in cardiovascular parameters occur in patients who have impaired ventricular function. When thiopental is given to patients with hypovolemia, there is a significant reduction in CO (69%) and a large decrease in BP, which indicate that patients without adequate compensatory mechanisms may have serious hemodynamic depression with a thiopental induction. Thiopental produces greater changes in BP

Table 7.1 Induction Agents and Hemodynamic Changes

Parameter	Thiopental (%)	Midazolam (%)	Etomidate (%)	Propofol (%)	Ketamine (%)
Heart rate	0 to 36	−14 to +21	0 to +22	−6 to +12	0 to +59
MAP	−18 to +8	−12 to −26	0 to −20	0 to −47	0 to +40
Systemic vascular resistance	0 to +19	0 to −20	0 to −17	−9 to −25	0 to +33
Pulmonary artery pressure	Unchanged	Unchanged	0 to −17	−4 to +8	+44 to +47
Pulmonary vascular resistance	Unchanged	Unchanged	0 to +27	—	0 to +33
LAP or PAOP	Unchanged	0 to −25	—	—	—
Left ventricular end-diastolic pressure or PAOP	—	—	0 to −11	+13	Unchanged
Right atrial pressure	0 to +33	Unchanged	Unchanged	−8 to −21	+15 to +33
Cardiac index	0 to +24	0 to −25	0 to +14	−6 to −26	0 to +42
Stroke volume	−12 to −35	0 to −18	0 to −15	−8 to −18	0 to −21
Left ventricular stroke work index	0 to −26	−28 to −42	0 to −27	−15 to −40	0 to +27
Right ventricular stroke work index	NR	−41 to −57	—	—	—
dP/dt	−14	0 to −12	0 to −18	—	Unchanged
1/PEP[2]	−18 to −28	—	—	—	—
Systolic time interval	—	—	Unchanged	—	NR

dP/dt, Rate of left ventricular pressure rise in early systole; LAP, left atrial pressure; MAP, mean arterial pressure; NR, not reported; PAOP, pulmonary artery occlusion pressure; PEP, pre-ejection period.

and HR than midazolam when used for induction of American Society of Anesthesiologists (ASA) class III (ie, severe systemic disease) and class IV (ie, severe systemic disease that is life-threatening) patients.

Uses in Cardiac Anesthesia

Thiopental can be used safely for the induction of anesthesia in normal patients and in those who have compensated cardiac disease. Because of the negative inotropic effects, increase in venous capacitance, and dose-related decrease in CO, caution should be used when thiopental is given to patients who have left or right ventricular failure, cardiac tamponade, or hypovolemia. The development of tachycardia is a potential problem in patients with ischemic heart disease.

A controversial additional use for thiopental infusion is for putative cerebral protection during CPB in patients undergoing selected cardiac operations. However, the cerebral protective effect of thiopental during CPB has been challenged. It has been demonstrated that no differences exist in outcome between thiopental and control patients undergoing hypothermic CPB for CABG. Although the administration of a barbiturate during CPB may result in myocardial depression necessitating additional inotropic support, suggested beneficial effects of a thiopental infusion during CPB include maintaining peripheral perfusion, which allowed more uniform warming, decreased base deficit, and decreased requirements for postoperative pressor support.

Midazolam

General Characteristics

Midazolam, a water-soluble benzodiazepine, was synthesized in the United States in 1975. It is unique among benzodiazepines because of its rapid onset, short duration of action, and relatively rapid plasma clearance. The dose for induction of general anesthesia is between 0.05 and 0.2 mg/kg and depends on the premedication and speed of injection.

The pharmacokinetic variables of midazolam reveal that it is cleared significantly more rapidly than diazepam and lorazepam. The rapid redistribution of midazolam and high rate of liver clearance account for its relatively short hypnotic and hemodynamic effects. The $t_{1/2}\beta$ is about 2 hours, which is at least tenfold less than for diazepam.

Cardiovascular Effects

The hemodynamic effects of midazolam have been investigated in healthy subjects, in ASA class III patients, and in patients who have ischemic and valvular heart disease (VHD). Table 7.1 summarizes the hemodynamic changes after induction of anesthesia with midazolam. Only small hemodynamic changes occur after intravenous administration of midazolam (0.2 mg/kg) in premedicated patients who have CAD. Potentially important changes include a decrease in MAP of 20% and an increase in HR of 15%. The CI is maintained. Filling pressures are unchanged or decreased in patients who have normal ventricular function, but they are significantly decreased in patients who have an increased pulmonary capillary wedge pressure (PCWP = 18 mm Hg).

Midazolam appears to affect the capacitance vessels more than diazepam does, at least during CPB, when decreases in venous reservoir volume of the pump are greater with midazolam than with diazepam. Diazepam decreases SVR more than midazolam during CPB.

Midazolam (0.15 mg/kg) and ketamine (1.5 mg/kg) have proved to be a safe and useful combination for rapid-sequence induction for emergency surgery. This combination was superior to thiopental alone because it caused less cardiovascular depression, more amnesia, and less postoperative somnolence. If midazolam is given to patients who have received fentanyl, significant hypotension may occur, as seen with diazepam and fentanyl. However, midazolam routinely is combined with fentanyl for induction and maintenance of general anesthesia during cardiac surgery without adverse hemodynamic sequelae.

Uses

Midazolam is distinctly different from the other benzodiazepines because of its rapid onset, short duration, water solubility, and failure to produce significant thrombophlebitis. It is therefore one of the mainstays of anesthesia in the cardiac operating room.

Etomidate

General Characteristics

Etomidate is a carboxylated imidazole derivative. It was found that etomidate had a safety margin four times greater than that of thiopental. The recommended induction dose of 0.3 mg/kg has pronounced hypnotic effects. Etomidate is moderately lipid soluble and has a rapid onset (ie, 10 to 12 seconds) and a brief duration of action. It is hydrolyzed primarily in the liver and in the blood.

Etomidate infusion and single injections directly suppress adrenocortical function, which interferes with the normal stress response. Blockade of 11β-hydroxylation mediated by the imidazole radical of etomidate results in decreased biosynthesis of cortisol and aldosterone. The clinical significance of etomidate-induced adrenal suppression remains undetermined.

Cardiovascular Effects

In comparative studies with other anesthetic drugs, etomidate is usually described as the drug that changes hemodynamic variables the least. Studies of noncardiac patients and those who have heart disease document the remarkable hemodynamic stability after administration of etomidate (see Table 7.1). Compared with other anesthetics, etomidate produces the least change in the balance of myocardial oxygen demand and supply. Systemic BP remains unchanged in most series but may be decreased 10% to 19% in patients who have VHD.

Intravenous etomidate (0.3 mg/kg), used to induce general anesthesia in patients with acute myocardial infarction (AMI) undergoing percutaneous coronary angioplasty, did not alter the HR, MAP, and rate-pressure product, demonstrating the remarkable hemodynamic stability of this agent. However, VHD may influence the hemodynamic responses to etomidate. Whereas most patients can maintain their BP, patients with aortic and mitral VHD had significant decreases of 17% to 19% in systolic and diastolic BP and had decreases of 11% and 17% in pulmonary artery pressure (PAP) and PCWP, respectively. CI in patients who had VHD and received 0.3 mg/kg remained unchanged or decreased 13%. There was no difference in response to etomidate between patients who had aortic valve disease and those who had mitral valve disease.

Uses

In certain situations, the advantages of etomidate outweigh the disadvantages. Emergency uses include situations in which rapid induction is essential. Patients who have hypovolemia, cardiac tamponade, or low CO probably represent the population for whom etomidate is better than other drugs, with the possible exception of ketamine. The brief hypnotic effect means that additional analgesic or hypnotic drugs, or both, must be administered. Etomidate offers no real advantage over most other induction drugs for patients undergoing elective surgical procedures.

Ketamine

General Characteristics

Ketamine is a phencyclidine derivative whose anesthetic actions differ so markedly from barbiturates and other CNS depressants that its effect has been labeled *dissociative anesthesia*. Although ketamine produces rapid hypnosis and profound analgesia, respiratory and cardiovascular functions are not depressed as much as with most other induction agents. Disturbing psychotomimetic activity (ie, vivid dreams, hallucinations, or emergence phenomena) remains a problem.

Cardiovascular Effects

The hemodynamic effects of ketamine have been examined in noncardiac patients, critically ill patients, geriatric patients, and patients who have a variety of heart diseases. Table 7.1 contains the range of hemodynamic responses to ketamine. A unique feature of ketamine is stimulation of the CVS. The most prominent hemodynamic changes are significant increases in HR, CI, SVR, PAP, and systemic artery pressure. These circulatory changes increase $M\dot{V}O_2$, with an apparently appropriate increase in coronary blood flow (CBF). A second dose of ketamine produces hemodynamic effects opposite to those of the first. The cardiovascular stimulation seen after ketamine induction of anesthesia (2 mg/kg) in a patient who has VHD is not observed with the second administration, which is accompanied instead by decreases in the BP, PCWP, and CI.

Ketamine produces similar hemodynamic changes in healthy patients and those who have ischemic heart disease. In patients who have increased PAP (eg, mitral valvular disease), ketamine appears to cause a more pronounced increase in pulmonary vascular resistance (PVR) than in SVR. Marked tachycardia after administration of ketamine and pancuronium also can complicate the induction of anesthesia in patients who have CAD or VHD with atrial fibrillation.

One of the most common and successful approaches to blocking ketamine-induced hypertension and tachycardia is prior administration of benzodiazepines. Diazepam, flunitrazepam, and midazolam successfully attenuate the hemodynamic effects of ketamine. For example, with VHD, ketamine (2 mg/kg) does not produce significant hemodynamic changes when preceded by diazepam (0.4 mg/kg). The HR, MAP, and rate-pressure product remain unchanged, however, with a significant decrease in CI.

The combination of diazepam and ketamine rivals the high-dose fentanyl technique with regard to hemodynamic stability. No patient had hallucinations, although 2% had dreams and 1% had recall of events in the operating room.

Studies have demonstrated the safety and efficacy of induction with ketamine (2 mg/kg) in hemodynamically unstable patients who required emergency operations. Most patients were hypovolemic because of trauma or massive hemorrhage. Ketamine induction was accompanied in most patients by the maintenance of BP and presumably of CO. In patients who have an accumulation of pericardial fluid with or without constrictive pericarditis, induction with ketamine (2 mg/kg) maintains CI and increases BP, SVR, and right atrial pressure (RAP). The HR in this group of patients was unchanged by ketamine, probably because cardiac tamponade already produced a compensatory tachycardia.

Uses

In adults, ketamine is probably the safest and most efficacious drug for patients who have decreased blood volume or cardiac tamponade. Undesired tachycardia, hypertension, and emergence delirium may be attenuated with benzodiazepines.

7

Propofol

Propofol was introduced into clinical practice in 1986. It is an alkylphenol with hypnotic properties.

Cardiovascular Effects

The hemodynamic effects of propofol have been investigated in ASA class I and class II patients, elderly patients, patients with CAD and good left ventricular function, and patients with impaired left ventricular function (see Table 7.1). Numerous studies have compared the cardiovascular effects of propofol with the most commonly used induction drugs, including the thiobarbiturates and etomidate. It is clear that systolic arterial pressure declines 15% to 40% after intravenous induction with 2 mg/kg and maintenance infusion with 100 µg/kg per minute of propofol. Similar changes are seen in diastolic arterial pressure and MAP.

The effect of propofol on HR varies. Most studies have demonstrated significant reductions in SVR (ie, 9% to 30%), CI, SV, and left ventricular stroke work index (LVSWI) after propofol. Although controversial, the evidence points to a dose-dependent decrease in myocardial contractility.

Uses

When given during nonpulsatile CPB, propofol produces statistically significant reductions in cerebral blood flow and cerebral metabolic rate in a coupled manner without adverse effects on the cerebral arteriovenous oxygen content difference or jugular bulb venous saturation. The coupled reductions in cerebral blood flow and cerebral metabolic rate suggest the potential for propofol to reduce cerebral exposure to emboli during CPB.

The effect of propofol on hypoxic pulmonary vasoconstriction was minimal in thoracic surgical patients undergoing one-lung ventilation. Compared with isoflurane, maintenance of anesthesia with propofol resulted in a lower CI and right ventricular ejection fraction but avoided the threefold increase in shunt fraction observed with isoflurane on commencement of one-lung ventilation.

Dexmedetomidine

Dexmedetomidine, the pharmacologically active D-isomer of medetomidine, is a highly selective, specific, and potent adrenoreceptor agonist. Medetomidine has a considerably greater α_2/α_1 selectivity ratio than does the classic prototype α_2-adrenergic agonist clonidine in receptor-binding experiments. Compared with clonidine, it is more efficacious as an α_2-adrenoreceptor agonist. It has effectively reduced volatile anesthetic requirements as measured by the minimal alveolar concentration (MAC), and it can be a complete anesthetic in sufficiently high doses. The exact mechanisms of function and reduced anesthetic requirement are unknown but are thought to involve actions at presynaptic and postsynaptic α_2-adrenoreceptors in the CNS.

Cardiovascular Effects

The cardiovascular effects of dexmedetomidine are dose related. In studies, women who were ASA class I who received low-dose premedication with 0.5 µg/kg of dexmedetomidine demonstrated modest decreases in BP and HR. The use of perioperative intravenous infusions of low-dose dexmedetomidine in vascular patients at risk for CAD produced lower preoperative HR and systolic BP and less postoperative tachycardia, but it also resulted in a greater intraoperative requirement for pharmacologic intervention to support BP and HR. The precise cause of this effect is unknown, but it may reflect the attenuation of sympathetic outflow from the CNS.

Some controversy exists about whether the hemodynamic effects of dexmedetomidine are influenced by the background anesthetic. In conscious animals, the hypotensive effect of the drug dominates, but with the addition of potent inhalation anesthetics, MAP remains unchanged or increased, which implies a different mechanism of interaction of inhalation agents for this class of anesthetics. Dexmedetomidine has little effect on respiration, with minimal increase in arterial carbon dioxide tension ($PaCO_2$) after administration to spontaneously ventilating dogs. It has a potential advantage over other respiratory depressant anesthetics. Antinociceptive effects of medetomidine are mediated by suppression of responses of the pain-relay neurons in the dorsal horn of the spinal cord.

Uses

Clinical studies have suggested that α_2-adrenergic agonists can safely reduce anesthetic requirements and improve hemodynamic stability. These agents may enhance sedation and analgesia without producing respiratory depression or prolonging the recovery period.

The use of dexmedetomidine as a sedative adjunct in the management of patients after surgery in the intensive care unit is becoming increasingly popular. The idea that the type and amount of agent used intraoperatively can influence the postoperative course, specifically neuropsychologic events, is emerging as an important paradigm. Pharmacologic evidence suggests dexmedetomidine may be useful as an adjuvant in cardiac anesthesia.

OPIOIDS IN CARDIAC ANESTHESIA

Terminology and Classification

Various terms are commonly used to describe morphine-like drugs that are potent analgesics. The word *narcotic* is derived from the Greek word for "stupor" and refers to any drug that produces sleep. In legal terminology, it refers to any substance that produces addiction and physical dependence. Its use to describe morphine or morphine-like drugs is misleading and should be discouraged.

Opiates refer to alkaloids and related synthetic and semisynthetic drugs that interact stereospecifically with one or more of the opioid receptors to produce a pharmacologic effect. The more encompassing term, *opioid*, also includes the endogenous opioids and is used in this chapter. Opioids may be agonists, partial agonists, or antagonists.

Opioid Receptors

The existence of separate opioid receptors was shown by correlating analgesic activity with the chemical structure of many opioid compounds (Box 7.4). The concept of multiple opioid receptors is accepted, and several subtypes of each class of opioid receptors have been identified. Through biochemical and pharmacologic methods, the μ, δ, and κ receptors have been characterized. Pharmacologically, the δ-opioid receptors consist of two subtypes: δ_1 and δ_2.

Opioid receptors involved in regulating the CVS have been localized centrally to the cardiovascular and respiratory centers of the hypothalamus and brainstem and peripherally to cardiac myocytes, blood vessels, nerve terminals, and the adrenal medulla.

7

BOX 7.4 *Opioids*

The μ-, κ-, and δ-opioid receptors and endogenous opioid precursors have been identified in cardiac and vascular tissue.

The functional roles of opioid precursors and opioid receptors in the cardiovascular system of persons with pathophysiologic conditions (eg, congestive heart failure, arrhythmia) are areas of ongoing investigation.

The predominant cardiovascular effect of exogenously administered opioids is attenuation of central sympathetic outflow.

Endogenous opioids and opioid receptors (especially the δ_1-opioid receptor) are likely important contributors to early and delayed preconditioning in the heart.

Plasma drug concentrations are profoundly altered by cardiopulmonary bypass as a result of hemodilution, altered plasma protein binding, hypothermia, exclusion of the lungs from the circulation, and altered hemodynamics that likely modulate hepatic and renal blood flow. The specific effects are drug dependent.

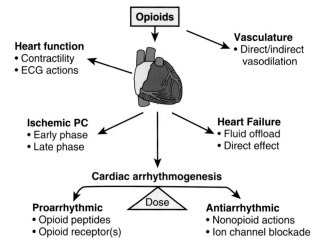

Fig. 7.4 Actions of opioids on the heart and cardiovascular system. Actions may involve direct opioid receptor–mediated actions, such as the involvement of the δ-opioid receptor in ischemic preconditioning (*PC*), or indirect, dose-dependent, nonopioid-receptor–mediated actions, such as ion channel blockade associated with the antiarrhythmic actions of opioids. *ECG,* Electrocardiogram.

Opioid receptors are differentially distributed between atria and ventricles. The highest specific receptor density for binding of κ-opioid agonists is in the right atrium and least in the left ventricle. As with the κ-opioid receptor, distribution of the δ-opioid receptor favors atrial tissue and the right side of the heart more than the left.

Cardiac Effects of Opioids

At clinically relevant doses, the cardiovascular actions of opioid analgesics are limited. The actions opioids exhibit are mediated by opioid receptors located centrally in specific areas of the brain and nuclei that regulate the control of cardiovascular function and peripherally by tissue-associated opioid receptors. Opioids exhibit a variety of complex pharmacologic actions on the CVS (Fig. 7.4).

Most of the hemodynamic effects of opioids in humans can be related to their influence on sympathetic outflow from the CNS. Pharmacologic modulation of the sympathetic activity by centrally or peripherally acting drugs elicits cardioprotective effects. Opioid–receptor agonists such as fentanyl exhibit significant central sympathoinhibitory effects.

With the exception of meperidine, all opioids produce bradycardia, although morphine given to unpremedicated, healthy persons may cause tachycardia. The mechanism of opioid-induced bradycardia is central vagal stimulation. Premedication with atropine can minimize but not totally eliminate opioid-induced bradycardia, especially in patients taking β-adrenoceptor antagonists. Although severe bradycardia should be avoided, moderate slowing of the HR may be beneficial in patients with CAD by decreasing myocardial oxygen consumption.

Hypotension can occur after even small doses of morphine and is primarily related to decreases in SVR. The most important mechanism responsible for these changes is histamine release. The amount of histamine release is reduced by slow administration (<10 mg/min). Pretreatment with a histamine H_1 or H_2 antagonist does not block these reactions, but they are significantly attenuated by combined H_1 and H_2 antagonist pretreatment. Opioids may directly act on vascular smooth muscle, independent of histamine release.

Cardioprotective Effects of Exogenous Opioid Agonists

In 1996, it was first demonstrated that an opioid could attenuate ischemia-reperfusion damage in the heart. Morphine at the dose of 300 μg/kg was given before left anterior descending coronary artery occlusion for 30 minutes in rats in vivo. The infarct area or area at risk was diminished from 54% to 12% by this treatment. The infarct-reducing effect of morphine has been shown in hearts in situ, isolated hearts, and cardiomyocytes. Morphine also improved postischemic contractility. It is now accepted that morphine provides protection against ischemia-reperfusion injury.

Fentanyl has been studied in a limited fashion and has had mixed results as far as its ability to protect the myocardium. This may be because of differences in species studied or fentanyl concentrations, or both.

Opioids in Cardiac Anesthesia

A technique of anesthesia for cardiac surgery involving high doses of morphine was developed in the late 1960s and early 1970s. The technique was based on the observation that patients requiring mechanical ventilation after surgery for end-stage VHD tolerated large doses of morphine for sedation without discernible circulatory effects. When they attempted to administer equivalent doses of morphine as the anesthetic for patients undergoing cardiac surgery, they discovered serious disadvantages, including inadequate anesthesia (even at doses of 8 to 11 mg/kg), episodes of hypotension related to histamine release, and increased intraoperative and postoperative blood and fluid requirements. Attempts to overcome these problems by combining lower doses of morphine with a variety of supplements (eg, N_2O, halothane, diazepam) proved unsatisfactory, resulting in significant myocardial depression, with decreases in CO and hypotension.

Because of the problems associated with the use of morphine, other opioids were investigated in an attempt to find a suitable alternative. The use of fentanyl in cardiac anesthesia was first reported in 1978. Since then, there have been extensive investigations of fentanyl, sufentanil, and alfentanil in cardiac surgery. The fentanyl group of opioids has proved to be the most reliable and effective for producing anesthesia for patients with valvular disorders and CABG.

A major advantage of fentanyl and its analogs for patients undergoing cardiac surgery is their lack of cardiovascular depression, which is important during anesthesia induction, when episodes of hypotension can be critical. Cardiovascular stability may be less evident during surgery; in particular, the period of sternotomy, pericardiectomy, and aortic root dissection may be associated with significant hypertension and tachycardia. During and after sternotomy, arterial hypertension increases in SVR and decreases in CO frequently occur. Variability in hemodynamic responses to surgical stimulation, even with similar doses of fentanyl, probably reflects differences in the patient populations studied by different investigators. One factor is the influence of β-blocking agents. In patients anesthetized with fentanyl while undergoing CABG, 86% of those not taking β-blockers became hypertensive during sternal spread compared with only 33% of those who were taking β-blockers.

The degree of myocardial impairment influences the response. Critically ill patients or patients with significant myocardial dysfunction appear to require lower doses of opioid for anesthesia. This may reflect altered pharmacokinetics in the patients. A decrease in liver blood flow resulting from decreased CO and congestive heart failure (CHF) reduces plasma clearance. Patients with poor left ventricular function may develop greater plasma and brain concentrations for a given loading dose or infusion rate than patients with good left ventricular function. Patients with depressed myocardial function may lack the ability to respond to surgical stress by increasing CO in the face of progressive increases in SVR.

EFFECTS OF CARDIOPULMONARY BYPASS ON PHARMACOKINETICS AND PHARMACODYNAMICS

Institution of CPB has profound effects on the plasma concentration, distribution, and elimination of administered drugs. The major factors responsible are hemodilution and altered plasma protein binding, hypotension, hypothermia, pulsatile versus nonpulsatile flow, isolation of the lungs from the circulation, and uptake of anesthetic drugs by the bypass circuit. These changes result in altered blood concentrations, which also depend on the particular pharmacokinetics of the drug administered.

Hemodilution

At the onset of CPB, the circuit priming fluid is mixed with the patient's blood. In adults, the priming volume is 1.5 to 2 L, and the prime may be crystalloid or crystalloid combined with blood or colloid. The overall result is a reduction in the patient's hematocrit to approximately 25%, with an increase in plasma volume of 40% to 50%. This decreases the total blood concentration of any free drug in the blood. When CPB is initiated, there is an immediate reduction in the levels of circulating proteins such as albumin and α_1-acid glycoprotein. This affects the protein binding of drugs because of alteration in the ratio of bound-to-free drug in the circulation

In the blood, free (ie, unbound) drug exists in equilibrium with bound (ie, bound to plasma proteins) drug. The free drug interacts with the receptor to produce the drug effect. Drugs primarily are bound to the plasma protein albumin and α_1-acid glycoprotein. Changes in protein binding are of clinical significance only for drugs that are highly protein bound. The degree of drug-protein binding depends on the total drug concentration, the affinity of the protein for the drug, and other substances that may compete with the drug or alter the drug's binding site. If the drug has a high degree of plasma protein binding, hemodilution results in a relatively larger increase in the free fraction than for a drug with a low affinity for plasma protein binding.

Blood Flow

Hepatic, renal, cerebral, and skeletal perfusion is reduced during CPB, and the use of vasodilators and vasoconstrictor agents to regulate arterial pressure may further change regional blood flow. Alterations in regional blood flow distribution have implications for drug distribution and metabolism. The combination of hypotension, hypothermia, and nonpulsatile blood flow significantly affects distribution of the circulation, with a marked reduction in peripheral flow and relative preservation of the central circulation.

CPB may be conducted with or without pulsatile perfusion. Nonpulsatile perfusion is associated with altered tissue perfusion. Nonpulsatile flow and decreased peripheral perfusion from CPB, hypothermia, and administration of vasoconstrictors may result in cellular hypoxia and probable intracellular acidosis. This may affect the tissue distribution of drugs whose tissue binding is sensitive to pH. On reperfusion, rewarming, and reestablishment of normal cardiac (pulsatile) function, redistribution of drugs from poorly perfused tissue is likely to add to the systemic plasma concentration because basic drugs have been trapped in acidic tissue.

Hypothermia

Hypothermia commonly is used and can reduce hepatic and possibly renal enzyme function. Hypothermia depresses metabolism by inhibiting enzyme function and reduces tissue perfusion by increasing blood viscosity and activation of autonomic and endocrine reflexes to produce vasoconstriction. Hepatic enzymatic activity is decreased during hypothermia, and there is marked intrahepatic redistribution of blood flow with the development of significant intrahepatic shunting. Hypothermia reduces metabolic drug clearance and has been shown to reduce the metabolism of propranolol and verapamil. Altered renal drug excretion occurs as a result of decreased renal perfusion, glomerular filtration rate (GFR), and tubular secretion. In dogs, GFR is decreased by 65% at 25°C.

Sequestration

When normothermia is reestablished, reperfusion of tissue may lead to washout of drugs sequestered during the hypothermic CPB period, which may explain the increase in opioid plasma levels during the rewarming period.

Many drugs bind to components of the CPB circuit, and their distribution may be affected by changes in circuit design, such as the use of oxygenators (ie, gas exchange devices) from different manufacturers. In vitro, various oxygenators bind lipophilic agents such as volatile anesthetic agents, propofol, opioids, and barbiturates. This phenomenon has never been demonstrated to be important in vivo, likely because any drug removed by the circuit is replaced from the much larger tissue reservoir.

During CPB, the lungs are isolated from the circulation, with the pulmonary artery blood flow being interrupted. Basic drugs (eg, lidocaine, propranolol, fentanyl) that are taken up by the lungs are sequestered during CPB, and the lungs can serve as a reservoir for drug release when systemic reperfusion is established. After the onset of CPB, plasma fentanyl concentrations decrease acutely and then plateau. However, when mechanical ventilation of the lungs is instituted before separation from CPB, plasma fentanyl concentrations increase. During CPB, pulmonary artery fentanyl concentrations exceed radial artery levels, but when mechanical ventilation resumes, the pulmonary artery-to-radial ratio is reversed, suggesting that fentanyl is being washed out from the lungs.

7

Specific Agents

Opioids

The total drug concentration of all opioids decreases on commencing CPB. The degree of decrease is greater with fentanyl, because a significant proportion of the drug adheres to the surface of the CPB circuit. Inadequate anesthesia has been described when fentanyl was used as the major anesthetic agent. There is high first-pass uptake of fentanyl by the lungs, and reperfusion of the lungs at the end of CPB results in increased fentanyl concentrations.

Benzodiazepines

The total concentration of benzodiazepines decreases on commencing CPB. Because the drugs are more than 90% protein bound, changes in free concentrations are greatly influenced by changes in protein concentrations or factors such as acid-base balance that influence protein binding. This is particularly pertinent in the context of CPB, but no studies have commented on free versus total concentrations of benzodiazepines.

Intravenous Anesthetic Agents

Total drug concentrations of thiopental and methohexital decrease on commencing CPB, but the active free concentrations are remarkably stable. Conflicting results have been obtained for propofol. The total concentration of propofol may decrease on commencing CPB with an increase in the free fraction, or the total concentration may remain unchanged. The free active concentrations of these drugs usually remain unchanged, but their actions may be prolonged.

Volatile Anesthetic Agents

The effect of CPB on MAC remains uncertain. Some researchers have shown that CPB reduces the MAC of enflurane by as much as 30%, whereas others have failed to demonstrate any reduction. Several groups have shown variation in MAC with temperature and found reduced volatile concentrations were required at lower temperatures.

The effect of CPB with cooling on the uptake of volatile anesthetics administered to the oxygenator depends on three factors: the blood/gas solubility of the agent and opposing effects of cooling in increasing blood/gas solubility of blood compared with hemodilution, which decreases the solubility of volatile anesthetics; the increased solubility in tissue of volatile anesthetics due to hypothermia; and uptake by the oxygenator. CPB produces changes in the blood/gas partition coefficient that depend on the prime used and the temperature. Volatile agents can bind to a variety of plastics, which may account for some of the decrease in concentrations on commencing CPB. A volatile agent started during hypothermic CPB takes longer to equilibrate, and agents already in use need to equilibrate, potentially changing the depth of anesthesia, until equilibration is complete. Because these agents are metabolized to a small degree and washout is fast, the duration of action is not prolonged after CPB.

Neuromuscular Blockers

CPB influences the concentrations and response relationships of neuromuscular blockers during hypothermia. The requirements for neuromuscular blockade are significantly reduced as a result of several pharmacokinetic and pharmacodynamic effects. Cooling affects cholinesterase enzyme activity, which is temperature dependent. The most important effect of cooling is decreased mobilization of acetylcholine. During hypothermia, less muscle relaxant is needed to obtain the same amount of muscle relaxation obtained in normothermic conditions. Cooling alters the mechanical properties of the muscle and has potentially significant effects on electrolytes, which modulate the contractile response.

CPB causes hemodilution, which may result in an initial decrease in the free drug concentration. The albumin concentration is also decreased during CPB, and although the total drug concentration may be decreased as a result of hemodilution, the free drug concentration may be increased if the drug is partially bound to albumin. This phenomenon may occur with neuromuscular blockers such as rocuronium.

SUGGESTED READINGS

Barletta JF, Miedema SL, Wiseman D, et al. Impact of dexmedetomidine on analgesic requirements in patients after cardiac surgery in a fast-track recovery room setting. *Pharmacotherapy*. 2009;29:1427–1432.

Bendel S, Ruokonen E, Polonen P, et al. Propofol causes more hypotension than etomidate in patients with severe aortic stenosis: a double-blind, randomized study comparing propofol and etomidate. *Acta Anaesthesiol Scand*. 2007;51:284–289.

Gerlach AT, Murphy C, Dasta JF. An updated focused review of dexmedetomidine in adults. *Ann Pharmacother*. 2009;43:2064–2074.

Healy DA, Kahn WA, Wong CS, et al. Remote preconditioning and major clinical complications following adult cardiovascular surgery: systematic review and meta-analysis. *Int J Cardiol*. 2014;176(1):20–31.

Hudetz JA, Patterson KM, Iqbal Z, et al. Ketamine attenuated delirium after cardiac surgery with cardio-pulmonary bypass. *J Cardiothorac Vasc Anesth*. 2009;23:651–657.

Kloner RA, Jennings RB. Consequences of brief ischemia: stunning, preconditioning, and their clinical implications: part 2. *Circulation*. 2001;104(25):3158–3167.

Kondo U, Kim SO, Nakayama M, et al. Pulmonary vascular effects of propofol at baseline, during elevated vasomotor tone, and in response to sympathetic alpha- and beta-adrenoreceptor activation. *Anesthesiology*. 2001;94(5):815–823.

Landoni G, Biondi-Zoccai G, Zangrillo A, et al. Desflurane and sevoflurane in cardiac surgery: a meta-analysis of randomized clinical trials. *J Cardiothorac Vasc Anesth*. 2007;21:502–511.

Landoni G, Fochi O, Torri G. Cardiac protection by volatile anaesthetics: a review. *Curr Vasc Pharmacol*. 2008;6:108–111.

Neuhauser C, Preiss V, Feurer MK, et al. Comparison of S-(+)-ketamine with sufentanil-based anaesthesia for elective coronary artery bypass graft surgery: effect on troponin T levels. *Br J Anaesth*. 2008;100:765–771.

Sprung J, Ogletree-Hughes ML, McConnell BK, et al. The effects of propofol on the contractility of failing and nonfailing human heart muscles. *Anesth Analg*. 2001;93(3):550–559.

Tanaka K, Ludwig LM, Kersten JR, et al. Mechanisms of cardioprotection by volatile anesthetics. *Anesthesiology*. 2004;100(3):707–721.

Thielmann M, Kottenberg E, Kleinbongard P, et al. Cardioprotective and prognostic effects of remote ischaemic preconditioning, double-blind, controlled trial. *Lancet*. 2013;382(9892):597–604.

Warltier DC, Kersten JR, Pagel PS, et al. Editorial view: anesthetic preconditioning: serendipity and science. *Anesthesiology*. 2002;97(1):1–3.

Zangrillo A, Musu M, Greco T, et al. Additive effects on survival of anaesthetic cardiac protection and remote ischemic preconditioning in cardiac surgery: a Bayesian meta-analysis of randomized trials. *PLoS ONE*. 2015;10(7):e0134264.

7

Chapter 8

Cardiovascular Pharmacology

Roger L. Royster, MD • Leanne Groban, MD •
Adair Q. Locke, MD • Benjamin N. Morris, MD •
Thomas F. Slaughter, MD

Key Points

1. Ischemia during the perioperative period demands immediate attention by the anesthesiologist.
2. Nitroglycerin is indicated in most cases of perioperative myocardial ischemia. Mechanisms of action include coronary vasodilation and favorable alterations in preload and afterload. Nitroglycerin is contraindicated in cases of hypotension.
3. Perioperative β-blockade may reduce the incidence of perioperative myocardial ischemia by several mechanisms when initiated at an appropriate time in the preoperative period. Favorable hemodynamic changes associated with β-blockade include blunting of the stress response and reduced heart rate, blood pressure, and contractility. All of these conditions improve myocardial oxygen supply-to-demand ratios.
4. Calcium channel blockers reduce myocardial oxygen demand by depression of contractility, reduction of heart rate, and decrease in arterial blood pressure. Calcium channel blockers are often administered in the perioperative period for long-term antianginal symptomatic control.
5. Mild or moderate hypertension does not represent an independent risk factor for perioperative complications, but a diagnosis of hypertension necessitates preoperative assessment for target organ damage.
6. Patients with poorly controlled preoperative hypertension experience more labile blood pressures in the perioperative setting with a greater potential for hypertensive and hypotensive episodes.
7. The signs, symptoms, and treatment of chronic heart failure are related to the neurohormonal response and underlying ventricular dysfunction.
8. Treatments for chronic heart failure are aimed at prolonging survival, along with relief of symptoms.
9. The pathophysiology, treatment, and prognosis of low cardiac output syndrome seen after cardiac surgery are different from those of chronic heart failure, with which it is sometimes compared.
10. Physicians must be cautious in administering antiarrhythmic drugs because their proarrhythmic effects can increase mortality for certain subgroups of patients.
11. Amiodarone has become a popular intravenous antiarrhythmic drug for use in the operating room and critical care areas because it has a broad range of effects for ventricular and supraventricular arrhythmias.
12. β-Receptor antagonists are effective but underused antiarrhythmics in the perioperative period because many arrhythmias are adrenergically mediated owing to the stress of surgery and critical illness.
13. Managing electrolyte abnormalities and treating underlying disease processes such as hypervolemia and myocardial ischemia are critical treatment steps before the administration of any antiarrhythmic agent.

■ ANTIISCHEMIC DRUG THERAPY

Perioperative myocardial ischemia is an anesthetic emergency that should be treated promptly with appropriate therapy. All events of myocardial ischemia involve an alteration in the oxygen supply-to-demand balance. For the anesthetized patient with evidence of myocardial ischemia, initiation of antiischemic drug therapy is the primary intervention.

Nitroglycerin

Nitroglycerin (NTG) is clinically indicated as initial therapy for most types of myocardial ischemia. During therapy with intravenous NTG, if blood pressure (BP) drops and ischemia is not relieved, the addition of phenylephrine allows coronary perfusion pressure to be maintained while allowing higher doses of NTG to be used for ischemia relief. If reflex increases in heart rate and contractility occur, combination therapy with β-adrenergic blockers may be indicated to blunt the undesired increase in heart rate. Combination therapy with nitrates and calcium channel blockers may be an effective antiischemic regimen in selected patients.

Mechanism of Action

NTG enhances myocardial oxygen delivery and reduces myocardial oxygen demand. NTG is a smooth muscle relaxant that causes vasculature dilation. Nitrate-mediated vasodilation occurs with or without intact vascular endothelium. Nitrites, organic nitrites, nitroso compounds, and other nitrogen oxide–containing substances (eg, nitroprusside) enter the smooth muscle cell and are converted to reactive nitric oxide (NO) or S-nitrosothiols, which stimulate guanylate cyclase metabolism to produce cyclic guanosine monophosphate (cGMP)(Fig. 8.1). A cGMP-dependent protein kinase is stimulated with resultant protein phosphorylation in the smooth muscle. This leads to a dephosphorylation of the myosin light chain and smooth muscle relaxation. Vasodilation is also associated with a reduction of intracellular calcium. Sulfhydryl (SH) groups are required for formation of NO and the stimulation of guanylate cyclase. When excessive amounts of SH groups are metabolized by prolonged exposure to NTG, vascular tolerance occurs. The addition of N-acetylcysteine, an SH donor, reverses NTG tolerance. The mechanism by which NTG compounds are uniquely better venodilators, especially at lower serum concentrations, is unknown but may be related to increased uptake of NTG by veins compared with arteries.

Physiologic Effects

Two important physiologic effects of NTG are systemic and regional venous dilation. Venodilation can markedly reduce venous pressure, venous return to the heart, and cardiac filling pressures. Prominent venodilation occurs at lower doses and does not increase further as the NTG dose increases. Venodilation results primarily in pooling of blood in the splanchnic capacitance system. Mesenteric blood volume increases as ventricular size, ventricular pressures, and intrapericardial pressure decrease.

NTG increases the distensibility and conductance of large arteries without changing systemic vascular resistance (SVR) at low doses. At higher doses, NTG dilates smaller arterioles and resistance vessels, reducing afterload and BP. Reductions in cardiac dimension and pressure reduce myocardial oxygen consumption ($M\dot{V}O_2$) and improve myocardial ischemia. NTG may preferentially reduce cardiac preload while maintaining systemic perfusion pressure, an important hemodynamic effect in myocardial ischemia. However, in hypovolemic states, higher doses of NTG may reduce systemic BP to dangerous levels. A reflex increase in heart rate may occur at arterial vasodilating doses.

8

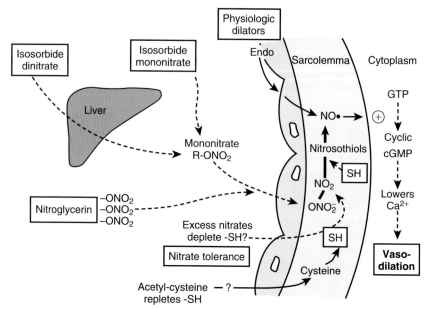

Fig. 8.1 Mechanisms of nitrates *(ONO₂)* in the generation of the free radical nitric oxide *(NO•)* and stimulation of guanylate cyclase cyclic guanosine monophosphate *(cGMP)*, which mediates vasodilation. Sulfhydryl *(SH)* groups are required for the formation of NO• and stimulation of guanylate cyclase. Isosorbide dinitrate is metabolized by the liver, whereas this route of metabolism is bypassed by the mononitrates. *Endo,* Endothelium; *GTP,* guanosine triphosphate. (Modified from Opie LH. *Drugs for the Heart.* 4th ed. Philadelphia: Saunders; 1995:33.)

NTG causes vasodilation of pulmonary arteries and veins and predictably decreases right atrial, pulmonary artery, and pulmonary capillary wedge pressures (PCWP). Pulmonary artery hypertension may be reduced by NTG in various disease states and in congenital heart disease. Renal arteries, cerebral arteries, and cutaneous vessels also dilate with NTG.

NTG has several important effects on the coronary circulation (Box 8.1). It is a potent epicardial coronary artery vasodilator in normal and diseased vessels. Stenotic lesions dilate with NTG, reducing the resistance to coronary blood flow (CBF) and improving myocardial ischemia. Smaller coronary arteries may dilate relatively more than larger coronary vessels, but the degree of dilation may depend on the baseline tone of the vessel. NTG effectively reverses or prevents coronary artery vasospasm.

Intravenous Nitroglycerin

NTG has been available since the early 1980s as a parenteral drug with a stable shelf half-life in a 400-µg/mL solution of 5% dextrose in water (D₅W). Blood levels are achieved instantaneously, and arterial dilating doses with resulting hypotension may quickly occur. If the volume status of the patient is unknown, initial doses of 5 to 10 µg/min are recommended. The dose necessary for relieving myocardial ischemia may vary from patient to patient, but relief is usually achieved with 75 to 150 µg/min. Arterial dilation becomes clinically apparent at doses around 150 µg/min. Drug offset after discontinuation of an infusion is rapid (2–5 minutes).

NTG remains a first-line agent for the treatment of myocardial ischemia. Special care must be taken in patients with signs of hypovolemia or hypotension because vasodilating effects of the drug may worsen the clinical condition (Box 8.2). The 2014

> ### BOX 8.1 *Effects of Nitroglycerin and Organic Nitrates on the Coronary Circulation*
>
> Epicardial coronary artery dilation: small arteries dilate proportionately more than larger arteries
> Increased coronary collateral vessel diameter and enhanced collateral flow
> Improved subendocardial blood flow
> Dilation of coronary atherosclerotic stenoses
> Initial short-lived increase in coronary blood flow; later reduction in coronary blood flow as myocardial oxygen consumption decreases
> Reversal and prevention of coronary vasospasm and vasoconstriction
>
> Modified from Abrams J. Hemodynamic effects of nitroglycerin and long-acting nitrates. *Am Heart J.* 1985;110(pt 2):216.

> ### BOX 8.2 *ACC/AHA Guidelines for Early Use of Nitroglycerin After STEMI*
>
> **Class I**
>
> 1. Patients with ongoing ischemic discomfort should receive sublingual nitroglycerin (0.4 mg) every 5 minutes for a total of three doses, after which an assessment should be made about the need for intravenous nitroglycerin (level of evidence [LOE] C).
> 2. Intravenous nitroglycerin is indicated for relief of ongoing ischemic discomfort, control of hypertension, or management of pulmonary congestion (LOE C).
>
> **Class III**
>
> 1. Nitrates should not be administered to patients with systolic blood pressure less than 90 mm Hg or greater than or equal to 30 mm Hg below baseline, severe bradycardia (<50 beats/min), tachycardia (>100 beats/min), or suspected right ventricular infarction (LOE C).
> 2. Nitrates should not be administered to patients who have received a phosphodiesterase inhibitor for erectile dysfunction within the last 24 hours (48 hours for tadalafil) (LOE B).
>
> *ACC,* American College of Cardiology; *AHA,* American Heart Association; *STEMI,* ST-segment elevation myocardial infarction.

8

American College of Cardiology/American Heart Association (ACC/AHA) guidelines address the prophylactic intraoperative use of NTG and state there is no benefit in preventing myocardial ischemia and cardiac morbidity in high-risk patients undergoing noncardiac surgery and that NTG use could be harmful.

β-Adrenergic Blockers

β-Adrenergic blockers have multiple favorable effects in treating the ischemic heart during anesthesia (Box 8.3). β-Adrenergic blockers reduce oxygen consumption by

BOX 8.3 *Effects of β-Adrenergic Blockers on Myocardial Ischemia*

Reductions in myocardial oxygen consumption
Improvements in coronary blood flow
Prolonged diastolic perfusion period
Improved collateral flow
Increased flow to ischemic areas
Overall improvement in the supply-to-demand ratio
Stabilization of cellular membranes
Improved oxygen dissociation from hemoglobin
Inhibition of platelet aggregation
Reduced mortality rate after myocardial infarction

decreasing heart rate, BP, and myocardial contractility. Heart rate reduction increases diastolic CBF. Increased collateral blood flow and redistribution of blood to ischemic areas may occur with β-blockers. β-Blockers should be started early in ischemic patients in the absence of contraindications. If hemodynamics prevent concomitant NTG and β-blocker use, β-blockers should receive precedence. Many patients at high risk for perioperative cardiac morbidity should be started on β-blockers before surgery and continued for up to 30 days after surgery. Adequate time in initiating β-blocker therapy should be allowed to adjust dosing before surgical procedures.

Many studies have shown that perioperative administration of β-adrenergic blockers reduces mortality and morbidity when given to patients at high risk for coronary artery disease (CAD) who must undergo noncardiac surgery. These data suggest that intermediate- and high-risk patients undergoing noncardiac surgery should receive perioperative β-adrenergic blockade to reduce postoperative cardiac mortality and morbidity.

Pharmacology of Intravenous β-Adrenergic Blockers

PROPRANOLOL

Propranolol has an equal affinity for β_1- and β_2-receptors, lacks intrinsic sympathomimetic activity (ISA), and has no β-adrenergic receptor activity (Table 8.1). It is the most lipid-soluble β-blocker and has the most central nervous system (CNS) side effects. Because the rate of first-pass liver metabolism is very high (90%), it requires much higher oral doses than intravenous doses for pharmacodynamic effect. The usual intravenous dose of propranolol initially is 0.5 to 1.0 mg titrated to effect. A titrated dose resulting in maximal pharmacologic serum levels is 0.1 mg/kg.

METOPROLOL

Metoprolol was the first clinically used cardioselective β-blocker. Its affinity for β_1-receptors is 30 times higher than its affinity for β_2-receptors. As with any cardioselective β-blocker, higher serum levels may result in greater incidence of β_2-blocking effects. Metoprolol is administered intravenously in 1- to 2-mg doses, titrated to effect. The potency of metoprolol is approximately one-half that of propranolol. Maximal β-blocker effect is achieved with 0.2 mg/kg given intravenously.

Table 8.1 Properties of β-Blockers in Clinical Use

Drug	Selectivity	Partial Agonist Activity	Usual Dose for Angina
Propranolol	None	No	20–80 mg bid
Metoprolol	β_1	No	50–200 mg bid
Atenolol	β_1	No	50–200 mg/d
Nadolol	None	No	40–80 mg/d
Timolol	None	No	10 mg bid
Acebutolol	β_1	Yes	200–600 mg bid
Betaxolol	β_1	No	10–20 mg/d
Bisoprolol	β_1	No	10 mg/d
Esmolol (infusion)	β_1	No	50–300 $\mu g \cdot kg^{-1} \cdot min^{-1}$
Labetalol[a]	None	Yes	200–600 mg tid
Pindolol	None	Yes	2.5–7.5 mg tid

[a]Labetalol is a combined α- and β-blocker.
Modified from Gibbons RJ, Chatterjee K, Daley J, Douglas JS. ACC/AHA/ACP-ASIM guidelines for the management of patients with chronic stable angina: a report of the American College of Cardiology/American Heart Association Task Force on Practice Guidelines (Committee on Management of Patients with Chronic Stable Angina). *J Am Coll Cardiol.* 1999;33:2092–2197.

ESMOLOL

The chemical structure of esmolol is similar to that of metoprolol and propranolol, except that it has a methyl ester group in the para-position of the phenyl ring, making it susceptible to rapid hydrolysis by red blood cell esterases (ie, 9-minute half-life). Esmolol is not metabolized by plasma cholinesterase. Hydrolysis results in an acid metabolite and methanol with clinically insignificant levels. Ninety percent of the drug is eliminated in the form of the acid metabolite, normally within 24 hours. A loading dose of 500 µg/kg given intravenously followed by a 50 to 300 µg/kg per minute infusion reaches steady-state concentrations within 5 minutes. Without the loading dose, steady-state concentrations are reached in 30 minutes.

Esmolol is cardioselective, blocking primarily β_1-receptors. It lacks ISA and membrane-stabilizing effects and is mildly lipid soluble. Esmolol produced significant reductions in BP, heart rate, and the cardiac index after a loading dose of 500 µg/kg and an infusion of 300 µg/kg per minute in patients with CAD, and the effects were completely reversed 30 minutes after discontinuation of the infusion. Initial therapy during anesthesia may require significant reductions in the loading and infusion doses.

Hypotension is a common side effect of intravenous esmolol. The incidence of hypotension was higher with esmolol (36%) than with propranolol (6%) at equal therapeutic end points. The cardioselective drugs may cause more hypotension because of β_1-induced myocardial depression and the failure to block β_2 peripheral vasodilation. Therefore administering a test dose of 20 mg IV is a good clinical practice.

LABETALOL

Labetalol is an equal mixture of four stereoisomers with various α- and β-blocking properties. Labetalol provides selective α_1-receptor blockade and nonselective β_1- and β_2-blockade. The potency of β-adrenergic blockade is 5- to 10-fold greater than α_1-adrenergic blockade. Labetalol has partial β_2-agonist effects that promote vasodilation. It is moderately lipid soluble and is completely absorbed after oral administration. First-pass hepatic metabolism is significant, with production of inactive metabolites.

Renal excretion of the unchanged drug is minimal. Elimination half-life is approximately 6 hours.

In contrast to other β-blockers, labetalol should be considered a peripheral vasodilator that does not cause a reflex tachycardia. BP and systolic vascular resistance decrease after an intravenous dose. Stroke volume (SV) and cardiac output (CO) remain unchanged, with the heart rate decreasing slightly. The reduction in BP is dose related, and acutely hypertensive patients usually respond within 3 to 5 minutes after a bolus dose of 100 to 250 μg/kg. However, the more critically ill or anesthetized patients should have their BP titrated, beginning with 5- to 10-mg intravenous increments. The BP reduction may last as long as 6 hours after intravenous dosing.

Summary

β-Adrenergic blockers are first-line agents in the treatment of myocardial ischemia. These agents effectively reduce myocardial work and oxygen demand. Although perioperative β-blockers may decrease perioperative cardiovascular events in noncardiac surgery, the benefit may come at an increased short-term risk for severe complications, including stroke and death if started too close to the time of surgery.

Calcium Channel Blockers

Calcium channel blockers reduce myocardial oxygen demands by depression of contractility, heart rate, and arterial BP. Myocardial oxygen supply may be improved by dilation of coronary and collateral vessels. In an acute ischemic situation, calcium channel blockers (ie, verapamil and diltiazem) may be used for rate control when β-blockers cannot be used.

The most important effects of calcium channel blockers may be the treatment of variant angina. These drugs can attenuate ergonovine-induced coronary vasoconstriction in patients with variant angina, suggesting protection by coronary dilation. Most episodes of silent myocardial ischemia, which may account for 70% of all transient ischemic episodes, are not related to increases in myocardial oxygen demands (ie, heart rate and BP); instead, intermittent obstruction of coronary flow is likely caused by coronary vasoconstriction or spasm. All calcium channel blockers are effective at reversing coronary spasm, reducing ischemic episodes, and reducing NTG consumption in patients with variant or Prinzmetal angina.

Combinations of NTG and calcium channel blockers, which also effectively relieve and possibly prevent coronary spasm, are rational therapy for variant angina. β-Blockers may aggravate anginal episodes in some patients with vasospastic angina and should be used with caution. Preservation of CBF with calcium channel blockers is a significant difference from the predominant β-blocker antiischemic effects of reducing $M\dot{V}O_2$.

Physiologic Effects

HEMODYNAMIC EFFECTS

Systemic hemodynamic effects of calcium channel blockers in vivo represent a complex interaction among myocardial depression, vasodilation, and reflex activation of the autonomic nervous system (Table 8.2).

Nifedipine, like all dihydropyridines (DHPs), is a potent arterial dilator with few venodilating effects. Reflex activation of the sympathetic nervous system (SNS) may increase heart rate. The intrinsic negative inotropic effect of nifedipine is offset by potent arterial dilation, which lowers BP and increases CO in patients. DHPs are excellent antihypertensive agents because of their arterial vasodilatory effects. Antianginal effects result from reduced myocardial oxygen requirements owing to

Table 8.2 Calcium Channel Blocker Vasodilator Potency and Inotropic, Chronotropic, and Dromotropic Effects on the Heart

Characteristic	Amlodipine	Diltiazem	Nifedipine	Verapamil
Heart rate	↑/0	↓	↑/0	↓
Sinoatrial node conduction	0	↓↓	0	↓
Atrioventricular node conduction	0	↓	0	↓
Myocardial contractility	↓/0	↓	↓/0	↓↓
Neurohormonal activation	↑/0	↑	↑	↑
Vascular dilatation	↑↑	↑	↑↑	↑
Coronary flow	↑	↑	↑	↑

0, No effect.
From Eisenberg MJ, Brox A, Bestawros AN. Calcium channel blockers: an update. *Am J Med.* 2004;116:35–43.

the afterload-reducing effect and to coronary vascular dilation resulting in improved myocardial oxygen delivery.

Verapamil is a less potent arterial dilator than the DHPs and results in less reflex sympathetic activation. In vivo, verapamil usually results in moderate vasodilation without significant changes in heart rate, CO, or SV. Verapamil can significantly depress myocardial function in patients with preexisting ventricular dysfunction.

Diltiazem is a less potent vasodilator and has fewer negative inotropic effects compared with verapamil. Clinical studies reveal reductions in SVR and BP, with increases in CO, pulmonary arterial wedge pressure, and ejection fraction (EF).

CORONARY BLOOD FLOW

Coronary artery dilation occurs with the calcium channel blockers, along with increases in total CBF. Nifedipine is the most potent coronary vasodilator, especially in epicardial vessels, which are prone to coronary vasospasm. Diltiazem is effective in blocking coronary artery vasoconstriction caused by a variety of agents, including α-agonists, serotonin, prostaglandin, and acetylcholine.

Pharmacology

NICARDIPINE

Nicardipine is a DHP agent with vascular selectivity for coronary and cerebrovascular beds. Nicardipine may be the most potent overall relaxant of vascular smooth muscle among the DHPs. Peak plasma levels are reached 1 hour after oral administration, with bioavailability of 35%. Plasma half-life is approximately 8 to 9 hours. Although the drug undergoes extensive hepatic metabolism, with less than 1% of the drug excreted renally, greater renal elimination occurs in some patients. Plasma levels may increase in patients with renal failure, and reduction of the dose is recommended in these patients.

CLEVIDIPINE

Clevidipine is a DHP agent with a unique chemical structure that renders it inactive by cleavage of an ester linkage by nonspecific esterases in the blood and in tissues.

This unique property renders it extremely short acting, similar to other drugs (eg, esmolol) that are metabolized through this pathway. Its initial phase half-life is 1 minute, with 90% of the drug eliminated. Its clinical effects are fully reversed in 5 to 15 minutes for most patients after discontinuing the infusion.

Clevidipine is a potent arterial vasodilator whose primary use is as a parenteral antihypertensive agent. A reflexive tachycardia may be seen with its use in healthy volunteers and patients with essential hypertension that, combined with possible hypotension, would limit its role in treating ongoing myocardial ischemia. In studies looking at perioperative and postoperative cardiac surgical patients, clevidipine was effective in decreasing mean arterial pressure but did not affect heart rate or filling pressures.

VERAPAMIL

The structure of verapamil is similar to that of papaverine. Verapamil exhibits significant first-pass hepatic metabolism, with a bioavailability of only 10% to 20%. One hepatic metabolite, norverapamil, is active and has a potency approximately 20% of that of verapamil. Peak plasma levels are reached within 30 minutes. Bioavailability markedly increases in hepatic insufficiency, mandating reduced doses. Intravenous verapamil achieves hemodynamic and dromotropic effects within minutes, peaking at 15 minutes and lasting up to 6 hours. Accumulation of the drug occurs with prolonged half-life during long-term oral administration.

DILTIAZEM

After oral dosing, the bioavailability of diltiazem is greater than that of verapamil, varying between 25% and 50%. Peak plasma concentration is achieved between 30 and 60 minutes, and the elimination half-life is 2 to 6 hours. Protein binding is approximately 80%. As with verapamil, hepatic clearance is flow dependent, and major hepatic metabolism occurs, with metabolites having 40% of the clinical activity of diltiazem. Hepatic disease may require decreased dosing, whereas renal failure does not affect dosing.

▓ DRUG THERAPY FOR SYSTEMIC HYPERTENSION

Systemic hypertension, long recognized as a leading cause of cardiovascular morbidity and mortality, accounts for enormous health-related expenditures. Almost one-fourth of the US population has hypertensive vascular disease, but 30% of these individuals are unaware of their condition, and another 30% to 50% are inadequately treated. On a worldwide basis, almost 1 billion individuals are hypertensive. Hypertension management comprises the most common reason underlying adult visits to primary care physicians, and antihypertensive drugs are the most prescribed medication class. Despite the asymptomatic nature of hypertensive disease, with symptom onset delayed 20 to 30 years after development of systemic hypertension, substantial and incontrovert-ible evidence demonstrates a direct association between systemic hypertension and increased morbidity and mortality. The World Health Organization (WHO) estimates that hypertension underlies one in eight deaths worldwide, making elevated BP the third leading cause of mortality.

Hypertension is the single most treatable risk factor for myocardial infarction (MI), stroke, peripheral vascular disease, congestive heart failure (CHF), renal failure, and aortic dissection. In prospective, randomized trials, over the course of adult lifetimes, successful treatment of hypertension has been associated with a 35% to 40% reduction in the incidence of stroke, 50% reduction in CHF, and 25% reduction in MIs. Improved treatment of hypertension has been credited with the major reductions in stroke and cardiovascular mortality occurring in the United States during the past 30 years.

The Eighth Report of the Joint National Committee on Prevention, Detection, Evaluation, and Treatment of High Blood Pressure (JNC8) provided significant modifications to prior recommendations for the management of high BP. In contrast to prior guidelines, JNC8 recommendations are derived from evidence-based guidelines drawn only from randomized, controlled trials (RCTs). Specific recommendations emanating from the new guidelines include lifestyle interventions and pharmacologic treatment as needed to attain systolic BPs less than 150 mm Hg and diastolic BPs less than 90 mm Hg for adults 60 years of age and older. For younger patients and those with diabetes or chronic kidney disease, treatment goals include systolic BPs less than 140 mm Hg and diastolic BPs less than 90 mm Hg.

Although antihypertensive drug therapy is widely regarded as essential for BPs greater than 150/90 mm Hg, evidence suggests benefits to more aggressive BP reduction for certain patient subsets. The association between systemic BP and cardiovascular risk has been described as a J curve, with progressive cardiovascular risk reductions accompanying BP reductions until a critical threshold, after which the potential for myocardial ischemia and other organ injury increases. Risk for cardiovascular disease appears to increase at BPs greater than 115/75 mm Hg, with a doubling in risk associated with each 20/10-mm Hg increment in systemic pressure.

Medical Treatment for Hypertension

Almost 80 distinct medications are marketed for the treatment of hypertension. Combined therapy with two or more classes of antihypertensive medications is often needed to achieve treatment goals. Although the specific drug selected for initial therapy is deemed less important than in the past, recognition that specific antihypertensive drug classes alleviate end-organ damage beyond that associated with reductions in systemic BP has led to targeted selection of antihypertensive drug combinations on the basis of coexisting risk factors such as recent MI, chronic renal insufficiency, or diabetes.

Management of Severe Hypertension

Severe hypertension may be characterized as a *hypertensive emergency,* with target organ injury (eg, myocardial ischemia, stroke, pulmonary edema), or as *hypertensive urgency,* with severe elevations in BP not yet associated with target organ damage. Specific BPs associated with these conditions prove somewhat arbitrary, but BPs exceeding 220/125 mm Hg pose an immediate risk for life-threatening end-organ damage. A hypertensive emergency necessitates immediate therapeutic intervention, most often with intravenous antihypertensive therapy and invasive arterial BP monitoring. In the most extreme cases of *malignant hypertension,* severe elevations in BP may be associated with retinal hemorrhages, papilledema, and evidence of encephalopathy, which may include headache, vomiting, seizure, and coma. Progressive renal failure and cardiac decompensation may characterize the most severe hypertensive urgencies.

Sodium nitroprusside, long favored as a parenteral treatment for hypertensive urgencies in intraoperative settings (Table 8.3), acts as an NO donor to induce arterial and venous dilation. A rapid physiologic response and relatively predictable titratable effect prove useful for intraoperative settings. However, the potency of sodium nitroprusside and the potential for prolonged administration to be associated with

8

Table 8.3 Parenteral Drugs for Treating Hypertensive Emergencies[a]

Drug	Dose	Onset of Action	Duration of Action	Adverse Effects[b]	Special Indications
Nicardipine hydrochloride	5–15 mg/h IV	5–10 min	15–30 min, may exceed 4 h	Tachycardia, headache, flushing, local phlebitis	Most hypertensive emergencies except acute heart failure; caution with coronary ischemia
Clevidipine	1–2 mg/h IV	2–4 min	5–15 min	Headache, nausea, vomiting, soy and egg allergy cross-reactivities	Most hypertensive emergencies except severe aortic stenosis
Sodium nitroprusside	0.25–10 µg/kg per minute as IV infusion[c]	Immediate	1–2 min	Nausea, vomiting, muscle twitching, sweating, thiocyanate and cyanide intoxication	Most hypertensive emergencies; caution with high intracranial pressure or azotemia
Fenoldopam mesylate	0.1–0.3 µg/kg per min IV infusion	<5 min	30 min	Tachycardia, headache, nausea, flushing	Most hypertensive emergencies; caution with glaucoma
Nitroglycerin	5–100 µg/min as IV infusion	2–5 min	5–10 min	Headache, vomiting, methemoglobinemia, tolerance with prolonged use	Coronary ischemia
Enalaprilat	1.25–5 mg every 6 h IV	15–30 min	6–12 h	Precipitous fall in pressure in high-renin states; variable response	Acute left ventricular failure; avoid in acute myocardial infarction
Hydralazine hydrochloride	10–20 mg IV / 10–40 mg IM	10–20 min IV / 20–30 min IM	1–4 h IV / 4–6 h IM	Tachycardia, flushing, headache, vomiting, aggravation of angina	Eclampsia

Adrenergic Inhibitors

Labetalol hydrochloride	20–80 mg IV bolus every 10 min	5–10 min	3–6 h	Vomiting, scalp tingling, dizziness, nausea, heart block, orthostatic hypotension, bronchoconstriction	Most hypertensive emergencies except acute heart failure
Esmolol hydrochloride	0.5–2.0 mg/min IV infusion 250–500 µg/kg per minute IV bolus, then 50–100 µg/kg per minute by infusion; may repeat bolus after 5 min or increase infusion to 300 µg/min	1–2 min	10–30 min	Hypotension, nausea, asthma, first-degree heart block, heart failure	Aortic dissection, perioperative
Phentolamine	5–15 mg IV bolus	1–2 min	10–30 min	Tachycardia, flushing, headache	Catecholamine excess

[a]Doses may vary from those in the *Physicians Desk Reference* (PDR).
[b]Hypotension may occur with all agents.
[c]Requires special delivery system.
IM, Intramuscular route; *IV*, intravenous route.
Modified from Chobanian AV, Bakris GL, Black HR, et al. Seventh Report of the Joint National Committee on Prevention, Detection, Evaluation, and Treatment of High Blood Pressure. *Hypertension.* 2003;42:1206.

8

cyanide or thiocyanate toxicity have provided an opportunity for newer parenteral antihypertensive drugs.

Nicardipine and clevidipine, parenteral DHP calcium channel blockers, have proved particularly applicable for hypertensive urgencies in perioperative settings. Although less potent and predictable than sodium nitroprusside, NTG, another NO donor, may be preferable in the setting of myocardial ischemia or after coronary artery bypass graft (CABG) surgery.

PHARMACOTHERAPY FOR ACUTE AND CHRONIC HEART FAILURE

Chronic heart failure (HF) is a major cardiovascular disorder that continues to increase in incidence and prevalence in the United States and worldwide. It affects almost 5.7 million persons in the United States, with 870,000 new cases annually among those 55 years of age or older. Currently, 1% to 2% of those between 40 and 59 years of age and 11% to 14% of individuals older than 80 years have HF. Because HF is primarily a disease of the elderly, its prevalence is projected to increase 46% from 2012 to 2030, resulting in more than 8 million people with HF, paralleling the substantial increase in growth of this population sector.

The increasingly prolonged survival of patients with various cardiovascular disorders that culminate in ventricular dysfunction (eg, patients with CAD are living longer rather than dying acutely with MI), and the greater diagnostic awareness further compound the HF epidemic. By age 40, the lifetime risk of developing HF for men and women is one in five, and this risk remains constant into the 80s, even in the face of a much shorter life expectancy. Despite improvements in the understanding of the neurohormonal mechanisms underlying its pathophysiology and remarkable advances made in pharmacologic therapy, HF continues to cost the United States an estimated $31 billion annually in medical expenditures, and it is projected to increase 127% (almost $70 million) by 2030.

The pharmacologic management of HF was revised in the 2013 guidelines published by the American College of Cardiology Foundation and the American Heart Association (ACCF/AHA). The focus is primarily on chronic HF with a reduced EF (HFrEF) and HF with a preserved EF (HFpEF), although acute HF is also discussed.

Heart Failure Classification

The ACCF/AHA guidelines for evaluating and managing HF include the four-stage classification system, which emphasizes the evolution and progression of the disease (Fig. 8.2), and the New York Heart Association (NYHA) classification (Table 8.4), which focuses on exercise capacity and symptomatic severity of the disease. The four-stage classification system calls attention to patients with preclinical stages of HF to focus on halting disease progression. By recognizing its progressive course and identifying those who are at risk (ie, the first two stages, A and B, are clearly not HF), it reinforces the importance of determining the optimal strategy for neurohormonal antagonism in an attempt to improve the natural history of the syndrome.

Pathophysiologic Role of the Renin-Angiotensin System in Heart Failure

The renin-angiotensin system (RAS) is one of several neuroendocrine systems that are activated in patients with HF. The RAS is also an important mediator in the

Table 8.4   Comparison of ACCF/AHA Stages of Heart Failure and New York Heart Association (NYHA) Functional Classifications

ACCF/AHA Stages of Heart Failure		NYHA Functional Classification	
Stage	Definition	Class	Definition
A	At high risk for HF but without structural heart disease or symptoms of HF	None	
B	Structural heart disease but without signs or symptoms of HF	I	No limitation of physical activity; ordinary physical activity does not cause HF symptoms
C	Structural heart disease with prior or current HF symptoms	I	No limitation of physical activity; ordinary physical activity does not cause HF symptoms
		II	Slight limitation of physical activity; comfortable at rest, but ordinary physical activity results in HF symptoms
		III	Marked limitation of physical activity; comfortable at rest, but less than ordinary activity causes HF symptoms
		IV	Unable to carry on any physical activity without HF symptoms or symptoms of HF at rest
D	Refractory HF requiring specialized interventions		Unable to carry on any physical activity without HF symptoms or symptoms of HF at rest

ACCF/AHA, American College of Cardiology Foundation/American Heart Association; HF, heart failure; NYHA, New York Heart Association.
From Yancy CW, Jessup M, Bozkurt B, et al. 2013 ACCF/AHA Guideline for the Management of Heart Failure: a report of the American College of Cardiology Foundation/American Heart Association Task Force on Practice Guidelines. Circulation. 2013;128:e240.

progression of HF. In the short term, the juxtaglomerular cells of the kidney release the proteolytic enzyme renin in response to a decrease in BP or renal perfusion (eg, hemorrhage), generating angiotensin (Ang) I from circulating angiotensinogen. Angiotensin-converting enzyme (ACE) cleavage of Ang II from Ang I in the lung produces circulating Ang II. Acutely, Ang II acts as a potent arteriolar and venous vasoconstrictor to return BP and filling pressure to baseline, respectively. Ang II also stimulates the release of aldosterone from the adrenal cortex and antidiuretic hormone from the posterior pituitary. Both contribute to increases in blood volume through their effects on the kidney to promote salt and water reabsorption, respectively. In the long term, elevations in Ang II lead to sodium and fluid retention and increases in SVR, which contribute to symptoms of HF, pulmonary congestion, and hemodynamic decompensation.

In addition to the cardiorenal and cardiocirculatory effects, most of the hormones and receptors of the RAS are expressed in the myocardium, where they contribute to maladaptive growth or remodeling, a key factor in the progression of HF. Increased

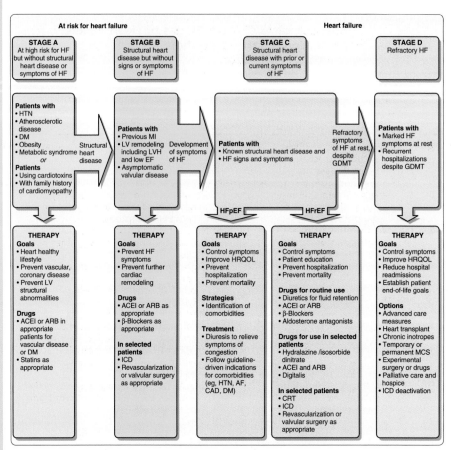

Fig. 8.2 Stages in the development of heart failure *(HF)* and recommended therapy by stage. *ACEI*, Angiotensin-converting enzyme inhibitor; *AF*, atrial fibrillation; *ARB*, angiotensin-receptor blocker; *CAD*, coronary artery disease; *CRT*, cardiac resynchronization therapy; *DM*, diabetes mellitus; *EJ*, ejection fraction; *GDMT*, guideline-directed medical therapy; *HFpEF*, heart failure with preserved ejection fraction; *HFrEF*, heart failure with reduced ejection fraction; *HRQOL*, heart-related quality of life; *HTN*, hypertension; *ICD*, implantable cardioverter-defibrillator; *LV*, left ventricular; *LVH*, left ventricular hypertrophy; *MCS*, mechanical circulatory system; *MI*, myocardial infarction. (From Yancy CW, Jessup M, Bozkurt B, et al. 2013 ACCF/AHA Guideline for the Management of Heart Failure: a report of the American College of Cardiology Foundation/American Heart Association Task Force on practice guidelines. *Circulation.* 2013;128:e240.)

expression of mRNA for angiotensinogen, ACE, and Ang II has been identified in the failing human heart. Moreover, progressive increases in coronary sinus Ang II production correlated with increases in NYHA functional classification of HF. These data provide evidence that intracardiac RAS is involved in the evolution of the disease process (Fig. 8.3).

The Ang II that is formed locally in the heart acts primarily through AT_1 receptors located on myocytes and fibroblasts, where it participates in the regulation of cardiac remodeling. The long-term effects of intracardiac Ang II on the AT_1 receptor result in cardiomyocyte hypertrophy, fibroblast proliferation, and extracellular matrix deposition (Fig. 8.3). These processes contribute to progressive left ventricular (LV) remodeling and LV dysfunction characteristic of HF.

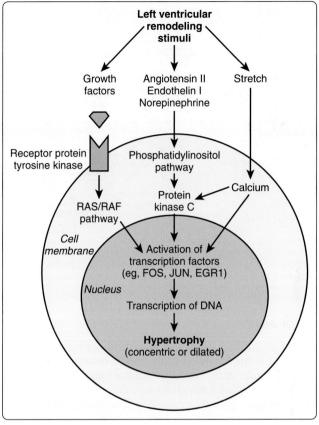

Fig. 8.3 Left ventricular remodeling stimuli.

Angiotensin-Converting Enzyme Inhibitors

CLINICAL EVIDENCE

Evidence supporting the beneficial use of ACE inhibitors in HF patients comes from various randomized, placebo-controlled clinical trials. Patients with NYHA class II to IV HF treated with ACE inhibitors had reductions in mortality ranging from 16% to 31%. ACE inhibitors were also found to improve outcomes for asymptomatic patients with LV systolic dysfunction in the following categories: patients with EFs less than 35% due to cardiomyopathy, patients within 2 weeks after MI with EFs less than 40%, and patients within the first 24 hours of MI regardless of EF.

Results from the Heart Outcomes Prevention Evaluation (HOPE) study further expanded the indications for this class of agents to include asymptomatic, high-risk patients to prevent new-onset HF. In patients with diabetes or peripheral vascular disease and an additional atherosclerotic risk factor but without clinical HF or systolic dysfunction, ramipril (10 mg/day) reduced the HF risk by 23%. Since the commencement of these trials, the rationale for the use of ACE inhibitors has expanded from a reduction in the progression of clinical HF through ACE inhibitor–mediated vasodilatory action to acknowledgment that ACE inhibitors also directly affect the cellular mechanisms responsible for progressive myocardial pathology.

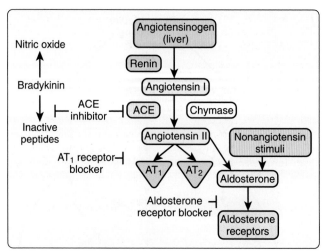

Fig. 8.4   Activation of the renin-angiotensin-aldosterone system (RAAS). *ACE,* Angiotensin-converting enzyme; *AT₁,* angiotensin I receptor; *AT₂,* angiotensin II receptor. (Modified from Mann DL. *Heart Therapy: A Companion to Braunwald's Heart Disease.* Philadelphia: Saunders; 2004.)

MECHANISMS OF ACTION

ACE inhibitors act by inhibiting one of several proteases responsible for cleaving the decapeptide Ang I to form the octapeptide Ang II. Because ACE is also the enzyme that degrades bradykinin, ACE inhibitors increase circulating and tissue levels of bradykinin (Fig. 8.4). ACE inhibitors have several useful effects in chronic HF. They are potent vasodilators through decreasing Ang II and norepinephrine and increasing bradykinin, NO, and prostacyclin. By reducing the secretion of aldosterone and antidiuretic hormone, ACE inhibitors also reduce salt and water reabsorption from the kidney. ACE inhibitors reduce release of norepinephrine from sympathetic nerves by acting on AT_1 receptors at the nerve terminal. In tissue, ACE inhibitors inhibit Ang II production and attenuate Ang II–mediated cardiomyocyte hypertrophy and fibroblast hyperplasia.

Angiotensin II Receptor Blockers for Heart Failure

PATHOPHYSIOLOGY AND MECHANISM OF ACTION

Although ACE inhibitors reduce mortality, many patients do not tolerate their side effects. ACE inhibitors incompletely antagonize Ang II. These factors have prompted the development of specific Ang II receptor blockers (ARBs) for the pharmacologic treatment of HF. Non–ACE-generated Ang II within the myocardium contributes to LV remodeling and HF progression through AT_1 receptor effects. Selective AT_1 blockers prevent Ang II from acting on the cell, preventing vasoconstriction, sodium retention, release of norepinephrine, and delaying or preventing LV hypertrophy and fibrosis. AT_2 receptors remain unaffected, and their actions, including NO release, remain intact.

CLINICAL PRACTICE

ARBs are used as alternatives to ACE inhibitors for the treatment of patients with symptomatic HF if there are side effects to ACE inhibitors (eg, persistent cough, angioedema, hyperkalemia, worsening renal dysfunction). An ARB may be used as an alternative to an ACE inhibitor in patients who are already taking an ARB for another reason, such as hypertension, and who subsequently develop HF. Because ARBs do not affect bradykinin levels, cough and angioedema are rare side effects.

Aldosterone Receptor Antagonists

Aldosterone, a mineralocorticoid, is another important component of the neurohormonal hypothesis of HF. Although it was previously assumed that treatment with an ACE inhibitor (or ARB) would block the production of aldosterone in patients with HF, elevated levels of aldosterone have been measured despite inhibition of Ang II.

Adverse effects of elevated aldosterone levels on the cardiovascular system include sodium retention, potassium and magnesium loss, ventricular remodeling (eg, collagen production, myocyte growth, hypertrophy), myocardial norepinephrine release, and endothelial dysfunction.

Given the multiple endocrine and autocrine or paracrine contributions of aldosterone to the neurohormonal hypothesis of HF, the possibility that aldosterone receptor antagonism might halt disease progression became an increasingly attractive hypothesis. Besides the traditional mechanisms of mineralocorticoid receptor blockade, including natriuresis, diuresis, and kaliuresis, beneficial nonrenal effects of aldosterone antagonism include decreased myocardial collagen formation, increased myocardial norepinephrine uptake and decreased circulating norepinephrine levels, normalization of baroreceptor function, increased heart rate variability, and improved endothelial vasodilator dysfunction and basal NO bioactivity at the vascular level.

CLINICAL PRACTICE

Evidence supports aldosterone antagonists for patients with symptomatic HF and patients with LV dysfunction after MI. Aldosterone receptor antagonists should be considered in addition to standard therapy (including ACE inhibitors and β-blockers) in patients with NYHA II disease who have prior cardiovascular hospitalization or elevated brain natriuretic peptide (BNP) levels and those with NYHA IV HF and an EF of 35% or less, unless contraindicated. Class I recommendations also pertain to patients after an acute MI with an EF of 40% or less who develop HF symptoms or who have a history of diabetes, unless contraindicated.

Combination Approaches With Renin-Angiotensin System Inhibition

Angiotensin receptor–neprilysin inhibitors (ARNIs) offer treatment for HF that involves neprilysin inhibition and AT_1 receptor blockade. ARNIs can modulate two counter-regulatory neurohormonal systems in HF: the renin-angiotensin-aldosterone system (RAAS) and natriuretic peptide system (Fig. 8.5). Drugs that inhibit the RAAS have been foundational to cardiovascular drug therapy for almost three decades. RAAS inhibitors moderate vasoconstriction, myocyte hypertrophy, and myocardial fibrosis, an effect that has translated into clinically meaningful improvements in functional status and survival. Natriuretic peptides, which include atrial natriuretic peptide, BNP, and urodilatin, are secreted by the heart, vasculature, kidney, and CNS in response to increased cardiac wall stress and other stimuli. Natriuretic peptides have potent natriuretic and vasodilatory properties, inhibit the RAAS, reduce sympathetic drive, and have antiproliferative and antihypertrophic effects. Neprilysin inhibition results in an increased concentration of natriuretic peptides. The beneficial effects of RAAS inhibition are likely to be augmented by the enhancement of natriuretic peptide activity.

Entresto (LCZ696) is the first and most clinically developed agent in the new class of ARNI compounds. The chemical entity comprises anionic moieties of the neprilysin inhibitor prodrug AHU377 and the ARB valsartan in a fixed-dose combination in a 1 : 1 ratio. It was recently reported that LCZ696 was more effective than enalapril in

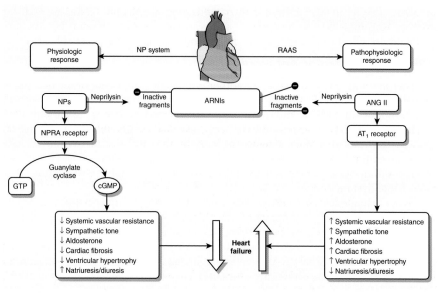

Fig. 8.5 Angiotensin receptor–neprilysin inhibitors *(ARNIs)* can modulate two counterregulatory neurohormonal systems in heart failure: the renin-angiotensin-aldosterone system *(RAAS)* and the natriuretic peptide *(NP)* system (eg, atrial NP, B-type NP). *ANG,* angiotensin; *AT$_1$,* angiotensin I receptor; *cGMP,* cyclic guanosine monophosphate; *GTP,* guanosine-5'-triphosphate; *NPRA,* natriuretic peptide receptor A; ↑, increased; ↓, decreased. (From Langenickel TH. Angiotensin receptor–neprilysin inhibition with LCZ696: a novel approach for the treatment of heart failure. *Drug Discov Today Ther Strateg.* 2012;9:e131.)

reducing the risks of cardiovascular death (by an incremental 20%), HF hospitalization (by an incremental 21%), and all-cause mortality (by an incremental 16%). In 2015, the US Food and Drug Administration (FDA) approved the combination valsartan/sacubitril tablet for the treatment of patients with stage C HF with reduced EF (ie, NYHA class II or IV).

β-Adrenergic Receptor Antagonists

Sympathetic Nervous System Activation and Its Role in the Pathogenesis of Heart Failure

Activation of the SNS (eg, after MI, for long-standing hypertension), much like increases in RAS activity, contributes to the pathophysiology of HF. SNS activation leads to pathologic LV growth and remodeling. Myocytes thicken and elongate, with eccentric hypertrophy and increases in sphericity. Wall stress is increased by this architecture, promoting subendocardial ischemia, cell death, and contractile dysfunction. The activated SNS can also harm myocytes directly through programmed cell death. As myocytes are replaced by fibroblasts, heart function deteriorates from this remodeling. The threshold for arrhythmias may also be lowered, contributing in a deteriorating cycle.

β-Adrenergic Receptor Blockers Influence on Heart Failure Pathophysiology

In chronic HF, the beneficial effects of long-term β-blockade include improved systolic function and myocardial energetics and reversal of pathologic remodeling. A shift in substrate use from free fatty acids to glucose, a more efficient fuel in the face of myocardial ischemia, may partly explain the improved energetics and mechanics in the failing heart treated with β-blockade. Heart rate, a major determinant of $M\dot{V}o_2$, is reduced by β_1-receptor blockade.

CLINICAL EVIDENCE

The use of β-blockers in patients with HF was initially accepted with skepticism because of the perceived risk of decompensation from transient negative inotropic effects. However, data from human studies have shown that β-blockers improve energetics and ventricular function and reverse pathologic chamber remodeling. Randomized trials show that metoprolol, bisoprolol, and carvedilol (in conjunction with ACE inhibitors) reduce morbidity in patients with symptomatic, stage C and D HF.

CLINICAL PRACTICE

Evidence suggests that β-blockers should be given to all patients with HF who have reduced EFs (<0.40) and who are on ACE inhibitors or ARBs unless there is a contraindication. This recommendation is endorsed by the ACC/AHA and the European Society of Cardiology. Patients with ongoing decompensation (ie, requiring intravenous inotropic or vasodilator therapy), overt fluid retention, or symptomatic hypotension should not receive β-blockers.

The three agents with clinical trial evidence for improved morbidity and mortality for patients with HF are carvedilol, metoprolol, and bisoprolol. Starting doses of β-blockers should be small to minimize worsening of HF symptoms, hypotension, and bradycardia. The dose should be doubled every 1 to 2 weeks, as tolerated, until the target doses shown to be effective in large trials are achieved. Although it is recommended that β-blocker therapy be continued indefinitely in patients with HF, if it is to be electively stopped, a slow titration period is preferred. Acute withdrawal of β-blocker therapy in the face of high adrenergic tone may result in sudden cardiac death.

Adjunctive Drugs

In addition to ACE inhibitors and β-blockers, diuretics and digoxin are often prescribed for patients with LV systolic dysfunction and symptomatic HF.

Diuretics

For most patients, volume status should be optimized before introduction of β-blockers and ACE inhibitors. Patients with pulmonary congestion often require a loop diuretic in addition to standard therapy. Diuretics relieve dyspnea, decrease heart size and wall stress, and correct hyponatremia from volume overload. However, overly aggressive and especially unmonitored diuretic therapy can lead to metabolic abnormalities, intravascular depletion, hypotension, and neurohormonal activation.

Digoxin

Digoxin continues to be useful for patients with symptomatic HF and LV systolic dysfunction despite receiving ACE inhibitor, β-blocker, and diuretic therapy. Digoxin is the only positive inotropic drug approved for the management of chronic HF. Its indirect mechanism of positive inotropy begins with inhibition of the myocardial sarcolemmal Na^+/K^+-ATPase, resulting in increased intracellular Na^+. This prompts the Na^+/Ca^{2+} exchanger to extrude Na^+ from the cell, increasing the intracellular concentration of Ca^{2+}. The increased Ca^{2+} available to the contractile proteins increases contractile function.

The efficacy of digoxin for symptomatic HF was shown in RCTs. The Digitalis Investigators Group (DIG) trial, enrolling more than 6500 patients with an average follow-up of 37 months, showed that digoxin reduced the incidence of HF exacerbations. Although the study showed no difference in survival in patients with EFs less than 45% receiving digoxin or placebo, the combined end point of death or hospitalization for HF was significantly reduced in patients who received digoxin (27% vs 35%; relative risk = 0.72; 95% confidence interval [CI], 0.66 to 0.79).

Anticoagulation

Patients with chronic HFrEF are at an increased risk for thromboembolic events owing to stasis of blood in dilated hypokinetic cardiac chambers and in peripheral blood vessels and possibly because of increased activation of procoagulant factors. Even so, there are no large-scale data to support the routine use of anticoagulants in patients with HFrEF without atrial fibrillation (AF), a prior thromboembolic event, or a cardioembolic source (class III). However, a class I recommendation does exist for its use in patients with HF who have permanent, persistent, or paroxysmal AF and an additional risk factor for cardiometabolic stroke, including a history of hypertension, diabetes, previous stroke or transient ischemic attack, or age of at least 75 years.

I_F Current Inhibitors

The funny current (I_F current) is the most important current for SA node depolarization. The inward current affects Na^+ and K^+ channels and has a significant effect on heart rate. Ivabradine is the first I_F current inhibitor available for oral use (usually 5 mg daily) in the United States. It has been approved by the FDA for treatment of angina pectoris as an adjunct to other drugs for patients with an increased heart rate, for those who have a contraindication to β-receptor blockers, and for CHF in patients with an increased heart rate.

Ivabradine appears to be very effective in patients with HF. In a study of 6558 patients with an EF less than 35% and heart rate greater than 70 beats/min, compared with placebo the drug significantly reduced the incidence of HF death and the readmission rate for HF treatment. All patients were also receiving β-blocker treatment for HF. The most impressive responses were in patients who had the fastest heart rates. Heart rate is a marker for a bad outcome in HF, and reducing the heart rate appears to improve outcomes, likely by reducing ventricular loading conditions.

Pharmacologic Treatment of Heart Failure With Preserved Ejection Fraction or Diastolic Heart Failure

Abnormal diastolic ventricular function is a common cause of clinical HF. The incidence of HF with a normal or near-normal EF (≥50%) includes up to 50% of the general HF population. The risk of HFpEF increases with age, approaching 50% among patients older than 70 years. HFpEF is also more common in women and in those with multiple comorbidities, such as hypertension, diabetes, vasculopathy, renal disease, AF, and metabolic syndrome.

In terms of morbidity and mortality, the prognosis associated with the diagnosis of HFpEF is similar to that of HFrEF. Because this syndrome carries substantial morbidity (eg, exercise intolerance, poor quality of life, frequent hospitalizations) and reduced survival and results in substantial annual health care expenditures, pharmacotherapy for HFpEF represents one of the current frontiers of clinical cardiovascular medicine.

In contrast to the large, randomized trials that led to the treatment guidelines for HFrEF, the randomized, double-blind, placebo-controlled, multicenter trials enrolling

Table 8.5	Diastolic Heart Failure Treatments	
Goal	Management Strategy	Recommended Doses
Reduce the Congestive State		
Prevent fluid retention and reduce blood pressure	Salt restriction	Sodium, <2 g/day
	Diuretics (avoid reductions in cardiac output)	Furosemide, 10–120 mg
		Hydrochlorothiazide, 12.5–25 mg
	ACE inhibitors	Enalapril, 2.5–40 mg
		Lisinopril, 10–40 mg
	Angiotensin II receptor blockers	Candesartan, 4–32 mg
		Losartan, 25–100 mg
Target Underlying Cause		
Control hypertension (<130/80 mm Hg)	Antihypertensive agents	β-Blockers, ACE inhibitors, all receptor blockers: dose according to published guidelines
Restore sinus rhythm	Atrioventricular sequential pacing	—
Prevent tachycardia	β-Blockers, calcium channel blockers	Atenolol, 12.5–100 mg
		Metoprolol, 25–100 mg
		Diltiazem, 120–540 mg
Treat aortic stenosis	Aortic valve replacement	—
Target Underlying Mechanisms		
Promote regression of hypertrophy and prevent myocardial fibrosis	Renin-angiotensin axis blockade (theoretical)	Enalapril, 2.5–40 mg
		Lisinopril, 10–40 mg
		Captopril, 25–150 mg
		Candesartan, 4–32 mg
		Losartan, 50–100 mg
		Spironolactone, 25–75 mg
		Eplerenone, 25–50 mg

ACE, Angiotensin-converting enzyme.

patients with diastolic HF have resulted in neutral results for primary outcomes. Consequently, the treatment of HFpEF remains empiric.

The general pharmacologic approach to treating HFpEF has three main components (Table 8.5). First, treatment should reduce symptoms, primarily by lowering pulmonary venous pressure during rest and exercise by carefully reducing LV volume and maintaining atrial-ventricular synchrony or tachycardia control. Second, treatment should target the underlying diseases that cause HFpEF. Ventricular remodeling (eg, myocardial hypertrophy, fibrosis) should be reversed by controlling hypertension, treating ischemia, and controlling glycemia in diabetic patients. Third, treatment should attempt to target the underlying mechanisms that are altered by the disease processes. However, owing to our lack of understanding of the pathogenesis of HFpEF, the third goal remains elusive.

Many of the drugs used to treat HFrEF are also used to treat HFpEF. However, the reason for their use and the doses used may be different for diastolic HF. For instance, in diastolic HF, β-blockers may be used to prevent tachycardia and thereby prolong diastolic filling and reduce left atrial pressure; whereas in systolic HF, β-blockers (eg, carvedilol) are used to reverse heart remodeling. Metoprolol may be a better β-blocker choice than carvedilol for HFpEF because an excessively low BP (as a consequence of carvedilol) may be detrimental for the patient with diastolic HF.

Class I recommendations for patients with HFpEF include control of systolic and diastolic BP in accordance with clinical practice guidelines and use of diuretics to relieve symptoms from pressure overload. β-Blockers and ACE inhibitors or ARBs are considered reasonable to use to control BP. Coronary revascularization is considered reasonable in patients with CAD in whom angina or demonstrable myocardial ischemia has an adverse effect on symptomatic HFpEF despite optimal medical therapy. AF is managed according to clinical practice guidelines. The use of an ARB can be considered for these patients to decrease hospitalizations.

Management of Acute Exacerbations of Chronic Heart Failure

Despite good medical management, patients with chronic HF may experience episodes of pulmonary edema or other signs of acute volume overload. Other patients may experience exacerbations of HF associated with acute myocardial ischemia or infarction, hypertension, arrhythmia, worsening valvular dysfunction, infections (including myocarditis), or failure to maintain an established drug or dietary regimen. These patients may require hospitalization for intensive management if initial treatments fail to relieve their symptoms.

Vasodilators

In the absence of systemic hypotension, intravenous vasodilators may be used to treat dyspnea in patients with decompensated chronic HF. Vasodilators reduce ventricular filling pressures and SVR while increasing SV and CO. NTG is commonly used for this purpose and has been studied in numerous clinical trials.

NESIRITIDE

Nesiritide, a recombinant BNP, was approved in 2001 and is indicated for patients with acute HF and dyspnea with minimal activity. Nesiritide produces arterial and venous dilation through increasing cGMP levels. Nesiritide does not increase heart rate and has no effect on cardiac inotropy. It has a rapid onset of action and a short elimination half-life (ie, 15 minutes). Initial studies showed that nesiritide reduced dyspnea associated with acute decompensated HF similar to NTG but without development of acute tolerance and with fewer adverse events than NTG.

Inotropes

Positive inotropic drugs, principally dobutamine or milrinone, have long been used to treat decompensated HF despite the lack of data showing an outcome benefit for their use. In the past, some chronic HF patients received intermittent infusions of positive inotropic drugs as part of their maintenance therapy. Small studies consistently demonstrate improved hemodynamic values and reduced symptoms after administration of these agents to patients with HF. Studies comparing dobutamine with milrinone for advanced decompensated HF showed large differences in drug costs, favoring dobutamine, and only small hemodynamic differences, favoring milrinone.

Nevertheless, placebo-controlled studies suggest there may be no role for discretionary administration of positive inotropes to patients with chronic HF. Positive inotropic drug support can be recommended only when there is no alternative. Dobutamine and milrinone continue to be used to treat low CO in selected patients with decompensated HF.

Alternative Therapies

When drug treatment proves unsuccessful, HF patients may require invasive therapy, including ultrafiltration for diuresis, ventricular assist devices, biventricular pacing, coronary bypass with or without surgical remodeling, or cardiac orthotopic transplantation.

Low-Output Syndrome

Acute HF is a frequent concern of the cardiac anesthesiologist, particularly at the time of separation from cardiopulmonary bypass (CPB). New-onset ventricular dysfunction with a low CO after aortic clamping and reperfusion is a condition with more pathophysiologic similarity to cardiogenic shock than to chronic HF, and it is typically treated with positive inotropic drugs, vasopressors (or vasodilators) if needed, or mechanical assistance.

Causes

Most patients undergoing cardiac surgery with CPB experience a temporary decline in ventricular function, with a recovery to normal function in roughly 24 hours. Pathophysiologic explanations acknowledge the usually temporary nature of the low-output syndrome after CPB. It likely results from one of three processes, all related to inadequate oxygen delivery to the myocardium: acute ischemia, hibernation, or stunning. All three processes can be expected to improve with adequate revascularization and moderate doses of positive inotropic drugs, consistent with the typical progress of the cardiac surgery patient. All three processes can be expected to be more troublesome in patients with preexisting chronic HF, pulmonary hypertension, or arrhythmias.

Risk Factors for Low-Output Syndrome After Cardiopulmonary Bypass

The need for inotropic drug support after CPB can often be anticipated based on data available in the preoperative medical history, physical examination, and imaging studies. In a series of consecutive patients undergoing elective CABG, it was observed that increasing age, decreasing left ventricular ejection fragment (LVEF), female sex, cardiac enlargement on the chest radiograph, and prolonged duration of CPB were associated with an increased likelihood that the patient would be receiving positive inotropic drugs on arrival in the intensive care unit. Similarly, in a study of patients undergoing mitral valve surgery, independent predictors of low-CO syndrome were urgency of the case, LVEF less than 40%, NYHA class IV, a body surface area of 1.7 m^2 or less, ischemic mitral valve pathology, and CPB time. Another study of patients undergoing aortic valve surgery identified renal failure, LVEF less than 40%, shock, female gender, and increasing age as independent risk factors. Data from an intraoperative transesophageal echocardiographic examination may also help identify patients who are more likely to need inotropic support. Patients with a decreased wall motion score index or those with moderate or severe mitral regurgitation may need inotropic support.

Drugs for Treating Low-Output Syndrome

Although all positive inotropic drugs increase the strength of contraction in noninfarcted myocardium, the mechanisms of action are different. The drugs can be divided into those that increase cyclic adenosine monophosphate (cAMP) (directly or indirectly) as their mechanism of action and those that do not. The agents that do not depend on cAMP form a diverse group, including cardiac glycosides, calcium salts, calcium sensitizers, and thyroid hormone. In contrast to chronic HF, cardiac glycosides are not used for this indication owing to their limited efficacy and narrow margin of safety. Calcium salts continue to be administered for ionized hypocalcemia and hyperkalemia, common occurrences during and after cardiac surgery.

Levosimendan is an inodilator that increases cardiac contractility by calcium sensitization of troponin C. Because levosimendan does not increase the intracellular Ca^{2+} concentration, it does not impair diastolic cardiac function. Peripheral and coronary vasodilation due to its effects on ATP-sensitive K^+ channels provides afterload reduction and improved coronary perfusion. These combined effects result in improvement of myocardial contractility without an increase in $M\dot{V}O_2$. Another attractive feature of this inotropic agent is that its effects are not diminished by β-blockade. It is indicated for the short-term treatment of severe chronic HF when conventional therapy is not sufficient, but it is being increasingly studied in cardiac surgical settings with favorable results.

Levosimendan is an acceptable choice for patients with acutely decompensated HF after hypovolemia has been corrected. Suggested dosing includes an infusion with or without a loading dose of 6 to 12 µg/kg for 10 minutes, followed by 0.005 to 2 µg/kg per minute for no more than 24 hours. Loading doses are not recommended for patients with low-normal BP (eg, systolic blood pressure [SBP] <100 mm Hg). Without a loading dose, maximal effect of the drug occurs after 4 hours. Infusions should not continue for longer than 24 hours due to levosimendan's active metabolites, which can accumulate and produce refractory hypotension and tachycardia.

Intravenous thyroid hormone (liothyronine [T_3]) has been studied extensively as a positive inotrope in cardiac surgery. There are multiple studies that support the existence of euthyroid sick syndrome with persistent reduced concentrations of T_3 in blood after cardiac surgery in children and adults. Data suggest that after ischemia and reperfusion, T_3 increases inotropy faster than and as potently as isoproterenol.

cAMP-dependent agents are the mainstays of positive inotropic drug therapy after cardiac surgery. There are two main classes of agents: phosphodiesterase enzyme (PDE) inhibitors and β-adrenergic receptor agonists. PDEs in clinical use around the world include enoximone, inamrinone, milrinone, olprinone, and piroximone. Comparisons among the agents have failed to demonstrate important hemodynamic differences.

PDE inhibitors produce rapid increases in contractile function and CO and decreases in SVR. The effect on BP depends on the pretreatment state of hydration and hemodynamics, but the typical response is a small decrease in BP. There is no effect on heart rate or a small increase.

Among the many β-adrenergic receptor agonists, the agents most often given to patients recovering from cardiac surgery are dopamine, dobutamine, and epinephrine. Dopamine has long been assumed to have dose-defined receptor specificity. This makes it unlikely that the dose-response relationship is as consistent as has been described in textbooks for the past 20 years. Moreover, dopamine is a relatively weak inotrope that has a predominant effect on heart rate rather than on SV.

Dobutamine is a selective β-adrenergic receptor agonist. Most studies suggest that it causes less tachycardia and hypotension than isoproterenol. It has been frequently compared with dopamine, in which dobutamine's greater tendency for pulmonary and systemic vasodilation is evident. Dobutamine has a predominant effect on heart rate compared with SV, and as the dose is increased more than 10 µg/kg per minute there are further increases in heart rate without changes in SV.

Epinephrine is a powerful adrenergic agonist, and, like dopamine, it demonstrates different effects depending on the dose. At small doses (10–30 ng/kg per minute), despite an almost pure β-adrenergic receptor stimulus, there is almost no increase in heart rate. Clinicians have long assumed that epinephrine increases heart rate more than dobutamine administered at comparable doses. In patients recovering from cardiac surgery, the opposite is true; dobutamine increases heart rate more than epinephrine.

Other β-adrenergic agonists are used in specific circumstances. For example, isoproterenol is often used after cardiac transplantation to exploit its powerful chronotropy and after correction of congenital heart defects to exploit its pulmonary vasodilatory effects. Norepinephrine is used to counteract profound vasodilation. Outside of North America, dopexamine, a weak dopaminergic and β-agonist with a pronounced tendency for tachycardia, is sometimes used.

PHARMACOTHERAPY FOR CARDIAC ARRHYTHMIAS

The most widely used electrophysiologic and pharmacologic classification of antiarrhythmic drugs is that proposed by Vaughan Williams (Table 8.6). There is, however, substantial overlap in pharmacologic and electrophysiologic effects of specific agents among the classes, and the linkage between observed electrophysiologic effects and the clinical antiarrhythmic effect is often tenuous. Likewise, especially in class I, there may be considerable diversity within a single class. Other antiarrhythmic drugs are not included in this classification, such as digitalis, the classic antiarrhythmic for chronic AF, or adenosine, a drug with potent antiarrhythmic effects mediated by a specific class of membrane receptors.

Although the class I and especially subclass IC agents are most commonly known for their proarrhythmic effects, the other classes are not devoid of this side effect.

Table 8.6 Classification of Antiarrhythmic Drugs

Effects	Type of Antiarrhythmic Drug			
	I (Membrane Stabilizers)	II (β-Adrenergic Receptor Antagonists)	III (Drugs Prolonging Repolarization)	IV (Calcium Antagonists)
Pharmacologic	Fast channel (Na$^+$) blockade	β-Adrenergic receptor blockade	Uncertain: possible interference with Na$^+$ and Ca^{2+} exchange	Decreased slow–channel calcium conductance
Electrophysiologic	Decreased rate of V_{max}	Decreased V_{max}, increased APD, increased ERP, and increased ERP:APD ratio	Increased APD, increased ERP, increased ERP:APD ratio	Decreased slow–channel depolarization; decreased APD

APD, Action potential duration; *ERP*, effective refractory period; V_{max}, maximal rate of depolarization.

BOX 8.4 *Drugs That Can Produce Torsades De Pointes*

Amiodarone	Procainamide
Disopyramide	Quinidine
Dofetilide	Sotalol
Ibutilide	

Table 8.7 Subgroup of Class I Antiarrhythmic Drugs

Electrophysiologic Activity	Subgroup		
	IA	IB	IC
Phase 0	Decreased	Slight effect	Marked decrease
Depolarization	Prolonged	Slight effect	Slight effect
Conduction	Decreased	Slight effect	Markedly slowed
ERP	Increased	Slight effect	Slight prolongation
APD	Increased	Decreased	Slight effect
ERP:APD ratio	Increased	Decreased	Slight effect
QRS duration	Increased	No effect during sinus rhythm	Marked increase
Prototype drugs	Quinidine, procainamide, disopyramide, diphenylhydantoin	Lidocaine, mexiletine, tocainide	Lorcainide, encainide, flecainide, aprindine

APD, Action potential duration; *ERP,* effective refractory period.

For the first week after initiation of sotalol, a nonspecific β-adrenergic blocker that is considered a class III arrhythmic agent, there is an increased incidence of torsades de pointes. The proarrhythmic effects appear to be increased in the setting of hypokalemia, bradycardia, CHF, and a history of sustained ventricular dysfunction (Box 8.4).

Chronic antiarrhythmic therapy should be initiated only after careful evaluation of the risks and benefits of the intervention. The appropriate use of intravenous antiarrhythmic agents with sudden-onset arrhythmias is not clear. Life-threatening ventricular arrhythmias must be treated. High-risk patients may be treated more safely in some cases by implantation of internal cardioverter-defibrillators.

Class I Antiarrhythmic Drugs: Sodium Channel Blockers

Class I drugs inhibit the fast inward depolarizing current carried by sodium ions. Because of the diversity of other effects of the class I drugs, a subgroup of the class has been proposed (Table 8.7). Whether the depression of fast inward current of the sodium channel produces the primary antiarrhythmic effect of all class I drugs is controversial.

Class IA Drugs

PROCAINAMIDE

Electrophysiologic effects of procainamide include decreased maximal velocity (V_{max}) and amplitude during phase 0, decreased rate of phase 4 depolarization, and prolonged effective refractory period (ERP) and action potential duration (APD). Clinically, procainamide prolongs conduction and increases the ERP in atrial and His-Purkinje portions of the conduction system, which may prolong PR interval and QRS complex durations.

Procainamide is used to treat ventricular arrhythmias and to suppress atrial premature beats to prevent the occurrence of AF and atrial flutter. It has been useful for chronic suppression of premature ventricular contractions (PVCs). Procainamide reduces the frequency of the short-coupling interval (<400 ms) PVCs and thereby reduces the frequency of ventricular tachycardia (VT) or ventricular fibrillation (VF) created by the R-on-T phenomenon.

Administered intravenously, procainamide is an effective emergency treatment for ventricular arrhythmias, especially after lidocaine failure, but amiodarone has become a more popular drug for intravenous suppression of ventricular arrhythmias. Dosage is 100 mg, or approximately 1.5 mg/kg given at 5-minute intervals until the therapeutic effect is obtained or a total dose of 1 g or 15 mg/kg is given (Tables 8.8 and 8.9). Arterial pressure and the electrocardiogram should be monitored continuously during loading and administration stopped if significant hypotension occurs or if the QRS complex is prolonged by 50% or more. Maintenance infusion rates are 2 to 6 mg/min to maintain therapeutic plasma concentrations of 4 to 8 µg/mL.

Class IB Drugs

LIDOCAINE

First introduced as an antiarrhythmic drug in the 1950s, lidocaine has become the clinical standard for the acute intravenous treatment of ventricular arrhythmias except those precipitated by an abnormally prolonged QT interval. Lidocaine may be one of the most useful drugs in clinical anesthesia because it has local and general anesthetic properties in addition to an antiarrhythmic effect.

The direct electrophysiologic effects of lidocaine produce virtually all of its antiarrhythmic action. Lidocaine depresses the slope of phase 4 diastolic depolarization in Purkinje fibers and increases the VF threshold.

The clinical pharmacokinetics of lidocaine are well described. The distribution and elimination half-lives of lidocaine are short, approximately 60 seconds and 100 minutes, respectively. Hepatic extraction of lidocaine is about 60% to 70%, and essentially all lidocaine is metabolized because the urine contains negligible amounts of unchanged lidocaine. Therapeutic plasma levels of lidocaine range from 1.5 to 5 µg/mL; signs of toxicity are common with concentrations greater than 9 µg/mL.

An initial bolus dose of 1 to 1.5 mg/kg should be followed immediately by a continuous infusion of 20 to 50 µg/kg per minute to prevent the therapeutic hiatus produced by the rapid redistribution half-life of lidocaine.

Class IC Drugs

PROPAFENONE

Propafenone blocks the fast sodium current in a use-dependent manner. Propafenone blocks β-receptors and is a weak potassium channel blocker. This drug usually slows

8

Table 8.8 Intravenous Supraventricular Antiarrhythmic Therapy

Class I Drugs

Procainamide (IA): converts acute atrial fibrillation, suppresses PACs and precipitation of atrial fibrillation or flutter, converts accessory pathway SVT; 100 mg IV loading dose every 5 minutes until arrhythmia subsides or total dose of 15 mg/kg (rarely needed) with continuous infusion of 2 to 6 mg/min.

Class II Drugs

Esmolol: converts or maintains slow ventricular response in acute atrial fibrillation; 0.5 to 1 mg/kg loading dose with each 50 μg/kg per minute increase in infusion, with infusions of 50 to 300 μg/kg per minute. Hypotension and bradycardia are limiting factors.

Class III Drugs

Amiodarone: converts acute atrial fibrillation to sinus rhythm; 5 mg/kg IV over 15 minutes.

Ibutilide (Convert): converts acute atrial fibrillation and flutter.
    Adults (>60 kg): 1 mg IV given over 10 minutes; may repeat once.
    Adults (<60 kg) and children: 0.01 mg/kg IV given over 10 minutes; may repeat once.

Vernakalant: 3 mg/kg over 10 minutes in acute-onset atrial fibrillation; if no conversion; wait 15 minutes and then repeat with 2 mg/kg over 10 minutes. Hypotension may occur in a few patients.

Class IV Drugs

Verapamil: slow ventricular response to acute atrial fibrillation; converts AV node reentry SVT; 75–150 μg/kg IV bolus.

Diltiazem: slow ventricular response in acute atrial fibrillation; converts AV node reentry SVT; 0.25 μg/kg bolus, then 100–300 μg/kg/h infusion.

Other Therapy

Adenosine: converts AV node reentry SVT and accessory pathway SVT; aids in diagnosis of atrial fibrillation and flutter. Increased dosage required with methylxanthines, decreased use required with dipyridamole.
    Adults: 3–6 mg IV bolus, repeat with 6–12 mg bolus.
    Children: 100 μg/kg bolus, repeat with 200 μg/kg bolus.

Digoxin: maintenance IV therapy for atrial fibrillation and flutter; slows ventricular response.
    Adults: 0.25 mg IV bolus followed by 0.125 mg every 1–2 hours until rate is controlled; not to exceed 10 μg/kg in 24 hours.
    Children (<10 years): 10–30 μg/kg load given in divided doses over 24 hours.
    Maintenance: 25% of loading dose.

AV, Atrioventricular; *IV,* intravenous; *PACs,* premature atrial contractions; *SVT,* supraventricular tachycardia.

conduction and prolongs refractoriness of most cardiac conduction system tissue. Propafenone is indicated for life-threatening ventricular arrhythmias, various supraventricular arrhythmias, and AF. In one study, a single 600-mg oral dose of propafenone converted 76% of patients in AF. Propafenone was more effective than placebo in preventing atrial tachyarrhythmias after cardiac surgery with combined intravenous and oral therapy.

Propafenone is well absorbed orally and is highly protein bound, with an elimination half-life of 6 to 8 hours. Therapeutic serum levels are 0.2 to 1.5 μg/mL. The metabolites of propafenone are active and demonstrate significant action potential and β-blocking effects. The drug has few proarrhythmic problems, likely because of the β-blocking effects, which tend to decrease arrhythmic traits of antiarrhythmic drugs.

Table 8.9 Intravenous Ventricular Antiarrhythmic Therapy

Class I Drugs

Procainamide (IA): 100 mg IV loading dose every 5 minutes until arrhythmia subsides or total dose of 15 mg/kg (rarely needed) with continuous infusion of 2 to 6 mg/min.

Lidocaine (IB): 1.5 mg in divided doses given twice over 20 minutes with continuous infusion of 1 to 4 mg/min.

Class II Drugs

Propranolol: 0.5 to 1 mg given slowly up to a total β-blocking dose of 0.1 mg/kg; repeat bolus as needed.

Metoprolol: 2.5 mg given slowly up to a total β-blocking dose of 0.2 mg/kg; repeat bolus as needed.

Esmolol: 0.5 to 1.0 mg/kg loading dose with each 50 μg/kg/min increase in infusion, with infusions of 50 to 300 μg/kg/min. Hypotension and bradycardia are limiting factors.

Class III Drugs

Bretylium: 5 mg/kg loading dose given slowly with a continuous infusion of 1 to 5 mg/min. Hypotension may be a limiting factor.

Amiodarone: 150 mg over 10 minutes IV; then 1 mg/min for 6 hours; then 0.5 mg/min for the next 18 hours. Repeat bolus as needed.

Other Therapy

Magnesium: 2 g of $MgSO_4$ over 5 minutes; then continuous infusion of 1 g/h for 6–10 hours to restore intracellular magnesium levels.

From Royster RL. *Diagnosis and Management of Cardiac Disorders.* ASA Refresher Course Lectures. Park Ridge, IL: American Society of Anesthesiologists; 1996.

Class II Drugs: β-Adrenergic Receptor Antagonists

PROPRANOLOL

Propranolol was the first major β-receptor–blocking drug to be used clinically. Propranolol is very potent but is nonselective for β_1- and β_2-receptor subtypes. It possesses essentially no ISA. Because it interferes with the bronchodilating actions of epinephrine and the sympathetic stimulating effects of hypoglycemia, propranolol is less useful in patients with diabetes or bronchospasm. These difficulties with propranolol stimulated the search for β-receptor–blocking drugs with receptor subtype specificity, such as metoprolol, esmolol, and atenolol.

The electrophysiologic effects of β-receptor antagonism are decreased automaticity, increased APD (primarily in ventricular muscle), and a substantially increased ERP in the atrioventricular (AV) node. β-Blockade decreases the rate of spontaneous (phase 4) depolarization in the sinoatrial (SA) node; the magnitude of this effect depends on the background sympathetic tone. Although resting heart rate is decreased by β-blockade, inhibition of the increase of heart rate in response to exercise or emotional stress is much more marked. Automaticity in the AV node and more distal portions of the conduction system is also depressed. β-Blockade affects VF threshold variably, but it consistently reverses the fibrillation threshold–lowering effect of catecholamines.

An appropriate intravenous dose for acute control of arrhythmias is 0.5 to 1.0 mg titrated to therapeutic effect up to a total of 0.1 to 0.15 mg/kg. Stable therapeutic plasma concentrations of propranolol can be obtained with a continuous intravenous infusion. However, with the availability of esmolol, a propranolol infusion is no longer necessary.

METOPROLOL

Metoprolol is a relatively selective β-receptor antagonist. The potency of metoprolol for β_1-receptor blockade is equal to that of propranolol, but metoprolol exhibits only 1% to 2% of the effect of propranolol at β_2-receptors.

Metoprolol is useful for treating supraventricular and ventricular arrhythmias that are adrenergically driven. The primary advantage of metoprolol is its relative lack of most of the bronchoconstrictive effects in patients with chronic obstructive pulmonary disease. Acute intravenous dosage is 1.0 mg titrated to therapeutic effect up to 0.1 to 0.2 mg/kg.

ESMOLOL

Esmolol is a cardioselective β_1-receptor antagonist with an extremely brief duration of action. Electrophysiologic effects of esmolol are those of β-adrenergic receptor antagonism. Esmolol is rapidly metabolized in blood by hydrolysis of its methyl ester linkage. Its half-life in whole blood is 12.5 to 27.1 minutes in humans. The acid metabolite possesses a slight degree (1500 times less than esmolol) of β-antagonism. Esmolol is not affected by plasma cholinesterase; the esterase responsible is located in erythrocytes and is not inhibited by cholinesterase inhibitors. Of importance to clinical anesthesia, no metabolic interactions between esmolol and other ester molecules are known.

In a multicenter trial that compared esmolol with propranolol for the treatment of paroxysmal supraventricular tachyarrhythmia (PSVT), esmolol was equally efficacious and had the advantage of a much faster termination of the β-blockade. Esmolol has become a useful agent in controlling sinus tachycardia in the perioperative period, a time when a titratable and brief β-blockade is highly desirable. Dosing begins at 25 μg/kg per minute and is titrated to effect up to 250 μg/kg per minute. Doses greater than this may cause significant hypotension because of reduced CO in patients. Esmolol is especially effective in treating acute-onset AF or flutter perioperatively, and it results in acute control of the ventricular response and conversion of the arrhythmia to sinus rhythm.

Class III Drugs: Potassium Channel Blockers and Agents That Prolong Repolarization

AMIODARONE

Amiodarone is a benzofuran derivative that was initially introduced as an antianginal drug and was subsequently found to have antiarrhythmic effects. The drug has a wide spectrum of effectiveness, including supraventricular, ventricular, and preexcitation arrhythmias. It also may be effective against VT and VF refractory to other treatment. Amiodarone has been approved by the AHA as the first-line antiarrhythmic in cardiopulmonary resuscitation. Amiodarone may be effective prophylactically in preventing AF after surgery. It also can decrease the number of shocks in patients who have implantable cardioverter-defibrillators compared with other antiarrhythmic drugs.

Amiodarone increases the amount of electric current required to elicit VF (ie, increase in the VF threshold). In most patients, refractory VT is suppressed by acute intravenous use of amiodarone. This effect has been attributed to a selectively increased activity in diseased tissue, as has been seen with lidocaine.

Hemodynamic effects of intravenous amiodarone (10 mg/kg) include decreased LV dP/dt, maximal negative dP/dt, mean aortic pressure, heart rate, and peak LV pressure after coronary artery occlusion in dogs. CO was increased despite the negative inotropic effect as a result of the more marked decrease in LV afterload. A 5-mg/kg intravenous dose during cardiac catheterization decreased BP, LV end-diastolic pressure, and SVR and increased CO, but it did not affect heart rate. Chronic amiodarone therapy is not associated with clinically significant depression of ventricular function in patients without LV failure.

In acute situations with stable patients, a 150-mg intravenous bolus is followed by a 1.0-mg/min infusion for 6 hours and then 0.5 mg/min thereafter. In cardiopulmonary resuscitation (CPR), a 300-mg intravenous bolus is given and repeated with multiple boluses as needed if defibrillation is unsuccessful.

Despite relatively widespread use of amiodarone, anesthetic complications infrequently have been reported. In case reports, bradycardia and hypotension were prominent. The slow decay of amiodarone in plasma and tissue makes such adverse reactions possible long after discontinuing its administration. Epinephrine is more effective than dobutamine or isoproterenol in reversing amiodarone-induced cardiac depression.

An RCT of amiodarone administered 6 days before and 6 days after cardiac surgery demonstrated significant reductions in atrial tachyarrhythmias and ventricular arrhythmias in patients of different ages and in different types of cardiac surgical procedures. There were no differences in hospital mortality rates between groups.

SOTALOL

Sotalol is classified as a class III agent, but it also has class II β-adrenergic–blocking properties. It prolongs refractoriness in atrial and ventricular tissues because of blockade of the delayed rectifier potassium current. The β-blocking effects result in decreased heart rate and increased refractory periods at the atrial and ventricular levels. It is indicated for life-threatening ventricular arrhythmias and AF.

Sotalol has been used to treat supraventricular and ventricular tachyarrhythmias. It was found to be superior to class I agents in preventing the recurrence of ventricular arrhythmias.

Sotalol administration is associated with increased risk for torsades de pointes and QT-interval prolongation. Female patients and patients with renal failure are at increased risk for the proarrhythmic side effects.

8

Class IV Drugs: Calcium Channel Antagonists

Although the principal direct electrophysiologic effects of the three main chemical groups of calcium antagonists (ie, verapamil, a benzoacetonitrite; nifedipine, a DHP; and diltiazem, a benzothiazepine) are similar, verapamil and diltiazem are the primary antiarrhythmics.

VERAPAMIL AND DILTIAZEM

Verapamil and diltiazem have been used extensively in the treatment of supraventricular arrhythmias, AF, and atrial flutter. They are especially effective at preventing or terminating PSVT by blocking impulse transmission through the AV node by prolonging AV nodal conduction and refractoriness. They are also useful in the treatment of AF and atrial flutter by slowing AV nodal conduction and decreasing the ventricular response. The effect on ventricular response is similar to that of the cardiac glycosides, although the onset is more rapid and acutely effective for control of tachycardia in patients.

In the perioperative period, verapamil is a useful antiarrhythmic agent. In one study of anesthetized patients, it successfully controlled a variety of supraventricular and ventricular arrhythmias. However, verapamil should be used with caution intraoperatively because significant cardiac depression may occur in conjunction with inhalation anesthetics.

Verapamil dosage for acute intravenous treatment of PSVT is 0.07 to 0.15 mg/kg over 1 minute, with the same dose repeated after 30 minutes if the initial response is inadequate (10 mg maximum). Because the cardiovascular depressant effects of the inhalation anesthetics involve inhibition of calcium-related intracellular processes, the interaction of verapamil and these anesthetics is synergistic.

Diltiazem in doses of 0.25 to 0.30 mg/kg administered intravenously and followed by a titratable intravenous infusion of 10 to 20 mg/h is rapid acting and efficacious in controlling ventricular response rate in new-onset AF and atrial flutter. The prophylactic use of intravenous diltiazem can reduce the incidence of postoperative supraventricular arrhythmias after pneumonectomy and cardiac surgery. Diltiazem also may have a role in treating ventricular arrhythmias.

Other Antiarrhythmic Agents

DIGOXIN

The primary therapeutic use of digitalis drugs is to slow the ventricular response during AF or atrial flutter, which occurs because of a complex combination of direct and indirect actions on the AV node. The primary direct pharmacologic effect of digitalis is inhibition of the membrane-bound Na^+/K^+-ATPase. This enzyme provides the chemical energy necessary for the transport of sodium (out) and potassium (in) during repolarization. The glycosides bind to the enzyme in a specific saturable way that inhibits enzyme activity and impairs the active transport of sodium and potassium. The net result is a slight increase in intracellular sodium and a corresponding decrease in intracellular potassium concentration. The sodium exchanges for calcium, resulting in a relatively weak inotropic effect.

The main preparation of cardiac glycosides available is digoxin. Digoxin reaches peak effects in 1.5 to 2 hours but has a significant effect within 5 to 30 minutes. For undigitalized patients, the initial dose is 0.5 to 0.75 mg of digoxin, with subsequent doses of 0.125 to 0.25 mg. The usual total digitalizing dose is 0.75 to 1.0 mg administered by the intravenous route.

ADENOSINE

The important cardiac electrophysiologic effects of adenosine are mediated by the A_1 receptor and consist of negative chronotropic, dromotropic, and inotropic actions. Adenosine decreases SA node activity, AV node conductivity, and ventricular automaticity. In many ways, these effects mimic those of acetylcholine.

For clinical use, adenosine must be administered by a rapid intravenous bolus in a dose of 100 to 200 µg/kg, although continuous intravenous infusions of 150 to 300 µg/kg per minute have been used to produce controlled hypotension. For practical purposes, in adults, a dose of 3 to 6 mg is given by intravenous bolus followed by a second dose of 6 to 12 mg after 1 minute if the first dose was not effective. This therapy rapidly interrupts narrow-complex tachycardia caused by AV nodal reentry. Comparison with verapamil has shown adenosine to be equally effective as an antiarrhythmic, but with the advantages of fewer adverse hemodynamic effects, a faster onset of action, and a more rapid elimination so that undesired effects are short-lived.

POTASSIUM

Because of the close relationship between extracellular pH and potassium, the primary mechanism of pH-induced arrhythmias may be alteration of potassium concentration. Hypokalemia and hyperkalemia are associated with cardiac arrhythmias, but hypokalemia is more common perioperatively in cardiac surgical patients and is more often associated with arrhythmias. Decreasing the extracellular potassium concentration increases the peak negative diastolic potential, which appears to decrease the likelihood of spontaneous depolarization. However, because the permeability of the myocardial cell membrane to potassium is directly related to extracellular potassium concentration, hypokalemia decreases cellular permeability to potassium. This prolongs the action potential by slowing repolarization, which slows conduction, increases the dispersion of recovery of excitability, and predisposes to the development of arrhythmias. ECG correlates of hypokalemia include appearance of a U wave and increased P-wave amplitude. The arrhythmias most commonly associated with hypokalemia are premature atrial contractions, atrial tachycardia, and supraventricular tachycardia. Hypokalemia also accentuates the toxicity of cardiac glycosides.

With chronic potassium deficiency, the plasma level poorly reflects the total body deficit. Because only 2% of total body potassium is in plasma and total body potassium stores may be 2000 to 3000 mEq, a 25% decline in serum potassium from 4 to 3 mEq/L indicates an equilibrium total body deficiency of 500 to 800 mEq, replacement of which should be undertaken slowly.

Acute hypokalemia frequently occurs after CPB as a result of hemodilution, urinary losses, and intracellular shifts, with the latter perhaps relating to abnormalities of the glucose-insulin system seen with nonpulsatile hypothermic CPB. With frequent assessment of serum potassium concentrations and continuous ECG monitoring, potassium infusion at rates of up to 10 to 15 mEq/h may be administered to treat serious hypokalemia.

MAGNESIUM

Magnesium deficiency is a relatively common electrolyte abnormality in critically ill patients, especially in chronic situations. Hypomagnesemia is associated with a variety of cardiovascular disturbances, including arrhythmias. Functionally, magnesium is required for the membrane-bound Na^+/K^+-ATPase, which is the principal enzyme that maintains normal intracellular potassium concentration. Not surprisingly, the ECG findings seen with magnesium deficiency mimic those seen with hypokalemia: prolonged PR and QT intervals, increased QRS duration, and ST-segment abnormalities. As with hypokalemia, magnesium deficiency predisposes to the development of the arrhythmias produced by cardiac glycosides. Magnesium is effective as an adjuvant in the treatment of patients with a prolonged QT syndrome and torsades de pointes.

Arrhythmias induced by magnesium deficiency may be refractory to treatment with antiarrhythmic drugs and electrical cardioversion or defibrillation. Adjunctive treatment of refractory arrhythmias with magnesium has been advocated even when magnesium deficiency has not been documented. Magnesium deficiency is common in cardiac surgery patients because of the diuretic agents these patients are often receiving and because magnesium levels decrease with CPB because of hemodilution of the pump. Magnesium lacks a counterregulatory hormone to increase magnesium levels during CPB, in contrast to the hypocalcemia that is corrected by parathyroid hormone. The results of magnesium administration trials involving CABG have been conflicting. Some studies have shown a benefit, and others have not in regard to reducing the incidence of postoperative arrhythmias.

8

SUGGESTED READINGS

Antman EM, Hand M, Armstrong PW, et al. 2007 Focused update of the ACC/AHA 2004 guidelines for the management of patients with ST-elevation myocardial infarction: a report of the American College of Cardiology/American Heart Association Task Force on Practice Guidelines: developed in collaboration with the Canadian Cardiovascular Society endorsed by the American Academy of Family Physicians: 2007 Writing Group to review new evidence and update the ACC/AHA 2004 guidelines for the management of patients with ST-elevation myocardial infarction, writing on behalf of the 2004 Writing Committee. *Circulation.* 2008;117:296.

Dabrowski W, Rzecki Z, Sztanke M, et al. The efficiency of magnesium supplementation in patients undergoing cardiopulmonary bypass: changes in serum magnesium concentrations and atrial fibrillation episodes. *Magnes Res.* 2008;21:205.

Eisenberg MJ, Brox A, Bestawros AN. Calcium channel blockers: an update. *Am J Med.* 2004;116:35.

Fleisher LA, Fleischmann KE, Auerbach AD, et al. 2014 ACC/AHA guideline on perioperative cardiovascular evaluation and management of patients undergoing noncardiac surgery: a report of the American College of Cardiology/American Heart Association Task Force on practice guidelines. *J Am Coll Cardiol.* 2014;64:e77.

Gupta A, Lawrence AT, Krishnan K, et al. Current concepts in the mechanisms and management of drug-induced QT prolongation and torsade de pointes. *Am Heart J.* 2007;153:891.

Harrison RW, Hasselblad V, Mehta RH, et al. Effect of levosimendan on survival and adverse events after cardiac surgery: a meta-analysis. *J Cardiothorac Vasc Anesth.* 2013;27:1224.

James PA, Oparil S, Carter BL, et al. 2014 Evidence-based guideline for the management of high blood pressure in adults: report from the panel members appointed to the Eighth Joint National Committee (JNC8). *JAMA.* 2014;311:507.

London MJ, Hur K, Schwartz GG, et al. Association of perioperative β-blockade with mortality and cardiovascular morbidity following major noncardiac surgery. *JAMA.* 2013;309:1704.

Lund LH, Benson L, Dahlström U, et al. Association between use of renin-angiotensin system antagonists and mortality in patients with heart failure and preserved ejection fraction. *JAMA.* 2012;308:2108.

McMurray JJ, Packer M, Desai AS, et al. Angiotensin-neprilysin inhibition versus enalapril in heart failure. *N Engl J Med.* 2014;371:993.

Mitchell LB, Exner DV, Wyse DG, et al. Prophylactic oral amiodarone for the prevention of arrhythmias that begin early after revascularization, valve replacement, or repair: PAPABEAR: a randomized controlled trial. *JAMA.* 2005;294:3093.

Mozaffarian D, Benjamin EJ, Go AS, et al. Executive summary: heart disease and stroke statistics—2015 update: a report from the American Heart Association. *Circulation.* 2015;131:434.

Nordlander M, Sjöquist PO, Ericsson H, et al. Pharmacodynamic, pharmacokinetic and clinical effects of clevidipine, an ultrashort-acting calcium antagonist for rapid blood pressure control. *Cardiovasc Drug Rev.* 2004;22:227.

O'Connor CM, Starling RC, Hernandez AF, et al. Effect of nesiritide in patients with acute decompensated heart failure. *N Engl J Med.* 2011;365:32.

Reil J-C, Tardif J-C, Ford I, et al. Selective heart rate reduction with ivabradine unloads the left ventricle in heart failure patients. *J Am Coll Cardiol.* 2013;62:1977.

Schroten NF, Gaillard CA, van Veldhuisen DJ, et al. New roles for renin and prorenin in heart failure and cardiorenal crosstalk. *Heart Fail Rev.* 2012;17:191.

Tiryakioglu O, Demirtas S, Ari H, et al. Magnesium sulphate and amiodarone prophylaxis for prevention of postoperative arrhythmia in coronary by-pass operations. *J Cardiothorac Surg.* 2009;4:8.

Wijeysundera DN, Duncan D, Nkonde-Price C, et al. Perioperative beta blockade in noncardiac surgery: a systematic review for the 2014 ACC/AHA guideline on perioperative cardiovascular evaluation and management of patients undergoing noncardiac surgery: a report of the American College of Cardiology/American Heart Association Task Force on Practice Guidelines. *J Am Coll Cardiol.* 2014;64:2406.

Yancy CW, Jessup M, Bozkurt B, et al. 2013 ACCF/AHA guideline for the management of heart failure: a report of the American College of Cardiology Foundation/American Heart Association Task Force on Practice Guidelines. *J Am Coll Cardiol.* 2013;62:e147.

Zimetbaum P. Antiarrhythmic drug therapy for atrial fibrillation. *Circulation.* 2012;125:381.

Section III

Monitoring

Chapter 9

Electrocardiographic Monitoring

Leon Freudzon, MD • Shamsuddin Akhtar, MBBS •
Martin J. London, MD • Paul G. Barash, MD

Key Points

1. The electrocardiogram reflects differences in transmembrane voltages in myocardial cells that occur during depolarization and repolarization within each cycle.
2. Processing of the electrocardiogram occurs in a series of steps.
3. Where and how electrocardiographic (ECG) electrodes are placed on the body are critical determinants of the morphology of the ECG signal.
4. ECG signals must be amplified and filtered before display.
5. How accurately the clinician places ECG leads on the patient's torso is probably the single most important factor influencing clinical utility of the electrocardiogram.
6. The ST segment is the most important portion of the QRS complex for evaluating ischemia.
7. Use of inferior leads (II, III, aVF) allows superior discrimination of P-wave morphology and facilitates visual diagnosis of arrhythmias and conduction disorders.
8. Electrolyte abnormalities typically cause changes in repolarization (ST-T-U waves).

Despite the introduction of more sophisticated cardiovascular monitors such as the pulmonary artery catheter and echocardiography, the electrocardiogram (coupled with blood pressure measurement) serves as the foundation for guiding cardiovascular therapeutic interventions in the majority of anesthetic cases. It is indispensable for diagnosing arrhythmias, acute coronary syndromes, and electrolyte abnormalities (particularly of serum potassium and calcium) and in the detection of some forms of genetically mediated electrical or structural cardiac abnormalities (eg, Brugada syndrome).

One of the most important changes in electrocardiography is the widespread use of computerized systems for recording electrocardiograms. Bedside units are capable of recording diagnostic-quality 12-lead electrocardiograms that can be transmitted over a hospital network for storage and retrieval. Most of the electrocardiograms in the United States are recorded by digital, automated devices, equipped with software that can measure electrocardiographic (ECG) intervals and amplitudes and can provide virtually instantaneous interpretation.

▧ THE 12-LEAD SYSTEM

Where and how ECG electrodes are placed on the body are critical determinants of the morphology of the ECG signal. Lead systems have been developed based on

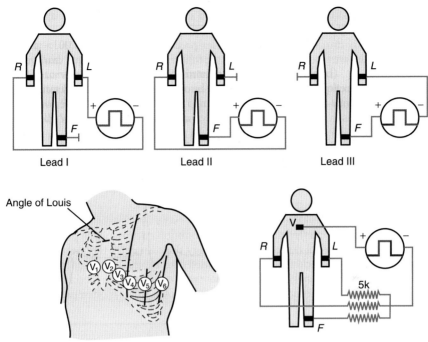

Fig. 9.1 *(Top)* Electrode connections for recording the three standard limb leads I, II, and III. R, L, and F indicate locations of electrodes on the right arm, the left arm, and the left foot, respectively. *(Bottom)* Electrode locations and electrical connections for recording a precordial lead. *(Left)* The positions of the exploring electrode (V) for the six precordial leads. *(Right)* Connections to form the Wilson central terminal for recording a precordial (V) lead. (From Mirvis DM, Goldberger AL. Electrocardiography. In: Bonow RO, Mann DL, Zipes DP, Libby P, eds. *Braunwald's Heart Disease: A Textbook of Cardiovascular Medicine.* 8th ed. Philadelphia: Saunders; 2008:153.)

theoretical considerations and references to anatomic landmarks that facilitate consistency among individual patients (eg, standard 12-lead system). Einthoven established electrocardiography using three extremities as references: the left arm (LA), right arm (RA), and left leg (LL). He recorded the difference in potential between the LA and RA (lead I), between the RA and LL (lead II), and between the LA and LL (lead III) (Fig. 9.1). Because the signals recorded were differences between two electrodes, these leads were called bipolar. The right leg (RL) served only as a reference electrode. Because the Kirchhoff loop equation states that the sum of the three voltage differential pairs must equal zero, the sum of leads I and III must equal lead II.

The positive or negative polarity of each of the limbs was chosen by Einthoven to result in positive deflections of most of the waveforms and has no innate physiologic significance. He postulated that the three limbs defined an imaginary equilateral triangle with the heart at its center. Wilson refined and introduced the precordial leads into clinical practice. To implement these leads, he postulated a mechanism whereby the absolute level of electrical potential could be measured at the site of the exploring precordial electrode (the positive electrode). A negative pole with zero potential was formed by joining the three limb electrodes in a resistive network in which equally weighted signals cancel each other out. He called this the central terminal, and in a fashion similar to Einthoven's vector concepts, he postulated that it was located at the electrical center of the heart, representing the mean electrical potential of the body throughout the cardiac cycle. He described three additional limb leads

9

(aVL, aVR, and aVF). These leads measured new vectors of activation, and in this way the hexaxial reference system for determination of the electrical axis was established. He subsequently introduced the six unipolar precordial V leads in 1935.

Six electrodes are placed on the chest in the following locations: V_1, fourth intercostal space at the right sternal border; V_2, fourth intercostal space at the left sternal border; V_3, midway between V_2 and V_4; V_4, fifth intercostal space in the midclavicular line; V_5, in the horizontal plane of V_4 at the anterior axillary line, or, if the anterior axillary line is ambiguous, midway between V_4 and V_6; and V_6, in the horizontal plane of V_4 at the midaxillary line (see Fig. 9.1).

▥ ELECTROCARDIOGRAPHIC ARTIFACT

Electrical Power–Line Interference

Electrical power–line interference (60 Hz) is a common environmental problem. Power lines and other electrical devices radiate energy that can enter the monitor by poor electrode contact or cracked or poorly shielded lead cables. Interference can also be induced electromagnetically as these signals radiate through the loop formed by the body, lead cables, and monitor. A line frequency "notch" filter is often used to remove 60-Hz noise.

Electrocautery

Electrocautery units generate radiofrequency currents at very high frequencies (800–2000 kHz) and high voltages (1 kV, which is 100 times greater than the ECG signal). Older units used a modulation frequency of 60 Hz, which spread substantial electrical noise into the QRS frequency range of the ECG signal. Newer units use a modulation frequency of 20 kHz, thus minimizing this problem; however, reports still exist of electrocautery as a cause of artifactual ST-segment changes in intraoperative electrocardiograms. To minimize electrocautery artifact, the RL reference electrode should be placed as close as possible to the return plate, and the ECG monitor should be plugged into a different power outlet from the electrosurgical unit.

Clinical Sources of Artifact

Clinical devices in physical contact with the patient, particularly through plastic tubing, may at times cause clinically significant ECG artifact. Although the exact mechanism is uncertain, two leading explanations are either a piezoelectric effect secondary to mechanical deformation of the plastic or buildup of static electricity between two dissimilar materials, especially those materials in motion (as in the case of cardiopulmonary bypass [CPB] tubing and the roller pump head). In this situation, the electricity generated in the pump flows into the patient through the tubing and is picked up by the electrodes. This artifact is not related to the electricity used to power the CPB pump because it has been reproduced by manually turning the pump heads.

ECG interference during CPB has been recognized for many years. It is manifested by marked irregularity of the baseline, similar to ventricular fibrillation, with a frequency of 1 to 4 Hz and a peak amplitude up to 5 mV. Uncorrected, it may make effective diagnosis of arrhythmias and conduction disturbances very difficult (Fig. 9.2), especially during the critical period of weaning from CPB, and it may also make accurate determination of asystolic arrest from cardioplegia difficult. Accumulation of static

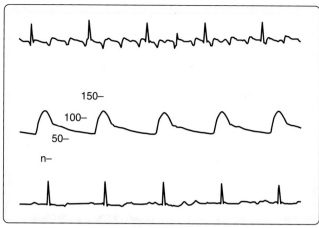

Fig. 9.2 *(Top)* Baseline artifact simulates atrial flutter in a cannulated patient. *(Middle)* This patient had stable arterial pressure just before institution of full cardiopulmonary bypass, similar to that described by Kleinman and associates. *(Bottom)* The "pseudo-flutter waves" are corrected by application of the grounding cable. (From London MJ, Kaplan JA. Advances in electrocardiographic monitoring. In: Kaplan JA, Reich DL, Konstadt SN, eds. *Cardiac Anesthesia*. 4th ed. Philadelphia: Saunders; 1999.)

electricity is assumed to be the major etiologic factor. Khambatta and colleagues recommended maintaining ambient temperature higher than 20°C.

ELECTROCARDIOGRAPHIC CHANGES WITH MYOCARDIAL ISCHEMIA

Detection of Myocardial Ischemia

The ST segment is the most important portion of the QRS complex for evaluating ischemia. It may come as a surprise that no gold standard criteria exist for the ECG diagnosis of myocardial ischemia. Many anesthesiologists, when evaluating an electrocardiogram for signs of ischemia, look for signs of repolarization or ST-segment abnormalities. Many other signs of myocardial ischemia may also be seen in the electrocardiogram, including T-wave inversion, QRS and T-wave axis alterations, R- or U-wave changes, or the development of previously undocumented arrhythmias or ventricular ectopy. None of these, however, is as specific for ischemia as ST-segment depression or elevation. Depending on the location of the infarction, and the observed leads, the ST-segment changes have a specificity of 84% to 100% and a sensitivity of 12% to 66% for myocardial ischemia.

The origin of the ST segment, at the J point, is easy to locate. However, J-point termination, which is generally accepted as the beginning of any change of slope of the T wave, is more difficult to determine. Physiologically normal persons may have no discernible ST segment because the T wave starts with a steady slope from the J point, especially at rapid heart rates. The TP segment has been used as the isoelectric baseline from which changes in the ST segment are evaluated, but with tachycardia, this segment is eliminated, and, during exercise testing, the PR segment is used. The PR segment is used in all ST-segment analyzers.

Repolarization of the ventricle proceeds from the epicardium to the endocardium, opposite to the vector of depolarization. The ST segment reflects the midportion, or phase 2, of repolarization during little change in electrical potential. It is usually

9

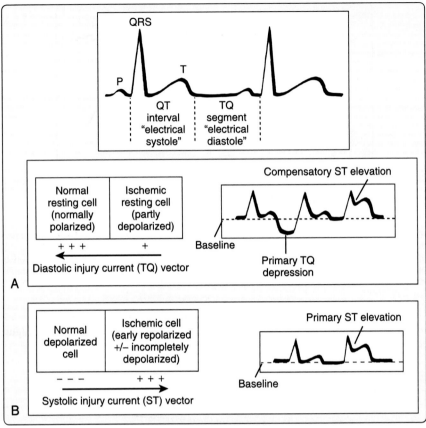

Fig. 9.3 Pathophysiology of ischemic ST-segment elevation. Two basic mechanisms have been advanced to explain the elevation seen with acute myocardial injury. (A) Diastolic current of injury. In this case (first QRS-T complex), the ST-segment vector is directed away from the relatively negative, partly depolarized, ischemic region during electrical diastole (TQ interval), and the result is primary TQ-interval depression. Conventional alternating current electrocardiograms compensate for the baseline shift, and an apparent ST-segment elevation (second QRS-T complex) results. (B) Systolic current of injury. In this case, the ischemic zone is relatively positive during electrical systole because the cells are repolarized early and the amplitude and upstroke velocity of their action potentials may be decreased. This injury current vector is oriented toward the electropositive zone, and the result is primary ST-segment elevation. (From Mirvis DM, Goldberger AL. Electrocardiography. In: Bonow RO, Mann DL, Zipes DP, Libby P, eds. *Braunwald's Heart Disease: A Textbook of Cardiovascular Medicine.* 8th ed. Philadelphia: Saunders; 2008:174.)

isoelectric. Ischemia causes a loss of intracellular potassium, resulting in a current of injury. With subendocardial injury, the ST segment is depressed in the surface leads. With epicardial or transmural injury, the ST segment is elevated (Figs. 9.3 and 9.4). Although myocardial ischemia may manifest in PR-segment, QRS complex, ST-segment, or T-wave changes, the earliest ECG signs of ischemia are typically T-wave and ST-segment changes. With myocardial ischemia, repolarization is affected, resulting in downsloping or horizontal ST-segment depression. Various local effects and differences in vectors during repolarization result in different ST-segment morphologic features that are recorded by the different leads. It is generally accepted that ST-segment changes in multiple leads are associated with more severe degrees of coronary artery disease (CAD).

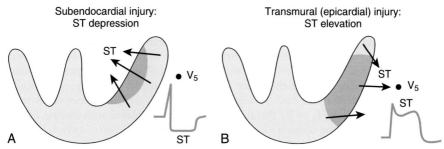

Fig. 9.4 Current of injury patterns with acute ischemia. (A) With predominant subendocardial ischemia the resultant ST-segment vector is directed toward the inner layer of the affected ventricle and the ventricular cavity. Overlying leads therefore record ST-segment depression. (B) With ischemia involving the outer ventricular layer (transmural or epicardial injury), the ST-segment vector is directed outward. Overlying leads record ST-segment elevation. Reciprocal ST-segment depression can appear in contralateral leads. (From Mirvis DM, Goldberger AL. Electrocardiography. In: Bonow RO, Mann DL, Zipes DP, Libby P, eds. *Braunwald's Heart Disease: A Textbook of Cardiovascular Medicine*. 8th ed. Philadelphia: Saunders; 2008:174.)

The criteria for myocardial infarction (MI) are divided into two categories: ST-segment elevation MI (STEMI), and ST-segment depression/T-wave change MI (NSTEMI). The J point is located at the juncture of the QRS complex and the ST segment, and it is used to measure the magnitude of the ST-segment deflection as compared with the baseline of the electrocardiogram. A new J-point elevation of 0.1 mV or greater is required in all leads except V_2 and V_3 to meet the criteria for STEMI. J-point elevations of up to 0.25 mV may be seen in leads V_2 and V_3 in healthy men younger than 40 years of age; however, this finding decreases with age and is less prominent in women. The J-point elevations must be seen in two or more contiguous leads for the satisfaction of ST-segment elevation criteria. New horizontal or downsloping ST-segment depressions of 0.05 mV or greater or T-wave inversion of 0.1 mV or greater in two contiguous leads with an R-wave–to–S-wave ratio greater than 1 satisfy the criteria for NSTEMI. However, ST-segment elevations are more specific than ST-segment depressions and/or T-wave inversions for localizing the site of ischemia. ST-segment elevation generally suggests greater degrees of myocardial damage than ST-segment depression or T-wave changes. Previously inverted T waves may pseudonormalize during episodes of acute myocardial ischemia (Appendix 9.1).

Nonspecific ST-segment depression can be related to drug use, particularly digoxin. Interpretation of ST-segment changes in patients with left ventricular hypertrophy is particularly controversial given the tall R-wave baseline, J-point depression, and steep slope of the ST segment.

ST-segment elevation is rarely reported in the setting of noncardiac surgical procedures. However, it is commonly observed during weaning from CPB in cardiac operations and during CABG procedures (on and off pump) with interruption of coronary flow in a native or graft vessel. ST-segment elevation in a lead with a Q wave should not be analyzed for acute ischemia, although it may indicate the presence of a ventricular aneurysm.

Anatomic Localization of Ischemia With the Electrocardiogram

As noted earlier, ST-segment depression is a common manifestation of subendocardial ischemia. From a practical clinical standpoint, it has a single major strength and limitation. Its strength is that it is almost always present in one or more of the anterolateral precordial leads (V_4–V_6). However, it fails to "localize" the offending coronary lesion and has little relation to underlying segmental asynergy.

In contrast, ST-segment elevation correlates well with segmental asynergy and localizes the offending lesion relatively well. Reciprocal ST-segment depression often is present in one or more of the other 12 leads. In patients with angiographically documented single-vessel disease, ST-segment elevation (as well as Q waves or inverted T waves) in leads I, aVL, or V_1 through V_4 is closely correlated with disease of the left anterior descending coronary artery, whereas similar findings in leads, I, III, and aVF indicate disease of the right coronary or left circumflex arteries (surprisingly, the latter two cannot be differentiated by ECG criteria).

Clinical Lead Systems for Detecting Ischemia

Early clinical reports of intraoperative monitoring using the V_5 lead in high-risk patients were based on observations during exercise testing, in which bipolar configurations of V_5 demonstrated high sensitivity for myocardial ischemia detection (up to 90%). Subsequent studies using 12-lead monitoring (torso-mounted for stability during exercise) confirmed the sensitivity of the lateral precordial leads. Some studies, however, reported higher sensitivity for leads V_4 or V_6 compared with V_5, followed by the inferior leads (in which most false-positive responses were reported).

Intraoperative Lead Systems

The cardiac anesthesiologist encounters a variety of ECG changes consistent with myocardial ischemia or infarction at many phases of the perioperative period in patients undergoing cardiac operations. In the majority of these patients (ie, those with known CAD), the sensitivity and specificity of the major signs described are high, and few false-positive or false-negative changes are encountered. However, the abnormal physiology of CPB, including acute changes in temperature, electrolyte concentrations, and catecholamine levels can significantly influence sensitivity and specificity. In addition, patients undergoing valve replacement, even those without coronary artery lesions, can develop significant subendocardial and transmural ischemia (ie, coronary artery embolus of valve calcification, vegetations, or air).

Detecting and recognizing the clinical significance of various ECG signs of ischemia or infarction and coordinating the findings with transesophageal echocardiography (TEE) can enhance patient care in the acute setting, as in emergency treatment of coronary artery spasm or air embolus, or by alerting the surgeon that myocardial revascularization may have been inadequate. This may lead to reexploration of a saphenous vein or internal mammary artery anastomosis, especially if the TEE data support the diagnosis of ischemia.

The early reports recommending routine intraoperative monitoring of V_5 in high-risk patients cited exercise tolerance tests as the source of their recommendations. Subsequently, the recommended leads for intraoperative monitoring, based on several clinical studies, did not differ substantially from those used during exercise testing, although considerable controversy on the optimal leads persists in both clinical settings. The use of continuous ECG monitoring in the coronary care unit has received increasing attention. A clinical study using continuous, computerized 12-lead ECG analysis in a mixed cohort reported that almost 90% of changes involved ST-segment depression alone (75% in V_5 and 61% in V_4). In approximately 70% of patients, significant changes were observed in multiple leads. The sensitivity of each of the 12 leads in

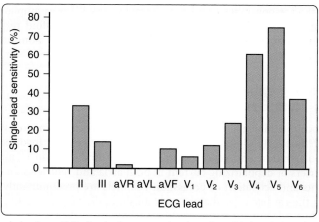

Fig. 9.5 Single-lead sensitivity for the intraoperative detection of ischemia based on 51 episodes detected in 25 patients undergoing noncardiac surgical procedures. Sensitivity was calculated by dividing the number of episodes detected in that electrocardiographic (ECG) lead by the total number of episodes. Sensitivity was greatest in lead V5, and the lateral leads (I, aVL) were insensitive. (Reproduced with permission from London MJ, Hollenberg M, Wong MG, et al. Intraoperative myocardial ischemia: localization by continuous 12-lead electrocardiography. *Anesthesiology.* 1988;69:232.)

that study is shown in Fig. 9.5. When considered in combination, sensitivity for the standard clinical combination of leads II and V_5 was 80%.

ELECTROCARDIOGRAPHIC CHANGES WITH PACEMAKERS, RESPIRATIONS, ELECTROLYTES, AND MEDICATIONS

Use of the inferior leads (II, III, aVF) allows superior discrimination of P-wave morphology and facilitates the visual diagnosis of arrhythmias and conduction disorders (Appendix 9.1).With the increasing use of implantable defibrillators and automatic external defibrillators to treat ventricular fibrillation and ventricular tachycardia, considerable interest exists in the refinement of arrhythmia detection algorithms and their validation. As expected, the accuracy of these devices for detecting ventricular arrhythmias is high, but it is much lower for detecting atrial arrhythmias. Detection of pacemaker spikes may be complicated by very low-amplitude signals related to bipolar pacing leads, amplitude varying with respiration, and total body fluid accumulation. Most critical care and ambulatory monitors incorporate pacemaker spike enhancement for small high-frequency signals (typically 5–500 mV with 0.5- to 2-ms pulse duration) to facilitate recognition. However, this can cause artifact if high-frequency noise is present within the lead system.

A promising application of the electrocardiogram is to correlate respiratory variation in wave amplitude with patients' volume responsiveness. The R wave, especially in lead II (RII), shows consistent respiratory amplitude variation during positive-pressure mechanical ventilation. This variation is likely caused by the "Brody effect," a theoretical analysis of left ventricular volume and electrical conductance. RII-wave amplitude variation may be used as a dynamic index of volume responsiveness in a mechanically ventilated patient, similar to the use of arterial pulse contour analysis and esophageal Doppler monitoring to derive pulse-pressure and stroke volume variation as dynamic measures of fluid responsiveness. Real-time, intraoperative RII-wave amplitude variation has the potential to become a truly noninvasive monitor for fluid responsiveness; however, at present, no commercially available intraoperative monitoring systems provide ECG R-wave amplitude variation measures.

Electrocardiographic Changes Resulting From Electrolyte Disorders

Cardiac myocytes exhibit a long action potential (200–400 ms) compared with neurons and skeletal muscle (1–5 ms). Multiple different channels are involved in cardiac muscle depolarization and repolarization. Sodium and calcium channels are the primary carriers of depolarizing current in both atria and ventricles. Inactivation of these currents and activation of potassium channels are predominantly involved in repolarizing the cardiac cells, thereby reestablishing the negative resting membrane potential. Thus it is not surprising that perturbations in the plasma concentrations of potassium and calcium ions lead to changes in the finely tuned cardiac electrical activity and the surface electrocardiogram. They typically cause changes in repolarization (ST-T-U waves) and can also lead to QRS complex prolongation.

Hyperkalemia

Hyperkalemia is not an uncommon occurrence in patients undergoing cardiac surgical procedures with CPB. Hyperkalemia affects repolarization of cardiac cells. Although progressive changes in the surface electrocardiogram with increasing levels of potassium have been described, the correlation between serum potassium levels and ECG changes is not strong. Typically, ECG changes start with narrowing and peaking of the T waves. Further elevation of extracellular potassium leads to prolongation of the QRS complex. The reason is delayed AV conduction, and an AV block may appear. These changes are typically followed by prolongation of the PR interval, flattening of the P waves, and loss of the P wave because the high potassium levels delay the spread of the cardiac activating impulse through the myocardium. Further increase in plasma potassium levels cause sine waves, which can progress to asystole or ventricular fibrillation. Hyperkalemia may also reduce the myocardial response to artificial pacemaker stimulation. These changes are all seen with use of potassium cardioplegia.

Hypokalemia

Because potassium channels and ions are significantly involved in cardiac repolarization, it is not surprising that hypokalemia prolongs ventricular repolarization. This results in characteristic reversal in the relative amplitudes of the T and U waves. T-wave flattening or inversion is noted, whereas U waves become more prominent. The U-wave prominence is caused by the prolongation of the recovery phase of the cardiac action potential. This can lead to the life-threatening torsades de pointes type of ventricular arrhythmia. Slight depression of the ST segment may also occur, as well as increased amplitude and width of the P waves with prolongation of the PR interval.

Hypocalcemia and Hypercalcemia

The ventricular recovery time, as represented on the electrocardiogram by the QTc interval, is altered by the extremes of serum calcium. Hypocalcemia can cause a prolonged QTc interval (ST portion), whereas hypercalcemia shortens the QTc interval. In hypocalcemia, the prolonged QT interval may be accompanied by terminal T-wave inversions. In extreme hypercalcemia, an increase in QRS complex, biphasic T waves, and Osborn waves has been described.

Medications

Many antiarrhythmic medications are used in the perioperative period in patients undergoing cardiac surgical procedures. Generally, drugs that increase the duration of the cardiac action potential prolong the QT interval. These include class Ia and Ic antiarrhythmic drugs (eg, quinidine, procainamide), phenothiazines, antidepressants, haloperidol, and atypical antipsychotic agents. Intravenous amiodarone, commonly used in the management of perioperative arrhythmias, also causes QT-interval prolongation. Other class III antiarrhythmic drugs (eg, sotalol) cause QT-interval prolongation as well. Unlike class Ia and III antiarrhythmic drugs, digitalis glycosides shorten the QT interval and often cause "scooping" of the ST-T wave complex.

ELECTROCARDIOGRAPHIC MONITORING

SUGGESTED READINGS

Balaji S, Ellenby M, McNames J, et al. Update on intensive care ECG and cardiac event monitoring. *Card Electrophysiol Rev.* 2002;6:190–195.

Carley SD. Beyond the 12 lead: review of the use of additional leads for the early electrocardiographic diagnosis of acute myocardial infarction. *Emerg Med (Fremantle).* 2003;15:143–154.

Horacek BM, Wagner GS. Electrocardiographic ST-segment changes during acute myocardial ischemia. *Card Electrophysiol Rev.* 2002;6:196–203.

Jain A, Kaur Makkar J, Mangal K. Electrocautery-induced artifactual ST-segment depression in a patient with coronary artery disease. *J Electrocardiol.* 2010;43:336–337.

Katz AM. The electrocardiogram. In: *Physiology of the Heart.* Philadelphia: Lippincott Williams & Wilkins; 2006:427–461.

Kligfield P, Gettes LS, Bailey JJ, et al. Recommendations for the standardization and interpretation of the electrocardiogram: part I. The electrocardiogram and its technology: a scientific statement from the American Heart Association Electrocardiography and Arrhythmias Committee, Council on Clinical Cardiology; the American College of Cardiology Foundation; and the Heart Rhythm Society: endorsed by the International Society for Computerized Electrocardiology. *Circulation.* 2007;115:1306–1324.

Landesberg G, Mosseri M, Wolf Y, et al. Perioperative myocardial ischemia and infarction: identification by continuous 12-lead electrocardiogram with online ST-segment monitoring. *Anesthesiology.* 2002;96:264–270.

Levkov C, Mihov G, Ivanov R, et al. Removal of power-line interference from the ECG: a review of the subtraction procedure. *Biomed Eng Online.* 2005;4:50.

London MJ. Multilead precordial ST-segment monitoring: "the next generation. *Anesthesiology.* 2002;96:259–261.

Lorne E, Mahjoub Y, Guinot PG, et al. Respiratory variations of R-wave amplitude in lead II are correlated with stroke volume variations evaluated by transesophageal Doppler echocardiography. *J Cardiothorac Vasc Anesth.* 2012;26:381–386.

Martinez EA, Kim LJ, Faraday N, et al. Sensitivity of routine intensive care unit surveillance for detecting myocardial ischemia. *Crit Care Med.* 2003;31:2302–2308.

Montague BT, Ouellette JR, Buller GK. Retrospective review of the frequency of ECG changes in hyperkalemia. *Clin J Am Soc Nephrol.* 2008;3:324–330.

Moss AJ. Long QT syndrome. *JAMA.* 2003;289:2041–2044.

Ringborn M, Pettersson J, Persson E, et al. Comparison of high-frequency QRS components and ST-segment elevation to detect and quantify acute myocardial ischemia. *J Electrocardiol.* 2010;43:113–120.

Rubart M, Zipes DP. Genesis of cardiac arrhythmias: electrophysiological considerations. In: Libby P, Bonow RO, Mann DL, et al, eds. *Braunwald's Heart Disease: A Textbook of Cardiovascular Medicine.* 8th ed. Philadelphia: Saunders; 2008:727–762.

Said SA, Bloo R, de Nooijer R, et al. Cardiac and non-cardiac causes of T-wave inversion in the precordial leads in adult subjects: a Dutch case series and review of the literature. *World J Cardiol.* 2015;7:86–100.

Solanki SL, Kishore K, Goyal VK, et al. Electrocautery induced artifactual ST segment depression in leads II, III and aVF on intra-operative 5-lead electrocardiogram. *J Clin Monit Comput.* 2013;27:97–98.

Thygesen K, Alpert JS, Jaffe AS, et al. Third universal definition of myocardial infarction. *Circulation.* 2012;126:2020–2035.

Wagner GS, Macfarlane P, Wellens H, et al. AHA/ACCF/HRS recommendations for the standardization and interpretation of the electrocardiogram. Part VI. Acute ischemia/infarction: a scientific statement from the American Heart Association Electrocardiography and Arrhythmias Committee, Council on Clinical Cardiology; the American College of Cardiology Foundation; and the Heart Rhythm Society. Endorsed by the International Society for Computerized Electrocardiology. *J Am Coll Cardiol.* 2009;53:1003–1011.

Zimetbaum PJ, Josephson ME. Use of the electrocardiogram in acute myocardial infarction. *N Engl J Med.* 2003;348:933–940.

9

Appendix 9.1

Electrocardiogram Atlas: A Summary of Important Changes on the Electrocardiogram

Gina C. Badescu, MD • Benjamin Sherman, MD • James R. Zaidan, MD, MBA • Paul G. Barash, MD

Lead Placement		
	Electrode	
Lead Placement	Positive	Negative
Bipolar Leads		
I	LA	RA
II	LL	RA
III	LL	LA
Augmented Unipolar Leads		
aVR	RA	LA, LL
aVL	LA	RA, LL
aVF	LL	RA, LA
Precordial Leads		
V1	4 ICS–RSB	
V2	4 ICS–LSB	
V3	Midway between V2 and V4	
V4	5 ICS–MCL	
V5	5 ICS–AAL	
V6	5 ICS–MAL	

AAL, Interaxillary line; *ICS,* intercostal space; *LA,* left arm; *LL,* left leg; *LSB,* left sternal border; *MAL,* midaxillary line; *MCL,* midclavicular line; *RA,* right arm; *RSB,* right sternal border.

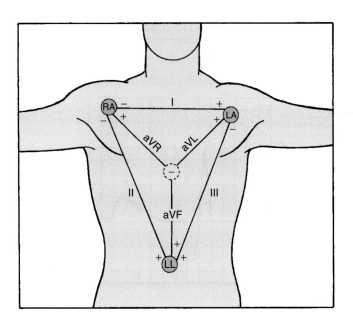

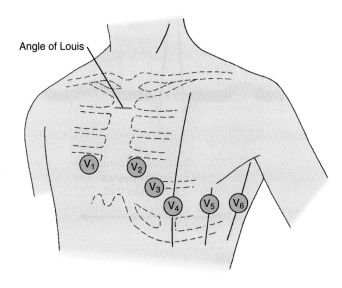

NORMAL ELECTROCARDIOGRAM: CARDIAC CYCLE

The normal electrocardiogram is composed of waves (P, QRS, T, and U) and intervals (PR, QRS, ST, and QT).

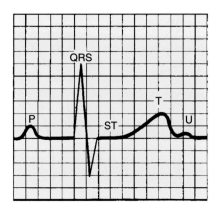

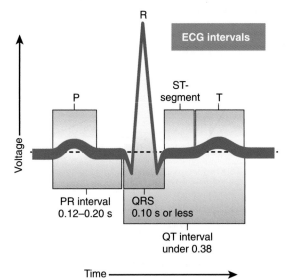

ATRIAL FIBRILLATION

Rate: Variable (~150–200 beats/min)
Rhythm: Irregular
PR interval: No P wave; PR interval not discernible
QT interval: QRS normal

Note: This must be differentiated from atrial flutter: (1) absence of flutter waves and presence of fibrillatory line; (2) flutter usually associated with higher ventricular rates (>150 beats/min). Loss of atrial contraction reduces cardiac output (10–20%). Mural atrial thrombi may develop. It is considered controlled if the ventricular rate is <100 beats/min.

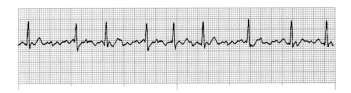

ATRIAL FLUTTER

Rate: Rapid, atrial usually regular (250–350 beats/min); ventricular usually regular (<100 beats/min)
Rhythm: Atrial and ventricular regular
PR interval: Flutter (F) waves saw-toothed; PR interval cannot be measured
QT interval: QRS usually normal; ST segment and T waves not identifiable

Note: Carotid massage slows the ventricular response, thus simplifying recognition of the F waves.

II

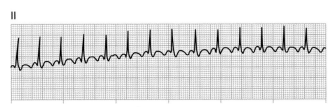

ATRIOVENTRICULAR BLOCK

First-Degree

Rate: 60–100 beats/min
Rhythm: Regular
PR interval: Prolonged (>0.20 second) and constant
QT interval: Normal

Note: It is usually clinically insignificant; it may be an early harbinger of drug toxicity.

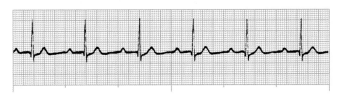

9

Second-Degree: Mobitz Type I/Wenckebach Block

Rate: 60–100 beats/min
Rhythm: Atrial regular; ventricular irregular
PR interval: P-wave normal; PR interval progressively lengthens with each cycle until QRS complex is dropped (dropped beat); PR interval following dropped beat is shorter than normal.
QT interval: QRS complex normal but dropped periodically

Note: It is commonly seen in (1) trained athletes and (2) patients with drug toxicity.

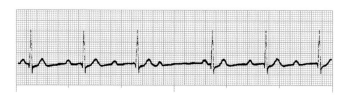

Second-Degree: Mobitz Type II Block

Rate: <100 beats/min
Rhythm: Atrial regular; ventricular regular or irregular
PR interval: P waves normal, but some not followed by QRS complex
QT interval: Normal but may have widened QRS complex if block is at level of bundle branch. ST segment and T wave may be abnormal, depending on location of block

Note: In contrast to Mobitz type I block, the PR and RR intervals are constant and the dropped QRS occurs without warning. The wider the QRS complex (block lower in the conduction system), the greater is the amount of myocardial damage.

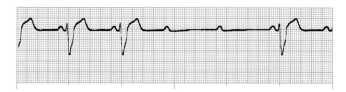

Third-Degree: Complete Heart Block

Rate: <45 beats/min
Rhythm: Atrial regular; ventricular regular; no relationship between P wave and QRS complex
PR interval: Variable because atria and ventricles beat independently
QT interval: QRS morphology variable, depending on the origin of the ventricular beat in the intrinsic pacemaker system (atrioventricular [AV] junctional vs ventricular pacemaker); ST segment and T wave normal

Note: AV block represents complete failure of conduction from atria to ventricles (no P wave is conducted to the ventricle). The atrial rate is faster than the ventricular rate. P waves have no relation to QRS complexes (eg, they are electrically disconnected). In contrast, with AV dissociation, the P wave is conducted through the AV node, and the atrial and ventricular rates are similar. Immediate treatment with atropine or isoproterenol is required if cardiac output is reduced. Consideration should be given to insertion of a pacemaker. This is seen as a complication of mitral valve replacement.

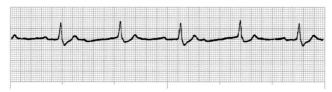

■ ATRIOVENTRICULAR DISSOCIATION

Rate: Variable
Rhythm: Atrial regular; ventricular regular; ventricular rate faster than atrial rate; no relation between P wave and QRS complex
PR interval: Variable because atria and ventricles beat independently
QT interval: QRS morphology dependent on location of ventricular pacemaker; ST segment and T wave abnormal

Note: In AV dissociation, the atria and ventricles beat independently. The P wave is conducted through the AV node, and the atrial and ventricular rate are similar. In contrast, AV block represents complete failure of conduction from atria to ventricles (no P wave is conducted to the ventricle). The atrial rate is faster than the ventricular rate. P waves have no relation to QRS complexes (eg, they are electrically disconnected). Digitalis toxicity can manifest as AV dissociation.

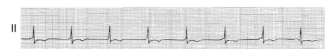

9

■ BUNDLE BRANCH BLOCK

Left Bundle Branch Block

Rate: <100 beats/min
Rhythm: Regular
PR interval: Normal
QT interval: Complete left bundle branch block (LBBB; QRS >0.12 second); incomplete LBBB (QRS = 0.10–0.12 second); lead V_1 negative RS complex; I, aVL, V_6 wide R wave without Q or S component; ST-segment and T-wave defection opposite direction of the R wave

Note: LBBB does not occur in healthy patients and usually indicates serious heart disease with a poorer prognosis. In patients with LBBB, insertion of a pulmonary artery catheter may lead to complete heart block.

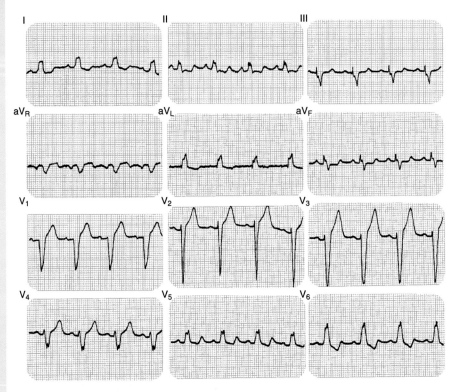

Right Bundle Branch Block

Rate: <100 beats/min

Rhythm: Regular

PR interval: Normal

QT interval: Complete right bundle branch block (RBBB; QRS >0.12 second); incomplete RBBB (QRS = 0.10–0.12 second); varying patterns of QRS complex; rSR (V₁); RS, wide R with M pattern; ST-segment and T-wave opposite direction of the R wave

Note: In the presence of RBBB, Q waves may be seen with a myocardial infarction (MI).

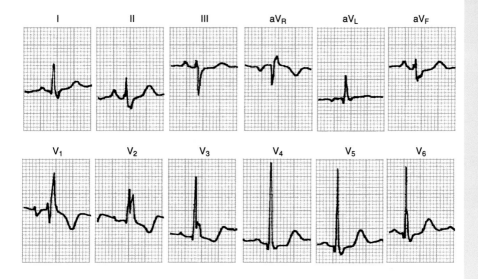

▦ CORONARY ARTERY DISEASE

Transmural Myocardial Infarction

Q waves seen on the electrocardiogram, useful in confirming diagnosis, are associated with poorer prognosis and more significant hemodynamic impairment. Arrhythmias frequently complicate the course. Small Q waves may be a normal variant. For MI, Q waves last longer than 0.04 second, and depth exceeds one-third of the R wave (inferior wall MI). For inferior wall MI, differentiate it from right ventricular hypertrophy by axis deviation.

Anatomic Site	Leads	ECG Changes	Coronary Artery
Inferior	II, III, AVF	Q, ↑ST, ↑T	Right
Anatomic Site	**Leads**	**ECG Changes**	**Coronary Artery**
Posterior	V1–V2	↑R, ↓ST, ↓T	Left circumflex
Anatomic Site	**Leads**	**ECG Changes**	**Coronary Artery**
Lateral	I, aVL, V5, V6	Q, ↑ST, ↑T	Left circumflex
Anatomic Site	**Leads**	**ECG Changes**	**Coronary Artery**
Anterior	I, aVL, V1–V4	Q, ↑ST, ↑T	Left anterior descending
Anatomic Site	**Leads**	**ECG Changes**	**Coronary Artery**
Anteroseptal	V1–V4	Q, ↑ST, ↑T	Left anterior descending

9

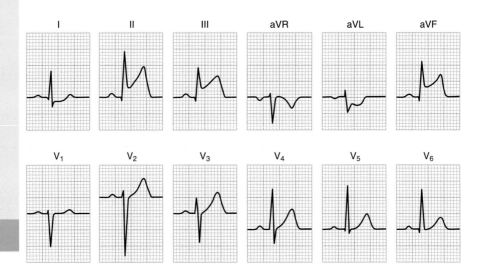

Aorta

Left main
coronary artery

Dominant right
coronary artery (RCA)

Septal artery

Circumflex artery

a

b

Obtuse
marginal artery

Right ventricular
marginal branch

Diagonal artery

Posterior
descending artery

Left anterior
descending
artery (LAD)

Posterolateral branch
of the circumflex artery

I   II   III   aVR   aVL   aVF

V₁   V₂   V₃   V₄   V₅   V₆

III

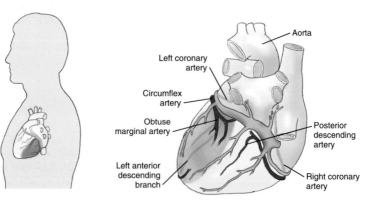

Aorta

Left coronary
artery

Circumflex
artery

Obtuse
marginal artery

Posterior
descending
artery

Left anterior
descending
branch

Right coronary
artery

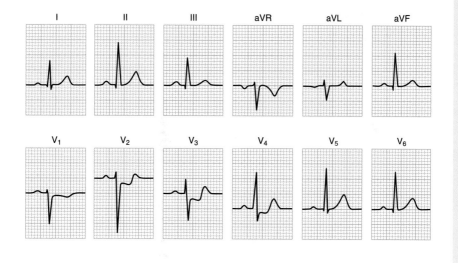

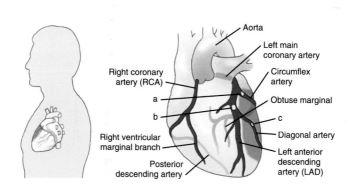

9

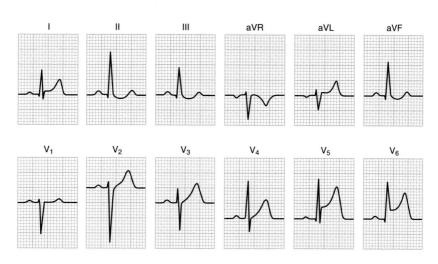

187

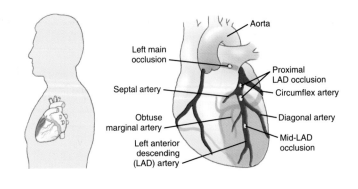

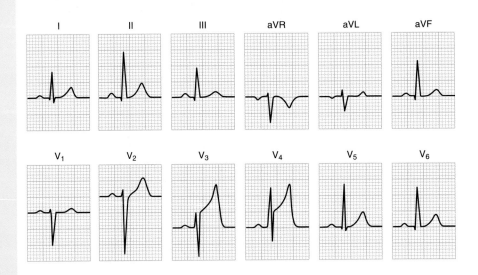

III

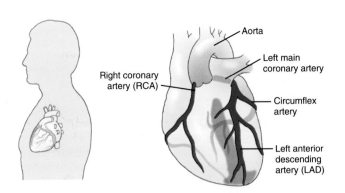

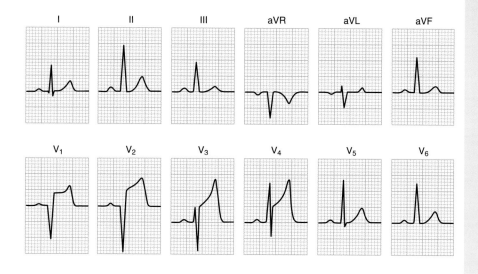

Subendocardial Myocardial Infarction

Persistent ST-segment depression or T-wave inversion occurs in the absence of a Q wave. This usually requires additional laboratory data (eg, isoenzymes) to confirm the diagnosis. The anatomic site of the coronary lesion is similar to that of transmural MI electrocardiographically.

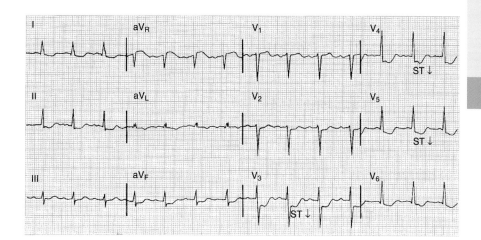

Myocardial Ischemia

Rate: Variable
Rhythm: Usually regular, but may show atrial and/or ventricular arrhythmias
PR interval: Normal
QT interval: ST segment depressed; J-point depression; T-wave inversion; conduction
   disturbances; coronary vasospasm (Prinzmetal) ST-segment elevation; (A) TP
   and PR intervals baseline for ST-segment deviation, (B) ST-segment elevation,
   (C) ST-segment depression

Note: Intraoperative ischemia usually is seen in the presence of "normal" vital signs
(eg, ±20% of preinduction values).

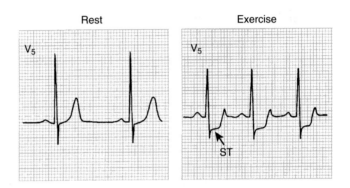

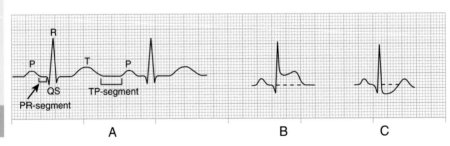

DIGITALIS EFFECT

Rate: <100 beats/min
Rhythm: Regular
PR interval: Normal or prolonged
QT interval: ST-segment sloping ("digitalis effect")

Note: Digitalis toxicity can be the cause of many common arrhythmias (eg, premature ventricular contractions, second-degree heart block). Verapamil, quinidine, and amiodarone cause an increase in serum digitalis concentration.

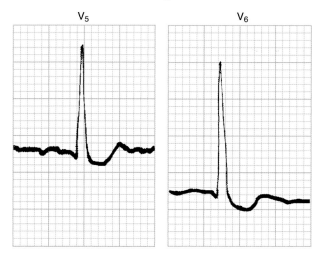

V_5 V_6

◼ ELECTROLYTE DISTURBANCES

	↓ Calcium	↑ Calcium	↓ Potassium	↑ Potassium
Rate	<100 beats/min	<100 beats/min	<100 beats/min	<100 beats/min
Rhythm	Regular	Regular	Regular	Regular
PR interval	Normal	Normal/increased	Normal	Normal
QT interval	Increased	Decreased	Normal	Increased
Other			T wave flat U wave	T wave peaked

Note: Electrocardiographic (ECG) changes usually do not correlate with serum calcium. Hypocalcemia rarely causes arrhythmias in the absence of hypokalemia. In contrast, abnormalities in serum potassium concentration can be diagnosed by electrocardiogram. Similarly, in the clinical range, magnesium concentrations rarely are associated with unique ECG patterns. The presence of a "u" wave (>1.5 mm in height) also is seen in left main coronary artery disease, certain medications, and long QT syndrome.

9

Calcium

Hypocalcemia	Normal	Hypercalcemia

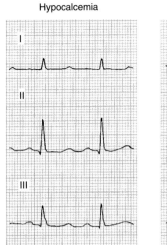 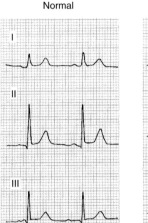 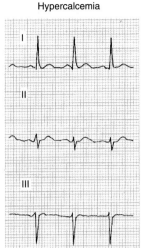

Potassium

Hypokalemia (K⁺ = 1.9 mEq/L)

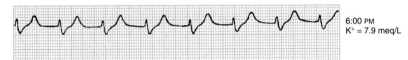

11:00 AM
K^+ = 1.9 meq/L

Hyperkalemia (K⁺ = 7.9 mEq/L)

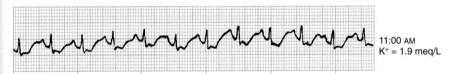

6:00 PM
K^+ = 7.9 meq/L

▨ HYPOTHERMIA

Rate: <60 beats/min
Rhythm: Sinus
PR interval: Prolonged
QT interval: Prolonged

Note: This is seen at temperatures less than 33°C with ST-segment elevation (J-point or Osborn wave). Tremor caused by shivering or Parkinson disease may interfere with ECG interpretation and may be confused with atrial flutter. This may represent a normal variant of early ventricular repolarization. (The *arrow* indicates J-point or Osborn waves.)

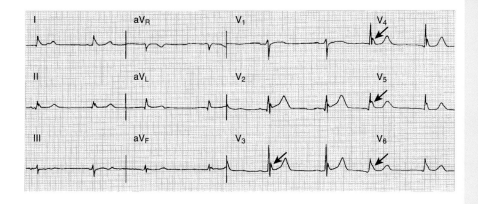

▣ MULTIFOCAL ATRIAL TACHYCARDIA

Rate: 100–200 beats/min
Rhythm: Irregular
PR interval: Consecutive P waves are of varying shape
QT interval: Normal

Note: This is seen in patients with severe lung disease. Carotid massage has no effect. At heart rates lower than 100 beats/min, it may appear as wandering atrial pacemaker. It may be mistaken for atrial fibrillation. Treatment is of the causative disease process.

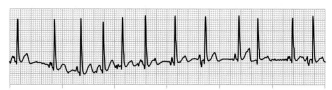

▣ PAROXYSMAL ATRIAL TACHYCARDIA

Rate: 150–250 beats/min
Rhythm: Regular
PR interval: Difficult to distinguish because of tachycardia obscuring P wave; P wave may precede, be included in, or follow QRS complex
QT interval: Normal, but ST segment and T wave may be difficult to distinguish

Note: Therapy depends on the degree of hemodynamic compromise. Carotid sinus massage may terminate the rhythm or decrease heart rate. In contrast to management of paroxysmal atrial tachycardia (PAT) in awake patients, synchronized cardioversion rather than pharmacologic treatment is preferred in hemodynamically unstable anesthetized patients.

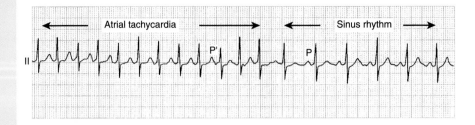

PERICARDITIS

Rate: Variable
Rhythm: Variable
PR interval: Normal
QT interval: Diffuse ST- and T-wave changes with no Q wave, and seen in more leads than an MI

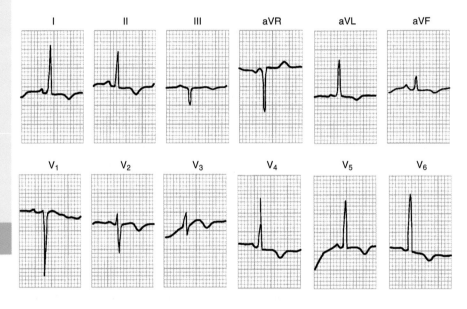

PERICARDIAL TAMPONADE

Rate: Variable
Rhythm: Variable
PR interval: Low-voltage P wave
QT interval: Seen as electrical alternans with low-voltage complexes and varying amplitude of P, QRS, and T waves with each heartbeat

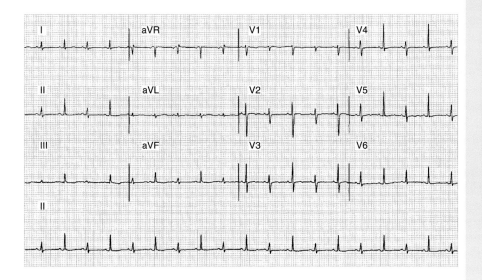

PNEUMOTHORAX

Rate: Variable
Rhythm: Variable
PR interval: Normal
QT interval: Normal

Note: Common ECG abnormalities include right-axis deviation, decreased QRS amplitude, and inverted T waves in leads V_1 to V_6. Differentiate from pulmonary embolus. It may manifest as electrical alternans; thus, pericardial effusion should be ruled out.

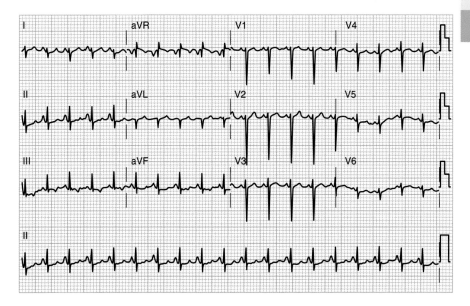

9

▣ PREMATURE ATRIAL CONTRACTION

Rate: <100 beats/min
Rhythm: Irregular
PR interval: P waves may be lost in preceding T waves; PR interval variable
QT interval: QRS normal configuration; ST segment and T wave normal

Note: Nonconducted premature atrial contraction (PAC) appearance is similar to that of sinus arrest; T waves with PAC may be distorted by inclusion of a P wave in the T wave.

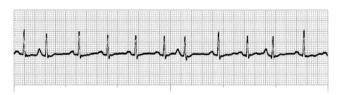

▣ PREMATURE VENTRICULAR CONTRACTION

Rate: Usually <100 beats/min
Rhythm: Irregular
PR interval: P wave and PR interval absent; retrograde conduction of P wave can be seen
QT interval: Wide QRS (>0.12 second); ST segment cannot be evaluated (eg, ischemia); T wave opposite direction of QRS with compensatory pause; fourth and eighth beats premature ventricular contractions

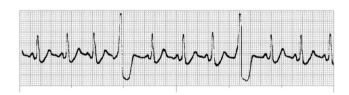

▣ PULMONARY EMBOLUS

Rate: >100 beats/min
Rhythm: Sinus
PR interval: P-pulmonale waveform
QT interval: Q waves in leads III and AV$_F$

Note: Classic ECG signs of S$_1$Q$_3$T$_3$ with T-wave inversion are also seen in leads V$_1$ to V$_4$ and right ventricular strain (ST-segment depression in V$_{1-4}$). It may manifest with atrial fibrillation or flutter.

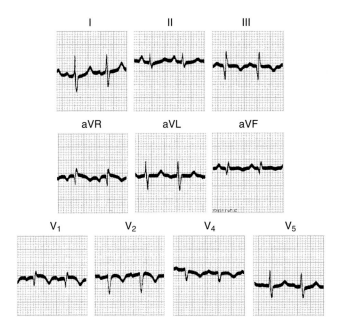

SINUS BRADYCARDIA

Rate: <60 beats/min
Rhythm: Sinus
PR interval: Normal
QT interval: Normal

Note: This is seen in trained athletes as a normal variant.

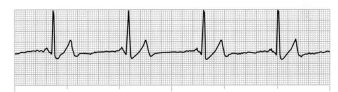

SINUS ARRHYTHMIA

Rate: 60–100 beats/min
Rhythm: Sinus
PR interval: Normal
QT interval: R-R interval variable

Note: Heart rate increases with inhalation and decreases with exhalation are ±10% to 20% (respiratory). Nonrespiratory sinus arrhythmia is seen in older adults with heart disease. It is also seen with increased intracranial pressure.

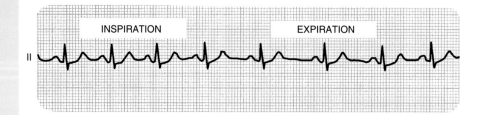

SINUS ARREST

Rate: <60 beats/min
Rhythm: Varies
PR interval: Variable
QT interval: Variable

Note: Rhythm depends on the cardiac pacemaker's firing in the absence of sinoatrial stimulus (atrial pacemaker, 60–75 beats/min; junctional, 40–60 beats/min; ventricular, 30–45 beats/min). Junctional rhythm is most common. Occasional P waves may be seen (retrograde P wave).

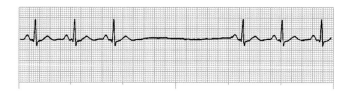

SINUS TACHYCARDIA

Rate: 100–160 beats/min
Rhythm: Regular
PR interval: Normal; P wave may be difficult to see
QT interval: Normal

Note: This should be differentiated from PAT. With PAT, carotid massage terminates the arrhythmia. Sinus tachycardia may respond to vagal maneuvers but reappears as soon as vagal stimulus is removed.

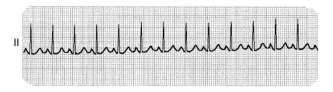

SUBARACHNOID HEMORRHAGE

Rate: <60 beats/min
Rhythm: Sinus
PR interval: Normal
QT interval: T-wave inversion deep and wide, prominent U waves; sinus arrhythmias; Q waves may be seen and may mimic acute coronary syndrome

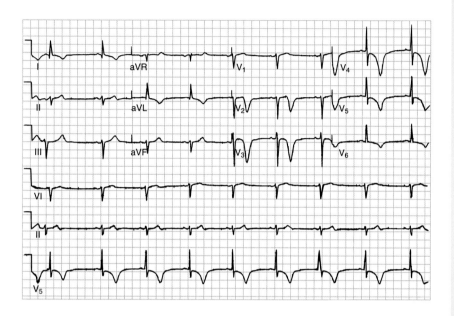

TORSADES DE POINTES

Rate: 150–250 beats/min
Rhythm: No atrial component seen; ventricular rhythm regular or irregular
PR interval: P wave buried in QRS complex
QT interval: QRS complexes usually wide and with phasic variation twisting around a central axis (a few complexes point upward, then a few point downward); ST segments and T waves difficult to discern

Note: This type of ventricular tachycardia (VT) is associated with a prolonged QT interval. It is seen with electrolyte disturbances (eg, hypokalemia, hypocalcemia, and hypomagnesemia) and bradycardia. Administering standard antiarrhythmic agents (eg, lidocaine, procainamide) may worsen torsades de pointes. Prevention includes treatment of the electrolyte disturbance. Treatment includes shortening of the QT interval, pharmacologically or by pacing; unstable polymorphic VT is treated with immediate defibrillation.

Torsades de Pointes: Sustained

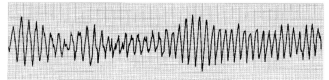

9

199

VENTRICULAR FIBRILLATION

Rate: Absent
Rhythm: None
PR interval: Absent
QT interval: Absent

Note: "Pseudoventricular fibrillation" may be the result of a monitor malfunction (eg, ECG lead disconnect). Always check for the carotid pulse before instituting therapy.

Coarse Ventricular Fibrillation

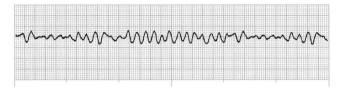

Fine Ventricular Fibrillation

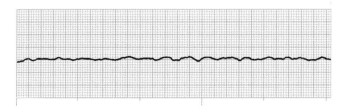

VENTRICULAR TACHYCARDIA

Rate: 100–250 beats/min
Rhythm: No atrial component seen; ventricular rhythm irregular or regular
PR interval: Absent; retrograde P wave may be seen in QRS complex
QT interval: Wide, bizarre QRS complex; ST segment and T wave difficult to determine

Note: In the presence of hemodynamic compromise, immediate direct current synchronized cardioversion is required. If the patient is stable, with short bursts of ventricular tachycardia, pharmacologic management is preferred. This should be differentiated from supraventricular tachycardia with aberrancy (SVT-A). A compensatory pause and AV dissociation suggest a premature ventricular contraction. P waves and SR' (V_1) and slowing to vagal stimulus also suggest SVT-A.

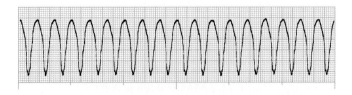

▣ WOLFF-PARKINSON-WHITE SYNDROME

Rate: <100 beats/min

Rhythm: Regular

PR interval: P wave normal; PR interval short (<0.12 second)

QT interval: Duration (>0.10 second) with slurred QRS complex; type A has delta wave, RBBB, with upright QRS complex V_1; type B has delta wave and downward QRS-V_1; ST segment and T wave usually normal

Note: Digoxin should be avoided in the presence of Wolff-Parkinson-White syndrome because it increases conduction through the accessory bypass tract (bundle of Kent) and decreases AV node conduction; consequently, ventricular fibrillation can occur.

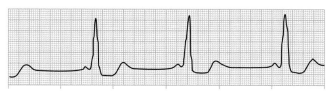

▣ PACING

Atrial Pacing

Atrial pacing, as demonstrated in this figure, is used when the atrial impulse can proceed through the AV node. Examples are sinus bradycardia and junctional rhythms associated with clinically significant decreases in blood pressure. (The *arrows* are the pacemaker spike.)

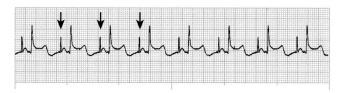

Ventricular Pacing

In this tracing, ventricular pacing is evident by absence of an atrial wave (P wave) and the pacemaker spike preceding the QRS complex. Ventricular pacing is used in the presence of bradycardia secondary to AV block or atrial fibrillation. (The *arrows* are the pacemaker spike.)

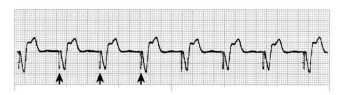

9

DDD Pacing

The DDD pacemaker (generator), one of the most commonly used, paces and senses both the atrium and the ventricle. Each atrial and ventricular complex is preceded by a pacemaker spike.

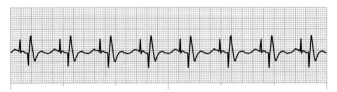

■ ACKNOWLEDGMENTS

Illustrations in this appendix are reprinted from Aehlert B. *ECGs Made Easy.* 4th ed. St. Louis: Mosby; 2011; Goldberger AL. *Clinical Electrocardiography: A Simplified Approach.* 7th ed. Philadelphia: Mosby; 2006; Groh WJ, Zipes DP. Neurological disorders and cardiovascular disease. In: Bonow RO, Mann DL, Zipes DP, et al, eds. *Braunwald's Heart Disease: A Textbook of Cardiovascular Medicine.* 9th ed. Philadelphia: Saunders; 2012; Huszar RJ. *Basic Dysrhythmias: Interpretation and Management.* 2nd ed. St. Louis: Mosby Lifeline; 1994; and Soltani P, Malozzi CM, Saleh BA, et al. Electrocardiogram manifestation of spontaneous pneumothorax. *Am J Emerg Med.* 2009;27:750.e1–5.

BIBLIOGRAPHY

Aehlert B. *ECGs Made Easy.* 4th ed. St. Louis: Mosby; 2011:337.
Drew BJ, Ackerman MJ, Funk M, et al. Prevention of torsade de pointes in hospital settings: a scientific statement from the American Heart Association and the American College of Cardiology Foundation. *Circulation.* 2010;121:1047–1060.
Goldberger AL. *Clinical Electrocardiography: A Simplified Approach.* 7th ed. Philadelphia: Mosby; 2006:337.
Groh WJ, Zipes DP. Neurological disorders and cardiovascular disease. In: Libby P, Bonow RO, Mann DL, et al, eds. *Braunwald's Heart Disease: A Textbook of Cardiovascular Medicine.* 8th ed. Philadelphia: Saunders; 2008:2135–2154.
Huszar RJ. *Basic Dysrhythmias: Interpretation and Management.* 2nd ed. St. Louis: Mosby Lifeline; 1994:453.
Mirvis DM, Goldberger AL. Electrocardiography. In: Libby P, Bonow RO, Mann DL, et al, eds. *Braunwald's Heart Disease: A Textbook of Cardiovascular Medicine.* 8th ed. Philadelphia: Saunders; 2008:149–194.
Salonti J, Malozzi CM, Saleh BA, et al. Electrocardiogram manifestation of spontaneous pneumothorax. *Am J Emerg Med.* 2009;27:750.e1–750.e5.
Thaler MS. *The Only EKG Book You'll Ever Need.* 6th ed. Philadelphia: Wolters Kluwer/Lippincott Williams & Wilkins; 2010:326.

III

Chapter 10

Monitoring of the Heart and Vascular System

Alexander J.C. Mittnacht, MD • David L. Reich, MD •
Michael Sander, MD • Joel A. Kaplan, MD, CPE, FACC

Key Points

1. Patients with severe cardiovascular disease and those undergoing surgery associated with rapid hemodynamic changes should be adequately monitored at all times.
2. Standard monitoring for cardiac surgery patients includes invasive blood pressure, electrocardiography, central venous pressure, urine output, temperature, capnometry, pulse oximetry, and intermittent blood gas analysis.
3. Additional monitoring is based on specific patient, surgical, and environmental factors.
4. The Society of Cardiovascular Anesthesiologists and the American Society of Echocardiography have published recommendations for intraoperative transesophageal echocardiography (TEE). TEE is recommended for all patients undergoing cardiac surgery, unless contraindications to probe insertion apply.
5. Ultrasound-guided vascular access is now routinely practiced in many institutions.
6. The use of pulmonary artery catheters (PACs) has been steadily declining. Guidelines for PAC use have been published. Many practitioners still use PACs to guide treatment in patients with low cardiac output or pulmonary arterial hypertension.
7. The use of additional highly invasive monitoring techniques, such as coronary sinus pressures and cerebrospinal fluid pressures, are restricted to very specific indications.

HEMODYNAMIC MONITORING

The availability of monitoring devices is increasing continually. These devices range from those that are completely noninvasive to those that are highly invasive, such as the pulmonary artery catheter (PAC). Limitations to less invasive monitoring technologies often apply, and interventions based on information gained from noninvasive monitoring carry intrinsic risks. To make the best use of any monitoring technology, the potential benefits to be gained from the information must outweigh the potential complications. This risk-benefit ratio is highly variable and must be evaluated for each clinical scenario individually. Although outcome changes are difficult to prove, the assumption that appropriate hemodynamic monitoring should reduce the incidence of major cardiovascular complications is reasonable. This is based on

BOX 10.1 *Standard Monitoring for Cardiac Surgical Patients*

(Invasive) blood pressure
Electrocardiogram
Pulse oximetry
Capnometry
Temperature
Central venous pressure
Transesophageal echocardiography
Urine output
Intermittent arterial blood sampling for blood gas and laboratory analyses
Neuromonitoring (cerebral oximetry, processed electroencephalography)

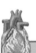

BOX 10.2 *Extended Monitoring for Patients Based on Case-Specific Factors*

Retrograde cardioplegia pressure
Pulmonary artery catheter
Cardiac output measurements
Left atrial pressure
Cerebrospinal fluid (intrathecal) pressure

the presumption that the data obtained from these monitors are interpreted correctly and that therapeutic interventions known to improve outcomes are implemented in a timely fashion.

Standard monitoring for all patients undergoing surgery has been defined by the American Society of Anesthesiologists (ASA) practice guidelines. In patients undergoing cardiac or major noncardiac surgery with expected large fluid shifts or hemodynamic instability, invasive blood pressure (BP) monitoring is nearly universally employed, which also enables frequent arterial blood sampling. Transesophageal echocardiography (TEE), a less invasive technology, provides extensive hemodynamic data and other diagnostic information. The Society of Cardiovascular Anesthesiologists and the American Society of Echocardiography have published recommendations for intraoperative TEE use. Unless contraindications to probe insertion apply, TEE is now recommended for all patients undergoing cardiac surgery. Box 10.1 summarizes monitoring typically used in cardiac surgeries.

The next tier of monitoring is typically more invasive, including PACs with thermodilution cardiac output (CO). The interpretation of these complex data requires an astute clinician who is aware of the patient's overall condition and the limitations of the monitors. Additionally, with the expansion of less invasive surgical techniques, the anesthesiologist is getting more involved in guiding cardiopulmonary bypass (CPB) cannulation and adequacy of cardioprotection techniques. This includes retrograde cardioplegia cannula positioning in the coronary sinus (CS) and pressure monitoring. Advanced monitoring is summarized in Box 10.2.

Anesthesia for cardiac and major noncardiac surgeries is frequently complicated by rapid and sudden changes in BP. Sudden losses of large amounts of blood, direct compression of the heart, impaired venous return attributable to retraction and cannulation of the vena cavae and aorta, arrhythmias, and manipulations that may impair right ventricular outflow and pulmonary venous return all contribute to hemodynamic instability. Therefore a safe and reliable method of measuring acute changes in BP is indispensable. Direct intraarterial monitoring remains the gold standard, providing a continuous, beat-to-beat indication of the arterial pressure and waveform and allowing frequent sampling of arterial blood for laboratory analyses.

The magnitude of BP is directly related to CO and systemic vascular resistance (SVR). This is conceptually similar to Ohm's law of electricity (voltage = current × resistance), in which BP is analogous to voltage, CO to current flow, and SVR to resistance. An increase in BP may reflect an increase in CO or SVR, or both.

Mean arterial pressure (MAP) is probably the most useful parameter when assessing overall end-organ perfusion. MAP is measured directly by integrating the arterial waveform tracing over time or using the formula: MAP = (SBP + [2 × DBP]) ÷ 3 (where SBP is systolic blood pressure and DBP is diastolic blood pressure). Perfusion of the heart differs from most other organs, with coronary perfusion of the left ventricle mostly occurring during diastole. Coronary blood flow to the normal right ventricle (RV) is maintained during systole and diastole.

Arterial Cannulation Sites

Factors that influence the site of arterial cannulation include the location of surgery, the possible compromise of arterial flow attributable to patient positioning or surgical manipulations, CPB cannulation and perfusion techniques, and any history of ischemia or prior surgery on the limb to be cannulated. Monitoring arterial BP at two or more sites may be warranted in complex cases with complex perfusion techniques.

Temporary central aortic pressure monitoring can be achieved by using a needle (attached to pressure tubing) that is placed in the aorta or by pressure tubing connected to the aortic CPB cannula or the anterograde cardioplegia cannula. Central aortic monitoring is usually only necessary for several minutes until the problem resolves; in rare cases, a femoral arterial cannula is placed from the surgical field.

The radial artery is the most commonly used artery for continuous BP monitoring because it is easy to cannulate, readily accessible during surgery, and the collateral circulation is usually adequate and easy to check. The ulnar artery provides most of the blood flow to the hand in approximately 90% of patients. The radial and ulnar arteries are connected by a palmar arch, which provides collateral flow to the hand in the event of radial artery occlusion. Some clinicians perform the Allen test before radial artery cannulation to assess the adequacy of collateral circulation to the hand; however, the predictive value of the Allen test has been challenged.

The brachial artery lies medial to the bicipital tendon in the antecubital fossa in close proximity to the median nerve. Brachial artery pressure tracings resemble those in the femoral artery with less systolic augmentation than radial artery tracings. Brachial arterial pressures were found to reflect central aortic pressures more accurately than radial arterial pressures before and after CPB. A few series of patients with perioperative brachial arterial monitoring have documented the relative safety of this technique.

The femoral artery may be cannulated for monitoring purposes and typically provides a more reliable central arterial pressure after discontinuation of CPB. In

10

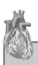

BOX 10.3 *Indications for Intraarterial Monitoring*

Major surgical procedures involving large fluid shifts or blood loss
Surgery requiring cardiopulmonary bypass
Surgery of the aorta
Patients with pulmonary disease requiring frequent arterial blood gases
Patients with recent myocardial infarctions, unstable angina, or severe coronary artery disease
Patients with decreased left ventricular function (congestive heart failure) or significant valvular heart disease
Patients in hypovolemic, cardiogenic, or septic shock, or with multiple organ failure
Procedures involving the use of prolonged deliberate hypotension or deliberate hypothermia
Massive trauma cases
Patients with right-sided heart failure, chronic obstructive pulmonary disease, pulmonary hypertension, or pulmonary embolism
Patients requiring inotropes or intraaortic balloon counterpulsation
Patients with electrolyte or metabolic disturbances requiring frequent blood samples
Inability to measure arterial pressure noninvasively (eg, extreme morbid obesity)

patients undergoing thoracic aortic surgery, distal aortic perfusion (using partial CPB, left-sided heart bypass, or a heparinized shunt) may be performed during aortic cross-clamping to preserve spinal cord and visceral organ blood flow. In these situations, measuring the distal aortic pressure at the femoral artery or a branch vessel is useful (ie, dorsalis pedis or posterior tibial artery) to optimize the distal perfusion pressure. Consulting the surgeon before cannulating the femoral vessels is necessary, because these vessels may be used for extracorporeal perfusion or placement of an intraaortic balloon pump during the surgical procedure.

The indications for invasive arterial monitoring are provided in Box 10.3.

Insertion Techniques

Direct Cannulation

Proper technique is helpful in obtaining a high degree of success in arterial catheterization. The wrist is often placed in a dorsiflexed position on an armboard over a pack of gauze and immobilized in a supinated position. Overextension of the wrist should be avoided, since this flattens and decreases the cross-sectional area of the radial artery and may cause median nerve damage by stretching the nerve over the wrist. When the artery is entered, the angle between the needle and skin is reduced to 10 degrees, the needle is advanced another 1 to 2 mm to ensure that the tip of the catheter also lies within the lumen of the vessel, and the outer catheter is then threaded off the needle. If blood ceases flowing while the needle is being advanced, then the needle has penetrated the back wall of the vessel.

Alternatively, the artery can be transfixed by the passage of the catheter-over-needle assembly "through-and-through" the artery. The needle is then completely withdrawn. As the catheter is slowly withdrawn, pulsatile blood flow emerges from the catheter when its tip is within the lumen of the artery. At this point the catheter can either be advanced in the lumen of the artery or a guidewire advanced into the lumen first,

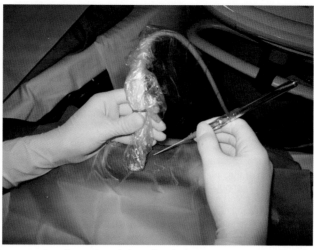

Fig. 10.1 Demonstration of aseptic technique for ultrasonic guidance of radial artery cannulation.

followed by advancing the catheter over the wire (modified Seldinger technique). Compared with a direct cannulation method, using the Seldinger technique increases the success rate of arterial catheter placement.

Ultrasound and Doppler-Assisted Techniques

An ultrasound-guided (UG) technique is probably most useful in patients with severe peripheral vasculopathy, as well as in infants and small children. The use of ultrasound in guiding arterial catheter placement is easy to learn when proper training in this technique is provided. There is, however, a significant learning curve. Fig. 10.1 shows a proper full-sterile set up for UG arterial cannulation. Fig. 10.2 demonstrates the "triangulation" technique typically applied with UG arterial cannulation. The ultrasound imaging plane and the needle plane can be viewed as the two sides of a triangle that should meet and intersect at the depth of the structure (eg, radial artery) for which cannulation is attempted. The experienced operator will choose the distance (needle insertion site vs imaging plane) and insertion angle, depending on the depth of the target vessel. After perforating the skin, the ultrasound plane and the needle insertion angle both have to be adjusted further to follow the needle tip when viewed in the transverse (short-axis) approach. Failure to align the ultrasound plane accurately with the needle tip results in viewing the needle shaft instead. Fig. 10.3 shows a typical ultrasound image obtained during short-axis (transverse) cannulation. After puncturing the vessel, the catheter can be advanced into the lumen. A significantly higher success rate can usually be achieved using the through-and-through and modified Seldinger techniques.

If a longitudinal ("in-plane") approach is chosen (ie, the vessel is viewed in its long axis), the needle tip can be followed more easily as it is advanced; however, structures adjacent to the ultrasound plane (lateral to the vessel) cannot be viewed simultaneously. Exactly aligning the needle and vessel axis together in a 2D echo plane, particularly with a tortuous atherosclerotic artery, is technically more difficult. Fig. 10.4 shows the arterial catheter entering the radial artery using the longitudinal (in-plane) approach. A high-frequency linear array ultrasonic transducer (8 to 12 MHz) is optimal for UG arterial catheter placement, since higher frequencies are needed

10

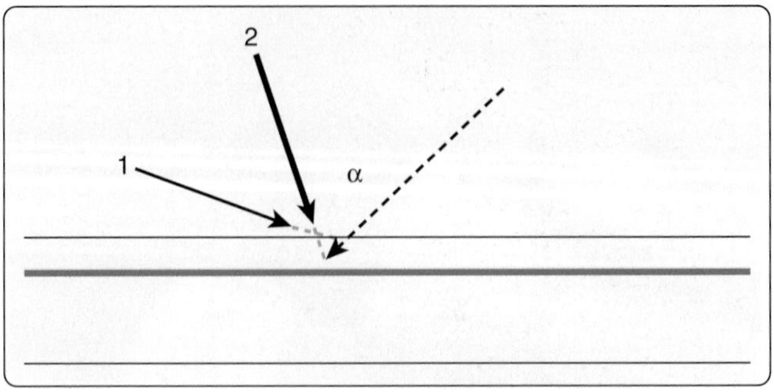

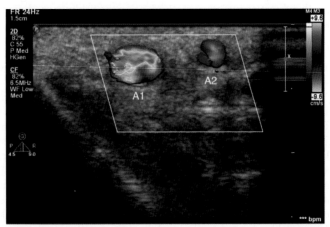

Fig. 10.2 Demonstration of the "triangulation" technique typically applied with ultrasound-guided (UG) venous and/or arterial cannulation in the transverse imaging approach. The echo imaging plane and the needle plane can be viewed as the two sides of a triangle that should meet and intersect at the depth of the structure (eg, radial artery *[red line]*) for which cannulation is attempted. The experienced operator will change the angle *(α)* between the two planes (ultrasound and needle) and the distance (needle insertion site vs imaging plane), depending on the depth of the structure. To follow the needle tip in the transverse approach (vessel viewed in short axis), the echo plane or needle insertion angle has to be further adjusted from needle entry through the skin to the perforation of the vessel. A greater angle is used (echo plane angled toward the skin *[1]*) to visualize the needle tip after it penetrates the skin, and then a more perpendicular angle relative to the skin is applied to see the needle tip entering the vessel lumen (*2*).

Fig. 10.3 A typical ultrasound image with color Doppler during short-axis (transverse) cannulation. Note the anatomic variation with a larger radial artery (*A1*) next to a smaller artery (*A2*) positioned laterally.

for high-resolution imaging of the near field. Box 10.4 summarizes the potential benefits and concerns related to UG arterial catheter placement.

CENTRAL VENOUS PRESSURE MONITORING

Central venous pressure (CVP) catheters are used to measure the filling pressure of the RV, give an estimate of the intravascular volume status, assess right ventricular function, and serve as a site for volume or drug infusions. For accurate pressure measurement, the distal end of the catheter must lie within one of the large intrathoracic

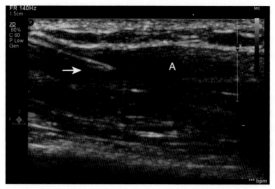

Fig. 10.4 Catheter entering the radial artery using the longitudinal (in-plane) approach.

BOX 10.4 *Ultrasound-Guided Arterial Cannulation*

Benefits

- Higher success rate on first attempt
- Fewer overall attempts
- Increased patient comfort (fewer attempts)
- Fewer complications (eg, anticoagulated patients)
- Demonstration of vessel patency, anatomic variants
- Low pulsatile or nonpulsatile flow (eg, nonpulsatile assist devices, extracorporeal membrane oxygenation, shock)
- Nonpalpable or weakly palpable pulses (eg, peripheral edema, hematoma)
- Emergency access (eg, catheter placement during resuscitation)

Concerns

- Risk of catheter-related infections if poor aseptic technique is applied
- Additional training required
- Costs involved with equipment required

10

veins or the right atrium (RA). As in any pressure monitoring system, having a reproducible landmark, such as the midaxillary line with a closed chest or the left atrium (LA) during surgery, as a zero reference is necessary. Frequent changes in patient positioning without proper leveling of the transducers relative to the heart produce proportionately larger errors compared with arterial pressure monitoring.

The normal CVP waveform consists of three upward deflections (A, C, and V waves) and two downward deflections (X and Y descents). The A wave is produced by right atrial contraction and occurs just after the P wave on the electrocardiogram (ECG). The C wave occurs because of the isovolumic ventricular contraction, forcing the tricuspid valve (TV) to bulge upward into the RA. The pressure within the RA then decreases as the TV is pulled away from the atrium during right ventricular ejection, forming the X descent. Right atrial filling continues during late ventricular systole, forming the V wave. The Y descent occurs when the TV opens and blood from the RA empties rapidly into the RV during early diastole. The CVP waveform may be useful in the diagnosis of pathologic cardiac conditions. For example, the onset of an irregular rhythm and loss of the A wave suggest atrial flutter or fibrillation.

Cannon A waves occur as the RA contracts against a closed TV, as occurs in junctional (atrioventricular [AV] nodal) rhythm, complete heart block, and ventricular arrhythmias. This occurrence is clinically relevant because nodal rhythms are frequently seen during anesthesia and may produce hypotension attributable to a decrease in stroke volume (SV).

The CVP is a useful monitor if the factors affecting it are recognized and its limitations are understood. Thromboses of the vena cavae and alterations of intrathoracic pressure, such as those induced by positive end-expiratory pressure (PEEP), also affect measurement of the CVP. The correlation with left-sided heart filling pressures and assessment of left ventricular preload is poor. Clinically, following serial measurements (trends) rather than individual numbers is often more relevant. The response of the CVP to a volume infusion, however, is a useful test.

Internal Jugular Vein

Cannulation of the internal jugular vein (IJV) has multiple advantages, including the high success rate as a result of the relatively predictable relationship of the anatomic structures: a short, straight course to the RA that almost always ensures RA or superior vena cava (SVC) localization of the catheter tip; and easy access from the head of the surgical table. The IJV is located under the medial border of the lateral head of the sternocleidomastoid (SCM) muscle (Fig. 10.5). The carotid artery is usually deep and medial to the IJV; however, this spatial relationship can vary, and puncture of the carotid artery is best avoided by using an UG technique. The right IJV is preferred, because this vein takes the straightest course into the SVC, the right cupola of the lung may be lower than the left, and the thoracic duct is on the left side.

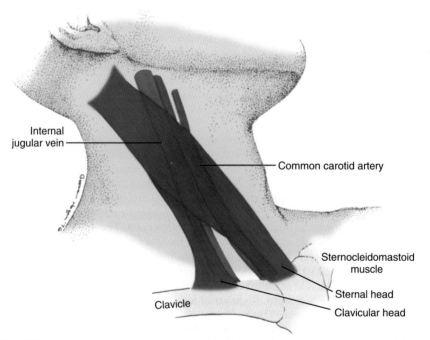

Internal jugular vein

Common carotid artery

Sternocleidomastoid muscle

Sternal head

Clavicular head

Clavicle

Fig. 10.5 The internal jugular vein is usually located deep to the medial border of the lateral head of the sternocleidomastoid muscle, just lateral to the carotid pulse.

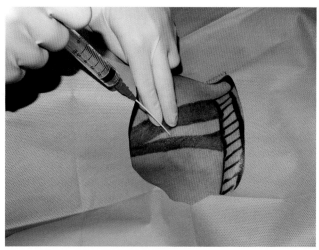

Fig. 10.6 Preferred middle approach to the right internal jugular vein. The needle enters the skin at the apex of the triangle formed by the sternal and clavicular heads of the sternocleidomastoid muscle. The needle is held at a 30- to 45-degree angle to the skin and directed toward the ipsilateral nipple.

The *middle approach* to the right IJV is shown in Fig. 10.6. The Trendelenburg position is chosen to distend the IJV. The head is then turned toward the contralateral side, and the fingers of the left hand are used to palpate the two heads of the SCM muscle and the carotid pulse. The needle is inserted slightly lateral to the carotid pulse at a 45-degree angle to the skin and directed toward the ipsilateral nipple until venous blood return is obtained. Alternatively, the use of a small-gauge *finder* needle can be used to avoid carotid puncture with a large-bore needle. When venous return is present, the whole assembly is lowered to prevent the needle from going through the posterior wall of the central vein and advanced an additional 1 to 2 mm until the tip of the catheter is within the lumen of the vein. Aspiration of blood must be confirmed before the catheter is then threaded into the vein. It is recommended by the ASA practice guidelines, and often mandated by institutional protocols, that the correct intravenous catheter position be confirmed before placing a large-bore introducer sheath. Various techniques have been suggested. The small-bore catheter can be attached to a transducer by sterile tubing to observe the pressure waveform. Another option is to attach the cannula to sterile tubing and allow blood to flow retrograde into the tubing. The tubing is then held upright as a venous manometer, and the height of the blood column is observed. If the catheter is in a vein, then it will stop rising at a level consistent with the CVP and demonstrate respiratory variation. Despite its reported use in the past, color comparison and observation of nonpulsatile flow are notoriously inaccurate methods of determining that the catheter is not in the carotid artery. A guidewire is then passed through the 18-gauge catheter, and the catheter is exchanged for the wire. With the more widespread use of echocardiography, the correct intravenous position can also be confirmed by following the Seldinger wire along its course in the IJV more distally by handheld transcutaneous probes or demonstrated within the RA if the TEE probe was inserted before IJV cannulation. The use of more than one technique to confirm the venous location of the guidewire may provide additional reassurance of correct placement before cannulation of the vein with a larger catheter or introducer. Once it is certain that the guidewire is in the venous circulation, the CVP catheter is passed over it and the wire is removed.

Ultrasound-Guided Internal Jugular Vein Cannulation

Ultrasound has been increasingly used for central venous access, in particular to guide IJV cannulation and to define the anatomic variations of the IJV. Using ultrasound to guide central venous cannulation increases the success rate and helps prevent complications and thus may ultimately help improve patient outcomes. Most studies have demonstrated that 2D UG IJV cannulation has a higher success rate on the first attempt and fewer complications. Those findings also were confirmed in pediatric patients.

Box 10.5 lists some of the recognized benefits and concerns of UG central venous cannulation. Circumstances in which ultrasound guidance of IJV cannulation can be particularly advantageous include patients with difficult neck anatomy (eg, short neck, obesity), prior neck surgery, anticoagulated patients, and infants.

Ultrasound provides instantaneous and patient-specific information regarding the structural relationship between the IJV, the carotid artery, and adjacent anatomic structures (Fig. 10.7). The spatial relationships can vary significantly, and the IJV may be absent or completely or partially overlapping the carotid artery. Box 10.6 summarizes some of the positional considerations in UG IJV cannulation.

For central venous catheterization, full aseptic technique is mandatory. Although the long-axis (in-plane) approach allows better visualization of the true needle tip throughout the insertion and vessel penetration, the simultaneous display of the IJV and its relationship to the carotid artery is lost. Additionally, the size of the ultrasound probe in patients with short neck anatomy often does not provide adequate room for an in-plane approach to the IJV. Most practitioners therefore choose the short-axis (out-of-plane) approach to UG IJV cannulation. The most important aspect of imaging a needle out of plane is avoiding the mistake of visualizing the needle shaft rather than the needle tip. Otherwise, the needle tip could be in a structure not being imaged, such as the carotid artery or pleura. With training and experience, the practitioner learns to sweep the ultrasonic plane inferiorly along the course of the needle shaft until the needle tip is identified. Adjusting the ultrasonic plane and the angle of the needle insertion enables visualization of the needle tip as it enters the IJV. An extremely

III

BOX 10.5   *Ultrasound-Guided Central Venous Cannulation*

Benefits

- Higher success rate on first attempt
- Fewer overall attempts
- Facilitates access with difficult neck anatomy (obesity, prior surgery)
- Fewer complications (eg, carotid artery puncture, anticoagulated patients)
- Demonstration of vessel patency, anatomic variants
- Relatively inexpensive technology

Concerns

- Training personnel to maintain aseptic technique when using sterile probe sheaths
- Additional training required
- Lack of observation of surface anatomy
- Potential loss of landmark-guided skills when needed for emergency central venous catheterization.

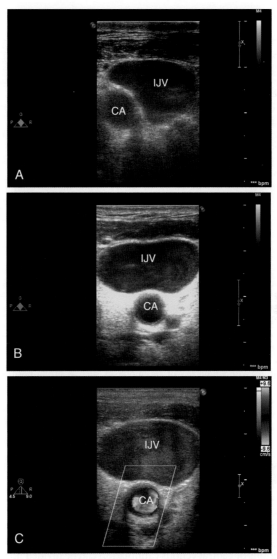

Fig. 10.7 Anatomic relationship between the internal jugular vein (*IJV*) and the carotid artery (*CA*) in two patients. (A) The IJV partially overlies the CA. (B) The CA is situated deep to the IJV. (C) Color Doppler demonstrates the flow in the CA.

favorable sign of needle tip visualization during needle advancement is indentation of the anterior wall of the IJV as the needle tip encounters the vessel wall.

It is important to realize that UG IJV cannulation has reduced, but not eliminated, inadvertent carotid arterial cannulation, and that the insertion of large catheters into the carotid artery with ultrasound guidance has been reported. Venous cannulation always should be confirmed before advancing the dilators or inserting the large-bore catheter and introducer sheath.

In addition to hemodynamic monitoring, central venous access is typically warranted to establish a secure venous access route for the administration of vasoactive or irritating

BOX 10.6 *Positional Considerations in Ultrasound-Guided Right Internal Jugular Venous Cannulation*

Slight Trendelenburg position

Head turned slightly away from the cannulation side (turning too far may flatten the internal jugular vein [IJV] and rotate the IJV above the carotid artery)

Overextension of the head should be avoided; mild head elevation can be advantageous (overextension flattens IJV)

Minimal neck pressure by manual palpation and/or ultrasonic probe to avoid compression of the IJV

Ultrasound probe should scan the course of the IJV to find the best cannulation site (largest IJV diameter and least overlap with the carotid artery)

BOX 10.7 *Indications for Central Venous Catheter Placement*

Major operative procedures involving large fluid shifts or blood loss in patients with good heart function

Intravascular volume assessment when urine output is not reliable or unavailable (eg, renal failure)

Major trauma

Surgical procedures with a high risk of air embolism, such as sitting-position craniotomies during which the central venous pressure catheter may be used to aspirate intracardiac air

Frequent venous blood sampling

Venous access for vasoactive or irritating drugs

Chronic drug administration

Inadequate peripheral intravenous access

Rapid infusion of intravenous fluids (only when using large-bore cannulae)

Total parenteral nutrition

drugs, the rapid infusion of intravenous fluids, and total parenteral nutrition. Perioperative indications for the insertion of a central venous catheter are listed in Box 10.7.

The complications of central venous cannulation can be divided into three categories: vascular access, catheter insertion, and catheter presence. These complications are summarized in Box 10.8.

PULMONARY ARTERIAL PRESSURE MONITORING

At the time of the introduction of the flow-directed PAC in 1970, the amount of diagnostic information that could be obtained at the bedside dramatically increased. Some of the earlier studies showed that clinicians were often unaware of hemodynamic problems or incorrectly predicted preload and CO without PAC monitoring. Although PAC-derived data can help in the differential diagnosis of hemodynamic instability and guide treatment, the clinical significance has been questioned.

Between 1993 and 2004 PAC use in the United States alone decreased by 65% for all medical admissions. The most significant decrease in PAC use was documented

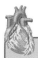

BOX 10.8   *Complications of Central Venous Catheterization*

Complications of Central Venous Access and Cannulation

- Arterial puncture with hematoma
- Arteriovenous fistula
- Hemothorax
- Chylothorax
- Pneumothorax
- Nerve injury
- Brachial plexus injury
- Stellate ganglion injury (Horner syndrome)
- Air embolus
- Catheter or wire shearing
- Guidewire loss and embolization
- Right atrial or right ventricular perforation

Complications of Catheter Presence

- Thrombosis, thromboembolism
- Infection, sepsis, endocarditis
- Arrhythmias
- Hydrothorax

in patients with acute myocardial infarction, whereas those patients diagnosed with septicemia showed the least decline in use. These findings were almost identical to the surgical patient population, in which PAC use decreased by 63% in the same observed period.

Currently, the incidence of right heart (PAC) catheterization is highly variable among hospitals. A recent survey among the members of the Society of Cardiovascular Anesthesiologists found that a majority of practitioners (68.2%) still frequently (>75%) use a PAC for cases with CPB. However, the use of a PAC differed significantly between private (79.2%), academic (64.5%), and governmental (34%) practice settings. With decreasing exposure to PACs, clinicians may become less likely to make the best use of PAC-derived hemodynamic data.

Placing a PAC is a highly invasive procedure. Vascular structures are accessed with large-bore introducer sheaths with all the possible complications listed. Most important, even in the best of all circumstances with uncomplicated PAC placement and correct data collection and interpretation, it has to be recognized that a PAC is only a monitoring tool. As such, a change in patient outcome cannot be expected unless the treatment that is initiated based on the PAC measurements is effective for improving patient outcome. In some of the most critically ill patients, mortality remains high despite efforts to find new treatment strategies. Furthermore, diagnoses often can be made on clinical grounds only, and treatment strategies once thought to improve patient outcome actually may be harmful.

Technical Aspects of Pulmonary Artery Catheter Use

Considerations for the insertion site of a PAC are the same as for CVP catheters. Infection guidelines list specific recommendations regarding PAC use, strongly recommending use of a sterile sleeve to protect the PAC during insertion (category IB). The right IJV approach remains the preferred access route for many practitioners. This is because of the direct path between this vessel and the RA during IJV approach and the frequent kinking of the introducers during sternal retraction when subclavian access is chosen.

Passage of the PAC from the vessel introducer to the PA can be accomplished by monitoring the pressure waveform from the distal port of the catheter or under fluoroscopic or echocardiographic (TEE) guidance. Waveform monitoring is the most common technique for perioperative right-sided heart catheterization. First, the catheter must be advanced through the vessel introducer (15 to 20 cm) before inflating the balloon. The inflation of the balloon facilitates further advancement of the catheter through the RA and RV into the pulmonary artery (PA). Normal intracardiac pressures are shown in Table 10.1. The pressure waveforms seen during advancement of the PAC are illustrated in Fig. 10.8. Catheter manipulation and positional changes may be useful. Trendelenburg positioning places the RV more superior to the RA and thus may aid in advancing the PAC past the TV. TEE guidance can prove invaluable in these cases. The experienced echocardiographer can assist in guiding the catheter tip toward the TV orifice by directing catheter and positional manipulations. The right atrial waveform is seen until the catheter tip crosses the TV and enters the RV. In the RV, there is a sudden increase in SBP but little change in DBP, compared with the right atrial tracing. Arrhythmias, particularly premature ventricular complexes, usually

Table 10.1	Normal Intracardiac Pressures	
Location	Mean (mm Hg)	Range (mm Hg)
Right atrium	5	1–10
Right ventricle	25/5	15–30/0–8
Pulmonary arterial systolic and diastolic pressures	23/9	15–30/5–15
Mean pulmonary arterial	15	10–20
Pulmonary capillary wedge pressure	10	5–15
Left atrial pressure	8	4–12
Left ventricular end-diastolic pressure	8	4–12
Left ventricular systolic pressure	130	90–140

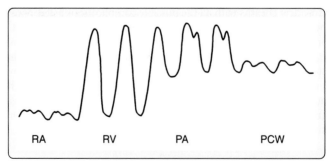

Fig. 10.8 The waveforms encountered during the flotation of a pulmonary artery catheter from the venous circulation to the pulmonary capillary wedge *(PCW)* position. Notice the sudden increase in systolic pressure as the catheter enters the right ventricle *(RV)*, the sudden increase in diastolic pressure as the catheter enters the pulmonary artery *(PA)*, and the decrease in mean pressure as the catheter reaches the PCW position. *RA,* Right atrium.

occur at this point, but they almost always resolve without treatment once the catheter tip has crossed the pulmonary valve. The catheter is advanced through the RV toward the PA. As the catheter crosses the pulmonary valve, a dicrotic notch appears in the pressure waveform, and the diastolic pressure suddenly increases. The pulmonary capillary wedge pressure (PCWP; also termed *pulmonary capillary occlusion pressure*) tracing is obtained by advancing the catheter approximately 3 to 5 cm farther until a change in the waveform associated with a drop in the measured mean pressure occurs. Deflation of the balloon results in the reappearance of the PA waveform and an increase in the mean pressure value. Using the right IJV approach, the RA is entered at 25 to 35 cm, the RV at 35 to 45 cm, the PA at 45 to 55 cm, and the PCWP at 50 to 60 cm in most patients.

If the catheter does not enter the PA by 60 cm (from the right IJV approach), the balloon should be deflated and the catheter should be withdrawn into the RA or the inflow portion of the RV. Further attempts can then be made to advance the catheter into proper position using the techniques previously described. Excessive coiling of the catheter in the RA or RV should be avoided to prevent catheter knotting. The balloon should be inflated only for short periods to measure the PCWP. The PA waveform should be monitored continually to be certain that the catheter does not advance into a constant wedge position, which may lead to PA rupture or pulmonary infarction. Not infrequently, the PAC must be withdrawn a short distance because the catheter softens and advanced more peripherally into the PA over time, or on CPB attributable to the decreased size of the heart.

Specific information that can be gathered with the PAC and the quantitative measurements of cardiovascular function that can be derived from this information are listed in Table 10.2. One of the primary reasons that clinicians measure PCWP and PA diastolic (PAD) pressure is that these parameters are estimates of left atrial

Table 10.2   Derived Hemodynamic Parameters

Formula	Normal Values
Cardiac index (CI) CI = CO/BSA	2.6–4.2 L/min/m²
Stroke volume (SV) SV = CO*1000/HR	50–110 mL (per beat)
Stroke index (SI) SI = SV/BSA	30–65 mL/beat/m²
Left ventricular stroke work index (LVSWI) LVSWI = 1.36* (MAP–PCWP)* SI/100	45–60 gram-meters/m²
Right ventricular stroke work index (RVSWI) RVSWI = 1.36* (MPAP–CVP)* SI/100	5–10 gram-meters/m²
Systemic vascular resistance (SVR) SVR = (MAP–CVP)* 80/CO	900–1400 dynes·s·cm^{-5}
Systemic vascular resistance index (SVRI) SVRI = (MAP–CVP)* 80/CI	1500–2400 dynes·s·cm^{-5}/m²
Pulmonary vascular resistance (PVR) PVR = (MPAP–PCWP)* 80/CO	150–250 dynes·s·cm^{-5}
Pulmonary vascular resistance index (PVRI) PVRI = (MPAP–PCWP)* 80/CI	250–400 dynes·s·cm^{-5}/m²

BSA, Body surface area; *CO*, cardiac output; *CVP*, central venous pressure; *HR*, heart rate; *MAP*, mean arterial pressure; *MPAP*, mean pulmonary artery pressure; *PAP*, pulmonary arterial pressure; *PCWP*, pulmonary capillary wedge pressure.

10

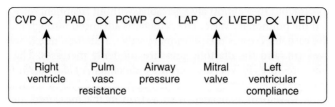

Fig. 10.9 The left ventricular end-diastolic volume (*LVEDV*) is related to left ventricular end-diastolic pressure (*LVEDP*) by the left ventricular compliance. The LVEDP is related to the left atrial pressure (*LAP*) by the diastolic pressure gradient across the mitral valve. The pulmonary capillary wedge pressure (*PCWP*) is related to the LAP by the pulmonary capillary resistance. The pulmonary artery diastolic (*PAD*) pressure is an estimate of the PCWP. The central venous pressure (*CVP*) will reflect the PAD pressure if right ventricular function is normal.

pressure (LAP), which can serve as an estimate of left ventricular preload. The relationship between left ventricular end-diastolic pressure (LVEDP) and left ventricular end-diastolic volume (LVEDV) is described by the left ventricular compliance curve. This nonlinear curve is affected by many factors, such as ventricular hypertrophy and myocardial ischemia. The relationship of these parameters is illustrated in the diagram in Fig. 10.9. In the echo era, left ventricular preload in the surgical unit is better evaluated using TEE measures, such as end-diastolic area or volume. However, elevation of either PCWP or LAP is still a useful criterion in estimating acute exacerbation of heart failure.

The indications for using a PAC are assessing hemodynamic parameters such as loading conditions of the heart (preload, afterload), CO, and indices useful in assessing oxygen delivery and demand (ie, SvO$_2$). In 2003, the American Society of Anesthesiologists Task Force on Pulmonary Artery Catheterization published updated practice guidelines for PA catheterization. These guidelines emphasized that the patient, surgery, and practice setting had to be considered when deciding on the use of a PAC. Generally, the routine use of PACs is indicated in high-risk patients (eg, ASA IV or V) and high-risk procedures, during which large fluid changes or hemodynamic disturbances are expected. The practice setting is important, because evidence suggests that inadequate training or experience may increase the risk for perioperative complications associated with the use of a PAC. The recommendation is that the routine use of a PAC should be confined to centers with adequate training and experience in the perioperative management of patients with PACs (Box 10.9). The authors of this chapter have composed a list of possible procedural indications (Box 10.10). Contraindications to PA catheterization are summarized in Box 10.11.

Complications

The complications associated with PAC placement include almost all of those of CVP placement. Additional complications that are unique to the PAC are detailed. The ASA Task Force on Pulmonary Artery Catheterization concluded that serious complications attributable to PAC catheterization occur in 0.1% to 0.5% of patients monitored with a PAC.

Arrhythmias

The most common complications associated with PAC insertion are transient arrhythmias, especially premature ventricular contractions. However, fatal arrhythmias have rarely been reported. A positional maneuver entailing 5-degree head-up and

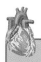

BOX 10.9 *American Society of Anesthesiologists' Practice Guidelines for Pulmonary Artery Catheter Use*

Opinions

- PA catheterization provides new information that may change therapy, with poor clinical evidence of its effect on clinical outcome or mortality.
- There is no evidence from large, controlled studies that preoperative PA catheterization improves outcome regarding hemodynamic optimization.
- Perioperative PAC monitoring of hemodynamic parameters leading to goal-directed therapy has produced inconsistent data in multiple studies and clinical scenarios.
- Having immediate access to PAC data allows important preemptive measures for selected subgroups of patients who encounter hemodynamic disturbances that require immediate and precise decisions about fluid management and drug treatment.
- Experience and understanding are the major determinants of PAC effectiveness.
- PA catheterization is inappropriate as routine practice in surgical patients and should be limited to cases in which the anticipated benefits of catheterization outweigh the potential risks.
- PA catheterization can be harmful.

Recommendations

- The appropriateness of PA catheterization depends on a combination of patient-, surgery-, and practice setting–related factors.
- Perioperative PA catheterization should be considered in patients with significant organ dysfunction or major comorbidities that pose an increased risk for hemodynamic disturbances or instability (eg, ASA IV or V patients).
- Perioperative PA catheterization in surgical settings should be considered based on the hemodynamic risk of the individual case rather than generalized surgical setting–related recommendations. High-risk surgical procedures are those during which large fluid changes or hemodynamic disturbances can be anticipated and procedures that are associated with a high risk of morbidity and mortality.
- Because of the risk of complications from PA catheterization, the procedure should not be performed by clinicians or nursing staff or in practice settings in which competency in safe insertion, accurate interpretation of results, and appropriate catheter maintenance cannot be guaranteed.
- Routine PA catheterization is not recommended when the patient, procedure, or practice setting poses a low or moderate risk for hemodynamic changes.

ASA, American Society of Anesthesiologists; PA, pulmonary artery; PAC, pulmonary artery catheter.
From American Society of Anesthesiologists. Practice guidelines for pulmonary artery catheterization. Available at: http://www.asahq.org/~/media/sites/asahq/files/public/resources/standards-guidelines/practice-guidelines-for-pulmonary-artery-catheterization.pdf

10

right lateral tilt was associated with a statistically significant decrease in malignant arrhythmias (compared with the Trendelenburg position) during PAC insertion.

Complete Heart Block

Complete heart block may develop during PA catheterization in patients with preexisting left bundle branch block. This potentially fatal complication is most likely due to electrical irritability from the PAC tip causing transient right bundle branch block as it passes through the right ventricular outflow tract. The incidence of developing right bundle branch block was 3% in a prospective series of patients undergoing PA

BOX 10.10 *Possible Clinical Indications for Pulmonary Artery Catheter Monitoring*

Major procedures involving large fluid shifts or blood loss in patients with:
- Right-sided heart failure, pulmonary hypertension
- Severe left-sided heart failure not responsive to therapy
- Cardiogenic or septic shock or with multiple-organ failure
- Orthotopic heart transplantation
- Left ventricular–assist device implantation

BOX 10.11 *Contraindications for Pulmonary Artery Catheterization*

Absolute Contraindications

- Severe tricuspid or pulmonary stenosis
- Right atrial or right ventricular mass
- Tetralogy of Fallot

Relative Contraindications

- Severe arrhythmias
- Left bundle branch block (consider pacing PAC)
- Newly inserted pacemaker wires, AICD, or CRT
- Severe coagulopathy

AICD, Automatic implantable cardioverter defibrillator; *CRT,* cardiac resynchronization therapy; *PAC,* pulmonary artery catheter.

catheterization. Having an external pacemaker immediately available or using a pacing PAC when placing a PAC in patients with left bundle branch block is imperative.

Endobronchial Hemorrhage

The incidence of PAC-induced endobronchial hemorrhage in one large series was 0.064% to 0.20%. The ASA PAC guidelines report an incidence of 0.03% to 1.5% from the reviewed literature. Regardless of the exact incidence, this rare complication is associated with a high mortality rate. From these reports, several risk factors have emerged: advanced age, female sex, pulmonary hypertension, mitral stenosis, coagulopathy, distal placement of the catheter, and balloon hyperinflation. Balloon inflation in distal PAs is probably accountable for most episodes of PA rupture because of the high pressures generated by the balloon. Hypothermic CPB also may increase risk attributable to distal migration of the catheter tip with movement of the heart and hardening of the PAC. Pulling back the PAC approximately 3 to 5 cm when CPB is instituted is common practice.

Consideration of the cause of the hemorrhage when forming a therapeutic plan is important. If the hemorrhage is minimal and a coagulopathy coexists, then correction of the coagulopathy may be the only necessary therapy. Protection of the uninvolved lung is of prime importance. Tilting the patient toward the affected side and placing a double-lumen endotracheal tube, as well as other lung-separation maneuvers, should protect the contralateral lung. Strategies proposed to stop the hemorrhage include the application of PEEP, the placement of bronchial blockers, and pulmonary resection. The clinician is obviously at a disadvantage unless the site of hemorrhage is known. A chest radiograph will usually indicate the general location of the lesion. Although the cause of endobronchial hemorrhage may be unclear, the bleeding site must be unequivocally located before surgical treatment is attempted. A small amount of radiographic contrast dye may help pinpoint the lesion if active hemorrhage is present. In severe hemorrhage and with recurrent bleeding, transcatheter coil embolization has been used and may emerge as the preferred treatment method.

Pulmonary Infarction

Pulmonary infarction is a rare complication of PAC monitoring. An early study suggested that a 7.2% incidence of pulmonary infarction was reported with PAC use. However, continuously monitoring the PA waveform and keeping the balloon deflated when not determining the PCWP (to prevent inadvertent wedging of the catheter) were not standard practice at that time. Distal migration of PACs may also occur intraoperatively as a result of the action of the RV, uncoiling of the catheter, and softening of the catheter over time. Inadvertent catheter wedging occurs during CPB because of the diminished right ventricular chamber size and retraction of the heart to perform the operation. Embolization of thrombus formed on a PAC also could result in pulmonary infarction.

Catheter Knotting and Entrapment

Knotting of a PAC usually occurs as a result of coiling of the catheter within the RV. Insertion of an appropriately sized guidewire under fluoroscopic guidance may aid in unknotting the catheter. Alternatively, the knot may be tightened and withdrawn percutaneously along with the introducer if no intracardiac structures are entangled. If cardiac structures, such as the papillary muscles, are entangled in the knotted catheter, then surgical intervention may be required. Sutures placed in the heart may inadvertently entrap the PAC. Reports of such cases and the details of the percutaneous removal have been described.

Valvular Damage

Withdrawal of the catheter with the balloon inflated may result in injury to the tricuspid or pulmonary valves. Placement of the PAC with the balloon deflated may increase the risk of passing the catheter between the chordae tendineae. Septic endocarditis has also resulted from an indwelling PAC.

Pacing Pulmonary Artery Catheters

Electrode-coated PACs and pacing wire catheters are available commercially. The possible indications for placement of a pacing PAC are shown in Box 10.12.

The multipurpose PAC (Edwards Lifesciences Corp., Irvine, CA) contains three atrial and two ventricular electrodes for atrial, ventricular, or AV sequential pacing. The intraoperative success rates for atrial, ventricular, and AV sequential capture have been reported as 80%, 93%, and 73%, respectively.

The Paceport and A-V Paceport PA catheters (Edwards Lifesciences Corp., Irvine, CA) have lumens for the introduction of a ventricular wire or both atrial and ventricular wires for temporary transvenous pacing. The success rate for ventricular and AV capture with Paceport PACs is higher, compared with electrode-pacing PACs.

BOX 10.12 *Indications for Perioperative Placement of Pacing Pulmonary Artery Catheters*

Sinus node dysfunction or symptomatic bradycardia
Hemodynamically relevant second-degree (Mobitz II) atrioventricular block
Complete (third-degree) atrioventricular block
Need for atrioventricular sequential pacing
Left bundle branch block

Mixed Venous Oxygen Saturation Catheters

Monitoring the Svo2 is a means of providing a global estimation of the adequacy of oxygen delivery relative to the needs of the various tissues (oxygen supply-demand ratio). The formula for SvO_2 calculation can be derived by modifying the Fick formula and assuming that the effect of dissolved oxygen in the blood is negligible:

$$SvO_2 = SaO_2 - \frac{\dot{V}O_2}{CO \cdot 1.34 \cdot Hb}$$

A decrease in the SvO_2 can indicate one of the following situations: decreased CO, increased oxygen consumption, decreased arterial oxygen saturation, or decreased hemoglobin (Hb) concentration. To measure SvO_2 in the laboratory, blood is aspirated from the distal port of the PAC slowly, so as not to contaminate the sample with oxygenated alveolar blood.

The addition of fiberoptic bundles to PACs has enabled the continuous monitoring of SvO_2 using reflectance spectrophotometry. The catheter is connected to a device that includes a light-emitting diode and a sensor to detect the light returning from the PA. SvO_2 is calculated from the differential absorption of various wavelengths of light by the saturated and desaturated Hb. The values obtained with various fiberoptic catheter systems showed good agreement with in vitro (co-oximetry) SvO_2 measurements.

▓ CARDIAC OUTPUT MONITORING

The CO is the amount of blood delivered to the tissues by the heart each minute. This measurement reflects the status of the entire circulatory system, not just the heart, because it is governed by autoregulation from the tissues. The CO is equal to the product of the SV and the HR. Preload, afterload, HR, and contractility are the major determinants of the CO.

Thermodilution

Intermittent Thermodilution Cardiac Output

The thermodilution method, using the PAC, is the most commonly used method at present for invasively measuring CO in the clinical setting. With this technique, multiple CO measurements can be obtained at frequent intervals using an inert indicator and without blood withdrawal. A bolus of cold fluid is injected into the RA, and the resulting temperature change is detected by the thermistor in the PA. When a thermal indicator is used, the modified Stewart–Hamilton equation is used to calculate CO:

$$CO = \frac{V(T_B - T_I) \times K_1 \times K_2}{\int_0^\infty \Delta T_B(t)dt}$$

in which CO is the cardiac output (L/min), V is the volume of injectate (mL), T_B is the initial blood temperature (degrees Celsius), T_I is the initial injectate temperature (degrees Celsius), K_1 is the density factor, K_2 is the computation constant, and $\int_0^\infty \Delta T_B(t)dt$ is the integral of blood temperature change over time.

A computer that integrates the area under the temperature versus time curve is used to perform the calculation. CO is inversely proportional to the area under the curve.

The temperature-versus-time curve is the crux of this technique, and any circumstances that affect it have consequences for the accuracy of the CO measurement. Specifically, anything that results in less "cold" reaching the thermistor, more "cold" reaching the thermistor, or an unstable temperature baseline will adversely affect the accuracy of the technique. Less "cold" reaching the thermistor would result in overestimation of the CO, which could be caused by a smaller amount of indicator, an indicator that is too warm, a thrombus on the thermistor, or partial wedging of the catheter. Conversely, underestimation of the CO will occur if excessive volume of injectate or injectate that is too cold is used to perform the measurement. In patients with large intracardiac shunts, PAC-derived thermodilution CO is not recommended for accurate CO measurement. Box 10.13 lists common errors in PAC thermodilution CO measurements.

Continuous Thermodilution Cardiac Output

Pulmonary arterial catheters with the ability to measure CO continuously were introduced into clinical practice in the 1990s. The method that has gained the

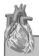

> **BOX 10.13** *Common Errors in Pulmonary Artery Catheter Thermodilution Cardiac Output Measurements*
>
> **Underestimation of True Cardiac Output**
> - Injectate volume greater than programmed volume (typically 10 mL)
> - Large amounts of fluid administered simultaneous to cardiac output measurement (rapid infusions should be stopped)
> - Injectate colder than measured temperature injectate (injectate temperature probe next to heat-emitting hardware instead of injectate fluid)
>
> **Overestimation of True Cardiac Output**
> - Injectate volume less than programmed volume
> - Injectate warmer than measured temperature injectate
>
> **Other Considerations**
> - Surgical manipulation of the heart
> - Fluid administration from aortic cardiopulmonary bypass cannula
> - Arrhythmias

10

most clinical use functions by mildly heating the blood. Good correlations exist between this method and other measures of CO. Unfortunately, the correlation with CO measurements using the intermittent thermodilution method is inconsistent, particularly with rapidly changing hemodynamics; for example, in the initial phase after separating from CPB. In contrast, an excellent correlation exists between intermittent and continuous CO measurements obtained in more physiologically stable periods. Perhaps the reason for this observation lies in the unstable thermal baseline after hypothermic CPB.

CORONARY SINUS CATHETERIZATION

In some centers, an endovascular CS catheter is placed to enable the administration of retrograde cardioplegia during minimally invasive cardiac surgical procedures. It is usually the responsibility of the cardiac anesthesiologist to place the CS catheter via the right IJV while being guided by TEE and fluoroscopy. The CS pressure and waveform can be measured during insertion and cardioplegia infusion. This procedure raises a number of issues, including how deep to place the catheter and what pressures and flows to use with the administration of the cardioplegia. Retrograde cardioplegia flow rate is usually set at 150 to 200 mL/min with CS pressure over 30 mm Hg.

The insertion of the CS catheter can be difficult even with TEE and fluoroscopic monitoring. A modified bicaval view at approximately 110 degrees allows visualization of the catheter from the SVC to the CS. After the catheter enters the CS, its final position is usually guided by fluoroscopy. The balloon is then inflated while looking for a change in the pressure tracing from a typical venous pressure tracing to a pulsatile tracing attributable to the transmission of the pressure back from the left ventricle (ventricularizaton).

SUGGESTED READINGS

American Society of Anesthesiologists Task Force on Pulmonary Artery Catheterization. Practice guidelines for pulmonary artery catheterization: an updated report by the American Society of Anesthesiologists Task Force on Pulmonary Artery Catheterization. *Anesthesiology.* 2003;99:988.

Brouman EY, Gabriel RA, Dutton RP, et al. Pulmonary artery catheter use during cardiac surgery in the United States, 2010 to 2014. *J Cardiothorac Vasc Anesth.* 2016;30:579–584.

Dilisio R, Mittnacht AJ. The "medial-oblique" approach to ultrasound-guided central venous cannulation–maximize the view, minimize the risk. *J Cardiothorac Vasc Anesth.* 2012;26:982–984.

Ezaru CS, Mangione MP, Oravitz TM, et al. Eliminating arterial injury during central venous catheterization using manometry. *Anesth Analg.* 2009;109:130–134.

Fletcher N, Geisen M, Meeran H, et al. Initial clinical experience with a miniaturized transesophageal echocardiography probe in a cardiac intensive care unit. *J Cardiothorac Vasc Anesth.* 2015;29:582–587.

Gravlee GP, Wong AB, Adkins TG, et al. A comparison of radial, brachial, and aortic pressures after cardiopulmonary bypass. *J Cardiothorac Anesth.* 1989;3:20–26.

Greenhow DE. Incorrect performance of Allen's test: ulnar artery flow erroneously presumed inadequate. *Anesthesiology.* 1972;37:356.

Haddad F, Zeeni C, El Rassi I, et al. Can femoral artery pressure monitoring be used routinely in cardiac surgery? *J Cardiothorac Vasc Anesth.* 2008;22:418–422.

Haglund NA, Maltais S, Bick JS, et al. Hemodynamic transesophageal echocardiography after left ventricular assist device implantation. *J Cardiothorac Vasc Anesth.* 2014;28(5):1184–1190.

Handlogten KS, Wilson GA, Clifford L, et al. Brachial artery catheterization: an assessment of use patterns and associated complications. *Anesth Analg.* 2014;118:288–289.

Judge O, Ji F, Fleming N, et al. Current use of the pulmonary artery catheter in cardiac surgery: a survey study. *J Cardiothorac Vasc Anesth.* 2015;29:69–75.

Marik PE, Flemmer M, Harrison W. The risk of catheter-related bloodstream infection with femoral venous catheters as compared to subclavian and internal jugular venous catheters: a systematic review of the literature and meta-analysis. *Crit Care Med.* 2012;40:2479–2485.

Reuter DA, Huang C, Edrich T, et al. Cardiac output monitoring using indicator-dilution techniques: basics, limits, and perspectives. *Anesth Analg.* 2010;110:799–811.

Shiver S, Blaivas M, Lyon M. A prospective comparison of ultrasound-guided and blindly placed radial arterial catheters. *Acad Emerg Med.* 2006;13:1275–1279.

Sotomi Y, Sato N, Kajimoto K, et al; Investigators of the Acute Decompensated Heart Failure Syndromes (ATTEND) Registry. Impact of pulmonary artery catheter on outcome in patients with acute heart failure syndromes with hypotension or receiving inotropes: from the ATTEND Registry. *Int J Cardiol.* 2014;172:165–172.

Vernick WJ, Szeto WY, Li RH, et al. The utility of atrioventricular pacing via pulmonary artery catheter during transcatheter aortic valve replacement. *J Cardiothorac Vasc Anesth.* 2015;29:417–420.

Weiner MM, Geldard P, Mittnacht AJ. Ultrasound-guided vascular access: a comprehensive review. *J Cardiothorac Vasc Anesth.* 2013;27:345–360.

Wiener RS, Welch HG. Trends in use of the pulmonary artery catheter in the United States, 1993–2004. *JAMA.* 2007;298:423–429.

Zollner C, Goetz AE, Weis M, et al. Continuous cardiac output measurements do not agree with conventional bolus thermodilution cardiac output determination. *Can J Anaesth.* 2001;48:1143.

10

Chapter 11

Basic Intraoperative Transesophageal Echocardiography

Ronald A. Kahn, MD • Timothy Maus, MD, FASE •
Ivan Salgo, MD, MBA • Menachem M. Weiner, MD •
Stanton K. Shernan, MD • Stuart J. Weiss, MD, PhD •
Joseph S. Savino, MD • Jared W. Feinman, MD

Key Points

1. An ultrasound beam is a continuous or intermittent train of sound waves emitted by a transducer or wave generator that is composed of density or pressure. Ultrasound waves are characterized by their wavelength, frequency, and velocity.
2. Doppler frequency shift analysis can be used to obtain blood-flow velocity, direction, and acceleration of red blood cells, in which the magnitude and direction of the frequency shift are related to the velocity and direction of the moving target. These velocity flow measurements may be used to determine gradients and blood-flow volumes.
3. *Axial resolution* is the minimum separation between two interfaces located in a direction parallel to the ultrasound beam, enabling them to be imaged as two different interfaces. *Lateral resolution* is the minimum separation of two interfaces aligned along a direction perpendicular to the beam. *Elevational resolution* refers to the ability to determine differences in the thickness of the imaging plane.
4. Absolute contraindications to transesophageal echocardiography in intubated patients include esophageal stricture, diverticula, tumor, recent suture lines, and known esophageal interruption. Relative contraindications include symptomatic hiatal hernia, esophagitis, coagulopathy, esophageal varices, and unexplained upper gastrointestinal bleeding.
5. Horizontal imaging planes are obtained by moving the transesophageal echocardiography probe up and down (upper esophageal: 20–25 cm; midesophageal: 30–40 cm; transgastric: 40–45 cm; deep transgastric: 45–50 cm). Multiplane probes may further facilitate the interrogation of complex anatomic structures by allowing up to 180 degrees of axial rotation of the imaging plane without manual probe manipulation.
6. Aortic stenosis may be evaluated by planimetry, transaortic gradients, or the continuity equation. The use of planimetry is usually limited by the presence of aortic valvular calcifications. Peak, as well as mean, gradients may be measured using continuous-wave Doppler over the aortic valve in either the deep transgastric or transgastric long-axis view. The continuity equation uses measurement of flow through the left ventricular outflow tract and the aortic valve to determine aortic valve area.
7. Quantification of aortic regurgitation is usually based on the analysis of color-flow Doppler patterns in the left ventricular outflow tract during diastole. The most reliable measurements are the vena contracta width and the ratio of proximal jet width to the width of the left ventricular outflow tract.

8. Mitral stenosis may be evaluated by planimetry of the valve in the transgastric basal short-axis view. Transmitral Doppler spectral analysis may be used to calculate mean transmitral gradient and mitral valve area using the pressure half-time measurement of the E wave.

9. Mitral regurgitation may be quantified by the analysis of color-flow Doppler spectra in the left atrium during ventricular systole. The severity of regurgitation may be further quantified using an analysis of pulmonary venous blood-flow velocities and measurements of regurgitant orifice areas using proximal isovelocity surface area. The vena contracta width measurement is easily deployed and is a reproducible technique for assessing mitral regurgitation.

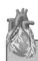

BOX 11.1 *Common Applications of Transesophageal Echocardiography*

Assessment of valvular anatomy and function
Evaluation of the thoracic aorta
Detection of intracardiac defects
Evaluation of pericardial effusions
Detection of intracardiac air, clots, or masses
Assessment of biventricular systolic and diastolic function
Evaluation of myocardial ischemia

Few areas in cardiac anesthesia have developed as rapidly as the field of intraoperative echocardiography. In the early 1980s, when transesophageal echocardiography (TEE) was first used in the surgical unit, its primary application was the assessment of global and regional left ventricular (LV) function. Since that time, there have been numerous technical advances: biplane and multiplane probes; multifrequency probes; enhanced scanning resolution; color-flow Doppler (CFD), pulsed-wave Doppler (PWD), and continuous-wave Doppler (CWD); automatic edge detection; Doppler tissue imaging (DTI); three-dimensional (3D) reconstruction; and digital image processing. With these advances, the number of clinical applications of TEE has significantly increased. The common applications of TEE include (1) assessment of valvular anatomy and function, (2) evaluation of the thoracic aorta, (3) detection of intracardiac defects, (4) detection of intracardiac masses, (5) evaluation of pericardial effusions, (6) detection of intracardiac air and clots, and (7) assessment of biventricular systolic and diastolic function. In many of these evaluations, TEE is able to provide unique and critical information that was not previously available in the surgical unit (Box 11.1).

BASIC CONCEPTS

Properties of Ultrasound

In echocardiography, the heart and great vessels are insonated with ultrasound, which is sound above the human audible range. The ultrasound is sent into the thoracic cavity and is partially reflected by the cardiac structures. From these reflections, distance, velocity, and density of objects within the chest are derived.

11

An ultrasound beam is a continuous or intermittent train of sound waves emitted by a transducer or wave generator. It comprises density or pressure waves and can exist in any medium with the exception of a vacuum. Ultrasound waves are characterized by their wavelength, frequency, and velocity. Wavelength is the distance between the two nearest points of equal pressure or density in an ultrasound beam, and velocity is the speed at which the waves propagate through a medium. As the waves travel past any fixed point in an ultrasound beam, the pressure cycles regularly and continuously between a high and low value. The number of cycles per second (measured in hertz [Hz]) is called the frequency of the wave. Ultrasound is sound with frequencies above 20,000 Hz, which is the upper limit of the human audible range. The relationship among the frequency (f), wavelength (λ), and velocity (v) of a sound wave is defined by the following formula:

$$v = f \times \lambda \qquad \text{[Eq. 11.1]}$$

Piezoelectric crystals convert between ultrasound and electrical signals. When presented with a high-frequency electrical signal, these crystals produce ultrasound energy; conversely, when they are presented with an ultrasonic vibration, they produce an alternating current electrical signal. Commonly, a short ultrasound signal is emitted from the piezoelectric crystal, which is directed toward the areas to be imaged. After ultrasound wave formation, the crystal "listens" for the returning echoes for a given period and then pauses before repeating this cycle. This cycle length is known as the pulse repetition frequency (PRF). This cycle length must be long enough to provide enough time for a signal to travel to and return from a given object of interest. When reflected ultrasound waves return to these piezoelectric crystals, they are converted into electrical signals, which may be appropriately processed and displayed. Electronic circuits measure the time delay between the emitted and received echoes. Since the speed of ultrasound through tissue is constant, this time delay may be converted into the precise distance between the transducer and tissue. The amplitude or strength of the returning ultrasound signal provides information about the characteristics of the insonated tissue.

IMAGING TECHNIQUES

M Mode

The most basic form of ultrasound imaging is M-mode echocardiography. In this mode, the density and position of all tissues in the path of a narrow ultrasound beam (ie, along a single line) are displayed as a scroll on a video screen. The scrolling produces an updated, continuously changing time plot of the studied tissue section several seconds in duration. Because this is a timed *motion display* (normal cardiac tissue is always in motion), it is called *M mode*. Because only a very limited part of the heart is being observed at any one time and because the image requires considerable interpretation, M mode is not currently used as a primary imaging technique. M mode is, however, useful for the precise timing of events within the cardiac cycle and is often used in combination with CFD for the timing of abnormal flows

Two-Dimensional Mode

By rapid, repetitive scanning along many different radii within an area in the shape of a fan (sector), echocardiography generates a two-dimensional (2D) image of a section of the heart. This image, which resembles an anatomic section, can be more easily interpreted than an M-mode display. Information on structures and motion in the plane of a 2D scan is updated 20 to 40 times per second. This repetitive update produces a live (real-time) image of the heart. Scanning 2D echocardiographic devices usually image the heart using an electronically steered ultrasound beam (phased-array transducer).

Doppler Techniques

Most modern echocardiographic scanners combine Doppler capabilities with their 2D imaging capabilities. After the desired view of the heart has been obtained with 2D echocardiography, the Doppler beam, represented by a cursor, is superimposed on the 2D image. The operator positions the cursor as parallel as possible to the assumed direction of blood flow and then empirically adjusts the direction of the beam to optimize the audio and visual representations of the reflected Doppler signal. At the present time, Doppler technology can be used in at least four different ways to measure blood velocities: pulsed, high-repetition frequency, continuous-wave, and color-flow.

Color-Flow Doppler

Advances in electronics and computer technology have allowed the development of CFD ultrasound scanners capable of displaying real-time blood flow within the heart as colors while also showing 2D images in black and white. In addition to showing the location, direction, and velocity of cardiac blood flow, the images produced by these devices allow the estimation of flow acceleration and differentiation of laminar from turbulent blood flow. CFD echocardiography is based on the principle of multigated PWD in which blood-flow velocities are sampled at many locations along many lines covering the entire imaging sector. At the same time, the sector is also scanned to generate a 2D image.

A location in the heart where the scanner has detected flow toward the transducer (the top of the image sector) is assigned the color red. Flow away from the direction of the top is assigned the color blue. This color assignment is arbitrary and determined by the equipment's manufacturer and the user's color mapping. In the most common color-flow coding scheme, the faster the velocity (up to a limit), the more intense the color. Flow velocities that change by more than a preset value within a brief time interval (flow variance) may have an additional hue added to either the red or the blue. Both rapidly accelerating laminar flow (change in flow speed) and turbulent flow (change in flow direction) satisfy the criteria for rapid changes in velocity. In summary, the brightness of the red or blue colors at any location and time is usually proportional to the corresponding flow velocity, whereas the hue is proportional to the temporal rate of change of the velocity.

▦ EQUIPMENT

All TEE probes share several common features. All of the currently available probes use a multifrequency transducer that is mounted on the tip of a gastroscope housing. The majority of the echocardiographic examination is performed using ultrasound between 3.5 and 7 MHz. The tip can be directed by the adjustment of knobs placed at the proximal handle. There are two knobs in most probes for adults; one allows anterior and posterior movement, and the other permits side-to-side motion. Multiplane probes also include a control to rotate the echocardiographic array mechanically from

11

0 to 180 degrees. Thus in combination with the ability to advance and withdraw the probe and to rotate it, many echocardiographic windows are possible. Another feature common to most probes is the inclusion of a temperature sensor to warn of possible heat injury from the transducer to the esophagus.

Currently, most adult echocardiographic probes are multiplane (variable orientation of the scanning plane), whereas pediatric probes are either multiplane or biplane (transverse and longitudinal orientation, parallel to the shaft). The adult probes usually have a shaft length of 100 cm and are between 9 and 12 mm in diameter. The tips of the probes vary slightly in shape and size but are generally 1 to 2 mm wider than the shaft. The size of these probes requires the patient to weigh at least 20 kg. Depending on the manufacturer, the adult probes contain between 32 and 64 elements per scanning orientation. In general, the image quality is directly related to the number of elements used. The pediatric probes are mounted on a narrower, shorter shaft with smaller transducers. These probes may be used in patients weighing as little as 1 kg.

An important feature that is often available is the ability to alter the scanning frequency. A lower frequency, such as 3.5 MHz, has greater penetration and is more suited for the transgastric (TG) view. It also increases the Doppler velocity limits. Conversely, the higher frequencies yield better resolution for detailed imaging. One of the limitations of TEE is that structures very close to the probe are seen only in a very narrow sector. Newer probes may also allow a broader near-field view. Finally, newer probes possess the ability to scan simultaneously in more than one plane. Nonmechanical matrix array probes use a diced crystal stack that can scan both laterally and elevationally. This 2D array can create a 3D ultrasound image and can also create simultaneous intersecting 2D images.

▦ COMPLICATIONS

Complications resulting from intraoperative TEE can be separated into two groups: injury from direct trauma to the airway and esophagus and indirect effects of TEE (Box 11.2). In the first group, potential complications include esophageal bleeding, burning, tearing, dysphagia, and laryngeal discomfort. Many of these complications could result from pressure exerted by the tip of the probe on the esophagus and the airway. Although maximum flexion of the probe will not result in pressure above 17 mm Hg in most patients, occasionally, even in the absence of esophageal disease, pressures greater than 60 mm Hg will result.

> **BOX 11.2** *Complications From Intraoperative Transesophageal Echocardiography*
>
> Injury from direct trauma to the airway and esophagus
> - Esophageal bleeding, burning, tearing
> - Dysphagia
> - Laryngeal discomfort
> - Bacteremia
> - Vocal cord paralysis
>
> Indirect effects
> - Hemodynamic and pulmonary effects of airway manipulation
>
> Distraction from patient care

Further confirmation of the low incidence of esophageal injury from TEE is apparent in the few case reports of complications. In the literature there are only a few reports of a fatal esophageal perforation and benign Mallory-Weiss tear after intraoperative TEE. Therefore, if resistance is met while advancing the probe, then the procedure should be aborted to avoid potentially lethal complications.

The second group of complications that results from TEE includes hemodynamic and pulmonary effects of airway manipulation and, particularly for new TEE operators, distraction from patient care. Fortunately, in the anesthetized patient, hemodynamic consequences to esophageal placement of the probe are rare, and no studies specifically address this issue. More important for the anesthesiologist are the problems of distraction from patient care. Although these reports have not appeared in the literature, the authors have heard of several endotracheal tube disconnections that went unnoticed to the point of desaturation during TEE examination. Additionally, instances during which severe hemodynamic abnormalities have been missed because of a fascination with the images or the controls of the echocardiograph machine have been reported. Clearly, new echocardiographic operators should enlist the assistance of an associate to watch the patient during the echocardiographic examination. This second anesthesiologist will become unnecessary after sufficient experience is gained. Ensuring that all respiratory and hemodynamic alarms are activated during the echocardiographic examination is also important.

SAFETY GUIDELINES AND CONTRAINDICATIONS

To ensure the continued safety of TEE, the following recommendations are made. The probe should be inspected before each insertion for cleanliness and structural integrity. If possible, the electrical isolation should also be checked. The probe should be inserted gently; if resistance is met, then the procedure should be aborted. Minimal transducer energy should be used, and the image should be frozen when not in use. Finally, when not imaging, the probe should be left in the neutral, unlocked position to avoid prolonged pressure on the esophageal mucosa.

Absolute contraindications to TEE in intubated patients include esophageal stricture, diverticula, tumor, recent suture lines, and known esophageal interruption. Relative contraindications include symptomatic hiatal hernia, esophagitis, coagulopathy, esophageal varices, and unexplained upper gastrointestinal bleeding. Notably, despite these relative contraindications, TEE has been used in patients undergoing hepatic transplantation without reported sequelae.

TECHNIQUE OF PROBE PASSAGE

The passage of a TEE probe through the oral and pharyngeal cavities in anesthetized patients may be challenging at times. The usual technique is to place the well-lubricated probe in the posterior portion of the oropharynx with the transducer element pointing inferiorly and anteriorly. The remainder of the probe may be stabilized by looping the controls and the proximal portion of the probe over the operator's neck and shoulder. The operator's left hand then elevates the mandible by inserting the thumb behind the teeth, grasping the submandibular region with the fingers, and then gently lifting. The probe is then advanced against a slight but even resistance, until a loss of resistance is detected as the tip of the probe passes the inferior constrictor muscle of the pharynx, which usually occurs 10 cm past the lips in neonates to 20 cm past the lips in adults. Further manipulation of the probe is performed under echocardiographic guidance.

Difficult TEE probe insertion may be caused by the probe tip abutting the pyriform sinuses, vallecula, posterior tongue, or an esophageal diverticulum. Overinflation of the endotracheal tube cuff could also obstruct passage of the probe. Maneuvers that might aid the passage of the probe include changing the neck position, realigning the TEE probe, and applying additional jaw thrust by elevating the angles of the mandible. The probe may also be passed with the assistance of laryngoscopy. The probe should never be forced past an obstruction. This could result in airway trauma or esophageal perforation.

COMPREHENSIVE INTRAOPERATIVE MULTIPLANE TRANSESOPHAGEAL ECHOCARDIOGRAPHIC EXAMINATION

Probe Manipulation: Descriptive Terms and Technique

The process of obtaining a comprehensive intraoperative multiplane TEE examination begins with a fundamental understanding of the terminology and technique for probe manipulation (Fig. 11.1). Efficient probe manipulation minimizes esophageal injury and facilitates the process of acquiring and sweeping through 2D image planes. Horizontal imaging planes are obtained by moving the TEE probe up and down (proximal and distal) in the esophagus at various depths relative to the incisors (*upper esophageal [UE]*: 20–25 cm; *midesophageal [ME]*: 30–40 cm; *TG*: 40–45 cm; *deep TG*: 45–50 cm) (Table 11.1). Vertical planes are obtained by manually turning the probe to the patient's left or right. Further alignment of the imaging plane can be obtained by manually rotating one of the two control wheels on the probe handle, which flexes the probe tip to the left or right direction or in the anterior or posterior plane. Multiplane probes may further facilitate interrogation of complex anatomic structures, such as the mitral valve (MV), by allowing up to 180 degrees of axial rotation of the imaging plane without manual probe manipulation.

Text continued on p. 239

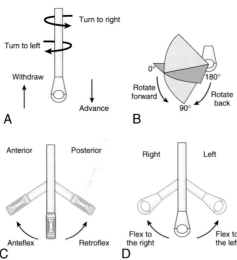

Fig. 11.1 Ways to adjust the probe. (A) Probe movement in the esophagus. (B) Scanning angles obtained by crystal rotation. (C) Movement of the tip forward and back. (D) Movement of the tip from side to side.

Table 11.1 Comprehensive Intraoperative Multiplane Transesophageal Echocardiographic Examination

View	Midesophageal Five-Chamber
Multiplane angle range	0–20 degrees
Anatomy imaged	Left ventricular outflow tract
	Left ventricle and atrium
	Right ventricle and atrium
	Mitral and tricuspid valves
	Interatrial and interventricle septa
Clinical utility	Ventricle function: global and regional
	Intracardiac chamber masses: thrombus, tumor, air; foreign bodies
	Mitral and tricuspid valve evaluation: pathologic and pathophysiologic conditions
	Congenital or acquired interatrial and ventral septal defects
	Hypertrophic obstructive cardiomyopathy evaluation
	Ventricular diastolic evaluation via transmitral and pulmonary vein
	Doppler-flow profile analysis
	Pericardial evaluation: pericarditis; pericardial effusion

View	Midesophageal Four-Chamber
Multiplane angle range	0–20 degrees
Anatomy imaged	Left ventricle and atrium
	Right ventricle and atrium
	Mitral and tricuspid valves
	Interatrial and interventricle septa
	Left pulmonary veins
	Right pulmonary veins
	Coronary sinus
Clinical utility	Ventricle function: global and regional
	Intracardiac chamber masses: thrombus, tumor, air; foreign bodies
	Mitral and tricuspid valve evaluation: pathologic and pathophysiologic conditions
	Congenital or acquired interatrial and ventral septal defects
	Hypertrophic obstructive cardiomyopathy evaluation
	Ventricular diastolic evaluation via transmitral and pulmonary veins
	Doppler-flow profile analysis
	Pericardial evaluation: pericarditis; pericardial effusion
	Coronary sinus evaluation: coronary sinus catheter placement; dilation secondary to persistent left superior vena cava

View	Midesophageal Mitral Commissural
Multiplane angle range	60–70 degrees
Anatomy imaged	Left ventricle and atrium
	Mitral valve
Clinical utility	Left ventricle function: global and regional
	Left ventricle and atrial masses: thrombus, tumor, air; foreign bodies
	Mitral valve evaluation: pathologic and pathophysiologic conditions
	Ventricular diastolic evaluation via transmitral Doppler-flow profile analysis

Continued

233

Table 11.1 Comprehensive Intraoperative Multiplane Transesophageal Echocardiographic Examination—cont'd

View	Midesophageal Two-Chamber
Multiplane angle range	80–100 degrees
Anatomy imaged	Left ventricle, atrium, atrial appendage
	Mitral valve
	Left pulmonary veins
	Coronary sinus
Clinical utility	Left ventricle function: global and regional
	Left ventricle and atrial masses: thrombus, tumor, air; foreign bodies
	Mitral valve evaluation: pathologic and pathophysiologic conditions
	Ventricular diastolic evaluation via transmitral and pulmonary vein Doppler-flow profile analysis
	Coronary sinus evaluation: coronary sinus catheter placement; dilation secondary to persistent left superior vena cava
View	**Midesophageal Long Axis**
Multiplane angle range	120–160 degrees
Anatomy imaged	Left ventricle and atrium
	Left ventricular outflow tract
	Aortic valve
	Mitral valve
	Ascending aorta
Clinical utility	Left ventricle function: global and regional
	Left ventricle and atrial masses: thrombus, tumor, air; foreign bodies
	Mitral valve evaluation: pathologic and pathophysiologic conditions
	Ventricular diastolic evaluation via transmitral Doppler-flow profile analysis
	Aortic valve evaluation: pathologic and pathophysiologic conditions
	Ascending aorta pathologic conditions: atherosclerosis, aneurysms, dissections
	Hypertrophic obstructive cardiomyopathy evaluation
View	**Midesophageal Aortic Valve Long Axis**
Multiplane angle range	120–160 degrees
Anatomy imaged	Aortic valve
	Proximal ascending aorta
	Left ventricular outflow tract
	Mitral valve
	Right pulmonary artery
Clinical utility	Aortic valve: pathologic and pathophysiologic conditions
	Ascending aorta pathologic conditions: atherosclerosis, aneurysms, dissections
	Mitral valve evaluation: pathologic and pathophysiologic conditions
View	**Midesophageal Ascending Aorta Long Axis**
Multiplane angle range	100–150 degrees
Anatomy imaged	Ascending aorta
	Right pulmonary artery
Clinical utility	Ascending aorta pathologic conditions: atherosclerosis, aneurysms, dissections
	Anterograde cardioplegia delivery evaluation
	Pulmonary embolus, thrombus

III

Table 11.1	Comprehensive Intraoperative Multiplane Transesophageal Echocardiographic Examination—cont'd
View	**Midesophageal Ascending Aortic Short Axis**
Multiplane angle range	0–60 degrees
Anatomy imaged	Ascending aorta
	Superior vena cava (short axis)
	Main pulmonary artery
	Right pulmonary artery
	Left pulmonary artery
	Pulmonic valve
Clinical utility	Ascending aorta pathologic conditions: atherosclerosis, aneurysms, dissections
	Pulmonic valve: pathologic and pathophysiologic conditions
	Pulmonary embolus, thrombus evaluation
	Superior vena cava pathologic conditions: thrombus, sinus venosus atrial septal defect
	Pulmonary artery catheter placement
View	**Midesophageal Right Pulmonary Vein**
Multiplane angle range	0–30 degrees
Anatomy imaged	Midascending aorta
	Superior vena cava
	Right pulmonary vein
Clinical utility	Ascending aorta dissection, aneurysm, plaque
	Superior vena cava thrombus
	Right pulmonary vein Doppler-flow velocity
View	**Midesophageal Aortic Valve Short Axis**
Multiplane angle range	30–60 degrees
Anatomy imaged	Aortic valve
	Interatrial septum
	Coronary ostia and arteries
	Right ventricular outflow tract
	Pulmonary valve
Clinical utility	Aortic valve: pathologic and pathophysiologic conditions
	Ascending aorta pathologic conditions: atherosclerosis, aneurysms, dissections
	Left and right atrial masses: thrombus, embolus, air, tumor, foreign bodies
	Congenital or acquired interatrial septal defects evaluation
View	**Midesophageal Right Ventricular Inflow-Outflow ("Wraparound")**
Multiplane angle range	60–90 degrees
Anatomy imaged	Right ventricle and atrium
	Left atrium
	Tricuspid valve
	Aortic valve
	Right ventricular outflow tract
	Pulmonic valve and main pulmonary artery
Clinical utility	Right ventricle and atrial masses and left atrial: thrombus, embolus, tumor, foreign bodies
	Pulmonic valve and subpulmonic valve: pathologic and pathophysiologic conditions
	Pulmonary artery catheter placement
	Tricuspid valve: pathologic and pathophysiologic conditions
	Aortic valve: pathologic and pathophysiologic conditions

11

Continued

235

Table 11.1 Comprehensive Intraoperative Multiplane Transesophageal Echocardiographic Examination—cont'd

View	Midesophageal Modified Bicaval Tricuspid Valve
Multiplane angle range	50–70 degrees
Anatomy imaged	Right and left atria
	Superior vena cava (long axis)
	Inferior vena cava orifice
	Interatrial septum
	Right pulmonary veins
	Coronary sinus and Thebesian valve
	Eustachian valve
	Tricuspid valve
Clinical utility	Right and left atrial masses: thrombus, embolus, air, tumor, foreign bodies
	Superior vena cava pathologic conditions: thrombus, sinus venosus atrial septal defect
	Inferior vena cava pathologic conditions: thrombus, tumor
	Femoral venous line placement
	Coronary sinus catheter line placement
	Right pulmonary vein evaluation: anomalous return, Doppler evaluation for left ventricular diastolic function
	Congenital or acquired interatrial septal defects evaluation
	Pericardial effusion evaluation
	Tricuspid valve evaluation for stenosis, regurgitation, and calculated estimation of pulmonary artery pressures from regurgitant
	Doppler-flow velocity profile
View	Midesophageal Bicaval
Multiplane angle range	80–110 degrees
Anatomy imaged	Right and left atria
	Superior vena cava (long axis)
	Inferior vena cava orifice: advance probe and turn to right to visualize inferior vena cava in the long axis, liver, hepatic and portal veins
	Interatrial septum
	Right pulmonary veins: turn probe to right
	Coronary sinus and Thebesian valve
	Eustachian valve
Clinical utility	Right and left atrial masses: thrombus, embolus, air, tumor, foreign bodies
	Superior vena cava pathologic conditions: thrombus, sinus venosus atrial septal defect
	Inferior vena cava pathologic conditions: thrombus, tumor
	Femoral venous line placement
	Coronary sinus catheter line placement
	Right pulmonary vein evaluation: anomalous return, Doppler evaluation for left ventricular diastolic function
	Congenital or acquired interatrial septal defects evaluation
	Pericardial effusion evaluation

III

Table 11.1 Comprehensive Intraoperative Multiplane Transesophageal Echocardiographic Examination—cont'd

View	Upper Esophageal Right and Left Pulmonary Veins
Multiplane angle range	90–100 degrees
Anatomy imaged	Pulmonary veins
	Pulmonary artery
	Ascending aorta
Clinical utility	Pulmonary vein pathologic condition
	Ascending aortic aneurysm, dissection
	Pulmonary embolism, thrombus
View	**Midesophageal Left Atrial Appendage**
Multiplane angle range	90–110 degrees
Anatomy imaged	Left pulmonary veins
	Left atrial appendage
Clinical utility	Left pulmonary vein Doppler-flow velocity
	Left atrial appendage thrombus
View	**Midesophageal Ascending Aortic Short Axis**
Multiplane angle range	0–60 degrees
Anatomy imaged	Ascending aorta
	Superior vena cava (short axis)
	Main pulmonary artery
	Right pulmonary artery
	Left pulmonary artery
	Pulmonic valve
Clinical utility	Ascending aorta pathologic conditions: atherosclerosis, aneurysms, dissections
View	**Transgastric Basal Short Axis**
Multiplane angle range	0–20 degrees
Anatomy imaged	Left and right ventricles
	Mitral valve
	Tricuspid valve
Clinical utility	Mitral valve evaluation ("fish-mouth view"): pathologic, pathophysiologic conditions
	Tricuspid valve evaluation: pathologic, pathophysiologic conditions
	Basal left ventricular regional function
	Basal right ventricular regional function
View	**Transgastric Midpapillary**
Multiplane angle range	0–20 degrees
Anatomy imaged	Left and right ventricles
	Papillary muscles
Clinical utility	Mid left and right ventricular regional and global functions
	Intracardiac volume status
View	**Transgastric Apical Short Axis**
Multiplane angle range	0–20 degrees
Anatomy imaged	Left and right ventricles
Clinical utility	Apical left and right ventricular regional functions
	Ventricular aneurysm
View	**Transgastric Right Ventricular Basal**
Multiplane angle range	0–20 degrees
Anatomy imaged	Left and right ventricle
	Right ventricular outflow tract
	Tricuspid valve (short axis)
	Pulmonic valve

11

Continued

Table 11.1 Comprehensive Intraoperative Multiplane Transesophageal Echocardiographic Examination—cont'd

Clinical utility	Left and right ventricular regional and global functions
	Intracardiac volume status
	Tricuspid valve pathologic condition
	Pulmonic valve regurgitation and stenosis evaluation
View	**Transgastric Right Ventricular Inflow-Outflow**
Multiplane angle range	60–90 degrees
Anatomy imaged	Right ventricle and right atrium
	Left atrium
	Tricuspid valve
	Aortic valve
	Right ventricular outflow tract
	Pulmonic valve and main pulmonary artery
Clinical utility	Right ventricle and atrial masses and left atrial: thrombus, embolus, tumor, foreign bodies
	Pulmonic valve and subpulmonic valve: pathologic, pathophysiologic conditions
	Pulmonary artery catheter placement
	Tricuspid valve: pathologic, pathophysiologic conditions
	Aortic valve: pathologic, pathophysiologic conditions
View	**Transgastric Two-Chamber**
Multiplane angle range	80–100 degrees
Anatomy imaged	Left ventricle and left atrium
	Mitral valve: chordae and papillary muscles
	Coronary sinus
Clinical utility	Left ventricular regional and global functions (including apex)
	Left ventricular and atrial masses: thrombus, embolus, air, tumor, foreign bodies
	Mitral valve: pathologic, pathophysiologic conditions
View	**Transgastric Right Ventricular Inflow**
Multiplane angle range	100–120 degrees
Anatomy imaged	Right ventricle and right atrium
	Tricuspid valve: chordae and papillary muscles
Clinical utility	Right ventricular regional and global functions
	Right ventricular and atrial masses: thrombus, embolus, tumor, foreign bodies
	Tricuspid valve: pathologic, pathophysiologic conditions
View	**Transgastric Long Axis**
Multiplane angle range	90–120 degrees
Anatomy imaged	Left ventricle and outflow tract
	Aortic valve
	Mitral valve
Clinical utility	Left ventricular regional and global functions
	Mitral valve: pathologic, pathophysiologic conditions
	Aortic valve: pathologic, pathophysiologic conditions
View	**Deep Transgastric Long Axis**
Multiplane angle range	0–20 degrees (anteflexion)
Anatomy imaged	Left ventricle and outflow tract
	Interventricular septum
	Aortic valve and ascending aorta
	Left atrium
	Mitral valve
	Right ventricle
	Pulmonic valve

Table 11.1	Comprehensive Intraoperative Multiplane Transesophageal Echocardiographic Examination—cont'd
Clinical utility	Aortic and subaortic valve: pathologic, pathophysiologic conditions
	Mitral valve: pathologic, pathophysiologic conditions
	Left and right ventricular global functions
	Left and right ventricular masses: thrombus, embolus, tumor, foreign bodies
	Congenital or acquired interventricular septal defect evaluation
View	Upper Esophageal Aortic Arch: Long Axis
Multiplane angle range	0 degrees
Anatomy imaged	Aortic arch; left brachiocephalic vein; left subclavian and carotid arteries; right brachiocephalic artery
Clinical utility	Ascending aorta and arch pathologic conditions: atherosclerosis, aneurysms, dissections; aortic cannulation site evaluation for cardiopulmonary bypass
View	Upper Esophageal Aortic Arch: Short Axis
Multiplane angle range	90 degrees
Structures imaged	Aortic arch; left brachiocephalic vein; left subclavian and carotid arteries; right brachiocephalic artery
	Main pulmonary artery and pulmonic valve
Clinical utility	Ascending aorta and arch pathologic conditions: atherosclerosis, aneurysms, dissections
	Pulmonary embolus; pulmonary valve evaluation (insufficiency, stenosis, Ross procedure); pulmonary artery catheter placement
View	Descending Aorta Short Axis
Multiplane angle range	0 degrees
Anatomy imaged	Descending thoracic aorta
	Left pleural space
Clinical utility	Descending aorta pathologic conditions: atherosclerosis, aneurysms, dissections
	Intraaortic balloon placement evaluation
	Left pleural effusion
View	Descending Aorta Long Axis
Multiplane angle range	90–110 degrees
Anatomy imaged	Descending thoracic aorta
	Left pleural space
Clinical utility	Descending aorta pathologic conditions: atherosclerosis, aneurysms, dissections
	Intraaortic balloon placement evaluation
	Left pleural effusion

11

Comprehensive Intraoperative Transesophageal Echocardiographic Examination: Imaging Planes and Structural Analysis

Left and Right Ventricles

The left ventricle should be examined carefully for global and regional function using multiple transducer planes, depths, and rotational and angular orientations (Fig. 11.2). Analysis of segmental function is based on a qualitative visual assessment that includes the following grading system of both LV wall thickness and motion (endocardial border excursion) during systole: 1 = normal (>30% thickening); 2 = mild hypokinesis (between 10% and 30% thickening); 3 = severe hypokinesis

(<10% thickening); 4 = akinesis (no thickening); 5 = dyskinesis (paradoxic motion). The recently recommended ME five-chamber view enables visualization of the septal and lateral walls (slightly anterior) of the left ventricle at 0 to 20 degrees from its base to the apex, along with the left ventricular outflow tract (LVOT), right ventricle and both atria (see Fig. 11.2). Slight TEE probe advancement eliminates the LVOT from the image window and permits the development of the *ME four-chamber* view (see Fig. 11.2), demonstrating a slightly more mid-to-inferior plane. TEE probe rotation to approximately 80 to 100 degrees develops the ME *two-chamber* view (see Fig. 11.2), which removes the right-sided chambers from the imaging window but enables visualization of the inferior and anterior LV walls at the basal, mid, and apical levels segments. The *ME long-axis (LAX)* view at 120 to 160 degrees (see Fig. 11.2) allows evaluation of the remaining anteroseptal and inferolateral (posterior) LV segments. Because the left ventricle is usually oriented inferiorly to the true horizontal plane, slight retroflexion of the probe tip may be required to minimize LV foreshortening. The *TG midpapillary SAX* view *(TG mid-SAX)* at 0 to 20 degrees (see Fig. 11.2) is the most commonly used view for monitoring LV function, because it allows a midpapillary assessment of the LV segments supplied by the corresponding coronary arteries (right coronary artery, left circumflex, and left anterior descending [LAD]). This view also enables qualitative and quantitative evaluation of pericardial effusions. Advancing or withdrawing the probe at the TG depth enables LV evaluation at the respective newly recommended *TG apical SAX* and basal levels *(TG basal SAX)* (see Fig. 11.2), respectively. Further evaluation of the left ventricle can be obtained at the midpapillary TG depth by rotating the probe forward to the *TG two-chamber* view (80 to 100 degrees) (Fig. 11.2) and *TG LAX* (90 to 120 degrees) (see Fig. 11.2).

Right ventricular (RV) regional and global function can be assessed from the *ME five-chamber* and *four-chamber* views (see Fig. 11.2), which allows visualization of the septal and free walls. Although a formal segmental scheme has not been developed for the RV free wall, regional assessment of the septum can be performed. Turning the probe to the right and advancing slightly from the ME depth allows visualization of the tricuspid valve (TV), coronary sinus (CS), and RV apex. Rotating the probe between 60 and 90 degrees reveals the *ME RV inflow-outflow* view (see Fig. 11.2), in which the right atrium (RA), TV, inferior RV free wall, right ventricular outflow tract (RVOT), pulmonic valve (PV), and main pulmonary artery (PA) can be viewed wrapping around the centrally oriented aortic valve (AV). This view often allows optimal Doppler beam alignment to evaluate the TV and can also be helpful for directing PA catheter floating and positioning. The same right-sided structures can also be visualized from a different perspective by advancing the probe to the TG depth to obtain the newly recommended *TG RV inflow-outflow* view (see Fig. 11.2). The *TG midpapillary SAX* view (see Fig. 11.2) displays the crescent-shaped, thinner-walled right ventricle to the left of the left ventricle. Slightly withdrawing the probe reveals the right ventricle at a more basal level along with the PV in the newly recommended TG RV basal view (see Fig. 11.2). The *TG RV inflow* view (see Fig. 11.2) is developed by turning the probe to the right to center the right ventricle at this depth and rotating the multiplane angle forward to 100 to 120 degrees, thereby revealing the inferior RV free wall.

Mitral Valve

The echocardiographic evaluation of the MV requires a thorough assessment of its leaflets (anterior and posterior), annulus, and the subvalvular apparatus (chordae tendineae, papillary muscles, and adjacent LV walls) to locate lesions and to define the cause and severity of the pathophysiologic condition. The mitral leaflets can be

Text continued on p. 245

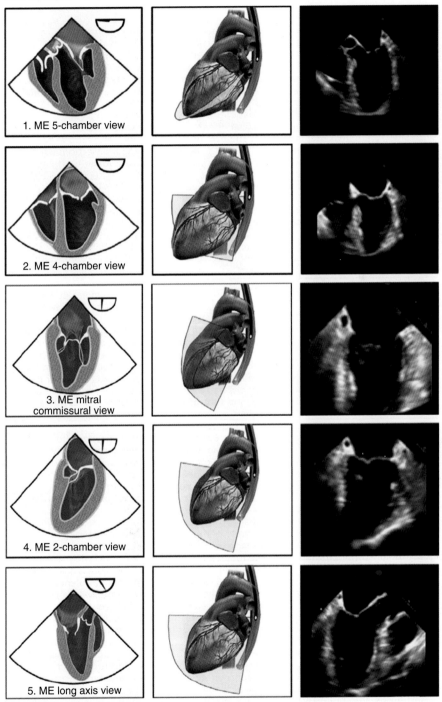

1. ME 5-chamber view

2. ME 4-chamber view

3. ME mitral commissural view

4. ME 2-chamber view

5. ME long axis view

Fig. 11.2 Schematic drawings of the comprehensive examination. *AV,* Aortic valve; *LAX,* long axis; *ME,* midesophageal; *RV,* right ventricle; *SAX,* short axis; *TG,* transgastric; *UE,* upper esophageal. (Adapted with permission. From Hahn RT, Abraham T, Adams MS, et al. Guidelines for performing a comprehensive transesophageal echocardiographic examination: recommendations from the American Society of Echocardiography and the Society of Cardiovascular Anesthesiologists. *J Am Soc Echocardiogr.* 2013;9:921–964.)

Midesophageal views

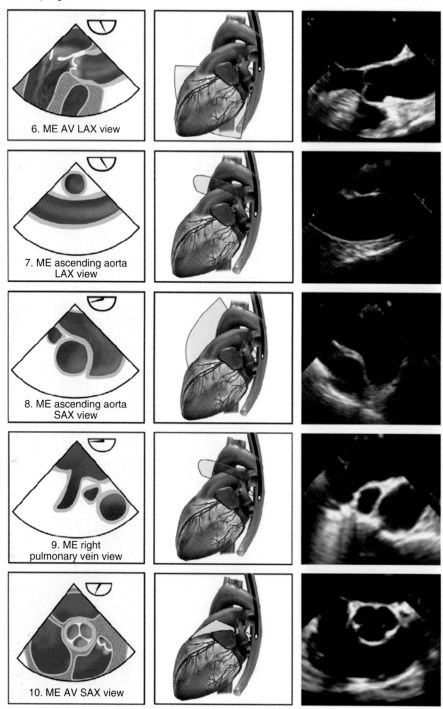

6. ME AV LAX view

7. ME ascending aorta LAX view

8. ME ascending aorta SAX view

9. ME right pulmonary vein view

10. ME AV SAX view

Fig. 11.2, cont'd

Continued

Midesophageal views

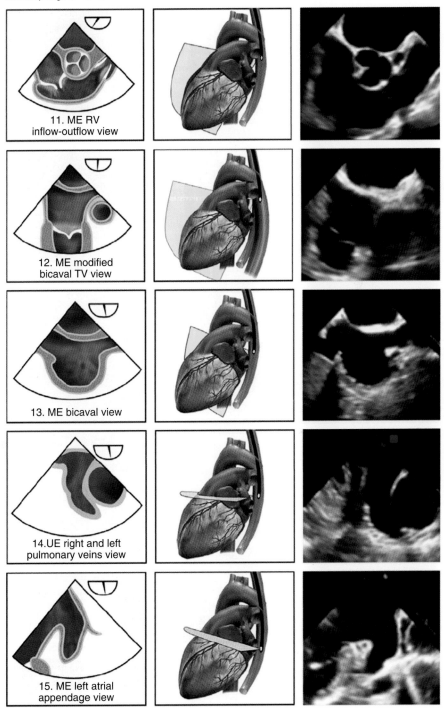

11. ME RV inflow-outflow view

12. ME modified bicaval TV view

13. ME bicaval view

14. UE right and left pulmonary veins view

15. ME left atrial appendage view

Fig. 11.2, cont'd

11

Transgastric views

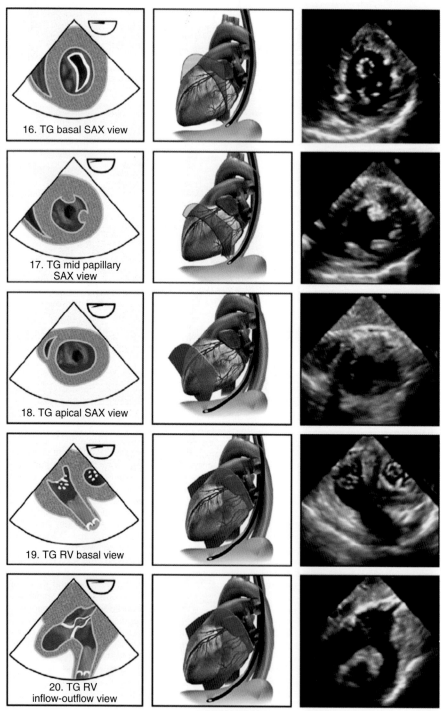

16. TG basal SAX view

17. TG mid papillary SAX view

18. TG apical SAX view

19. TG RV basal view

20. TG RV inflow-outflow view

III

Fig. 11.2, cont'd

Continued

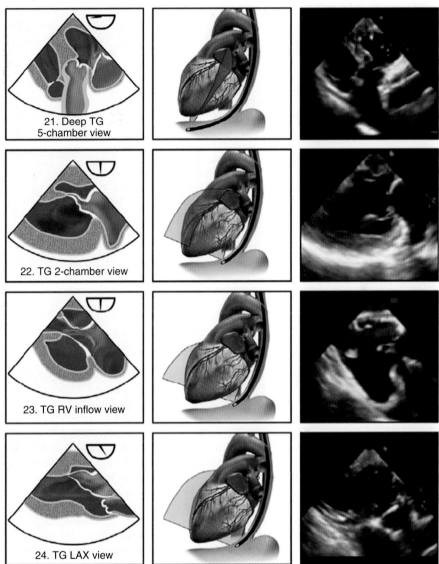

21. Deep TG 5-chamber view

22. TG 2-chamber view

23. TG RV inflow view

24. TG LAX view

Fig. 11.2, cont'd

further divided into posterior leaflet scallops: lateral (P1), middle (P2), and medial (P3), which correspond with respective anterior leaflet sections: lateral third (A1), middle third (A2), and medial third (A3). The leaflets are united at the anterolateral and posteromedial commissures. The *ME four-chamber* view (see Fig. 11.2) displays the larger appearing anterior leaflet (A2,3) to the left of the posterior leaflet (P2,1), whereas the *ME five-chamber* view reveals more of A1 and P1. Anteflexing the probe provides imaging of the anterolateral aspect of the MV, whereas gradual advancement of the probe and retroflexion shift the image plane to the posteromedial aspect of MV. Maintaining the probe at the ME depth and rotating the multiplane angle forward to 60 to 70 degrees develops the *ME mitral commissural* view (see Fig. 11.2), in which

MONITORING

25. Descending aorta SAX view

26. Descending aorta LAX view

27. UE aortic arch LAX view

28. UE aortic arch SAX view

Fig. 11.2, cont'd

A2 is flanked by P1 on the right and P3 on the left, giving A2 the appearance of a "trap-door" as it moves in and out of the imaging plane throughout the cardiac cycle. Farther forward rotation of the probe to 80 to 100 degrees develops the *ME two-chamber* view (see Fig. 11.2), revealing P3 to the left and A1 on the right. Final forward probe rotation to 120 to 160 degrees reveals the *ME LAX* view (see Fig. 11.2), which images P2 on the left and A2 on the right. The *TG basal SAX* view (see Fig. 11.2) enables visualization of both MV leaflets ("fish-mouth view") if the probe is anteflexed and withdrawn slightly from the midpapillary level of the left ventricle. In this view, the posteromedial commissure is in the upper left, the anterolateral commissure is in the lower right, the posterior leaflet is to the right, and the anterior leaflet is to the left of the displayed image. Rotation of the probe to 80 to 100 degrees develops the *TG two-chamber* view (see Fig. 11.2) that is especially useful for evaluating the chordae tendineae and corresponding papillary muscles.

Aortic Valve, Aortic Root, and Left Ventricular Outflow

The three cusps of the semilunar AV are best visualized simultaneously in the *ME AV SAX* view (see Fig. 11.2), which is obtained by rotating the probe forward to 30 to 60 degrees. The noncoronary cusp is superior, lying adjacent to the atrial septum; the right cusp is inferior; and the left cusp lies to the right, pointing in the direction of the left atrial appendage (LAA). This view permits planimetry of the AV orifice, evaluation of congenital anomalies of the AV (eg, bicuspid AV), and qualitative assessment of aortic insufficiency (AI) when CFD is used. The *ME AV LAX* view (see Fig. 11.2) can be obtained at the same depth while rotating the probe to 120 to 160 degrees, allowing for visualization of the LVOT, AV annulus, and leaflets (right and either noncoronary or left), sinuses of Valsalva, sinotubular junction, and proximal ascending aorta. This view is particularly useful for evaluating AI with CFD, systolic anterior motion of the MV, and proximal aortic pathologic conditions (eg, dissections, aneurysms). Rotating the probe back to 90 to 120 degrees and advancing into the stomach to TG level develops the *TG LAX* view (see Fig. 11.2). In this view, the LVOT and AV are oriented to the right and inferiorly in the displayed image, thereby providing an optimal window for parallel Doppler beam alignment for the assessment of flows and pressure gradients (aortic stenosis [AS], hypertrophic obstructive cardiomyopathy). Rotating the probe back farther to 0 to 20 degrees, advancing deep into the stomach, and anteflexing the tip so that it lies adjacent to the LV apex, allows for the development of the *deep TG LAX* view, now referred to as the *deep TG five-chamber* view (see Fig. 11.2), which also provides optimal Doppler beam alignment for measuring transaortic valve and LVOT flow velocities and may provide an additional window for assessing flows through muscular ventricular septal defects and LV apical pathologic conditions (thrombus, aneurysms).

Tricuspid Valve

The echocardiographic evaluation of the TV requires a thorough assessment of its three leaflets (anterior, posterior, and septal), annulus, chordae tendineae, papillary muscles, and the corresponding RV walls. In the *ME five-chamber* view, the septal TV leaflet is displayed on the right side, and the anterior leaflet is usually on the left side of the annulus. Advancing the probe slightly reveals the *ME four-chamber* view (see Fig. 11.2), with the septal TV leaflet on the right side and the posterior TV leaflet usually on the left side of the annulus. Rotating the multiplane angle to 50 to 70 degrees develops the *ME RV inflow-outflow* view (see Fig. 11.2), which displays the posterior TV leaflet on the left side of the image and the anterior TV leaflet on the right side of the image adjacent to the AV. Slightly turning the probe rightward from the *ME bicaval* view permits the development of the newly recommended *ME-modified bicaval TV* view (see Fig. 11.2) with the anterior leaflet on the right and the posterior leaflet on the left. The ME-modified bicaval view often provides better alignment of a CWD beam with a tricuspid regurgitation (TR) jet for estimating PA pressures. The *TG RV inflow* view (see Fig. 11.2) is obtained by advancing the probe into the stomach and rotating to 100 to 120 degrees. This view is ideal for visualizing the chordae tendineae and papillary muscles in the right ventricle. Rotating back to the *TG mid-SAX* at 0 to 20 degrees and slightly withdrawing the probe to obtain the *TG RV basal* view provides a cross-sectional, SAX view of the TV, displaying the anterior leaflet in the far field, the posterior leaflet to the left in the near field, and the septal leaflet on the right side of the image.

247

11

Pulmonic Valve and Pulmonary Artery

The PV is a trileaflet, semilunar valve. The *ME AV SAX* view (see Fig. 11.2) displays the transition between the RVOT and PV. Rotating the probe back toward 0 degrees and withdrawing slightly develops the *ME ascending aortic SAX* view (see Fig. 11.2) displaying the transition between the PV and the main PA and its bifurcation. Although the right PA is usually easy to visualize by turning the probe to the right, the left PA is often obscured by the interposing, air-filled, left mainstem bronchus. The *ME RV inflow-outflow* view (see Fig. 11.2) can also be used to assess the PV and main PA, which lie on the right side of the image adjacent to the AV. However, the newly recommended *TG RV inflow-outflow* view (see Fig. 11.2), with the PV on the right side of the screen and the more reliable *UE aortic arch SAX* view (see Fig. 11.2), displays the PV oriented to the left of the cross-sectional view of the aortic arch and usually provides a more parallel Doppler beam orientation through for the evaluation of pulmonic regurgitation or stenosis.

Left Atrium, Left Atrial Appendage, Pulmonary Veins, and Atrial Septum

The left atrium is the closest cardiac structure to the TEE probe when positioned in the esophagus. Consequently, the left atrium is usually easily displayed in the superior aspect of the 2D image sector. The *ME five-chamber* and *four-chamber* views (see Fig. 11.2) display the left atrium almost in its entirety with the LAA oriented to its superior and lateral aspects when the probe is slightly withdrawn. The muscular ridges of the pectinate muscles within the LAA should not be confused with thrombi. A slightly farther withdrawal of the probe, turning it to the left, and rotating the array to approximately 90 degrees, develops the newly defined *UE left pulmonary vein view* (see Fig. 11.2), which allows the left upper pulmonary vein (LUPV) to be imaged as it enters the left atrium from the anterior-to-posterior direction and separated from the lateral border of the LAA by the *warfarin ridge*. Turning the probe to the right at this depth reveals the newly defined *UE right pulmonary* view (see Fig. 11.2), and a slight advancement and rotation of the array to 0 degrees permits visualization of the newly defined *ME right pulmonary vein* view (see Fig. 11.2), which both reveal the right upper pulmonary vein (RUPV) entering the left atrium in an anterior-to-posterior direction and the right PA or superior vena cava (SVC), respectively.

The interatrial septum (IAS), consisting of thicker limbus regions flanking the thin fossa ovalis, can also be imaged in the *ME four-chamber* view (see Fig. 11.2). Benign lipomatous hypertrophy of the IAS must be distinguished from pathologic lesions such as atrial myxomas. The patency of the IAS and the presence of a patent foramen ovale (PFO) or congenital atrial septal defects should be assessed with Doppler echocardiography and intravenous injections of agitated saline. Advancing and rotating the probe to 80 to 100 degrees develops the *ME two-chamber* view (see Fig. 11.2), which allows for further imaging of the left atrium from left to right. The LAA and LUPV can be seen by turning the probe slightly to the left to develop the newly defined *ME LAA* view (see Fig. 11.2). Rotating the probe to the right at this level and adjusting the multiplane angle to 80 to 110 degrees will develop the *ME bicaval* view (see Fig. 11.2), which delineates the SVC entering the RA to the right of the image and the inferior vena cava (IVC) entering from the left. The IAS can be seen in the middle of the image separating the left and right atria.

Right Atrium and Coronary Sinus

The RA can be most easily visualized in the *ME five-chamber* and *ME four-chamber* views (see Fig. 11.2) by turning the probe to the patient's right side, as well as in the

ME RV inflow-outflow view (see Fig. 11.2). In these views, the entire RA can be visualized for size, overall function, and the presence of masses (thrombi, tumors). Rotating the multiplane angle to 80 to 110 degrees develops the *ME bicaval* view (see Fig. 11.2), which displays the RA and its internal structures (Eustachian valve, Chiari network, crista terminalis). The SVC can be imaged entering the RA on the right, superior to the right atrial appendage, and the IVC enters the RA on the left of the display. Advancing and turning the probe to the right will allow for a qualitative evaluation of the intrahepatic segment of the IVC and hepatic veins. At the TG depth, both the *TG RV inflow-outflow* and *TG RV inflow* views may provide more optimal imaging windows for visualizing the RA and collateral structures. Pacemaker electrodes and central venous catheters for hemodynamic monitoring or cardiopulmonary bypass (CPB) can be easily imaged in this view.

The CS lies posteriorly in the atrioventricular groove, emptying into the RA at the inferior extent of the atrial septum. The CS can be viewed in LAX entering the RA just superior to the tricuspid annulus by advancing and slightly retroflexing the probe from *ME four-chamber* view (see Fig. 11.2). The CS can be imaged cross-sectionally in the SAX in the *ME two-chamber* view (see Fig. 11.2) in the upper left of the display. The CS and Thebesian valve can also be visualized in the *ME-modified bicaval* view (see Fig. 11.2) on the upper left of the image as it enters the RA at an obtuse angle. Echocardiographic visualization of the CS can be useful for directing the placement of CS catheters used for CPB.

Thoracic Aorta

The proximal and midascending thoracic aorta can be visualized in the SAX in the *ME ascending aortic SAX* view (see Fig. 11.2). Advancing and withdrawing the probe should enable visualization of the thoracic aorta from the sinotubular junction to a point 4- to 6-cm superior to the AV and allow an inspection for aneurysms and dissections. Rotating the multiplane angle to 100 to 150 degrees develops the *ME ascending aortic LAX* view (see Fig. 11.2), which optimally displays the parallel anterior and posterior walls for measuring proximal and midascending aortic diameters. This display can also be obtained from the *ME AV LAX* view (see Fig. 11.2) by slightly withdrawing and turning the probe to the left.

TEE imaging of the aortic arch is often obscured by the interposing, air-filled trachea. The most optimal views of the aortic arch are obtained by withdrawing the probe from the *ME ascending aortic SAX* view at 0 degrees and rotating to the left to obtain the *UE aortic arch LAX* view (see Fig. 11.2), which displays the proximal arch followed by the mid-arch, the great vessels (brachiocephalic, left carotid artery, and left subclavian artery), and the distal arch before it joins the proximal descending thoracic aorta imaged in cross-section. Alternatively, rotating the probe to 90 degrees develops the *UE aortic arch SAX* view (see Fig. 11.2). Turning the probe to the left in this view delineates the transition of the distal arch with the proximal descending thoracic aorta. Turning the probe to the right and slightly withdrawing it will allow for the mid-arch and great vessels to be imaged on the right side of the screen, followed by the distal ascending aorta when the probe is subsequently advanced and rotated forward to the 120-degree *ME ascending aortic LAX* view (see Fig. 11.2). Epiaortic aortic scanning may be particularly useful for assessing the extent of ascending aortic and arch pathologic conditions (ie, aneurysms, dissection, atherosclerosis) to determine cross-clamping and cannulation sites for CPB.

A SAX image of the descending thoracic aorta is obtained by turning the probe leftward from the *ME four-chamber* view to produce the *descending aortic SAX* view (see Fig. 11.2). Rotating the multiplane angle of the probe from 0 to 90 to 110 degrees produces an LAX image, the *descending aortic LAX* view (see Fig. 11.2). The descending

11

thoracic aorta should be interrogated in its entirety, beginning at the distal aortic arch, by continually advancing the probe and turning slightly to the left until the celiac and superior mesenteric arteries are visualized branching tangentially from the anterior surface of abdominal aorta when the probe is in the stomach. A thorough examination of the descending thoracic aorta may be necessary to evaluate the distal extent of an aneurysm or dissection. In addition, the *descending aortic SAX* and *LAX* views can be useful for confirming appropriate intraaortic balloon positioning.

CLINICAL APPLICATIONS

Left Ventricular Assessment

Assessment of Left Ventricular Size

LV volume measurements may be with biplane disk summary or area-length measurements using 2D echocardiography or using 3D data sets. Since the biplane disk summation method (modified Simpson method) corrects for shape distortions, it is currently the recommended method of 2D volume measurements. With biplane disk summation, the total LV volume is calculated from the summation of a stack of elliptical disks. The height of each disk is calculated as a fraction of the LV LAX, based on the longer of the two lengths from the two- and four-chamber views. The cross-sectional area (CSA) of the disk is based on the diameters obtained, and the volume of the disk is estimated. The volume is obtained by the summation of these values.

Left Ventricular Preload by End-Diastolic Dimensions

Preload is often estimated by measuring left-sided heart filling pressures (pulmonary capillary wedge pressure [PCWP], left atrial pressure [LAP], or left ventricular end-diastolic pressure [LVEDP]) in conventional hemodynamics, measuring LV end-diastolic dimensions. It has been proposed that end-diastolic dimensions provide a better index of preload than the PCWP. When PCWP and end-diastolic volume (EDV), derived from SAX areas at the level of the papillary muscles, were compared as predictors of cardiac index (CI) in patients undergoing coronary artery bypass grafting (CABG) surgery, a strong correlation was observed between end-diastolic area (EDA) or EDV and CI, whereas no significant correlation was found between PCWP and CI.

TEE is often, for practical reasons, limited to a single SAX view at the level of the papillary muscles. Some evidence suggests that SAX EDAs measured at this level correlate reasonably well with measurements obtained by on-heart echocardiography and with EDVs measured simultaneously using radionuclides. There are two main echocardiographic signs of decreased preload:

1. Decrease in EDA (<5.5 cm^2/m^2) invariably reflects hypovolemia.
2. Obliteration of the end-systolic area (the "kissing ventricle sign") that accompanies the decrease in EDA in severe hypovolemia.

Left Ventricular Systolic Function

The echocardiographic assessment of global and regional LV function consists of 2D, 3D, or Doppler evaluation of cardiac structures. Using echocardiography, contractility has most frequently been estimated utilizing end-diastolic and end-systolic dimensions.

With 2D echocardiography, multiple tomographic cuts can be obtained and used to calculate ventricular volumes using a variety of formulas such as the modified Simpson formula. Using the ventricular volumes, ejection fraction (EF) can be calculated using the standard formula:

$$EF = (LVEDV - LVESV)/LVEDV \qquad \textbf{[Eq. 11.2]}$$

where LVEDV is LV end-diastolic volume, and LVESV is LV end-systolic volume.

During intraoperative TEE, it is most convenient to monitor a single, SAX view at the level of the midpapillary muscles. Once the end-diastolic and end-systolic endocardial areas have been delineated with the help of tracing software, contractility may be estimated using the fractional area of contraction (FAC) or the ejection fraction area (EFA):

$$FAC = (LVEDA - LVESA)/LVEDA \qquad \textbf{[Eq. 11.3]}$$

where LVEDA is LV end-diastolic area, and LVESA is LV end-systolic area.

▨ MYOCARDIAL ISCHEMIA MONITORING

Regional Wall Motion

Echocardiography has been used for decades in assessing regional wall motion abnormalities (RWMAs) associated with myocardial ischemia. The ability to reliably detect RWMAs is clinically relevant because of its diagnostic and therapeutic implications. Consequently, it is important to note that RWMAs detected by TEE must always be interpreted within the clinical context, because not every RWMA is diagnostic for myocardial ischemia. Myocarditis, ventricular pacing, and bundle-branch blocks can easily lead to wall motion abnormalities that can potentially lead to mismanagement of the patient.

By understanding coronary anatomy, the echocardiographer can make assumptions regarding localization of a potential coronary artery lesion based on the region of abnormal wall motion.

Wall Motion

The simplest assessment of wall motion is performed by eyeballing the motion of the individual segments of the left ventricle. This qualitative assessment is classified as being normal, hypokinetic, akinetic, dyskinetic, or aneurismal. In addition to movement, the normal myocardium thickens during systole. Wall thickening can be assessed qualitatively.

$$PSWT = SWT - DWT/SWT \times 100 \qquad \textbf{[Eq. 11.4]}$$

where PSWT is the percentage of systolic wall thickening, SWT represents end-systolic wall thickening, and DWT is end-diastolic wall thickening.

The degree of thickening can also be used to assess overall function of the observed segment. A thickening greater than 30% is normal, 10% to 30% represents mild hypokinesia, 0% to 10% is severe hypokinesia, no thickening is akinesia; if the segment bulges during systole, then dyskinesia is present.

Diagnosis of Ischemia

The precise sequence of functional changes that occur in the myocardium after interruption of flow has been studied in models of acute ischemia, including percutaneous transluminal coronary angioplasty (PTCA). Abnormalities in diastolic function usually precede abnormal changes in systolic function. Normal function is critical for LV filling and is dependent on ventricular relaxation, compliance, and atrial

11

contraction. Diastolic ventricular function can be assessed by monitoring the rate of filling associated with changes in the chamber dimensions (see earlier discussion). Regional systolic function can be estimated by echocardiographic determination of wall thickening and wall motion during systole in both LAX and SAX views of the ventricle. The SAX view of the left ventricle at the papillary muscle level displays myocardium perfused by the three main coronary arteries and is therefore very useful. However, because the SAX view does not image the ventricular apex, which is a very common location of ischemia, the LAX and longitudinal ventricle views are also clinically important.

Although wall thickening is probably a more specific marker of ischemia than wall motion, its measurement requires visualization of the epicardium, which is not always possible. Alternatively, by observing the movement of the endocardium toward the center of the cavity during systole, systolic wall motion can almost always be assessed. As the myocardial oxygen supply-demand balance worsens, graded systolic wall motion abnormalities progress from mild hypokinesia to severe hypokinesia, akinesia, and finally dyskinesia. Normal contraction is defined as greater than 30% shortening of the radius from the center to the endocardial border. Mild hypokinesia refers to inward contraction that is slower and less vigorous than normal during systole, with radial shortening of 10% to 30%. Severe hypokinesia is defined as less than 10% radial shortening. The precise distinction between varying degrees of hypokinesia can be difficult. Akinesia refers to the absence of wall motion or no inward movement of the endocardium during systole. Dyskinesia refers to paradoxic wall motion or movement outward during ventricular systole.

Limitations

Although TEE appears to have many advantages over traditional intraoperative monitors of myocardial ischemia, potential limitations remain as well. The most obvious limitation of TEE monitoring is the fact that ischemia cannot be detected during critical periods, such as induction, laryngoscopy, intubation, emergence, and extubation. In addition, the adequacy of RWMA analysis may be influenced by artifact.

The septum, in particular, must be given special consideration with respect to wall motion and wall thickness assessment. The septum comprises two parts: the lower muscular portion and the basal membranous portion. The basal septum does not exhibit the same degree of contraction as the lower muscular part. At the most superior basal portion, the septum is attached to the aortic outflow track. Its movement at this level is normally paradoxic during ventricular systole. The septum is also a unique region of the left ventricle because it is a region of the right ventricle as well and is therefore influenced by forces from both ventricles. In addition, sternotomy, pericardiotomy, and CPB have been found to alter the translational and rotational motion of the heart within the chest, which may cause changes in ventricular septal motion.

Another potential problem of RWMA assessment is the evaluation of the discoordinated contraction that occurs as a result of a bundle-branch block or ventricular pacing. In these situations, the system used to assess RWMAs must compensate for global motion of the heart (usually accomplished with a floating frame of reference) and evaluate not only regional endocardial wall motion but also myocardial thickening.

Not all RWMAs are indicative of myocardial ischemia or infarction. Clearly, under normal conditions, all hearts do not contract in a homogeneous and consistent manner. It is reasonable to assume, however, that most of the time an acute change in the regional contraction pattern of the heart during surgery is likely attributable to myocardial ischemia. An important exception to this rule may apply in models of acute coronary artery occlusion. In these models, it has been established that myocardial function becomes abnormal in the center of an ischemic zone, but it is also true that the myocardial regions adjacent to the ischemic zones become dysfunctional as well. Several studies have reported that the total area of dysfunctional myocardium commonly exceeds the area of ischemic or infarcted myocardium. The impairment of function in nonischemic tissue has been thought to be caused by a *tethering effect*. Tethering, or the attachment of noncontracting tissue that is normally perfused, probably accounts for the consistent overestimation of infarction size by echocardiography when compared with postmortem studies.

Another limitation of RWMA analysis during surgery is that it does not differentiate stunned or hibernating myocardium from acute ischemia, nor does it differentiate the cause of ischemia between increased oxygen demand and decreased oxygen supply. Finally, it should be noted that areas of previous ischemia or scarring may become unmasked by changes in afterload and appear as new RWMAs. This is particularly important in vascular surgery, during which major abrupt changes in afterload occur.

Outcome Significance

Data regarding the significance of intraoperative detection of RWMAs suggest that transient abnormalities unaccompanied by hemodynamic or electrocardiogram (ECG) evidence of ischemia may not represent significant myocardial ischemia and are usually not associated with postoperative morbidity. Hypokinetic myocardial segments appear to be associated with minimal perfusion defects compared with the significant perfusion defects that accompany akinetic or dyskinetic segments. Therefore hypokinesia may be a less predictive marker for postoperative morbidity.

Intraoperative TEE has helped predict the results of CABG surgery. After CABG to previously dysfunctional segments, immediate improvement of regional myocardial function (which is sustained) has been demonstrated. In addition, prebypass compensatory hypercontracting segments have been reported to revert toward normal immediately after successful CABG. Persistent RWMAs after CABG appear to be related to adverse clinical outcomes, and lack of evidence of RWMAs after CABG has been shown to be associated with a postoperative course without cardiac morbidity.

Right Ventricular Function

The right ventricle is a complex structure that pumps venous blood to the normally low pressure–low resistance pulmonary arterial circuit. When RV function and loading conditions are normal, the right ventricle is typically triangular when viewed in the ME four-chamber view, yet crescent-shaped when viewed in the TG mid-SAX view. The right ventricle consists of three portions: (1) the inflow portion near the TV, chordae tendineae, and papillary muscles; (2) the trabeculated apical myocardium; and (3) the RVOT near the ventricular septum and PV. These three portions of the right ventricle create a *wrap-around* appearance, which is apparent in an ME RV inflow-outflow view. Unlike the left ventricle, which has a piston-like contraction, the right ventricle contracts in a peristaltic-like manner with contraction of the inflow, followed in sequence by the apical and outflow portion. RV dysfunction is often in response to increased pulmonary vascular afterload and pulmonary hypertension, which leads to increased RV wall tension and an imbalance of RV oxygen supply and demand. When increased afterload and/or RV ischemia occur, these result in decreased systolic function with a rise in RV diastolic pressures and chamber dilatation.

As previously described, the right ventricle is particularly sensitive to increases in afterload. The presentation of this response to chronic increases in afterload may be volume- or pressure-related changes such as RV dilation, hypertrophy, septal wall

11

abnormalities, and RV failure. RV dilation is readily identified by echocardiography and may be assessed qualitatively or quantitatively. Qualitatively, the RV size is compared with the LV size in the ME four-chamber view in which its CSA normally occupies two-thirds of the *normal* LV CSA. Mild enlargement is an increase greater than two-thirds; moderate enlargement is present when the chambers are equal in size, whereas severe enlargement is present when the RV area is larger than the LV area.

RV pressure or volume overload may cause distortion or flattening of the inter-ventricular septum, most easily identified in the TG mid-SAX view. The overload of the right ventricle, as well as the underfilled left ventricle from reduced RV cardiac output (CO), leads to a leftward deviation of the septum and a *D-shaped* LV chamber appearance.

Although the right ventricle contracts in a peristaltic-like manner from the base through the apex to the outflow portion, the largest contributor to its systolic function is the longitudinal basal contraction. Therefore one of the easily deployed and widely used measurement tools is tricuspid annular plane systolic excursion, which is a measurement of the longitudinal contraction of the lateral tricuspid annulus toward the apex during systole. Because the septal segment of the tricuspid annulus is fixed, the longitudinal contraction of the right ventricle causes a hinge-like movement of the lateral annulus. This movement can be measured in the ME four-chamber view as the change in distance from annulus to apex in diastole and systole. Current guidelines suggest that a value less than 17 mm is suggestive of RV systolic dysfunction.

▦ HEMODYNAMIC ASSESSMENT

Intravascular Pressures

Echocardiographic techniques may be used to estimate intracardiac and intravascular gradients. Newton's conservation of energy states that the energy within a closed system must remain the same. If blood passes through an area of stenosis, then the potential energy (as represented by high pressure) must be converted into kinetic energy as observed as high blood-flow velocities. Utilizing the measurement of a blood velocity, a clinically relevant estimation of pressure gradient may be obtained.

The simplified Bernoulli equation is:

$$p_1 - p_2 = 4v_2{}^2 \qquad \text{[Eq. 11.5]}$$

where, p_1 is the pressure proximal to the obstruction; p_2 is the pressure proximal to the obstruction; $p_1 - p_2$ is the pressure difference over the obstruction; v_2 is the velocity proximal to the obstruction.

With this formula, the pressure gradient across a fixed orifice can be approximated. It may be applied to the measurement of intravascular pressures, as well as the gradient across a stenotic orifice.

Determination of Intravascular Pressures

The velocity of blood traveling through a regurgitant valve is a direct application of pressure gradient calculations and can be used to calculate intracardiac pressure. For example, TR velocity reflects systolic pressure differences between the right ventricle and the RA. RV systolic pressure can be obtained by adding estimated or measured RA pressure (RAP) to the systolic pressure gradient across TV during systole. This systolic gradient may be estimated as 4(TR velocity)^2. In the absence of RVOT obstruction, PA systolic pressure will be the same as RV end-systolic pressure (RVESP). For example,

$$\text{If TR velocity} = 3.8 \ \frac{m}{\text{secand}} \ \text{RAP} = 10 \ \text{mm Hg,} \quad \text{then,}$$

$$\text{RVESP} = (\text{TRvelocity})^2 \times 4 + \text{RAP}$$

$$4(3.8)^2 = 58 \ \text{mm Hg} + 10 \ \text{mm Hg}$$

$$\text{RVESP} = \text{PA systolic} = 68 \ \text{mm Hg}$$

CARDIAC OUTPUT

Doppler Measurements

In addition to measuring gradients, the measurements of blood-flow velocity may be used to estimate flow with a given structure. A CWD velocity profile is a display of velocity versus time. If this velocity profile is integrated between two time points, that is, calculates the area under the curve, then the distance traversed of a "region of blood" during this period may be estimated. This integration of flow velocities in a given period is called the *velocity-time integral* (VTI) and has the units centimeters.

VTI may then be used to calculate flow. The CSA for a circular orifice, such as the LVOT is:

$$\text{CSA} = \pi(D/2)^2 \qquad \text{[Eq. 11.6]}$$

where D represents the diameter obtained by 2D imaging. Flow across a given orifice or stroke volume (SV) is equal to the product of the CSA of the orifice and distance traversed during a single cardiac cycle, as calculated by the VTI. SV and CO may thus be calculated as:

$$\text{SV} = \text{CSA} \times \text{VTI} \qquad \text{[Eq. 11.7]}$$

$$\text{CO} = \text{SV} \times \text{HR} \qquad \text{[Eq. 11.8]}$$

where HR is heart rate.

CONTRAST APPLICATIONS

Hand-agitated saline solutions are useful to enhance right-sided structures. These saline solutions can be easily prepared by hand agitation of saline between two 10-mL Luer lock syringes connected by a three-way stopcock; small amounts of blood may be added to improve right-sided opacification. This technique is most commonly used to opacify the RA and right ventricle, assisting in the diagnosis of intraatrial and ventricular shunts and to enhance pulmonary arterial Doppler signals. The most common indication is the detection of a PFO. After obtaining a bicaval view, a Valsalva maneuver is induced, and hand-agitated saline is injected into a large vein. After the RA is opacified, the Valsalva is released, and the left atrium is examined for contrast.

The commercially available contrast agents allow for left ventricular opacification (LVO) as well. The LVO allows enhancement of LV endocardial borders in patients whose normal studies are challenging. Such challenging studies include patients who are obese, with pulmonary disease, are critically ill, or are on a ventilator. Underestimation

11

of LV volume measurements, which is common with standard echocardiography, may be virtually eliminated with the use of LVO. Finally, LVO provides greater visualization of structural abnormalities such as apical hypertrophy, noncompaction, ventricular thrombus, endomyocardial fibrosis, LV apical ballooning (Takotsubo cardiomyopathy), LV aneurysms or pseudoaneurysms, and myocardial rupture.

Echocardiographic contrast may be used to diagnosis aortic dissections. Artifacts may be distinguished from true aortic dissection and artifact by the homogeneous distribution of contrast within the aortic lumen. The intimal flap may be visualized, the entry and exit points may be identified, and the extension into major aortic branches may be more easily defined. The use of contrast further increases the successful differentiation between the true and false lumen.

VALVULAR EVALUATION

Aortic Valve Evaluation

Two-dimensional TEE provides information on valve area, leaflet structure, and mobility. The valve has three fibrous cusps, right, left, and noncoronary, that are attached to the root of the aorta. The spaces between the attachments of the cusps are called the *commissures*, and the circumferential connection of these commissures is the *sinotubular junction*. The aortic wall bulge behind each cusp is known as the *sinus of Valsalva*. The sinotubular junction, the sinuses of Valsalva, the valve cusps, the junction of the AV with the ventricular septum, and the anterior MV leaflet comprise the AV complex. The aortic ring is at the level of the ventricular septum and is the lowest and narrowest point of this complex. The three leaflets of the AV are easily visualized, and vegetations or calcifications can be identified on basal transverse imaging or longitudinal imaging.

Aortic Stenosis

AS may be caused by congenital unicuspid, bicuspid, tricuspid, or quadricuspid valves; rheumatic fever; or degenerative calcification of the valve in older adults. Valvular AS is characterized by thickened, echogenic, calcified, immobile leaflets and is usually associated with concentric LV hypertrophy and a dilated aortic root. The valve leaflets may be domed during systole; this finding is sufficient for a diagnosis of AS.

Aortic valve area (AVA) may be measured by planimetry (Fig. 11.3). A cross-sectional view of the AV orifice may be obtained by using the ME AV SAX view, which

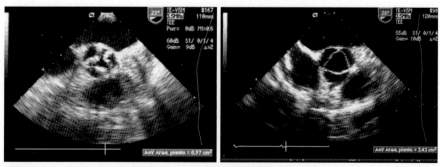

Fig. 11.3 Aortic valve stenosis by planimetry. The panel on the *left* illustrates a stenotic aortic valve, whereas the panel on the *right* illustrates a normal aortic valve. Because calcification is not significant, planimetry may be used to estimate aortic valve area.

corresponds well to measurements of the AVA obtained by transthoracic echocardiography (TTE) and cardiac catheterization, assuming the degree of calcification is not severe. With severe calcification, echocardiographic shadowing is significant, which limits the accuracy of this measurement.

Alternatively, AS may be quantified using CWD echocardiography. The evaluation of severity, however, is contingent on the alignment of the ultrasonic beam with the direction of blood flow through the LVOT. This alignment may be obtained using either a deep TG or TG LAX view. Because severe stenosis limits AV opening, the imaging of the actual AV orifice may be challenging. Superimposition of a CFD spectrum over the calcific AV may guide accurate CWD cursor placement. Normal Doppler signals across the AV have a velocity of less than 1.5 m/s and have peak signals during early systole. With worsening AS, the flow velocity increases and the peak signal is later in systole. Severe AS is characterized by a peak velocity of greater than 4 m/s, which will usually correspond to a mean gradient greater than 40 mm Hg.

Alternatively, AVA may be calculated using the continuity equation by comparing blood flow through the LVOT with blood through the AV. As previously discussed in greater detail, SV may be estimated by multiplying the CSA of a particular orifice by the VTI over one cardiac cycle through that orifice. The continuity equation describes the conservation of a physical quantity; that is, energy and mass. Blood flow in one portion of the heart must be equal to the blood flow in another portion of the heart. This application of the continuity equation is commonly used to calculate the AVA. In this case, it is assumed that the blood flow as measured at the level of the LVOT must be equal to the blood flow through the AV. Using either a deep TG or TG LAX view, the Doppler spectrum of the AV and LVOT is displayed. The diameter of the LVOT is measured in an ME LAX view. Remembering,

$$SV = CSA * VTI \qquad \text{[Eq. 11.9]}$$

where SV is stroke volume, CSA is cross-sectional area, and VTI represents velocity time integral, the continuity equation states that:

$$SV_{LVOT} = SV_{AV} \qquad \text{[Eq. 11.10]}$$

where LVOT represents left ventricular outflow tract, and AV is aortic valve.

Substituting the SV equation into the continuity equation,

$$CSA_{LVOT} * VTI_{LVOT} = CSA_{AV} * VTI_{AV} \qquad \text{[Eq. 11.11]}$$

Rearranging the terms,

$$CSA_{AV} = CSA_{LVOT} * VTI_{LVOT}/VTI_{AV} \qquad \text{[Eq. 11.12]}$$

Because the LVOT is essentially cylindrical, the CSA_{LVOT} may be estimated by

$$CSA_{LVOT} = \pi(radius_{LVOT})^2 \qquad \text{[Eq. 11.13]}$$

Because CSA_{LVOT}, VTI_{LVOT}, and VTI_{AV} are known, the CSA_{AV} or AVA may be calculated.

AS severity should be described by maximum velocity, mean gradient, and AVA. Aortic velocity allows classification of stenosis as mild (2.6 to 2.9 m/s), moderate (3 to 4 m/s), or severe (greater than 4 m/s). Normal AVA is 3 to 4 cm². AVA consistent with mild AS is greater than 1.5 cm². An AVA of 1.0 to 1.5 cm² is consistent with

11

moderate AS, and an area less than 1 cm² or 0.6 cm²/m² is consistent with severe disease.

Aortic Regurgitation

AR may result from either diseases of the aortic leaflets or the aortic root. Valvular lesions that may result in AR include leaflet vegetations and calcifications, perforation, or prolapse. AR may be caused by annular dilation secondary to a variety of causes, including annuloaortic ectasia, Marfan syndrome, aortic dissection, collagen vascular disease, and syphilis. Leaflet movement (excessive, restricted, or normal), origin of jet (central or peripheral), and direction of regurgitant jet (eccentric or central) should be determined to provide insight into the underlying pathologic conditions.

The mechanism of AR may be classified according to leaflet movement. Type I dysfunction is a result of dilation of the aortic annulus, sinuses of Valsalva, or sinotubular junction without any other causes of regurgitation. This dilation results in the tethering of the AV cusps as a result of a mismatch between AV annular and the sinotubular junction diameters. Type II lesions result in eccentric jets. The cusp tissue quality and quantity is good. Cusp prolapse or flail is classified as type IIa dysfunction. Type IIb dysfunction is a free-edge fenestration. In these cases, there is an eccentric AR jet without definite evidence of a cusp prolapse. Finally, type III dysfunction is a result of a poor quality or quantity of leaflet tissue. This may be a result of thickened, rigid, or destroyed valves attributable to endocarditis or calcification.

CFD has traditionally been the major method of assessing the severity of valvular regurgitation. Aortic regurgitant flow through the LVOT is characteristically a high-velocity, turbulent jet extending through the LVOT and left ventricle during diastole. In addition to providing the regurgitant jet area, the origin and width of the jet and the spatial orientation should be carefully defined. The severity of AR may be assessed by examining the width of the jet by CFD measurements.

The vena contracta is the narrowest portion of a regurgitant jet that usually occurs at or immediately upstream from the valve. This jet width is directly proportional to the severity of the AR, and is usually characterized by high-velocity and laminar flow, and is slightly smaller than the regurgitant orifice. A vena contracta diameter less than 0.3 cm is consistent with mild AR, and a diameter greater than 0.6 cm is consistent with severe AR (Fig. 11.4). An eccentric jet may be confined to a wall of the LVOT and thus appear very narrow, underestimating the severity of regurgitation. Similarly, central jets may expand fully in the LVOT and may overestimate the severity of regurgitation. The accuracy of the measurement may be improved by normalizing

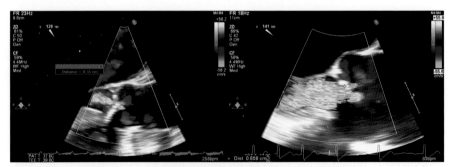

Fig. 11.4 Color-flow Doppler spectrum of a regurgitant aortic valve. Midesophageal aortic valve long-axis view visualizes an aortic regurgitant jet in the left ventricular outflow tract. *(Left)* The vena contracta is approximately 3 mm, which is consistent with mild regurgitation. *(Right)* The vena contracta is greater than 8 mm, which is consistent with severe aortic regurgitation.

the jet width to the LVOT diameter by an examination of the ratio of the proximal jet width within the LVOT to the LVOT width (w_J/w_{LVOT}). A w_J/w_{LVOT} value of 0.25 discriminates mild from moderate regurgitation, and a valve of 0.65 discriminates moderate from severe regurgitation.

Mitral Valve Evaluation

The MV consists of two leaflets, chordae tendineae, two papillary muscles, and a valve annulus. The anterior leaflet is larger than the posterior and is semicircular; however, the posterior MV leaflet has a longer circumferential attachment to the MV annulus. The posterior valve leaflet may be divided into three scallops: lateral (P1), middle (P2), and medial (P3). The leaflets are connected to each other at junctures of continuous leaflet tissue called the *anterolateral* and *posteromedial commissures*. Primary, secondary, and tertiary chordal structures arise from the papillary muscle, subdividing as they extend and attach to the free edge and several millimeters from the margin on the ventricular surface of both the anterior and posterior valve leaflets. The annulus of the MV primarily supports the posterior MV leaflet, whereas the anterior MV leaflet is continuous with the membranous ventricular septum, AV, and aorta.

Mitral Stenosis

The most common cause of mitral stenosis (MS) is rheumatic heart disease; other causes are congenital valvular stenosis, vegetations and calcifications of the leaflets, parachute MV, and annular calcification. In addition to structural valvular abnormalities, MS may be caused by nonvalvular causative factors such as intraatrial masses (myxomas or thrombus) or extrinsic constrictive lesions. Generally, MS is characterized by restricted leaflet movement, a reduced orifice, and diastolic doming. The diastolic doming occurs when the MV is unable to accommodate all the blood flowing from the left atrium into the left ventricle; consequently, the body of the leaflets separates more than the edges. In rheumatic disease, calcification of the valvular and subvalvular apparatus, as well as thickening, deformation, and fusion of the valvular leaflets at the anterolateral and posteromedial commissures, produces a characteristic fish mouth–shaped orifice. Other characteristics that may be associated with chronic obstruction to left atrial outflow include an enlarged left atrium, spontaneous echocardiographic contrast or smoke (which is related to low-velocity blood flow with subsequent rouleaux formation by red blood cells), thrombus formation, and RV dilation.

The leaflets, annulus, chordae, and papillary muscles may be assessed in the ME four-chamber, commissural, two-chamber, and LAX views. If annular calcification is significant, then the TG views may be necessary to assess the subvalvular apparatus. Because of the propensity for thrombus formation, the entire left atrium and the LAA should be carefully interrogated for thrombus.

A transmitral Doppler spectrum is measured along the axis of transmitral blood flow, which usually may be obtained in an ME four- or two-chamber view. Transmitral valve flow is characterized by two peaked waves of flow away from the transducer. The first wave (E) represents early diastolic filling, whereas the second wave (A) represents atrial systole. Transvalvular gradient may be estimated using the modified Bernoulli equation (pressure gradient = $4 \times$ velocity^2). Because peak gradient is heavily influenced by LA compliance and ventricular diastolic function, the mean gradient is the relevant clinical measurement.

Mitral Regurgitation

Mitral regurgitation (MR) may be classified as primary or secondary. Primary causes of regurgitation are structural or organic, whereas secondary causes are functional

11

without evidence of structural abnormalities on the MV. The most common causes of primary MR are degenerative (Barlow disease, fibroelastic degeneration, Marfan syndrome, Ehlers-Danlos syndrome, annular calcification), rheumatic disease, toxic valvulopathies, and endocarditis. MR may be caused by disorders of any component of the MV apparatus, specifically, the annulus, the leaflets and chordae, or the papillary muscles. With chronic regurgitation, the annulus and atrium dilate and the annulus loses its normal elliptical shape, becoming more circular. Annular dilation, in turn, leads to poor leaflet coaptation and worsening of valve incompetence. Although increased LA and LV dimensions may suggest severe MR, smaller dimensions do not exclude the diagnosis.

The most common cause of chronic primary MR in developed countries is MV prolapse. Younger individuals exhibit Barlow syndrome, whereas older populations have fibroelastic deficiency disease. A Barlow valve is usually characterized by gross redundancy of multiple segments of the anterior or posterior leaflets and chordal apparatus. The leaflets are bulky and billowing with multiple areas of prolapse. In contrast, fibroelastic deficiency usually affects only a single segment. The nonaffected leaflets tend to be thin, with a thickening of the affected segment. Excessively mobile structures near the leaflet tips during diastole may represent elongated chords or ruptured minor chords. A flail leaflet segment generally points in the direction of the left atrium; this directionality of leaflet pointing is the main criterion for distinguishing a flailed leaflet from severe valvular prolapse. Flail leaflets are most commonly caused by ruptured chordae and less commonly caused by papillary muscle rupture.

With secondary or functional MR, the MV is structurally normal. LV dilation, secondary to another process such as myocardial infarction or idiopathic-dilated cardiomyopathies, results in papillary muscle displacement and annular dilation with resultant tethering of the MV leaflets with incomplete leaflet coaption. Since the valvular regurgitation is only one component of the disease process, its progress is worse than primary MR, and its treatment is less clear.

Qualitative Grading Using Color-Flow Doppler

The diagnosis of MR is made primarily by the use of color-flow mapping (Fig. 11.5). Because flow is best detected when it is parallel to the ultrasonic beam and because some MR jets may be thin and eccentric, multiple views of the left atrium should be interrogated for evidence of MR. Eccentric jet direction provides corroborative evidence of structural leaflet abnormalities, which may include leaflet prolapse, chordal elongation, chordal rupture, or papillary muscle rupture.

Atrioventricular valve regurgitation is graded semiquantitatively as mild, moderate, or severe. Regurgitation less than mild may be classified as either trivial or trace. The most common method of grading the severity of MR is CFD mapping of the left

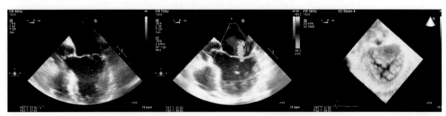

Fig. 11.5 Mitral regurgitation type I. *(Left and center)* Midesophageal five-chamber view reveals the anterior and posterior leaflets coapt at the level of the mitral valve annulus, but the space between the two leaflets is significant. *(Center)* Application of color-flow Doppler reveals a central jet. *(Right)* In addition to the poor coaption of the anterior and posterior leaflet, this three-dimensional reconstruction visualizes a large cleft in the posterior leaflet, which contributes to the regurgitation.

atrium. With the Nyquist limit set at 50 to 60 cm/s, jet areas less than 4 cm² or 20% of the left atrial size are usually classified as mild, whereas jets greater than 10 cm² or 40% of the atrial volume are classified as severe. In addition, jet direction should be considered when grading regurgitation, because eccentric jets that cling to the atrial wall (Coanda effect) have a smaller area than central (free) jets with similar regurgitant volumes and regurgitant fractions. An alternative method of grading MR is based on the vena contracta width. Although the vena contracta is commonly circular, it may be elliptical in shape with secondary causes or functional regurgitation. In these cases, multiple views of the vena contracta along different axes should be obtained and averaged. A vena contracta width of less than 0.3 cm is associated with mild MR, whereas a width greater than 0.7 cm is associated with severe MR.

Tricuspid Valve

The TV consists of three leaflets, an annular ring, chordae tendineae, and multiple papillary muscles. The anterior leaflet is usually the largest, followed by the posterior and septal leaflets. The septal leaflet of the TV is usually farther apical than the septal attachments of the MV. Chordae arise from a large single papillary muscle, double or multiple septal papillary muscles, and several small posterior papillary muscles, attached to the corresponding walls of the right ventricle.

Although TR may have primary causative factors, most causes are secondary or functional as a result of either tricuspid annular dilation (>40 mm) or RV dilation. RV enlargement results in annular dilation and papillary muscle displacement with tethering of the TV leaflets. This tethering may result in poor leaflet coaption. TR results in additional RV enlargement and further leaflet tethering with worsening TR.

The apparent severity of TR is exquisitely sensitive to right-sided heart loading conditions. Thus during the intraoperative evaluation of TR, PA, and right atrial pressures should be kept near levels observed in the awake resting state. Some authors suggest that the severity of TR can be estimated by the apparent size of the color-flow disturbance of TR relative to right atrial size. A central jet area of less than 5 cm² is consistent with mild regurgitation, whereas a jet area greater than 10 cm² is consistent with severe regurgitation. Additionally, a vena contracta width less than 0.3 mm is consistent with mild regurgitation, whereas a vena contracta greater than 0.7 cm is consistent with severe regurgitation.

INTRAOPERATIVE TRANSESOPHAGEAL ECHOCARDIOGRAPHY: INDICATIONS

The first decision by the echocardiographer is whether TEE is indicated. Application of intraoperative TEE in the care of the patient with mitral disease is widely accepted. Even in this area, however, there is a paucity of data supporting an improved outcome for intraoperative patients cared for with TEE compared with no TEE. The decision to perform TEE during cardiac surgery is substantiated by practice expectations and consensus opinion. In an attempt to develop an evidence-based approach to this expanding technology, the American Society of Anesthesiologists and the Society of Cardiovascular Anesthesiologists cosponsored a task force to develop guidelines for defining the indications for perioperative TEE. Despite the scarcity of outcome data to support the application of TEE in the perioperative period, TEE had rapidly been adopted by cardiac surgeons and cardiac anesthesiologists as a routine monitoring and diagnostic modality during cardiac surgery. In 1996, the task force published their guidelines designed to establish the scientific merit of TEE and justification of its use in defined patient cohorts. The indications were grouped into three categories based on the strength of the supporting evidence/expert opinion that TEE improves outcome (Box 11.3). Category I indications suggested strong evidence/expert opinion that TEE was useful in improving clinical outcome. Category II indications suggested there was weak evidence/expert opinion that TEE improves outcome in these settings. Category III indications suggested there was little or no scientific merit or expert support for the application of TEE in these settings. There were updated recommendations from the American Society of Anesthesiology in 2010 (Box 11.4).

> **BOX 11.3** *Indications for the Use of Transesophageal Echocardiography*
>
> **Category I**
>
> - Heart valve repair
> - Congenital heart surgery
> - Hypertrophic obstructive cardiomyopathy
> - Endocarditis
> - Acute aortic dissection
> - Acute, unstable aortic aneurysm
> - Aortic valve function in the setting of aortic dissection
> - Traumatic thoracic aortic disruption
> - Pericardial tamponade
>
> **Category II**
>
> - Myocardial ischemia and coronary artery disease
> - Increased risk of hemodynamic disturbances
> - Heart valve replacement
> - Aneurysms of the heart
> - Intracardiac masses
> - Intracardiac foreign bodies
> - Air emboli
> - Intracardiac thrombi
> - Massive pulmonary emboli
> - Traumatic cardiac injury
> - Chronic aortic dissection
> - Chronic aortic aneurysm
> - Detection of aortic atheromatous disease as a source of emboli
> - Evaluating the effectiveness of pericardiectomies
> - Heart-lung transplantation
> - Mechanical circulatory support
>
> **Category III**
>
> - Other cardiomyopathy
> - Emboli during orthopedic procedures
> - Uncomplicated pericarditis
> - Pleuropulmonary disease
> - Placement of intra-aortic balloon pump, pulmonary artery catheter
> - Monitoring the administration of cardioplegia
>
> Modified from the Practice guidelines for perioperative transesophageal echocardiography: a report by the American Society of Anesthesiologists and the Society of Cardiovascular Anesthesiologists Task Force on Transesophageal Echocardiography. *Anesthesiology.* 1996;84:986.

> ### BOX 11.4 *2010 Updated Recommendations for Transesophageal Echocardiography*
>
> **Cardiac and Thoracic Aortic Surgery**
>
> - *All* adult open-heart (eg, valves) and thoracic aortic surgical procedures
> - Consider in coronary artery bypass grafting procedures
> - Transcatheter intracardiac procedures
>
> **Critical Care**
>
> - When diagnostic information that is expected to alter management cannot be obtained by transthoracic echocardiography or other modalities
>
> Modified from Practice guidelines for perioperative transesophageal echocardiography: an updated report by the American Society of Anesthesiologists and the Society of Cardiovascular Anesthesiologists Task Force on Transesophageal Echocardiography. *Anesthesiology.* 2010;112:1084.

CASE STUDIES OF INTRAOPERATIVE TRANSESOPHAGEAL ECHOCARDIOGRAPHY

Case Study 1	CARDIAC FUNCTION AND REGIONAL WALL MOTION ABNORMALITIES

FRAMING

Ventricular function is a predictor of outcome after heart surgery and a predictor of long-term outcome in patients with cardiovascular disease. Patients with compensated congestive heart failure may have severely decreased EF with minimal symptoms. Regional ventricular dysfunction is most commonly caused by myocardial ischemia or infarction. Hence, there is an imperative to detect ventricular dysfunction and institute treatment in an attempt to prevent acute or long-term consequences.

Is ventricular function normal or abnormal? Is the abnormal function global or regional? What is the coronary distribution that relates to an RWMA? Is the ventricle big or small? Is the myocardium thinned or hypertrophied? Is the abnormal function new or old? Does the medical or surgical intervention improve or deteriorate ventricular function?

DATA COLLECTION

LV systolic function is assessed echocardiographically based on regional and global wall motion. Methods of assessment include changes in regional wall thickness, radial shortening with endocardial excursion, fractional area change, and systolic displacement of the mitral annulus. Off-line measurements of EF can be calculated using Simpson's rule. Fractional area change is the most common metric used to assess global LV function. Other measures include EDA, end-systolic area (ESA), and meridional wall stress.

Regional assessment provides an index of myocardial well-being that can be linked to coronary anatomy and blood flow. Although the measurement of coronary blood flow is not achieved by TEE, the perfusion beds and corresponding myocardium for the LAD, left circumflex (LCX), and right coronary (RCA) arteries are relatively distinct and can be scrutinized by TEE using multiplane imaging. The

Continued

11

TG and LAX imaging views of the LV are the most widely used for evaluating wall motion abnormalities. Digital archival systems have gained popularity for their ability to capture a single cardiac cycle that can then be examined more closely as a continuous cine loop. Cine loops can also permit side-by-side display of images obtained under varying conditions (eg, prebypass and postbypass). Regional myocardial ischemia produces focal changes in the corresponding ventricular walls before changes occur on the ECG. Changes progress from normal wall motion to hypokinesis or akinesis. Dyskinesis, thinning, and calcification of the myocardium suggest a nonacute process, likely a prior infarction.

DISCUSSION

Preexisting ventricular dysfunction suggests increased risk for surgery and poorer long-term outcome. The presence of such ventricular dysfunction may deteriorate intraoperatively, requiring the need for marked pharmacologic or mechanical support. A patient with a preoperative EF of 10% scheduled for CABG and MV repair is at increased risk of intraoperative ischemia, acute heart failure, and difficulty maintaining hemodynamic stability during the immediate postbypass period. Anticipating such problems, placement of an intra-aortic balloon pump or femoral arterial catheter is considered during the prebypass period (Fig. 11.6). The same patient is likely to benefit from the administration of inotropic agents.

A marked decrement or unexpected decrease in global cardiac function after release of the aortic cross-clamp can be caused by poor myocardial preservation during cross-clamping or distension of the heart during bypass. The risk of such incidents can be reduced by the monitoring of the electrical activity of the heart and PA pressures and for distension of the RV and LV. Effective venting of the heart is often difficult to discern by visual inspection alone, especially with the use of minimally invasive surgery through small incisions. TEE imaging can diagnose ventricular distension produced by AV insufficiency.

Not all preexisting RWMAs benefit from coronary revascularization. Regions of akinesia and dyskinesia are usually the result of a myocardial infarction and may reflect nonviable myocardium, although "hibernating" myocardium is possible. Hypokinetic segments are generally viable and may represent active ischemia. Preoperative positron emission tomography (PET) scanning can detect hibernating myocardium and may be cost-effective to guide CABG. The detection of hibernating myocardium in an area of chronic ischemia and regional hypokinesis will direct the surgeon to revascularize the corresponding stenosed coronary artery. In contrast, an occluded coronary artery with downstream infarction may not benefit from revascularization, as contractile function may be irreversibly lost. However, in this latter scenario, revascularization postinfarction may provide some benefit in decreasing the risk of ventricular aneurysm formation.

If the intraoperative examination reveals new ventricular dysfunction, the intraoperative team must determine the etiology and severity and plan a treatment. Other causes of RWMAs such as conduction abnormalities (left bundle-branch block or ventricular pacing) can be difficult to distinguish. Treatment of myocardial ischemia may include optimizing hemodynamics; administering anticoagulants, nitrates, calcium channel blockers, or β-blockers; inserting an intra-aortic balloon pump; or instituting CPB and coronary revascularization. The presence of a new-onset RWMA after separation from bypass is worrisome for myocardial ischemia. Even the patient without coronary artery disease remains at risk because of hypotension, shower of air or debris into the coronary circulation, or coronary spasm. The patient with coronary artery disease undergoing coronary revascularization may have all the above risks, technical difficulties at the anastomotic site, injury to the native coronary artery (eg, stitch caught the back wall), or occlusion of the coronary graft by thrombosis or aortic dissection. The coronary arteries, grafts, and anastomoses should be carefully inspected for patency and flow. Graft patency in the operating room is difficult to determine. Techniques include manual stripping and refill, measuring coronary flow by hand-held Doppler, or administration of echocardiographic contrast agents. A new RWMA in the distribution of a new coronary graft can prompt the decision-making strategies listed in Table 11.2.

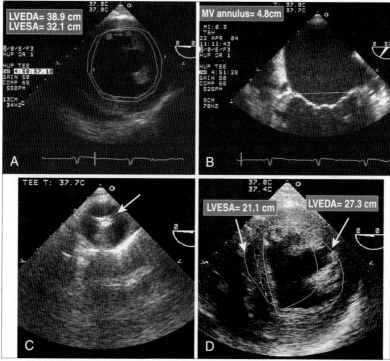

Fig. 11.6 The prebypass transesophageal echocardiography (TEE) examination may have predictive value for postbypass circulatory management. A 63-year-old woman with a past medical history of hypertension, congestive heart failure, pulmonary edema, dilated cardiomyopathy, diabetes, and obesity was scheduled for coronary artery bypass grafting (CABG) and mitral valve (MV) repair. The preoperative evaluation documented moderate to severe mitral regurgitation (MR) with reversal of systolic pulmonary vein blood-flow velocity. (A) The prebypass TEE midesophageal four-chamber view showed a markedly dilated left ventricle (LV) and mildly dilated right ventricle (RV) with mildly decreased global dysfunction. The transgastric view was characterized by severe global dysfunction and an LV end-diastolic diameter of 6.6 cm. The fractional area change (FAC) was 17% [FAC = (LV end-diastolic area − LV end-systolic area)/LV end-diastolic area × 100]. Revascularization alone was unlikely to significantly improve MV function. (B) The midesophageal bicommissural view of the MV demonstrated marked dilation of the MV annulus (major axis = 4.8 cm) and tethering of the leaflets below the valve plane that was caused by LV chamber dilation. A femoral arterial catheter was inserted for monitoring of central aortic pressure and/or possibly placing an intra-aortic balloon pump. The patient underwent a CABG × 3 and MV annuloplasty for moderate MR. The separation from bypass was difficult, requiring milrinone, epinephrine, vasopressin, and placement of an intra-aortic balloon pump. (C) TEE, which was used to initially confirm the location of the femoral guidewire, was later used to position the balloon pump just downstream to the left subclavian artery. (D) Worsening of RV function that was characterized by increased central venous pressure, new-onset tricuspid regurgitation, and a hypokinetic RV can be appreciated by ventricular septal flattening and dilation of the RV. The LV ejection fraction did not decrease as might be expected; after correcting MR, the FAC improved slightly from 17% to 22% postbypass. Cardiac function continued to improve, and the counterpulsation device was removed without complication on the first day after surgery. The infusions of milrinone and epinephrine were continued for several days.

11

Table 11.2 Management Strategies for New-Onset Myocardial Ischemia After Bypass

Diagnosis	Plausible Treatment
Coronary graft occlusion	Revise coronary graft
Coronary air emboli	Increase coronary perfusion pressure, administer coronary dilators
Coronary calcium/atheroma emboli	Support circulation
Dissection of the aortic root	Repair dissection
Coronary spasm	Administer coronary dilators

Case Study 2   MANAGEMENT OF ISCHEMIC MITRAL REGURGITATION

FRAMING

Ischemic heart disease is the most common cause of mitral insufficiency in the United States. Mechanisms of valve incompetence are varied and include annular dilatation, papillary muscle dysfunction from active ischemia or infarction, papillary muscle rupture, or ventricular remodeling from scar, often leading to a tethering effect of the subvalvular apparatus. Mitral regurgitation leads to pulmonary hypertension, pulmonary vascular congestion, and pulmonary edema with functional disability. Ventricular function deteriorates as the left ventricle becomes volume-overloaded with corresponding chamber dilatation. Left untreated, severe MR from ischemic heart disease has a poor prognosis, hence the imperative for diagnosis and treatment. Patients presenting for surgical coronary revascularization often have concomitant MR of a mild or moderate degree. The intraoperative team is confronted with the decision of whether to surgically address the MV during the coronary operation.

Does MR warrant mitral surgery? What is the mechanism of the regurgitation? What is the grade of the MR? Is the MR likely to improve by coronary revascularization alone?

DATA COLLECTION

Pertinent data, including preoperative functional status and evaluation, need to be considered to appropriately interpret and place the intraoperative data in context. The preoperative echocardiogram and ventriculogram need to be reviewed. The intraoperative hemodynamic data are coupled with TEE information to complete the data set needed to move forward with the decision-making process. The severity of MR on TEE is measured by the vena contracta, maximum area of the regurgitant jet, regurgitant orifice area, and pulmonary vein blood-flow velocities. Wall motion assessment and the ECG are used for detecting reversible myocardial dysfunction that may benefit from revascularization. The hemodynamic and TEE data are coupled with provocative testing of the MV in an attempt to emulate the working conditions of the MV in an awake, unanesthetized state. It is not uncommon that preoperative mild to moderate MR with a structurally normal valve totally resolves under the unloading conditions of general anesthesia.

DISCUSSION

Most cases of ischemic MR are categorized as "functional" rather than structural. In a study of 482 patients with ischemic MR, 76% had functional ischemic MR, compared with 24% having significant papillary muscle dysfunction. The mechanism of ischemic MR is attributed to annular dilatation, secondary to LV enlargement and regional LV remodeling with papillary muscle displacement, causing apical tethering and restricted systolic leaflet motion. The importance of local LV remodeling with papillary muscle displacement as a mechanism for ischemic MR has been reproduced in an animal model.

The MR is prioritized in accordance with principal diagnosis (eg, coronary artery disease), comorbidities, functional disability, and short- and long-term outcome. Ischemic MR is quantitated and the mechanism of valve dysfunction is defined. Intraoperative MR is compared with preoperative findings. Discrepancies between the preoperative and intraoperative assessment of the valve may reflect the pressure and volume unloading effects of general anesthesia. In patients with functional ischemic MR who have 1 to 2+ MR, the MV is often not repaired or replaced. However, the need for surgical intervention in patients with 2+ MR under anesthesia remains a point of debate and has not been definitively answered by prospective studies. MV surgery is typically recommended to improve functional status and long-term outcome for patients with 3+ ischemic MR or greater. Ignoring significant ischemic MR at the time of CABG can limit the functional benefit derived from surgery.

The risks to the patient of not surgically altering the MV and anticipated residual regurgitation is weighed against the risk of atriotomy, mitral surgery, extending cardiopulmonary and aortic cross-clamp times, and the likelihood that the coronary surgery will be successful at decreasing the severity of MR. Added risk includes commitment to a mechanical prosthesis should a reparative procedure prove unsuccessful. MR due to acute ischemia may resolve after restoration of coronary blood flow (Fig. 11.7). The reversibility of the regurgitation is difficult to predict: factors supporting reversibility (and hence no immediate need to surgically address the valve) include a structurally normal MV, normal left atrium and LV dimension, including the mitral annulus, and RWMAs associated with transient regurgitation and pulmonary edema. Revascularization of the culprit myocardium with improvement in regional function may be all that is necessary to restore normal mitral coaptation. Myocardial infarction with a fixed wall motion defect or aneurysm, chronically dilated left-sided heart, dilated annulus, or other structural abnormalities that are not reversible (ruptured papillary muscle or chordae, leaflet prolapse, leaflet perforation) suggest myocardial revascularization is unlikely to correct the valvular incompetence.

The decision to proceed or not to proceed with mitral surgery in the setting of ischemic heart disease is institution- and surgeon-dependent. Centers may elect to surgically address any degree of MR detected during the preoperative or intraoperative workup of a patient scheduled for coronary surgery. Less aggressive sites elect to proceed with coronary revascularization, followed by repeat scrutiny of the ventricular wall motion and MV. If revascularization has not corrected the MR, the surgeon proceeds with CPB and mitral surgery. With the advent of off-pump coronary artery bypass surgery, this process has gained another level of complexity, because decisions to proceed with mitral repair will commit the patient to CPB. Off-pump mitral surgical procedures may be possible in the near future.

11

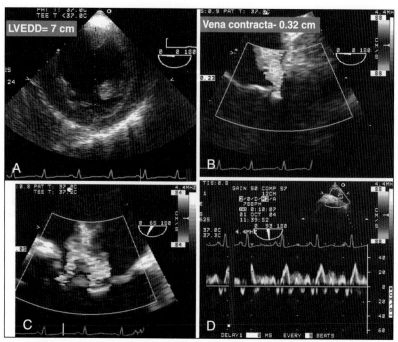

Fig. 11.7 Evaluation of mitral regurgitation (MR) in a patient undergoing coronary artery bypass grafting. A 63-year-old man was scheduled to undergo off-pump coronary artery revascularization. The patient had a history of progressive congestive heart failure without evidence of acute pulmonary edema. The physical examination was significant for diffuse laterally displaced point of maximum impulse and a systolic murmur at the apex that radiated to the axilla. The patient received an intraoperative transesophageal echocardiography (TEE) examination to evaluate the severity of MR. (A) The left ventricle (LV) was significantly dilated with an LV end-diastolic dimension of 7 cm and had depressed systolic function with an estimated ejection fraction of 40%. The MR was characterized by color-flow Doppler imaging to be a central jet of mild to moderate severity. (B) The grading of MR was based on the area of the regurgitant jet and the vena contracta viewed in a bicommissural view. The pathogenesis of MR was believed to be functional and resulted from restricted leaflet mobility caused by the dilated LV. (C) The coaptation of the anterior and posterior leaflets was below the valve plane. (D) The absence of reversal of pulmonary vein blood flow measured in the left lower pulmonary vein supported the assessment of moderate MR. Because the annulus was not significantly dilated (the minor axis measured 2.97 cm) and the MR graded as only mild to moderate, the surgeon proceeded with his initial plan of off-pump coronary artery bypass grafting. The MR decreased immediately after revascularization, and the patient's symptoms were expected to further improve with afterload reduction.

| Case Study 3 | MANAGEMENT OF PREVIOUSLY UNDIAGNOSED AORTIC VALVE DISEASE |

FRAMING

A relatively common clinical scenario for the echocardiographer is to assess the significance of previously unrecognized AV pathology. This discussion has pertinence for the echocardiographer faced with the new diagnosis of a bicuspid valve, AS, or insufficiency.

What are the symptoms that brought the patient to medical attention? What is the patient's baseline function? What is the anatomy of the AV? What is the severity of AR or of AS? How do the intraoperative findings of AV disease differ from the preoperative assessment? Would surgical repair or replacement of the AV benefit the patient's short- or long-term outcome? What is the planned procedure, and how would the risks be changed if the procedure was altered to address the new finding? Does another health care provider need to be involved in the decision of whether to surgically address the valve? Is the pathology of the AV significant enough to require surgical intervention at this time?

DATA COLLECTION AND CHARACTERIZATION OF THE AORTIC VALVE

Multiplane TEE permits an accurate assessment of AV area, valvular pathology, severity of regurgitation and stenosis, and detection of secondary cardiac changes. In the case of AS, the severity of valvular dysfunction is determined by measuring the transvalvular pressure gradient, by calculating the AV area using the continuity equation, and by planimetry of the AV systolic orifice. Planimetry of the AV orifice with TEE is more closely correlated with the catheterization-determined valve area (using the Gorlin formula) than the value derived from TTE ($r = 0.91$ vs. 0.84). The severity of AR by TEE is generally graded with CFD imaging with measurement of the width of the regurgitant jet relative to the width of the LV outflow tract. TEE is sensitive to even the most trivial amount of AR. Jet areas measured by TEE tend to be larger, and their severity is graded as greater compared with AR assessed by TTE. Determining the clinical significance of AR typically requires assessment of more than just regurgitant grade, although severe 4+ AR is never left unaddressed.

The etiology and extent of AV disease can be best delineated by TEE, as shown in Fig. 11.8. The relatively high resolution of the AV and associated structures in the near field of the ME SAX and LAX views permits an accurate assessment of the severity and mechanism of valvular disease. The aortic leaflets should be inspected in the ME LAX view for the presence of vegetations, perforation, restriction, thickening/calcification, malcoaptation, and leaflet prolapse. The presence of subvalvular disease, such as a discrete fibrous subaortic membrane, can also be reliably excluded. The ascending aorta from the valve to the right PA also should be viewed in LAX. This view is usually optimal for examining associated pathology of the aortic root and ascending aorta (eg, aortoannular ectasia, bicuspid valve, type A aortic dissection).

AS is caused by calcification of the AV and rheumatic heart disease. Bicuspid AVs are at greater risk compared with the general population. AS produces a systolic pressure gradient between the left ventricle and aorta. Secondary findings are dependent on where the patient's condition is along the natural course of the disease. Secondary findings often contribute to the decision-making process, because they infer the effects or consequences of the disease. AS is commonly associated with LV hypertrophy and abnormal filling of the left ventricle. The diastolic function is often impaired owing to a thickened, noncompliant left ventricle. Hence, MV and pulmonary vein blood-flow velocities would demonstrate a blunted passive filling phase of the ventricle. Systolic function is often normal or hyperdynamic. The LV chamber size is normal or small. However, long-standing AS results in progressive ventricular systolic dysfunction and heart failure. The left ventricle becomes dilated with compromised contractile function. As the ventricle fails, CO decreases with a resultant decrease in trans-AV pressure gradient. Hence, the pressure gradient across an AV may be misleading as a measure for severity of AS.

NATURAL COURSE OF AORTIC STENOSIS

The natural course of AS in the adult begins with a prolonged asymptomatic period associated with minimal mortality. Progression of the disease is manifested by a reduction in the valve area and an increase in the transvalvular systolic pressure gradient. The progression is quite variable, exhibiting a decrease in effective valve area ranging from 0.1 to 0.3 cm^2/year. AV calcification, as depicted by echocardiography, has been suggested to be an independent predictor of

Continued

outcome. Patients with no or mild valvular calcification, compared with those with moderate or severe calcification, had significantly increased rates of event-free survival at 1 and 4 years (92% vs. 60% and 75% vs. 20%, respectively). Decisions regarding valve replacement for mild or moderate AV disease in the setting of cardiac surgery for another cause are complicated by the variability in the natural progression of the disease. The pathogenesis of AS is an active process having many similarities to the progression of atherosclerosis. AV calcification is not a random degenerative process but an actively regulated disease associated with hypercholesterolemia, inflammation, and osteoblast activity. More aggressive medical control of these processes might be expected to have a positive impact on outcome by retarding the degenerative process.

ASSESSMENT OF MILD AND MODERATE AORTIC STENOSIS

The intraoperative management of mild to moderate AS at the time of cardiac surgery remains controversial. A patient arrives in the operating room scheduled for a CABG but is discovered to also have mild or moderate AS that was unappreciated preoperatively. The operative team must decide whether to surgically address the AV. The American College of Cardiology/American Heart Association (ACC/AHA) task force recommends valve replacement at the time of coronary surgery if the asymptomatic patient has severe AS but acknowledges there are very limited data to support intervention in the case of mild or moderate AS. It is in this exact scenario that the rate of progression of AS is of value, but it is rarely obtainable. A rapidly calcifying valve in a young patient that is becoming rapidly stenotic would sway the operative team to perform an aortic valve replacement (AVR). A combined double cardiac procedure (CABG/AVR) increases the initial perioperative risk, as well as those risks associated with long-term prosthetic valve implantation. A delay in AVR and commitment to a second heart operation in the future subjects the patient to the risk of a repeated sternotomy in the setting of patent coronary grafts and its associated morbidities. If the AV is not operated on during the initial presentation for CABG, the development of symptomatic AS may be quite delayed or may not happen.

A review of 1,344,100 patients in the national database of the Society of Thoracic Surgeons having CABG, CABG/AVR, or AVR alone culminated in a decision paradigm recommendation. The study assumed rates of AV disease progression (pressure gradient of 5 mm Hg/year), valve-related morbidity, and age-adjusted mortality rates that were obtained from published reports. The authors proposed three factors in the consideration of CABG or AVR/CABG: age (life expectancy), peak pressure gradient, and rate of progression of the AS (if known). Since the latter is difficult to discern, the analysis assumed an average rate of disease progression and recommended patients should undergo AVR/CABG when the pressure gradient exceeds 30 mm Hg. The threshold (AS pressure gradient) to perform both procedures is increased for patients older than 70 years of age because the reduced life expectancy diminishes the likelihood that they will become symptomatic from the AV disease. Whether to perform a concomitant AVR at the time of revascularization was also addressed by Rahimtoola, who advocated a less aggressive approach. One problem with both studies is that they analyzed the transvalvular pressure gradient, which may be a misleading measure of the degree of stenosis of the AV, as its value is dependent on CO. A low CO and flow rate will produce a low transvalvular pressure gradient, even in the setting of a severely stenotic AV. However, in the setting of preserved ventricular systolic function and mild or moderate AS, a pressure gradient is a useful metric. The variable rate of disease progression and the controversy regarding the indications for "prophylactic" AVR preclude a simple algorithm for dealing with this patient cohort. Increased age, lack of symptoms, minimal LV hypertrophy, with a valve area suggesting milder disease, and a pressure gradient less than 30 mm Hg would sway the decision to not replace the AV. In an asymptomatic young patient, a severely calcified valve, bicuspid valve, and LV hypertrophy in the setting of moderate stenosis, and a pressure gradient greater than 30 mm Hg would suggest that an AVR might be beneficial in the long term. It is often useful to include the patient's primary cardiologist and family in the decision-making process.

ASSESSMENT OF LOW PRESSURE GRADIENT AORTIC STENOSIS

Patients with LV dysfunction and decreased CO in the setting of AS often present with only modest transvalvular pressure gradients (<30 mm Hg). Distinguishing patients with a low CO and severe AS from patients with mild to moderate AS can be challenging (Fig. 11.9). The standard for assessing severity of AS is AV area, typically calculated using either a continuity method or by planimetry. Patients with low-gradient AS with severe LV dysfunction who received an AVR had improved survival and functional status compared with patients who did not have a valve replacement.

A low pressure gradient related to LV dysfunction may not open the AV to its maximum capacity. Dobutamine challenge in a patient with low pressure gradient AS can be useful in establishing true AV area. The ability to distinguish between true AV stenosis and a state of "pseudostenosis" relies on characteristic changes in hemodynamic and structural measurements in response to the augmented CO. The test is not typically performed in the operative setting but rather as a preoperative evaluation. The increase in calculated AV area is related to the increase in the CO and is attributed to partial reversal of primary cardiac dysfunction. If dobutamine improves CO and increases AV area, it is likely the baseline calculations overestimated the severity of the AS. The dobutamine challenge is conducted as follows: patients with low-gradient AS receive intravenous dobutamine at 5 µg/kg/min with stepwise increases in dose. Patients may exhibit a significant increase in AV area (0.8 cm² to 1.1 cm²) and a decline in valve resistance after dobutamine challenge. Patients with fixed, high-grade AS would demonstrate no change in valve area and an increase in valve resistance. The 2003 ACC/AHA/ASE (American Society of Echocardiography) Task Force gave a class IIb recommendation (usefulness/efficacy is less well established by evidence/ opinion) for the use of dobutamine echocardiography in the evaluation of patients with low-gradient AS and ventricular dysfunction. In addition to its role in distinguishing between true stenosis and pseudostenosis, low-dose dobutamine echocardiography is helpful in risk-stratifying of patients with severe true AS. Patients with augmented contractile function after dobutamine administration have an improved outcome after surgery.

11

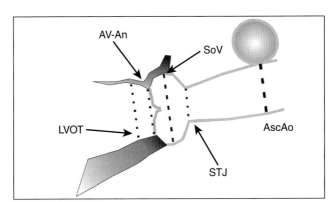

Fig. 11.8   Anatomy of the aortic root. This schematic figure of the aortic valve in long axis shows the components of the aortic root, which include sinotubular junction (*STJ*), sinus of Valsalva (*SoV*), and the annulus of the aortic valve (*AV-An*). *AscAo,* Ascending aorta; *LVOT,* left ventricular outflow tract.

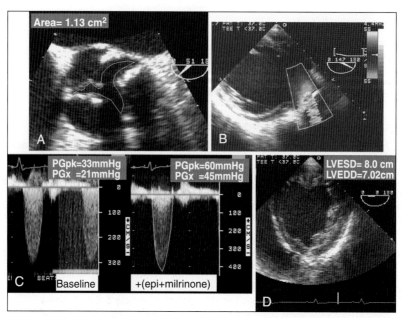

Fig. 11.9 Low pressure gradient severe aortic stenosis. A 76-year-old cachetic man was scheduled to undergo corrective surgery for severe mitral regurgitation (MR) and possibly clinically significant aortic stenosis (AS). (A) The midesophageal short-axis view of the aortic valve (AV) showed a highly calcified trileaflet valve with restricted mobility. The measurement of AV area, 1.13 cm², which was obtained by planimetry, was believed to underestimate the severity of AS because of the shadowing artifacts related to the severity of calcification. (B) The transgastric long axis view of the left ventricle (LV) was obtained, and the velocity profiles of blood flow within the LV outflow tract and the AV were measured. (C) Although the patient had a diagnosis of severe AS, the maximal *(PGpk)* and mean *(PGx)* pressure gradients were 33 mm Hg and 21 mm Hg, respectively. The area of the AV was calculated to be 0.83 cm² using the continuity equation. (D) The LV function was characterized by a severe dilated cardiomyopathy with an ejection fraction of 8%, LV end-systolic dimension *(LVESD)* of 8 cm, and LV end-diastolic dimension *(LVEDD)* of 7 cm. The diagnosis of low pressure gradient AS was considered, and infusions of epinephrine and milrinone were started. Cardiac performance improved from 2.4 L/min to 4.5 L/min, and the pressure gradients increased to 60 mm Hg, peak, and 45 mm Hg, mean (C). Although the calculated valve area that was recorded under conditions of inotrope support slightly increased to 0.9 cm², transesophageal echocardiography *(TEE)* clarified that the marked increase in the pressure gradient was consistent with a diagnosis of low-gradient AS and confirmed the presence of cardiac reserve.

Case Study 4   ACUTE AORTIC SYNDROMES

FRAMING

The unstable patient with suspected acute aortic disease or injury is often the most challenging of TEE cases. There are few more crucially important decisions that are posed to the intraoperative echocardiographer than to quickly and accurately diagnose the nature and extent of acute aortic injury. Hypotension and respiratory distress may prevent a complete and comprehensive evaluation before surgery. Patient history is often unobtainable. The echocardiographer becomes a detective. Clues are quickly gathered from the available clinical presentation, past history, and associated physical findings. The TEE is often the only modality used to establish the diagnosis and define the surgical plan.

It is midnight on a gloomy rainy night. The hospital helicopter pilot calls in "young woman, unrestrained driver, deceleration injury, steering wheel impact, chest contusion, unconscious, hypotensive. She is intubated with bilateral breath sounds. Her blood pressure is 70/40 mm Hg with an HR=125 sinus tachycardia. She is being fluid-resuscitated and being transported directly to the cardiac operating room." The patient is too unstable for magnetic resonance imaging (MRI) or computed tomography (CT). The patient arrives with a portable chest radiograph obtained as she traveled through the emergency department, showing a widened mediastinum. The vital signs have not changed except that she is receiving dopamine at 10 μg/kg/min. Pulses are palpable in the groin and the neck (Fig. 11.10). The attending surgeon turns to the echocardiographer-anesthesiologist and asks, "I need to know whether this is an anterior injury with heart contusion, injury to the ascending aorta, tamponade with blood in the pericardium, or a transected aorta, or does the patient have a nonoperable injury? The former will require a sternotomy. The transections will require a left thoracotomy. If we make the incorrect decision, the patient will surely die." The patient is stabilized in the operating room, and the TEE probe is inserted. After the diagnosis is made, the patient is positioned and prepped accordingly for the definitive surgery.

The sensitivity and specificity of TEE to detect and diagnose injury or disease of the thoracic aorta are significantly better than the sensitivity and specificity of TTE and are comparable to findings on CT and MRI. TEE provides information regarding cardiac performance and the presence of other critically important sequelae that may be important in determining the approach and timing for surgical intervention. Hence, TEE is indicated even if MRI or CT has confirmed the diagnosis.

Can consent be obtained from the patient or family members? In these emergency circumstances, it may be more prudent to proceed with the TEE examination rather than delaying diagnosis and treatment in an attempt to find family members. What is the differential diagnosis of a widened mediastinum? How does TEE discriminate the different causes of a widened mediastinum? Is the TEE performed in the awake, distressed patient, or is the TEE done under more controlled conditions of an anesthetized, intubated patient? Is there a risk of cervical spine injury? Is there a risk of esophageal injury? Can insertion of the TEE probe further compromise the patency of mediastinal structures? Is there fluid in the pericardium? What is the biventricular function? Is there myocardial rupture? Is there aortic rupture? Is the thoracic aorta intact? Is there an intimal flap and a dissection? Is there a transection? Is there a pleural or periaortic effusion/hematoma? What factors determine the urgency of intervention and strategies for management?

DATA COLLECTION

Because the diagnosis and cause for instability are not established, the entire mediastinum, including the left pleural space, is interrogated before definitive therapy is initiated. Rarely is there not enough time to do a complete TEE examination. The operative team can often proceed with confidence in the management of these critically ill patients with only TEE to guide the treatment. The primary event in aortic dissection is a tear and separation of the aortic intima. It is uncertain whether the inciting event is a primary rupture of the intima with secondary dissection of the media, or hemorrhage within the media and subsequent rupture of the overlying intima. Systolic ejection forces blood into the aortic media through a tear that leads to the separation of the intima from the surrounding media, creating a false lumen. Blood flow may exist in both the false and true lumens through communicating fenestrations. Aortic dissections are classified by one of two anatomic schemes (the DeBakey and Stanford classifications). Transection is diagnosed through the detection of para-aortic hematoma near the isthmus and a "step-up" in the internal media wall.

DISCUSSION

Acute dissections (Stanford type A or DeBakey type I or type II) involving the ascending aorta or arch are considered acute surgical emergencies. In contrast, dissections confined to the descending aorta (distal to the left subclavian artery; Stanford type B or DeBakey type III) are treated medically unless the patient

Continued

demonstrates proximal extension, hemorrhage, or malperfusion. From the International Registry of Acute Aortic Dissection (IRAD), 73% of the 384 patients with type B dissections were managed medically; in-hospital mortality was 10%. The long-term survival rate after applying medical therapy is 60% to 80% at 4 to 5 years and 40% to 45% at 10 years. Survival is best in patients with noncommunicating and retrograde dissections. From the IRAD registry, in-hospital mortality for surgical patients was significantly higher (32%). The increased rate of mortality for surgically treated patients is likely influenced by selecting a cohort of patients with more advanced disease and complicated course (malperfusion, leakage, extension). The overall reported short- and long-term outcomes are similar for medically treated patients with type B dissections. Of 142 patients with type aortic dissections, there was a trend toward lower mortality with medical therapy compared with surgical treatment at 1 year (15% vs. 33%). Both groups had similar survival at 5 and 10 years (60% and 35%).

Ascending aortic dissections (involving the aortic root, ascending aorta, or arch) are acute surgical emergencies, because of the high risk for a life-threatening complication such as AR, cardiac tamponade, myocardial infarction, rupture, and stroke. The mortality rate is as high as 1% to 2% per hour early after symptom onset. Neither acute myocardial ischemia nor cerebral infarction should contraindicate urgent intervention. Although patients with stroke in progress may be at increased risk for hemorrhagic cerebral infarction due to intraoperative anticoagulation, leading to hemorrhagic stroke, the authors have seen several patients who experienced dramatic neurologic recovery. Operative mortality for ascending aortic dissections at experienced centers varies from 7% to 36%, well below the greater than 50% mortality with medical therapy.

Traumatic aortic rupture is a life-threatening vascular injury that often results in lethal hemorrhage. In a multicenter trial of 274 patients, the overall mortality rate reached 31%, with 63% of deaths attributable to aortic rupture. Aortic transection and rupture usually occur at the aortic isthmus (between the left subclavian and the first intercostal arteries) and result from shear forces generated by unrestrained frontal collisions. Although aortography had been considered the gold standard for the diagnosis of transection, TEE and contrast-enhanced spiral CT and MRI are currently favored, especially for patients with renal insufficiency. Intravascular ultrasonography has been proposed as a potential diagnostic tool for the identification of limited aortic injuries. Traumatic aortic rupture needs to be distinguished from an aortic dissection. Imaging of a dissected aorta typically reveals true and false lumens at multiple levels. The focal aortic injury of aortic transection is quite localized and may be overlooked when performing a cursory examination. A second potential diagnostic problem is that protuberant atherosclerotic changes of the aorta may be difficult to differentiate from partial aortic tears. The thick and irregular intraluminal flap, which corresponds to disruption of both intimal and medial aortic layers, can be imaged in both the short- and long-axis planes in the vicinity of the isthmus. In the longitudinal view, the medial flap is nearly perpendicular to the aortic wall because traumatic lesions are usually confined within a few centimeters distal to the left subclavian artery. The formation of a localized contained rupture of the false aneurysm is common. CFD imaging and spectral Doppler imaging can be used to detect turbulence associated with nonlaminar flow at the aortic defect and the presence of a pressure gradient. Traditional treatment includes immediate surgical intervention using a right lateral decubitus approach and resection of the aorta with insertion of a tube graft. Deployment of endovascular stent grafts has been successful. Two series that included a total of 16 patients having aortic transection reported successful repair with no mortality or serious morbidity. However, the application of this device under such conditions poses a high risk for left subclavian malperfusion and paraplegia. The decision regarding appropriate management and time course of therapy will depend on the technical availability and expertise within the institution and the forthcoming results of clinical trials that use newer, less invasive technologies.

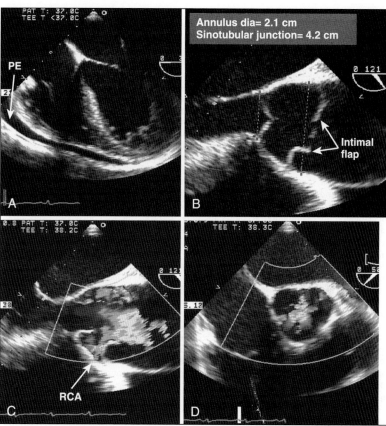

Fig. 11.10 Acute aortic syndrome as the etiology of hemodynamic compromise. A 62-year-old previously healthy, unrestrained driver had a motor vehicle accident. On arrival to the emergency department, the patient was hypotensive (blood pressure = 90/45) and tachycardic (heart rate = 120). He described an episode of loss of consciousness that was associated with severe chest pain but could not recall if the syncopal episode preceded the accident. The chest radiograph was significant for several fractured ribs, widened mediastinum, and a pleural effusion. The patient became progressively more unstable and was transferred to the operating room to perform diagnostic transesophageal echocardiography (TEE) and definitive surgical procedure if necessary. The echo-cardiographer performed a quick transthoracic echocardiographic examination that confirmed the presence of pericardial effusion with findings that were consistent for tamponade. After fluid resuscitation and induction of anesthesia, a TEE examination was performed. (A) The midesophageal four-chamber view showed presence of a pericardial effusion *(PE)* that compromised right atrial filling. (B) The midesophageal long-axis view of the aortic valve revealed a type A dissection that was characterized by intimal flaps within the aortic root and that extended distally into the descending thoracic aorta. The annulus of the aortic valve was of normal size, but the sinus and root were markedly enlarged (diameter of sinotubular junction = 4.22 cm). (C) The dissection extended into the noncoronary and right coronary sinus segments, narrowing blood flow at the coronary ostia *(arrow).* Although the ECG did not show acute ischemia, the right ventricular function and inferior wall of the left ventricle were mildly hypokinetic. (D) Although an effaced aortic root, ascending aortic aneurysm, and acute dissection in this age group are suggestive of congenital bicuspid valve, the short-axis view of the aortic valve showed a trileaflet valve with a coaptation defect with aortic insufficiency at the noncoronary cusp. The surgeon resuspended the aortic valve and replaced the ascending aorta and hemiarch with a tube graft. The valve repair was successful with only +1 aortic insufficiency and cardiac return to normal after surgery. *RCA,* Right coronary artery.

SUGGESTED READINGS

American Society of Anesthesiologists and Society of Cardiovascular Anesthesiologists Task Force on Transesophageal Echocardiography. Practice guidelines for perioperative transesophageal echocardiography. An updated report by the American Society of Anesthesiologists and the Society of Cardiovascular Anesthesiologists Task Force on Transesophageal Echocardiography. *Anesthesiology*. 2010;112:1084–1096.

Anyanwu AC, Adams DH. Etiologic classification of degenerative mitral valve disease: Barlow's disease and fibroelastic deficiency. *Semin Thorac Cardiovasc Surg*. 2007;19:90–96.

Baumgartner H, Hung J, Bermejo J, et al. Echocardiographic assessment of valve stenosis: EAE/ASE recommendations for clinical practice. *J Am Soc Echocardiogr*. 2009;22:1–23.

Bonow RO, Carabello BA, Chatterjee K, et al. 2008 focused update incorporated into the ACC/AHA 2006 guidelines for the management of patients with valvular heart disease: a report of the American College of Cardiology/American Heart Association Task Force on Practice Guidelines (Writing Committee to Revise the 1998 Guidelines for the Management of Patients With Valvular Heart Disease). Endorsed by the Society of Cardiovascular Anesthesiologists, Society for Cardiovascular Angiography and Interventions, and Society of Thoracic Surgeons. *Circulation*. 2008;118(15):e523–e661.

Hahn RT, Abraham T, Adams MS, et al. Guidelines for performing a comprehensive transesophageal echocardiographic examination: recommendations from the American Society of Echocardiography and the Society of Cardiovascular Anesthesiologists. *J Am Soc Echocardiogr*. 2013;9:921–964.

Itagaki S, Hosseinian L, Varghese R. Right ventricular failure after cardiac surgery: management strategies. *Semin Thorac Cardiovasc Surg*. 2012;24:188–194.

Lancellotti P, Tribouilloy C, Hagendorff A, et al. Recommendations for the echocardiographic assessment of native valvular regurgitation: an executive summary from the European Association of Cardiovascular Imaging. *Eur Heart J Cardiovasc Imaging*. 2013;14(7):611–644.

Lang RM, Badano LP, Mor-Avi V, et al. Recommendations for cardiac chamber quantification by echocardiography in adults: an update from the American Society of Echocardiography and the European Association of Cardiovascular Imaging. *J Am Soc Echocardiogr*. 2015;28:1–39.

Mathew JP, Glas K, Troianos CA, et al. ASE/SCA recommendations and guidelines for continuous quality improvement in perioperative echocardiography. *Anesth Analg*. 2006;103:1416–1425.

Min JK, Spencer KT, Furlong KT, et al. Clinical features of complications from transesophageal echocardiography: a single-center case series of 10,000 consecutive examinations. *J Am Soc Echocardiogr*. 2005;18:925–929.

Minhaj M, Patel K, Muzic D, et al. The effect of routine intraoperative transesophageal echocardiography on surgical management. *J Cardiothorac Vasc Anesth*. 2007;21(6):800–804.

Movsowitz HD, Levine RA, Hilgenberg AD, et al. Transesophageal echocardiographic description of the mechanisms of aortic regurgitation in acute type A aortic dissection: implications for aortic valve repair. *J Am Coll Cardiol*. 2000;36:884–890.

Nishimura RA, Otto CM, Bonow RO, et al. 2014 AHA/ACC guideline for the management of patients with valvular heart disease: executive summary: a report of the American College of Cardiology/American Heart Association Task Force on Practice Guidelines. *J Am Coll Cardiol*. 2014;63(22):2438–2488.

Parra V, Fita G, Rovira I, et al. Transoesophageal echocardiography accurately detects cardiac output variation: a prospective comparison with thermodilution in cardiac surgery. *Eur J Anaesthesiol*. 2008;25(2):135–143.

Pibarot P, Dumesnil JG. Low-flow, low-gradient aortic stenosis with normal and depressed left ventricular ejection fraction. *J Am Coll Cardiol*. 2012;60:1845–1853.

Piercy M, McNicol L, Dinh DT, et al. Major complications related to the use of transesophageal echocardiography in cardiac surgery. *J Cardiothorac Vasc Anesth*. 2009;23:62–65.

Rudski LG, Lai WW, Afilalo J, et al. Guidelines for the echocardiographic assessment of the right heart in adults: a report from the American Society of Echocardiography endorsed by the European Association of Echocardiography, a registered branch of the European Society of Cardiology, and the Canadian Society of Echocardiography. *J Am Soc Echocardiogr*. 2010;23:685–713, quiz 786–788.

Tan CO, Harley I. Perioperative transesophageal echocardiographic assessment of the right heart and associated structures: a comprehensive update and technical report. *J Cardiothorac Vasc Anesth*. 2014;28:1112–1133.

Vlahakes GJ. Right ventricular failure after cardiac surgery. *Cardiol Clin*. 2012;30:283–289.

Zoghbi WA, Enriquez-Sarano M, Foster E, et al. Recommendations for evaluation of the severity of native valvular regurgitation with two-dimensional and Doppler echocardiography. *J Am Soc Echocardiogr*. 2003;16:777–802.

Chapter 12

Central Nervous System Monitoring

Harvey L. Edmonds, Jr., PhD • Emily K. Gordon, MD • Warren J. Levy, MD

Key Points

1. Electroencephalography can detect both cerebral ischemia or hypoxia and seizures and can measure hypnotic effect.
2. Middle-latency auditory-evoked potentials objectively document inadequate hypnosis.
3. Somatosensory-evoked potentials may detect developing injury in cortical and subcortical brain structures and peripheral nerves.
4. Transcranial electric motor–evoked potentials monitor function of the descending motor pathways.
5. Transcranial Doppler ultrasound examination assesses the direction and character of blood flow through large intracranial arteries and identifies microemboli.
6. Cerebral oximetry, using spatially resolved transcranial near-infrared spectroscopy, provides a continuous measure of change in the balance of cerebral oxygen supply and demand.
7. Used in concert, these technologies can reduce the incidence of brain injury and ensure the adequacy of hypnosis.

Yearly, nearly one-half of the 1 million patients undergoing cardiac surgical procedures worldwide will likely experience transient neurologic, cognitive, or neuropsychological dysfunction; in one-quarter of these patients, the changes will be persistent. The direct annual cost to US insurers for brain injury from just one type of cardiac operation, myocardial revascularization, is estimated at $2 billion. Furthermore, the same processes that injure the central nervous system (CNS) also appear to influence dysfunction of other vital organs. Thus, enormous clinical and economic incentives exist to improve CNS protection during cardiac surgical procedures.

Historically, neurophysiologic monitoring during cardiac surgical procedures has elicited little enthusiasm because of the presumed key role of macroembolization. It is widely assumed that most brain injuries during cardiac operations in adults result from cerebral embolization of atheromatous or calcified material dislodged from sclerotic blood vessels during the manipulation of these vessels. Until the introduction of myocardial revascularization without cardiopulmonary bypass (CPB) or aortic clamp application, these injuries often were viewed as unavoidable and untreatable.

Technical developments are altering this perception. First, CNS injuries still occur despite reductions in aortic manipulation with the newer approaches to coronary

III

BOX 12.1 *Factors Contributing to Brain Injury During Cardiac Surgical Procedures*

Atheromatous emboli from aorta manipulation
Lipid microemboli from recirculation of unwashed cardiotomy suction
Gaseous microemboli from air leakage and cavitation
Cerebral hypoperfusion or hyperperfusion
Cerebral hyperthermia
Cerebral dysoxygenation

artery bypass grafting (CABG) and aortic surgical procedures. Second, neurophysiologic studies have implicated hypoperfusion and dysoxygenation as major causative factors in CNS injury (Box 12.1). Because these functional disturbances are often detectable and correctable, the impetus is to examine the role of neurophysiologic monitoring in organ protection.

ELECTROENCEPHALOGRAPHY

Electroencephalographic (EEG) monitoring for ischemia detection has been performed since the first CPB procedures. However, its widespread use has previously been limited by a number of factors.

First, small, practical, and affordable EEG monitors have only recently become available.

Second, the traditional diagnostic approach to EEG analysis depended on complex pattern recognition of 21-channel analog waveforms to identify focal ischemic changes. This analytic format necessitated extensive training and constant vigilance. Therefore, EEG monitoring during cardiac operations by anesthesia providers was viewed as impractical. However, reduced electrode array perioperative EEG recordings that include bilateral activity appear to be effective in identifying cortical ischemia and seizure activity in the perioperative and critical care settings. In addition, computerized processing of EEG signals provides simplified trend displays that have helped to overcome many of the earlier interpretational complexities.

Third, EEG analysis during cardiac surgical procedures was often confounded by anesthetic agents, hypothermia, and roller pump artifacts. Fortunately, these technical problems have now been overcome by: (1) elimination or replacement of the troublesome roller pumps with centrifugal pumps, (2) routine use of mild hypothermic or normothermic bypass, and (3) adoption of fast-track anesthesia protocols that avoid marked EEG suppression.

Physiologic Basis of Electroencephalography

Electroencephalographically directed interventions designed to correct cerebral hypoperfusion during cardiac surgical procedures require an appreciation of the underlying neurophysiologic substrate. Scalp-recorded EEG signals reflect the temporal and spatial summation of long-lasting (10–100 milliseconds) postsynaptic potentials that arise from columnar cortical pyramidal neurons (Fig. 12.1).

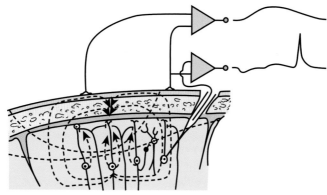

Fig. 12.1 Production of electroencephalographic (EEG) waves. Scalp electrodes record potential differences that are caused by postsynaptic potentials in the cell membrane of cortical neurons. The *closed loop dashed lines* represent the summation of extracellular currents produced by the postsynaptic potentials. *Open segment dashed lines* connect all points having the same voltage level. The two scalp electrodes record changes in the voltage difference over time *(top trace at upper right).* The *lower trace* from a microelectrode inserted in a single cortical neuron has little direct relationship with the summated EEG wave. (Modified from Fisch BJ. *EEG Primer.* 3rd ed. New York: Elsevier, 1999:6.)

Table 12.1	**Electroencephalographic Frequency Bands**
Delta (δ)	0.1–4 Hz
Theta (θ)	4–8 Hz
Alpha (α)	8–14 Hz
Beta (β)	14–25 Hz
Gamma (γ)	25–55 Hz

EEG rhythms represent regularly recurring waveforms of similar shape and duration. These signal oscillations depend on the synchronous excitation of a neuronal population. The descriptive nature of conventional EEG findings characterizes the oscillations (measured in cycles per second [cps] or Hertz [Hz]) as sinusoids that were classified according to their amplitude and frequency. The terminology used to describe the frequency bands of the most common oscillatory patterns is illustrated in Fig. 12.2. In addition, a high-frequency (25–55 Hz) gamma band is recognized (Table 12.1).

Practical Considerations of Electroencephalographic Recording and Signal Processing

Standardized electrode placement is based on the International 10–20 System (Fig. 12.3). It permits uniform spacing of electrodes, independent of head circumference, in scalp regions known to correlate with specific areas of cerebral cortex. Four anatomic landmarks are used—the nasion, inion, and preauricular points.

The frequency range involved in production of the EEG waveform is termed its *bandwidth.* The upper and lower bandwidth boundaries are controlled by filters that reject frequencies above and below the EEG bandwidth. Both the appearance of the unprocessed EEG waveform and the value of univariate numeric EEG descriptors such as the mean dominant frequency (MDF) may be heavily influenced by signal

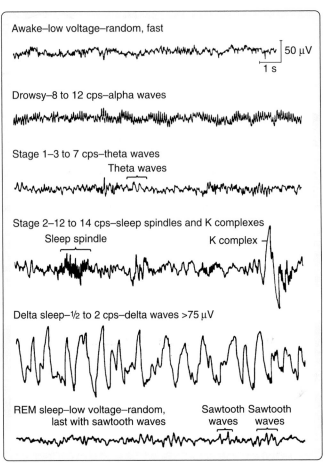

Fig. 12.2 Specific electroencephalographic characteristics of human sleep-wakefulness cycle stages. Note the appearance of the four most common frequency bands, from the lowest frequency delta through theta and alpha to high-frequency beta. An even higher gamma frequency band (25 to 55 cps) is also described. *REM,* Rapid-eye-movement. (Courtesy GE Healthcare.)

bandwidth that is often user-controlled by high- and low-frequency filter settings. Similarly, the same cerebral biopotential recorded by different EEG devices may result in dissimilar waveforms and numeric values.

Display of Electroencephalographic Information

Time-Domain Analysis

Traditional display of the electroencephalogram is a graph of biopotential voltage (*y*-axis) as a function of time and consequently is described as a time-domain process. The objective of a diagnostic electroencephalogram is to identify the most likely cause of a detected abnormality at one moment in time. Typically, a diagnostic electroencephalogram is obtained under controlled conditions, using precisely defined protocols. Recorded EEG appearance is visually compared with reference patterns. Interpretation is based on recognition of unique waveform patterns that are pathognomonic for

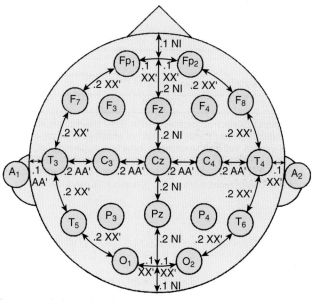

Fig. 12.3 Electroencephalographic electrode positions in the International 10–20 system. The sagittal hemicircumference (labeled *AA'*) is measured from the root of one zygoma (just anterior to the ear) to the other, across the vertex. The third measurement is the ipsilateral hemicircumference (*XX'*) measured from a point 10% of the coronal hemicircumference above the zygoma. Through these intersecting lines, all the scalp electrodes may be located, except the frontal (*F_3, F_4*) and parietal (*P_3, P_4*). The frontal and parietal electrodes are placed along the frontal or parietal coronal line midway between the middle electrode and the electrode marked in the circumferential ring.

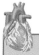

BOX 12.2 *Law of the Electroencephalogram*

In the absence of disease, electroencephalographic amplitude and frequency are inversely related
Simultaneous decrease may indicate ischemia, anoxia, or excessive hypnosis
Simultaneous increase may indicate seizure or artifact

12

specific clinical conditions. In contrast, the goal of EEG monitoring is to identify clinically important change from an individualized baseline. Unlike diagnostic EEG interpretation, monitoring requires immediate assessment of continuously fluctuating signals in an electronically hostile, complex, and poorly controlled recording environment. Therefore, of necessity, interpretation relies less on pattern recognition and more on statistical characterization of change. Numeric descriptors thus may appropriately form an integral part of EEG monitoring.

Both EEG diagnostic and monitoring interpretations are based in part on the "law of the electroencephalogram" (Box 12.2). It states that amplitude and dominant frequency are inversely related. The inverse relationship between amplitude and frequency generally is maintained during unchanging cerebral metabolic states. Parallel increases in both may occur in some hypermetabolic states such as seizure activity, whereas decreases may be seen in hypometabolic states such as hypothermia. In the absence of these influences, simultaneous decreases in both amplitude and frequency

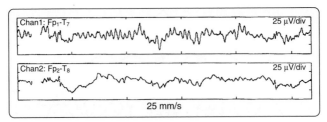

Fig. 12.4 The importance of electroencephalographic (EEG) baseline recording. This two-channel EEG recording was made immediately after induction of anesthesia, before head repositioning for insertion of a central venous catheter. Anesthetic induction apparently uncovered a preexisting asymmetry that was not evident in the waking electroencephalogram. Although the patient had a history of an earlier mild cerebrovascular accident and transient ischemic attacks, he appeared neurologically normal at preoperative assessment. (Courtesy GE Healthcare.)

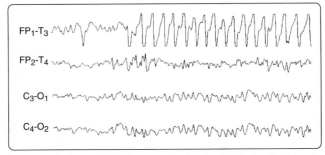

Fig. 12.5 Electroencephalographic (EEG) contamination by electrical artifact. The large-amplitude 2-Hz triangular waves in the left frontotemporal derivation *(top trace)* are the result of temporalis muscle activation with a nerve stimulator. Current spread from the stimulating to the EEG recording electrodes may be minimized with use of the appropriate facial nerve stimulation site at the jaw angle. (Courtesy GE Healthcare.)

may indicate ischemia or anoxia (Fig. 12.4); a parallel increase may represent artifact (Fig. 12.5).

Time-domain analysis of traditional electroencephalography uses linear signal amplitude (ie, voltage) and time scales. The amplitude range of EEG signals is quite large (several hundred microvolts), and univariate statistical measures of its central tendency and dispersion may contain clinically useful information. Furthermore, amplitude variation may show clinically significant changes in reactivity that can be obscured by frequency-domain analysis. Advances in the technology of EEG amplitude integration have prompted a resurgent interest in this attractively simple approach, particularly in pediatrics.

Frequency-Domain Analysis

An alternative method, frequency-domain analysis, is exemplified by the prismatic decomposition of white light into its component frequencies (ie, color spectrum). As the basis of spectral analysis, the Fourier theorem states that a periodic function can be represented in part by a sinusoid at the fundamental frequency and an infinite series of integer multiples (ie, harmonics). The Fourier function at a specific frequency equals the amplitude and phase angle of the associated sinusoid. Graphs of amplitude and phase angle as functions of frequency are called Fourier spectra (ie, spectral analysis). The EEG amplitude spectral scale (Fig. 12.6) squares voltage values to eliminate troublesome negative values. Squaring changes the unit of amplitude measure from microvolts

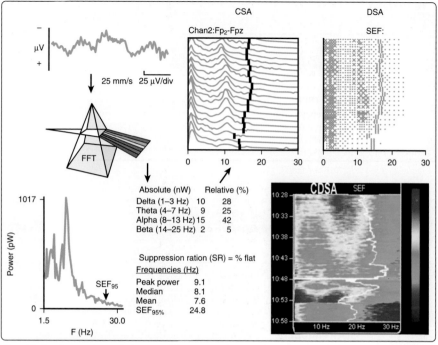

Fig. 12.6 Comparison of time- and frequency-domain electroencephalographic (EEG) displays. The traditional analog EEG signal shown in the *upper left* is a time-domain graph of scalp-recorded amplitude (μV) as a function of time. Digitized EEG segments (epochs) are computer-processed using the fast Fourier transform *(FFT)*, which, like a prism, decomposes a complex electromagnetic signal into a series of sinusoids, each with a discrete frequency. The instantaneous relationship is then graphically depicted by the power spectrum *(lower left)*, a frequency–domain plot of power (μV^2 or *pW*) as a function of frequency. The spectral edge frequency *(SEF)* defines the signal amplitude upper boundary. The three-dimensional compressed spectral array *(CSA)* plots successive power spectra with time on the z-axis *(upper middle)*. The density-modulated spectral array *(DSA; upper right)* improves data compression by using dot density to represent signal amplitude (ie, power). Amplitude resolution is improved through color coding in the color density spectral array *(CDSA)* shown at the *lower right*. The SEF is shown as the *white vertical line*. Note the EEG suppression at the bottom of each spectral trend.

to either picowatts (pW) or nanowatts (nW). However, a power amplitude scale tends to overemphasize large-amplitude changes. Clinically important changes in low-amplitude components that are readily discernible in the linearly scaled unprocessed EEG waveform may become invisible in power spectral displays.

Simplification of the large amount of spectral information generally has been achieved through the use of univariate numeric descriptors. Most commonly, the power contained in a specified traditional EEG frequency band (delta, theta, alpha, or beta) is calculated in absolute, relative, or normalized terms.

The most widely used univariate frequency descriptors (Box 12.3) are as follows:

1. Total power (TP).
2. Peak power frequency (PPF), the single frequency of the spectrum that contains the highest amplitude.
3. Mean dominant frequency (MDF), the sum of power contained at each frequency of the spectrum times its frequency divided by the TP.

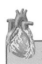

BOX 12.3 *Common Univariate Electroencephalographic Descriptors Detecting Ischemia*

Total power (TP)
Peak power frequency (PPF)
Mean dominant frequency (MDF)
95% spectral edge frequency (SEF)
Suppression ratio (SR)

Table 12.2 Commercial Multivariate Quantitative Electroencephalographic Descriptors of Hypnotic Effect

Acronym	Index Name	Mode	Manufacturer
BIS	Bispectral	Bilateral	Covidien, Boulder, CO
CSI	Cerebral state	Unilateral	Danmeter A/S, Odense, Denmark
NT	Narcotrend	Bilateral	MonitorTechnik, Bad Bramstedt, Germany
PSI	Patient state	Bilateral	Masimo, Irvine, CA
SE	State entropy	Unilateral	GE Healthcare/Datex-Ohmeda, Helsinki, Finland
SNAP II	SNAP II	Unilateral	Stryker Instruments, Kalamazoo, MI

4. Spectral edge frequency (SEF), the frequency below which a predetermined fraction, usually 90% or 95%, of the spectral power occurs.
5. Suppression ratio (SR), the percentage of flat-line electroencephalogram contained within sampled epochs.

Multivariate (ie, composed of several variables) descriptors have been developed to improve simple numeric characterization of clinically important EEG changes. With this approach, algorithms are used to generate a single number that represents the pattern of amplitude-frequency-phase relationships occurring in a single epoch. Several commercially available monitors provide unitless numbers that have been transformed to arbitrary (ie, 0–100) scales. Each monitor provides a different probability estimate of a patient's response to verbal instruction. Current monitors designed for use by anesthesia providers are listed in Table 12.2. BIS (bispectral index, Covidien, Boulder, CO), NT (NarcoTrend, Monitor Technik, Bad Bramstedt, Germany), PSI (Sedline, Masimo, Irvine, CA), and SNAP II (Stryker Instruments, Kalamazoo, MI) are rule-based proprietary indices empirically derived from patients' data. In contrast, CSI (Danmeter A/S, Odense, Denmark) uses a fuzzy logic–based algorithm, whereas SE applies standard entropy equations to EEG analysis. Each product is designed to require the use of proprietary self-adhesive forehead sensors. Collectively, these products are now in widespread use as objective measures of hypnotic effect.

Scalp-recorded cerebral biopotentials are complex physiologic signals. They represent the algebraic summation of voltage changes produced from cortical synaptic activity (ie, electroencephalogram), upper facial muscle activity (ie, facial electromyogram [fEMG]), and eye movement (ie, electro-oculogram [EOG]). During consciousness and light sedation, high-frequency gamma power (ie, 25–55 Hz) is a mixture of electroencephalography and subcortically influenced facial electromyography. Muscle activity makes a larger contribution because of the closer proximity of signal generators to the recording electrodes. Hypnotic and analgesic agents typically suppress both cerebral and muscle activities, with resulting reduced gamma power. Because the upper facial muscles are relatively insensitive to moderate neuromuscular blockade, they may remain reactive to noxious stimuli. Nociception results in sudden gamma power increase, independent of activity in the lower-frequency classic EEG bands.

The EEG analyzers just described either provide separate quantitative estimates of the high-frequency information or incorporate this information into the hypnotic index. For example, the Datex-Ohmeda Entropy Module (GE Healthcare/Datex-Ohmeda, Helsinki, Finland) separately analyzes the 32- to 47-Hz band and terms the signal Response Entropy (RE). Addition of RE to the lower-frequency state entropy (SE) is claimed by the manufacturer to facilitate distinction between changes in hypnosis and analgesia, although supporting evidence for this proposition awaits carefully designed and adequately powered randomized, prospective studies. EEG suppression decreases both entropy indices because noise-free flat-line EEG segments are generally thought to have near-zero entropy. However, during cardiac surgical procedures, EEG signals that appear to be totally suppressed may be associated with paradoxically very high entropy values. To minimize this problem, SE uses a special algorithm that assigns zero entropy to totally suppressed EEG epochs.

In addition to the quantitative EEG numeric indices, many monitors also display pseudo-three-dimensional plots of successive power spectra as a function of time. This frequency-domain approach was originated by Joy and was popularized by Bickford, who coined the term "compressed spectral array" (CSA). Its popularity stems in part from enormous data compression. For example, the essential information contained in a 4-hour traditional EEG recording consuming more than 1000 pages of unprocessed waveforms can be displayed in CSA format on a single page.

With CSA (see Fig. 12.6), successive power spectra of brief (2- to 60-second) EEG epochs are displayed as smoothed histograms of amplitude as a function of frequency. Spectral compression is achieved by partially overlaying successive spectra, with time represented on the z-axis. Hidden-line suppression improves clarity by avoiding overlap of successive traces. Although the display is aesthetically attractive, it has limitations. The extent of data loss resulting from spectral overlapping depends on the nonstandard axial rotation that varies among EEG monitors.

An alternative to the CSA display to reduce data loss is the diversity-modulated spectral array (DSA) that uses a two-dimensional monochrome dot matrix plot of time as a function of frequency (see Fig. 12.6). The density of dots indicates the amplitude at a particular time-frequency intersection (eg, an intense large spot indicates high amplitude). Clinically significant shifts in frequency may be detected earlier and more easily than with CSA. However, the resolution of amplitude changes is reduced. Therefore color DSA (CDSA) was developed to enhance amplitude resolution (see Fig. 12.6). The CSA, DSA, and CDSA displays are not well suited for the detection of nonstationary or transient phenomena such as burst suppression or epileptiform activity.

In summary, a quick assessment of EEG change in either the time- or frequency-domain focuses on (1) maximal peak-to-peak amplitude, (2) relation of maximal amplitude to dominant frequency, (3) amplitude and frequency variability, and (4) new or growing asymmetry between homotopic (ie, same position on each cerebral hemisphere) EEG derivations. These objectives are generally best achieved through the viewing of both unprocessed and processed displays with a clear understanding of the characteristics and limitations of each (Box 12.4).

12

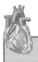

BOX 12.4 *Measures That Define Electroencephalographic Changes*

Maximum peak-to-peak amplitude (or total power)
Relation of maximum amplitude to dominant frequency
Amplitude and frequency variability
Right-to-left symmetry

AUDITORY-EVOKED POTENTIALS

Auditory-evoked potentials (AEPs) assess specific areas of the brainstem, midbrain, and auditory cortices. Because of their simplicity and reproducibility, AEPs are suitable for monitoring patients during cardiovascular surgical procedures. Specific applications of AEP monitoring in this environment are the assessment of temperature effects on brainstem function and the evaluation of hypnotic effect. Direct involvement of cardiac anesthesia providers with AEP monitoring is likely to increase following the introduction of EEG/AEP modules designed for use with available operating room physiologic monitors.

Acoustic stimuli trigger a neural response integrated by a synchronized neuronal depolarization that travels from the auditory nerve to the cerebral cortex. Scalp-recorded signals, obtained from electrodes located at the vertex and earlobe, contain both the AEPs and other unrelated EEG and electromyographic activity. Extraction of the relatively low-amplitude AEP from the larger-amplitude background activity requires signal-averaging techniques. Because the AEP character remains constant for each stimulus repetition, averaging of many repetitions increases the signal amplitude linearly. Thus increases in the signal-to-noise ratio of 10-fold to 30-fold are commonly achieved. For the AEP sensory stimulus, acoustic clicks are the most commonly used. These broadband signals are generated by unidirectional rectangular short pulses (40–500 microseconds) with frequency spectra lower than 10 kHz.

Brainstem auditory-evoked potentials (BAEPs) are useful in assessing brainstem and subcortical function during surgical procedures, in part because of their relative resistance to the suppressant effects of most anesthetic agents.

The middle-latency AEPs (MLAEPs), with poststimulus latencies between 10 and 100 milliseconds, are generated in the midbrain and primary auditory cortex. Latency and amplitude changes allow reliable detection of consciousness and nociception during cardiac surgical procedures. In addition, parallel monitoring of MLAEP and quantitative EEG descriptors (ie, BIS) may permit distinction between the hypnotic and antinociceptive anesthetic components. This approach has also been used successfully in pediatric cardiac surgical patients to assess postoperative sedation objectively.

Somatosensory-Evoked Potentials

In many ways, the somatosensory-evoked potential (SSEP) is similar to the AEP. An electrical stimulus is applied peripherally to the arms or legs, or both, and the progression of the neuronal transmission through the spinal cord and subcortical structures is tracked, with various neurogenerators producing specific positive or negative deflection of the recorded signal at various times. In this way, SSEPs provide an objective measure

III

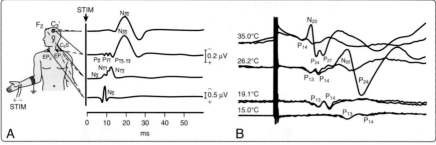

Fig. 12.7 Upper limb somatosensory-evoked potential (SSEP) waveforms. (A) The waveforms show ascending responses to median nerve electrical stimulation. With the aid of noncephalic reference electrodes, the N_9 clavicular (Erb point) potential reflects signal passage through the brachial plexus, whereas the N_{13} potential represents activation of the cervical and brainstem lemniscal structures. Signals passing through the cortical radiations and sensory cortex result in the N_{20} potential when recorded between a scalp active electrode and cephalic reference. (B) Each pair of upper limb SSEP waveforms is created by the superimposition of parietal recordings ipsilateral and contralateral to single limb median nerve stimulation. The *shaded area* represents signal generated within the cortical mantle. Cooling to 26.2°C increases the latency of both subcortical and cortical waveform components and results in the emergence of a second (ie, P_{13}) brainstem potential. Although the deep hypothermia at 19.1°C suppressed cortical activity, brainstem P_{13} and P_{14} responsiveness persists. (A, From Misulis KE, Fakhoury T. *Spehlmann's Evoked Potential Primer.* 3rd ed. Boston: Butterworth–Heinemann; 2001:98, with permission of the publisher. B, Modified from Guérit JM. Intraoperative monitoring during cardiac surgery. In: Nuwer MR, ed. *Handbook of Clinical Neurophysiology. Vol. 8. Intraoperative Monitoring of Neural Function.* New York: Elsevier; 2008:834.)

of ascending sensory pathway function. Like AEPs, they are recorded by signal averaging over a large number of stimuli, with the duration of recording after each stimulus being somewhat longer and thus the frequency of stimulation somewhat lower. SSEPs are moderately sensitive to depression from inhaled anesthetic agents, but they do not generally preclude the use of potent agents in a balanced technique or as supplement to a high-dose narcotic approach. Fig. 12.7 illustrates the key neural structures involved in a prominent upper limb sensory pathway suitable for cardiac surgical neuromonitoring.

Motor-Evoked Potentials

By relying on the delivery of a rapid stimulus pulse train, it is now possible to monitor the integrity of descending motor pathways continuously by using transcranial electric motor-evoked potentials (MEPs). The most frequent application of this emerging monitoring modality for cardiothoracic surgical procedures currently is during open surgical or endovascular repair of the descending aorta. The need for improved spinal cord protection remains critical because, even with modern spinal cord preservation techniques, the infarction rate during type I and II aneurysm repairs in patients remains disturbingly high.

The neurophysiologic basis for the MEP is illustrated in Fig. 12.8. Individual high-intensity transcranial stimuli depolarize cortical motor neurons directly in the axon hillock region or indirectly by activation of interneurons. Synaptic transmission of individual impulses to segmental α-motor neurons lowers the postsynaptic membrane potential, but it is often insufficient to initiate cell firing. Instead, this goal is achieved through use of a pulse train that triggers lower motor neuron discharge by temporal summation of individual subthreshold responses.

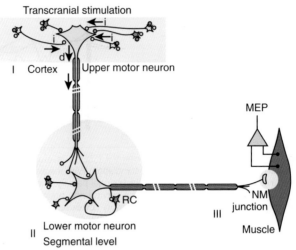

Transcranial stimulation

I Cortex — Upper motor neuron

MEP

NM junction

III

II Lower motor neuron
Segmental level

RC

Muscle

Fig. 12.8 Neural generators of transcranial motor-evoked potentials *(MEP)*. High-intensity transcranial electric or magnetic stimulation results in direct *(d)* activation of upper motor neurons. In addition, indirect motor neuron activation *(i)* results from transcranial activation of horizontally oriented excitatory (light) and inhibitory (dark) neuronal axons. Descending motor potentials are conducted unidirectionally through the corticospinal, rubrospinal, tectospinal, vestibulospinal, and cerebellospinal tracts to lower (alpha) motor neurons in the lateral and anterior spinal cord. In the absence of complete pharmacologic neuromuscular *(NM)* blockade, alpha motor neuron action potentials then produce muscle fiber contraction that is recorded by electromyography. (Modified from Journee JL. Motor EP physiology, risks and specific anesthetic effects. In: Nuwer MR, ed. *Handbook of Clinical Neurophysiology. Vol. 8. Intraoperative Monitoring of Neural Function.* New York: Elsevier; 2008:219.)

Even though lower limb MEPs are necessary to document the functional integrity of motor pathways in the thoracolumbar spinal cord, upper limb recording is also important. The upper limb responses identify generalized MEP suppression. Its causes include anesthetic-induced synaptic inhibition, hypocapnia, and hypothermia, as well as position-related ischemia involving cerebral or upper limb motor pathways, or both (Fig. 12.9). The effects of anesthetic agents on evoked potentials are summarized in Table 12.3. In addition to these generalized effects, volatile anesthetic agents suppress both cortical and spinal cord motor neurons. Thus the use of these drugs should be avoided or minimized during attempted MEP monitoring.

Correct interpretation of MEP amplitude change requires precise monitoring and control of neuromuscular blockade. Information on the extent of neuromuscular blockade obtained from evoked electromyographic train-of-four responses in both upper and lower limb muscles bilaterally helps guide relaxant administration and detects limb ischemia.

▣ TRANSCRANIAL DOPPLER ULTRASOUND

Ultrasound Technology

Ultrasonic probes of a clinical transcranial Doppler (TCD) sonograph contain an electrically activated piezoelectric crystal that transmits low-power 1- to 2-MHz acoustic vibrations (ie, insonation) through the thinnest portion of temporal bone (ie, acoustic window) into brain tissue. Blood constituents (predominantly erythrocytes) contained in large arteries and veins reflect these ultrasonic waves back to the probe,

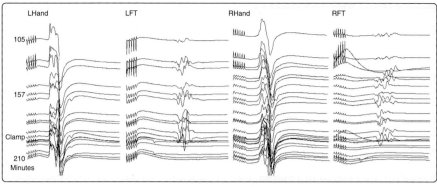

Fig. 12.9 Motor-evoked potential (MEP) detection of spinal cord hypoperfusion. Changes are shown in hand (*LHand* and *RHand*) and foot (*LFT* and *RFT*) MEP responses to clamping of the descending aorta during surgical repair of a thoracoabdominal aneurysm. Note the bilateral loss of lower limb MEP with clamp application. MEP monitoring helped guide management of left-sided heart bypass and reimplantation of the superior mesenteric and renal arteries into the aortic graft.

Table 12.3	Anesthetic[a] Effects on Sensory- and Motor-Evoked Responses			
Pharmacologic Class	Agent	SSEP	AEP	MEP
Nonspecific inhibitor	Isoflurane	Suppression	Suppression	Suppression
	Sevoflurane	Suppression	Suppression	Suppression
	Desflurane	Suppression	Suppression	Suppression
	Barbiturates	Suppression	Suppression	Suppression
GABA-specific agonist	Propofol	Suppression[b]	Suppression	Suppression[b]
α₂ Agonist	Clonidine	Suppression[b]	?	Suppression[b]
	Dexmedetomidine	Suppression[b]	?	Suppression[b]
NMDA antagonist	Nitrous oxide	Suppression	—	Suppression
	Ketamine	Increase	—	Suppression[b]
	Xenon	Suppression[b]	Suppression[b]	Suppression[b]

[a]1 MAC-equivalent dose.
[b]Slight to minimal effect.
AEP, Auditory-evoked potential; *GABA,* γ-aminobutyric acid; *MAC,* minimum alveolar concentration; *MEP,* motor-evoked potential; *NMDA,* N-methyl-D-aspartate; *SSEP,* somatosensory-evoked potential.
Modified from Sloan TB, Jäntti V. Anesthetic effects on evoked potentials. In: Nuwer MR, ed. *Handbook of Clinical Neurophysiology. Vol. 8. Intraoperative Monitoring of Neural Function.* New York: Elsevier; 2008:94–126.

12

which also serves as a receiver. Because of laminar blood flow, erythrocytes traveling in the central region of a large blood vessel move with higher velocity than those near the vessel wall. Thus, within each vascular segment (ie, sample volume), a series of echoes associated with varying velocities is created. The frequency differences between the insonation signal and each echo in the series are proportional to the associated velocity, and this velocity is determined from the Doppler equation. Although several large intracranial arteries may be insonated through the temporal window, the middle cerebral artery is generally monitored during cardiac operations because it carries approximately 40% of the hemispheric blood flow.

Pulsed-Wave Spectral Display

Pulsed-wave Doppler examination samples the ultrasonic echoes at a user-selected distance (ie, single gate) below the scalp. The frequency composition of these Doppler-shifted echoes is analyzed by Fourier analysis, the same technique used to quantify EEG frequency patterns. The analysis produces a momentary amplitude spectrum displayed as a function of blood flow velocity (eg, Doppler-shift frequency). This relationship is mapped as one vertical strip in the spectrogram display (Fig. 12.10, *upper right*). Amplitude at each frequency is expressed as log change (ie, decibels [dB]) from the background composed of random echoes. The momentary analysis is repeated 100 times per second to produce a scrolling spectrogram of time-related changes in flow velocity.

The maximum velocity, the upper edge (envelope) of the velocity spectrum, represents the maximum Doppler shift (erythrocyte velocity) in the vessel center. Peak-systolic and end-diastolic velocities are derived from this spectral edge. Intensity-weighted mean velocity is calculated by weighted averaging of the intensity of all Doppler spectral signals in a vessel cross-section. Sampling echoes at multiple loci (multigating) produces spectrograms for each of the different probe-to-sample site distances (Fig. 12.11).

Power M-Mode Doppler Display

An alternative method for processing pulsed-wave Doppler echoes is nonspectral power M-mode Doppler (PMD) (Fig. 12.12). Unlike the series of spectra generated with multigating, PMD creates one image with each depth represented by a plot of signal amplitude (ie, power) and depth as functions of time. A color scale signifies

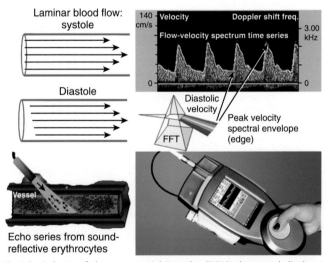

Fig. 12.10 Physiologic basis of the transcranial Doppler (TCD) ultrasound display. Large-vessel laminar flow results in a cross-sectional series of erythrocyte velocities, with the lowest values nearest the vessel wall. Ultrasonic vessel insonation produces a series of erythrocyte echoes. The frequency differences (ie, Doppler-shift frequencies) between the insonating signal and its echoes are proportional to erythrocyte velocity and flow direction. Fast Fourier transform *(FFT)* analysis of this complex echo produces an instantaneous power spectrum analogous to that used in electroencephalographic analysis. The time-series of successive Doppler-shift spectra *(upper right)* resembles an arterial pressure waveform but represents fluctuating erythrocyte velocities during each cardiac cycle. Some modern TCD sonographs are small enough to be handheld or incorporated into multimodal neurophysiologic signal analyzers. (Image of the 500P Pocket Transcranial Doppler courtesy Multigon Industries, Inc, Yonkers, NY.)

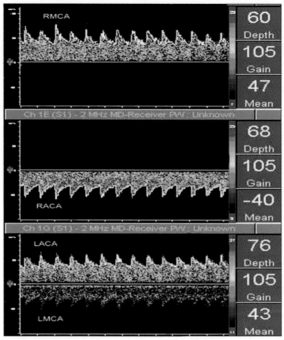

Fig. 12.11 Multigated transcranial Doppler ultrasound display. Multigating of pulsed-wave Doppler signals permits simultaneous display of echo spectra generated at several different intracranial loci. *LACA,* Left anterior cerebral artery; *LMCA,* left middle cerebral artery; *RACA,* right anterior cerebral artery; *RMCA,* right middle cerebral artery.

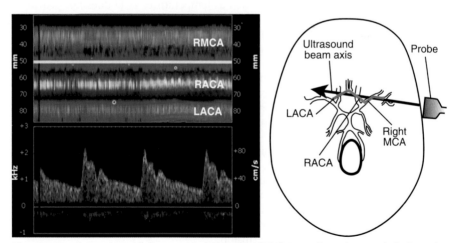

Fig. 12.12 Comparison of the transcranial Doppler (TCD) M-mode and spectral displays. The TCD continuous wave M-mode *(upper left)* and pulsed-wave spectral *(lower left)* displays are compared. The horizontal bands of the M-mode display represent a series of Doppler-shift echoes. Signals in the 30- to 50-mm depth range *(upper red band)* represent flow in the right middle cerebral artery *(right MCA)* ipsilateral to the ultrasonic probe. The *red color* signifies flow directed toward the probe *(right diagram).* Echoes arising between 55 and 70 mm from the probe emanate from the ipsilateral (right) anterior cerebral artery *(RACA)* are shown in the *middle blue band* of the M-mode display. Signals in the 72- to 85-mm range arise from the contralateral (left) ACA *(LACA)* with flow directed toward the probe *(lower red band).* The M-mode *yellow line* at a depth of 50 mm indicates the measurement site for the TCD frequency spectral display shown at the *lower left.* (Courtesy Dr. Mark Moehring, Spencer Technologies, Seattle, WA.)

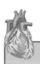

BOX 12.5 *Transcranial Doppler Ultrasonography*

Detects change in intracranial blood flow
Detects particulate or gaseous emboli

flow direction (red is flow directed toward the probe; blue is flow away from the probe), whereas color intensity is directly related to signal power.

Embolus Detection

Erythrocytes (approximately 5 million/mL) are the most acoustically reflective nonpathologic blood elements (ie, have the greatest acoustic impedance). However, gaseous and particulate emboli are better reflectors of sound than are erythrocytes. The presence of high-intensity transient signals (HITS) within either the PMD or spectral TCD display may signify the presence of an embolus.

Currently available spectral or PMD TCD monitors can determine neither the size nor the composition of emboliform material responsible for HITS (Box 12.5). Nevertheless, the HITS aggregate has been shown to be predictive of neurodeficit following aortic surgical procedures.

Intervention Threshold

Because erythrocyte velocity and flow may be differentially influenced by vessel diameter, blood viscosity, and pH, as well as temperature, TCD does not provide a reliable measure of cerebral blood flow. However, in the absence of hemodilution, *change* in TCD velocity does correlate closely with *change* in blood flow. Sudden large changes in velocity or direction are readily detected by continuous TCD monitoring. The clinical significance of velocity changes has been assessed in conscious patients during implantable cardioverter-defibrillator and tilt-table testing. In both circumstances, clinical evidence of cerebral hypoperfusion was accompanied by a mean velocity decline of greater than 60% and absent diastolic velocity. During vascular operations, the ischemia threshold appears to be an 80% decrease below the preincision baseline.

In general, reduction of flow velocity indicating severe ischemia is associated with profound depression of EEG activity. However, with adequate leptomeningeal collateral flow, cerebral function may remain unchanged in the presence of a severely decreased or absent middle cerebral artery flow velocity. Together, these findings form the rationale for a TCD-based intervention threshold. During cardiac surgical procedures, mean velocity reductions of greater than 80% or velocity losses during diastole suggest clinically significant cerebral hypoperfusion.

JUGULAR BULB OXIMETRY

Oximeter catheters transmitting three wavelengths of light may be inserted into the cerebral venous circulation to measure cerebral (jugular) venous oxygen saturation (S_{jvo_2}) directly and continuously. Commercially available devices are modifications of the catheter oximeter originally developed for the pulmonary circulation. Reflected light signals are averaged, filtered, and displayed. Conditions affecting the accuracy of these measurements include catheter kinking, blood flow around the catheter, changes in hematocrit, fibrin deposition on the catheter, and changes in temperature. The normal $SjvO_2$ range is widely assumed to be between 55% and 70%. However, a study using radiographically confirmed catheter placement observed a much wider 45% to 70% range in healthy subjects.

This technology has two major limitations. First, $SjvO_2$ represents a global measure of venous drainage from unspecified cranial compartments. Because cerebral and extracranial venous anatomy is notoriously varied, clinical interpretation of measured change is a major challenge. Second, accurate measurement using jugular oximetry requires continuous adequate flow past the catheter. Low-flow or no-flow states such as profound hypoperfusion or complete ischemia render $SjvO_2$ unreliable.

CEREBRAL OXIMETRY

Near-Infrared Technology

Because the human skull is translucent to infrared light, intracranial intravascular rSO_2 may be measured noninvasively with transcranial near-infrared spectroscopy (NIRS). An infrared light source contained in a self-adhesive patch affixed to glabrous skin of the scalp transmits photons through underlying tissues to the outer layers of the cerebral cortex. Adjacent sensors separate photons reflected from the skin, muscle, skull, and dura from those of the brain tissue (Fig. 12.13). NIRS measures all hemoglobin, pulsatile and nonpulsatile, in a mixed microvascular bed composed of gas–exchanging vessels with a diameter of less than 1 mm. The measurement is thought to reflect approximately 70% venous blood. Cerebral oximetry appears both to quantify

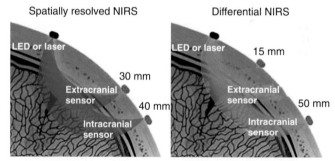

Fig. 12.13 Comparison of transcranial spatially resolved near-infrared spectroscopy *(spatially resolved NIRS)* and differential NIRS. Unabsorbed photons travel a parabolic (ie, banana-shaped) path through the adult cranium from scalp-mounted infrared sources to nearby sensors. The average penetration depth of these reflected photons is given by the square root of the source-detector separation. Spatially resolved NIRS uses a pair of sensors located at sufficient distances from the light source to ensure that both signals detect photons reflected from extracranial and intracranial tissue *(left panel)*. Two-point extracranial and intracranial measurement permits partial suppression of both the extracranial signal and the interpatient variance in intracranial photon scatter. The resultant cerebral oxygen saturation measurement appears to be approximately 65% intracranial. In contrast, differential NIRS uses a sensor placed very near the light source to record exclusively extracranial signal and another more distant sensor for extracranial and intracranial measurement *(right panel)*. Single-point subtraction suppresses much of the extracranial signal, but not the intersubject variation in intracranial photon scatter. Mitigation of this confounding influence is attempted through the use of additional infrared wavelengths. The proportion of the differential regional hemoglobin oxygen saturation signal that represents intracranial tissue has not been established. *LED,* Light-emitting diode. (Spatially resolved NIRS diagram courtesy of Covidien, Boulder, CO.)

change reliably from an individualized baseline and to offer an objective measure of regional hypoperfusion. Unlike pulse and jugular bulb oximetry, cerebral oximetry may be used during nonpulsatile CPB and circulatory arrest.

Similar to TCD monitoring, cerebral oximetry is primarily used to quantify change because the substantial NIRS intersubject baseline variability makes it difficult to establish a reliable threshold value signifying tissue injury. An adverse shift in oxygen supply-demand balance is indicated by a decreasing oxyhemoglobin fraction. The clinical significance of the decline has been demonstrated in conscious subjects and patients during G-force studies with high-speed centrifugation, implantable cardioverter-defibrillator testing, tilt-table testing, carotid artery occlusion, and intracranial artery balloon occlusion. In each setting, a decline of greater than 20% was associated with syncope or signs of focal cerebral ischemia. During adult and pediatric cardiac surgical procedures, the magnitude and duration of cerebral dysoxygenation are associated with hospital cost-driver increase as well as the incidence and severity of adverse clinical outcomes.

The clinical performance of cerebral oximetry systems appears to be device-specific. Supporting evidence for one device does not necessarily apply to competing products. Objective comparison of these devices remains difficult because of the lack of a universally accepted direct reference standard measure of regional brain microcirculatory oxygen saturation.

Validation

The rSo_2 value has been validated from arterial and jugular bulb oxygen saturation measurements in adults and children. Hypoxemia involving cerebral tissue proximate to the cranial optodes was consistently detected. Except during ischemia and CPB, $Sjvo_2$ and rSo_2 generally correlate in the midrange saturation, although discrepancies may appear at the extremes. The validity of rSo_2 also has been assessed by comparison with direct microprobe measurement of brain tissue oxygen partial pressure. The two measures appear to be directly and significantly related; however, the invasive monitoring of tissue oxygenation would be appropriate in few cardiac surgical situations.

MULTIMODALITY NEUROMONITORING

Because each monitoring modality may evaluate only a portion of the CNS, multimodal monitoring would appear to be desirable to monitor neurologic wellness more completely (Table 12.4).

Surgery on the Aorta

Circulatory Arrest

When the planned technique includes circulatory arrest, with or without retrograde cerebral perfusion, the first imperative is to ensure that the brain is adequately cooled to withstand the necessary period of cerebral ischemia. Optimal protection of cerebral cortical tissue by cooling occurs when electrical silence has occurred on the electroencephalogram because more than 60% of the brain's metabolic effort is expended in the generation of electrical signals. Cooling slows the electroencephalogram in a dose-dependent fashion (Fig. 12.14), with recovery following a similar pattern but not necessarily following the same curve or returning completely to baseline. The actual temperature at which electrical silence occurs can vary from 11° to 18°C, and therefore reliance on temperature alone may prolong cooling (and therefore rewarming and bypass) unnecessarily.

Table 12.4	Multimodality Neuromonitoring for Cardiac Surgical Procedures	

Modality	Function
Electroencephalography	Cortical synaptic activity
Brainstem auditory-evoked potentials	Cochlear, auditory nerve, and brainstem auditory pathway function
Middle latency auditory-evoked potentials	Subcortical-cortical afferent auditory pathway function
Somatosensory-evoked potentials	Peripheral nerve, spinal cord, and brain somatosensory afferent pathway function
Transcranial motor-evoked potentials	Cortical, subcortical, spinal cord, and peripheral nerve efferent motor pathway function
Transcranial Doppler ultrasonography	Cerebral blood flow change and emboli detection
Tissue oximetry	Regional tissue oxygen balance

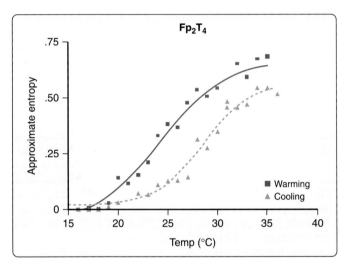

Fig. 12.14   Cooling and rewarming in circulatory arrest. The approximate entropy was calculated from a single channel of the electroencephalogram during cooling to 18°C for circulatory arrest and subsequent rewarming. The delay in the resumption of electroencephalographic activity as a function of nasal temperature is clearly evident. (From Levy WJ, Pantin E, Mehta S, et al. Hypothermia and the approximate entropy of the electroencephalogram. *Anesthesiology*. 2003;98:53–57, with permission of the publisher.)

Cooling prolongs SSEP peak and interpeak latencies and suppresses amplitude of the cortical response predominantly (see Fig. 12.7B). Consequently, SSEP responses can also be used to assess cooling. However, because subcortical SSEP responses involve far fewer synapses than the electroencephalogram, these responses often persist when cortical neuronal activity is totally cold-suppressed. Thus detection of cerebral ischemia by SSEPs can be achieved during EEG quiescence. Because clinical results with EEG guidance of cooling are quite good, it is not clear that SSEP monitoring offers any advantage.

A subset of patients undergoing circulatory arrest has aortic dissections and, in this population, evidence indicates that TCD monitoring may be beneficial. One prospective investigation demonstrated that TCD monitoring during acute aortic dissection repair reduced the incidence of transient neurologic deficit from 52% to 15%, although no significant change was observed in the incidence of stroke or in-hospital or 30-day mortality rates.

Antegrade Cerebral Perfusion

Management of aortic surgical procedures using antegrade cerebral perfusion through the right subclavian artery typically involves only moderate hypothermia. However, the potential for cerebral ischemia secondary to an incomplete circle of Willis emphasizes the need for the early detection of ischemia with some form of neuromonitoring. The circle of Willis is completely normal in only a small fraction (25%) of patients, although many of the anomalies consist of hypoplasia (not absence) of a single segment and may not predispose patients to ischemia. Theoretic arguments favor a multichannel EEG montage because the region of malperfusion cannot be predicted with certainty. The acute occurrence of asymmetry in any monitored modality coincident with initiation of perfusion through the right subclavian artery would suggest a need to change surgical technique.

The use of only moderate hypothermia with antegrade cerebral perfusion potentially predisposes patients to another neurologic complication: spinal cord ischemia. Because the brain is perfused but the body is not, a theoretic concern exists about the integrity of the spinal neurons that could justify SSEP monitoring. Clinical reports of spinal cord complications following aortic repair using antegrade cerebral perfusion are infrequent, a finding suggesting that this complication is more theoretic than real.

Descending Aorta Surgery

Surgical procedures on the descending thoracic aorta may involve partial (left atrial to left femoral) bypass, complete circulatory arrest, or entirely endovascular techniques. If circulatory arrest is used because proximal cross-clamping is not possible, the issues already discussed regarding circulatory arrest remain considerations. In addition, and regardless of the management of bypass, operations on the descending aorta impose significant risk of spinal cord ischemia and warrant consideration of neurologic monitoring for early diagnosis and treatment. Three modalities have the potential to provide this information—SSEPs, MEPs, and tissue oxygenation, although the last is currently viewed as highly experimental. Anatomic considerations of the vascular supply to the spinal cord suggest that the anterior structures, perfused by radicular arteries from the aorta, are at greater risk than are the posterior columns, whose perfusion is derived as an extension of the vertebral artery. These considerations would suggest that MEP monitoring would be the preferred technology. Comparative studies of MEP and SSEP monitoring have shown very high predictive values for ischemia if the changes are permanent. However, SSEP monitoring is relatively resistant to potent agents and muscle relaxants, thereby allowing intraoperative use. By comparison, exclusion of these common techniques greatly complicates the anesthetic management of patients when MEP monitoring is planned.

Routine Coronary Artery Bypass Graft and Valve Procedures

NIRS monitoring has been the most thoroughly studied of the neuromonitoring techniques in recent years. The profusion of interest comes both from the (apparent) simplicity of the device and the stimulus of commercial enterprises to justify their use. Different devices use different proprietary techniques to extract the signal, and they may result in different values of rSo_2 under identical clinical conditions. This renders the determination of the threshold for treatment somewhat arbitrary and results in the assessment of value on the basis of improvement in surrogate measures (eg, improvement in rSo_2) and not on the prevention of complications.

Extracorporeal Membrane Oxygenation

Extracorporeal membrane oxygenation (ECMO) is becoming more common for the support of patients with failing cardiac or pulmonary function. The magnitude of the support can encompass complete bypass of the native cardiopulmonary function; however, some cardiac ejection commonly occurs even though ECMO flows are providing essentially all systemic needs. This small cardiac output consists of blood that has gone through the lungs and may be inadequately oxygenated if the patient has respiratory failure. This blood preferentially perfuses the innominate artery, and thus the right side of the brain may be receiving hypoxic blood even though arterial blood gas measurements (obtained from an indwelling catheter in the groin or left radial artery) appear normal. Although application of pulse oximeters to fingers of both hands may detect such right-sided desaturation, the pulse waveform during ECMO is often inadequate for detection of the saturation by pulse oximetry. Cerebral oximetry is well suited for assessing the development of unilateral desaturation in these patients, who may need to be monitored continuously for days or weeks.

Depth of Anesthesia

For assessment of anesthetic depth, BIS or other processed EEG methods are the most commonly used technologies. These hypnotic indices appear to provide clinically useful information. However, their *fundamental differences may result in monitor-specific performance, so agreement among these measures during surgical procedures should not be expected.* Reported rates of intraoperative awareness during cardiac operations range from 0.2% to 2%, a 10-fold increase in risk compared with the general surgical population. The American Society of Anesthesiologists Practice Advisory on Awareness and Brain Monitoring made the recommendation that the decision to use a brain monitor, including a BIS monitor, should be made on a case-by-case basis and should not be considered standard of care.

12

☒ SUMMARY

Cardiac surgical procedures vary significantly in their associated risk of neurologic injury, the portion of the nervous system at risk, and the options for treatment if injury is identified. Aggressive treatment of clinically insignificant or ambiguous changes may carry unrecognized risks that effectively counter the expected benefit of treatment. An understanding of the methodologies, the underlying physiology, and the therapeutic options is necessary for appropriate application of these technologies during cardiac surgical procedures.

SUGGESTED READINGS

American Society of Anesthesiologists Task Force on Intraoperative Awareness. Practice advisory for intraoperative awareness and brain function monitoring: a report by the American Society of Anesthesiologists Task Force on Intraoperative Awareness. *Anesthesiology.* 2006;104:847–864.

Avidan MS, Jacobsohn E, Glick D, et al. Prevention of intraoperative awareness in a high-risk surgical population. *N Engl J Med.* 2011;365:591–600.

Avidan MS, Zhang L, Burnside BA, et al. Anesthesia awareness and the bispectral index. *N Engl J Med.* 2008;358:1097–1108.

Bickler PE, Feiner JR, Rollins MD. Factors affecting the performance of 5 cerebral oximeters during hypoxia in healthy volunteers. *Anesth Analg.* 2013;117:813.

Bismuth J, Garami Z, Anaya-Ayala JE, et al. Transcranial Doppler findings during thoracic endovascular aortic repair. *J Vasc Surg.* 2011;54:364.

Dabrowski W, Rzecki Z, Pilat J, et al. Brain damage in cardiac surgery patients. *Curr Opin Pharmacol.* 2012;12:1.

Deschamps A, Lambert J, Cuture P, et al. Reversal of decreases in cerebral saturation in high-risk cardiac surgery. *J Cardiothorac Vasc Anesth.* 2013;27:1260.

Ferrari M, Quaresima V. Near infrared brain and muscle oximetry: from the discovery to current applications. *J Near Infrared Spectrosc.* 2012;20:1.

Hunter GRW, Young GB. Seizures after cardiac surgery. *J Cardiothorac Vasc Anesth.* 2011;25:299.

Levy WJ, Pantin E, Mehta S, et al. Hypothermia and the approximate entropy of the electroencephalogram. *Anesthesiology.* 2003;98:53–57.

McCarthy RJ, McCabe AE, Walker R, et al. The value of transcranial Doppler in predicting cerebral ischaemia during carotid endarterectomy. *Eur J Vasc Endovasc Surg.* 2001;21:408.

Papantchev V, Hristove S, Todorova D, et al. Some variations of the circle of Willis, important for cerebral protection in aortic surgery: a study in Eastern Europeans. *Eur J Cardiothorac Surg.* 2007;31(27):982.

Samra SK, Rajajee V. Monitoring of jugular venous oxygen saturation. In: Koht A, Sloan TB, Toleikis JR, eds. *Monitoring the Nervous System for Anesthesiologists and Other Health Care Professionals.* New York: Springer; 2012:255–277.

Seubert CN, Herman M. Auditory evoked potentials. In: Koht A, Sloan TB, Toleikis JR, eds. *Monitoring the Nervous System for Anesthesiologists and Other Health Care Professionals.* New York: Springer; 2012:47–68.

Sloan TB, Jameson LC. Surgery on thoracoabdominal aortic aneurysms. In: Koht A, Sloan TB, Toleikis JR, eds. *Monitoring the Nervous System for Anesthesiologists and Other Health Care Professionals.* New York: Springer; 2012:705–722.

Sloan TB. General anesthesia for monitoring. In: Koht A, Sloan TB, Toleikis JR, eds. *Monitoring the Nervous System for Anesthesiologists and Other Health Care Professionals.* New York: Springer; 2012:319–336.

Stecker MM, Cheung AT, Pochettino A, et al. Deep hypothermic circulatory arrest. I. Effects of cooling on electroencephalogram and evoked potentials. *Ann Thorac Surg.* 2001;71:14–21.

Tsai JY, Pan W, Lemaire SA, et al. Moderate hypothermia during aortic arch surgery is associated with reduced risk of early mortality. *J Thorac Cardiovasc Surg.* 2013;146:662.

Werther T, Olischar M, Giordano V, et al. Bispectral index and lower margin amplitude of the amplitude-integrated electroencephalogram in neonates. *Neonatology.* 2015;107:34.

Zheng F, Sheinberg R, Yee M-S, et al. Cerebral near-infrared spectroscopy monitoring and neurologic outcomes in adult cardiac surgery patients: a systematic review. *Anesth Analg.* 2013;116:198.

III

Chapter 13

Coagulation Monitoring

Linda Shore-Lesserson, MD • Liza J. Enriquez, MD •
Nathaen Weitzel, MD

Key Points

1. Monitoring the effect of heparin is done using the activated coagulation time (ACT), a functional test of heparin anticoagulation. The ACT is susceptible to prolongation because of hypothermia and hemodilution and to reduction because of platelet activation or thrombocytopathy.
2. Heparin resistance can be congenital or acquired. Pretreatment heparin exposure predisposes a patient to altered heparin responsiveness because of antithrombin III depletion, platelet activation, or activation of extrinsic coagulation.
3. Before considering a transfusion of plasma, it is important to document that the effect of heparin has been neutralized. This can be done using a heparinase-neutralized test or a protamine-neutralized test.
4. Point-of-care tests are available for use in transfusion algorithms that can measure coagulation factor activity (normalized ratio, activated partial thromboplastin time) and platelet function.
5. Newer thrombin inhibitor drugs are available for anticoagulation in patients who cannot receive heparin. These can be monitored using the ecarin clotting time or a modified ACT. Bivalirudin and hirudin are the two direct thrombin inhibitors that have been used most often in cardiac surgical procedures.
6. Platelet dysfunction is the most common reason for bleeding after cardiopulmonary bypass. Point-of-care tests can be used to measure specific aspects of platelet function.
7. The degree of platelet inhibition as measured by standard or point-of-care instruments has been shown to correlate with decreased ischemic outcomes after coronary intervention. However, cardiac surgical patients who are receiving antiplatelet medication are at increased risk for postoperative bleeding.

The need to monitor anticoagulation during and after surgical procedures is the reason that the cardiac surgical setting has evolved into a major area for the evaluation and use of hemostasis monitors. The rapid and accurate identification of abnormal hemostasis has been the major impetus toward the development of point-of-care (POC) tests that can be performed at the bedside or in the operating room. The detection and treatment of specific coagulation disorders in a timely and cost-efficient manner are major goals in hemostasis monitoring for the cardiac surgical patient.

MONITORING HEPARIN EFFECT

Cardiac surgical procedures had been performed for decades with empiric heparin dosing in the form of a bolus and subsequent interval dosing. Empiric dosing continued because of the lack of an easily applicable bedside test to monitor the anticoagulant effects of heparin.

The first clotting time used to measure heparin effect was the whole-blood clotting time (WBCT) or the Lee-White WBCT. This test simply requires whole blood to be placed in a glass tube, maintained at 37°C, and manually tilted until blood fluidity is no longer detected. This test fell out of favor for monitoring cardiac surgical patients because it was so labor intensive and required the undivided attention of the person performing the test for up to 30 minutes. Although the glass surface of the test tube acts as an activator of factor XII, the heparin doses used for cardiac surgical procedures prolong the WBCT to such a profound degree that the test is impractical as a monitor of the effect of heparin during cardiac operations. To speed the clotting time so that the test was appropriate for clinical use, activators were added to the test tubes, and the activated coagulation time (ACT) was introduced into practice.

Activated Coagulation Time

The ACT was first introduced by Hattersley in 1966 and is still the most widely used monitor of heparin effect during cardiac surgical procedures. Whole blood is added to a test tube containing an activator, either diatomaceous earth (Celite) or kaolin. The presence of activator augments the contact activation phase of coagulation, which stimulates the intrinsic coagulation pathway. The ACT can be performed manually, whereby the operator measures the time interval from when blood is injected into the test tube to when clot is seen along the sides of the tube. More commonly, the ACT is automated, as it is in the Hemochron (International Technidyne Corp., Edison, NJ) and ACT Plus (Medtronic Perfusion Services, Minneapolis, MN) systems. In the automated systems, the test tube is placed in a device that warms the sample to 37°C. The Hemochron device rotates the test tube, which contains Celite activator and a small iron cylinder, to which 2 mL of whole blood is added. Before clot forms, the cylinder rolls along the bottom of the rotating test tube. When clot forms, the cylinder is pulled away from a magnetic detector, interrupts a magnetic field, and signals the end of the clotting time. Normal ACT values range from 80 to 120 seconds. The Hemochron ACT also can be performed using kaolin as the activator in a similar manner.

The ACT Plus (formerly Hemotec [Hepcon] ACT) device is a cartridge with two chambers that contain kaolin activator and are housed in a heat block. Blood (0.4 mL) is placed into each chamber, and a daisy-shaped plunger is raised and passively falls into the chamber. The formation of clot slows the rate of descent of the plunger. This decrease in velocity of the plunger is detected by a photo-optical system that signals the end of the ACT test. The Hemochron and Hemotec ACT tests have been compared in several investigations and have been found to differ significantly at low heparin concentrations. However, differences in heparin concentration, activator concentration, and the measurement technique make comparison of these tests difficult and have led to the realization that the results of the Hemochron and Hemotec ACT tests are not interchangeable. In adult patients given 300 IU/kg of heparin for cardiopulmonary bypass (CPB), the Hemochron and Hemotec ACTs were both therapeutic at all time points, although the Hemochron ACT was statistically longer at two time points.

The ACT test can be modified by the addition of heparinase. With this modification, the coagulation status of the patient can be monitored during CPB while the anti-coagulant effects of heparin are eliminated. Because this test is a side-by-side comparison of the untreated ACT with the heparinase ACT, it also has the advantage of being a rapid test for assessment of a circulating heparin-like substance or for residual heparinization after CPB.

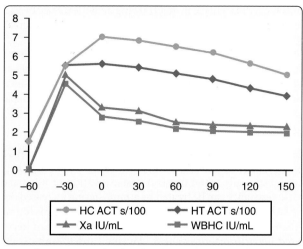

Fig. 13.1 Anticoagulation measured at baseline (−60 minutes), at heparinization (−30 minutes), and six time points after institution of cardiopulmonary bypass. Note the close correlation between the anti–factor Xa *(Xa; triangles)* activity and whole-blood heparin concentration *(WBHC; squares)*, which does not parallel the change in Hemochron (International Technidyne Corp., Edison, NJ) activated coagulation time (ACT) *(HC ACT; circles)* or Hemotec (Medtronic Perfusion Services, Minneapolis, MN) ACT *(HT ACT; diamonds)*. (Modified from Despotis GJ, Summerfield AL, Joist JH. Comparison of activated coagulation time and whole blood heparin measurements with laboratory plasma anti-Xa heparin concentration in patients having cardiac operations. *J Thorac Cardiovasc Surg.* 1994;108:1076–1082.)

With the introduction of ACT monitoring into cardiac surgical practice, clinicians have been able to titrate heparin and protamine dosages more accurately. As a result, many investigators report reductions in blood loss and transfusion requirements, although many of these studies used retrospective analyses. The improvements in postoperative hemostasis documented with ACT monitoring are potentially attributable to better intraoperative suppression of microvascular coagulation and improved monitoring of heparin reversal with protamine.

ACT monitoring of heparinization is not without pitfalls, and its use has been criticized because of the extreme variability of the ACT and the absence of a correlation with plasma heparin levels (Fig. 13.1). Many factors have been suggested to alter the ACT, and these factors are prevalent during cardiac surgical procedures. When the extracorporeal circuit prime is added to the patient's blood volume, hemodilution occurs and may theoretically increase the ACT. Evidence suggests that this degree of hemodilution alone is not enough to alter the ACT. Hypothermia increases the ACT in a "dose-related" fashion. Although hemodilution and hypothermia significantly increase the ACT of a heparinized blood sample, similar increases do not occur in the absence of added heparin. The effects of platelet alterations are more problematic. At mild-to-moderate degrees of thrombocytopenia, the baseline and heparinized ACTs are not affected. It is not until platelet counts are reduced to less than 30,000 to 50,000/µL that the ACT may be prolonged. Patients treated with platelet inhibitors such as prostacyclin, aspirin, or platelet membrane receptor antagonists have a prolonged heparinized ACT compared with patients not treated with platelet inhibitors. This ACT prolongation is not related exclusively to decreased levels of platelet factor 4 (PF4; PF4 is a heparin-neutralizing substance) because it also occurs when blood is anticoagulated with substances that are not neutralized by PF4. Platelet lysis, however, significantly shortens the ACT because of the release of PF4 and other platelet membrane

13

components, which may have heparin-neutralizing activities. Anesthesia and operation decrease the ACT and create a hypercoagulable state, possibly by creating a thromboplastic response or through activation of platelets.

During CPB, heparin decay varies substantially, and its measurement is problematic because hemodilution and hypothermia alter the metabolism of heparin. In a CPB study, the consumption of heparin varied from 0.01 to 3.86 IU/kg/min, and no correlation was noted between the initial sensitivity to heparin and the rate of heparin decay.

Heparin Resistance

Heparin resistance is documented by an inability to increase the ACT of blood to expected levels despite an adequate dose and plasma concentration of heparin. In many clinical situations, especially when heparin desensitization or a heparin inhibitor is suspected, heparin resistance can be treated by administering increased doses of heparin in a competitive fashion. If an adequately prolonged clotting time is ultimately achieved using greater-than-expected doses of heparin, a better term than heparin resistance would be "altered heparin responsiveness." During cardiac surgical procedures, the belief that a safe minimum ACT value of 300 to 400 seconds is required for CPB is based on a few clinical studies and a relative paucity of scientific data. However, an inability to attain this degree of anticoagulation in the heparin-resistant patient engenders the fear among cardiac surgical providers that the patient will experience microvascular consumptive coagulopathy or that clots will form in the extracorporeal circuit.

Many clinical conditions are associated with heparin resistance. Sepsis, liver disease, and pharmacologic agents represent just a few. Many investigators have documented decreased levels of antithrombin III (AT III) secondary to heparin pretreatment. Patients receiving preoperative heparin therapy traditionally require larger heparin doses to achieve a given level of anticoagulation when that anticoagulation is measured by the ACT. Presumably, this "heparin resistance" is the result of deficiencies in the level or activity of AT III. Other possible causes include enhanced factor VIII activity and platelet dysfunction leading to a decrease in ACT response to heparin. In vitro addition of AT III enhances the ACT response to heparin. AT III concentrate is available as a heat-treated human product or in recombinant form, and its use is a reasonable method of treating patients with documented AT III deficiency (Box 13.1).

Measurement of Heparin Sensitivity

Even in the absence of heparin resistance, patients' responses to an intravenous bolus of heparin are extremely variable. The variability stems from different concentrations of various endogenous heparin-binding proteins such as vitronectin and PF4. This variability exists whether measuring heparin concentration or the ACT; however,

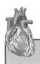

BOX 13.1 *Heparin Resistance*

It is primarily caused by antithrombin III deficiency in pediatric patients.
It is multifactorial in adult cardiac surgical patients.
The critical activated coagulation time value necessary in patients who demonstrate acquired heparin resistance is not yet determined.
Heparin resistance also can be a sign of heparin-induced thrombocytopenia.

variability seems to be greater when measuring the ACT. Because of the large interpatient variation in heparin responsiveness and the potential for heparin resistance, it is critical that a functional monitor of heparin anticoagulation (with or without a measure of heparin concentration) be used in the cardiac surgical patient. Bull documented a threefold range of ACT response to a 200 IU/kg heparin dose and similar discrepancy in heparin decay rates and thus recommended the use of individual patient dose-response curves to determine the optimal heparin dose. This is the concept on which POC individual heparin dose-response (HDR) tests are based.

An HDR curve can be generated manually by using the baseline ACT and the ACT response to an in vivo or in vitro dose of heparin. Extrapolation to the desired ACT provides the additional heparin dose required for that ACT. Once the actual ACT response to the heparin dose is plotted, further dose-response calculations are made based on the average of the target ACT and the actual ACT (Fig. 13.2). This method was first described by Bull and forms the scientific basis for the automated

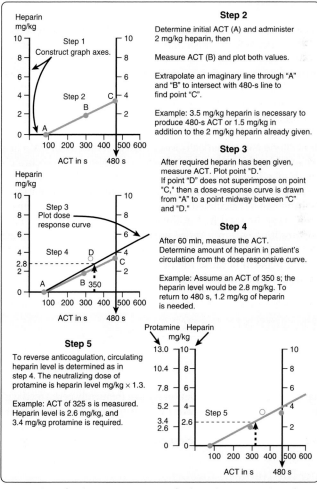

Fig. 13.2 Construction of a dose-response curve for heparin. *ACT*, Activated coagulation time. (From Bull BS, Huse WM, Brauer FS, et al. Heparin therapy during extracorporeal circulation. II. The use of a dose-response curve to individualize heparin and protamine dosage. *J Thorac Cardiovasc Surg.* 1975;69:685–689.)

dose-response systems in the proprietary Hemochron and Hemotec devices. The Hemochron RxDx (International Technidyne Corp., Edison, NJ) system uses the heparin-response test, which is an ACT with a known quantity of in vitro heparin (3 IU/mL). A dose-response curve is generated that enables calculation of the heparin dose required to attain the target ACT by using an algorithm that incorporates the patient's baseline ACT, estimated blood volume, and heparin-response test. The patient's heparin sensitivity can be calculated in seconds per international units per milliliter (s/IU/mL) by dividing the heparin-response test by 3 IU/mL.

The Hemochron RxDx system also provides an individualized protamine dose based on the protamine-response test (PRT). This is an ACT with one of two specific quantities of protamine, depending on the amount of circulating heparin suspected (2 or 3 IU/mL). The protamine dose needed to return the ACT to baseline can be calculated on the basis of a protamine-response curve using the patient's heparinized ACT, the PRT, and an estimate of the patient's blood volume.

Heparin Concentration

Proponents of ACT measurement to guide anticoagulation for CPB argue that a functional assessment of the anticoagulant effect of heparin is mandatory and that the variability in ACT represents a true variability in the coagulation status of the patient. Opponents argue that during CPB, the sensitivity of the ACT to heparin is altered, and ACT does not correlate with heparin concentration or with anti–factor Xa activity measurement. Heparin concentration can be measured using the Hepcon HMS system, which uses an automated protamine titration technique. With a cartridge with four or six chambers containing tissue thromboplastin and a series of known protamine concentrations, 0.2 mL of whole blood is automatically dispensed into the chambers. The first channel to clot is the channel in which the protamine concentration most accurately neutralizes the heparin without a heparin or a protamine excess. Because protamine neutralizes heparin in the ratio of 1 mg protamine per 100 IU heparin, the concentration of heparin in the blood sample can be calculated. A cartridge that monitors heparin concentration over a wide range can be used first, followed by another cartridge that can measure heparin concentrations within a more narrow range. The maintenance of a stable heparin concentration rather than a specific ACT level usually results in administration of larger doses of heparin because the hemodilution and hypothermia during CPB increase the sensitivity of the ACT to heparin.

HEPARIN NEUTRALIZATION

Protamine Effects on Coagulation Monitoring

Reversal of heparin-induced anticoagulation is most frequently performed with protamine. Different successful dosing plans have been proposed. The recommended dose of protamine for heparin reversal is 1 to 1.3 mg protamine per 100 IU heparin; however, this dose often results in a protamine excess.

Monitoring for Heparin Rebound

The phenomenon referred to as heparin rebound describes the re-establishment of a heparinized state after heparin has been neutralized with protamine. The most commonly postulated explanation is that rapid distribution and clearance of protamine occur shortly after protamine administration, thus leaving unbound heparin remaining after protamine clearance. Furthermore, endogenous heparin antagonists have an even shorter life span than protamine and are eliminated rapidly, resulting in free heparin concentrations. Also possible is the release of heparin from tissues considered heparin storage sites (endothelium, connective tissues). Endothelial cells bind and depolymerize heparin through PF4. Uptake into the cells of the reticuloendothelial system, vascular smooth muscle, and extracellular fluid may account for the storage of heparin that contributes to the reactivation of heparin anticoagulation referred to as heparin rebound.

Residual low levels of heparin can be detected by sensitive heparin concentration monitoring in the first hour after protamine reversal and can be present for up to 6 hours postoperatively. Without careful monitoring for heparin rebound in the postoperative period, increased bleeding as a result of heparin rebound may occur, specifically when larger doses of heparin have been administered. Monitoring for heparin rebound can be accomplished using tests that are sensitive to low levels of circulating heparin. These tests are also useful monitors for confirmation of heparin neutralization at the conclusion of CPB.

Heparin Neutralization Monitors

To administer the appropriate dose of protamine at the conclusion of CPB, it would be ideal to measure the concentration of heparin present and give the dose of protamine necessary to neutralize only the circulating heparin. As a result of heparin metabolism and elimination, which vary considerably among individual patients, the dose of protamine required to reverse a given dose of heparin decreases over time. Furthermore, protamine antagonizes the anti–factor IIa effects of heparin more effectively than the anti–factor Xa effects and thus varies in its potency depending on the source of heparin and its anti–factor IIa properties. Administration of a large fixed dose of protamine or a dose based on the total heparin dose given is no longer the standard of care and may result in an increased incidence of protamine-related adverse effects. An optimal dose of protamine is desired because unneutralized heparin results in clinical bleeding, and an excess of protamine may produce undesired coagulopathy. The use of individualized protamine dose-response curves uniformly results in a reduced protamine dose and has been shown to reduce postoperative bleeding. One such dose-response test, the Hemochron PRT test, is an ACT performed on a heparinized blood sample that contains a known quantity of protamine. With knowledge of the ACT, PRT, and the estimated blood volume of the patient, the protamine dose needed to neutralize the existing heparin level can be extrapolated. The Hepcon instrument also has a PRT, which is the protamine titration assay. The chamber that clots first contains the dose of protamine that most closely approximates the circulating dose of heparin. The protamine dose required for heparin neutralization is calculated on the basis of a specified heparin/protamine dose ratio by measuring the circulating heparin level.

At the levels of heparinization needed for cardiac surgical procedures, tests that are sensitive to heparin become unclottable. The ACT is relatively insensitive to heparin and is ideal for monitoring anticoagulation at high heparin levels, but it is too insensitive to detect incomplete heparin neutralization accurately. The ACT has a high predictive value for adequate anticoagulation (confirmed by laboratory activated partial thromboplastin time [aPTT]) when the ACT is longer than 225 seconds but is poorly predictive for inadequate anticoagulation when the ACT is shorter than 225 seconds. The low levels of heparin present when heparin is incompletely neutralized are best measured by other, more sensitive tests of heparin-induced anticoagulation, such as heparin

13

BOX 13.2   *Heparin Neutralization*

BOX 13.2   *Heparin Neutralization*

The most benign form of bleeding after cardiac surgical procedures results from residual heparinization.

Treatment is with either protamine or another heparin-neutralizing product.

Transfusion of allogeneic blood products is rarely indicated.

Residual heparin can be measured by using the following:

- A protamine titration assay
- A heparin-neutralized thrombin time assay
- A heparinase-activated coagulation time (ACT) compared with ACT
- Any other heparinase test that compares itself with the test without heparinase added.

---

concentration, aPTT, and TT. Thus, after CPB, confirmation of return to the unanticoagulated state should be performed with a sensitive test for heparin anticoagulation (Box 13.2).

TESTS OF COAGULATION

Standard tests of coagulation, the prothrombin time (PT) and the aPTT, are performed on plasma to which the anticoagulant citrate has been added. Because these tests are performed on plasma, they require centrifugation of blood and generally are not feasible for use at the bedside. The aPTT tests the integrity of the intrinsic and the final coagulation pathways and is more sensitive to low levels of heparin than the ACT. Factors IX and X are most sensitive to heparin effects, and thus the aPTT is prolonged even at very low heparin levels. The test uses a phospholipid substance to simulate the interaction of the platelet membrane in activating factor XII. (Thromboplastin is a tissue extract containing tissue factor and phospholipid. The term *partial thromboplastin* refers to the use of the phospholipid portion only.) The aPTT is prolonged in the presence of the following deficiencies: factors XII, XI, IX, and VIII; HMWK (high-molecular-weight kininogen); and kallikrein. The aPTT reaction is considerably slower than the PT, and an activator such as Celite or kaolin is added to the assay to speed activation of factor XII. After incubation of citrated plasma with phospholipid and activator, calcium is added, and the time to clot formation is measured. Normal aPTT is 28 to 32 seconds, which often is expressed as a ratio with a control plasma sample from the same laboratory. This is important because partial thromboplastin reagents have different sensitivities to heparin, and many have nonlinear responses to heparin in various concentration ranges.

The PT measures the integrity of the extrinsic and common coagulation pathways. The PT is prolonged in the presence of factor VII deficiency, warfarin sodium (Coumadin) therapy, or vitamin K deficiency. Large doses of heparin also prolong the PT because of factor II inactivation. The addition of thromboplastin to citrated plasma results in activation of extrinsic coagulation. After a 3-minute incubation and recalcification, the time to clot formation is measured and is recorded as the PT. Normal PT is 12 to 14 seconds; however, because of differences in the quality and lot of the thromboplastin used, absolute PT values are not standardized and are difficult to compare across different testing centers. The international normalized ratio (INR) has been adopted as the standard for coagulation monitoring. The INR is an

III

internationally standardized laboratory value that is the ratio of the patient's PT to the result that would have been obtained if the International Reference Preparation had been used instead of the laboratory reagents. Each laboratory uses reagents with a specific sensitivity (International Sensitivity Index [ISI]) relative to the International Reference Preparation. The ISI of a particular set of reagents is provided by each manufacturer so that the INR can be reported.

Bedside Tests of Coagulation

The PT and aPTT tests performed on whole blood are available for use in the operating room or at the bedside. The Hemochron PT test tube contains acetone-dried rabbit brain thromboplastin to which 2 mL of whole blood is added, and the tube is inserted into a standard Hemochron machine. Normal values range from 50 to 72 seconds and are automatically converted by a computer to the plasma-equivalent PT and INR. The Hemochron aPTT contains kaolin activator and a platelet factor substitute and is performed similarly to the PT. The aPTT is sensitive to heparin concentrations as low as 0.2 IU/mL and displays a linear relationship with heparin concentration up to 1.5 IU/mL.

A comparison of bedside coagulation monitors after cardiac surgical procedures documented acceptable accuracy and precision levels for the Hemochron and Ciba Corning Biotrack PTs in comparison with the standard laboratory plasma PT, thus making them potentially valuable for use in the perioperative period. Neither the Hemochron aPTT nor the Ciba Corning aPTT reached this level of clinical competence compared with standard laboratory tests. Because of rapid turnaround times, these POC coagulation monitors may be useful in predicting which patients will bleed after cardiac surgical procedures, and they have also been used successfully in transfusion algorithms to decrease the number of allogeneic blood products given to cardiac surgical patients.

Fibrinogen Level

A whole-blood POC fibrinogen assay is available using the Hemochron system. The specific test tube contains a lyophilized preparation of human thrombin, snake venom extract, protamine, buffers, and calcium stabilizers. The test tube is incubated with 1.5 mL of distilled water and is heated in the Hemochron instrument for 3 minutes. Whole blood is placed into a diluent vial, where it is 50% diluted, and from this vial, 0.5 mL of diluted whole blood is placed into the specific fibrinogen test tube. The clotting time is measured using standard Hemochron technology, as described previously. The fibrinogen concentration is determined by comparison with a standard curve for this test. Normal fibrinogen concentration of 180 to 220 mg/dL correlates with a clotting time of 54 ± 2.5 seconds. Fibrinogen deficiency of 50 to 75 mg/dL correlates with a clotting time of 150 ± 9.0 seconds.

◾ MONITORING THE THROMBIN INHIBITORS

A newer class of drugs, the selective thrombin inhibitors, provides a viable alternative to heparin anticoagulation for CPB. These agents include hirudin, argatroban, bivalirudin, and experimental agents. A major advantage of these agents over heparin is that they can effectively inhibit clot-bound thrombin in an AT III–independent fashion. They are also useful in patients with heparin-induced thrombocytopenia (HIT), in whom the administration of heparin and subsequent antibody-induced

13

platelet aggregation would be dangerous. The lack of a potent antidote (eg, protamine) and a prolonged duration of action are the major reasons that hirudin and other thrombin inhibitors have not found widespread clinical acceptance for use in CPB procedures.

Bivalirudin

Bivalirudin is a small, 20–amino acid molecule with a plasma half-life of 24 minutes. It is a synthetic derivative of hirudin and thus acts as a direct thrombin inhibitor. Bivalirudin binds to both the catalytic binding site and the anion-binding exosite on fluid-phase and clot-bound thrombin. The part of the molecule that binds to thrombin is actually cleaved by thrombin itself, so the elimination of bivalirudin activity is independent of specific organ metabolism. Bivalirudin has been used successfully as an anticoagulant agent in interventional cardiology procedures as a replacement for heparin therapy (Box 13.3).

Multicenter clinical trials comparing bivalirudin with heparin anticoagulation in off-pump coronary artery bypass operations and in CPB demonstrated "noninferiority" of bivalirudin. Efficacy of anticoagulation and markers of blood loss were similar in the two groups, a finding suggesting that bivalirudin can be a safe and effective anticoagulant agent in CPB. These multicenter trials used the ACT as the monitor of anticoagulant activity intraoperatively, but ideal monitoring is performed using the ecarin clotting time. The ecarin clotting time has a closer correlation with anti–factor IIa activity and plasma drug levels than does the ACT. For this reason, standard ACT monitoring during antithrombin therapy is not preferred if ecarin clotting time can be measured. A plasma-modified ACT can be used to assay the anticoagulant effects of the thrombin inhibitor drugs more accurately than ACT. This test requires the addition of exogenous plasma and thus is not readily available as a POC assay.

▦ MONITORING PLATELET FUNCTION

Platelet Count

Numerous events during cardiac surgical procedures predispose patients to platelet-related hemostasis defects. The two major categories are thrombocytopenia and qualitative platelet defects. Thrombocytopenia commonly occurs during cardiac surgical procedures as a result of hemodilution, sequestration, and destruction by nonendothelial surfaces. Platelet counts commonly decline to 100,000/μL or less; however, the final

III

BOX 13.4   *Platelet Function*

The platelet count does not correlate with bleeding after cardiac surgical procedures.

Patients frequently have extreme degrees of thrombocytopenia but do not bleed because they have adequate platelet function.

The measure of platelet function correlates temporally with the bleeding course seen after cardiac surgical procedures.

The thromboelastogram maximal amplitude, mean platelet volume, and other functional platelet tests are useful in transfusion algorithms.

platelet count greatly depends on the starting value and the duration of platelet-destructive interventions (ie, CPB). Between 10,000 and 100,000/µL, the bleeding time (BT) decreases directly; however, at platelet counts greater than 50,000/µL, neither the BT nor the platelet count has any correlation with postoperative bleeding in cardiac surgical patients

Qualitative platelet defects occur more commonly than thrombocytopenia during CPB. The range of possible causes of platelet dysfunction includes traumatic extracorporeal techniques, pharmacologic therapy, hypothermia, and fibrinolysis; the hemostatic insult increases with the duration of CPB. The use of bubble oxygenators (although infrequent), noncoated extracorporeal circulation, and cardiotomy suctioning causes various degrees of platelet activation, initiates the release reaction, and partly depletes platelets of the contents of their α granules.

Protamine-heparin complexes and protamine alone also contribute to platelet depression after CPB. Mild-to-moderate degrees of hypothermia are associated with reversible degrees of platelet activation and platelet dysfunction. Overall, the potential coagulation benefits of normothermic CPB compared with hypothermic CPB require further study in well-conducted randomized trials (Box 13.4).

BEDSIDE COAGULATION AND PLATELET FUNCTION TESTING

Viscoelastic Tests

Thromboelastography

The Thrombelastograph (TEG, Haemonetics, Braintree, MA) can be used on-site either in the operating room or in a laboratory and provides rapid whole-blood analysis that yields information about clot formation and clot dissolution (Table 13.1 and Fig. 13.3). Within minutes, information on the integrity of the coagulation cascade, platelet function, platelet-fibrin interactions, and fibrinolysis is obtained. The principle is as follows: whole blood (0.36 mL) is placed into a plastic cuvette into which a plastic pin is suspended; this plastic pin is attached to a torsion wire that is coupled to an amplifier and recorded; the cuvette then oscillates through an arc of 4 degrees, 45 minutes at 37°C. When the blood is liquid, movement of the cuvette does not affect the pin. However, as clot begins to form, the pin becomes coupled to the motion of the cuvette, and the torsion wire generates a signal that is recorded. The recorded tracing can be stored by computer, and the parameters of interest are calculated using a simple software package. Alternatively, the tracing can be generated online with a

Table 13.1 Mechanisms of Point-of-Care Platelet Function Monitors

Instrument	Mechanism	Platelet Agonist	Clinical Utility
Thrombelastograph (Haemonetics, Braintree, MA)	Viscoelastic	Thrombin (native), ADP, arachidonic acid	Post CPB, liver transplant, pediatrics, obstetrics, drug efficacy
Sonoclot (Sienco, Arvada, CO)	Viscoelastic	Thrombin (native)	Post CPB, liver transplant
ROTEM (TEM Systems, Durham, NC)	Viscoelastic	Thrombin (native)	Post CPB, transfusion algorithm
HemoSTATUS (Medtronic Perfusion Services, Minneapolis, MN)	ACT reduction	PAF	Post CPB, DDAVP, transfusion algorithm
Plateletworks (Helena Laboratories, Beaumont, TX)	Platelet count ratio	ADP, collagen	Post CPB, drug therapy
PFA-100 (Siemens Medical Solutions USA, Malvern, PA)	In vitro bleeding time	ADP, epinephrine	vWD, congenital disorder, aspirin therapy, post CPB
VerifyNow (Accriva Diagnostics, Accumetrics, San Diego, CA)	Agglutination	TRAP, ADP	GpIIb/IIIa receptor blockade therapy, drug therapy, post CPB
Clot Signature Analyzer (Xylum, Scarsdale, NY)	Shear-induced in vitro bleeding time	Collagen (one channel only)	Post CPB, drug effects
Whole-blood aggregometry	Electrical impedance	Multiple	Post CPB
Impact Cone and Plate(let) Analyzer (Matis Medical, Beersel, Belgium)	Shear-induced platelet function	None	Post CPB, congenital disorder, drug effects
Multiplate Analyzer (Roche Diagnostics, Indianapolis, IN)	Electrical impedance	ADP, arachidonic acid, collagen, ristocetin, TRAP-6	Drug therapy, congenital disorder, post CPB

ACT, Activated clotting time; *ADP,* adenosine diphosphate; *CPB,* cardiopulmonary bypass; *DDAVP,* desmopressin; *Gp,* glycoprotein; *PAF,* platelet-activating factor; *ROTEM,* rotational thrombelastometry; *TRAP,* thrombin receptor agonist peptide; *vWD,* von Willebrand disease.

recording speed of 2 mm/min. The tracing generated has a characteristic conformation that is the signature of the TEG. The most current commercially available TEG incorporates this viscoelastic measurement into a cartridge-based hemostasis test, thus eliminating the need for blood pipetting and reducing the instrument sensitivity to motion.

The specific parameters measured by TEG include the reaction time (R value), coagulation time (K value), "α" angle, maximal amplitude (MA), amplitude 60 minutes after the maximal amplitude (A60), and clot lysis indices at 30 and 60 minutes after MA (LY30 and LY60, respectively) (Fig. 13.4). The R value represents the time for initial fibrin formation and measures the intrinsic coagulation pathway, the extrinsic

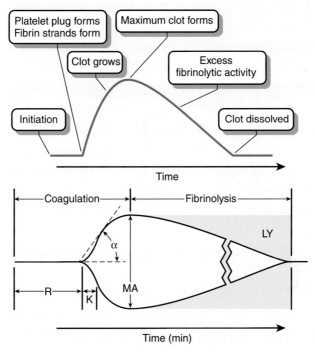

Fig. 13.3 Normal Thrombelastograph (TEG, Haemonetics, Braintree, MA) tracing with standard parameters. *R,* The reaction time or the latency time from placing blood in the cup until the clot begins to form and the tracing opens to 2 mm (typically relates to function or amount of coagulation factors); *K,* a parameter arbitrarily assigned as the time between the TEG trace reaching 2 mm and going up to 20 mm (thought to reflect fibrinogen levels); *α,* the angle between the line in the middle of the TEG tracing and the line tangential to the developing TEG tracing (predictive of maximal amplitude); *MA,* maximal amplitude (largest measured width on the TEG tracing) and is considered to represent maximal thrombin-induced platelet activity and clot formation (total clot strength representing platelet function and clot interactions); *LY,* lysis index, which is the percent of lysis, typically measured as LY30 or 30 minutes after achieving MA.

13

coagulation pathway, and the final common pathway. R is measured from the start of the bioassay until fibrin begins to form, and the amplitude of the tracing is 2 mm. Normal values vary by activator, but they range from 7 to 14 minutes using Celite activator, or in the rapid TEG from 1 to 3 minutes using tissue factor activator. The K value is a measure of the speed of clot formation and is measured from the end of the R time to the time the amplitude reaches 20 mm. Normal values (3–6 minutes) also vary with the type of activators used. The α angle, another index of speed of clot formation, is the angle formed between the horizontal axis of the tracing and the tangent to the tracing at 20-mm amplitude. The α values normally range from 45 to 55 degrees. Because both the K value and the α angle are measures of the speed of clot strengthening, each is improved by high levels of functional fibrinogen. MA (normal is 50–60 mm) is an index of clot strength as determined by platelet function, the cross-linkage of fibrin, and the interactions of platelets with polymerizing fibrin. The peak strength of the clot, or the shear elastic modulus "G," has a curvilinear relation with MA and is defined as follows: $G = (5000\ MA)/(96 - MA)$. The percentage reduction in MA after 30 minutes reflects the fibrinolytic activity present and normally is not more than 7.5%.

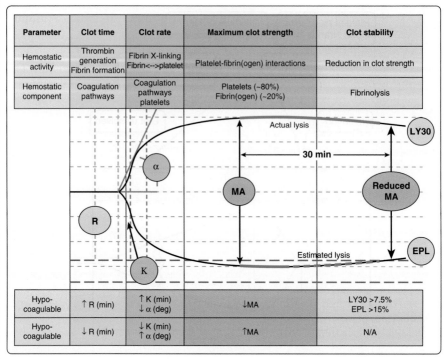

Parameter	Clot time	Clot rate	Maximum clot strength	Clot stability
Hemostatic activity	Thrombin generation Fibrin formation	Fibrin X-linking Fibrin<-->platelet	Platelet-fibrin(ogen) interactions	Reduction in clot strength
Hemostatic component	Coagulation pathways	Coagulation pathways platelets	Platelets (~80%) Fibrin(ogen) (~20%)	Fibrinolysis
Hypo-coagulable	↑ R (min)	↑ K (min) ↓ α (deg)	↓MA	LY30 >7.5% EPL >15%
Hypo-coagulable	↓ R (min)	↓ K (min) ↑ α (deg)	↑MA	N/A

Fig. 13.4 Normal Thrombelastograph (TEG, Haemonetics, Braintree, MA) tracing with standard parameters. α, An angle between the line in the middle of the TEG tracing and the line tangential to the developing TEG tracing (predictive of maximal amplitude); K, a parameter arbitrarily assigned as the time between the TEG trace reaching 2 mm and going up to 20 mm (may represent fibrinogen levels); LY, lysis index; MA, maximal amplitude, considered to represent maximal thrombin-induced platelet activity and clot formation (total clot strength representing platelet function and clot interactions); R, reaction time or the latency time from placing blood in the cup until the clot begins to form, reaching a TEG tracing amplitude of 2 mm (typically relates to function or amount of coagulation factors).

Characteristic TEG tracings can be recognized to indicate particular coagulation defects. A prolonged R value indicates a deficiency in coagulation factor activity or level and is seen typically in patients with liver disease and in patients receiving anticoagulant agents such as warfarin or heparin. MA and the α angle are reduced in states associated with platelet dysfunction or thrombocytopenia and are reduced even further in the presence of a fibrinogen defect. LY30, or the lysis index at 30 minutes after MA, is increased in conjunction with fibrinolysis. These particular signature tracings are depicted in Fig. 13.5.

TEG is a useful tool for diagnosing and treating perioperative coagulopathy in patients undergoing cardiac surgical procedures because of a variety of potential coagulation defects that may exist. Within 15 to 30 minutes, on-site information is available regarding the integrity of the coagulation system, the platelet function, fibrinogen function, and fibrinolysis. With the addition of heparinase, TEG can be performed during CPB and can provide valuable and timely information regarding coagulation status. Because TEG is a viscoelastic test and evaluates whole-blood hemostasis interactions, proponents suggest that TEG is a more accurate predictor of postoperative hemorrhage than are routine coagulation tests. Detractors of POC testing point to variance in the results with the earlier instruments and to some evidence that standard parameters have better correlation with bleeding.

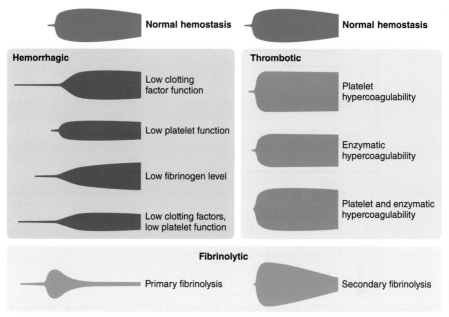

Fig. 13.5 Thrombelastograph (TEG, Haemonetics, Braintree, MA) tracings in various coagulation states.

Thromboelastography Modifications

PlateletMapping is a modification of TEG that assesses platelet function by comparing the MA tracing induced by activation with arachidonic acid (AA) or adenosine diphosphate (ADP) receptors (MA_{pi} [platelet inhibitor]) to the MA achieved with no platelet activity (MA_f), and with maximal platelet activation (MA_{kh}). For PlateletMapping, the reaction is carried out in the setting of heparinized blood, thus inhibiting thrombin platelet activation. The MA produced in this setting, when reptilase and factor XIII are used to form the clot, is the MA with "no platelet activity," or MA_f (fibrin). The MA_{pi} is the maximal activation of platelets and fibrin and is the largest amplitude that can be achieved with the specific platelet activators (ADP or AA). MA_{pi} tracings are compared with the MA_f. In addition, a standard kaolin-heparinase–activated TEG tracing is created to demonstrate maximal platelet activation that occurs when thrombin is present (MA_{kh}) (Fig. 13.6). The following formula calculates the percentage reduction in platelet activity using this assay:

$$\% \text{ inhibition} = 100 - [(MA_{pi} - MA_f)/(MAkh - MA_f) \times 100]$$

PlateletMapping has demonstrated consistent correlation with optical platelet aggregation assays. PlateletMapping studies demonstrate sensitivity in detecting aspirin resistance, as well as updated timeframes on when platelet function returns following cessation of clopidogrel therapy. The Timing Based on Platelet Function Strategy to Reduce Clopidogrel-Associated Bleeding Related to coronary artery bypass grafting (CABG) (TARGET-CABG) study investigated the utility of PlateletMapping in stratifying the waiting period for patients needing CABG who were taking clopidogrel. Results indicated not only that PlateletMapping could be used to individualize this waiting period based on platelet activity, but also that a 50% reduction in these wait times occurred without any increased bleeding complications. PlateletMapping has been

13

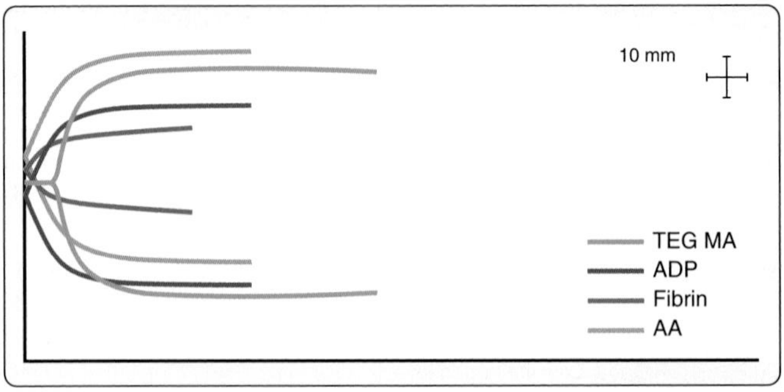

TEG Analysis results

Fig. 13.6 Multitracing displaying standard four reactions involved in the PlateletMapping modification of the Thrombelastograph (TEG, Haemonetics, Braintree, MA). The percentage of inhibition (% inhibition) of platelets is calculated according to the following equation: % inhibition = $100 - [(MA_{pi} - MA_f) / (TEG\ MA - MA_f) \times 100]$ where MA_f is maximum amplitude of *fibrin*-activated curve, MA_{pi} is maximum amplitude by specific platelet activators (either adenosine diphosphate [*ADP*] or arachidonic acid [*AA*], and *TEG MA* is maximum amplitude of kaolin-activated TEG.

shown to be useful in prediction of post-CPB bleeding in multiple small-scale studies, mostly in patients receiving antiplatelet medications. The percentage of inhibition, as well as the MA_{ADP}, was shown to predict postoperative chest tube output, which was the strategy used in the TARGET-CABG trial.

ROTEM (Rotational Thrombelastometry)

Rotational Thrombelastometry (ROTEM, TEM Systems, Durham, NC) gives a viscoelastic measurement of clot strength in whole blood. A small amount of blood and coagulation activators are added to a disposable cuvette that is then placed in a heated cuvette holder. A disposable pin (sensor) that is fixed on the tip of a rotating shaft is lowered into the whole-blood sample. The loss of elasticity on clotting of the sample leads to changes in the rotation of the shaft that is detected by the reflection of light on a small mirror attached to the shaft. A detector records the axis rotation over time, and this rotation is translated into a graph or thromboelastogram. ROTEM functions to measure changes in viscoelastic properties of clot formation in a fashion similar to that of TEG, but with some key differences.

The main descriptive parameters associated with the standard ROTEM tracing (Fig. 13.7) are the following:

- Clotting time: corresponding to the time in seconds from the beginning of the reaction to an increase in amplitude of the tracing of 2 mm. It represents the initiation of clotting, thrombin formation, and start of clot polymerization.
- CFT (clotting formation time): the time in seconds of an increase in amplitude from 2 to 20 mm. This identifies the fibrin polymerization and stabilization of the clot with platelets and factor XIII.
- Alpha (α) angle: the tangent to the clotting curve through the 2-mm point. It reflects the kinetics of clotting. Therefore, a larger α angle reflects the rapid clot formation mediated by thrombin-activated platelets, fibrin, and activated factor XIII [factor XIIIa]); CFT becomes shorter as the α angle becomes larger, and the two parameters are closely linked.
- A10 (amplitude obtained at 10 minutes): this directly relates to maximum clot firmness (MCF) and can be used to predict MCF and platelet function.

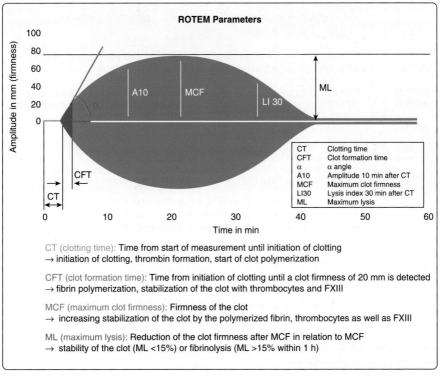

ROTEM Parameters

CT	Clotting time
CFT	Clot formation time
α	α angle
A10	Amplitude 10 min after CT
MCF	Maximum clot firmness
LI30	Lysis index 30 min after CT
ML	Maximum lysis

CT (clotting time): Time from start of measurement until initiation of clotting
→ initiation of clotting, thrombin formation, start of clot polymerization

CFT (clot formation time): Time from initiation of clotting until a clot firmness of 20 mm is detected
→ fibrin polymerization, stabilization of the clot with thrombocytes and FXIII

MCF (maximum clot firmness): Firmness of the clot
→ increasing stabilization of the clot by the polymerized fibrin, thrombocytes as well as FXIII

ML (maximum lysis): Reduction of the clot firmness after MCF in relation to MCF
→ stability of the clot (ML <15%) or fibrinolysis (ML >15% within 1 h)

Fig. 13.7 Rotational thrombelastometry (ROTEM, TEM Systems, Durham, NC) parameters.

- MCF: the maximum amplitude in millimeters reached in the tracing that correlates with platelet count, platelet function, and with the concentration of fibrinogen.
- LI30 (lysis index % at 30 minutes): a parameter representing fibrinolysis at a determined time point (typically 30 minutes). It correlates to the MCF (clot % remaining).
- ML (maximum lysis): this is the ratio of the lowest amplitude after reaching the maximum clot firmness to the maximum clot firmness. Like the LI30, this parameter can evaluate for hyperfibrinolysis.

ROTEM has been used extensively in Europe and increasingly in the United States after receiving approval from the US Food and Drug Administration (FDA) in 2011. ROTEM tests coagulation by using various reagents (Table 13.2), and the most common tests include INTEM (intrinsic system), EXTEM (extrinsic system), HEPTEM (intrinsic system in presence of heparin), FIBTEM (measures fibrinogen activity), and APTEM (tissue factor activation + tranexamic acid or aprotinin). Fig. 13.8 provides an example of a series of ROTEM reactions for a hematologically normal patient, compared with a patient with platelet dysfunction.

In 2015 ROTEM released a module that attaches to the standard platform that adds the capability to monitor platelet aggregation function in response to three platelet agonists (ADP, AA, and thrombin receptor agonist peptide [TRAP]) called the ADPTEM, ARATEM, and TRAPTEM, respectively. This system functions using the same concept as standard whole-blood aggregometry and is similar to the Multiplate aggregometer.

Table 13.2	**Standard Rotational Thrombelastometry Reagents and Assessment Pattern**
EXTEM	Tissue factor activation; factors VII, X, V, II, I, platelets, and fibrinolysis
INTEM	Contact phase activation; factors XII, XI, IX, VIII, II, I, platelets, and fibrinolysis
FIBTEM	EXTEM + cytochalasin D (platelet blocking); assessment of fibrinogen
APTEM	EXTEM plus aprotinin; useful to rule out fibrinolysis when compared to EXTEM
HEPTEM	INTEM plus heparinase; useful to detect residual heparin

APTEM, Tissue factor activation + tranexamic acid/aprotinin; *EXTEM*, extrinsic system; *FIBTEM*, measure of fibrinogen activity; *HEPTEM*, intrinsic system in presence of heparin; *INTEM*, intrinsic system.

Point-of-Care Tests of Platelet Response to Agonists

In contrast to viscoelastic testing, various platforms are now available as POC devices that allow for platelet function testing in response to agonists. Each system uses unique concepts, although most have been well validated with laboratory-based light transmission aggregometry (LTA), and some have been validated with the previously described viscoelastic tests.

VerifyNow

VerifyNow (Accumetrics, San Diego, CA) is a POC monitor approved by the FDA for use as a platelet function assay. In whole blood, it measures TRAP activation–induced platelet agglutination of fibrinogen-coated beads by using an optical detection system. After anticoagulated whole blood is added to the mixing chamber, the platelets become activated if they are responsive to the agonist. The activated glycoprotein (Gp)IIb/IIIa receptors on the platelets bind to adjacent platelets through the fibrinogen on the beads and cause agglutination of the blood and the beads. Light transmittance through the chamber is measured and increases as agglutination increases, much as in standard aggregometry. Antithrombotic drug effects cause diminished agglutination (measured by light transmittance); the degree of platelet inhibition can thus be quantified. VerifyNow has agonists to examine the antiplatelet activity of GpIIb/IIIa inhibitors, aspirin, and clopidogrel and can report and quantify the degree of platelet inhibition with good correlation with LTA.

Platelet Function Analyzer

The Platelet Function Analyzer (PFA-100; Siemens Medical Solutions USA, Malvern, PA) is a monitor of platelet adhesive capacity that is currently approved by the FDA and is valuable to identify drug-induced platelet abnormalities, platelet dysfunction of von Willebrand disease and other acquired and congenital platelet defects. The test is conducted as a modified in vitro BT. Whole blood is drawn through a chamber by vacuum and is perfused across an aperture in a collagen membrane coated with an agonist (epinephrine or ADP). Platelet adhesion and formation of aggregates seal the aperture, thus indicating the "closure time" measured by the PFA-100. In cardiac surgical patients, the preoperative PFA-100 closure time significantly correlated with postoperative blood loss (Box 13.5).

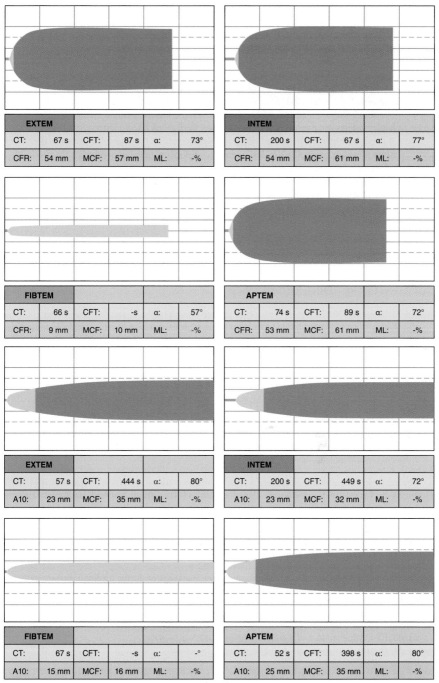

EXTEM			
CT:	67 s	CFT:	87 s	α:	73°
CFR:	54 mm	MCF:	57 mm	ML:	-%

INTEM			
CT:	200 s	CFT:	67 s	α:	77°
CFR:	54 mm	MCF:	61 mm	ML:	-%

FIBTEM			
CT:	66 s	CFT:	-s	α:	57°
CFR:	9 mm	MCF:	10 mm	ML:	-%

APTEM			
CT:	74 s	CFT:	89 s	α:	72°
CFR:	53 mm	MCF:	61 mm	ML:	-%

EXTEM			
CT:	57 s	CFT:	444 s	α:	80°
A10:	23 mm	MCF:	35 mm	ML:	-%

INTEM			
CT:	200 s	CFT:	449 s	α:	72°
A10:	23 mm	MCF:	32 mm	ML:	-%

FIBTEM			
CT:	67 s	CFT:	-s	α:	-°
A10:	15 mm	MCF:	16 mm	ML:	-%

APTEM			
CT:	52 s	CFT:	398 s	α:	80°
A10:	25 mm	MCF:	35 mm	ML:	-%

Fig. 13.8 *Left,* Normal tracings for the four standard parameters in the rotational thrombelastometry (ROTEM, TEM Systems, Durham, NC) system. *Right,* Platelet dysfunction, which is demonstrated by the prolonged clot formation time *(CFT)*, as well as a decreased maximum clot firmness *(MCF)* in both the extrinsic system *(EXTEM)* and the intrinsic system *(INTEM)* tests. *A10,* Amplitude 10 min after CT; *APTEM,* tissue factor activation + tranexamic acid/aprotinin; *CFR,* clot formation rate; *CT,* clotting time; *FIBTEM,* measure of fibrinogen activity.

BOX 13.5 *Platelet Function Tests*

The appropriate test to measure platelet function depends on the suspected platelet defect.
The Thrombelastograph (TEG, Haemonetics, Braintree, MA), Rotational
  Thromboelastometry (ROTEM, TEM Systems, Durham, NC), and
  thromboelastometry, and possibly other viscoelastic tests, are useful to measure
  platelet defects after cardiopulmonary bypass. VerifyNow (Accumetrics, San Diego,
  CA) and Multiplate (Helena Laboratories, Beaumont, TX) are useful to measure the
  effects of glycoprotein IIb/IIIa and adenosine diphosphate receptor-blocker therapy
  and aspirin therapy.
The PFA-100 test (Siemens Medical Solutions USA, Malvern, PA) is useful to measure the
  effects of aspirin on platelet adhesion.
It is important to understand the platelet defect being sought to use the proper test
  accurately.

SUGGESTED READINGS

Avidan MS, Levy JH, Scholz J, et al. A phase III, double-blind, placebo-controlled, multicenter study on
  the efficacy of recombinant human antithrombin in heparin-resistant patients scheduled to undergo
  cardiac surgery necessitating cardiopulmonary bypass. *Anesthesiology*. 2005;102:276–284.

Carroll RC, Craft RM, Chavez JJ, et al. Measurement of functional fibrinogen levels using the Thrombelastograph. *J Clin Anesth*. 2008;20:186–190.

Chitlur M, Sorensen B, Rivard GE, et al. Standardization of thromboelastography: a report from the
  TEG-ROTEM working group. *Haemophilia*. 2011;17:532–537.

Chowdhury M, Shore-Lesserson L, Mais AM, et al. Thromboelastograph with PlateletMapping(TM) predicts
  postoperative chest tube drainage in patients undergoing coronary artery bypass grafting. *J Cardiothorac
  Vasc Anesth*. 2014;28:217–223.

Dyke CM, Smedira NG, Koster A, et al. A comparison of bivalirudin to heparin with protamine reversal
  in patients undergoing cardiac surgery with cardiopulmonary bypass: the EVOLUTION-ON study.
  J Thorac Cardiovasc Surg. 2006;131:533–539.

Espinosa A, Stenseth R, Videm V, et al. Comparison of three point-of-care testing devices to detect hemostatic
  changes in adult elective cardiac surgery: a prospective observational study. *BMC Anesthesiol*. 2014;14:80.

Gorlinger K, Dirkmann D, Hanke AA. Potential value of transfusion protocols in cardiac surgery.
  Curr Opin Anaesthesiol. 2013;26:230–243.

Lemmer JH Jr, Despotis GJ. Antithrombin III concentrate to treat heparin resistance in patients undergoing
  cardiac surgery. *J Thorac Cardiovasc Surg*. 2002;123:213.

Lincoff AM, Bittl JA, Kleiman NS, et al. Comparison of bivalirudin versus heparin during percutaneous
  coronary intervention (the Randomized Evaluation of PCI Linking Angiomax to Reduced Clinical
  Events [REPLACE] trial). *Am J Cardiol*. 2004;93:1092.

Lobato RL, Despotis GJ, Levy JH, et al. Anticoagulation management during cardiopulmonary bypass: a
  survey of 54 North American institutions. *J Thorac Cardiovasc Surg*. 2010;139:1665–1666.

Mahla E, Suarez TA, Bliden KP, et al. Platelet function measurement-based strategy to reduce bleeding
  and waiting time in clopidogrel-treated patients undergoing coronary artery bypass graft surgery: the
  timing based on platelet function strategy to reduce clopidogrel-associated bleeding related to CABG
  (TARGET-CABG) study. *Circ Cardiovasc Interv*. 2012;5:261–269.

Merry AF. Bivalirudin, blood loss, and graft patency in coronary artery bypass surgery. *Semin Thromb
  Hemost*. 2004;30:337.

Merry AF, Raudkivi PJ, Middleton NG, et al. Bivalirudin versus heparin and protamine in off-pump coronary
  artery bypass surgery. *Ann Thorac Surg*. 2004;77:925.

Preisman S, Kogan A, Itzkovsky K, et al. Modified thromboelastography evaluation of platelet dysfunction
  in patients undergoing coronary artery surgery. *Eur J Cardiothorac Surg*. 2010;37:1367–1374.

Raymond PD, Ray MJ, Callen SN, et al. Heparin monitoring during cardiac surgery. Part 1: validation of
  whole-blood heparin concentration and activated clotting time. *Perfusion*. 2003;18:269–276.

Solomon C, Sorensen B, Hochleitner G, et al. Comparison of whole blood fibrin-based clot tests in
  thrombelastography and thromboelastometry. *Anesth Analg*. 2012;114:721–730.

Tanaka KA, Bolliger D, Vadlamudi R, et al. Rotational thromboelastometry (ROTEM)–based coagulation management in cardiac surgery and major trauma. *J Cardiothorac Vasc Anesth.* 2012;26:1083–1093.

Thiele RH, Raphael JA. 2014 Update on coagulation management for cardiopulmonary bypass. *Semin Cardiothorac Vasc Anesth.* 2014;18:177–189.

Weber CF, Klages M, Zacharowski K. Perioperative coagulation management during cardiac surgery. *Curr Opin Anaesthesiol.* 2013;26:60–64.

Weitzel NS, Weitzel LB, Epperson LE, et al. Platelet mapping as part of modified thromboelastography (TEG(R)) in patients undergoing cardiac surgery and cardiopulmonary bypass. *Anaesthesia.* 2012;67:1158–1165.

Welsby IJ, McDonnell E, El-Moalem H, et al. Activated clotting time systems vary in precision and bias and are not interchangeable when following heparin management protocols during cardiopulmonary bypass. *J Clin Monit Comput.* 2002;17:287–292.

13

Section IV

Anesthesia for Cardiac Surgical Procedures

Chapter 14

Anesthesia for Myocardial Revascularization

Alexander J.C. Mittnacht, MD • Martin J. London, MD • John D. Puskas, MD • Joel A. Kaplan, MD, CPE, FACC

Key Points

1. Guideline updates emphasize the efficacy of surgical approaches to myocardial revascularization in patients with multivessel coronary artery disease.
2. Perioperative risk reduction includes careful consideration of all of the patient's relevant antihypertensive, antiplatelet, and antianginal medications.
3. Significant valvular abnormalities in patients scheduled for coronary revascularization should be evaluated and considered in surgical planning.
4. Off-pump coronary artery bypass surgery is an established alternative to on-pump myocardial revascularization (ie, coronary artery bypass grafting [CABG]). The choice and outcomes of either approach are highly surgeon dependent. Despite apparent advantages of avoiding cardiopulmonary bypass (CPB), evidence from large prospective trials enrolling mostly low-risk patients has not shown clear reductions in mortality with an off-pump approach.
5. Possible indications for pulmonary artery catheter use in CABG surgery include patients with pulmonary hypertension, right-sided heart failure, or severely impaired ventricular function, particularly those who require postoperative cardiac output monitoring.
6. Fast-tracking, including early extubation and mobilization, has been almost universally adopted for patients undergoing myocardial revascularization.
7. Anesthetic drugs, especially inhaled anesthetic agents, may help to ameliorate myocardial injury associated with CPB and aortic cross-clamping by their preconditioning and postconditioning effects. However, the magnitude of these effects on outcome remains controversial.

The role of the cardiac anesthesiologist in the perioperative care of patients undergoing myocardial revascularization continues to evolve. Achievements of the past two decades include providing safe anesthesia that allows rapid recovery and optimizing monitoring that includes the establishment of transesophageal echocardiography (TEE) as a standard of care in the cardiac operating room. More recent developments in patient care include the introduction of a perioperative surgical home, which affects the management of patients undergoing myocardial revascularization. The anesthesiologist is vitally important in the multidisciplinary approach to patient care. Optimal perioperative care requires close collaboration and coordination between the various specialties involved on the heart team. The process begins with the decision to proceed to surgery and continues with preoperative optimization, state-of-the-art perioperative and postoperative care, and rehabilitation after hospital discharge. Beyond safe anesthesia technique, the anesthesiologist must be well versed in all areas of perioperative management for patients with coronary artery disease (CAD). This includes advances in pharmacologic risk reduction, new surgical techniques, and anesthetic management and monitoring techniques to improve patient outcomes.

EPIDEMIOLOGY

According to the American Heart Association Heart Disease and Stroke Statistics, most recently updated in 2014, epidemiologic data relevant to cardiovascular disease can be summarized as follows. Overall rates of death attributable to cardiovascular disease have declined 31%; for CAD, there was a 39.2% decrease from 2000 to 2010. This was partially attributed to improvements in acute treatment of patients with acute coronary syndromes (ACSs), secondary preventive therapies after myocardial infarction (MI), treatment of acute heart failure (HF), revascularization of chronic CAD, and other preventive therapies. However, the prevalence remains high, with cardiovascular disease accounting for 31.9% of all deaths in the United States. Based on current estimates, by 2030 43.9% of the US population will have some form of cardiovascular disease. Similarly, 15.4 million individuals had CAD in 2010; and ischemic heart disease causes approximately one of every six deaths in the United States. In 2010, 379,559 Americans died of CAD, and statistically, every 34 seconds one person in the United States has a coronary event.

Between 2000 and 2010 the total number of inpatient cardiovascular procedures in the United States increased by 28%, with a total of 7,588,000 cardiovascular procedures performed in 2010. In 2010 an estimated 219,000 patients underwent 397,000 coronary artery bypass graft (CABG) procedures (Fig. 14.1). The in-hospital mortality rate for CABG declined by 50% despite an increase in the comorbidity index. CAD alone resulted in more than $44 billion in expenses, making it the most expensive condition treated. The total direct and indirect cost of cardiovascular disease and stroke was estimated to be $315.4 billion in 2010, more than for any other diagnostic group.

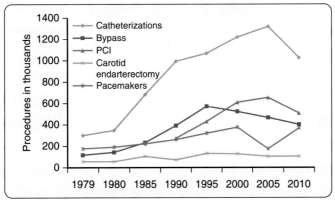

Fig. 14.1 Trends in cardiovascular operations and procedures from 1979 to 2010 for inpatient procedures only. *PCI*, Percutaneous coronary intervention. (From Mozaffarian D, Benjamin EJ, Go AS, et al. American Heart Association Statistics Committee and Stroke Statistics Subcommittee. Heart disease and stroke statistics: 2015 update. A report from the American Heart Association. *Circulation*. 2015;131:e29.)

▓ PATHOPHYSIOLOGY OF CORONARY ARTERY DISEASE

Anatomy

The anesthesiologist should be familiar with coronary anatomy if only to interpret the significance of angiographic findings. The coronary circulation and common sites for placement of distal anastomoses during CABG are shown in Figs. 14.2 through 14.4.

The right coronary artery (RCA) arises from the right sinus of Valsalva and is best seen in the left anterior oblique view on coronary cine angiography. It passes anteriorly for the first few millimeters and then follows the right atrioventricular (AV) groove and curves posteriorly within the groove to reach the crux of the heart, the area where the interventricular septum (IVS) meets the AV groove. In 84% of cases, it terminates as the posterior descending artery (PDA), which is its most important branch because it is the sole supply to the posterosuperior IVS. Other important branches are those to the sinus node in 60% of patients and the AV node in approximately 85% of patients. Anatomists consider the RCA to be dominant when it crosses the crux of the heart and continues in the AV groove regardless of the origin of the PDA. Angiographers, however, ascribe dominance to the artery—right coronary or left coronary (ie, circumflex)—that gives rise to the PDA.

The vertical and superior orientation of the RCA ostium allows easy passage of air bubbles during aortic cannulation, cardiopulmonary bypass (CPB), or open valve surgery. In sufficient volume, myocardial ischemia involving the inferior left ventricular (LV) wall segments and the right ventricle may occur (Fig. 14.5). In contrast, the

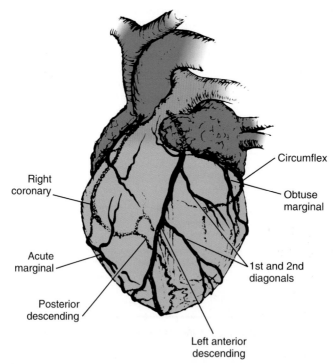

Fig. 14.2 Thirty-degree left anterior oblique angiographic view of the heart, which best shows the right coronary artery. *Lines* indicate common sites of distal vein graft anastomoses. (From Stiles QR, Tucker BL, Lindesmith GG, et al. *Myocardial Revascularization: A Surgical Atlas.* Boston, Little, Brown; 1976.)

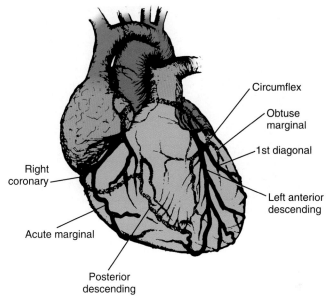

Fig. 14.3 Ten-degree right anterior oblique angiographic view of the heart, which best shows the left main coronary artery dividing into the circumflex and left anterior descending arteries. *Lines* indicate common sites of distal vein graft anastomoses. (Modified from Stiles QR, Tucker BL, Lindesmith GG, et al. *Myocardial Revascularization: A Surgical Atlas.* Boston: Little, Brown; 1976.)

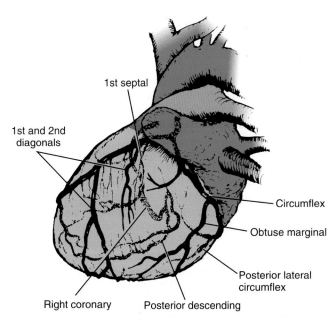

Fig. 14.4 Seventy-five–degree left anterior oblique angiographic view of the heart, which best shows branches of the left anterior descending and circumflex coronary arteries. *Lines* indicate common sites of distal vein graft anastomoses. (Modified from Stiles QR, Tucker BL, Lindesmith GG, et al. *Myocardial Revascularization: A Surgical Atlas.* Boston: Little, Brown; 1976.)

14

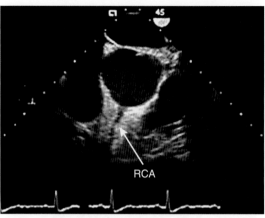

Fig. 14.5 The vertical and superior orientation of the right coronary artery *(RCA)* arising from the aortic root is identified by transesophageal echocardiography (TEE). The TEE transducer in the esophagus is at the top of the screen, and the patient's chest wall is at the bottom. Retained air preferentially enters the RCA, which may cause inferior ischemia, depending on the amount of air and the coronary perfusion pressure. Elevation of perfusion pressure using phenylephrine is often used to treat coronary air embolus. The left main coronary artery (not visible) arises at approximately 3 o'clock on this image. (Courtesy Martin J. London, MD, University of California, San Francisco, CA *[www.ucsf.edu/teeecho].)*

near-perpendicular orientation of the left main coronary ostium makes air embolization much less common.

The left coronary artery arises from the left sinus of Valsalva as the left main coronary artery. It is best seen in a shallow right anterior oblique projection (see Fig. 14.3). The left main coronary artery courses anteriorly and to the left, where it divides in a space between the aorta and pulmonary artery. Its branches are the left anterior descending (LAD) artery and circumflex artery. The LAD passes along the anterior interventricular groove. It may reach only two-thirds of the distance to the apex or extend around the apex to the diaphragmatic portion of the left ventricle. Major branches of the LAD are the diagonal branches, which supply the free wall of the left ventricle; and septal branches, which course posteriorly to supply the major portion of the IVS. Although there may be many diagonal and septal branches, the first diagonal and first septal branches serve as important landmarks in the descriptions of lesions of the LAD.

The circumflex artery arises at a sharp angle from the left main coronary artery and courses toward the crux of the heart in the AV groove. When the circumflex artery gives rise to the PDA, the circulation is left dominant, and the left coronary circulation supplies the entire IVS and the AV node. In approximately 40% of patients, the circumflex artery supplies the branch to the sinoatrial node. Up to four obtuse marginal (OM) arteries arise from the circumflex artery and supply the lateral wall of the left ventricle.

All of the previously described epicardial branches give rise to small vessels that supply the outer third of the myocardium and penetrating vessels that anastomose with the subendocardial plexus. The capillary plexus is unique in that it functions as an end-arterial system. Each epicardial arteriole supplies a capillary plexus that forms an end loop rather than anastomosing with an adjacent capillary from another epicardial artery. Significant collateral circulation does not exist at the microcirculatory level. The capillary anatomy explains the distinct areas of myocardial ischemia or infarction that can be related to disease in a discrete epicardial artery. CAD most commonly

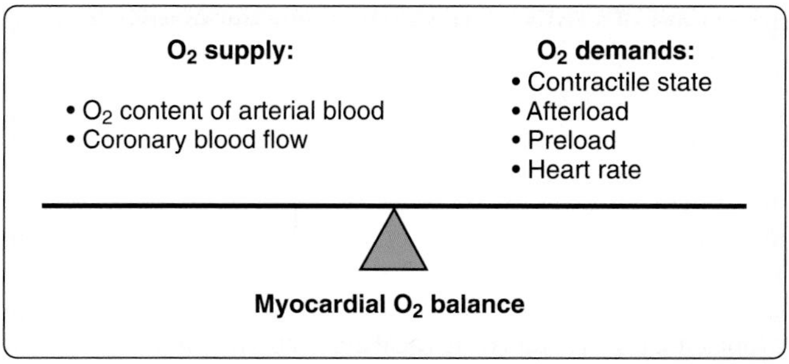

| O₂ supply: | O₂ demands: |

O_2 supply:

- O_2 content of arterial blood
- Coronary blood flow

O_2 demands:
- Contractile state
- Afterload
- Preload
- Heart rate

Myocardial O₂ balance

Fig. 14.6 Factors determining myocardial oxygen supply and demand.

affects the epicardial muscular arteries with rare intramyocardial lesions (with the exception of the transplanted heart). However, severe disorders of the microcirculation and primary impairment of coronary vascular reserve in normal coronary arteries have been described, especially in patients with diabetes, females, and those with variant angina. Epicardial lesions can be single but are more often multiple. A combined lesion of the RCA and both branches of the left coronary artery is referred to as *triple-vessel disease*. Venous drainage of the myocardium primarily occurs through the coronary sinus, which enters the right atrium between the inferior vena cava and the tricuspid valve. A small fraction enters the cardiac chambers directly through the Thebesian veins.

Myocardial Ischemia and Infarction

In patients with CAD, myocardial ischemia usually results from increases in myocardial oxygen demand exceeding the capacity of the stenosed coronary arteries to increase oxygen supply (Fig. 14.6). In atherosclerotic heart disease, the fundamental lesion is an intimal lipid plaque in the epicardial portion of a coronary artery that causes chronic stenosis and episodic thrombosis and sudden plaque rupture that results in almost complete occlusion. Characteristics of the vulnerable plaque include a high lipid content, a thin fibrous cap, a reduced number of smooth muscle cells, and increased macrophage activity. Chronic inflammation and acute processes such as a plaque rupture result in the release of vasoactive substances from platelets and leukocytes producing endothelial dysfunction and vasoconstriction and further reducing coronary blood flow (CBF). A larger plaque disruption and prolonged thrombosis produce a Q-wave infarction with transmural myocardial necrosis.

Collateral vessels exist in normal hearts, but in the setting of CAD, they are increased in size and number. Collaterals may develop between the ischemic zone and an adjacent nonischemic area supplied by a different vessel. Although beneficial at rest, during exercise or periods of increased oxygen demand, CBF may be shunted away from the ischemic myocardium to areas with intact autoregulation able to vasodilate; this is referred to as a *coronary steal*.

ANESTHESIA FOR CORONARY ARTERY BYPASS GRAFTING

The practitioner providing anesthesia care for patients undergoing coronary revascularization has to implement an anesthetic plan that takes patient- and surgery-specific factors into consideration, but it should also include the most recent recommendations and guidelines regarding the perioperative care of patients with CAD.

14

In the earlier days of cardiac surgery, the focus on anesthesia management for patients undergoing CABG was mainly on maintaining hemodynamic stability and preventing ischemia. This reflected the lack of anesthetic agents with minimal hemodynamic effects. Later reports supported a lack of effect of the technique, suggesting that hemodynamic control was more important (ie, it is not what you use, but how you use it). With the introduction of modern anesthetic agents, the focus shifted to investigating how the various regimens and techniques could help to improve outcomes of patients undergoing myocardial revascularization. For example, considerable data demonstrate the beneficial effects of using potent inhalation agents or sympathetic blockade on markers of myocardial ischemia and postoperative MI, such as improved recovery and shorter length of stay (LOS).

Premedication

The concept of premedication has been evolving beyond the traditional ordering of sedative-hypnotics or related agents to reduce patient anxiety and promote amnesia. The cardiac anesthesiologist must be familiar with the potential benefits of administering or hazards of not administering a variety of medications, including antianginal, β-blocker, and antiplatelet drugs.

Anxiolysis, Amnesia, and Analgesia

The purposes of premedication are to pharmacologically reduce apprehension and fear, to provide analgesia for potentially painful events before induction (eg, vascular cannulation), and to produce some degree of amnesia. In patients with CAD, premedication may help prevent preoperative anginal episodes that are relatively commonly observed and may be elicited by tachycardia due to anxiety or painful stimuli. Short-acting benzodiazepines are the mainstay of drugs administered for this purpose. When given intravenously in the preoperative holding area to patients with CAD, supplemental oxygen should be administered and the patients monitored by pulse oximetry, an electrocardiogram (ECG), and noninvasive blood pressure (BP) methods.

Management of Preoperative Medications

Patients undergoing myocardial revascularization routinely take medications aiming to prevent acute coronary events, worsening of ischemia, or HF symptoms. Many of these drugs have implications for anesthesia management, and the anesthesiologist should be familiar with the current guidelines and recommendations outlining their use in the perioperative setting (Box 14.1).

β-BLOCKING AGENTS

β-Blocking agents are routinely administered to many patients with CAD. As early as the mid-1970s, Kaplan suggested that it was safe to continue β-blockade in patients with ischemic heart disease undergoing cardiac or noncardiac surgery, even those with poor ventricular function. This was confirmed in many prospective, randomized trials that established the safety of continuing β-blockade in the perioperative period.

In a metaanalysis, Wiesbauer et al. found that perioperative β-blockers reduced perioperative arrhythmias after cardiac surgery, but they were unable to show an effect on MI or mortality. Based on the existing evidence from a few randomized, controlled trials, retrospective studies, and metaanalyses, β-blocker use was recommended by many specialty societies for patients undergoing CABG.

The 2011 American College of Cardiology Foundation and American Heart Association (ACCF/AHA) guideline for CABG surgery recommended that β-blockers should be administered for at least 24 hours before CABG to all patients without

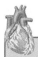

BOX 14.1 *Preoperative Medication Management*

1. β-Adrenergic blockers
   - Should be administered for at least 24 hours before coronary artery bypass grafting (CABG) to all patients without contraindications (eg, hypotension, third-degree heart block, bronchospasm).
   - After CABG surgery, should be reinstituted as soon as possible in all patients without contraindications.
2. Statins: All patients undergoing CABG should receive them unless contraindications apply.
3. Calcium channel blockers: Patients already on calcium channel blockers should continue them perioperatively.
4. Angiotensin-converting enzyme inhibitor:
   - Preoperative discontinuation is controversial (ie, increased risk of hypotension and vasoplegic syndrome).
   - Postoperatively, should be initiated and continued indefinitely in CABG patients who are stable unless contraindications apply.
5. Diuretics: No firm recommendations, but ensure adequate serum potassium levels.
6. Aspirin: Should be administered preoperatively. The decision about whether and when to discontinue aspirin before surgery depends on patient-specific factors such as individual risk for bleeding and presence of an acute coronary syndrome. Postoperatively, aspirin should be started as early as possible (ie, within 6 to 24 hours after surgery).
7. Antiplatelet agents such as oral inhibitors of purinergic receptor P2Y12: Because they are associated with an increased risk of bleeding, recommendations call for withholding for a few days before surgery. However, in high-risk patients and/or after placement of drug-eluting stents, recommendations may change, and intravenous glycoprotein IIb/IIIa inhibitors or cangrelor may be continued perioperatively despite increased risk of bleeding.
8. Heparin: Regimen often depends on the surgeon. Usually discontinued 4 hours preoperatively for stable patients, continued up to and through pre–cardiopulmonary bypass period for critical left main disease or acutely unstable angina patients.
9. Oral hypoglycemic agents: No firm recommendations; consider withholding administration. However, glucose control must be ensured.
10. Antibiotic prophylaxis: Optimal timing and weight adjustment (especially important with antibiotics that have slow tissue penetration such as vancomycin). Typically, a second-generation cephalosporin such as cephazolin (2 g IV) or cefuroxime (1.5 g IV) administered 20 to 60 minutes before incision; vancomycin (15 mg/kg) administered as a slow infusion to avoid hypotension and flushing (owing to slow tissue penetration, infusion should be completed 20 to 30 minutes before skin incision).

14

contraindications to reduce the incidence or clinical sequelae of postoperative atrial fibrillation (AF). The guidelines state that β-blockers in patients with CABG with an ejection fraction (EF) greater than 30% can be effective in reducing the risk of in-hospital mortality and the incidence of perioperative myocardial ischemia. In patients with severely depressed LV function (EF <30%), the effectiveness of preoperative β-blockers in reducing the in-hospital mortality rate is uncertain. After CABG, β-blockers should be reinstituted as soon as possible for all patients without contraindications.

In 2015, the AHA published a scientific statement complementing the existing guidelines that focused on secondary prevention measures after CABG. The expert statement supports the recommendation to give β-blockers starting before surgery, including administering them to patients with prior MI unless contraindicated (eg, bradycardia, severe reactive airway disease). In patients with previous MI, β-blockers are specifically recommended for patients with HF symptoms and an EF below 40%.

ANTIPLATELET DRUGS

In accordance with current guidelines, most patients undergoing CABG are treated with platelet inhibitors. Aspirin is a well-recognized component of primary and secondary prevention strategies for all patients with ischemic heart disease. Clopidogrel administration is established practice after coronary artery stent placement, and it is recommended in combination with aspirin for patients with ACS.

Guidelines summarizing the current evidence regarding antiplatelet drugs in patients undergoing surgery have been published by various specialty societies and are updated regularly. The most recent update of The Society of Thoracic Surgeons guidelines on the use of antiplatelet drugs in patients undergoing CABG was published in 2012. The highest level of evidence (class I recommendation, level A evidence) was found for aspirin administration within 6 to 24 hours after surgery in nonbleeding patients to optimize vein graft patency, and for dual antiplatelet therapy for patients undergoing CABG after ACS as soon as the bleeding risk is diminished to decrease adverse cardiovascular outcomes. The class I recommendation with level B evidence advised discontinuing inhibitors of the receptor P2Y12 for a few days before surgery to reduce the risk of bleeding and need for blood transfusion.

The 2011 ACCF/AHA guideline for CABG surgery recommended that aspirin should be administered to CABG patients preoperatively. For elective CABG, clopidogrel and ticagrelor should be discontinued for at least 5 days before surgery and prasugrel for at least 7 days to limit the need for blood transfusions. For urgent surgery, clopidogrel and ticagrelor should be discontinued for at least 24 hours to reduce major bleeding complications. Postoperatively, aspirin should be started within 6 hours after surgery. For those allergic to aspirin, clopidogrel should be used instead. Low-dose aspirin should be continued indefinitely. The 2015 AHA scientific statement on secondary prevention measures after CABG confirmed these recommendations and recommended dual antiplatelet therapy with aspirin and clopidogrel for 1 year.

HMG COA REDUCTASE INHIBITORS

Potent antiinflammatory and antithrombotic effects and beneficial effects on endothelial function and angiogenesis have been reported for 3-hydroxy-3-methyl-glutaryl–coenzyme A (HMG CoA) reductase inhibitors (ie, statins). Improved outcomes also have been described for patients undergoing CABG. This includes attenuation of myocardial reperfusion injury after CPB, reducing short- and long-term mortality rates, and decreasing early graft occlusion in patients with CABG.

Based on the accumulating evidence for the beneficial effects of statin therapy in patients undergoing myocardial revascularization, guidelines have been adjusted. The 2011 ACCF/AHA guideline for CABG surgery recommended that, unless contraindications apply, all patients undergoing CABG should receive statin therapy with the goal of lowering low-density lipoprotein (LDL) cholesterol by at least 30% or to less than 100 mg/dL. Even lower targets may be advisable (<70 mg/dL) for very high-risk patients. The most recent AHA scientific statement on secondary prevention measures after CABG confirmed these recommendations, and recommended statin therapy starting preoperatively and continued after surgery.

ANGIOTENSIN-CONVERTING ENZYME INHIBITORS

Angiotensin-converting enzyme (ACE) inhibitors are widely considered to be vasculoprotective, particularly with regard to ventricular remodeling after acute MI, and they appear to reduce damage after ischemic reperfusion. The role of ACE inhibitors in improving major outcomes for patients with ischemic heart disease and those undergoing myocardial revascularization has been investigated.

The 2011 ACCF/AHA guideline for CABG surgery recommended that preoperative use of ACE inhibitors and angiotension II receptor blockers (ARBs) should prompt reinstitution postoperatively after the patient is stable unless contraindicated. Independent of preoperative use, ACE inhibitors and ARBs should be initiated postoperatively and continued indefinitely in patients with CABG who are stable unless contraindications apply. The task force also acknowledges that the safety of the preoperative ACE inhibitors or ARBs in patients on chronic therapy is uncertain. The most recent AHA scientific statement on secondary prevention measures after CABG confirmed these recommendations and recommended administering ACE inhibitors or ARB therapy after CABG to all patients with LV dysfunction.

Monitoring

Electrocardiogram

On arrival in the operating room, the patient undergoing CABG should have routine monitors placed, including pulse oximetry, noninvasive BP, and the ECG. A five-lead system is standard for patients undergoing cardiac surgery. Monitoring leads V_5 and II allows detection of 90% of ischemic episodes and assessment of the rhythm to diagnose various atrial and ventricular arrhythmias (Box 14.2).

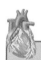

> BOX 14.2 *Intraoperative Monitoring for Myocardial Revascularization*
>
> 1. ECG: V_5 most sensitive for myocardial ischemia; inferior lead II for rhythm monitoring and inferior wall ischemia.
> 2. Arterial BP: Continuous invasive arterial BP monitoring and blood gas sampling by indwelling arterial catheter.
> 3. PAC: No evidence of improved outcome with PAC use. However, commonly used for treatment guidance in conjunction with TEE monitoring and for postoperative care in the ICU, particularly in patients with severely reduced ventricular function and those with pulmonary hypertension.
> 4. TEE: Recommended for all cardiac operations. TEE can assist in pre-CPB evaluation of cardiac function, associated valvular lesions, and evaluation of atheromatous plaques in the aorta.
> 5. Temperature monitoring: Bladder or esophageal (ie, core temperature) and nasopharyngeal or tympanic (ie, brain temperature) are recommended for all CPB cases to minimize temperature gradients and cerebral hyperthermia during rewarming. For OPCABs, bladder temperature only is sufficient.
> 6. Foley placement for all patients.
>
> *BP,* Blood pressure; *CPB,* cardiopulmonary bypass; *ECG,* electrocardiogram; *ICU,* intensive care unit; *OPCAB,* off-pump coronary artery bypass; *PAC,* pulmonary artery catheter; *TEE,* transesophageal echocardiography.

14

Arterial Pressure Monitoring

The radial artery usually is cannulated for BP monitoring during CABG. Choosing the best site for radial artery cannulation depends on surgery-specific considerations and institutional and practitioner preferences. Procedures such as previous transradial artery catheterization (TRAC), radial artery harvesting, or axillary CPB cannulation may influence the site chosen for invasive arterial pressure monitoring. The newer TRAC sheaths can be problematic for monitoring during emergency CABG, and they have been associated with many complications. The radial artery on the side of a previous TRAC procedure probably should not be used for monitoring purposes.

Radial arterial pressures have proved to be inaccurate immediately after hypothermic CPB. Substantial reductions in radial arterial pressure compared with aortic pressure have been reported in several clinical investigations and often require 20 to 60 minutes after CPB to resolve. Decreased forearm vascular resistance is thought to be responsible for this common phenomenon. This problem can be overcome by temporarily transducing the arterial pressure directly from the aorta by a needle or a cardioplegia cannula.

Central Venous Cannulation

Placement of a central venous pressure (CVP) catheter routinely is performed in cardiac anesthesia for right atrial pressure measurement and for infusing vasoactive drugs. Some centers routinely place two catheters (ie, large introducer and smaller CVP catheter) in the central circulation to facilitate volume infusion and vasoactive or inotropic drug administration.

Pulmonary Artery Catheterization

The use of a pulmonary artery catheter (PAC) in medical and surgical settings has declined steadily, mostly due to the increasing amount of data from large, randomized studies showing that major clinical outcomes (particularly death) are not changed by PAC use and that the adverse effects of PAC monitoring should be considered. During surgery for myocardial revascularization and in the intensive care unit (ICU) setting, patient outcomes are independent of PAC use despite the substantial amount of physiologic information obtained.

Judge and colleagues surveyed the members of the Society of Cardiovascular Anesthesiologists to assess current PAC use. The use of a PAC for myocardial revascularization was practice-dependent, with anesthesiologists in private practices using PACs for hemodynamic monitoring the most, followed by those in academic and government practice settings. Off-pump coronary artery bypass (OPCAB) and minimally invasive CABG procedures were more likely to be monitored with a PAC.

Patient risk factors that may warrant PAC placement include significant impairment of ventricular function, known pulmonary hypertension, and right-sided HF. The 2011 ACCF/ACC guideline for CABG surgery suggested that PAC placement can be useful in patients in cardiogenic shock or hemodynamically unstable patients.

Transesophageal Echocardiography

The earliest signs of myocardial ischemia include diastolic dysfunction followed by systolic regional wall motion abnormalities (RWMAs), which occur within seconds of acute coronary occlusion. Worsening of RWMAs after CABG is associated with an increased risk of long-term adverse cardiac morbidity and has been suggested as a prognostic indicator of adverse cardiovascular outcome. New RWMAs detected in the intraoperative period frequently may result from nonischemic or ischemic causes such as changes in loading conditions, alteration in electrical conduction in the heart, post-CPB pacing, myocardial stunning due to ischemia before or during weaning from CPB, or poor myocardial preservation. TEE is highly sensitive but lacks specificity for myocardial ischemia monitoring. Additional limitations apply because not all wall segments can be monitored continuously in real time and compared with preoperative findings.

Despite these limitations, TEE use in patients undergoing CABG can provide invaluable information beyond ischemia detection. TEE can assist in the pre-CPB evaluation of cardiac function, assessment and quantification of associated valvular lesions that may impact the surgical plan (eg, concomitant functional mitral regurgitation [MR], aortic stenosis), or CPB management (eg, aortic regurgitation).

The aorta can be assessed for the presence and severity of atheromatous plaques, and TEE can help to locate appropriate cannulation and cross-clamp sites or avoid the manipulation of the aorta altogether (ie, no-touch techniques). Cannulation techniques, including retrograde cardioplegia cannula positioning, a persistent left superior vena cava cannula (ie, retrograde cardioplegia problem), venous cannula positioning allowing unobstructed venous drainage, and an aortic cannula position in the aortic arch, can be assisted by TEE guidance. TEE can detect complications such as iatrogenic aortic dissection and can evaluate de-airing after release of the aortic cross-clamp. TEE monitoring can guide hemodynamic management after CPB, including the assessment of ventricular function, volume status, and the choice of and response to inotropic support.

The American Society of Anesthesiologists (ASA) and the Society of Cardiovascular Anesthesiologists (SCA) developed practice guidelines in 1996 for the perioperative use of TEE. The guidelines were updated in 2010, and the routine use of TEE was recommended for all cardiac or thoracic aortic surgery, including all CABG or OPCAB procedures. The ASA Task Force thereby acknowledged that TEE information could impact perioperative anesthesia, surgical management, and patient outcomes. A comprehensive TEE examination is recommended by the American Society of Echocardiography (ASA)/SCA Task Force before and after CPB or after completion of revascularization in OPCAB surgery.

Neuromonitoring

Stroke and neurocognitive dysfunction are feared complications associated with CABG, whether or not CPB is used, and they occur at a high enough rate that further improvements are needed. Although monitoring alone cannot change outcomes, early recognition of potentially harmful events and interventions with an associated outcome benefit may be useful. There is no consensus about which neuromonitoring modality should be selected. However, specialty societies have increasingly recommended neuromonitoring in an effort to decrease the incidence of poor neurologic outcomes associated with cardiac surgery, including CABG and OPCAB. The 2011 ACCF/AHA guideline for CABG surgery recommended central nervous system monitoring for patients undergoing myocardial revascularization (class IIb recommendation). However, they also recognized that more evidence demonstrating clear benefits was needed and that the effectiveness of detecting cerebral hypoperfusion based on the available data is uncertain.

Induction and Maintenance of General Anesthesia

The main considerations in choosing an induction technique for patients undergoing CABG are LV function and coronary pathology. No single approach to anesthesia for CABG is suitable for all patients. Most hypnotics, opioids, and volatile agents have

14

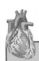

> **BOX 14.3** *Considerations for Anesthesia Induction and Maintenance During Myocardial Revascularization*
>
> 1. Anesthetic induction with tight control of hemodynamic parameters (ie, avoid tachycardia, hypotension), particularly in patients with left main or proximal LAD disease.
> 2. Fast-track anesthetic protocols aiming for early extubation are favored for most patients.
> 3. Given the increasing evidence for preconditioning effects, a potent volatile agent should be part of the anesthetic regimen. Avoid nitrous oxide because of the possibility of expanding gaseous emboli.
> 4. Maintain CPP without increasing myocardial oxygen demand (eg, phenylephrine, nitroglycerin; avoid tachycardia).
> 5. Antifibrinolytic therapy (ie, ε-aminocaproic acid or tranexamic acid) except in OPCAB patients. Aprotinin is no longer available in the United States.
> 6. Consider low tidal volume mechanical ventilation and no PEEP during LIMA dissection.
> 7. Heparin usually is administered before clamping the LIMA pedicle to avoid thrombosis. Papaverine, if injected retrograde into the LIMA by the surgeon, is frequently associated with hypotension.
> 8. Heparin administration (300–400 IU/kg) or as calculated by heparin titration (Hepcon) in CABG patients with CPB. ACT >480 seconds and/or heparin level >2.5 U/mL is required for institution of CPB.
>
> *ACT,* Activated coagulation time; *CABG,* coronary artery bypass grafting; *CPB,* cardiopulmonary bypass; *CPP,* coronary perfusion pressure; *LAD,* left anterior descending coronary artery; *LIMA,* left internal mammary artery; *OPCAB,* off-pump coronary artery bypass; *PEEP,* positive end-expiratory pressure.

been used in different combinations for the induction and maintenance of anesthesia, with good results in the hands of experienced clinicians. Limiting the amount of opioids or use of short-acting drugs is encouraged for patients eligible for fast-tracking and early extubation. With modern cardioplegia techniques and assuming an uneventful intraoperative course, cardiac function typically is well preserved, and the goal should be to extubate the patient within 6 hours postoperatively (Box 14.3).

Anesthetic Agents

The cardiac effects of commonly used induction agents have been investigated over many years. Unraveling the direct or indirect effects of a particular drug on the heart and circulation is complex because overall effects are based on contractility, vascular tone, and response of the autonomic nervous system and baroreceptors.

Etomidate is often the preferred induction agent in patients with depressed cardiac function because it has minimal or no direct negative inotropic or sympathomimetic effects. Despite the observed hemodynamic stability, unwanted side effects are common. Significant pain during injection, particularly in a small superficial vein, is unpleasant for the patient and causes tachycardia and hypertension, both of which increase myocardial oxygen demand. Unless combined with an adequate amount of opioids, blunting of the adrenergic response to intubation is poor and may result in hypertension and tachycardia. Even a single dose of etomidate can inhibit adrenal mitochondrial hydroxylase activity, resulting in reduced steroidogenesis; however, outcome differences in cardiac surgery patients have not been documented consistently.

Propofol is commonly used as an induction agent in patients undergoing CABG, for anesthesia maintenance, and for sedation postoperatively in the ICU. A load-independent measure of contractility, at four different plasma concentrations (0.6–2.6 mg/mL) found no direct effect on contractility, although it lowered preload and afterload. Although there seem to be well-documented advantages for using inhalation anesthetics in patients at risk for myocardial injury, benefits of propofol also have been reported. Propofol has strong free radical–scavenging properties that, in one CABG study, appeared to attenuate myocardial lipid peroxidation. In a multicenter, prospective study comparing an inhalation-based anesthetic with total intravenous anesthesia in patients undergoing combined valvular and CABG surgery, no observed beneficial effect of sevoflurane on the composite end point of mortality, prolonged ICU stay, and troponin levels was found. A large metaanalysis that included 133 studies and 14,516 cardiac and noncardiac surgery patients found no difference in mortality when propofol was used.

Benzodiazepines are commonly used in patients undergoing CABG for preoperative sedation and in combination with a narcotic to induce anesthesia. Midazolam is very well tolerated, with minimal hemodynamic effects even in patients with severe cardiac dysfunction.

In the late 1970s, Stanley first reported the use of high doses of fentanyl for CABG, with and without supplemental benzodiazepines. Clinicians worldwide perceived the lack of histamine release to be a very favorable property and rapidly adopted fentanyl into their clinical practice.

Reports on the use of the more potent sufentanil appeared at the same time as fentanyl, although most studies were not reported until the late 1980s. It was also widely adopted, although there was concern about its very potent bradycardic effects at high doses, particularly when administered with nonvagolytic muscle relaxants.

In the mid-1990s, remifentanil was introduced, and, fueled by intense interest in fast-tracking (promoted in the same time frame), it was intensively investigated.

The previously described opioids are pure opioid agonists, and none provides complete anesthesia as defined by predictable dose-response relationships for suppression of the stress response and release of endogenous catecholamines (particularly norepinephrine), even with high serum concentrations. Hypertension and tachycardia commonly have been reported in response to induction or intubation and surgical stimuli (particularly with sternotomy). In current practice, anesthesia using only a high-dose opioid is rarely practiced. To provide complete anesthesia, the usual practice is to supplement opioids with inhaled or other intravenous agents. This permits a reduction in the total dose of opioid and, particularly with volatile agents, more rapid return of respiratory drive, facilitating early extubation.

Neuromuscular blocking agents have been used to produce adequate intubating conditions and muscle relaxation during CABG. Traditionally, pancuronium was advocated for use with high-dose narcotic techniques because it offset opioid-induced bradycardia. Especially in fast-track cardiac surgery, shorter-acting neuromuscular blocking agents have completely replaced pancuronium, allowing earlier extubation and ICU discharge.

Inhalation Anesthetics and Myocardial Protection

Inhalation anesthetics are routinely used in patients undergoing CABG due to the shift from using a high-opioid anesthetic to fast-tracking and because of mounting evidence that potent inhalation anesthetics protect the myocardium against ischemia by eliciting protective cellular responses similar to those seen with ischemic preconditioning.

There is evidence that pharmacologic agents such as potent inhalation anesthetics and opioids mimic the effects seen with ischemic preconditioning, a concept called *pharmacologic or anesthetic preconditioning*.

14

Several metaanalyses looked at preconditioning and mortality rates or long-term outcomes for patients undergoing cardiac surgery. In a metaanalysis that included only studies with sevoflurane and desflurane, Landoni and coworkers showed a reduction in mortality rates and the incidence of MI after cardiac surgery. In two other metaanalyses that also included isoflurane, no such benefit was seen. De Hert and colleagues showed that the best results for myocardial protection were achieved when sevoflurane was administered throughout the intraoperative period rather than immediately before the planned myocardial ischemic event.

The 2011 ACCF/AHA guideline for CABG surgery provided level A evidence for using volatile-based anesthesia for patients undergoing myocardial revascularization to reduce the risk of perioperative myocardial ischemia and infarction.

Role of Central Neuraxial Blockade

A balanced general anesthetic is still the most commonly used technique for patients undergoing CABG. However, there are many publications on the use of neuraxial techniques, particularly from Europe and Asia, for patients undergoing cardiac surgery. It has been long appreciated that thoracic sympathectomy has favorable effects on the heart and coronary circulation.

In the United States, medicolegal concerns about the rare but real danger of a devastating neurologic injury, the substantial logistic issues regarding placement of the catheter the night before surgery (most patients undergoing nonemergent CABG in the United States are admitted on the morning of surgery), and the potential for cancellation of a procedure in the event of a bloody tap during epidural catheter placement have limited this technique. The ubiquitous use of potent antiplatelet drugs in patients with CAD and the insufficient data regarding when to safely discontinue those drugs before thoracic epidural anesthesia and before catheter removal postoperatively are major concerns. The advent of fast-tracking may be a driving force (ie, ability to extubate faster and have a more comfortable patient with thoracic epidural anesthesia), although most evidence suggests that a wide variety of techniques can be used effectively to facilitate early extubation. The cardioprotective effects of volatile agents may be as effective as the beneficial effects of thoracic sympathectomy.

Myocardial Ischemia in Patients Undergoing Revascularization Surgery

In addition to providing anesthesia, a major concern of the anesthesiologist is the prevention and treatment of myocardial ischemia. The 2011 ACCF/AHA guideline for CABG surgery recommended that determinants in coronary perfusion (ie, heart rate [HR], diastolic pressure or mean arterial pressure [MAP], and right ventricular [RV] or LV end-diastolic pressure [LVEDP]) should be monitored to reduce the risk of perioperative ischemia. Monitoring relevant hemodynamic parameters, detecting myocardial ischemia and prompt treatment are of paramount importance for patients undergoing myocardial revascularization.

The main hemodynamic goals are to ensure an adequate coronary perfusion pressure (CPP; ie, diastolic BP minus LVEDP) and HR control; HR is the single most important treatable determinant of myocardial oxygen consumption. Table 14.1 summarizes the treatment of acute perioperative myocardial ischemia.

Fig. 14.7 demonstrates how hypertension (ie, increase in wall stress), even in the absence of tachycardia, as a response to surgical stress (eg, skin incision) can be associated with pulmonary hypertension, elevated pulmonary capillary wedge pressure (PCWP), and prominent A and V waves on the PCWP waveform. Signs of myocardial

Table 14.1	Acute Treatments for Suspected Intraoperative Myocardial Ischemia[a]	
Associated Hemodynamic Finding	**Therapy**	**Dosage**
Hypertension, tachycardia[b]	Deepen anesthesia	
	Intravenous (IV) β-blockade	Esmolol, 20–100 mg ± 50–200 µg/kg/min prn
		Metoprolol, 0.5–2.5 mg
		Labetalol, 2.5–10 mg
	IV nitroglycerin	Nitroglycerin, 10–500 µg/min[c]
Normotension, tachycardia[b]	Ensure adequate anesthesia, change anesthetic regimen	
	IV β-blockade	β-Blockade, as above
Hypertension, normal heart rate	Deepen anesthesia	
	IV nitroglycerin or nicardipine	Nicardipine, 1–5 mg ± 1–10 µg/kg/min
		Nitroglycerin, 10–500 µg/min[c]
Hypotension, tachycardia[b]	IV α-agonist	Phenylephrine, 25–100 µg
		Norepinephrine, 2–4 µg
	Alter anesthetic regimen (eg, lighten)	
	IV nitroglycerin when normotensive	Nitroglycerin, 10–500 µg/min[c]
Hypotension, bradycardia	Lighten anesthesia	
	IV ephedrine	Ephedrine, 5–10 mg
	IV epinephrine	Epinephrine, 4–8 µg
	IV atropine	Atropine, 0.3–0.6 mg
	IV nitroglycerin when normotensive	Nitroglycerin, 10–500 µg/min[c]
Hypotension, normal heart rate	IV α-agonist/ephedrine	α-Agonist, as above
	IV epinephrine	Epinephrine, 4–8 µg
	Alter anesthesia (eg, lighten)	
	IV nitroglycerin when normotensive	Nitroglycerin, 10–500 µg/min[c]
No abnormality	IV nitroglycerin	Nitroglycerin, 10–500 µg/min[c]
	IV nicardipine	Nicardipine, 1–5 mg ± 1–10 µg/kg/min

[a]Ensure adequacy of oxygenation, ventilation, and intravascular volume status and consider surgical factors, such as manipulation of heart of coronary grafts.
[b]Tachyarrhythmias (eg, paroxysmal atrial tachycardia, atrial fibrillation) should be treated directly with synchronized cardioversion or specific pharmacologic agents.
[c]Bolus doses (25–50 µg) and a high infusion rate may be required initially.

ischemia (ie, ischemic MR) often resolve with administration of a nitroglycerin (NTG) infusion.

Intraoperative Treatment of Myocardial Ischemia

INTRAVENOUS NITROGLYCERIN

Since the introduction in 1976 by Kaplan of the V_5 lead to diagnose myocardial ischemia and intravenous NTG to treat it, the drug has been one of the mainstays for treating perioperative myocardial ischemia. Intravenous NTG acts immediately to reduce LV preload and wall tension, primarily by decreasing venous tone at lower

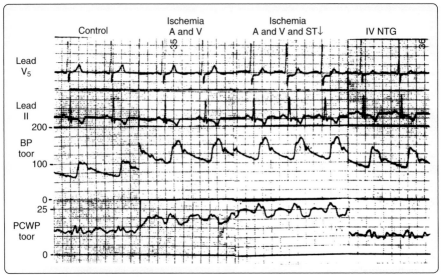

Fig. 14.7 Nitroglycerin *(NTG)* relieved postintubation intraoperative myocardial ischemia, as evidenced by large V waves in the pulmonary capillary wedge pressure *(PCWP)* tracing and then by ST-segment depression. *BP,* Blood pressure. (From Kaplan JA, Wells PH: Early diagnosis of myocardial ischemia using the pulmonary arterial catheter. *Anesth Analg.* 1981;60:789.)

BOX 14.4   *Intraoperative Use of Intravenous Nitroglycerin*

Hypertension
Elevated pulmonary artery pressure
New-onset AC and V waves (ischemic mitral regurgitation)
Acute ischemia (ST changes >1 mm)
New regional wall motion abnormalities on transesophageal echocardiography
Diastolic dysfunction
Systolic dysfunction (with adequate coronary perfusion pressure)
Coronary artery spasm

---

doses, and at larger doses, it decreases arterial and epicardial coronary arterial resistance. It is most effective in treating acute myocardial ischemia with ventricular dysfunction accompanied by sudden elevations in LV end-diastolic volume, LVEDP, and pulmonary arterial pressure (PAP). The elevations in LV preload and wall tension further exacerbate perfusion deficits in the ischemic subendocardium and usually respond immediately to NTG.

In the pre-CPB period and during OPCAB, NTG is used to treat signs of ischemia such as ST-segment depression, hypertension uncontrolled by the anesthetic technique, ventricular dysfunction, and coronary artery spasm (Box 14.4). During CPB, NTG can be used to control the MAP, but only about 60% of patients are responders because of alterations of the pharmacokinetics and pharmacodynamics of the drug with CPB. Factors contributing to the reduction of its effectiveness include adsorption to the plastic in the CPB system, alterations in regional blood flow, hemodilution, and hypothermia. After revascularization, NTG is used to treat residual ischemia or

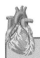

> **BOX 14.5** *Uses of Intravenous Nitroglycerin on Termination of Cardiopulmonary Bypass*
>
> Myocardial ischemia or stunning
> Diastolic dysfunction
> Elevated pulmonary artery pressure, pulmonary capillary wedge pressure, central venous pressure, pulmonary vascular resistance, systemic vascular resistance
> Increased coronary perfusion pressure along with a vasopressor
> Prevention of arterial graft spasm (ie, radial artery graft)
> Coronary artery spasm
> Reinfusion of oxygenator volume

coronary artery spasm, reduce preload and afterload, and it may be combined with vasopressors (eg, phenylephrine) to increase the CPP when treating coronary air embolism (Box 14.5).

Intravenous NTG has been compared with other vasodilators such as nitroprusside and calcium channel blockers. Kaplan and Jones first demonstrated that NTG was preferable to nitroprusside during CABG. Both drugs controlled intraoperative hypertension and decreased myocardial oxygen consumption, but NTG improved ischemic changes on the ECG, whereas nitroprusside did not. Nitroprusside decreased CPP or produced an intracoronary steal in about one-third of patients with myocardial ischemia.

CALCIUM CHANNEL ANTAGONISTS

Nicardipine is a short-acting dihydropyridine calcium antagonist similar to nifedipine, but it possesses a tertiary amine structure in the ester side chain. It has highly specific modes of action, which include coronary antispasmodic and vasodilatory effects and systemic vasodilation. Among the calcium antagonists, nicardipine is unique in its consistent augmentation of CBF and its ability to induce potent vasodilator responses in the coronary bed. Nicardipine produces minimal myocardial depression and significantly improves diastolic function in patients with ischemic heart disease. Despite these beneficial properties, nicardipine is typically not the primary choice in treating myocardial ischemia during CABG.

Clevidipine was introduced for the treatment of perioperative hypertension. It is an ultrashort-acting, intravenously administered, dihydropyridine calcium channel blocker that acts as an arterial-selective vasodilator, and its action is rapidly terminated by blood and tissue esterases. In a randomized, double-blind, placebo-controlled, multicenter trial of the drug in patients undergoing cardiac surgery, clevidipine effectively reduced arterial BP. Like nicardipine, it could be used if NTG does not control the BP.

β-BLOCKERS

Hypertension, tachycardia, arrhythmias, and myocardial ischemia from sympathetic stimulation are common occurrences in the perioperative period. Despite the benefits of early use of β-blockers in the treatment of myocardial ischemia, the relatively long half-life and prolonged duration of action of previously available β-blockers had significantly limited their use during surgery and the immediate postoperative period. However, with the introduction of esmolol in the late 1980s, an ultrashort-acting

14

cardioselective β_1-blocker with a half-life of 9 minutes became available. Esmolol was soon adopted by many clinicians for the prevention and treatment of myocardial ischemia. A mean esmolol dose of 17 ± 16 mg/min, with a range of 8 to 24 mg/min, was found to be effective in alleviating chest pain while increasing cardiac output in patients with unstable angina.

It was shown that esmolol was effective in treating acute myocardial ischemia, even in patients with poor LV function (ie, increased PCWP of 15–25 mm Hg). Esmolol was infused in doses up to 300 µg/kg per minute and produced decreases in HR, BP, and cardiac index. However, the PCWP was not significantly altered by the drug infusion. Even in the setting of moderate LV dysfunction, esmolol can safely reduce BP and HR in patients with acute myocardial ischemia.

Because of the favorable pharmacologic properties and encouraging clinical findings, esmolol was soon used frequently during CABG to treat hypertension and tachycardia and to prevent myocardial ischemia. It is usually given as a test dose of 20 mg IV. An infusion can then be used.

The Immediate Postoperative Period

Sedation

Patients usually are sedated to facilitate transport to the ICU and during the immediate postoperative period until extubation criteria are fulfilled. Dexmedetomidine, propofol, and midazolam are intravenously administered agents with favorable properties in this setting.

α_2-Adrenergic receptor agonists have unique properties (Box 14.6) that explain their increasing use in some cardiac surgery centers. In 1999, the FDA approved dexmedetomidine for continuous (up to 24 hours) intravenous sedation in the ICU. It is a more selective α_2-adrenoceptor agonist than clonidine, and exhibits central sympatholytic and peripheral vasoconstrictive effects. Intravenous bolus administration causes a transient increase in MAP and systemic vascular resistance due to stimulation of peripheral α- and β_2-adrenergic receptors in vascular smooth muscle. A continuous infusion (0.2–0.8 µg/kg per hour) has dose-dependent hemodynamic effects; most

IV

BOX 14.6   *α_2-Agonist Properties*

Sedation
Anxiolysis
Analgesia
Hemodynamic stability
Central sympatholytic effect
Decreased blood pressure and heart rate
Decreased perioperative oxygen consumption
Decreased plasma catecholamine levels
Decreased incidence of tachyarrhythmias
Prevention of histamine-induced bronchoconstriction
Treatment and prevention of postoperative shivering
Sedation in patients with postoperative delirium
Blunting of withdrawal symptoms in drug and alcohol addicts
Possible inhibition of inflammatory response

---

consistently decreases in HR, plasma catecholamine levels, and MAP. Dexmedetomidine may be a useful agent in the early postoperative period because its sedative properties are associated with minimal respiratory depression and appear to mimic natural sleep patterns. When administered continuously in postoperative patients, it caused no changes in respiratory rate, oxygen saturation, arterial pH, and arterial carbon dioxide (CO_2) tension compared with placebo. Patients usually were effectively sedated but still arousable and cooperative in response to verbal stimulation. Due to its analgesic properties, it significantly reduced additional opioid analgesia requirements in mechanically ventilated patients in the ICU.

Propofol has been used extensively intraoperatively and for sedation in the ICU. Several studies compared propofol and dexmedetomidine in the postoperative period after surgery. Dexmedetomidine reduced the requirement for opioid analgesia, but for patients after myocardial revascularization, it reduced HR more than propofol, whereas the arterial BP did not differ between the two groups.

A multicenter, randomized study compared a dexmedetomidine-based sedation regimen with propofol sedation after CABG in the ICU. Although there were no differences in time to extubation, the investigators found a significantly reduced need for additional analgesics (ie, propofol-sedated patients required four times the mean dose of morphine), antiemetics, and diuretics and they had fewer episodes of tachyarrhythmias requiring β-blockade (ie, ventricular tachycardia in 5% of the propofol-sedated group vs none in the dexmedetomidine group). However, hypotension was more common in the dexmedetomidine group compared with the propofol-sedated patients (24% vs 16%). Approximately 25% of the dexmedetomidine-associated hypotension occurred in the first hour of the study, particularly during or within 10 minutes after the loading infusion of 1 μg/kg. To avoid hypotension seen with a large loading dose of dexmedetomidine, loading doses are infrequently administered in clinical practice, but a continuous maintenance dose is started earlier to achieve appropriate plasma levels at the time of patient transfer from the operating room.

Coronary Artery and Arterial Conduit Spasm

There have been numerous descriptions of this complication. Spasm usually has been associated with profound ST-segment elevation on the ECG, hypotension, severe dysfunction of the ventricles, and myocardial irritability. Many hypotheses have been put forward to explain the origin of coronary artery spasm (Fig. 14.8). The underlying mechanism may be similar to the coronary spasm seen with Prinzmetal variant angina.

Therapy is usually effective with a wide range of vasodilators such as NTG, calcium channel blockers, milrinone, or combinations of NTG and calcium channel blockers. Arterial grafts with a vessel such as the left internal mammary artery (LIMA) and particularly radial artery grafts are prone to spasm after revascularization, and prevention and recognition are crucial to prevent serious complications.

Fast-Track Management for Coronary Artery Bypass Grafting

Although the fast-track clinical pathway encompasses a variety of perioperative and after-discharge management strategies, early extubation is the one that has received the greatest attention (Box 14.7). Early extubation is acknowledged as a key component of the fast-track clinical pathway and one that was considered the most radical change in practice during the peak of scrutiny of the fast-track pathway in the middle to late 1990s (Box 14.8).

The rigorous, randomized, controlled trial reported by Cheng and associates in 1996 ($N = 100$), in which mean time to extubation was 4.1 hours, is recognized as the most influential of the contemporary studies of early extubation. Reports of successful use of fast-tracking in a variety of patient populations have been reported

14

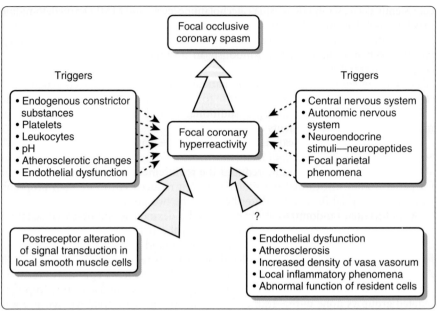

Fig. 14.8 Schematic representation of the pathogenesis of coronary artery spasm.

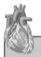

BOX 14.7   *Perioperative Goals of Fast-Track Management*

Preoperative education
Same-day admission whenever possible
Anesthetic technique tailored to early extubation
Effective postoperative analgesia
Flexibility in the use of recovery areas (eg, postanesthesia care unit instead of intensive care unit)
Protocol-driven care
Early mobilization
Early intensive care unit and hospital discharge
Follow-up (eg, telephone, office visits) after hospital discharge
Interdisciplinary continuous quality improvement strategies

since, including academic, private, elderly, rural settings, and Veterans Affairs patients from the United States and many other countries.

The first metaanalyses of early extubation reported were based on accumulated data from randomized, controlled trials. It reviewed studies in which fast-tracking was defined as use of reduced opioid dosing (ie, fentanyl ≤20 µg/kg) with stated intention to attempt extubation in less than 10 hours postoperatively. They identified 10 trials ($N = 1800$) with most involving CABG patients from 1989 to 2002. The fast-track groups had shorter times to extubation (by 8.1 hours), with no significant differences in major morbidity or mortality rates and only one instance of reintubation. ICU LOS was reduced by 5.4 hours, although hospital LOS was not shortened.

> **BOX 14.8** *Suggested Criteria for Early Extubation*
>
> Body temperature >35°C
> Normal acid-base status
> Stable hemodynamics on minimal inotropic support
> Adequate hemostasis with decreasing or stable mediastinal drainage
> Stable cardiac rhythm
> Spontaneous respiratory rate and adequate tidal volumes and inspiratory force
> Chest radiograph without major abnormalities (eg, minimal atelectasis)
> Adequate urine output
> Adequate reversal of neuromuscular blockade
> Awake, alert, cooperative, and moving all extremities

Some centers have adopted an even more aggressive form of fast-tracking. Walji and colleagues coined the term *ultrafast-tracking* to describe their practice and reported a 56% hospital discharge rate by postoperative day 4 and 23% discharge rate by postoperative day 2, although the readmission rate was 3.9%, but there was no early mortality. Ovrum and associates from Norway reported a cohort of 5658 patients with CABG, 99% of whom were extubated by 5 hours (median, 1.5 hours), with a 1.1% reintubation rate. More than 99% of patients were transferred to the ward the next morning.

CORONARY ARTERY BYPASS GRAFTING WITHOUT CARDIOPULMONARY BYPASS

The inherent risks of CPB and aortic cross-clamping continued to be a major factor in CABG morbidity and mortality. Avoiding CPB altogether seemed to offer a solution. It was not until the middle to late 1990s, when surgical researchers developed efficient mechanical stabilizer devices that minimized motion around the anastomotic site, that OPCAB surgery gained more widespread interest.

The pace and tempo of OPCAB surgery differs substantially from that of conventional CABG. Surgical manipulations involve a variety of geometric distortions of the cardiac anatomy, with resulting hemodynamic effects. Communication between all members of the surgical team and anticipation of these changes are vitally important to minimize resulting adverse hemodynamic effects on the heart and other organs. Significant hemodynamic changes that cannot be reversed may necessitate emergent conversion to CPB at any time during OPCAB surgery.

Cardiovascular Effects of Off-Pump Coronary Artery Bypass Grafting

Hemodynamic changes encountered during OPCAB involve the two independent variables of distortion of the right or left atria and ventricles by stabilizer and suspension devices and the effects of myocardial ischemia during anastomosis. The ability to expose the posterior surface of the heart to access the posterior descending and the circumflex vessels using suction devices placed on the apex or anterolateral wall of the heart, pericardial retraction sutures, slings, or other techniques without producing

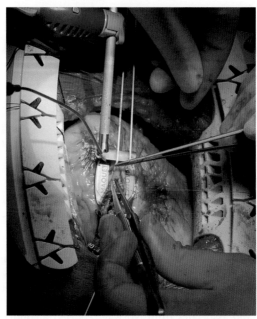

Fig. 14.9 Image depicting left anterior descending (LAD) artery anastomosis during off-pump coronary artery bypass grafting using a left internal mammary artery (LIMA) graft. The view is from the head of the patient. The Maquet mechanical stabilizer (Maquet, Wayne, NJ) is in place along with vascular snare sutures used to transiently occlude the artery. The LIMA is being anastomosed to the LAD, assisted by use of pressurized and heavily humidified carbon dioxide ("mister blower" metal cannula) to facilitate visualization of the vessel lumen. (Courtesy Alexander Mittnacht, MD, Mount Sinai School of Medicine, New York, NY.)

major hemodynamic compromise is critical for multivessel application of OPCAB surgery. Lifting of the heart to work on the posterior vessels commonly is referred to as *verticalization,* in contrast to *displacement* for the LAD and diagonal anastomoses (Figs. 14.9 through 14.11).

The effects of positional maneuvers, including verticalization of the heart, have been investigated. Most data have been obtained from patients with normal or only mildly depressed ventricular function without significant valvular disease with the Octopus stabilizer in the Trendelenburg position, right ventricular end-diastolic pressure increased in each position, with the greatest increase occurring with exposure of the circumflex vessels. This position was associated with the greatest deterioration of stroke volume (approximately 29% vs 22% for PDA and vs 18% for LAD). When comparing patients with EFs of more than or less than 40%, there were nonsignificant trends toward greater reductions in MAP and cardiac output with lower EF.

Mishra and colleagues have reported large-scale, prospective observational data on patients undergoing OPCAB surgery. TEE and PAC were used in all patients, and approximately 40% were considered high risk. Verticalization for exposure of the posterior wall was associated with a reduction in MAP of 18%, an increase in CVP of 66%, and a reduction in stroke volume of 36% and cardiac index of 45%. New RWMAs were common (60%), and global function decreased in a similar proportion. Their practice involved the use of inotropes during this period (79% vs 22% for the anterior wall). However, only 11% required intraaortic balloon pump (IABP), and 0.7% required CPB.

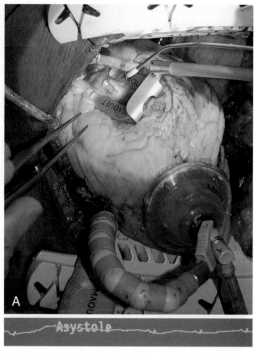

Fig. 14.10 (A) Posterior descending artery (PDA) anastomosis during off-pump coronary artery bypass grafting (CABG) uses a saphenous vein graft. The view is from the head of the patient. The Maquet access device (Maquet, Wayne, NJ) uses suction to position the heart (ie, verticalization) for easy access to the inferior surface of the left ventricle. The stabilizer is in place, and the anastomosis to the PDA is being performed. (B) Characteristic electrocardiographic (ECG) tracing during verticalization of the heart facilitates exposure of the PDA for anastomosis during off-pump CABG. Heart manipulations modify the positional relationship between the heart and surface electrodes. The shape of the tracing is altered, and the amplitude is reduced. The low-voltage electrocardiogram is interpreted by the device as asystole, an audible alarm sounds, and the practitioner is alerted with *Asystole* next to the ECG tracing. (Courtesy Alexander Mittnacht, MD, Mount Sinai School of Medicine, New York, NY.)

Specific Anesthetic Considerations in Patients Undergoing Off-Pump Coronary Artery Bypass Grafting

The anesthesia technique used for patients undergoing OPCAB surgery does not differ much from on-pump CABG (Box 14.9). The anesthesia technique should be tailored to the individual patient and, among other factors, it depends on the indication for OPCAB surgery. Fast-tracking, including early ICU and hospital discharge, is frequently a goal associated with OPCAB surgery, particularly for patients with adequate LV function. Patients with advanced age, significant ascending aortic disease, poor LV function, and multiple comorbidities may be scheduled for OPCAB surgery to avoid aortic cross-clamping, and a single LIMA-to-LAD anastomosis is sometimes performed.

A challenge during OPCAB surgery can be the hemodynamic changes encountered during positioning of the heart. PAP, PCWP, and CVP typically are increased during this phase; the occurrence of large V waves should alert the practitioner to acute ischemia or MR. Wall motion abnormalities and acute, significant MR frequently are seen on

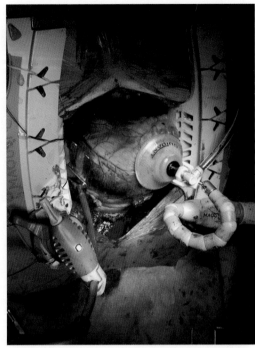

Fig. 14.11 First obtuse marginal anastomosis during off-pump coronary artery bypass grafting using a saphenous vein graft. The view is from the head of the patient. The previously completed left internal mammary artery to left anterior descending anastomosis is seen. The Maquet access device (Maquet, Wayne, NJ) uses suction to position the heart (ie, verticalization) for easy access to the circumflex coronary artery system. (Courtesy Alexander Mittnacht, MD, Mount Sinai School of Medicine, New York, NY.)

BOX 14.9   *Anesthetic Considerations for Off-Pump Coronary Artery Bypass Surgery*

1. Use standard monitoring, including invasive arterial blood pressure monitoring and central venous access.
2. A PAC should be considered in patients with poor LV function or significant mitral regurgitation.
3. TEE is recommended for all patients undergoing OPCAB surgery, unless contraindicated.
4. Use warming devices to maintain normothermia.
5. Dose of heparin according to institutional or surgeon's preference.
6. Fast-tracking, including early extubation, is often a goal in OPCAB surgery.
7. A neuraxial anesthesia technique may be used for postoperative analgesia or as the primary anesthetic technique. The patient must be carefully evaluated for absolute contraindications (eg, potent antiplatelet regimens).
8. Hemodynamic compromise may occur with positioning of the heart or stabilizer application. Positional maneuvers, volume administration, and vasoactive medications are used to maintain hemodynamic stability. CPB always should be immediately available.

CPB, Cardiopulmonary bypass; *LV,* left ventricular; *OPCAB,* off-pump coronary artery bypass grafting; *PAC,* pulmonary artery catheter; *TEE,* transesophageal echocardiography.

TEE. Exacerbation or new onset of MR may be related to structural changes from positioning the heart (eg, annular distortion), stabilizer application, or ischemia.

Hemodynamic compromise during OPCAB surgery can be managed with Trendelenburg positioning, volume administration, and temporary vasoconstrictor administration to maintain CPP during distal anastomosis. Opening of the right pleural space may accommodate the right ventricle, relieving the compression and improving hemodynamics. The right limb of the sternal retractor should be routinely elevated on a rolled towel to create space and avoid compressing of the right atrium or right ventricle against the right sternal border. Similarly, the right-sided pericardial traction sutures must be loosened when the heart is rotated to the right to avoid compression of the hemodynamically vulnerable right atrium and right ventricle against the right pericardial edge. Maintaining the CPP is critical during distal coronary anastomosis, and MAP is typically kept above 80 mm Hg during this phase.

Vasoconstrictor and volume therapy are preferred with inotrope use only in cases of severe hemodynamic compromise. In the setting of ongoing ischemia, the greater increase in oxygen demand with inotropes may place the patient at substantial risk for myocardial injury. In the setting of significant MR not responsive to antiischemic treatment, further increasing the afterload may worsen the clinical picture. Positive inotropic medications are then temporarily indicated if the surgeon cannot correct the position of the heart during critical phases of surgical anastomosis. The surgeon may or may not place temporary intracoronary shunts to allow distal coronary perfusion. There are controversial data and opinions about whether shunts have a clinical benefit in providing myocardial protection or instead cause endothelial damage.

CPB should always be immediately available during OPCAB surgery in case the hemodynamic situation cannot be managed pharmacologically. A lower arterial BP typically is preferred during the proximal (aortic) anastomosis to avoid complications seen with partial aortic clamping (ie, aortic side-clamp). Automated suture devices and techniques that eliminate aortic cross-clamping are being used. Avoidance of aortic partial clamping has been associated with a striking reduction in cerebral emboli and neurologic events during OPCAB. Regardless of the specific technique or device used, the MAP should be kept around 60 mm Hg during manipulation of the aorta and proximal anastomosis. Vasodilators such as NTG are frequently administered and titrated to achieve this goal.

Because CPB with a heat exchanger is not available for maintaining a target temperature, patients are at increased risk for hypothermia during OPCAB surgery. This is particularly problematic if fast-tracking with early extubation is the goal. The room temperature should be adjusted accordingly, and patient-warming devices should be applied.

Anticoagulation in patients undergoing OPCAB surgery is an area of controversy, and the topic always should be discussed with the surgeon before anesthesia induction. Some surgeons prefer low-dose heparinization (eg, 100–200 U/kg of heparin) with a target-activated coagulation time (ACT) of 250 to 300 seconds, whereas others may choose full heparinization (eg, 300 U/kg) during the procedure. The ACT is measured every 30 minutes, and heparin is administered accordingly to maintain the target ACT.

Outcomes for Off-Pump Coronary Artery Bypass Grafting

Although the literature base is increasing, the final word about differences in outcomes and which patients may benefit from OPCAB has not been written. This is not surprising given the technical challenges of OPCAB surgery and highly

14

operator-dependent outcomes, which are difficult to account for even in large, prospective, randomized trials.

A metaanalysis of randomized trials by Cheng and associates found no significant differences in 30-day or 1- to 2-year mortality rates, MI, stroke (at 30 days and 1 to 2 years), renal dysfunction, need for IABP, wound infection, or reoperation for bleeding or reintervention (for ischemia). OPCAB was associated with significant reductions in AF (odds ratio [OR] = 0.58), numbers of patients transfused (OR = 0.43), respiratory infections (OR = 0.41), need for inotropes (OR = 0.48), duration of ventilation (weighted mean difference [WMD] of 3.4 hours), ICU LOS (WMD of 0.3 day), and hospital LOS (WMD of 1.0 days). Changes in neurocognitive dysfunction were not different in the immediate postoperative period; they were significantly improved at 2 to 6 months (OR = 0.57), but there were no differences seen at 12 months.

The critical issue of graft patency was addressed in only four studies, which varied substantially with regard to when assessment occurred (ie, 3 months in two and 12 months in two studies). Only one study reported a difference (ie, reduction in circumflex patency with OPCAB). Because of the small numbers of patients, the overall data for this category were considered inadequate for metaanalysis.

A working group of the AHA Council on Cardiovascular Surgery and Anesthesia analyzed the then-current literature and several small metaanalyses, although not the same ones as Cheng and coworkers. In an informal manner, they concluded that OPCAB probably was associated with less bleeding, less renal dysfunction, less short-term neurocognitive dysfunction (especially in patients with calcified aortas), and shorter hospital LOS. However, they also observed that it is more technically demanding, has a greater learning curve, and may be associated with lower rates of long-term graft patency. Perhaps related to the greater technical demands, surgeons appear to place fewer grafts compared with on-pump CABG, and incomplete revascularization may influence long-term outcomes. Puskas and colleagues reviewed 12,812 patients with CABG (1997–2006) and compared in-hospital major adverse events and long-term survival after OPCAB versus on-pump CABG. Long-term (10-year follow-up) outcomes did not differ significantly between on-pump and off-pump patients. OPCAB was associated with significant reductions in short-term outcomes such as operative mortality, stroke, and major adverse cardiac events. Further data analysis showed that short-term outcome (ie, operative mortality rate) did not differ between the two groups for patients at low risk (ie, The Society of Thoracic Surgeons [STS] predicted risk of death), whereas lower mortality rates were found for OPCAB surgery in high-risk patients.

MINIMALLY INVASIVE CORONARY ARTERY SURGERY

First reported in 1967, minimally invasive direct coronary artery bypass (MIDCAB) was performed with a limited left thoracotomy and LIMA-to-LAD graft on a beating heart. In the subsequent five decades, coronary artery surgery through a midline sternotomy has become the most commonly used approach. In the earlier years of cardiac surgery, this involved a large midline incision with associated complications such as wound infection and brachial plexus injury. Less invasive techniques were sought and developed with the goals of avoiding these complications, faster patient recovery, earlier hospital discharge, and improved patient satisfaction (eg, cosmetically more appealing incision). The following terminology is a sample of what is being used to describe the various surgical approaches.

The original term *MIDCAB* refers to LIMA takedown and anastomosis to the LAD through a small anterior thoracotomy. It can be performed off-pump or on-pump with femoral cannulation. Thoracoscopic and robotic techniques have been developed to avoid chest wall retraction and associated complications. Experience with robotically assisted CABG is limited, and clear outcome benefits have not been reported. Because of limited access to the coronary artery system using this approach, the procedure is often combined with percutaneous revascularization using coronary stents (ie, hybrid coronary revascularization). The hybrid approach is gaining popularity for selected patients with complex proximal-ostial LAD stenosis and typically one other lesion in a non-LAD vessel that can be easily stented.

Totally endoscopic coronary revascularization (TECAB) describes complete surgical revascularization through small chest wall incisions using thoracoscopic instruments and a robot to access coronary lesions that are not close to the chest wall incision. The procedure can be performed with or without CPB; the latter is called *beating-heart TECAB*. Endoscopically assisted CABG (EndoACAB) was developed to avoid the high costs associated with robotic use. In place of expensive robotic equipment, EndoACAB uses thoracoscopic and nondisposable instruments to harvest the LIMA. The coronary anastomosis is performed on a beating heart.

Most minimally invasive coronary artery surgical techniques are technically demanding and require close cooperation by the multidisciplinary surgical team to plan the exact approach, including the type and location of surgical incision; on-pump versus off-pump, patient access during surgery (especially in robotic surgery); and goals of fast-tracking, including early extubation and adequate pain relief. Although a fast-track anesthesia technique often is preferred, anesthesia induction and maintenance do not differ from the approach used in a midline sternotomy (Box 14.10).

An important difference is the requirement for lung deflation on the side of the surgical incision during a beating-heart minimal thoracotomy or thoracoscopy approach. Lung separation techniques, including a double-lumen tube and bronchial blockers with a standard endotracheal tube, have been described. Alternatively, jet ventilation has been reported to facilitate surgical access. Additional challenges compared with thoracic surgery with one-lung ventilation are thoracic insufflation of CO_2, which is required for intrathoracic surgical instrument manipulation and access to surgical anastomosis on the heart, and its hemodynamic consequences. Insufflation pressures

14

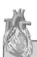

BOX 14.10 *Anesthetic Considerations for Minimally Invasive Coronary Artery Surgery*

1. Apply fast-track anesthesia techniques, including adequate postoperative pain management.
2. Intraoperative monitoring should include central venous access, invasive arterial pressure monitoring, and transesophageal echocardiography. In complex multivessel coronary artery revascularization, the benefits of pulmonary artery catheter monitoring may outweigh the risks.
3. Defibrillator pads are mandatory and need to be placed with regard to the exact location of surgical incisions.
4. Lung separation may be required for off-pump procedures.
5. Intrathoracic carbon dioxide insufflation can cause hemodynamic changes.
6. In prolonged procedures, measurements of adequate body perfusion and oxygen balance should be performed frequently.
7. Emergency conversion to an on-pump procedure and/or emergency sternotomy may be required.

are typically kept below 10 to 15 mm Hg; nevertheless, significant increases in CVP and PAP typically occur. RWMAs have been described with thoracic insufflation, as has decreased cardiac output at higher insufflation pressures. Fluid administration and vasoconstrictor or inotropic support are frequently used to maintain hemodynamic stability. Urine output, plasma lactate, and SvO_2 should be monitored frequently, especially during long procedures.

If hemodynamic stability cannot be maintained or is acutely compromised (including uncontrolled surgical bleeding), the use of femoral-femoral cannulation and prompt initiation of CPB can be lifesaving. Any otherwise unexplained rise in end-tidal CO_2 should alert the practitioner to increased CO_2 absorption from the positive-pressure thoracic insufflation. Sudden decreases in end-tidal CO_2 have been described with positive-pressure CO_2 insufflation in different settings and, if encountered, they should alert the practitioner to possible massive CO_2 embolization.

Due to the hemodynamic changes associated with thoracic inflation and prolonged one-lung ventilation in long surgical cases, adequate monitoring of hemodynamic and oxygenation parameters is considered prudent. TEE is recommended and, although outcome data are lacking, a PAC catheter is frequently inserted, especially if more than a single-vessel LIMA anastomosis is planned.

Access to the heart is limited, and defibrillator pads have to be placed before the patient is positioned and draped. This is further complicated by interference with surgical instruments and left chest wall incisions, and the defibrillator pad position may have to be modified accordingly. Because of the frequently cited advantages of early patient mobilization and hospital discharge, fast-track anesthesia is often part of the perioperative management strategy. A midline sternotomy is less painful for most patients compared with a small thoracoscopic incision with chest wall retraction. Adequate pain management is therefore mandatory in achieving fast-tracking goals for these patients. Long-acting intercostal nerve or other types of nerve blocks, administered before skin incision and redosed at the end of the surgical procedure, can facilitate overall anesthesia and pain management.

SUGGESTED READINGS

Bomb R, Oliphant CS, Khouzam RN. Dual antiplatelet therapy after coronary artery bypass grafting in the setting of acute coronary syndrome. *Am J Cardiol*. 2015;116:148.

Brinkman W, Herbert MA, O'Brien S, et al. Preoperative β-blocker use in coronary artery bypass grafting surgery: national database analysis. *JAMA Intern Med*. 2014;174:1320.

Cavallaro P, Rhee AJ, Chiang Y, et al. In-hospital mortality and morbidity after robotic coronary artery surgery. *J Cardiothorac Vasc Anesth*. 2015;29:27.

Chassot PG, van der Linden P, Zaugg M, et al. Off-pump coronary artery bypass surgery: physiology and anaesthetic management. *Br J Anaesth*. 2004;92:400.

Cheng DC, Bainbridge D, Martin JE, et al. Does off-pump coronary artery bypass reduce mortality, morbidity, and resource utilization when compared with conventional coronary artery bypass? A meta-analysis of randomized trials. *Anesthesiology*. 2005;102:188.

Collison SP, Agarwal A, Trehan N. Controversies in the use of intraluminal shunts during off-pump coronary artery bypass grafting surgery. *Ann Thorac Surg*. 2006;82:1559.

Coronary Revascularization Writing Group, Patel MR, Dehmer GJ, Hirshfeld JW, et al. ACCF/SCAI/STS/AATS/AHA/ASNC/HFSA/SCCT 2012 appropriate use criteria for coronary revascularization focused update: a report of the American College of Cardiology Foundation Appropriate Use Criteria Task Force, Society for Cardiovascular Angiography and Interventions, Society of Thoracic Surgeons, American Association for Thoracic Surgery, American Heart Association, American Society of Nuclear Cardiology, and the Society of Cardiovascular Computed Tomography. *J Thorac Cardiovasc Surg*. 2012;143:780.

Curtis JA, Hollinger MK, Jain HB. Propofol-based versus dexmedetomidine-based sedation in cardiac surgery patients. *J Cardiothorac Vasc Anesth*. 2013;27:1289.

Daniel WT 3rd, Kilgo P, Puskas JD, et al. Trends in aortic clamp use during coronary artery bypass surgery: effect of aortic clamping strategies on neurologic outcomes. *J Thorac Cardiovasc Surg*. 2014;147:652.

De Hert S, Vlasselaers D, Barbe R, et al. A comparison of volatile and non volatile agents for cardioprotection during on-pump coronary surgery. *Anaesthesia.* 2009;64:953.

De Hert SG, Cromheecke S, ten Broecke PW, et al. Effects of propofol, desflurane, and sevoflurane on recovery of myocardial function after coronary surgery in elderly high-risk patients. *Anesthesiology.* 2003;99:314.

de Waal BA, Buise MP, van Zundert AA. Perioperative statin therapy in patients at high risk for cardiovascular morbidity undergoing surgery: a review. *Br J Anaesth.* 2015;114:44.

Judge O, Ji F, Fleming N, et al. Current use of the pulmonary artery catheter in cardiac surgery: a survey study. *J Cardiothorac Vasc Anesth.* 2015;29:69.

Landoni G, Biondi-Zoccai GG, Zangrillo A, et al. Desflurane and sevoflurane in cardiac surgery: a meta-analysis of randomized clinical trials. *J Cardiothorac Vasc Anesth.* 2007;21:502.

Landoni G, Greco T, Biondi-Zoccai G, et al. Anaesthetic drugs and survival: a Bayesian network meta-analysis of randomized trials in cardiac surgery. *Br J Anaesth.* 2013;111:886.

Landoni G, Guarracino F, Cariello C, et al. Volatile compared with total intravenous anaesthesia in patients undergoing high-risk cardiac surgery: a randomized multicentre study. *Br J Anaesth.* 2014;113:955.

Mishra M, Shrivastava S, Dhar A, et al. A prospective evaluation of hemodynamic instability during off-pump coronary artery bypass surgery. *J Cardiothorac Vasc Anesth.* 2003;17:452.

Myles PS, Daly DJ, Djaiani G, et al. A systematic review of the safety and effectiveness of fast-track cardiac anesthesia. *Anesthesiology.* 2003;99:982.

Pasin L, Landoni G, Nardelli P, et al. Dexmedetomidine reduces the risk of delirium, agitation and confusion in critically ill patients: a meta-analysis of randomized controlled trials. *J Cardiothorac Vasc Anesth.* 2014;28:1459.

Puskas JD, Kilgo PD, Lattouf OM, et al. Off-pump coronary bypass provides reduced mortality and morbidity and equivalent 10-year survival. *Ann Thorac Surg.* 2008;86:1139.

Shahian DM, O'Brien SM, Sheng S, et al. Predictors of long-term survival after coronary artery bypass grafting surgery: results from the Society of Thoracic Surgeons Adult Cardiac Surgery Database (the ASCERT study). *Circulation.* 2012;125:1491.

Stenger M, Fabrin A, Schmidt H, et al. High thoracic epidural analgesia as an adjunct to general anesthesia is associated with better outcome in low-to-moderate risk cardiac surgery patients. *J Cardiothorac Vasc Anesth.* 2013;27:1301.

Wagner CE, Bick JS, Johnson D, et al. Etomidate use and postoperative outcomes among cardiac surgery patients. *Anesthesiology.* 2014;120:579.

Wiesbauer F, Schlager O, Domanovits H, et al. Perioperative beta-blockers for preventing surgery related mortality and morbidity: asystemic review and meta-analysis. *Anesth Analg.* 2007;104:27.

Zhang X, Zhao X, Wang Y. Dexmedetomidine: a review of applications for cardiac surgery during perioperative period. *J Anesth.* 2015;29:102.

14

Chapter 15

Valvular Heart Disease: Replacement and Repair

Harish Ramakrishna, MD, FASE, FACC •
Ryan C. Craner, MD • Patrick A. Devaleria, MD •
David J. Cook, MD • Philippe R. Housmans, MD, PhD •
Kent H. Rehfeldt, MD, FASE

Key Points

1. Although various valvular lesions generate different physiologic changes, all valvular heart disease is characterized by abnormalities of ventricular loading.
2. The left ventricle normally compensates for increases in afterload by increases in preload. This increase in end-diastolic fiber stretch or radius further increases wall tension in accordance with Laplace's law, resulting in a reciprocal decline in myocardial fiber shortening. The stroke volume is maintained because the contractile force is augmented at the higher preload level.
3. Treatment modalities for hypertrophic obstructive cardiomyopathy, a relatively common genetic malformation of the heart, include β-adrenoceptor antagonists, calcium channel blockers, and myectomy of the septum. Newer approaches include dual-chamber pacing and septal reduction (ie, ablation) therapy with ethanol.
4. The severity and duration of symptoms of aortic regurgitation may correlate poorly with the degree of hemodynamic and contractile impairment, delaying surgical treatment while patients are undergoing progressive deterioration.
5. Mitral regurgitation causes left ventricular volume overload. Treatment depends on the underlying mechanism and includes early reperfusion therapy, angiotensin-converting enzyme inhibitors, and surgical repair or replacement of the mitral valve.
6. Rheumatic disease and congenital abnormalities of the mitral valve are the main causes of mitral stenosis, a slowly progressive disease. Surgical treatment options include closed and open commissurotomy and percutaneous mitral commissurotomy.
7. Most tricuspid surgery occurs in the context of significant aortic or mitral disease, and anesthesia management primarily is determined by the left-sided valve lesion.
8. Innovations in surgical valve repair include aortic valve repair and closed- and open-chamber procedures for mitral regurgitation.

Valve surgery is very different from coronary artery bypass grafting (CABG). Over the natural history of valvular heart disease (VHD), the physiology changes markedly. In the operating room, physiologic conditions and hemodynamics are quite dynamic and are readily influenced by anesthesia. For some types of valve lesions, it can be relatively difficult to predict before surgery how the heart will respond to the altered loading conditions associated with valve repair or replacement.

It is essential to understand the natural history of adult-acquired valve defects and how the pathophysiology evolves. Clinicians must also understand surgical decision making for valve repair or replacement. A valve operated on at the appropriate stage of its natural history has a good and more predictable outcome compared with a heart operated on at a later stage, for which the perioperative result can be poor. The dynamic physiology and natural history of each valve defect govern the anesthesia plan, which must include the requirements for preload, pacing rate, and rhythm; use of inotropes or negative inotropes; and use of vasodilators or vasoconstrictors to alter loading conditions.

Although valvular lesions impose different physiologic changes, a unifying concept is that all VHD is characterized by abnormalities of ventricular loading. The status of the ventricle changes over time because ventricular function and the valvular defect itself are influenced by the progression of volume or pressure overload. The clinical status of patients with VHD can be complex and dynamic. It is possible to have clinical decompensation in the context of normal ventricular contractility or have ventricular decompensation and performance with normal ejection indices. The altered loading conditions characteristic of VHD may result in a divergence between the function of the heart as a systolic pump and the intrinsic inotropic state of the myocardium. The divergence between cardiac performance and inotropy results from compensatory physiologic mechanisms that are specific to each of the ventricular loading abnormalities.

AORTIC STENOSIS

Clinical Features and Natural History

Aortic stenosis (AS) is the most common cardiac valve lesion in the United States. Approximately 1% to 2% of people are born with a bicuspid aortic valve, which is prone to stenosis with aging. Clinically significant aortic valve stenosis occurs in 2% of unselected individuals older than 65 years and in 5.5% of those older than 85 years.

Calcific AS has several features in common with coronary artery disease (CAD). Both conditions are more common in men, older people, and patients with hypercholesterolemia, and both result in part from an active inflammatory process. Clinical evidence indicates that an atherosclerotic process is the cellular mechanism of aortic valve stenosis. There is a clear association between clinical risk factors for atherosclerosis and the development of AS: increased lipoprotein levels, increased low-density lipoprotein (LDL) cholesterol, cigarette smoking, hypertension, diabetes mellitus, increased serum calcium and creatinine levels, and male sex. The early lesion of aortic valve sclerosis may be associated with CAD and vascular atherosclerosis. Aortic valve calcification is an inflammatory process promoted by atherosclerotic risk factors.

The average rate of progression is a decrease in aortic valve area (AVA) of 0.1 cm²/year, and the peak instantaneous gradient increases by 10 mm Hg/year. The rate of progression of AS in men older than 60 is faster than in women, and it is faster in women older than 75 than in women 60 to 74 years old.

Angina, syncope, and congestive heart failure (CHF) are the classic symptoms of the disease, and their appearance is of serious prognostic significance because postmortem studies indicate that symptomatic AS is associated with a life expectancy of only 2 to 5 years.

There is evidence that patients with moderate AS (ie, valve areas of 0.7 to 1.2 cm²) are also at increased risk for complications, with the appearance of symptoms further increasing their risk.

15

Angina is a frequent and classic symptom of the disease, occurring in approximately two-thirds of patients with critical AS, and about one-half of symptomatic patients have anatomically significant CAD.

It is probably never too late to operate on patients with symptomatic AS. Unlike patients with aortic regurgitation (AR), most symptomatic patients undergo valve replacement when left ventricular function is still normal. Even when impaired left ventricular function develops in AS, the relief of pressure overload almost always restores normal function or produces considerable improvement. Morbidity rates, mortality rates, and clinical results are favorable even for the oldest surgical candidates. Advances in operative techniques and perioperative management have contributed to excellent results after aortic valve replacement (AVR) in patients 80 years of age or older, with minimal incremental postoperative morbidity.

Preoperative assessment of AS with Doppler echocardiography includes measurement of the AVA and the transvalvular pressure gradient. The latter is calculated from the Doppler-quantified transvalvular velocity of blood flow, which is increased in the setting of AS. The maximal velocity (v) is then inserted into the modified Bernoulli equation to determine the pressure gradient (PG) between the left ventricle (LV) and the aorta:

$$PG = P(\text{left ventricle}) - P(\text{aorta}) = 4(v^2)$$

The *pressure gradient* is the maximal difference between the LV and aortic pressures that occurs during ventricular systole.

Pressure gradients determined invasively or by Doppler echocardiography correctly classify AS severity in less than 50% of cases compared with estimates of AVA. The preferred method of obtaining AVA requires only two Doppler-generated velocities: those proximal or distal to the stenotic valve. These values are inserted into the continuity equation, which relates the respective velocities and cross-sectional areas proximal and distal to a stenotic area:

$$V_{max} \times AVA = \text{area}(LVOT) \times V(LVOT)$$

In the equation, AVA is the aortic valve area, V is the volume, and LVOT is the left ventricular outflow tract.

Pathophysiology

The normal AVA is 2.6 to 3.5 cm^2, with hemodynamically significant obstruction usually occurring at cross-sectional valve areas of 1 cm^2 or less. Accepted criteria for critical outflow obstruction include a systolic pressure gradient greater than 50 mm Hg, with a normal cardiac output, and an AVA of less than 0.4 cm^2. In view of the ominous natural history of severe AS (AVA <0.7 cm^2), symptomatic patients with this degree of AS are usually referred for immediate AVR. A simplification of the Gorlin equation to calculate the AVA is based on the cardiac output (CO) and the peak pressure gradient (PG) across the valve.

$$AVA = CO/\sqrt{(PG)}$$

An obvious corollary of the previously described relationship is that "minimal" pressure gradients may reflect critical degrees of outflow obstruction when the CO is significantly reduced (ie, generation of a pressure gradient requires some finite amount of flow). Clinicians have long recognized this phenomenon as a paradoxical decline in the intensity of the murmur (ie, minimal transvalvular flow) as the AS worsens.

Stenosis at the level of the aortic valve results in a pressure gradient from the LV to the aorta. The intracavitary systolic pressure generated to overcome this stenosis directly increases myocardial wall tension in accordance with Laplace's law:

$$\text{Wall tension} = P \times R/2h$$

In the equation, P is the intraventricular pressure, R is the inner radius, and h is the wall thickness.

The increase of wall tension is thought to be the direct stimulus for the further parallel replication of sarcomeres, which produces the concentrically hypertrophied ventricle characteristic of chronic pressure overload. The consequences of left ventricular hypertrophy (LVH) include alterations in diastolic compliance, potential imbalances in the myocardial oxygen supply and demand relationship, and possible deterioration of the intrinsic contractile performance of the myocardium.

Fig. 15.1 shows a typical pressure-volume loop for a patient with AS. Two differences from the normal curve are immediately apparent. First, the peak pressure generated during systole is much greater because of the high transvalvular pressure gradient. Second, the slope of the diastolic limb is steeper, reflecting the reduced left ventricular diastolic compliance that is associated with the increase in chamber thickness. Clinically, small changes in diastolic volume produce relatively large increases in ventricular filling pressure.

Increased chamber stiffness places a premium on the contribution of atrial systole to ventricular filling, which in patients with AS may account for up to 40% of the left ventricular end-diastolic volume (LVEDV) rather than the 15% to 20% characteristic of the normal LV. Echocardiographic and radionuclide studies have documented that diastolic filling and ventricular relaxation are abnormal in patients with hypertrophy

15

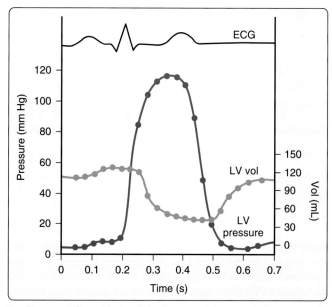

Fig. 15.1 Simultaneous left ventricular *(LV)* volume and pressure during one cardiac cycle. *ECG,* Electrocardiogram. (From Barash PG, Kopriva DJ. Cardiac pump function and how to monitor it. In: Thomas SJ, ed. *Manual of Cardiac Anesthesia.* New York: Churchill Livingstone; 1984:1.)

from a variety of causes, and significant prolongation of the isovolumic relaxation period is the most characteristic finding. This necessarily compromises the duration and amount of filling achieved during the early rapid diastolic filling phase and increases the relative contribution of atrial contraction to overall diastolic filling. A much greater mean left atrial pressure is necessary to distend the LV in the absence of the sinus mechanism. One treatment of junctional rhythm is volume infusion.

The systolic limb of the pressure-volume loop shows preservation of pump function, as evidenced by maintenance of the stroke volume (SV) and ejection fraction (EF). Use of preload reserve and adequate LVH are likely the principal compensatory mechanisms that maintain forward flow. Clinical studies have confirmed that ejection performance is preserved at the expense of myocardial hypertrophy, and the adequacy of the hypertrophic response has been related to the degree to which it achieves normalization of wall stress, in accordance with the Laplace relation. LVH can be viewed as a compensatory physiologic response; however, severe afterload stress and proportionately massive LVH could decrease subendocardial perfusion and superimpose a component of ischemic contractile dysfunction.

In AS, signs and symptoms of CHF usually develop when preload reserve is exhausted, not because contractility is intrinsically or permanently impaired. This contrasts with mitral regurgitation (MR) and AR, in which irreversible myocardial dysfunction may develop before the onset of significant symptoms.

The major threat to the hypertrophied ventricle is its exquisite sensitivity to ischemia. Ventricular hypertrophy directly increases basal myocardial oxygen demand ($M\dot{V}O_2$). The other major determinants of overall $M\dot{V}O_2$ are heart rate, contractility, and, most important, wall tension. Increases in wall tension occur as a direct consequence of Laplace's law in patients with relatively inadequate hypertrophy. The possibility of ischemic contractile dysfunction in the inadequately hypertrophied ventricle arises from increases in wall tension, which directly parallels the imbalance between the increased peak systolic pressure and the degree of mural hypertrophy. Although there is considerable evidence for supply-side abnormalities in the myocardial supply and demand relationship in patients with AS, clinical data also support increased $M\dot{V}O_2$ as important in the genesis of myocardial ischemia.

On the supply side, the greater left ventricular end-diastolic pressure (LVEDP) of the poorly compliant ventricle inevitably narrows the diastolic coronary perfusion pressure (CPP) gradient. With severe outflow obstruction, decreases in SV and resultant systemic hypotension may critically compromise coronary perfusion. A vicious cycle may develop because ischemia-induced abnormalities of diastolic relaxation can aggravate the compliance problem and further narrow the CPP gradient. This sets the stage for ischemic contractile dysfunction, additional decreases in SV, and worsening hypotension.

Difficulty of Low-Gradient, Low-Output Aortic Stenosis

A subset of patients with severe AS, left ventricular dysfunction, and low transvalvular gradient suffers a high operative mortality rate and poor prognosis. It is difficult to assess accurately the AVA in low-flow, low-gradient AS because the calculated valve area is proportional to forward SV and because the Gorlin constant varies in low-flow states. Some patients with low-flow, low-gradient AS have a decreased AVA as a result of inadequate forward SV rather than anatomic stenosis. Surgical therapy is unlikely to benefit these patients because the underlying pathology is a weakly contractile myocardium. However, patients with severe anatomic AS may benefit from valve replacement despite the increased operative risk associated with the low-flow,

Table 15.1	**Pressure-Overload Hypertrophy**
Beneficial Aspects	Detrimental Aspects
Increases ventricular work Normalizes wall stress Normalizes systolic shortening	Decreases ventricular diastolic distensibility Impairs ventricular relaxation Impairs coronary vasodilator reserve, leading to subendocardial ischemia

From Lorell BH, Grossman W. Cardiac hypertrophy: the consequences for diastole. *J Am Coll Cardiol.* 1987;9:1189.

low-gradient hemodynamic state. American College of Cardiology/American Heart Association (ACC/AHA) guidelines call for a dobutamine echocardiography evaluation to differentiate patients with fixed anatomic AS from those with flow-dependent AS with left ventricular dysfunction. Low-flow, low-gradient AS is defined as a mean gradient of less than 30 mm Hg and a calculated AVA less than 1.0 cm^2.

Timing of Intervention

For asymptomatic patients with AS, it appears to be relatively safe to delay surgery until symptoms develop, but outcomes vary widely. Moderate or severe valvular calcification along with a rapid increase in aortic-jet velocity identify patients with a very poor prognosis. They should be considered for early valve replacement rather than delaying until symptoms develop.

Echocardiography and exercise testing may identify asymptomatic patients who are likely to benefit from surgery. In a study of 58 asymptomatic patients, 21 had symptoms for the first time during exercise testing. Guidelines for AVR in patients with AS are shown in Table 15.1.

Functional outcome after AVR for patients older than 80 years is excellent, operative risk is limited, and late survival rates are good. For patients with severe left ventricular dysfunction and a low transvalvular mean gradient, the operative mortality rate was increased, but AVR was associated with improved functional status. Postoperative survival rates were best for younger patients and those with larger prosthetic valves, whereas medium-term survival rates were correlated with improved postoperative functional class.

Anesthesia Considerations

The described pathophysiologic principles dictate anesthesia management based on avoidance of systemic hypotension, maintenance of sinus rhythm and an adequate intravascular volume, and awareness of the potential for myocardial ischemia (Box 15.1). In the absence of CHF, adequate premedication may reduce the likelihood of undue preoperative excitement, tachycardia, and exacerbation of myocardial ischemia and the transvalvular pressure gradient. In patients with critical outflow tract obstruction, however, heavy premedication with an exaggerated venodilatory response can reduce the appropriately increased LVEDV (and LVEDP) needed to overcome the systolic pressure gradient. In these patients, the additional precaution of administering supplementary oxygen may obviate the possibility of a similarly pronounced response to the sedative effects of the premedicant.

357

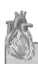

BOX 15.1 *Aortic Stenosis*

Maintain preload and diastolic filling
Maintain sinus rhythm
Maintain or increase afterload
Avoid myocardial depression
Avoid tachycardia, hypotension, and increased myocardial oxygen demand situations

Intraoperative monitoring should include a standard five-lead electrocardiographic (ECG) system, including a V_5 lead, because of the LV's vulnerability to ischemia. A practical constraint in terms of interpretation is that these patients usually exhibit ECG changes because of preoperative LVH. The associated ST-segment abnormalities (ie, strain pattern) may be indistinguishable from or very similar to those of myocardial ischemia, making the intraoperative interpretation difficult. Lead II and possibly an esophageal electrocardiogram should be readily obtainable for assessing the P-wave changes in the event of supraventricular arrhythmias.

Hemodynamic monitoring is controversial, and few prospective data are available on which to base an enlightened clinical decision. The central venous pressure (CVP) is a particularly poor estimate of left ventricular filling when left ventricular compliance is reduced. A normal CVP can significantly underestimate the LVEDP or pulmonary capillary wedge pressure (PCWP). The principal risks, although minimal, of using a pulmonary artery catheter (PAC) in the patient with AS are arrhythmia-induced hypotension and ischemia. Loss of synchronous atrial contraction or a supraventricular tachyarrhythmia can compromise diastolic filling of the poorly compliant LV, resulting in hypotension and the potential for rapid hemodynamic deterioration. The threat of catheter-induced arrhythmias is significant for the patient with AS. However, accepting a low-normal CVP as evidence of good ventricular function can lead to similarly catastrophic underfilling of the LV on the basis of insufficient replenishment of surgical blood loss. To some extent, even the PCWP can underestimate the LVEDP (and LVEDV) when ventricular compliance is markedly reduced. Placement of a PAC also allows measurement of CO, derived hemodynamic parameters, mixed venous oxygen saturation (SvO_2), and possible transvenous pacing.

Intraoperative fluid management should be aimed at maintaining appropriately increased left-sided filling pressures. This is one reason why many clinicians think that the PAC is worth its small arrhythmogenic risk. Keeping up with intravascular volume losses is particularly important in noncardiac surgery, in which the shorter duration of the operation may make inhalation or potentially vasodilating regional anesthesia preferable to a narcotic technique.

Patients with symptomatic AS are usually encountered only in the setting of cardiovascular surgery because of their ominous prognosis without AVR. Few studies have specifically addressed the response of these patients to the standard intravenous and inhalation induction agents; however, the responses to narcotic and nonnarcotic intravenous agents are apparently not dissimilar from those of patients with other forms of VHD. The principal benefit of a narcotic induction is assurance of an adequate depth of anesthesia during intubation, which reliably blunts potentially deleterious reflex sympathetic responses capable of precipitating tachycardia and ischemia.

Many clinicians also prefer a pure narcotic technique for maintenance. The negative inotropy of inhalation anesthetics is a theoretical disadvantage for a myocardium

IV

358

faced with the challenge of overcoming outflow tract obstruction. A more clinically relevant drawback may be the increased risk for arrhythmia-induced hypotension, particularly that associated with nodal rhythm and resultant loss of the atrium's critical contribution to filling of the hypertrophied ventricle.

Occasionally, surgical stimulation elicits a hypertensive response despite the impedance posed by the stenotic valve and a seemingly adequate depth of narcotic anesthesia. In these patients, a judicious trial of low concentrations of an inhalation agent, used purely for control of hypertension, may prove efficacious. The ability to concurrently monitor CO is useful in this situation. The temptation to control intraoperative hypertension with vasodilators should be resisted in most cases. Given the risk for ischemia, nitroglycerin seems to be a particularly attractive drug. Its effectiveness in relieving subendocardial ischemia in patients with AS is controversial; however, there is always the risk for transient episodes of overshoot. The hypertrophied ventricle's critical dependence on an adequate CPP may be unforgiving of even a momentary dip in the systemic arterial pressure.

Intraoperative hypotension, regardless of the primary cause, should be treated immediately and aggressively with a direct α-adrenergic agonist such as phenylephrine. The goal should be to immediately restore the CPP and then to address the underlying problem (eg, hypovolemia, arrhythmia). After the arterial pressure responds, treatment of the precipitating event should be equally aggressive, but rapid transfusion or cardioversion should not delay the administration of a direct-acting vasoconstrictor. Patients with severe AS in whom objective signs of myocardial ischemia persist despite restoration of the blood pressure should be treated extremely aggressively. This may mean the immediate use of an inotropic agent or accelerating the institution of cardiopulmonary bypass (CPB).

HYPERTROPHIC CARDIOMYOPATHY

Hypertrophic Obstructive Cardiomyopathy

Obstructive hypertrophic cardiomyopathy (HCM) is a relatively common genetic malformation of the heart with a prevalence of approximately 1 case in 500 births. The hypertrophy initially develops in the septum and extends to the free walls, often giving a picture of concentric hypertrophy. Asymmetric septal hypertrophy leads to a variable pressure gradient between the apical left ventricular chamber and the LVOT. The LVOT obstruction leads to increases in left ventricular pressure, which fuels a vicious cycle of further hypertrophy and increased LVOT obstruction.

Treatment modalities include β-adrenoceptor antagonists, calcium channel blockers, and surgical myectomy of the septum. For more than 40 years, the standard treatment has been the ventricular septal myotomy-myectomy of Morrow, in which a small amount of muscle from the subaortic septum is resected. Two new treatment modalities have gained popularity in recent years: dual-chamber pacing and septal reduction (ie, ablation) with ethanol.

Clinical Features and Natural History

The clinical presentation of patients varies widely. Echocardiography has unquestionably increased the number of asymptomatic patients who carry the diagnosis. Most patients with HCM are asymptomatic and have been seen by the echocardiographer because of relatives having clinical disease. Follow-up remains an important problem for cardiologists because sudden death or cardiac arrest may occur as the presenting symptom in slightly more than one-half of previously asymptomatic patients.

Less dramatic presenting complaints include dyspnea, angina, and syncope. The clinical picture is often similar to valvular AS. The symptoms may share a similar pathophysiologic basis (eg, poor diastolic compliance) in the two conditions. The prognostic implications of clinical disease, however, are less certain for patients with HCM. Although cardiac arrest may be an unheralded event, some patients may have a stable pattern of angina or intermittent syncopal episodes for many years. Palpitations are frequently described and may be related to a variety of underlying arrhythmias.

Pathophysiology

In HCM, the principal pathophysiologic abnormality is myocardial hypertrophy. The hypertrophy is a primary event in these patients and occurs independently of outflow tract obstruction. Unlike in AS, the hypertrophy begets the pressure gradient, not the other way around. Histologically, the hypertrophy consists of myocardial fiber disarray, and anatomically, there is usually disproportionate enlargement of the interventricular septum.

HCM is characterized by a broad spectrum of obstruction, which is absent in some patients and varies from mild to severe in others. The most distinctive qualities of obstruction are its dynamic nature (ie, depends on contractile state and loading conditions), its timing (ie, begins early and peaks variably), and its subaortic location. Subaortic obstruction arises from the hypertrophied septum's encroachment on the systolic outflow tract, which is bounded anteriorly by the interventricular septum and posteriorly by the anterior leaflet of the mitral valve. In most patients with obstruction, exaggerated anterior (ie, toward the septum) motion of the anterior mitral valve leaflet during systole accentuates the obstruction. The cause of systolic anterior motion (SAM) is unclear. One possibility is that the mitral valve is pulled toward the septum by contraction of the papillary muscles, whose orientation is abnormal because of the hypertrophic process. Another theory is that vigorous contraction of the hypertrophied septum results in rapid acceleration of the blood through a simultaneously narrowed outflow tract. The generated hydraulic forces (consistent with a Venturi effect) can cause the anterior leaflet of the mitral valve to be drawn close to or in contact with the interventricular septum (Fig. 15.2). After the obstruction is triggered, the mitral valve leaflet is forced against the septum by the pressure difference across the orifice. However, the pressure difference further decreases orifice size and further increases the pressure difference in a time-dependent, amplifying feedback loop. This analysis is consistent with observations that the measured gradient directly correlates with the duration of mitral-septal contact. Although still controversial, there appears to be good correlation between the degree of SAM and the magnitude of the pressure gradient. The SAM-septal contact also underlies the severe subaortic obstruction characteristic of HCM of the elderly, although the narrowing usually is more severe and the contribution of septal movement toward the mitral valve is usually greater.

In addition to SAM, approximately two-thirds of patients exhibit a constellation of structural malformations of the mitral valve. Malformations include increased leaflet area and elongation of the leaflets or anomalous papillary muscle insertion directly into the anterior mitral valve leaflet. HCM is not a disease process confined to cardiac muscle alone because these anatomic abnormalities of the mitral valve are unlikely to be acquired or caused by mechanical factors.

Three basic mechanisms—increased contractility, decreased afterload, and decreased preload—exacerbate the degree of SAM-septal contact and produce the dynamic

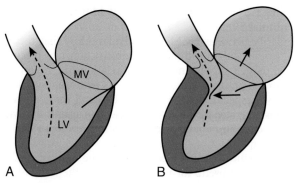

Fig. 15.2 Proposed mechanism of systolic anterior motion in hypertrophic cardiomyopathy. (A) Normally, blood is ejected from the left ventricle *(LV)* through an unimpeded outflow tract. (B) Thickening of the ventricular septum restricts the outflow tract, and the obstruction causes the blood to be ejected at a higher velocity and closer to the area of the anterior mitral valve *(MV)* leaflet. Owing to its proximity to the high-velocity fluid path, the anterior MV leaflet is drawn toward the hypertrophied septum by a Venturi effect *(left arrow)*. (From Wigle ED, Sasson Z, Henderson MA, et al. Hypertrophic cardiomyopathy: the importance of the site and the extent of hypertrophy—a review. *Prog Cardiovasc Dis.* 1985;28:1.)

obstruction characteristic of patients with HCM. The common pathway is a reduction in ventricular volume (actively by increased contractility directly or reflexively in response to vasodilation or passively by reduced preload), which increases the proximity of the anterior mitral valve leaflet to the hypertrophied septum. Factors that usually impair contractile performance, such as myocardial depression, systemic vasoconstriction, and ventricular overdistension, characteristically improve systolic function in patients with HCM and outflow tract obstruction.

Diagnostically, the paradoxes are exploited by quantifying the degree of subaortic obstruction after isoproterenol (eg, increased inotropy, tachycardia, decreased volume) and the Valsalva maneuver (eg, decreased venous return, ventricular volume), both of which reliably elicit increases in the pressure gradient. In the operating room, catheter-induced ectopy or premature ventricular contractions resulting from cardiac manipulation may transiently exacerbate the gradient by increased inotropy from postextrasystolic potentiation. Therapeutically, volume loading, myocardial depression, and vasoconstriction can minimize obstruction and augment forward flow.

Poor diastolic compliance is the most clinically apparent manifestation of the relaxation abnormalities. Left ventricular filling pressures are markedly increased despite enhanced systolic ejection and a normal or subnormal EDV. The reduced ventricular volume emphasizes the pivotal role played by the hypertrophied but intrinsically depressed myocardium. Reductions in afterload, which are mediated by hypertrophy, support the ventricle's systolic performance, resulting in increased emptying and a small diastolic volume. However, hypertrophy also impairs relaxation, resulting in poor diastolic compliance and an increased ventricular filling pressure. The high filling pressure does not reflect distension of a failing ventricle, although stress-volume relationships suggest that contractility is intrinsically depressed. This disease is characterized by systolic and diastolic dysfunction.

As in patients with valvular AS, relatively high filling pressures reflect the LVEDV (ie, degree of preload reserve) needed to overcome the outflow obstruction. Intervention with vasodilators is therefore inappropriate. The poor ventricular compliance also means that patients with HCM depend on a large intravascular volume and the maintenance of sinus rhythm for adequate diastolic filling. The atrial contribution

15

to ventricular filling is even more important in HCM than in valvular AS, and it may approach 75% of total SV.

Another similarity between HCM and valvular AS is that the combination of myocardial hypertrophy, with or without LVOT obstruction, may precipitate imbalances in the myocardial oxygen supply and demand relationship. Angina-like discomfort is a classic symptom of patients with HCM, and its pathogenesis has been attributed to increases in $M\dot{V}O_2$, specifically the increased overall muscle mass and the high systolic wall tension generated by the ventricle's ejection against the dynamic subaortic obstruction. However, as in patients with AS, there is evidence of a compromise in myocardial oxygen supply.

β-Blockers and calcium channel blockers form the basis of medical therapy for HCM. β-Blockade is most useful for preventing sympathetically mediated increases in the subaortic gradient and for the prevention of tachyarrhythmias, which can exacerbate outflow obstruction. Disopyramide also has been used to reduce contractility and for its antiarrhythmic properties. Calcium channel blockers often prove clinically effective in patients with HCM, regardless of the presence or absence of systolic obstruction. The mechanism of action involves improvement in diastolic relaxation, allowing an increase in LVEDV at a lower LVEDP. The negative inotropy may attenuate the subaortic pressure gradient, but in selected patients the gradient may worsen because of pronounced and unpredictable degrees of vasodilation.

Surgery (ie, septal myotomy or partial myomectomy by the aortic approach) is reserved for patients who remain symptomatic despite maximal pharmacologic therapy. In a long-term retrospective study, the cumulative survival rate was significantly better in surgically than in pharmacologically treated patients. However, it is likely that pharmacologic therapy may be more appropriate for the patient with a dynamic component to their degree of subaortic obstruction. Further improvement in the clinical outcome of surgically treated patients may be achieved with the addition of verapamil, presumably reflecting a two-pronged attack on the systolic (ie, myomectomy) and diastolic (ie, verapamil) components of the disease. Enthusiasm continues for the therapeutic use of dual-chamber pacing in this disease, with some patients demonstrating reductions in their subaortic gradients. It is not an option for patients with atrial fibrillation (AF).

Anesthesia Considerations

Priorities in anesthesia management are to avoid aggravating the subaortic obstruction while remaining aware of the derangements in diastolic function that may be somewhat less amenable to direct pharmacologic manipulation (Box 15.2). It is necessary to maintain an appropriate intravascular volume while avoiding direct or reflex increases in contractility or heart rate. The latter goals can be achieved with a deep level of general anesthesia and the associated direct myocardial depression. Regardless of the

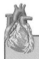

BOX 15.2 *Hypertrophic Cardiomyopathy*

Preload is increased
Afterload is increased
Goal is myocardial depression
Avoid tachycardia, inotropes, and vasodilators

IV

specific technique, preservation of an adequate CPP using vasoconstrictors rather than inotropes is necessary to avoid myocardial ischemia. Heavy premedication is advisable, with a view to avoiding anxiety-induced tachycardia or a reduction in ventricular filling. Chronic β-blockade or calcium channel blockade, or both, should be continued up to and including the day of surgery. These medications should be restarted immediately after surgery, particularly in patients undergoing noncardiac surgery.

Intraoperative monitoring should include an ECG system with the capability of monitoring a V_5 lead and each of the six limb leads. Inspection of lead II may be helpful in the accurate diagnosis of supraventricular and junctional tachyarrhythmias, which may precipitate catastrophic hemodynamic deterioration because of the potential for inadequate ventricular filling resulting from the reduction in diastolic time or loss of the atrial contribution to ventricular filling. The latter may be crucial in patients with significantly reduced diastolic compliance. Abnormal Q waves have been described on the electrocardiograms of 20% to 50% of patients with HCM. These waves should not raise concern about a previous myocardial infarction; instead, they probably represent accentuation of normal septal depolarization or delay in depolarization of electrophysiologically abnormal cells. Some patients exhibit a short PR interval with initial slurring of the QRS complex, and they may be at increased risk for supraventricular tachyarrhythmias due to preexcitation. Although the specific predisposing factors are unknown, patients with HCM are at increased risk for any type of arrhythmia in the operative setting.

Given the pronounced abnormalities in left ventricular diastolic compliance, the CVP is likely to be an inaccurate guide to changes in left ventricular volume. However, a CVP catheter is extremely useful for the prompt administration of vasoactive drugs if they become necessary. As in valvular AS, the information provided by insertion of a PAC is worth the small arrhythmogenic risk. The potential for hypovolemia-induced exacerbation of outflow tract obstruction makes it crucial that the clinician have an accurate gauge of intravascular filling. Reduced diastolic compliance means that the PCWP overestimates the patient's true volume status, and a reasonable clinical objective is to maintain the PCWP in the high-normal to elevated range. A PAC with pacing capability is ideal because atrial overdrive pacing can effect immediate hemodynamic improvement in the event of episodes of junctional rhythm. The absolute requirement of these patients for an adequate preload cannot be overemphasized because even abrupt positioning changes have resulted in acute hemodynamic deterioration, including acute pulmonary edema.

Intraoperative arrhythmias require aggressive therapy. During cardiac surgery, insertion of venous cannulas may precipitate atrial arrhythmias. Because the resultant hypotension may be severe, the surgeon should cannulate the aorta before atrial manipulation. Supraventricular or junctional tachyarrhythmias may require immediate cardioversion if they precipitate catastrophic degrees of hypotension. Although verapamil is one drug of choice for paroxysmal atrial and junctional tachycardia, it can disastrously worsen the LVOT obstruction if it elicits excessive vasodilation or it is used in the setting of severe hypotension. Cardioversion is preferable when the mean arterial pressure is already very low. The concurrent administration of phenylephrine also is advisable. This drug is typically a low-risk, high-yield choice for the hypotensive patient with HCM. It augments perfusion, may ameliorate the pressure gradient, and often elicits a potentially beneficial vagal reflex when used to treat tachyarrhythmia-induced hypotension.

The inhalation anesthetics commonly are used for patients with HCM. Their dose-dependent myocardial depression is ideal because negative inotropy reduces the degree of SAM-septal contact, which reduces LVOT obstruction. Hypotension is usually

15

the result of underlying hypovolemia, which is potentially exacerbated by anesthetic-induced vasodilation. Inotropes, β-adrenergic agonists, and calcium are contraindicated because they worsen the systolic obstruction and perpetuate the hypotension. In most cases, a beneficial response can be obtained with aggressive replenishment of intravascular volume and concurrent infusion of phenylephrine.

AORTIC REGURGITATION

Clinical Features and Natural History

AR may result from an abnormality of the valve itself, bicuspid anatomy, a rheumatic or infectious origin, or in association with any condition producing dilation of the aortic root and leaflet separation. Nonrheumatic valvular diseases commonly resulting in AR include infective endocarditis, trauma, and connective tissue disorders such as Marfan syndrome or cystic medial necrosis of the aortic valve. Aortic dissection from trauma, hypertension, or chronic degenerative processes also can result in dilation of the root and functional incompetence.

The natural history of chronic AR is that of a long asymptomatic interval during which the valvular incompetence and secondary ventricular enlargement become progressively more severe. When symptoms do appear, they are usually those of CHF, and chest pain, if it occurs, is often nonexertional in origin. The life expectancy for patients with significant disease has historically been about 9 years, and, in contrast with AS, the onset of symptoms because of AR does not portend an immediately ominous prognosis. In the absence of surgery, early recognition of AR and chronic use of vasodilators prolong the life span for this patient population.

A relatively unique and problematic feature of chronic AR is that the severity of symptoms and their duration may correlate poorly with the degree of hemodynamic and contractile impairment. The issue in surgical decision making is that many patients can remain asymptomatic, during which time they are undergoing progressive deterioration in myocardial contractility. Noninvasive diagnostic studies (ie, radionuclide cine angiography and two-dimensional and Doppler echocardiographic assessment of response to pharmacologic afterload stress) may facilitate the detection of early derangements in contractile function in relatively asymptomatic patients. These findings are important to the cardiologist when considering surgical referral because patients with depressed preoperative left ventricular function have greater perioperative mortality rates and are at increased risk for persistent postoperative heart failure (HF).

As in acute MR, the physiology of acute AR is quite different from chronic AR. Common causes include endocarditis, trauma, and acute aortic dissection. Because of a lack of chronic compensation, these patients usually have pulmonary edema and heart failure refractory to optimal medical therapy. Patients are often hypotensive and clinically appear to be on the verge of cardiovascular collapse.

Pathophysiology

Left ventricular volume overload is the pathognomonic feature of chronic AR. The degree of volume overload is determined by the magnitude of the regurgitant flow, which is related to the size of the regurgitant orifice, the aorta-ventricular pressure gradient, and the diastolic time.

Chronically, AR results in a state of left ventricular volume and pressure overload. Progressive volume overloading from AR increases end-diastolic wall tension (ie, ventricular afterload) and stimulates the serial replication of sarcomeres, producing

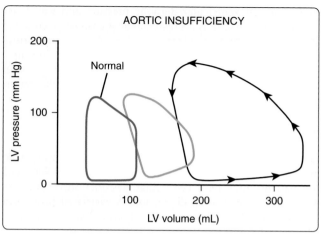

Fig. 15.3 Pressure-volume loop in aortic regurgitation (AR). Acute AR *(green loop)*; chronic AR *(black loop)*. *LV*, Left ventricular. (Modified from Jackson JM, Thomas SJ, Lowenstein E. Anesthetic management of patients with valvular heart disease. *Semin Anesth.* 1982;1:239.)

a pattern of eccentric ventricular hypertrophy. In accordance with Laplace's law, dilation of the ventricle increases the systolic wall tension, stimulating some concentric hypertrophy. The result is normalization of the ratio of ventricular wall thickness to cavitary radius. This process of eccentric hypertrophy results in the greatest absolute degrees of cardiomegaly seen in valve disease. EDV may be three to four times normal, and very high COs can be sustained.

Fig. 15.3 shows the pressure-volume loops for acute and chronic AR. In the chronic form, the diastolic pressure-volume curve is shifted far to the right. This permits a tremendous increase in LVEDV with minimal change in filling pressure, a property frequently described as high diastolic compliance.

Because the increase in preload is compensated for by ventricular hypertrophy, CO is maintained by the Frank-Starling mechanism, and cardiac failure is not seen despite probable decreases in contractility. There is virtually no isovolumic diastolic phase because the ventricle is filling throughout diastole. The isovolumic phase of systole also is brief because of the low aortic diastolic pressure. Minimal impedance to the forward ejection of a large SV allows performance of maximal myocardial work at a minimum of oxygen consumption. Eventually, however, progressive volume overload increases ventricular EDV to the point that compensatory hypertrophy is no longer sufficient to compensate, and a decline in systolic function occurs. As systolic function declines, the end-systolic dimension increases further, left ventricular wall stress increases, and left ventricular function is further compromised by the excessive ventricular afterload. At this point, the decline of ventricular function is progressive and can be quite rapid.

Despite the relatively normal $M\dot{V}O_2$, angina can occur in one-third of patients with severe AR, even in the absence of CAD. Patients with chronic AR may be at risk for myocardial ischemia caused by hypertrophy-induced abnormalities of the coronary circulation. The increase in total myocardial mass can increase baseline $M\dot{V}O_2$, and there is evidence that total coronary blood flow, although increased, fails to keep pace with the increase in myocardial mass. Evidence suggests that the insidious development of contractile dysfunction may in part have an ischemic basis.

Intraoperatively, patients with chronic AR may be at risk for acute ischemia with episodes of significant bradycardia. As bradycardia prolongs diastolic time, it increases

15

regurgitant flow, and left ventricular diastolic pressure and wall tension increase rapidly. Simultaneously, the CPP is decreased as aortic runoff occurs during diastole and diastolic ventricular pressure is increased. Under these conditions, myocardial perfusion pressure may be insufficient. Clinically, very rapid decompensation can occur. The ischemic ventricle can dilate rapidly such that progressively increased end-systolic dimensions are seen, and ischemia and ventricular failure become a positive feedback loop.

Surgical Decision Making

An accurate assessment of contractility is crucial to surgical decision making, because the clinical history of chronic AR may be an unreliable index of ventricular function. Asymptomatic patients may have ventricular dysfunction, whereas symptomatic patients may be free of myocardial depression. A variety of prognostic indicators have been used to identify early ventricular dysfunction as a trigger for surgical intervention. Clinical status, such as exercise capacity and New York Heart Association (NYHA) class, and noninvasive and invasive laboratory tests have been used. Hemodynamic parameters such as the end-systolic stress-volume relationship and estimates of the left ventricular contractile state have been evaluated as predictors of worsening left ventricular function.

Valve surgery is recommended for asymptomatic patients with left ventricular systolic dysfunction. Surgery also should be considered if ventricular dilation has occurred in the asymptomatic patient, even if the EF is normal. In patients who are symptomatic but have normal ventricular function, the ACC and AHA recommend further evaluation for an unrelated cause and observation. In these cases, serial echocardiographic assessment is appropriate. Symptomatic patients with left ventricular dysfunction should undergo surgery.

Acute Aortic Regurgitation

In acute AR, sudden diastolic volume overload of a nonadapted LV results in a precipitous increase in the EDP because the ventricle is operating on the steepest portion of the diastolic pressure-volume curve. In severe acute AR, the LVEDP can equilibrate with aortic diastolic pressure and exceed the left atrial pressure in late diastole. This may be sufficient to cause closure of the mitral valve before atrial systole. This is an important echocardiographic finding indicative of severe AR. Although this phenomenon initially shields the pulmonary capillaries from the full force of the dramatically increased LVEDP, the protection may be short lived. Severe left ventricular distension often follows and produces mitral annular enlargement and functional MR.

The inevitable decline in SV in acute decompensating AR elicits a reflex sympathetic response, making tachycardia and a high systemic vascular resistance common. Moderate tachycardia beneficially shortens the regurgitant time without reducing the transmitral filling volume. Vasoconstriction, however, preserves CPP at the expense of increasing the aortic-ventricular gradient and regurgitation.

Patients with acute AR may be at greater risk for myocardial ischemia. As with chronic AR and bradycardia, coronary perfusion may be compromised by the combination of a low diastolic arterial pressure and the precipitously increased LVEDP. Narrowing of CPP may be so severe that the phasic epicardial blood flow may change to a predominantly systolic pattern with severe acute AR. Dissection of the coronary ostia is rare but frequently causes the death of patients with acute AR. In addition to the structural impediment to myocardial oxygen delivery, catastrophic hypotension and

IV

high LVEDP combine to cause accentuated ischemia and ventricular dilation. Immediate surgical correction is the only hope for salvaging these patients, who often prove refractory to inotropes and vasodilators. Attempts at stabilizing the ischemic component of their injury with an intraaortic balloon are usually contraindicated because augmenting the diastolic pressure worsens regurgitation.

Acute AR most commonly results from infective endocarditis or aortic dissection, and intraoperative transesophageal echocardiography (TEE) has assumed increasing importance in the diagnosis of acute AR and in decisions regarding its surgical management. Transesophageal echocardiographic studies are highly sensitive and specific for the diagnosis of infective endocarditis and are significantly more sensitive than transthoracic echocardiography. TEE is particularly useful in the diagnosis of abscesses associated with endocarditis and may detect previously unsuspected abnormalities.

Anesthesia Considerations

Intraoperative monitoring should include an ECG system for monitoring a lateral precordial lead because ischemia is a potential hazard (Box 15.3). For most valvular procedures, a PAC provides useful information. A PAC allows determination of basal filling pressures and CO, which is particularly useful in chronic AR given the potential unreliability of the clinical history and EF. Equally important is the ability to accurately monitor ventricular preload and CO response to pharmacologic interventions. The aggressive use of vasodilators often is appropriate therapy perioperatively for the failing ventricle, but their use can compromise the preload to which the ventricle has chronically adjusted. Concurrent preload augmentation, guided by the diastolic pulmonary arterial pressure (PAP) or PCWP, may be crucial to optimize CO when afterload is pharmacologically manipulated. The other requirement for a PAC is to allow for pacing when it is anticipated. The deleterious effects of significant bradycardia in AR have been described. In patients who arrive in the operating room with heart rates less than 70 beats per minute or patients for whom rapid epicardial pacing may be difficult to establish (eg, reoperations), placement of a pacing wire probably is indicated. Typically, only a ventricular wire is appropriate. It is more reliable than atrial pacing, and in AR, the atrial contribution to ventricular diastolic volume usually is not essential. Capturing the ventricle with a PAC-based, transvenous wire can be difficult because of the very large ventricular cavity size in patients with chronic AR.

Because patients with AR may have widely different degrees of myocardial dysfunction, anesthesia management must be appropriately individualized. For cardiac or noncardiac surgery, the hemodynamic goals are a mild tachycardia, positive inotropic state, and controlled reduction in systemic vascular resistance. For cardiac surgery, dopamine or dobutamine, pancuronium, ketamine, and nitroprusside infusions are excellent choices. For the patient with acute AR, the goals are the same, but urgency

15

BOX 15.3   *Aortic Regurgitation*

Preload is increased
Afterload is decreased
Goal is augmentation of forward flow
Avoid bradycardia

must be stressed. It is essential to rapidly reduce end-diastolic and end-systolic ventricular volumes with the very aggressive use of inotropes (eg, epinephrine) and vasodilators. There is sometimes concern that inotropes may exacerbate the root dissection in acute AR by increasing the shear force on the aortic wall. Despite this theoretic concern, positive inotropes should not be withheld from the patient who deteriorates in the operating room because they may provide the precious additional minutes of hemodynamic stability needed to get on CPB.

In acute and chronic forms of AR, serial measurements of CO can indicate that ventricular size and CO have been optimized, regardless of the systemic pressure. TEE is useful to look at ventricular size, but probably maximizing CO under these conditions gets closer to the therapeutic goal than looking at ventricular size alone. With acute AR and premature closure of the mitral valve, PAPs may grossly underestimate the LVEDP, which continues to increase under the influence of the diastolic regurgitant jet from the aorta.

The early and late phases of CPB can be a problem, particularly in reoperations. Before cross-clamp placement, the ventricle is at risk for distension if it is not ejecting or being vented. If the ventricle dilates with AR during CPB, the intraventricular pressures may equilibrate with the aortic root pressures. Under these conditions, there is no coronary perfusion, and the ventricle may dilate rapidly and become profoundly ischemic. This can occur before cross-clamp placement with bradycardia, ventricular fibrillation, or tachycardia or with a rapid supraventricular rhythm that compromises organized mechanical activity. Correcting the rhythm, pacing, cross-clamping the aorta, or venting the ventricle addresses the problem. This also can occur in cardiac surgery for conditions other than AR. In patients with unknown or uncorrected AR, removal of the cross-clamp causes the same ventricular dilation and ischemia if the rhythm and ejection are not rapidly established. Ventricular venting or pacing may be essential until an organized, mechanically efficient, rhythm is established. This problem must be considered in patients referred for CABG alone, in those with mild or moderate AR not having AVR, and in patients for whom intraoperative TEE is not used.

■ MITRAL STENOSIS

Clinical Features and Natural History

Clinically significant MS in adult patients usually is a result of rheumatic disease. Congenital abnormalities of the mitral valve are a rare cause of MS in younger patients. Other uncommon conditions that do not directly involve the mitral valve apparatus but may limit left ventricular inflow and simulate the clinical findings of MS include cor triatriatum, large left atrial neoplasms, and pulmonary vein obstruction.

A decades-long asymptomatic period characterizes the initial phase of rheumatic MS. Symptoms rarely appear until the normal mitral valve area (MVA) of 4 to 6 cm^2 (Fig. 15.4) has been reduced to 2.5 cm^2 or less. When the MVA reaches 1.5 to 2.5 cm^2, symptoms usually occur only in association with exercise or conditions such as fever, pregnancy, or AF that lead to increases in heart rate or CO. After the MVA decreases to less than 1.5 cm^2, symptoms may develop at rest. Some patients are able to remain asymptomatic for long periods by gradually reducing their level of activity. Patients with MS commonly report dyspnea as their initial symptom, a finding reflective of increased left atrial pressure and pulmonary congestion. In addition to dyspnea, patients may report palpitations that signal the onset of AF. Systemic thromboembolization occurs in 10% to 20% of patients with MS and does not appear to be correlated

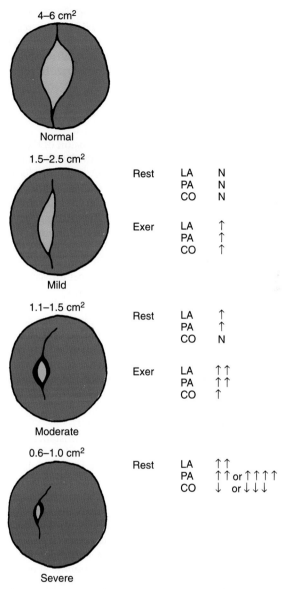

Fig. 15.4 Hemodynamic changes with progressive narrowing of the mitral valve. *CO*, Cardiac output; *Exer*, exercise; *LA*, left atrium; *N*, normal; *PA*, pulmonary artery; ↑, increased; ↓, decreased. (From Rapaport E. Natural history of aortic and mitral valve disease. *Am J Cardiol*. 1971;35:221.)

with the MVA or left atrial size. Chest pain that simulates angina occurs in a small number of patients with MS and may result from right ventricular hypertrophy (RVH) rather than CAD.

There has been a change in the typical age at which patients are diagnosed with MS. Previously, patients, often women, with MS were identified while in their 20s and 30s. Since the early 1990s, perhaps because of more slowly progressive disease in the United States, patients have been diagnosed in their 40s and 50s.

After symptoms develop, MS remains a slow, progressive disease. Patients often live 10 to 20 years with mild symptoms, such as dyspnea with exercise, before disabling NYHA class III and IV symptoms develop. The symptomatic state of the patient predicts the clinical outcome. For instance, the 10-year survival rate of patients with mild symptoms approaches 80%, but the 10-year survival rate of patients with disabling symptoms is only 15% without surgery.

Pathophysiology

Rheumatic MS results in valve leaflet thickening and fusion of the commissures. Later in the disease process, leaflet calcification and subvalvular chordal fusion may occur. These changes combine to reduce the effective MVA and limit diastolic flow into the LV. As a result of the fixed obstruction to left ventricular inflow, left atrial pressures increase. Elevated left atrial pressures limit pulmonary venous drainage and result in increased PAPs. Over time, pulmonary arteriolar hypertrophy develops in response to chronically increased pulmonary vascular pressures. Pulmonary hypertension may trigger increases in right ventricular end-diastolic volume (RVEDV) and pressure (RVEDP), and some patients may have signs of right ventricular failure such as ascites or peripheral edema. Left atrial enlargement is an almost universal finding in patients with established MS and is a risk factor for AF.

Patients with MS tolerate tachycardia particularly poorly. Left ventricular inflow, already limited by a mechanically abnormal valve, is further compromised by the disproportionate decline in the diastolic period that accompanies tachycardia. The flow rate across the stenotic valve must increase to maintain left ventricular filling in a shorter diastolic period. Because the valve area remains constant, the pressure gradient between the LA and LV increases by the square of the increase in the flow rate, according to the Gorlin formula, in which PG is the transvalvular pressure gradient:

$$\text{Valve area} = \text{Transvalvular flow rate}/\text{Constant} \times \sqrt{PG}$$

Tachycardia necessitates a significant increase in the transvalvular pressure gradient and may precipitate feelings of breathlessness in awake patients. In patients with AF, it is the increased ventricular rate that is most deleterious, rather than the loss of atrial contraction. Although coordinated atrial activity is always preferable, the primary goal in treating patients with MS and AF should be control of the ventricular rate.

MS results in diminished left ventricular preload reserve. As seen in the pressure-volume loop in Fig. 15.5, LVEDV and LVEDP are reduced, with an accompanying decline in SV. Controversy exists regarding the contractile state of the LV in these patients. Limited preload may contribute to a reduced EF in some of these patients. However, the observation that left ventricular contractile impairment persists after surgery in some patients suggests that other causes of left ventricular dysfunction may exist. Rheumatic myocarditis has been reported, although its role in producing left ventricular contractile dysfunction is uncertain.

Surgical Decision Making

Appropriate referral of patients for surgical intervention requires integration of clinical and echocardiographic data. Patients with severe symptoms (ie, NYHA class III and IV) should be immediately referred for surgery because the outcome is poor if treated medically. Patients with only mild MS and few or no symptoms may be treated conservatively with periodic evaluation. Patients who are asymptomatic but have

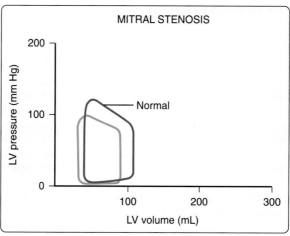

Fig. 15.5 Pressure-volume loop *(green)* for mitral stenosis. LV, Left ventricular. (From Jackson JM, Thomas SJ, Lowenstein E. Anesthetic management of patients with valvular heart disease. *Semin Anesth.* 1982;1:239.)

moderate MS (ie, MVA between 1.0 and 1.5 cm^2) require careful assessment. If significant pulmonary hypertension (ie, pulmonary artery systolic pressure >50 mm Hg) is identified, surgical intervention should be considered. Intervention also may be indicated if a patient becomes symptomatic or PAPs increase significantly during exercise testing.

The surgical options for treating MS continue to evolve. Closed commissurotomy, in which the surgeon fractures fused mitral commissures, was first performed in the 1920s. It became popular in the 1940s and still is used to treat MS in developing countries. With the advent of CPB in the 1950s, techniques of open commissurotomy developed, allowing the surgeon to directly inspect the valve before splitting the commissures. The common goals of closed and open mitral commissurotomy include increasing the effective MVA and decreasing the left atrial to left ventricular pressure gradient, with a resultant relief in the patient's symptoms.

Percutaneous mitral commissurotomy (PMC) allows a less invasive, catheter-based approach to MS. It was first reported by Inoue and coworkers in 1984, and clinicians worldwide perform PMC more than 10,000 times each year. The technique of PMC involves directing a balloon-tipped catheter across the stenotic mitral valve. Specifically designed balloons allow sequential inflation of the distal and proximal portions of the balloon, ensuring correct positioning across the mitral valve before the middle portion of the device is inflated to split the fused commissures. Patient selection for PMC requires careful echocardiographic evaluation.

Not all patients are candidates for surgical commissurotomy or PMC. Those with heavily calcified valves or significant MR are likely to experience suboptimal results after commissurotomy. Mitral valve anatomy unsuitable for PMC is more commonly encountered in Western countries, where patients with MS typically are diagnosed at an older average age. Mitral valve replacement commonly is recommended for these patients. The risk for mitral valve replacement depends on patient characteristics such as age, functional status, and other comorbid conditions. Surgical risk in younger patients with few coexisting medical problems usually is less than 5%. Conversely, surgical risk in elderly patients with severe symptoms related to MS and multiple comorbidities may be 10% to 20%.

15

◼ MITRAL REGURGITATION

Clinical Features and Natural History

Unlike mitral stenosis (MS), which is usually the result of rheumatic valve disease, MR may result from a variety of disease processes that affect the valve leaflets, chordae tendineae, papillary muscles, valve annulus, or LV. MR can be classified as organic or functional. Organic MR describes diseases that result in distortion, disruption, or destruction of the mitral leaflets or chordal structures. In Western countries, degenerative processes that lead to leaflet prolapse with or without chordal rupture are the most common cause of MR. Other causes of organic MR include infective endocarditis, mitral annular calcification, rheumatic valve disease, and connective tissue disorders such as Marfan or Ehlers-Danlos syndrome. Much less common causes of organic MR include congenital mitral valve clefts, diet-drug or ergotamine toxicity, and carcinoid valve disease with metabolically active pulmonary tumors or right-to-left intracardiac shunting.

Functional MR describes MR that occurs despite structurally normal leaflets and chordae tendineae. Resulting from altered function or geometry of the LV or mitral annulus, functional MR often occurs in the setting of ischemic heart disease, and the term *ischemic MR* is sometimes used interchangeably with *functional MR*. However, the functional form can occur in patients without demonstrable CAD, such as those with idiopathic dilated cardiomyopathy and mitral annular dilation. The term *ischemic MR* probably best applies to functional cases with a known ischemic cause. Rupture of a papillary muscle with acute, severe MR is somewhat more difficult to classify. Although usually a sequela of acute myocardial infarction (AMI) with normal leaflets and chordae, there is an obvious anatomic disruption of the mitral apparatus.

The natural history of MR varies because it can be caused by a wide variety of disease processes. Even among patients with acute-onset disease, the clinical course depends on the mechanism of regurgitation and the response to treatment. For instance, patients with acute, severe MR caused by a ruptured papillary muscle have a dismal outcome without surgery. However, the clinical course of acute MR caused by endocarditis can be favorable if the patient responds well to antibiotic therapy. Although those with chronic MR usually enter an initial, often asymptomatic, compensated phase, the time course for progression to left ventricular dysfunction and symptomatic heart failure is unpredictable. The literature reflects the wide variation in the natural history of MR, with 5-year survival rates for patients with MR of 27% to 97%.

Pathophysiology

MR causes left ventricular volume overload. The regurgitant volume combines with the normal left atrial volume and returns to the LV during each diastolic period. The increased preload leads to increased sarcomere stretch and, in the initial phases of the disease process, augmentation of LV ejection performance by the Frank-Starling mechanism. Systolic ejection into the relatively low-pressure left atrium (LA) further enhances the contractile appearance of the LV.

The clinical presentation of patients with MR depends on the pathophysiology of the specific condition, including the mechanism, severity, and acuity of the disease. In cases of acute, severe MR, such as in patients with a ruptured papillary muscle after AMI, the sudden increase in preload enhances left ventricular contractility by the Frank-Starling mechanism. Despite the increased preload, the size of the LV is initially normal. Normal left ventricular size combined with the ability to eject into a low-pressure circuit (ie, the LA) results in decreased afterload in the acute setting.

The measured left ventricular ejection fraction (LVEF) in cases of sudden, severe MR may approach 75%, although forward SV is reduced. However, because the LA has not yet dilated in response to the large regurgitant volume, left atrial pressure increases acutely and may lead to pulmonary vascular congestion, pulmonary edema, and dyspnea.

Many patients with MR, particularly those whose valvular incompetence develops more slowly, may enter a chronic, compensated phase. In this phase, chronic volume overload triggers left ventricular cavity enlargement by promoting eccentric hypertrophy. Increased preload continues to augment left ventricular systolic performance. At the same time, the LA dilates in response to the ongoing regurgitant volume. Although left atrial dilation maintains a low-pressure circuit that facilitates left ventricular systolic ejection, the increased radius of the left ventricular cavity leads to increased wall tension according to Laplace's law.

With the eventual decline in left ventricular systolic function, patients enter a decompensated phase. Progressive left ventricular dilation increases wall stress and afterload, causing further deterioration in left ventricular performance, mitral annular dilation, and worsening of the MR. Left ventricular end-systolic pressure increases. The increased left ventricular filling pressures result in increased left atrial pressures and, given time, pulmonary vascular congestion, pulmonary hypertension, and right ventricular dysfunction. In addition to fatigue and weakness, patients with decompensated, chronic MR also may report dyspnea and orthopnea. It is difficult to predict when a patient with MR is likely to decompensate clinically. Progression of disease in any patient depends on the underlying cause of MR, its severity, the response of the LV to volume overload, and possibly the effect of medical management. Because of the combination of increased preload and the ability to eject into the low-pressure LA, a normally functioning LV should display an increased EF in the setting of significant MR. Conversely, an EF considered normal in a patient with competent valves may represent diminished left ventricular function in the setting of MR. In patients with severe MR, an EF in the range of 50% to 60% likely represents significant left ventricular dysfunction and is an indication for surgery.

Ischemic Mitral Regurgitation

Ischemic MR represents MR occurring in the setting of ischemic heart disease in patients without significant abnormalities of the valve leaflets or chordal structures. Myocardial ischemia may result in focal or global left ventricular bulging and, with time, ventricular remodeling to a more spherical shape. Geometric changes cause outward migration of the papillary muscles. The finding most strongly correlated with chronic ischemic MR is outward papillary muscle displacement. When the papillary muscles are displaced outward, the point of mitral leaflet coaptation moves apically and away from the mitral annulus, resulting in the appearance of valve tenting. Besides outward bulging of the LV, scarring and retraction of the papillary muscles may produce mitral leaflet tethering, with the net effect of incomplete leaflet coaptation and valvular incompetence. An additional potential mechanism of ischemic MR is decreased contractility of the posterior mitral annulus. During systole, annular contraction reduces the mitral orifice area by 25%. Because the anterior portion of the mitral annulus is more fibrous, posterior annular contraction plays a greater role in reducing the size of the mitral orifice. Loss of posterior annular contraction may contribute to MR in the setting of myocardial ischemia.

The clinical approach to ischemic MR depends on its underlying mechanism. Timely surgical intervention often is warranted in cases of papillary muscle rupture. For patients with an intact mitral apparatus who have ischemic MR in

15

the setting of AMI, early reperfusion therapy improves regional and global left ventricular function, reduces ventricular dilation, and decreases the likelihood of adverse remodeling and associated papillary muscle displacement. The resultant improvements in ventricular function and geometry combine to reduce the incidence of ischemic MR.

Surgical Decision Making

The surgical approach to MR has evolved as its pathophysiology has been clarified. High operative mortality rates associated with the surgical correction of MR in the 1980s led many clinicians to treat patients conservatively. Because favorable loading conditions and high left atrial compliance allow patients with significant MR to remain asymptomatic for long periods, it is likely that many patients did not undergo surgery until the onset of disabling symptoms. More severe preoperative symptoms are associated with a lower EF and a greater incidence of postoperative CHF. Historically, poor outcomes after surgery for MR might have occurred because clinicians did not appreciate the true degree of left ventricular dysfunction at the time of surgery in symptomatic patients. An EF of less than 60% in the setting of severe MR represents significant left ventricular dysfunction and predicts a worse outcome with surgery or medical management. Surgical techniques common in the 1980s probably also contributed to unfavorable postoperative outcomes. For instance, although the mechanisms are incompletely understood, resection of the subvalvular apparatus contributes to decreased left ventricular systolic performance after mitral valve replacement.

In part because of improved surgical techniques, the operative mortality rate for patients with organic MR who are younger than 75 years is about 1% in some centers. Besides preservation of the subvalvular apparatus, valve repair is another surgical technique associated with improved postoperative outcome. Although not applicable to all patients, such as those with advanced rheumatic disease, the popularity of valve repairs continues to grow.

Studies indicate numerous benefits associated with mitral repair. For instance, after accounting for baseline characteristics, patients who undergo mitral repair instead of replacement have lower operative mortality rates and longer survival times, largely because of improved postoperative left ventricular function. The survival benefit that accompanies valve repair also is observed among patients undergoing combined valve and CABG surgery. Valve repair does not increase the likelihood of reoperation compared with replacement. Although originally used most often for posterior leaflet disease, surgeons now routinely repair anterior mitral leaflets with good success. When repairing anterior leaflet prolapse, surgeons may insert artificial chordae. The approach to flail or prolapsing posterior mitral leaflet segments often involves resection of a portion of the leaflet. In addition to resecting a portion of the leaflet and plicating the redundant tissue, an annuloplasty ring often is placed to reduce mitral orifice size and return the annulus to a more anatomic shape. Some surgeons favor a flexible, partial, posterior annuloplasty band, which may allow improved systolic contraction of the posterior annulus and better postoperative left ventricular function.

Minimally Invasive Mitral Valve Surgery

The concept of minimally invasive mitral surgery usually refers to valve repairs accomplished through a 3- or 4-cm right inframammary incision in the fourth or fifth intercostal space. Several additional 1-cm incisions around the primary incision facilitate placement of robotic arms or other thoracoscopic instruments. The arterial cannula for CPB may be inserted directly or by a chimney graft into the femoral artery or into the ascending aorta through a thoracic incision under direct visualization. Venous drainage is accomplished by the femoral route using TEE guidance with a multiple side hole peripheral access cannula. Supplementary venous drainage is used in some centers by inserting either a 15- to 17-Fr right internal jugular vein cannula or specialized PAC with multiple end holes that drains to the venous reservoir during CPB.

Cardioplegia may be given antegrade into the aortic root or retrograde through the coronary sinus. Surgeons typically administer antegrade cardioplegia by one of two methods. The first involves the placement of a catheter tip into the ascending aorta through a right parasternal stab incision under thoracoscopic vision. This method is similar to standard antegrade cardioplegia administration in median sternotomy cases. A long-shafted aortic cross-clamp placed through a stab incision in the right lateral chest wall is used to occlude the aorta distal to the cardioplegia cannula. The second method of antegrade cardioplegia administration uses a specialized endoaortic cannula inserted into the femoral artery. A balloon near the distal end of this cannula is positioned in the ascending aorta using TEE guidance. Inflation of the balloon occludes the ascending aorta while antegrade cardioplegia delivery commences at the distal tip of the device.

Although referred to as *robotic*, systems such as the da Vinci are probably more appropriately described as telemanipulators. These devices receive direct input from the hands and feet of the surgeon who is seated at a remote console that translates these motions to end-effectors within the chest of the patient. When seated at the remote console of a robotic device, the surgeon has near-stereoscopic vision compared with viewing a two-dimensional image on a television screen. Robotic devices provide motion scaling and tremor filtration to smooth movements. Because the robotic arms have articulating "wrists" at their distal ends, the surgeon can achieve 7 degrees of freedom of movement within the chest, similar to open surgery. By comparison, long-handled thoracoscopic instruments, which are often oriented almost parallel to one another, afford only 4 degrees of freedom. Both thoracoscopic and robotically assisted approaches use the same operative techniques as standard open repairs. Techniques such as leaflet resection, chordal insertion or transfer, sliding plasties, edge-to-edge repair, and annuloplasty band insertion may be used by experienced surgeons.

Just as catheter-based techniques have been developed to treat valvular AS, efforts are under way to develop percutaneous interventions for MR. The device with the largest clinical experience is the MitraClip system (Abbott Laboratories, Abbott Park, IL). Leaflet plication is based on the open mitral repair technique reported by Alfieri and colleagues. It entails the creation of a double-orifice mitral valve by suturing the free edges of the leaflets at the site of regurgitation together to improve leaflet coaptation and reduce MR. MitraClip uses a percutaneous femoral venous transseptal delivery system to deploy a cobalt-chromium clip to secure the mitral leaflets under fluoroscopic and echocardiographic guidance.

Percutaneous techniques attempt to correct annular pathology by indirectly pushing the posterior annulus anteriorly using devices that exploit the anatomic relationship of the coronary sinus and mitral annulus. One device is the Carillon Mitral Contour System. It consists of self-expandable nitinol (ie, nickel-titanium alloy) proximal and distal anchors connected by a nitinol bridge. The application of tension on the system pulls the posterior mitral annulus anteriorly, reducing septal–lateral annular diameter.

15

BOX 15.4 *Mitral Regurgitation*

Preload is increased
Afterload is decreased
Goal is mild tachycardia, vasodilation
Avoid myocardial depression

Anesthesia Considerations

Patients with MR may have significantly different risk factors for surgery, including duration of disease, symptoms, hemodynamic stability, ventricular function, and involvement of the right heart and pulmonary circulation (Box 15.4). For instance, a patient with severe MR caused by acute papillary muscle rupture may enter the operating room in cardiogenic shock with pulmonary congestion requiring intraaortic balloon pump augmentation. Another patient with a newly diagnosed flail posterior mitral leaflet may enter the surgical suite with relatively preserved left ventricular function and no symptoms; the compliance of the LA might have prevented pulmonary vascular congestion, pulmonary hypertension, and right ventricular dysfunction.

Despite differences in presentation, the general management goals remain similar and include maintenance of forward CO and reduction in the mitral regurgitant fraction. The anesthesiologist must optimize right ventricular function, in part by avoiding increases in pulmonary vascular congestion and pulmonary hypertension. Depending on the clinical presentation, various degrees of intervention are needed to achieve these hemodynamic management goals.

Invasive hemodynamic monitoring provides a wealth of important information. Arterial catheters are essential for monitoring beat-to-beat changes in blood pressure that occur in response to a variety of surgical and anesthesia manipulations. PACs facilitate many aspects of intraoperative patient management. Intraoperative use of a PAC allows careful optimization of left-sided filling pressures. Although the PCWP and diastolic PAP depend on left atrial and left ventricular compliance and filling, examination of intraoperative trends in these variables helps the anesthesiologist to provide appropriate levels of preload while avoiding volume overload. Periodic determination of CO allows a more objective assessment of the patient's response to interventions such as fluid administration or inotropic infusion. The presence or size of a v wave on a PCWP tracing does not reliably correlate with the severity of MR because this finding depends on left atrial compliance. As in the management of patients with AR, a benefit of PAC insertion is the ability to introduce a ventricular pacing wire to rapidly counteract hemodynamically significant bradycardia. In patients with right ventricular compromise, monitoring trends in the CVP recording may be helpful. Tricuspid regurgitation (TR) detected through analysis of the CVP tracing may suggest right ventricular dilation, which may be caused by pulmonary hypertension.

Intraoperative TEE provides invaluable information during the surgical correction of MR. It reliably identifies the mechanism of MR, thereby guiding the surgical approach, and it objectively demonstrates the size and function of the cardiac chambers. TEE can identify the cause of hemodynamic derangements, facilitating proper intervention. For instance, the appearance of SAM of the mitral apparatus immediately after valve repair allows the anesthesiologist to intervene with volume infusion and medications such as esmolol or phenylephrine as appropriate. In rare circumstances, when hemodynamically significant SAM persists despite these interventions, the surgeon may elect to further repair or replace the mitral valve. TEE also identifies concomitant pathology that may warrant surgical attention, such as atrial-level shunts and additional valve disease.

Intraoperative TEE is essential during minimally invasive and robotically assisted mitral valve surgery. The use of a right minithoracotomy for these procedures precludes bypass cannulation in the chest. Instead, femoral arterial and venous cannulation with or without supplementary venous drainage from the superior vena cava or pulmonary artery is used. Real-time TEE imaging typically guides cannulation for CPB. If an endoaortic balloon clamp is used, the echocardiographer ensures that the balloon is correctly positioned in the ascending aorta.

In addition to TEE considerations related to cannulation procedures, the selection of a minimally invasive or robotically assisted approach to mitral repair necessitates other changes in anesthesia management. Although not universally used, one-lung ventilation is preferred in many centers. This may be achieved by the usual methods, such as a double-lumen endotracheal tube or bronchial blocker. Impaired oxygenation can occur when one-lung ventilation is used during the termination of CPB during these procedures.

Intraoperative care of patients with MR before the institution of CPB focuses on optimizing forward CO, minimizing the mitral regurgitant volume, and preventing deleterious increases in PAPs. Maintaining adequate left ventricular preload is essential. An enlarged LV that operates on a higher portion of the Frank-Starling curve requires adequate filling. At the same time, excessive volume administration should be avoided because it may cause unwanted dilatation of the mitral annulus and worsening of the MR. Excessive fluid administration may precipitate right ventricular failure in patients with pulmonary vascular congestion and pulmonary hypertension. Optimization of preload is aided by analysis of data obtained from PAC measurements and TEE images. Because significant left ventricular dysfunction is seen in many patients with MR, specific induction and maintenance regimens are selected to avoid further depressing left ventricular function. Large doses of narcotics have been popular in the past. Others have shown that smaller doses of narcotics combined with vasodilating inhalation anesthetics produce acceptable intraoperative hemodynamics. By reducing the amount of narcotics administered, the addition of a vasodilating inhalation agent to the anesthetic regimen may allow for faster extubation of the trachea after surgery. With the current trend toward early referral of asymptomatic patients for mitral repair, anesthetic regimens that reduce the duration of postoperative mechanical ventilation may be advantageous.

In patients with severe left ventricular dysfunction, infusions of inotropic medications such as dopamine, dobutamine, or epinephrine may be required to maintain an adequate cardiac output. Phosphodiesterase inhibitors such as milrinone also may augment systolic ventricular performance and reduce pulmonary and peripheral vascular resistances. By reducing pulmonary and peripheral vascular resistance, forward CO is facilitated. Nitroglycerin and sodium nitroprusside represent two additional options for reducing the impedance to ventricular ejection. If patients prove refractory to inotropic and vasodilator therapy, insertion of an intraaortic balloon pump should be strongly considered.

Because severe MR may result in pulmonary hypertension and right ventricular dysfunction, intraoperative management strategies should avoid hypercapnia, hypoxia, and acidosis. Mild hyperventilation may be beneficial in some patients.

Patients with severe right ventricular dysfunction after CPB can prove exceptionally difficult to treat. Besides avoiding the factors known to increase pulmonary vascular resistance (PVR), only a few options exist for these patients. Inotropic agents with

15

vasodilating properties such as dobutamine, isoproterenol, and milrinone augment right ventricular systolic performance and decrease PVR, but their use often is confounded by systemic hypotension. Prostaglandin E_1 (PGE$_1$) reliably reduces PVR and undergoes extensive first-pass metabolism in the pulmonary circulation. Although PGE$_1$ reduces PAPs after CPB, systemic hypotension requiring infusions of vasoconstrictors through a left atrial catheter has occurred.

Inhaled nitric oxide is an alternative for the treatment of right ventricular failure in the setting of pulmonary hypertension. Nitric oxide reliably relaxes the pulmonary vasculature and is then immediately bound to hemoglobin and inactivated. Studies indicate that systemic hypotension during nitric oxide therapy is unlikely.

Left ventricular dysfunction may contribute to post-CPB hemodynamic instability. With mitral competence restored, the low-pressure outlet for left ventricular ejection is removed. The enlarged LV must then eject entirely into the aorta. Because left ventricular enlargement leads to increased wall stress, a condition of increased afterload often exists after CPB. At the same time, the preload augmentation inherent to MR is removed. The systolic performance of the LV often declines after surgical correction of MR. Treatment options in the immediate post-CPB period include inotropic and vasodilator therapy and, if necessary, intraaortic balloon pump augmentation.

Anesthesia Considerations

Several important goals should guide the anesthesia management of patients with significant MS. First, the anesthesiologist should prevent tachycardia or treat it promptly in the perioperative period (Box 15.5). Second, left ventricular preload should be maintained without exacerbation of pulmonary vascular congestion. Third, anesthesiologists should avoid factors that aggravate pulmonary hypertension and impair right ventricular function.

Prevention and treatment of tachycardia are central to perioperative management. Tachycardia shortens the diastolic filling period. An elevation in transvalvular flow rate is required, with a resultant increase in the left atrial–to–left ventricular pressure gradient to maintain left ventricular preload with a shortened diastolic period. Avoidance of tachycardia begins in the preoperative period. Anxiety-induced tachycardia may be treated with small doses of narcotics or benzodiazepines. However, excessive sedation is counterproductive because sedative-induced hypoventilation can result in hypoxemia or hypercarbia, potentially aggravating a patient's underlying pulmonary hypertension and because large doses of premedication can jeopardize the patient's already limited left ventricular preload. Appropriate monitoring and supplemental oxygen therapy should be considered for patients receiving preoperative narcotics or benzodiazepines. Medications taken by the patient before surgery to control heart rate, such as digitalis, β-blockers, calcium receptor antagonists, or amiodarone, should be continued in the perioperative period. Additional doses of β-blockers and calcium-receptor antagonists

BOX 15.5 *Mitral Stenosis*

Preload is normal or increased
Afterload is normal
Goal is controlled ventricular response
Avoid tachycardia, pulmonary vasoconstriction

may be required intraoperatively, particularly to control the ventricular rate in patients with AF. Control of the ventricular rate remains the primary goal in managing patients with AF, although cardioversion should not be withheld from patients with atrial tachyarrhythmias who become hemodynamically unstable. Narcotic-based anesthetics often are helpful in avoiding intraoperative tachycardia. However, clinicians should realize these patients may be receiving other vagotonic drugs and that profound bradycardia is possible in response to large doses of narcotics. The selection of a muscle relaxant such as pancuronium may help prevent the unwanted bradycardia associated with high-dose narcotics.

Maintenance of preload is an important goal for treating patients who have a fixed obstruction to left ventricular filling. Appropriate replacement of blood loss and prevention of excessive anesthetic-induced venodilation help preserve hemodynamic stability intraoperatively. Invasive hemodynamic monitoring allows the anesthesiologist to maintain adequate preload while avoiding excessive fluid administration that can aggravate pulmonary vascular congestion. Placement of an arterial catheter facilitates timely recognition of hemodynamic derangements. PACs can be invaluable in treating patients with significant MS. Although the PCWP overestimates left ventricular filling and the pulmonary artery diastolic pressure may not accurately reflect left-heart volume in patients with pulmonary hypertension, trends and responses to intervention can be more readily assessed. Tachycardia increases the pressure gradient between the LA and LV. Increased heart rates widen the discrepancy between the PCWP and the true LVEDP. Despite these limitations, the PAC remains a useful monitoring tool, providing information on CO and PAPs.

Many patients with MS have pulmonary hypertension. Anesthesia techniques that avoid increases in PVR are likely to benefit these patients and prevent additional right ventricular embarrassment. Meticulous attention to arterial blood gas results allows appropriate adjustment of ventilatory parameters. Vasodilator therapy for patients with pulmonary hypertension usually is ineffective because the venodilation produced further limits left ventricular filling and does not improve cardiac output. The only MS patients who may benefit from vasodilator therapy are those with concomitant MR or those with severe pulmonary hypertension and right ventricular dysfunction in whom pulmonary vasodilation can facilitate transpulmonary blood flow and improve left ventricular filling. The treatment of right ventricular dysfunction was discussed earlier.

15

TRICUSPID REGURGITATION

Clinical Features and Natural History

Tricuspid disease is caused by a structural defect in the valve apparatus or a functional lesion. Primary disorders of the tricuspid valve apparatus that may lead to more significant degrees of TR include congenital disease (ie, Ebstein anomaly), rheumatic valve disease, prolapse, irradiation, carcinoid syndrome, blunt chest trauma, endomyocardial biopsy–related trauma, and right ventricular pacemaker/defibrillator lead trauma. Despite numerous potential causes of primary tricuspid disease, they account for only 20% of TR cases. The remainder of TR disease is functional in nature. Left-sided valvular disease, usually MR, most commonly is responsible. Functional tricuspid incompetence also can result from MS, AR, or AS and from isolated pulmonary hypertension. Causes of functional TR include dilation of the annulus or leaflet tethering from right ventricular dilation and remodeling, global right ventricular dysfunction from cardiomyopathy and myocarditis or CAD with resulting ischemia, infarction, or rupture of the right ventricular papillary muscles. When mitral valve disease is severe enough to warrant valve repair or replacement, TR may be identified in 30% to 50% of patients.

Symptoms of isolated TR are usually minor in the absence of concurrent pulmonary hypertension. Intravenous drug abusers who develop tricuspid endocarditis are the classic example. In these patients, structural damage to the valve may be quite severe, but because they are free of other cardiac disease, they can tolerate complete excision of the tricuspid valve with few adverse effects. Excision of the tricuspid valve in endocarditis has been common because of the undesirability of placing a valve prosthesis in a region of infection. Surgical annuloplasty may be a better long-term option if the valve is structurally salvageable.

Another factor that broadly favors tricuspid repair rather than replacement is the high incidence of thrombotic complications with a valve in this position. The lower pressure and flow state on the right side of the heart are responsible for this phenomenon.

In chronic TR caused by right ventricular dilation, the clinical scenario often is much different from that of isolated tricuspid disease. The major hemodynamic derangements are usually those associated with mitral or aortic valve disease. The right ventricle (RV) dilates in the face of the afterload stress from long-standing pulmonary hypertension, and the resultant increase in end-diastolic fiber stretch (ie, preload reserve) promotes increases in SV mediated by the Starling mechanism. These increases are negated by a concurrently increasing right ventricular afterload because of relatively inadequate RVH. Regurgitation through the tricuspid valve reduces right ventricular wall tension at the price of a decrease in effective forward SV.

An important corollary to right ventricular chamber enlargement is the possibility of a leftward shift of the interventricular septum and encroachment on the left ventricular cavity. This phenomenon can reduce the left ventricular chamber size and the slope of the left ventricular diastolic pressure-volume curve, rendering the LV less compliant. Septal encroachment may mask left ventricular underfilling by decreasing left ventricular compliance, artificially increasing LVEDP. A failing RV underloads the left side by reduced effective SV and anatomic (ie, septal shift) mechanisms.

Surgical Decision Making

In cases of structural tricuspid insufficiency, the decision to repair or replace the valve is straightforward. The same cannot be said of functional TR. Because most functional cases are the consequence of left-sided valve lesions with right ventricular overload, the TR usually improves significantly (typically by at least one grade) after the aortic or mitral valve is repaired or replaced. It can be unclear in the operating room whether addition of a tricuspid procedure to the left-sided valve surgery is indicated. In this situation, intraoperative TEE plays an essential role. If the TR is severe in the pre-CPB assessment, tricuspid valve surgery is usually performed. The evidence is less clear when regurgitation is graded as moderate. Some surgeons choose to repair the tricuspid valve in cases of moderate TR, but others advocate observation. In the context of left-sided valve surgery, it is common with moderate or more severe TR to complete the left-sided procedure and then reassess the tricuspid valve with TEE when the heart is full and ejecting. If the TR remains more than moderate after the left-sided valve is fixed, many surgeons perform the tricuspid procedure. If regurgitation is moderate or less severe, the appropriate surgical course may remain unclear.

Some patients having left-sided valve procedures must return to the operating room for tricuspid surgery. Their morbidity and mortality rates are probably significantly higher than those for patients undergoing tricuspid valve repair at the time of the aortic or mitral valve procedure. Decision making for cases of functional TR is made more complicated by the inability to rigorously quantify the severity of the regurgitation and right ventricular dysfunction.

Anesthesia Considerations

Because most tricuspid surgery occurs in the context of significant aortic or mitral disease, anesthesia management primarily is determined by the left-sided valve lesion. The exception is when significant pulmonary hypertension and right ventricular failure exist. Under these conditions, the primary impediment to hemodynamic stability after surgery is right ventricular failure rather than the left-sided process.

If right ventricular dysfunction is predicted, it is useful to place a PAC, even if the tricuspid valve will be replaced. If the PAC must be removed because of tricuspid valve replacement, it still can be helpful to obtain CO and PAPs before CPB to get insight into right ventricular function and anticipate the hemodynamic support that may be required. A PAC is of greater use than CVP alone because the CVP is a poor index of intravascular filling and the degree of TR. The right atrium and vena cavae are highly compliant and accept large regurgitant volumes with relatively little change in pressure.

A PAC also is useful when intraoperative TEE is used. As in AR within the LV, the RV in chronic TR is volume-overloaded and dilated and requires a large EDV to maintain forward flow. Because of the unreliability of the CVP as an indicator of filling, it is possible to volume-overload patients with TR and right ventricular failure. CO in right ventricular failure often can be augmented with the use of vasodilators, and although right ventricular dimensions can be followed intraoperatively with TEE, maximizing CO (sometimes at the cost of systemic arterial pressure) is best done with serial CO measurements (as in AR). When there is significant right ventricular distension, the possibility of septal shift and secondary deterioration of left ventricular diastolic compliance should be carefully considered. Echocardiography is uniquely helpful for this assessment.

Post-CPB treatment of the patient undergoing an isolated tricuspid valve procedure is usually straightforward. Patients usually do not have significant right ventricular failure or pulmonary hypertension and typically require only a brief period of CPB without aortic cross-clamping. A larger group of patients, particularly those with TR related to AS, typically come off CPB with little need for support of the RV. These patients often do well because the improvement in left ventricular function after AVR for AS is usually sufficient to reduce PAPs significantly and offload the right heart. When left-sided valve surgery is for mitral disease, the improvement usually is not as marked, and greater degrees of inotropic support of the RV often are indicated. The combination of a phosphodiesterase inhibitor with a vasodilator and a catecholamine infusion is useful. Serial CO measurements to balance systemic pressure and right ventricular output and filling are critical.

A few other practical points on tricuspid valve repair and replacement should be made. First, because right-sided pressures can be chronically increased with TR, it is important to look for a patent foramen ovale and the potential for right-to-left shunting before initiation of CPB. Second, intravascular volume may be quite high in this patient population, and it is often practical to avoid red blood cell transfusion by hemofiltration during bypass. Third, if the patient has significant right ventricular dysfunction or peripheral edema or ascites, there is the potential for a coagulopathy related to liver congestion, and the patient should be treated accordingly. Fourth, central catheters, particularly PACs, should not be entrapped by right atrial suture lines.

15

◼ INNOVATIONS IN VALVE REPAIR

Interventional cardiology has had a significant impact on the volume of CABG, and it can be predicted that interventional cardiology will alter surgery for VHD over time. Many less invasive approaches to mitral valve repair are being assessed in animal studies or clinical trials, and tremendous inroads have been made in percutaneous replacement of the aortic valve. Innovations also are being made in surgical valve repair, including aortic valve repair and closed- and open-chamber procedures for MR.

Aortic Valve Repair

During the past several years, there has been a major shift from valve replacement to valve repair in patients with degenerative mitral valve disease. The same has not been true of the aortic valve because the valve disease is different in most patients and because of the high flow and pressure conditions across the aortic valve that make repair more prone to failure. However, aortic valve repair is being increasingly done as an appropriate patient population is defined. Although valve repair for AR has found broader use when regurgitation is associated with dissection or dilation of the aortic root, isolated valve repair has been less common. A growing body of data suggests that aortic valve repair may offer advantages over valve replacement in younger individuals with AR due to bicuspid valves. In contrast with AVR, aortic valve repair eliminates the need for anticoagulation for a mechanical valve and should delay the need for reoperation for a failed tissue valve. When regurgitation occurs with a bicuspid valve, the insufficiency usually is caused by retraction or prolapse, or both, of the conjoined cusp. Repair consists of a triangular incision to shorten and elevate the cusp to improve apposition. Although very long-term follow-up results have not been reported, late failure of the repair requiring reoperation does occur. Most of the failure was attributed to repairs done in the early experience of repairs.

As a result of this experience, aortic valve repair is likely to find increasing application in this patient population. For this group, anesthesia management usually is straightforward, although the clinical indications for valve repair in AR are the same as those for valve replacement. The compelling issue for the anesthesiologist in these cases is echocardiographic assessment of the valve for suitability of repair and the adequacy of the repair after the procedure.

Sutureless Valve Replacement

Surgical AVR continues to be the gold standard for patients with severe symptomatic aortic valve stenosis. Transcatheter aortic valve replacement (TAVR) reduced the rate of death and cardiac symptoms for patients deemed inoperable compared with medical therapy alone. These procedures have been associated with a decreased mortality rate at 1 year compared with open surgery in high-risk patients. However, these procedures are not without risk, including bradyarrhythmias requiring permanent pacemaker insertion, cardiac perforation, myocardial infarction, access-related complications, and other valve-related issues such as perivalvular leak and unknown long-term durability.

There is increased interest in the treatment of aortic valvular disease with sutureless AVR in patients who can benefit from a shorter cross-clamp time but are not truly inoperable. With the rapid technologic progress made in transcatheter valve technology and materials, sutureless AVR has been proposed as an additional therapeutic option for high-risk patients with severe AS. Potential advantages of sutureless AVR include removal of the diseased and often calcific native aortic valve and reduction in aortic cross-clamp and CPB times in the setting of a potentially minimally invasive surgical approach.

NEW TECHNIQUES FOR MITRAL VALVE REPAIR

MR frequently is associated with CHF. In dilated and ischemic cardiomyopathy, enlargement of the mitral annulus results in a failure of coaptation of the mitral leaflets and valve incompetence. Although cardiac surgery is an effective treatment, morbidity can be high. Three approaches have been developed to address MR occurring in the absence of structural mitral pathology. They address the failure of leaflet coaptation at the level of the valve leaflets or valve annulus or by altering the anatomic relationship of the septal and lateral walls of the LV.

Altering Ventricular Anatomy to Reduce Mitral Regurgitation

Valve leaflet and annulus repair techniques are described in earlier sections of this chapter. The approach to closed mitral valve repair consists of altering the geometry of the lateral and septal left ventricular walls to bring the valve leaflets together. The commercial Coapsys device has entered clinical trials. It consists of anterior and posterior epicardial pads connected by a cord. With an open chest, the cord is placed transventricularly in a subvalvular position, and the tension on the cord is adjusted before the opposing epicardial pad is fixed in place. This effectively brings the ventricular walls together and improves leaflet coaptation. TEE is used to optimize cord length and pad positioning. In contrast to the leaflet-based and annulus-based approaches, the Coapsys approach is surgical, requiring an open chest but not CPB.

SUGGESTED READINGS

Alfieri O, Maisano F, De Bonis M, et al. The double-orifice technique in mitral valve repair: a simple solution for complex problems. *J Thorac Cardiovasc Surg.* 2001;122:674–681.

Augoustides JG, Wolfe Y, Walsh EK, et al. Recent advances in aortic valve disease: highlights from a bicuspid aortic valve to transcatheter aortic valve replacement. *J Cardiothorac Vasc Anesth.* 2009;23:569–576.

Bonow RO, Carabello B, de Leon AC, et al. ACC/AHA guidelines for the management of patients with valvular heart disease: executive summary. A report of the American College of Cardiology/American Heart Association Task Force on Practice Guidelines (Committee on Management of Patients with Valvular Heart Disease). *J Heart Valve Dis.* 1998;7:672–707.

Carabello BA. Evaluation and management of patients with aortic stenosis. *Circulation.* 2002;105:1746–1750.

Chaliki HP, Brown ML, Sundt TM, et al. Timing of operation in asymptomatic severe aortic stenosis. *Expert Rev Cardiovasc Ther.* 2007;5:1065–1071.

Filsoufi F, Rahmanian PB, Castillo JG, et al. Excellent early and late outcomes of aortic valve replacement in people aged 80 and older. *J Am Geriatr Soc.* 2008;56:255–261.

Grayburn PA, Eichhorn EJ. Dobutamine challenge for low-gradient aortic stenosis. *Circulation.* 2002;106:763–765.

Karon BL, Enriquez-Sarano M. Valvular regurgitation. In: Lloyd MA, Murphy JG, eds. *Mayo Clinic Cardiology Review.* 2nd ed. Philadelphia: Lippincott Williams & Wilkins; 2000:303–330.

Levine RA. Dynamic mitral regurgitation: more than meets the eye. *N Engl J Med.* 2004;351:1681–1684.

Matsunaga A, Duran CM. Progression of tricuspid regurgitation after repaired functional ischemic mitral regurgitation. *Circulation.* 2005;112(9 suppl):I453–I457.

Mohty D, Orszulak TA, Schaff HV, et al. Very long-term survival and durability of mitral valve repair for mitral valve prolapse. *Circulation.* 2001;104:I1–I7.

Monchi M, Gest V, Duval-Moulin AM, et al. Aortic stenosis with severe left ventricular dysfunction and low transvalvular pressure gradients: risk stratification by low-dose dobutamine echocardiography. *J Am Coll Cardiol.* 2001;37:2101–2107.

15

Mueller XM, Tevaearai HT, Stumpe F, et al. Tricuspid valve involvement in combined mitral and aortic valve surgery. *J Cardiovasc Surg (Torino)*. 2001;42:443–449.

Nishimura RA, Grantham JA, Connolly HM, et al. Low-output, low-gradient aortic stenosis in patients with depressed left ventricular systolic function: the clinical utility of the dobutamine challenge in the catheterization laboratory. *Circulation*. 2002;106:809–813.

Nishimura RA, Otto CM, Bonow RO, et al. AHA/ACC guideline for the management of patients with valvular heart disease: executive summary. A report of the American College of Cardiology/American Heart Association Task Force on Practice Guidelines. *J Am Coll Cardiol*. 2014;2014(63):2438–2488.

Palep JH. Robotic assisted minimally invasive surgery. *J Minim Access Surg*. 2009;5:1–7.

Popovic AD, Stewart WJ. Echocardiographic evaluation of valvular stenosis: the gold standard for the next millennium? *Echocardiography*. 2001;18:59–63.

Roberts R, Sigwart U. New concepts in hypertrophic cardiomyopathies: part II. *Circulation*. 2001;104:2249–2252.

Roselli EE, Pettersson GB, Blackstone EH, et al. Adverse events during reoperative cardiac surgery: frequency, characterization, and rescue. *J Thorac Cardiovasc Surg*. 2008;135:316–323, 323 e1–6.

Shah PM, Raney AA. Tricuspid valve disease. *Curr Probl Cardiol*. 2008;33:47–84.

Siminiak T, Wu JC, Haude M, et al. Treatment of functional mitral regurgitation by percutaneous annuloplasty: results of the TITAN Trial. *Eur J Heart Fail*. 2012;14:931–938.

Skubas NJ, Shernan SK, Bollen B. An overview of the American College of Cardiology/American Heart Association 2014 Valve Heart Disease Practice Guidelines: what is its relevance to the anesthesiologist and perioperative medicine physician? *Anesth Analg*. 2015;121:1132–1138.

IV

Chapter 16

Congenital Heart Disease in Adults

Victor C. Baum, MD • Duncan G. de Souza, MD, FRCPC

Key Points

1. Because of successes in treating congenital cardiac lesions, there are currently as many or more adults than children with congenital heart disease (CHD).
2. These patients may require cardiac surgical intervention for primary cardiac repair, repair following prior palliation, revision of repair due to failure or lack of growth of prosthetic material, or conversion of a suboptimal repair to a more modern operation.
3. Noncardiac anesthesiologists will see these patients for a vast array of ailments and injuries requiring surgery.
4. If at all possible, noncardiac surgery on adult patients with moderate-to-complex CHD should be performed at an adult congenital heart center with the consultation of an anesthesiologist experienced with adult CHD.
5. Delegation of one anesthesiologist as the liaison with the cardiology service for preoperative evaluation and triage of adult patients with CHD is helpful.
6. All relevant cardiac tests and evaluations should be reviewed in advance.
7. Sketching out the anatomy and path(s) of blood flow is often an easy and enlightening aid in simplifying apparently very complex lesions.

Advances in perioperative care for children with congenital heart disease (CHD) over the past several decades have resulted in an ever-increasing number of these children reaching adulthood with their cardiac lesions palliated or repaired. The first paper on adult CHD (ACHD) was published in 1973. The field has grown such that several texts are now devoted to it, and a dedicated specialty society, the International Society for Adult Congenital Heart Disease (http://www.isachd.org), was formed in the 1990s. Each year an estimated 32,000 new cases of CHD occur in the United States and 1.5 million worldwide. More than 85% of infants born with CHD are expected to grow to adulthood. It is estimated that there are more than 1 million adults with CHD in the United States and 1.2 million in Europe, and this population is growing at approximately 5% per year; 55% of these adults remain at moderate-to-high risk, and more than 115,000 in the US have complex disease. These patients can be seen by anesthesiologists for primary cardiac repair, repair following a prior palliation, revision of repair due to failure or lack of growth of prosthetic material, or conversion of a suboptimal repair to a more modern operation (Box 16.1). In addition, these adults with CHD will be seen for the other common ailments of aging and trauma that require surgical intervention. Although it has been suggested that teenagers and adults can have repair of congenital cardiac defects with morbidity and mortality approaching that of surgery done during childhood, these data are limited and may reflect only a relatively young and acyanotic sampling. Other data suggest that, in

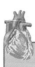

IV

> **BOX 16.1** *Indications for Cardiac Surgery in Adults With Congenital Heart Disease*
>
> Primary repair
> Total correction following palliation
> Revision of total correction
> Conversion of suboptimal obsolescent operation into more modern repair
> Heart transplantation

general, adults over 50 years of age represent an excessive proportion of the early postoperative mortality encountered, and the number of previous operations and cyanosis are both risk factors.

These patients bring with them anatomic and physiologic complexities of which physicians accustomed to caring for adults may be unaware, as well as medical problems associated with aging or pregnancy that might not be familiar to physicians used to caring for children. This has led to the establishment of the growing subspecialty of ACHD. The American College of Cardiology reviewed the available evidence and published superb guidelines for the care of these patients in 2008. A major recommendation was that adult patients with moderate or complex CHD be cared for in specialized adult congenital heart centers. An informed anesthesiologist is a critical member of the team required to care optimally for these patients. A specific recommendation was that noncardiac surgery on adult patients with moderate-to-complex CHD be done at an adult congenital heart center (regional centers) with the consultation of an anesthesiologist experienced with ACHD. In fact, one of the founding fathers of the subspecialty wrote, "A cardiac anesthesiologist with experience in CHD is pivotal…The cardiac anesthesiologist and the attending cardiologist are more important than the noncardiac surgeon." Despite this recommendation, the majority of adult patients with CHD having ambulatory surgery appear not to be having their surgery at ACHD centers.

GENERAL NONCARDIAC ISSUES WITH LONGSTANDING CONGENITAL HEART DISEASE

A variety of organ systems can be affected by long-standing CHD; these are summarized in Box 16.2. Because congenital cardiac disease can be one manifestation of a multiorgan genetic or dysmorphic syndrome, all patients require a full review of systems and examination.

CARDIAC ISSUES

The basic hemodynamic effects of an anatomic cardiac lesion can be modified by time and by the superimposed effects of chronic cyanosis, pulmonary disease, or the effects of aging. Although surgical cure is the goal, true universal cure, without residua, sequelae, or complications, is uncommon on a population-wide basis. Exceptions include closure of a nonpulmonary hypertensive patent ductus arteriosus (PDA) or atrial septal defect (ASD), probably in childhood. Although there have been reports of series of surgeries

BOX 16.2 *Potential Noncardiac Organ Involvement in Patients With Congenital Heart Disease*

Potential Respiratory Implications

- Decreased compliance (with increased pulmonary blood flow or impediment to pulmonary venous drainage)
- Compression of airways by large, hypertensive pulmonary arteries
- Compression of bronchioles
- Scoliosis
- Hemoptysis (with end-stage Eisenmenger syndrome)
- Phrenic nerve injury (prior thoracic surgery)
- Recurrent laryngeal nerve injury (prior thoracic surgery; very rarely from encroachment of cardiac structures)
- Blunted ventilatory response to hypoxemia (with cyanosis)
- Underestimation of $PaCO_2$ by capnometry in cyanotic patients

Potential Hematologic Implications

- Symptomatic hyperviscosity
- Bleeding diathesis
- Abnormal von Willebrand factor
- Artifactually elevated prothrombin/partial thromboplastin times with erythrocytic blood
- Artifactual thrombocytopenia with erythrocytic blood
- Gallstones

Potential Renal Implication

- Hyperuricemia and arthralgias (with cyanosis)

Potential Neurologic Implications

- Paradoxical emboli
- Brain abscess (with right-to-left shunts)
- Seizure (from old brain abscess focus)
- Intrathoracic nerve injury (iatrogenic phrenic, recurrent laryngeal, or sympathetic trunk injury)

16

on adults with CHD, the wide variety of defects and sequelae from prior surgery make generalizations difficult, if not impossible. Poor myocardial function can be inherent in the CHD but can also be affected by long-standing cyanosis or superimposed surgical injury, including inadequate intraoperative myocardial protection. This is particularly true of adults who had their cardiac repair several decades ago when myocardial protection may not have been as good and when repair was undertaken at an older age. Postoperative arrhythmias are common, particularly when surgery entails long atrial suture lines. Thrombi can be found in these atria precluding immediate cardioversion. Bradyarrhythmias can be secondary to surgical injury to the sinus node or conducting tissue or can be a component of the cardiac defect.

The number of cardiac lesions and subtypes, together with the large number of contemporary and obsolescent palliative and corrective surgical procedures, make a complete discussion of all CHD impossible. The reader is referred to one of the current texts on pediatric cardiac anesthesia for more detailed descriptions of these lesions, the available surgical repairs, and the anesthetic implications during primary repair. Some general perioperative guidelines to caring for these patients are offered in Box 16.3.

BOX 16.3 *General Approach to Anesthesia for Patients With Congenital Heart Disease*

General

- The best care for both cardiac and noncardiac surgery in adult patients with congenital heart disease (CHD) is afforded in a center with a multidisciplinary team experienced in the care of adults with CHD and knowledgeable about both the anatomy and physiology of CHD and the manifestations and considerations specific to adults with CHD.

Preoperative

- Review most recent laboratory data, catheterization, and echocardiogram, and other imaging data. The most recent office letter from the cardiologist is often most helpful. Obtain and review these in advance.
- Drawing a diagram of the heart with saturations, pressures, and direction of blood flow often clarifies complex and superficially unfamiliar anatomy and physiology.
- Avoid prolonged fast if patient is erythrocytotic to avoid hemoconcentration.
- No generalized contraindication to preoperative sedation.

Intraoperative

- Large-bore intravenous access for redo sternotomy and cyanotic patients.
- Avoid air bubbles in all intravenous catheters. There can be transient right-to-left shunting even in lesions with predominant left-to-right shunting (filters are available but will severely restrict ability to give volume and blood).
- Apply external defibrillator pads for redo sternotomies and patients with poor cardiac function.
- Appropriate endocarditis prophylaxis (orally or intravenously before skin incision).
- Consider antifibrinolytic therapy, especially for patients with prior sternotomy.
- Transesophageal echocardiography for cardiac operations.
- Modulate pulmonary and systemic vascular resistances as appropriate pharmacologically and by modifications in ventilation.

Postoperative

- Appropriate pain control (cyanotic patients have normal ventilatory response to hypercarbia and narcotics).
- Maintain hematocrit appropriate for arterial saturation.
- Maintain central venous and left atrial pressures appropriate for altered ventricular diastolic compliance or presence of beneficial atrial level shunting.
- PaO_2 may not increase significantly with the application of supplemental oxygen in the face of right-to-left shunting. Similarly, neither will it decrease much with the withdrawal of oxygen (in the absence of lung pathology).

Aortic Stenosis

Valvular aortic stenosis is the most common congenital heart defect but is often not seen in that light because it typically does not cause problems until adulthood. Most aortic stenosis in adults is due to a congenitally malformed bicuspid valve that does not become problematic until late middle age or beyond, although endocarditis risk is lifelong. Once symptoms (angina, syncope, near-syncope, heart failure) develop, survival is markedly shortened. Median survival is 5 years after the development of angina, 3 years after syncope, and 2 years after heart failure. Anesthetic management of aortic stenosis does not vary whether the stenosis is congenital (most common) or acquired.

Aortopulmonary Shunts

Depending on their age, adult patients may have had one or more of several aortopulmonary shunts to palliate cyanosis during childhood. These are shown in Fig. 16.1. Although lifesaving, these shunts had considerable shortcomings in the long term. All were inherently inefficient, because some of the oxygenated blood returning through the pulmonary veins to the left atrium and ventricle would then return to the lungs through the shunt, thus volume loading the ventricle. It was difficult to quantify the size of the earlier shunts, such as the Waterston (side-to-side ascending aorta to right pulmonary artery) and Potts (side-to-side descending aorta to left pulmonary artery). If too small, the patient was left excessively cyanotic; if too large, there was pulmonary overcirculation with the risk of developing pulmonary vascular disease. The Waterston, in fact, could on occasion stream blood flow unequally, resulting in a hyperperfused, hypertensive ipsilateral (right) pulmonary artery and a hypoperfused contralateral (left) pulmonary artery. There were also surgical issues when complete repair became possible. Takedown of Waterston shunts often required a pulmonary arterioplasty to correct deformity of the pulmonary artery at the site of the anastomosis, and the posteriorly located Potts anastomoses could not be taken down from a median sternotomy. Patients with a classic Blalock-Taussig shunt almost always lack palpable pulses on the side of the shunt, and arm length and strength can be mildly affected. Even if there is a palpable pulse (from collateral flow around the shoulder), blood pressure obtained from that arm will be artifactually low. Even after a modified Blalock-Taussig shunt (using a piece of GORE-TEX tubing instead of an end-to-side

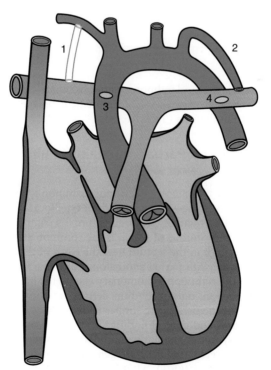

Fig. 16.1 The various aortopulmonary anastomoses. The illustrated heart is one with tetralogy of Fallot. The anastomoses are *(1)*, modified Blalock-Taussig, *(2)* classic Blalock-Taussig, *(3)* Waterston (Waterston-Cooley), and *(4)* Potts. (Reprinted with permission from Baum VC. The adult with congenital heart disease. *J Cardiothorac Vasc Anesth.* 1996;10:261.)

16

Table 16.1	Aortopulmonary Shunts	
Shunt	**Anatomy**	**Current Status**
Waterston	Ascending aorta → right pulmonary artery	No longer done
Potts	Descending aorta → left pulmonary artery	No longer done
Classic Blalock-Taussig	Subclavian artery → ipsilateral pulmonary artery	No longer done
Modified Blalock-Taussig	GORE-TEX tube subclavian artery → ipsilateral pulmonary artery	Current
Central shunt	GORE-TEX tube ascending aorta → main pulmonary artery	Current

BOX 16.4 *Complications of Atrial Septal Defect in Adulthood*

Paradoxical emboli
Effort dyspnea
Atrial tachyarrhythmias
Right-sided failure with pregnancy
Pulmonary hypertension
↑ Right-sided failure with ↓ left ventricular compliance with aging
Mitral insufficiency

anastomosis of the subclavian and pulmonary arteries), there can be a blood pressure disparity between the arms. To ensure a valid measurement, preoperative blood pressure should be measured in both arms (Table 16.1).

Atrial Septal Defect and Partial Anomalous Pulmonary Venous Return

There are several anatomic types of ASD. The most common type—and, if otherwise undefined, the presumptive type—is the secundum type located in the midseptum. The primum type at the lower end of the atrial septum is a component of endocardial cushion defects, the most primitive of which is the common atrioventricular canal. The sinus venosus type, high in the septum near the entry of the superior vena cava, is almost always associated with partial anomalous pulmonary venous return, most frequently drainage of the right upper pulmonary vein to the low superior vena cava. For purposes of this section, only secundum defects are considered, although the natural histories of all of the defects are similar (Box 16.4).

Because the symptoms and clinical findings of an ASD can be quite subtle and patients often remain asymptomatic until adulthood, ASDs represent approximately one-third of all CHD discovered in adults. Although asymptomatic survival to adulthood is common, significant shunts ($\dot{Q}_p/\dot{Q}_s$ >1.5:1) will probably cause symptoms over time, and paradoxical emboli can occur through defects with smaller shunts. Effort dyspnea occurs in 30% by the third decade, and atrial flutter or fibrillation in about 10% by age 40. The avoidance of complications developing in adulthood provides

IV

the rationale for surgical repair of asymptomatic children. The mortality for a patient with an uncorrected ASD is 6% per year over 40 years of age, and essentially all patients over 60 years of age are symptomatic. Large unrepaired defects can cause death from atrial tachyarrhythmias or right ventricular failure in 30- to 40-year-old patients. With the decreased left ventricular diastolic compliance accompanying the systemic hypertension or coronary artery disease that is common with aging, left-to-right shunting increases with age. Pulmonary vascular disease typically does not develop until after the age of 40, unlike ventricular or ductal level shunts, which can lead to it in early childhood. Paradoxical emboli remain a lifelong risk.

Late closure of the defect, after 5 years of age, has been associated with incomplete resolution of right ventricular dilation. Left ventricular dysfunction has been reported in some patients having defect closure in adulthood, and closure, particularly in middle age, may not prevent the development of atrial tachyarrhythmias or stroke. Survival of patients without pulmonary vascular disease has been reported to be best if operated on before 24 years of age, intermediate if operated on between 25 and 41 years of age, and worst if operated on thereafter. However, more recent series have shown that even at ages over 40, surgical repair provides an overall survival and complication-free benefit compared with medical management. Surgical morbidity in these patients is primarily atrial fibrillation, atrial flutter, or junctional rhythm. Current practice is to close these defects in adults in the catheterization laboratory via transvascular devices if anatomically practical (Fig. 16.2). Device closure is inappropriate if the defect is associated with anomalous pulmonary venous drainage. The indications for closure with a transvascular device are the same as for surgical closure.

Although some discussion is given to onset times with intravenous or inhalation induction agents, clinical differences are hard to notice with modern low-solubility volatile agents. Thermodilution cardiac output reflects pulmonary blood flow, which will be in excess of systemic blood flow. Pulmonary arterial catheters are not routinely indicated. Patients generally tolerate any appropriate anesthetic; however, particular care should be taken in patients with pulmonary arterial hypertension or right-sided failure.

Coarctation of the Aorta

Unrepaired coarctation of the aorta in the adult brings with it significant morbidity and mortality. Mortality is 25% by age 20, 50% by age 30, 75% by age 50, and 90% by age 60. Left ventricular aneurysms, rupture of cerebral aneurysms, and dissection of a postcoarctation aneurysm all contribute to the excessive mortality. Left ventricular failure can occur in patients over 40 with unrepaired lesions. If repair is not undertaken early, there is incremental risk for the development of premature coronary atherosclerosis. Even with surgery, coronary artery disease remains the leading cause of death 11 to 25 years after surgery. Coarctation is accompanied by a bicuspid aortic valve in the majority of patients. Although endocarditis of this abnormal valve is a lifelong risk, these valves often do not become stenotic until middle age or later. Coarctation can also be associated with mitral valve abnormalities (Box 16.5).

Aneurysms at the site of coarctation repair can develop years later, and restenosis as well can develop in adolescence or adulthood. Repair includes resection of the coarctation and end-to-end anastomosis. Because this sometimes resulted in recoarctation when done in infancy, for many years a common repair was the Waldhausen or subclavian flap operation, in which the left subclavian artery is ligated and the proximal segment opened and rotated as a flap to open the area of the coarctation. Aneurysms

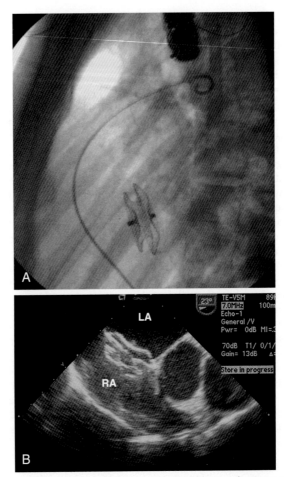

Fig. 16.2 Closure of an atrial septal defect in an adult with use of a transvascular device (the Amplatzer septal occluder). (A) Radiograph. (B) Transesophageal echocardiogram. The device is clearly visualized spanning and occluding the atrial septal defect. *RA*, Right atrium; *LA*, left atrium. (Courtesy Dr. Scott Lim.)

BOX 16.5   *Complications of Aortic Coarctation in Adulthood*

Left ventricular failure
Premature coronary atherosclerosis
Rupture of cerebral aneurysm
Aneurysm at site of coarctation repair
Complications of associated bicuspid aortic valve
Exacerbation of hypertension during pregnancy

in the area of repair are a particular concern in adolescents and adults following coarctectomy. Persistent systemic hypertension is common following coarctation repair. The risk of hypertension parallels the duration of unrepaired coarctation. Adult patients require continued periodic follow-up for hypertension. A pressure gradient of 20 mm Hg or more (less in the presence of extensive collaterals) is an indication for treatment. Recoarctation can be treated surgically or by balloon angioplasty with stenting. Surgical repair of recoarctation or aneurysm in adults is associated with increased mortality and can be associated with significant intraoperative bleeding due to previous scar or extensive collateral vessels. It requires lung isolation for optimal surgical exposure and placement of an arterial catheter in the right arm. Endovascular repair by ballooning/stenting has proven useful for these patients.

Blood pressure should be obtained in the right arm unless pressures in the left arm or legs are known to be unaffected by residual or recurrent coarctation. Postoperative hypertension is common after repair of coarctation and often requires treatment for some months. Postoperative ileus is also common, and patients should be maintained NPO for about 2 days.

Eisenmenger Syndrome

The term *Eisenmenger syndrome* has come to describe the clinical setting in which a large left-to-right cardiac shunt results in the development of pulmonary vascular disease and has been the subject of recent reviews. Although early on the pulmonary vasculature remains reactive, with continued insult pulmonary hypertension becomes fixed and does not respond to pulmonary vasodilators. Ultimately, the level of pulmonary vascular resistance (PVR) is so high that the shunt reverses and becomes right to left. Clinically, patients who are cyanotic from intracardiac right-to-left shunting are deemed to have Eisenmenger physiology even though their PVR may not yet truly be fixed. This is the intermediate phase of the disease before progression to a truly fixed PVR. The degree of reactivity can be determined in the catheterization laboratory by measuring the pulmonary blood flow on room air, pure oxygen, and pure oxygen with nitric oxide added.

Patients may be on chronic therapy with drugs such as intravenous prostacyclin, an oral phosphodiesterase 5 inhibitor such as sildenafil (eg, Revatio), an oral endothelin receptor antagonist such as bosentan (eg, Tracleer), a prostanoid, or a soluble guanylate cyclase stimulator such as riociguat (Adempas). Because of the risk of pulmonary thromboses, patients may be on chronic anticoagulants.

Eisenmenger physiology is compatible with survival into adulthood. Syncope, increased central venous pressure, and arterial desaturation to less than 85% are all associated with poor short-term outcome. Other factors associated with mortality include syncope, age at presentation, functional status, supraventricular arrhythmias, elevated right atrial pressure, renal insufficiency, severe right ventricular dysfunction, and trisomy 21. Most deaths are sudden cardiac deaths. Other causes of death include heart failure, hemoptysis, brain abscess, thromboembolism, and complications of pregnancy and noncardiac surgery. These patients face potentially significant perioperative risks. Findings of Eisenmenger syndrome are summarized in Box 16.6. Surgical closure of cardiac defects with fixed pulmonary vascular hypertension is associated with very high mortality. Lung or heart-lung transplantation is a surgical alternative.

When noncardiac surgery is deemed essential and time permits, a preoperative cardiac catheterization may be helpful to determine the presence of pulmonary reactivity to oxygen or nitric oxide. Fixed PVR precludes rapid adaptation to perioperative hemodynamic changes. Changes in systemic vascular resistance (SVR) are mirrored

16

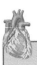

> ### BOX 16.6 *Findings in Eisenmenger Syndrome*
>
> Physical examination: Loud pulmonic component of the second heart sound, single or narrowly split second heart sound, Graham-Steell murmur of pulmonary insufficiency, pulmonic ejection sound ("click")
> Chest radiography: Decreased peripheral pulmonary arterial markings with prominent central pulmonary vessels ("pruning")
> Electrocardiogram: Right ventricular hypertrophy
> Impaired exercise tolerance
> Exertional dyspnea
> Palpitations (often due to atrial fibrillation or flutter)
> Complications from erythrocytosis/hyperviscosity
> Hemoptysis from pulmonary infarction, rupture of pulmonary vessels or aortopulmonary collateral vessels
> Complications from paradoxical embolization
> Syncope from inadequate cardiac output or arrhythmias
> Heart failure (usually end stage)

by changes in intracardiac shunting. A decrease in SVR is accompanied by increased right-to-left shunting and a decrease in systemic oxygen saturation. In addition, an acute fall in systemic resistance can impair left ventricular filling with the right ventricular encroachment. Systemic vasodilators, including regional anesthesia, should be used with caution, and close assessment of intravascular volume is important. Epidural analgesia has been used successfully in patients with Eisenmenger physiology, but the local anesthetic must be delivered slowly and incrementally with close observation of blood pressure and oxygen saturation. Postoperative postural hypotension can also increase the degree of right-to-left shunting, and these patients should change position slowly. All intravenous catheters must be maintained free of air bubbles.

Fixed PVR is by definition unresponsive to pharmacologic or physiologic manipulation, but, as previously mentioned, only patients at the true end stage of disease have fixed PVR. Thus the clinician must still avoid factors known to increase PVR, including cold, hypercarbia, acidosis, hypoxia, and α-adrenergic agonists. Although the last of these is commonly listed to be avoided, in the face of pulmonary vascular disease due to intracardiac shunting, the systemic vasoconstrictive effects predominate and systemic oxygen saturation increases.

Nerve blocks offer an attractive alternative to general anesthesia if otherwise appropriate.

If patients have general anesthesia, consideration should be given to postoperative observation in an intensive or intermediate care unit. Because of the increased perioperative risk, patients should be observed overnight, particularly if they have not had recent surgery or anesthesia, because their responses will be unknown. Ambulatory surgery is possible for patients having uncomplicated minor surgery with sedation or nerve block.

Although the perioperative mortality risk in the past has been estimated as high as 30%, estimates of mortality after noncardiac surgery in adulthood from more current series suggest that the mortality risk from noncardiac surgery and/or anesthetics is less than in the past.

Fontan Physiology

Fontan and colleagues proved that it was possible to deliver the entire systemic venous return to the lungs without the benefit of a ventricular pump. The Fontan operation was a landmark development in CHD because it established a "normal" series circulation in patients with a single ventricle. The price to be paid for a series circulation is the unique physiologic demand of passive pulmonary blood flow; Fontan's original operation was modified to an atriopulmonary connection (Fig. 16.3). Success of Fontan circulation was based on an unobstructed pathway from systemic veins to pulmonary artery, a pulmonary vasculature that was free from anatomic distortion (eg, from previous Blalock-Taussig shunt), low PVR, and good ventricular function without significant atrioventricular valve regurgitation. The incorporation of the atrium in the Fontan pathway proved disappointing. The atrium lost its contractile function, providing no assistance to pulmonary blood flow and causing serious complications. Understanding these complications and how the Fontan operation has evolved is the key to managing these challenging patients whose complex CHD has been palliated, not cured.

The Modern Fontan Operation

The atriopulmonary connection proved an inefficient method of pulmonary blood flow. Colliding streams of blood from the superior and inferior vena cavae resulted in energy loss and turbulence within the atrium. The energy required to propel blood forward into the pulmonary vasculature was lost as blood swirled sluggishly in the dilated atrium. The modern Fontan operation is a total cavopulmonary connection (Fig. 16.4). The lateral tunnel Fontan improved pulmonary blood flow, and only the lateral wall of the atrium was exposed to central venous hypertension. The extracardiac

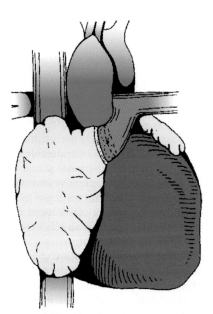

Fig. 16.3 The atriopulmonary modification of the Fontan operation. (Reprinted with permission from Kreutzer G, Galindez E, Bono H, et al. An operation for the correction of tricuspid atresia. *J Thorac Cardiovasc Surg.* 1973;66:613.)

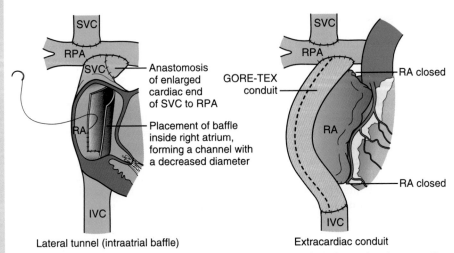

Fig. 16.4 Two variations of the modern Fontan operation, the lateral tunnel and extracardiac operations. *IVC,* Inferior vena cava; *RA,* right atrium; *RPA,* right pulmonary artery; *SVC,* superior vena cava. (Reprinted with permission from D'Udekem Y, Iyengar AJ, Cochrane AD, et al: The Fontan procedure: contemporary techniques have improved long-term outcomes. *Circulation.* 2007;116[11 Suppl]:I157.)

Fontan is a further modification of the total cavopulmonary connection. The extracardiac Fontan greatly reduces the number of atrial incisions and hopefully the long-term development of atrial arrhythmias. Has the modern Fontan improved outcomes? Reductions in arrhythmia and improvements in overall survival have been noted. Results for the extracardiac Fontan are even better than those of the lateral tunnel Fontan but are limited by the shorter duration of follow-up. It is not yet certain if the development of long-term complications has been truly reduced or only delayed.

Preoperative Assessment

IV

Patients with Fontan physiology are presenting in larger numbers for the entire array of noncardiac surgery. Patients with Fontan circulation have a low cardiac output state. This low output state exists despite the presence of good ventricular function, minimal atrioventricular valve regurgitation, and low PVR. Further compounding the issue is that patients' self-assessment grossly overestimates their objective exercise capacity. This places the anesthesiologist in a considerable dilemma when faced with a Fontan patient who rates his or her functional status as "good." Transthoracic echocardiography should be the initial preoperative investigation and is mandatory except in cases of very minor surgery. Further testing is guided by the results of the echocardiogram and in consultation with a cardiologist experienced in caring for adults with CHD. Normal ventricular function on echocardiogram would stratify the patient as "low risk" only within the context of patients with Fontan circulation.

A term that should immediately get the attention of the anesthesiologist is *failing Fontan.* Specific reasons for failing may differ, but the common denominator in these patients is a marked limitation of functional status. They will manifest some combination of refractory arrhythmias, liver dysfunction, hypoxemia, or congestive heart failure. Patients with a "failing Fontan" require a search for correctable lesions. First, any obstructions within the Fontan pathway should be treated, preferably with percutaneous techniques of dilation and stenting. Second, loss of sinus rhythm should be treated with pacing. If loss of sinus rhythm is accompanied by severe tachyarrhythmias, Fontan conversion surgery is indicated. Third, some patients develop collateral vessels. Aortopulmonary collaterals result in a progressive volume load on the single ventricle. The functional state of Fontan patients exists across a spectrum but generally falls into two groups. The first and largest group is made of those who report New York Heart Association (NYHA) I–II level of function but have been shown to possess much less cardiorespiratory reserve than age-matched two-ventricle controls. These patients will tolerate most surgical procedures with an acceptably low risk. The second group is smaller but consists of those patients who have manifested one of more of the "failing Fontan" criteria. Surgery in these patients carries much greater risk and should only be undertaken after careful consultation with physicians experienced in ACHD. When it comes to a discussion of anesthetic technique, the same lessons learned in caring for patients with acquired coronary artery disease apply. That is, there is no right drug for these patients, nor is there a single "best" anesthetic technique. Rather, the critical issue is to gain a clear and comprehensive understanding of the patient's pathophysiology. The key is not which drugs are used, but rather how they are used. Certain principles for patients with Fontan physiology are important and need to be stressed (Box 16.7).

Ventilatory Management

In an effort to minimize PVR, functional residual capacity should be maintained by the application of small amounts of positive end-expiratory pressure (PEEP) or continuous positive airway pressure (CPAP), and excessive lung volumes should be

---

BOX 16.7 *Management Principles for Patients With Fontan Physiology*

1. Maintenance of preload is essential. A prolonged NPO period without intravenous hydration should be avoided.
2. Regional and neuraxial techniques are attractive options, with appropriate attention to volume status. A neuraxial anesthetic is a poor choice if a high level of block is required. A slowly titrated epidural is preferable to a rapid-acting spinal anesthetic.
3. Airway management must be skilled to avoid hypercarbia and elevations in pulmonary vascular resistance (PVR).
4. Adequate levels of anesthesia must be established before stimulating events such as laryngoscopy. A surge of catecholamines may precipitate dangerous tachycardia.
5. Spontaneous ventilation that augments pulmonary blood flow is desirable but must not be pursued at all costs. Spontaneous ventilation under deep levels of anesthesia will result in significant hypercarbia. The benefit of spontaneous ventilation may be negated by the rise in PVR secondary to hypercarbia.
6. A plan must be in place to treat tachyarrhythmias.
7. Patients with pacemakers must have the device interrogated before surgery and a plan developed to avoid potential interference from electrocautery, particularly if the patient is pacemaker-dependent.
8. If large volume shifts are anticipated, invasive monitoring with central lines and transesophageal echocardiography is recommended.
9. An appropriate plan for postoperative pain management should be established. The need for anticoagulation in many Fontan patients may preclude the use of epidural analgesia.
10. A cardiologist experienced in caring for patients with congenital heart disease should be involved perioperatively.

16

avoided. PEEP or CPAP will not significantly impede cardiac output if less than 6 cm H_2O. Spontaneous ventilation has been assumed to be optimal for these patients to minimize intrathoracic pressure and encourage forward flow into the pulmonary circulation. Cardiac output should be optimized by limiting mean airway (intrathoracic) pressure: minimizing peak inspiratory pressure, limiting inspiratory time, using low respiratory rates, and applying judicious amounts of PEEP while using higher tidal volumes to maintain normocarbia. The benefits of very early postoperative tracheal extubation (in the operating room) have been considered particularly useful in these patients.

Tetralogy of Fallot

The classic description of tetralogy of Fallot includes (1) a large, nonrestrictive malaligned ventricular septal defect (VSD), with (2) an overriding aorta, (3) infundibular pulmonic stenosis, and (4) consequent right ventricular hypertrophy, all derived from an embryonic anterocephalad deviation of the outlet septum. However, there is a spectrum of disease with more severe defects, including stenosis of the pulmonary valve, stenosis of the pulmonary valve annulus, or stenosis and hypoplasia of the pulmonary arteries in the most severe cases. Pentalogy of Fallot refers to the addition of an ASD. With advances in genetics, up to one-third or more of cases of tetralogy have been ascribed to one of several genetic abnormalities, including trisomy 21, the 22q11 microdeletion, the genes NKX 2-5, JAG1, GATA4, and others. Tetralogy of Fallot is the most common cyanotic lesion encountered in the adult population. Unrepaired or nonpalliated, approximately 25% of patients survive to adolescence, after which the mortality is 6.6% per year. Only 3% survive to age 40. Unlike children, teenagers and adults with tetralogy do not develop "tet spells." Long-term survival with a good quality of life is expected after repair. The 32- to 36-year survival has been reported to be 85% to 86%, although symptoms, primarily arrhythmias and decreased exercise tolerance, occur in 10% to 15% at 20 years after the primary repair (Box 16.8).

It is uncommon to encounter an adolescent or adult with unrepaired tetralogy. However, it can be encountered in immigrants or in patients whose anatomic variation was considered to be inoperable when they were children. In tetralogy, the right ventricle "sees" the obstruction from the pulmonic stenosis. PVR is typically normal to low. Right-to-left shunting is caused by obstruction at the level of the right ventricular outflow tract and is unaffected by attempts at modulating PVR. Shunting is minimized, however, by pharmacologically increasing SVR. Because there is an unrestrictive VSD, in the unrepaired adult systemic hypertension developing in adult life imposes an

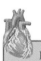

BOX 16.8   *Risk Factors for Sudden Death After Repair of Tetralogy of Fallot*

Repair requiring ventriculotomy
Older age at repair
Severe left ventricular dysfunction
Postoperative right ventricular hypertension (residual outflow tract obstruction)
Wide-open pulmonary insufficiency
Prolongation of the QRS

IV

additional load on both ventricles, not just the left. The increase in SVR decreases right-to-left shunting and diminishes cyanosis but at the expense of right ventricular or biventricular failure. Increases in the inotropic state of the heart increase the dynamic obstruction at the right ventricular infundibulum and worsen right-to-left shunting. β-Blockers are often used to decrease inotropy. Although halothane was the historic anesthetic of choice in children with tetralogy due to its myocardial depressant effects and ability to maintain SVR, current practice is to use sevoflurane, without undue consequence from a reduction in SVR. Anesthetic induction in adults can easily be achieved with any of the available agents, keeping in mind the principles of maintenance of systemic blood pressure, avoidance of hypovolemia, and preventing increases in inotropy.

Patients require closure of the VSD and resolution of the pulmonic stenosis. Although current practice is to repair the VSD through the right atrium in an effort to maintain competence of the pulmonary valve and limit any ventriculotomy, older patients will likely have had repair via a right ventriculotomy. A large right ventriculotomy increases the risks of arrhythmias and sudden death. Patients who have had a right ventriculotomy will have an obligate right bundle-branch block pattern on the ECG. However, unlike the more usual bundle-branch block in adults, this represents disruption of the His-Purkinje system only in the right ventricular outflow, in the area of the right ventricular incision. Because the vast majority of His-Purkinje conduction is intact, it does not carry increased risk for the development of complete heart block.

Some patients require repair of pulmonic stenosis by placement of a transannular patch, with obligate residual pulmonary insufficiency. Isolated mild-to-moderate pulmonary insufficiency is generally well tolerated, but in the long term, it can contribute to right ventricular dysfunction with a risk of ventricular tachycardia and sudden death.

Sudden death or ventricular tachycardia requiring treatment can occur in up to 5.5% of postoperative patients over 30 years, often years postoperatively. The foci for these arrhythmias are typically in the right ventricular outflow tract in the area that has had surgery, and they can be ablated in the catheterization laboratory. Older age at repair, severe left ventricular dysfunction, postoperative right ventricular hypertension from residual or recurrent outflow tract obstruction, wide-open pulmonary insufficiency, and prolongation of the QRS (to >180 milliseconds) are all predictors of sudden death. Premature ventricular contractions and even nonsustained ventricular tachycardia are not rare but do not seem to be associated with sudden death, making appropriate treatment options difficult.

Most adult patients require reoperation to repair the right ventricular outflow tract or to insert or replace a valve in the pulmonic position. Other reasons for reoperation include repair of an outflow tract aneurysm at the site of a patch, repair of a residual VSD, or repair of an incompetent tricuspid valve. These patients often have diminished right ventricular diastolic compliance and require higher-than-normal central venous pressure. Postoperative management includes minimizing PVR and maintaining central venous pressure. Patients often require treatment postbypass with an inotrope and afterload reduction.

Transposition of the Great Arteries (D-Transposition)

In D-transposition of the great arteries, there is a discordant connection of the ventricles and the great arteries. The aorta (with the coronary arteries) arises from the right ventricle, and the pulmonary artery arises from the left ventricle. Thus the two circulations are separate. Postnatal survival requires interchange of blood between the two circulations, typically via a patent foramen ovale and/or a PDA or VSD. With a 1-year

16

mortality approximating 100%, all adults with D-transposition have had some type of surgical intervention. Older adults will have had atrial-type repairs (Mustard or Senning), whereas children born after the mid-1980s will have had repair by arterial switch (the Jatene operation). Some will also have had repair of D-transposition with a moderate-to-large VSD by means of a Rastelli operation.

Atrial repairs result in a systemic right ventricle, and these patients consistently have abnormal right ventricular function that can be progressive with a right ventricular ejection fraction of about 40%. Mild tricuspid insufficiency is common, but severe tricuspid insufficiency suggests the development of severe right ventricular dysfunction. There is an 85% to 90% 10-year survival with these operations, but by 20 years, survival is less than 80%. Over 25 years, about half develop moderate right ventricular dysfunction and one-third develop severe tricuspid insufficiency. Although function always remains abnormal, it has been suggested that earlier surgery minimizes right ventricular dysfunction.

SUGGESTED READINGS

Andropoulos DB, Stayer SA, Skjonsby BS, et al. Anesthetic and perioperative outcome of teenagers and adults with congenital heart disease. *J Cardiothorac Vasc Anesth.* 2002;16:731.

Baum VC, Barton DM, Gutgesell HP. Influence of congenital heart disease on mortality following noncardiac surgery in hospitalized children. *Pediatrics.* 2000;105:332.

Baumgartner H, Bonhoeffer P, De Groot NM, et al. ESC guidelines for the management of grown-up congenital heart disease (new version 2010). *Eur Heart J.* 2010;31:2915.

Bennett JM, Ehrenfeld JM, Markham L, et al. Anesthetic management and outcomes for patients with pulmonary hypertension and intracardiac shunts and Eisenmenger syndrome: a review of institutional experience. *J Clin Anesth.* 2014;26:286.

Diller GP, Kempny A, Inuzuka R, et al. Survival prospects of treatment naïve patients with Eisenmenger: a systematic review of the literature and report of our own experience. *Heart.* 2014;100:1366.

d'Udekem Y, Iyengar AJ, Cochrane AD, et al. The Fontan procedure: contemporary techniques have improved long-term outcomes. *Circulation.* 2007;116:I157.

Marelli AJ, Mackie AS, Ionescu-Ittu R, et al. Congenital heart disease in the general population: changing prevalence and age distribution. *Circulation.* 2007;115:163.

Maxwell BG, Maxwell TG, Wong JK. Decentralization of care for adults with congenital heart disease in the United States: a geographic analysis of outpatient surgery. *PLoS ONE.* 2014;9:e106730.

Maxwell BG, Williams GD, Ramamoorthy C. Knowledge and attitudes of anesthesia providers about noncardiac surgery in adults with congenital heart disease. *Congenit Heart Dis.* 2014;9:45.

Maxwell BG, Wong JK, Kin C, et al. Perioperative outcomes of major noncardiac surgery in adults with congenital heart disease. *Anesthesiology.* 2013;119:762.

Maxwell BG, Wong JK, Lobato RL. Perioperative morbidity and mortality after noncardiac surgery in young adults with congenital or early acquired heart disease: a retrospective cohort analysis of the National Surgical Quality Improvement Program database. *Am Surg.* 2014;80:321.

Moons P, Engelfriet P, Kaemmerer H, et al. Delivery of care for adult patients with congenital heart disease in Europe: results from the Euro Heart Survey. *Eur Heart J.* 2006;27:1324.

Mutsuga M, Quiñonez LG, Mackie AS, et al. Fast-track extubation after modified Fontan procedure. *J Thorac Cardiovasc Surg.* 2012;144:547.

Mylotte D, Pilote L, Ionescu-Ittu R, et al. Specialized adult congenital heart disease care. The impact of policy on mortality. *Circulation.* 2014;129:1804.

O'Leary JM, Siddiqi OK, de Ferranti S, et al. The changing demographics of congenital heart disease hospitalizations in the United States, 1998 through 2010. *JAMA.* 2013;309:984.

Perloff JK, Warnes CA. Challenges posed by adults with repaired congenital heart disease. *Circulation.* 2001;103:2637.

Pillutla P, Shetty KD, Foster E. Mortality associated with adult congenital heart disease: trends in the US population from 1979 to 2005. *Am Heart J.* 2009;158:874.

Silversides CK, Marelli A, Beauchesne L, et al. Canadian Cardiovascular Society 2009 Consensus Conference on the management of adults with congenital heart disease: executive summary. *Can J Cardiol.* 2010;26:143.

Verheugt CL, Uiterwaal CS, van der Velde ET, et al. Mortality in adult congenital heart disease. *Eur Heart J.* 2010;31:1220.

IV

Warnes CA, Liberthson R, Danielson GK, et al. Task force 1: the changing profile of congenital heart disease in adult life. *J Am Coll Cardiol.* 2001;37:1170.

Warnes CA, Williams RG, Bashore TM, et al. ACC/AHA 2008 guidelines for the management of adults with congenital heart disease: a report of the American College of Cardiology/American Heart Association Task Force on Practice Guidelines (Writing Committee to Develop Guidelines on the Management of Adults With Congenital Heart Disease). Developed in collaboration with the American Society of Echocardiography, Heart Rhythm Society, International Society for Adult Congenital Heart Disease, Society for Cardiovascular Angiography and Interventions, and Society of Thoracic Surgeons. *J Am Coll Cardiol.* 2008;52:e143.

Webb GD, Williams RG. Care of the adult with congenital heart disease: introduction. *J Am Coll Cardiol.* 2001;37:1166.

Williams RG, Pearson GD, Barst RJ, et al. Report of the National Heart, Lung, and Blood Institute Working Group on research in adult congenital heart disease. *J Am Coll Cardiol.* 2006;47:701.

16

Chapter 17

Thoracic Aorta

Prakash A. Patel, MD • John G.T. Augoustides, MD, FASE, FAHA • Enrique J. Pantin, MD • Albert T. Cheung, MD

Key Points

1. Diseases of the thoracic aorta can occasionally be managed with medical treatment and surveillance, whereas others require surgical intervention. Depending on the disease process, some surgeries may be performed electively, whereas others are truly emergency operations.
2. Aortic surgery is complex, and therefore it requires an anesthetic tailored to the specific goals for hemodynamics, neuromonitoring, and cerebral/spinal cord perfusion.
3. Thoracic aortic aneurysms can cause compression of the trachea, left mainstem bronchus, right ventricular outflow tract, right pulmonary artery, or esophagus.
4. Deliberate hypothermia is the most important therapeutic intervention to prevent cerebral ischemia during temporary interruption of cerebral perfusion during aortic arch reconstruction.
5. Early detection and interventions to increase spinal cord perfusion pressure are effective for the treatment of delayed-onset spinal cord ischemia after thoracic or thoracoabdominal aortic aneurysm repair.
6. Severe atheromatous disease or thrombus in the thoracic or descending aorta is a risk factor for stroke.
7. Stanford type A dissection, involving the ascending aorta and aortic arch, is a surgical emergency. Stanford type B dissection, confined to the descending thoracic or abdominal aorta, should be managed medically when possible.
8. When adequate preoperative imaging is lacking, intraoperative transesophageal echocardiography can be used to diagnose type A dissection or traumatic aortic injuries that require emergency surgery.
9. Intraoperative transesophageal echocardiography and ultrasound imaging of the carotid arteries are useful for the diagnosis of aortic regurgitation, cardiac tamponade, myocardial ischemia, or cerebral malperfusion, complicating type A aortic dissection.
10. Newer endovascular approaches to the management of thoracic aortic disease continue to have a great impact on both elective and emergent aortic surgery.

Thoracic aortic diseases typically require surgical intervention (Box 17.1). Acute aortic dissections, rupturing aortic aneurysms, and traumatic aortic injuries are surgical emergencies. Subacute aortic dissection and expanding aortic aneurysms require urgent surgical intervention. Stable thoracic or thoracoabdominal aortic aneurysms (TAAAs), aortic coarctation, or atheromatous disease causing embolization may be addressed surgically on an elective basis. The volume of thoracic aortic procedures has grown steadily because of factors such as increased public awareness, an aging

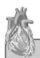

> **BOX 17.1** *Thoracic Aortic Diseases Amenable to Surgical Treatment*
>
> Aneurysm
> Congenital or developmental
> • Marfan syndrome, Ehlers-Danlos syndrome
> Degenerative
> • Cystic medial degeneration
> • Annuloaortic ectasia
> • Atherosclerotic
> Traumatic
> • Blunt and penetrating trauma
> Inflammatory
> • Takayasu arteritis, Behçet syndrome, Kawasaki disease
> Microvascular diseases (polyarteritis)
> Infectious (mycotic)
> • Bacterial, fungal, spirochetal, viral
> Mechanical
> • Poststenotic, associated with an arteriovenous fistula
> • Anastomotic (postarteriotomy)
> Pseudoaneurysm
> Aortic dissection
> • Stanford type A
> • Stanford type B
> Intramural hematoma
> Penetrating atherosclerotic ulcer
> Traumatic aortic injury
> Aortic coarctation
>
> Data from Kouchoukos NT, Dougenis D. Surgery of the aorta. *N Engl J Med.* 1997;336:1876–1878.

population, earlier diagnosis, multiple advances in imaging, and advances in surgical techniques, including endovascular stenting. Medical centers have emerged that specialize in thoracic aortic diseases, resulting in improved management and survival. This progress has created a set of patients who later require reoperation for long-term complications such as valve or graft failure, pseudoaneurysm at anastomotic sites, endocarditis, and/or progression of the original disease process into the residual native aorta.

The anesthetic management of thoracic aortic diseases has unique considerations, including the temporary interruption of blood flow, often resulting in ischemia of major organ systems. Critical components of anesthetic management include the maintenance of organ perfusion, protection of vital organs during ischemia, and monitoring and management of end-organ ischemia. As a result, the vigilant and skillful anesthesiologist contributes significantly to the overall success of these operations. The procedures performed by the thoracic aortic team for organ protection, such as partial left-heart bypass (PLHB) for distal aortic perfusion, cardiopulmonary bypass (CPB) with deep hypothermic circulatory arrest (DHCA), selective cerebral perfusion, and lumbar cerebrospinal fluid (CSF) drainage, are practiced routinely in no other area of medicine.

17

GENERAL CONSIDERATIONS FOR THE PERIOPERATIVE CARE OF AORTIC SURGICAL PATIENTS

Patients undergoing thoracic aortic surgery require the common considerations for the safe use of anesthesia and perioperative care that are addressed in this section (Box 17.2).

Preanesthetic Assessment

Identification of the aortic diagnosis is paramount because its extent and physiologic consequences dictate both anesthetic management and surgical approach. Aortic diseases proximal to the left carotid artery typically are approached via a median sternotomy, whereas aortic diseases distal to this point usually are approached via a left thoracotomy or thoracoabdominal incision. Although an aortic diagnosis often is established in advance, at times a definitive diagnosis must be verified after operating

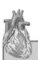

> **BOX 17.2** *Anesthetic Considerations for the Care of Thoracic Aortic Surgical Patients*
>
> **Preanesthetic Assessment**
>
> - Urgency of the operation (emergent, urgent, or elective)
> - Pathology and anatomic extent of the disease
> - Median sternotomy vs thoracotomy vs endovascular approach
> - Mediastinal mass effect
> - Airway compression or deviation
>
> **Preexisting or Associated Medical Conditions**
>
> - Aortic valve disease
> - Cardiac tamponade
> - Coronary artery stenosis
> - Cardiomyopathy
> - Cerebrovascular disease
> - Pulmonary disease
> - Renal insufficiency
> - Esophageal disease (contraindications to transesophageal echocardiography [TEE])
> - Coagulopathy
> - Prior aortic operations
>
> **Preoperative Medications**
>
> - Warfarin (Coumadin)
> - Antiplatelet therapy
> - Antihypertensive therapy
>
> **Anesthetic Management**
>
> - Hemodynamic monitoring
>   - Proximal aortic pressure
>   - Distal aortic pressure
>   - Central venous pressure
>   - Pulmonary artery pressure and cardiac output
>   - TEE

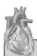

BOX 17.2   *Anesthetic Considerations for the Care of Thoracic Aortic Surgical Patients—cont'd*

- Neurophysiologic monitoring
  - Electroencephalography
  - Somatosensory-evoked potentials
  - Motor-evoked potentials
  - Jugular venous oxygen saturation
  - Lumbar cerebrospinal fluid pressure
  - Body temperature
- Single-lung ventilation for thoracotomy
  - Double-lumen endobronchial tube
  - Endobronchial blocker
- Potential for bleeding
  - Large-bore intravenous access
  - Blood product availability
  - Antifibrinolytic therapy
- Antibiotic prophylaxis

Postoperative Care Considerations and Complications

- Hypothermia
- Hypotension
- Hypertension
- Bleeding
- Spinal cord ischemia
- Stroke
- Renal insufficiency
- Respiratory insufficiency
- Phrenic nerve injury
- Diaphragmatic dysfunction
- Recurrent laryngeal nerve injury
- Pain management

room (OR) admission by direct review of diagnostic studies or by subsequent transesophageal echocardiography (TEE). In every case, a review of the operative plan with the surgical team facilitates thorough anesthetic preparation. Direct review of adequate aortic diagnostic imaging studies not only verifies the operative diagnosis but also determines the surgical possibilities. The anatomic details of an aortic disease permit the anesthesiologist to anticipate potential perioperative difficulties, including likely postoperative complications.

Anesthetic Management

Inherent in surgical procedure is the potential for massive bleeding and cardiovascular collapse. Therefore, it is essential to have immediate availability of packed red blood cells and clotting factors, large-bore vascular access, invasive blood pressure monitoring, and central venous access. Pulmonary artery catheterization assists in the management of cardiac dysfunction associated with CPB, DHCA, and PLHB. Intraoperative TEE is indicated in thoracic aortic procedures, including endovascular interventions, in which it assists in hemodynamic monitoring, procedural guidance, and endoleak detection A rationale exists for choosing to cannulate the left or right radial artery for intraarterial blood pressure monitoring. Right radial arterial pressure monitoring will often detect compromised flow into the brachiocephalic artery because of aortic cross-clamping too near its origin. Right radial arterial pressure monitoring also makes sense in procedures that require clamping of the left subclavian artery. Left radial arterial pressure monitoring is indicated when selective antegrade cerebral perfusion (ACP) is planned via the right axillary artery; however, a right-sided catheter may be preferred for ACP if direct brachiocephalic cannulation is used by the surgeon. At times, bilateral radial arterial pressure monitoring may be required. Femoral arterial pressure monitoring allows the assessment of distal aortic perfusion in procedures with PLHB.

Large-bore peripheral intravenous cannulation secures vascular access for rapid intravascular volume expansion. Rapid transfusion is desirable via an intravenous set with a fluid-warming device. Alternatively, large-bore central venous cannulation can be utilized for volume expansion. If a pulmonary artery catheter (PAC) is required, a second introducer sheath dedicated to volume expansion also can be placed in the same central vein. Central venous cannulation with ultrasound guidance often increases speed and safety, especially in emergencies. Both a urinary and a nasopharyngeal temperature probe are required for monitoring the absolute temperature of the periphery and core, as well as the rates of change during deliberate hypothermia and subsequent rewarming. The rectum is an alternative site for monitoring peripheral temperature, and the PAC can provide core temperature monitoring.

The induction of general anesthesia requires careful hemodynamic monitoring with anticipation of changes because of anesthetic drugs and tracheal intubation. Appropriate vasoactive drugs should be immediately available as required. Concomitant vasodilator infusions often are discontinued before anesthetic induction. Because etomidate does not attenuate sympathetic responses and has no direct effects on myocardial contractility, it may be preferred in the setting of hemodynamic instability. Thereafter, titration of a narcotic such as fentanyl and a benzodiazepine such as midazolam will provide maintenance of general anesthesia. In elective cases, anesthetic induction can proceed with routine intravenous hypnotics, followed by narcotic titration for attenuation of the hypertensive responses to tracheal intubation and skin incision. Antibiotic therapy optimally should be completed in most cases at least 30 minutes before skin incision to achieve adequate bactericidal tissue levels.

General anesthetic maintenance is typically with a balanced intravenous and inhalation anesthetic technique, and neuromuscular blockade is achieved by titration of a nondepolarizing muscle relaxant. Anesthetics can be reduced during moderate hypothermia and then discontinued during deep hypothermia. With concomitant electroencephalographic (EEG) and/or somatosensory-evoked potential (SSEP) monitoring, anesthetic signal interference is minimized with the avoidance of barbiturates, bolus propofol, and doses of inhaled anesthetic greater than 0.5 minimum alveolar concentration. Propofol infusion, narcotics, and neuromuscular blocking drugs do not interfere with SSEP monitoring. With intraoperative motor-evoked potential (MEP) monitoring, high-quality signals are obtained when the anesthetic technique comprises total intravenous anesthesia with propofol and a narcotic such as remifentanil without neuromuscular blockade.

The potential for significant bleeding and rapid transfusion is always relevant in thoracic aortic procedures. Consequently, it is prudent to have fresh frozen plasma and platelets available for ongoing replacement during massive red blood cell transfusion. The time delay associated with standard laboratory testing severely limits the intraoperative relevance of these data to guide transfusion; however, viscoelastic tests are being used with greater frequency to determine coagulation needs. Strategies to decrease bleeding and transfusion in these procedures include timely preoperative cessation of anticoagulants and platelet blockers, antifibrinolytic therapy, intraoperative cell salvage, biologic glue, activated factor VII, and avoidance of perioperative hypertension. The antifibrinolytic lysine analogs, epsilon-aminocaproic acid or tranexamic acid, are the commonly utilized blood conservation agents in thoracic aortic surgery with and without DHCA. Recombinant activated factor VII is a synthetic agent that accelerates thrombin production leading to hemostasis, and it may be considered for the management of intractable nonsurgical bleeding after CPB that is unresponsive to routine therapy. Although this agent has demonstrated efficacy in complex aortic surgery, concerns for arterial thrombotic events remain, requiring further trials to investigate perioperative safety. Finally, the use of fibrinogen concentrates in the management of coagulopathy continue to be investigated in cardiac surgery, with recent evidence suggesting decreased intraoperative bleeding when fibrinogen concentrates are used as a first-line therapy for coagulopathy after major aortic surgery.

Postoperative Care

With the exception of some endovascular aortic procedures, patients often remain intubated and sedated at the completion of the operation, when they are transported directly from the OR to the intensive care unit (ICU). The continuation of care from the OR to the ICU should be seamless and protocol-based. In the absence of complications, early anesthetic emergence is preferable for early assessment of neurologic function. If delayed anesthetic emergence is indicated, then sedation and analgesia can be provided. The chest roentgenogram allows confirmation of endotracheal tube and intravascular catheter position, as well as the diagnosis of acute intrathoracic pathologies. Common early complications include hypothermia, coagulopathy, delirium, stroke, hemodynamic lability, respiratory failure, metabolic disturbances, and renal failure. Frequent clinical and laboratory assessment is essential to manage this dynamic postoperative recovery, including the safe conduct of tracheal extubation. Given the risks associated with hyperglycemia after cardiac surgery, management of blood glucose levels should be standardized, with more recent data to suggest more liberal control (glucose less than 180 mg/dL) is acceptable with good outcomes. Antibiotic prophylaxis is typically continued for 48 hours after surgery to minimize surgical infection risk.

17

THORACIC AORTIC ANEURYSM

A thoracic aortic aneurysm is a permanent localized thoracic aortic dilatation that has at least a 50% diameter increase and three aortic wall layers. Localized dilatation of the thoracic aorta less than 150% of normal is termed *ectasis*. Annuloaortic ectasia is defined as isolated dilatation of the ascending aorta, aortic root, and aortic valve annulus. Pseudoaneurysm or a false aneurysm is a localized dilation of the aorta that does not contain all three layers of the vessel wall and instead consists of connective tissue and clot. Pseudoaneurysms are caused by a contained rupture of the aorta or arise from intimal disruptions, penetrating atheromas, or partial dehiscence of the suture line at the site of a previous aortic prosthetic vascular graft.

Thoracic aortic aneurysms are common and are the 15th most common cause of death in people older than 65. This disease process is virulent (Box 17.3) but indolent because it typically grows slowly at an approximate rate of 0.1 cm/year. The most common reason for more rapid degeneration is acute aortic dissection. Besides acquired risk factors such as hypertension, hypercholesterolemia, and smoking, current evidence points to the strong influence of genetic inheritance. The aneurysm's location and

BOX 17.3   *Complications of Thoracic Aortic Aneurysms*

Aortic rupture
Aortic regurgitation
Tracheobronchial and esophageal compression
Right pulmonary artery or right ventricular outflow tract obstruction
Systemic embolism from mural thrombus

extent determine the operative strategy and related perioperative complications. Aneurysms of the aortic root and/or ascending aorta commonly are associated with a bicuspid aortic valve. Dilation of the aortic valve annulus, aortic root, and ascending aorta pulls the aortic leaflets apart and causes central aortic regurgitation (AR). Aneurysms involving the aortic arch require temporary interruption of cerebral blood flow to accomplish the operative repair. Endovascular stent repair is an established therapy for aneurysms isolated to the descending thoracic aorta; however, ascending aorta stents have been employed in certain patients considered too high-risk for open surgery. Repair of descending thoracic aortic aneurysms requires the sacrifice of multiple segmental intercostal artery branches that compromises spinal cord perfusion and results in a significant risk for postoperative paraplegia from spinal cord ischemia.

Thoracic aortic aneurysms mostly are asymptomatic and frequently are discovered incidentally. Common symptoms of thoracic aortic aneurysm include chest and back pain caused by aneurysmal dissection, rupture, or bony erosion. The intrathoracic "mass effect" from a large thoracic aortic aneurysm can compress local structures to cause hoarseness (recurrent laryngeal nerve), dyspnea (trachea, mainstem bronchus, pulmonary artery), central venous hypertension (superior vena cava syndrome), and/or dysphagia (esophagus). Rupture of thoracic aortic aneurysms is a surgical emergency and is often accompanied with acute pain with or without hypotension. Although rupture of an ascending aortic aneurysm may cause cardiac tamponade, rupture in the descending thoracic aorta may cause hemothorax, aortobronchial fistula, or aortoesophageal fistula.

Surgical Considerations for Thoracic Aortic Aneurysms

Surgical repair aims to replace the aortic aneurysm with a tube graft to prevent further aneurysmal complications. For thoracic aortic aneurysm resection, indications include whenever the aneurysm is symptomatic regardless of size, evidence of rupture, an ascending aneurysm diameter greater than 5.5 cm, or descending aneurysm greater than 7.0 cm. Symptoms often herald the onset of rupture or dissection and should be interpreted as an urgent indication for surgery. A symptomatic presentation occurs in about 5% of patients. Unfortunately, the first symptom in the remaining 95% of patients often is death. Additionally, those patients who are undergoing open aortic valve procedures and who have an aortic root or ascending aortic diameter larger than 4.5 cm should be considered for concomitant aortic replacement (class I recommendation; level of evidence B).

Patients with aneurysms of the descending thoracic aorta should be considered for thoracic endovascular aortic repair (TEVAR) when technically feasible. Aneurysms of the ascending aorta and aortic arch are approached from a median sternotomy incision. Standard CPB can be used for the repair of aneurysms limited to the aortic root and ascending aorta that do not extend into the aortic arch by cannulating the distal ascending aorta or proximal aortic arch and applying an aortic cross-clamp between the aortic cannula and the aneurysm. Aneurysms that involve the aortic arch require CPB with temporary interruption of cerebral perfusion (DHCA). Neuroprotection strategies in this setting include deep hypothermia, selective ACP, and retrograde cerebral perfusion (RCP). Aortic aneurysms of the descending thoracic aorta require lateral thoracotomy for open surgical access. Aneurysmal resection requires cross-clamping with or without distal aortic perfusion.

Surgical Repair of Ascending Aortic and Arch Aneurysms

The type of surgical repair depends on aortic valve function and the aneurysm location and extent. Perioperative TEE can evaluate the aortic valve structure and function to guide and assess the surgical intervention (reimplantation, repair, replacement). Furthermore, TEE can assess the diameters of the aortic root, ascending aorta, and aortic arch to guide intervention. The most common aortic valve diseases associated with ascending aortic aneurysm are bicuspid aortic valve or AR caused by dilation of the aortic root (Fig. 17.1). If the aortic valve and aortic root are normal, a simple

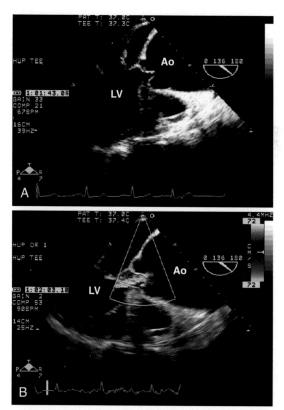

Fig. 17.1 Transesophageal echocardiographic midesophageal long-axis images of the aortic valve demonstrating aneurysmal dilation of the aortic root and ascending aorta (A). Doppler color-flow imaging (B) demonstrating severe aortic regurgitation caused by outward tethering of the aortic valve cusps by the aortic aneurysm. *Ao,* Aorta; *LV,* left ventricle.

17

tube graft can be used to replace the ascending aorta. If the aortic valve is diseased but the sinuses of Valsalva are normal, an aortic valve replacement combined with a tube graft for the ascending aorta without need for reimplantation of the coronary arteries can be performed. If disease involves both the aortic valve and the aortic root, the patient requires aortic root replacement and aortic valve intervention. If technically feasible, the aortic valve can be reimplanted, which includes graft reconstruction of the aortic root with reimplantation of the coronary arteries. If not feasible, aortic root replacement with a composite valve-graft conduit is indicated (Bentall procedure). Aortic root replacement requires coronary reimplantation or aortocoronary bypass grafting (Cabrol technique).

Anesthetic Management for Ascending Aorta and Arch Aneurysms

The conduct of general anesthesia in this setting has specific concerns. The imaging studies should be reviewed for aneurysm compression of mediastinal structures such as the right pulmonary artery and left mainstem bronchus. Prevention of hypertension increases forward flow in AR and minimizes the risk for aneurysm rupture. The preference for a left or right radial arterial catheter depends on the surgeon's approach to arch repair. Occasionally, bilateral radial arterial catheters can allow for simultaneous monitoring of cerebral and systemic perfusion pressures if arterial cannulation of the right axillary, subclavian, or brachiocephalic artery is planned for CPB and ACP. Nasopharyngeal, tympanic, and bladder temperatures are important for estimating brain and core temperatures for monitoring the conduct of DHCA. Monitoring of jugular bulb venous oxygen saturation and the electroencephalogram may reflect cerebral metabolic activity to guide the conduct of DHCA. Intraoperative TEE is essential to guide and assess the surgical interventions. In patients with AR, TEE can assist in the conduct of CPB by guiding placement of cannulae such as the retrograde cardioplegia cannula (coronary sinus) and by monitoring left ventricular (LV) volume to ensure that the LV drainage cannula keeps the ventricle collapsed. Intraoperative TEE is reasonable in thoracic aortic procedures, including endovascular interventions, in which it assists in hemodynamic monitoring, procedural guidance, and endoleak detection.

Neuroprotection Strategies for Temporary Interruption of Cerebral Blood Flow

The risk for stroke is substantial during the cerebral ischemia that accompanies aortic arch reconstruction. The first mechanism is cerebral ischemia due to hypoperfusion or temporary circulatory arrest during aortic arch repair. The second mechanism is cerebral ischemia due to embolization secondary to CPB and atheroma. Arterial embolic causes include air introduced into the circulation from open cardiac chambers, vascular cannulation sites, or arterial anastomosis. Atherosclerotic particulate debris may be released during clamping and unclamping of the aorta, the creation of anastomoses in the ascending aorta and aortic arch, or the excision of severely calcified and diseased cardiac valves. CPB may result in the microparticulate aggregates of platelets and fat. The turbulent high-velocity blood flow out of the aortic cannula used for CPB also may dislodge atherosclerotic debris within the aorta. Retrograde blood flow through a diseased descending thoracic aorta as a consequence of CPB conducted with femoral artery cannulation may cause retrograde cerebral embolization. For all these reasons, strategies to provide neurologic protection are essential in thoracic aortic operations (Box 17.4), and there exists a great degree of variation in the approaches used to protect and monitor brain function.

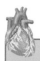

BOX 17.4 *Brain Protection for Aortic Arch Reconstruction*

Deep systemic hypothermia
Topical cerebral cooling
Retrograde cerebral perfusion
Selective antegrade cerebral perfusion
Cerebral hyperthermia prevention during rewarming

Deep Hypothermic Circulatory Arrest

The brain is extremely susceptible to ischemic injury within minutes after the onset of circulatory arrest because it has a high metabolic rate, continuous requirement for metabolic substrate, and limited reserves of high-energy phosphates. The physiologic basis for deep hypothermia as a neuroprotection strategy is to decrease cerebral metabolic rate and oxygen demands to increase the period that the brain can tolerate circulatory arrest. Existing evidence indicates that autoregulation of cerebral blood flow is maintained during deliberate hypothermia with alpha-stat blood gas management without compromise of clinical outcome. Direct measurement of cerebral metabolites and brainstem electrical activity in adults undergoing DHCA with RCP at 14°C indicated the onset of cerebral ischemia after only 18 to 20 minutes. Despite this observation, the large body of experimental evidence and clinical experience with deliberate hypothermia suggest that it is the single most important intervention for preventing neurologic injury in response to circulatory arrest.

Despite the proven efficacy of hypothermia for operations that require circulatory arrest, no consensus exists on an optimal protocol for the conduct of deliberate hypothermia for circulatory arrest. A strategy to protect the brain during aortic arch surgery must be a high priority in the perioperative management of these procedures to prevent stroke and optimize cognitive function. Although the average nasopharyngeal temperature for DHCA may be about 18°C, the optimal temperature for DHCA has not been established. A challenge in the selection of the ideal temperature for DHCA is the inability to directly measure the brain temperature. In an EEG-based approach to this question, the median nasopharyngeal temperature for electrocortical silence was 18°C, although a nasopharyngeal temperature of 12.5°C or cooling on CPB for at least 50 minutes achieved electrocortical silence in 99.5% of cases.

The conduct of DHCA extends CPB duration with consequent risks for coagulopathy and embolization. Rewarming increases cerebral metabolic rate and can aggravate neuronal injury during ischemia/reperfusion. Consequently, it is important to rewarm gradually by maintaining a temperature gradient of no more than 10°C in the heat exchanger and avoiding cerebral hyperthermia (nasopharyngeal temperature >37.5°C).

Retrograde Cerebral Perfusion

Although clinical studies would support the practice of limiting the duration of straight DHCA to shorter than 45 minutes to avoid the associated significant increases in stroke and mortality risks, the use of adjunct perfusion techniques for neuroprotection has allowed surgeons to work for longer periods of time in a safe manner. Similarly, these cerebral perfusion adjuncts have led to increased use of moderate degrees of hypothermia (20.1°C to 28.0°C). RCP is a cerebral perfusion technique performed by infusing cold oxygenated blood into the superior vena cava cannula at a temperature of 8°C to 14°C via CPB. The internal jugular venous pressure is maintained at less than 25 mm Hg to prevent cerebral edema. Internal jugular venous pressure is measured from the introducer port of the internal jugular venous catheter at a site proximal to the superior vena cava perfusion cannula and zeroed at the level of the ear. The patient is positioned in 10 degrees of Trendelenburg to decrease the risk for cerebral air embolism and prevent trapping of air within the cerebral circulation in the presence of an open aortic arch. RCP flow rates of 200 to 600 mL/minute usually can be achieved. The potential benefits of RCP include partial supply of cerebral metabolic substrate, cerebral embolic washout, and maintenance of cerebral hypothermia.

Selective Antegrade Cerebral Perfusion

Selective ACP should be considered for aortic arch repairs taking longer than 45 minutes. Compared with DHCA alone, the combined use of DHCA and selective ACP has been associated with superiority in terms of mortality outcomes. ACP typically is initiated during DHCA by selective cannulation of the right axillary artery, right subclavian artery, brachiocephalic artery, or left common carotid artery. In transverse aortic arch reconstruction procedures, ACP can be accomplished by inserting individual perfusion cannulae into the open end of the aortic branch vessels after opening the aortic arch. After reattachment of the aortic arch branch vessels to the vascular graft, ACP can be provided through a separate arm of the vascular graft or by direct cannulation of the graft. A functional circle of Willis may provide contralateral brain perfusion during interruption of antegrade perfusion in the brachiocephalic or left carotid arteries during construction of the vascular anastomoses. ACP with oxygenated blood at 10°C to 14°C at flow rates in the range of 250 to 1000 mL/minute typically achieves a cerebral perfusion pressure in the range of 50 to 80 mm Hg.

Unilateral ACP via right axillary arterial cannulation is a popular technique for adult aortic repair. This technique assumes an adequate circle of Willis; however, the anatomic completeness of the circle of Willis does not guarantee adequate cerebral cross-perfusion during aortic arch repair. Consequently, it remains essential to monitor the contralateral hemisphere in unilateral ACP with modalities such as cerebral oximetry, carotid artery scanning, and transcranial Doppler.

Pharmacologic Neuroprotection Strategies for Deep Hypothermic Circulatory Arrest

There are no proven pharmacologic regimens that have demonstrated effectiveness for decreasing the risk or severity of neurologic injury in the setting of thoracic aortic operations. The agents that have been reported in aortic arch series include thiopental, propofol, steroids, magnesium sulfate, and lidocaine. Furthermore, there is considerable variation in practice with these agents in aortic arch repair. In general, the existing evidence suggests that pharmacologic neuroprotection should be considered as a neuroprotective adjunct and not a substitute for hypothermia to protect against cerebral ischemia in the setting of hypoperfusion.

Descending Thoracic and Thoracoabdominal Aortic Aneurysms

Surgical therapy for descending thoracic and thoracoabdominal aortic aneurysms is to replace the aneurysmal aorta with a prosthetic tube graft. Surgical access is via lateral thoracotomy or thoracoabdominal incision. Despite recent advances, major

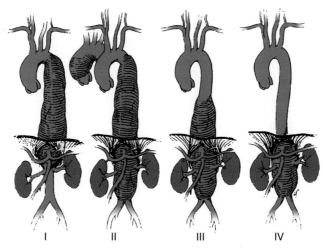

Fig. 17.2 Crawford classification of thoracoabdominal aortic aneurysm extent. (From Coselli JS, Bozinovski J, LeMaire SJ. Open surgical repair of 2286 thoracoabdominal aortic aneurysms. *Ann Thorac Surg.* 2007;83(2):S862–S864.)

I II III IV

surgical challenges remain because the typical patient is elderly with multiple significant comorbidities. The risks for spinal, mesenteric, renal, and lower extremity ischemia are significant because of thromboembolism, loss of collateral vascular networks, temporary interruption of blood flow, and reperfusion injury. The risks for wound dehiscence and respiratory failure remain significant because of the large incisions and diaphragmatic division, as well as injuries to the phrenic and recurrent laryngeal nerves. Consequently, TAAA repair is high risk.

Aneurysms of the thoracoabdominal aorta typically are defined by the Crawford classification (Fig. 17.2). Extent I TAAA begins at the left subclavian artery and ends below the diaphragm, but above the renal arteries. Extent II TAAA involves the entire descending thoracic aorta and ends below the diaphragm at the aortic bifurcation. Extent III TAAA begins in the lower half of the descending thoracic aorta and ends below the diaphragm at the aortic bifurcation. Extent IV TAAA is confined to the entire abdominal aorta. If an extent I or extent II TAAA involves the distal aortic arch, its surgical replacement often requires DHCA for the proximal anastomosis. The Crawford classification stratifies operative risk and guides perioperative management. Open repair of TAAA typically is accomplished by aortic cross-clamping with or without the addition of a shunt, PLHB, or partial CPB. The use of a shunt, PLHB or partial CPB is designed to provide distal perfusion during aortic cross-clamping,

Simple Aortic Cross-Clamp Technique

The major disadvantage of this technique, developed by Crawford, is the concomitant vital organ ischemia below the aortic clamp. Consequently, surgical speed is critical to achieve an ischemic time less than 30 minutes to limit the risk for vital organ dysfunction. Its further disadvantages include proximal aortic hypertension, bleeding, and hemodynamic instability on reperfusion. Despite anesthetic interventions, this proximal aortic hypertension may induce LV ischemia. Blood loss can be minimized with intraoperative red blood cell salvaging. Hemodynamic instability during reperfusion can be minimized with correction of metabolic acidosis, rapid intravascular volume expansion, vasopressor therapy, and/or gradual clamp release. Mild systemic hypothermia and selective spinal cooling protect against the ischemia associated with

17

> ### BOX 17.5 *Advantages and Disadvantages of Distal Perfusion Techniques*
>
> **Potential Advantages**
>
> * Control of proximal hypertension
> * Decrease left ventricular afterload
> * Less hemodynamic perturbations with aortic clamping and unclamping
> * Decrease duration of mesenteric ischemia
> * Decrease risk for paraplegia from spinal cord ischemia
> * Ability to control systemic temperature with heat exchanger
> * Vascular access for rapid volume expansion
> * Ability to oxygenate blood with extracorporeal oxygenator
> * Capability to selectively perfuse mesenteric organs or aortic branch vessels
> * Maintain lower extremity somatosensory-evoked potentials and motor-evoked potentials for neurophysiologic monitoring
>
> **Potential Disadvantages**
>
> * Require greater level of systemic anticoagulation
> * Increase risk for vascular injury at cannulation sites
> * Increase risk for thromboembolic events
> * Require perfusion team
> * Need to monitor and control upper and lower body arterial pressure and flow
> * Increase technical complexity of operation

this technique. Despite its physiologic consequences, this technique remains popular because it is simple and has proven clinical outcomes (Box 17.5).

Gott Shunt

Passive shunts allow for blood to be diverted from the proximal aorta to the distal aorta during aortic cross-clamping for thoracic aortic repair. One specific type is the heparin-coated Gott shunt. Blood flow from the proximal to distal aorta through the shunt depends on proximal aortic pressure, shunt length and diameter, and distal aortic pressure. Monitoring the femoral arterial pressure facilitates assessment of distal aortic perfusion and shunt flow. The advantages of the Gott shunt are its simplicity, its low cost, and its requirement for only partial anticoagulation. Its disadvantages include vessel injury, dislodgement, bleeding, and atheroembolism.

Partial Left-Heart Bypass

The control of both proximal and distal aortic perfusion during TAAA repair can be achieved with PLHB. This technique requires left atrial cannulation, usually via a left pulmonary vein. Oxygenated blood from the left atrium flows through the CPB circuit into the distal aorta or a major branch via the arterial cannula. The CPB circuit can include a heat exchanger, membrane oxygenator, and/or a venous reservoir. The degree of heparinization for PLHB is minimal with heparin-coated circuits without an oxygenator. Full systemic anticoagulation with ACT greater than 400 seconds is required for CPB circuits with membrane oxygenators and heat exchangers. During PLHB, the proximal mean arterial pressure (MAP; radial artery) is generally maintained in the 80 to 90 mm Hg range. Flow rates in the range of 1.5 to 2.5 L/minute typically maintain a distal aortic MAP in the 60 to 70 mm Hg range, monitored via a femoral

BOX 17.6 *Minimizing Paraplegic Risk After Thoracic or Thoracoabdominal Aortic Procedures*

Minimize Aortic Cross-Clamp Time

- Distal aortic perfusion
- Passive shunt (Gott)
- Partial left heart bypass
- Partial cardiopulmonary bypass

Deliberate Hypothermia

- Mild-to-moderate systemic hypothermia (32°C to 35°C)
- Deep hypothermic circulatory arrest (14°C to 18°C)
- Selective spinal cord hypothermia (epidural cooling, 25°C)

Increase Spinal Cord Perfusion Pressure

- Reimplantation of critical intercostal and segmental arterial branches
- Lumbar cerebrospinal fluid (CSF) drainage (CSF pressure ≤10 mm Hg)
- Arterial pressure augmentation (mean arterial pressure ≥85 mm Hg)

Intraoperative Monitoring of Lower Extremity Neurophysiologic Function

- Somatosensory-evoked potentials
- Motor-evoked potentials

Postoperative Neurologic Assessment for Early Detection of Delayed-Onset Paraplegia

- Serial neurologic examinations

Pharmacologic Neuroprotection

- Glucocorticoid
- Barbiturate or central nervous system depressants
- Magnesium sulfate
- Mannitol
- Naloxone
- Lidocaine
- Intrathecal papaverin

17

arterial catheter. Sequential advancement of the aortic cross-clamp during PLHB permits segmental aortic reconstruction with a decrease in end-organ ischemia. The advantages of PLHB include control of aortic pressures and systemic temperature, reliable distal aortic perfusion, and selective antegrade perfusion of important branch vessels. Its disadvantages include increased expense, increased complexity, and requirement for systemic anticoagulation (see Box 17.6). An alternative technique uses partial CPB by femoral vein to femoral artery perfusion with or without an oxygenator. This can allow for distal perfusion without the need for cannulation of the heart or aorta. However, it does not offer the control that is achieved with proper PLHB.

Cardiopulmonary Bypass With Deep Hypothermic Circulatory Arrest

When a TAAA involves the distal aortic arch, precluding an adequate cross-clamp site, CPB with DHCA is required to allow completion of the distal anastomosis. This technique has acceptable perioperative outcome for major reconstruction of the thoracoabdominal aorta because it also protects the spinal cord and mesenteric organs from ischemia. If CPB with DHCA is planned for TAAA repair through a left thoracotomy incision, TEE should monitor for aortic regurgitation so that any LV distension with the onset of asystole during deliberate hypothermia can be managed with insertion of a drainage cannula. The disadvantages of CPB with DHCA include the limited safe period for DHCA, risk for stroke from retrograde aortic perfusion, increased CPB duration, and bleeding. For TAAA with extension into the distal aortic arch, a two-stage elephant-trunk procedure can be performed instead of using CPB with DHCA. In the two-stage elephant-trunk procedure, the transverse aortic arch graft is performed first through a median sternotomy, leaving a short segment of graft extending into the descending aorta. The second stage of the repair is performed through a left thoracotomy incision to access and anastomose the distal end of the transverse arch graft to the proximal end of the descending thoracic aortic graft. This two-stage repair avoids the need for retrograde CPB perfusion through the diseased descending thoracic aorta and decreases the risk for injury to the recurrent laryngeal nerve, esophagus, and pulmonary artery located in the proximity of the distal aortic arch.

Endovascular Stent Graft Repair of Thoracic Aortic Aneurysms

Endovascular stent grafts are tube grafts reinforced by a wire frame that are collapsed within a catheter for delivery and deployment within the aortic lumen. The principle of TEVAR is that the deployed stent complex spans the length of diseased aorta to exclude blood flow into the aneurysm cavity. TEVAR requires a landing zone for each end of the tubular graft.

There are currently two major options for endovascular TAAA repair, namely, total TEVAR and hybrid TEVAR. Total endovascular TAAA repair requires customized stents that preserve major aortic branches with fenestrations or side branches. In hybrid TAAA repair, the landing zone for the nonfenestrated endovascular graft is created by aortic debranching procedures; for example, the renal and mesenteric arteries are anastomosed to the iliac arteries. This hybrid approach also has been used in aortic arch reconstruction for high-risk patients with aortic arch aneurysms. Furthermore, TEVAR recently has extended proximally for therapy of select aneurysms of the ascending aorta.

Anesthetic Management for Thoracoabdominal Aortic Aneurysm Repair

The anesthetic management of patients undergoing TAAA repair often requires selective right lung ventilation in the setting of a major left thoracotomy and anesthetic interventions to prevent spinal cord ischemia. Right radial arterial pressure monitoring typically is preferred, especially if the aortic repair involves clamping the left subclavian artery or surgical endovascular access via the left brachial artery. Femoral arterial pressure monitoring is required when distal aortic perfusion is planned either with PLHB or a passive shunt. Hemodynamic monitoring with a PAC usually is helpful for the management of the concomitant specialized perfusion techniques already discussed. The anesthetic plan must allow for spinal cord monitoring with SSEPs, MEPs, or both to account for decreases in renal function and decreases in spinal cord perfusion. Finally, a strategy for postoperative analgesia should be planned.

Lung Isolation Techniques

Selective ventilation of the right lung with concomitant left lung collapse during TAAA repair enhances surgical access and protects the right lung from left lung bleeding. Collapse of the left lung typically is achieved when the left main bronchus is intubated either with a double-lumen endobronchial tube (DLT) or a bronchial blocker. Routine fiberoptic bronchoscopic guidance guarantees the effectiveness of either technique. The increased length of the left mainstem bronchus facilitates placement of a left-sided DLT and subsequently anchors it during surgery. Endobronchial blockade is achieved with one of the following devices: the Arndt blocker, the Cohen blocker, or the Univent tube. Wire-guided endobronchial blocking catheters permit the balloon-tipped catheter to be guided and positioned precisely in the left mainstem bronchus with a fiberoptic bronchoscope. The advantages of a left DLT include the ability to apply selective continuous positive airway pressure to the left lung. Its disadvantages include increased difficulty in difficult airways and bronchial injury in distorted endobronchial anatomy. The major advantage of endobronchial blockade is its compatibility with an existing standard 8.0-mm endotracheal tube. This is advantageous in emergencies and in difficult airways. The disadvantages of endobronchial blockade include increased time for left-lung collapse and dislodgement during surgery. The majority of patients will require temporary postoperative mechanical ventilation, usually via a single-lumen endotracheal tube. ICU personnel often are unaccustomed to managing patients with DLTs with their risks for malposition, airway obstruction, and difficulty with airway secretions. Endotracheal tube exchange may be challenging if there is airway edema. An endotracheal tube exchange catheter in combination with direct laryngoscopy often facilitates safe endotracheal tube exchange.

Paraplegia After Thoracoabdominal Aortic Aneurysm Repair

Paraplegia after TAAA repair is a devastating complication. The temporary interruption of distal aortic perfusion and sacrifice of spinal segmental arteries during TAAA repair are central events in the pathogenesis of spinal cord ischemia and paraplegia. There are multiple contributing factors. The typical level of spinal cord ischemia after TAAA is midthoracic and is associated with a high perioperative mortality. There are many management strategies for prevention of this devastating complication after TAAA (Box 17.6).

The spinal cord arterial supply provides a partial explanation for the clinical features of paraplegia after TAAA repair. The anterior spinal artery supplies the anterior two-thirds of the spinal cord, and the posterior spinal arteries supply the posterior third. Branches from each vertebral artery join to form the anterior spinal artery that descends along the midline of the anterior surface of the spinal cord. The anterior spinal artery sometimes is discontinuous and fed in a variable extent by radicular arteries derived from ascending cervical, deep cervical, intercostal, lumbar, and sacral segmental arteries. The posterior spinal arteries also are derived from the vertebral arteries and receive collateral supply from posterior radicular arteries. The terminal cord segments are supplied by radicular arteries that arise from the internal iliac and sacral arterial network. The thoracolumbar spinal cord typically has multiple arterial sources with a clinical vulnerability to significant ischemia. In this watershed region, an important blood supply is derived from a large radicular artery (intercostal arteries T9–T12 in 75% of patients, T8–L3 in 15%, and L1–L2 in 10%). This important artery is known as the arteria magna or the artery of Adamkiewicz. Ischemia in the anterior spinal artery territory classically causes motor paralysis with preservation of proprioception. Clinical experience, however, has demonstrated that spinal cord ischemia after TAAA repair is variable, asymmetric, and can affect motor or sensory function, or both.

17

> **BOX 17.7** *Techniques to Decrease the Risk for Intraoperative Spinal Cord Ischemia*
>
> Mild systemic hypothermia
> Lumbar cerebrospinal fluid drainage
> Selective spinal cord cooling
> Distal aortic perfusion
> Minimizing the ischemic time
> Segmental aortic reconstruction
> Intercostal artery preservation
> Pharmacologic neuroprotection
> Intraoperative motor- or somatosensory-evoked potential monitoring
> Arterial pressure augmentation

Paraplegia is defined as lower extremity motor weakness with muscle strength weaker than gravity. Paraparesis is defined as lower extremity weakness with muscle power that allows movement at least against gravity. Spinal cord ischemia may have an immediate onset, defined as lower extremity weakness on emergence from anesthesia within 24 hours of the procedure. Delayed-onset spinal cord ischemia is defined as lower extremity weakness that follows a normal postoperative neurologic examination after emergence from anesthesia, and accounts for 37% of patients with postoperative paraplegia. Delayed-onset spinal cord ischemia can present days, weeks, or even months after TAAA repair. Immediate-onset paraplegia likely is a consequence of intraoperative spinal cord ischemia, leading to infarction that occurred during surgery. In contrast with delayed-onset paraplegia, recovery with intervention in immediate-onset paraplegia has not been consistently demonstrated. This lack of therapeutic response likely indicates that irreversible spinal cord injury has occurred. Consequently, strategies to prevent immediate-onset paraplegia are directed toward intraoperative spinal cord protection (Box 17.7). The objective of intraoperative spinal cord monitoring is to detect spinal cord ischemia for immediate intervention to improve spinal cord perfusion. Distal aortic perfusion maintains spinal cord function during aortic cross-clamping and improves the ability to monitor spinal cord integrity during surgery with SSEPs or MEPs.

Delayed-onset paraplegia indicates that, although the spinal cord was protected intraoperatively, it remains vulnerable to ischemia after surgery. Although the causes of this syndrome are incompletely understood, it often is preceded by hypotension. Strategies to minimize delayed-onset paraplegia include the prevention of perioperative hypotension, early anesthetic emergence for early and subsequent serial neurologic assessment, and lumbar CSF drainage (Box 17.8). Given the catastrophic sequelae of permanent paraplegia after TAAA repair, all reasonable attempts to treat delayed-onset paraplegia can be justified.

Lumbar Cerebrospinal Fluid Drainage

Lumbar CSF drainage is a strongly recommended spinal cord protective strategy for TAAA repair. The physiologic rationale is that reduction of CSF pressure improves spinal cord perfusion pressure (SCPP) and also may counter CSF pressure increases caused by aortic cross-clamping, reperfusion, increased central venous pressure, and/or spinal cord edema. Lumbar CSF drainage is performed by the insertion of a silicon elastomer ventriculostomy catheter via a 14-gauge Tuohy needle at the L3–L4 vertebral interspace. The catheter is advanced into the subarachnoid space and securely fastened to the skin at approximately 15 cm to prevent catheter movement while the patient is anticoagulated. The open end of the catheter is attached to a sterile reservoir, and CSF is drained when the lumbar CSF pressure exceeds 10 mm Hg. The lumbar CSF pressure is measured with a pressure transducer zero-referenced to the midline of the brain. Currently, the best strategy to manage a traumatic lumbar puncture or the drainage of blood-tinged CSF has not been determined. The lumbar CSF drainage catheter is inserted before or at the time of surgery for CSF drainage up to the first 24 hours after surgery. The lumbar drainage catheter subsequently can be capped and left in place for the next 24 hours. It then can be removed, assuming a normal neurologic examination and adequate coagulation.

The potential complications of lumbar CSF drainage include neuraxial hematoma, catheter fracture, meningitis, intracranial hypotension, and spinal headache. Neuraxial hemorrhage after lumbar drain insertion remains a risk in patients subsequently subjected to systemic anticoagulation for CPB. Despite this risk, the overall safety of this technique has been established in multiple case series. Measures to minimize neuraxial hematoma include establishing normal coagulation for both CSF catheter insertion and removal, as well as allowing a few hours between its insertion and heparinization for CPB. The complication rate associated with CSF drainage for thoracic aortic repair identified in two large series appears to be about 1%, with no spinal hematomas. Excessive CSF drainage is a principal risk factor for intracranial hypotension and subsequent subdural hematoma and suggests a limited CSF drainage protocol. For routine use, CSF only should be drained, using a closed circuit reservoir, when the lumbar CSF pressure exceeds 10 mm Hg. Meningitis is characterized by high fever, altered mentation, and CSF pleocytosis, often with bacteria. The risk for catheter fracture can be minimized by careful catheter removal.

Arterial Pressure Augmentation

The optimization of SCPP for spinal cord protection through arterial pressure augmentation is recognized. The principles of arterial pressure augmentation and CSF drainage for prevention and management of postoperative spinal cord ischemia are in relation to SCPP optimization. Spinal cord ischemia after TAAA repair is more likely in the setting of hypotension because the spinal arterial collateral network has been reduced due to factors such as intercostal artery sacrifice. Surgical techniques to preserve SCPP include selective intraoperative spinal cord perfusion and intercostal artery revascularization with interposition grafts. SCPP is estimated as the MAP minus the lumbar CSF pressure. In general, the SCPP should be maintained greater than 70 mm Hg after TAAA repair; that is, a MAP of 80 to 100 mm Hg.

Intraoperative Neurophysiologic Monitoring

Neurophysiologic monitoring of the spinal cord (SSEPs and/or MEPs) is recommended as a strategy for the diagnosis of spinal cord ischemia to allow immediate intraoperative neuroprotective interventions such as intercostal artery implantation, relative arterial hypertension, and CSF drainage. This management strategy may prevent immediate-onset postoperative paraplegia. SSEP monitoring is performed by applying electrical stimuli to peripheral nerves and recording the evoked potential that is generated at the level of the peripheral nerves, spinal cord, brainstem, thalamus, and cerebral cortex. Because SSEP monitors posterior spinal column integrity, MEPs have been advocated because they monitor the anterior spinal columns that are typically at risk during TAAA repair. MEP monitoring is performed by applying paired stimuli to the scalp and recording the evoked potential that is generated in the anterior tibialis muscle. Paraplegia caused by spinal cord ischemia significantly dampens lower extremity evoked potentials as compared with the upper extremity. Intraoperative comparison of upper and lower extremity evoked potentials distinguishes spinal cord ischemia from the generalized effects of anesthetics, hypothermia, and/or electrical interference. As discussed earlier, the anesthetic must be designed for minimal interference with the selected neuromonitoring strategy.

Spinal Cord Hypothermia

In addition to DHCA and moderate systemic hypothermia, topical spinal cord hypothermia is described with cold saline epidural infusion to avoid ischemia during TAAA repair. This technique may disseminate further, given its adjunctive benefit and the recent clinical development of a specialized countercurrent closed-lumen epidural catheter for epidural cooling during major distal aortic reconstructions.

Pharmacologic Protection of the Spinal Cord

Pharmacologic spinal cord protection with agents such as high-dose systemic gluco-corticoids, mannitol, intrathecal papaverine, and anesthetic agents has been described. Additional neuroprotective agents that have been studied in this regard include lidocaine, naloxone, and magnesium. Although there are multiple agents with potential benefit, only a few are utilized routinely in clinical practice.

Postoperative Analgesia After Thoracoabdominal Aortic Aneurysm Repair

It is well recognized that the extensive thoracoabdominal incision is very painful. Because epidural analgesia has proven outcome utility in this type of extensive incision, it typically is part of the analgesic plan after TAAA repair. The timing of epidural catheter placement and analgesia must take into account the perioperative anticoagulation status of the patient to minimize the risk for neuraxial hematoma. Furthermore, the epidural analgesia regimen should be formulated for a predominantly sensory block to allow serial motor assessment of the lower extremities and to minimize systemic vasodilation from a sympathectomy. For example, bupivacaine (0.05%), combined with fentanyl (2 µg/mL), can be initiated at a basal rate of 4 to 8 mL/hour after the patient exhibits normal neurologic function. Bolus administration of concentrated local anesthetic through the epidural catheter should be discouraged to avoid sympathetic blockade and associated hypotension. The epidural catheter can be inserted before surgery, at the time of surgery, or in the postoperative period.

Anesthetic Management for Thoracic Endovascular Aortic Repair

TEVAR has revolutionized the management of descending thoracic and TAAAs with significant clinical outcome benefit. The anesthetic management is based on the principles of care for patients undergoing endovascular abdominal aortic repair, but with the additional concerns of spinal cord ischemia and stroke. Typically, these patients undergo a balanced general anesthetic with invasive blood pressure monitoring and central venous access. Some centers have successfully performed these endovascular procedures using a local or regional anesthetic technique. However, it is important to differentiate neuraxial blockade effects from the effects of spinal cord ischemia. The right radial artery is preferred for blood pressure monitoring, given that the left subclavian artery frequently may be covered and/or the left brachial artery may be accessed as part of the procedure. TEE is reasonable in TEVAR in which it may assist in hemodynamic monitoring, procedural guidance, and endoleak detection. The risk factors for stroke after TEVAR include a history of prior stroke, mobile aortic arch atheroma, and TEVAR of the proximal or entire descending thoracic aorta. Therefore the detection of mobile atheroma in the aortic arch is an important TEE finding in TEVAR because it predicts a greater stroke risk. The risk factors for spinal cord ischemia after TEVAR include perioperative hypotension (decreased SCPP), prior abdominal/descending thoracic aortic procedures (compromised spinal collateral arterial network), and coverage of the entire descending thoracic aorta (significant loss of intercostal arteries). Consequently, indications for CSF lumbar drainage in TEVAR include planned extensive coverage of the descending thoracic aorta, history of prior abdominal/descending thoracic aortic procedures, and postoperative paraparesis/paraplegia despite relative hypertension.

▣ AORTIC DISSECTION

Aortic dissection results from an intimal tear that exposes the media to the pulsatile force of blood within the aortic lumen. Blood may exit the true aortic lumen and dissect the aortic wall to create a false lumen. The aortic dissection may remain localized at the primary entry site at the original intimal tear, or it may extend proximally, distally, or both. It also may extend into the aortic branch vessels to cause branch occlusion, or the intimal layer may shear at the site of branch vessels to result in intimal fenestrations. Propagation of the dissection into the aortic root can cause AR. The weakened aortic wall often results in acute aortic dilation, which can progress to rupture, resulting in pericardial tamponade, exsanguination, or both.

There are two generally accepted classifications of thoracic aortic dissections in regard to location and extent (Box 17.9).

Type A Aortic Dissection

Aortic dissections that involve the ascending aorta (Stanford type A) are considered surgical emergencies. The mortality rate without emergency surgery is about 1% per

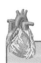

BOX 17.9 *Classification of Acute Aortic Dissection*

DeBakey Classification

- Type I: The entire aorta is involved (ascending, arch, and descending)
- Type II: Confined to the ascending aorta
- Type III: Intimal tear originating in the descending aorta with either distal or retrograde extension
- Type IIIA: Intimal tear originating in the descending aorta with extension distally to the diaphragm or proximally into the aortic arch
- Type IIIB: Intimal tear originating in the descending aorta with extension below the diaphragm or proximally into the aortic arch

Stanford Classification

- Type A: Involvement of the ascending aorta and/or aortic arch regardless of the site of origin or distal extent
- Type B: Confined to the descending aorta distal to the origin of the left subclavian artery

hour for the first 48 hours, 60% by about 1 week, 74% by 2 weeks, and 91% by 6 months. Immediate surgical intervention significantly improves the mortality rate, especially in patients younger than 80 years. The principal causes of mortality include rupture, cardiac tamponade, myocardial ischemia from coronary dissection, severe acute AR, stroke caused by brachiocephalic dissection, and malperfusion syndromes, including renal failure, ischemic bowel, and limb ischemia. An aortic dissection less than 2 weeks old is classified as acute and older than 2 weeks is classified as chronic. This distinction is clinically important because after 2 weeks, mortality risk has plateaued and thus emergency surgery is not necessarily indicated.

Type B Aortic Dissection

Aortic dissections confined to the descending thoracic aorta (Stanford type B) should be managed medically unless there are life-threatening complications present such as malperfusion and aortic rupture, as well as severe pain and/or hypertension despite aggressive medical therapy. Mortality with medical management in this type of aortic dissection is significantly lower than perioperative mortality. The greater operative mortality is due to the severe complications of type B aortic dissection and the operation itself. TEVAR for the therapy of complicated acute type B dissection is highly recommended.

Anesthetic Management for Aortic Dissection

Acute aortic dissection is a medical emergency. Initial medical management is directed at treatment of pain and decreasing the arterial pressure with antihypertensive agents. Vasodilator therapy should be initiated to decrease wall stress with control of heart rate and blood pressure. In the presence of acute AR, β-blockers should be used with caution because they block the compensatory tachycardia. In the absence of contraindications, β-blockers should be titrated to a heart rate of 60 beats/minute. Esmolol is a particularly useful β-blocker because it has a short pharmacologic half-life and can be rapidly titrated. In patients with β-blocker contraindications, heart rate control should be gained with titration of nondihydropyridine calcium channel blockers such as verapamil or diltiazem. If the systolic blood pressure remains greater than 120 mm Hg with adequate heart rate control, then vasodilators (eg, nitroprusside, clevidipine, or nicardipine) should be titrated for further reductions of blood pressure while still maintaining adequate vital organ perfusion. Vasodilator therapy should not be initiated before heart rate control to avoid the associated reflex tachycardia that might aggravate the aortic dissection.

In general, the anesthetic management of type A aortic dissection resembles the management of ascending aortic aneurysms that require DHCA. The anesthetic management of type B aortic dissections resembles the management of TAAA repair. Large-bore intravenous catheters are essential for intravenous medications and rapid volume expansion. A radial arterial catheter for invasive blood pressure monitoring is preferred over a femoral artery catheter to allow for CPB cannulation, depending on surgeon preference. If a pulse deficit is detected, the site for arterial pressure monitoring should be chosen to best represent the central aortic pressure. A central venous catheter or PAC to monitor CVP, pulmonary artery pressure, and cardiac output is useful. TEE insertion is performed after anesthetic induction, and it can be used to verify the diagnosis.

The induction of general anesthesia in hemodynamically stable patients with aortic dissection should proceed in a cautious manner. The dose of intravenous antihypertensive drugs may need to be reduced at the time of anesthetic induction to prevent severe hypotension when combined with anesthetic drugs. Hypotension may also occur on anesthetic induction in response to the attenuation of sympathetic nervous system tone or decreased cardiac preload caused by venodilation and positive pressure ventilation in patients with preexisting concentric LV hypertrophy. The hypertensive response to endotracheal intubation, TEE probe insertion, and sternotomy should be anticipated and attenuated with narcotic analgesics.

Surgical Treatment of Stanford Type A Aortic Dissection

Surgical repair for type A aortic dissection requires resection of the proximal extent of the dissection. The objective of surgical repair for type A dissections is to prevent death caused by AR, cardiac tamponade caused by rupture of the ascending aorta, myocardial infarction caused by dissection into the coronary ostia, and stroke caused by dissection into the aortic arch branches.

Although femoral arterial cannulation is popular for CPB, cannulation of the distal ascending aorta or the axillary artery (ideally with an end-to-end graft) has been associated with significantly enhanced clinical outcome. When central cannulation through dissected aorta is chosen, TEE is mandatory to verify initial wire placement in the true lumen. It remains important to monitor cerebral perfusion throughout the operative procedure for detection and correction of acute malperfusion. The use of selective cerebral perfusion techniques with circulatory arrest is reasonable to complete arch reconstructions to reduce neurologic complications.

In DeBakey type I dissections, the dissected descending thoracic aorta often undergoes aneurysmal degeneration and is responsible for significant aorta-related mortality in the long term. Consequently, long-term outcomes after extensive type A dissection would be significantly improved if this distal aortic degeneration could be prevented. Anterograde stenting of the descending thoracic aorta during

17

open aortic arch repair for DeBakey type I aortic dissection has been reported. This technique is also known as the endovascular stented elephant-trunk technique or the frozen elephant-trunk technique. The long-term aneurysmal degeneration of the descending thoracic aorta is prevented by immediate stenting in the acute dissection phase.

Integrated Management of Stanford Type B Aortic Dissection

Uncomplicated type B aortic dissection currently has the best clinical outcome when managed medically. Medical therapy for type B aortic dissection is directed at control of systemic hypertension to prevent aortic aneurysm formation, aortic rupture, and extension of the aortic aneurysm. In the presence of life-threatening complications, TEVAR has emerged as a preferred alternative therapy to surgery. Malperfusion syndromes associated with type B dissection also can be managed with intimal fenestration.

TRAUMATIC AORTIC INJURY

The most common cause of traumatic aortic injury is blunt chest trauma or rapid deceleration injuries associated with motor vehicle accidents or falls. Although this injury may be fatal, the majority of patients have injuries in the region of the aortic isthmus. Patients with traumatic aortic injury commonly will have associated significant injuries. TEE is helpful in the management of traumatic aortic injury because it is portable, is often available in the OR, provides a rapid diagnosis, and does not require aortic instrumentation or radiographic contrast injection. TEE also can detect cardiac tamponade, left pleural effusion, hypovolemia, ventricular dysfunction from myocardial contusion, or vascular injuries from penetrating chest wounds. Its disadvantages include limited imaging in the setting of facial injuries, suspected cervical spine injuries, and lesions in the distal ascending aorta. Injuries to the ascending aorta or aortic arch typically require CPB with DHCA for repair. Injuries to the aortic isthmus can be repaired via a left thoracotomy. The descending thoracic aorta usually is repaired with an interposition graft with the aid of PLHB. The risk for perioperative spinal cord ischemia is minimal when distal aortic perfusion is provided because only a short segment of the thoracic aorta is replaced. Although open repair is possible, TEVAR has emerged as the preferred intervention whenever possible.

SUGGESTED READINGS

Appoo JJ, Augoustides JG, Pochettino A, et al. Perioperative outcome in adults undergoing elective deep hypothermic circulatory arrest with retrograde cerebral perfusion in proximal aortic arch repair: evaluation of protocol-based care. *J Cardiothorac Vasc Anesth.* 2009;20:3–7.

Augoustides JG, Andritsos M. Innovations in aortic disease: the ascending aorta and aortic arch. *J Cardiothorac Vasc Anesth.* 2010;24:198–207.

Augoustides JG, Wolfe Y, Walsh EK, et al. Recent advances in aortic valve disease: highlights from a bicuspid aortic valve to transcatheter aortic valve replacement. *J Cardiothorac Vasc Anesth.* 2009;23:569–576.

Cheung AT, Pochettino A, Guvakov DV, et al. Safety of lumbar drains in thoracic aortic operations performed with extracorporeal circulation. *Ann Thorac Surg.* 2003;76:1190–1196.

Cheung AT, Weiss SJ, McGarvey ML, et al. Interventions for reversing delayed-onset postoperative paraplegia after thoracic aortic reconstruction. *Ann Thorac Surg.* 2002;74:413–419.

Davies RR, Gallo A, Coady MA, et al. Novel measurement of relative aortic size predicts rupture of thoracic aortic aneurysms. *Ann Thorac Surg.* 2006;81:169–177.

D'Elia P, Tyrrell M, Sobocinski J, et al. Endovascular thoracoabdominal aortic aneurysm repair: a literature review of early and midterm results. *J Cardiovasc Surg (Torino).* 2009;50:439–445.

Erbel R, Aboyans V, Boileau C, et al. 2014 ESC Guidelines on the diagnosis and treatment of aortic diseases: document covering acute and chronic aortic diseases of the thoracic and abdominal aorta of the adult; the task force for the diagnosis and treatment of aortic diseases of the European Society of Cardiology (ESC). *Eur Heart J.* 2014;35:2873–2926.

Estrera AL, Sheinbaum R, Miller CC, et al. Cerebrospinal fluid drainage during thoracic aortic repair: safety and current management. *Ann Thorac Surg.* 2009;88:9–15.

Etz CD, Weigang E, Hartert M, et al. Contemporary spinal cord protection during thoracic and thoracoabdominal aortic surgery and endovascular aortic repair: a position paper of the vascular domain of the European Association for Cardiothoracic Surgery. *Eur J Cardiothorac Surg.* 2015;47:943–957.

Frederick JR, Wang E, Trubelja A, et al. Ascending aortic cannulation in acute type A dissection repair. *Ann Thorac Surg.* 2013;95:1808–1811.

Gega A, Rizzo JA, Johnson MH, et al. Straight deep hypothermic arrest: experience in 394 patients supports its effectiveness as a sole means of brain preservation. *Ann Thorac Surg.* 2007;84:759–766.

Goldstein SA, Evangelista A, Abhara S, et al. Multimodality imaging of diseases of the thoracic aorta in adults: from the American Society of Echocardiography and the European Association of Cardiovascular Imaging: endorsed by the Society for Cardiovascular Computed Tomography and the Society for Cardiovascular Magnetic Resonance. *J Am Soc Echocardiogr.* 2015;28:119–182.

Gutsche JT, Cheung AT, McGarvey ML, et al. Risk factors for perioperative stroke after thoracic endovascular aortic repair. *Ann Thorac Surg.* 2007;84:1195–1200.

Gutsche JT, Szeto W, Cheung AT. Endovascular stenting of thoracic aneurysm. *Anesthesiol Clin.* 2008;26:481–499.

Hiratzka LF, Bakris GL, Beckman JA, et al. 2010 ACCF/AHA/AATS/ACR/ASA/SCA/SCAI/SIR/STS/SVM guidelines for the diagnosis and management of patients with thoracic aortic disease: executive summary. A report of the American College of Cardiology Foundation, American Heart Association Task Force on Practice Guidelines, American Association for Thoracic Surgery, American College of Radiology, American Stroke Association, Society of Cardiovascular Anesthesiologists, Society for Cardiovascular Angiography and Interventions, and Society for Vascular Medicine. *J Am Coll Cardiol.* 2010;55:1509–1544.

LeMaire SA, Price MD, Green SY, et al. Results of open thoracoabdominal aortic aneurysm repair. *Ann Cardiothorac Surg.* 2012;1:286–292.

Milewski RK, Szeto WY, Pochettino A, et al. Have hybrid procedures replaced open aortic arch reconstruction in high-risk patients? A comparative study of elective open arch debranching with endovascular stent graft placement and conventional elective open total and distal aortic arch reconstruction. *J Thorac Cardiovasc Surg.* 2010;140:590–597.

Patel AY, Eagle KA, Vaishnava P. Acute type B aortic dissection: insights from the International Registry of Acute Aortic Dissection. *Ann Cardiothorac Surg.* 2014;3:368–374.

Qian H, Hu J, Du L, et al. Modified hypothermic circulatory arrest for emergent repair of acute aortic dissection type A: a single center experience. *J Cardiothorac Surg.* 2013;8:125.

Sloan TB, Edmonds HL, Kohl A. Intraoperative electrophysiologic monitoring in aortic surgery. *J Cardiothorac Vasc Anesth.* 2013;27:1364–1373.

Svensson LG, Kouchoukos NT, Miller DC, et al. 2008 expert consensus document on the treatment of descending thoracic aortic disease using endovascular stent grafts. *Ann Thorac Surg.* 2008;85:S1–S41.

17

Chapter 18

Uncommon Cardiac Diseases

Jonathan F. Fox, MD • Mark M. Smith, MD • Gregory A. Nuttall, MD • William C. Oliver, Jr., MD

Key Points

1. Cardiac tumors are rare. In general, a cardiac mass is more likely a vegetation or a thrombus than a tumor. Secondary (metastatic) tumors are far more common than primary cardiac tumors. Among primary cardiac tumors, benign lesions are more common than malignant tumors.
2. Cardiac myxomas historically have been considered the most common benign cardiac tumor. Patients with myxomas typically exhibit signs and symptoms attributable to one of the triad of intracardiac obstruction, embolism, or constitutional symptoms.
3. Papillary fibroelastomas are the most common valvular cardiac tumor and may be the most common benign lesion as well. Typically solitary, fibroelastomas occur most frequently on the mitral and aortic valve leaflets. Once considered an incidental, benign finding, they have a high incidence of coronary and cerebral embolization.
4. Primary malignant cardiac tumors are less common than benign tumors. The overwhelming majority of primary malignant tumors are sarcomas.
5. Metastatic cardiac tumors are far more common than primary tumors. Pericardial involvement is the most common.
6. Carcinoid tumors are metastasizing neuroendocrine tumors. In patients with carcinoid syndrome, carcinoid heart disease is common and characterized by tricuspid regurgitation, mixed pulmonic regurgitation and stenosis, and right-sided heart failure. The mainstays of treatment are symptom management with somatostatin analogs, antitumor therapy, and cardiac surgical intervention.
7. Cardiomyopathies are a heterogeneous group of diseases that may be acquired or genetic and may be confined to the heart (primary) or may be part of a systemic disorder (secondary). The American Heart Association subclassifies primary processes as genetic, acquired, or mixed.
8. Dilated cardiomyopathy is the most common of the cardiomyopathies and may be acquired, hereditary, or idiopathic.
9. Hypertrophic cardiomyopathy is likely the most common inherited cardiac disease and may progress along one or more of three pathways: (1) sudden cardiac death, (2) heart failure, or (3) atrial fibrillation, with or without cardioembolic stroke.
10. The restrictive cardiomyopathies are heterogeneous and characterized by impaired myocardial relaxation and decreased ventricular compliance. Considering that their treatments are significantly different, restrictive cardiomyopathy and constrictive pericarditis must be distinguished.
11. The management of an incidental patent foramen ovale found during cardiac surgery via transesophageal echocardiography continues to evolve; however, few data suggest that closure offers morbidity or mortality benefit and may actually increase the risk of postoperative stroke.

Although some of the diseases discussed are quite rare and unlikely to be encountered regularly outside of large referral centers, other conditions, such as chronic kidney disease, are exceedingly common and likely to be routinely found in the patient population. Regardless of the prevalence of the disease or condition, however, optimal anesthetic management will depend both on a thorough understanding of the underlying pathologic and pathophysiologic findings, and on the recognition that the disease process may affect the anesthetic just as much as the anesthetic may exacerbate the disease process.

CARDIAC TUMORS

Cardiac tumors belong to the class of cardiac masses that includes vegetations and thrombi, for which tumors may be mistaken. Cardiac tumors may be classified as primary or secondary (metastatic). Primary tumors may be benign or malignant, whereas secondary tumors may involve the heart by direct extension (breast and lung), by venous extension (renal cell and hepatocellular carcinoma), or by hematogenous (melanoma, breast, and carcinoid) or lymphatic (lymphoma) spread.

In general, cardiac tumors are rare, and a cardiac mass encountered echocardiographically or radiographically is more likely to be a thrombus or a vegetation than a tumor. Metastatic tumors are more common than primary cardiac tumors, with an incidence at autopsy between 2.3% and 18.3%, whereas primary tumors have an incidence rate between 0.0014% and 0.33%. Among primary tumors, benign lesions are more common than malignant masses. In adults, the most common primary benign tumors are myxomas, although several series now suggest that papillary fibroelastomas may, in fact, be more common (Table 18.1). In children, rhabdomyomas are the most common benign tumor. Approximately 15% to 25% of primary cardiac tumors are malignant, with sarcomas being the most common in both adults and children. Tumors with high rates of cardiac metastases include pleural mesothelioma, melanoma, lung adenocarcinoma and squamous cell carcinoma, and breast carcinoma. Although metastases may involve the pericardium, epicardium, myocardium, or endocardium, pericardial involvement is most common.

18

Table 18.1 Incidence of Benign Cardiac Tumors in Adults and Children		
	Incidence (%)	
Neoplasms	Adults	Children
Myxoma	45	15
Lipoma	20	—
Papillary fibroelastoma	15	—
Angioma	5	5
Fibroma	3	15
Hemangioma	5	5
Rhabdomyoma	1	45
Teratoma	<1	15

Reproduced with permission from Shapiro LM. Cardiac tumors: diagnosis and management. *Heart.* 2001;85:218.

Although cardiac tumors may be clinically silent and diagnosed only at autopsy, advancements in imaging have facilitated both their often-incidental antemortem diagnosis and their characterization once detected. The increasing sophistication of two-dimensional echocardiography, the advent of three-dimensional echocardiographic imaging, and the continued refinement of computed tomography (CT) and magnetic resonance imaging (MRI) have all allowed earlier, more frequent, and more complete assessment of cardiac tumors. Although malignant primary lesions and metastatic tumors may produce constitutional symptoms, even histologically benign masses may cause concerning signs and symptoms associated with intracardiac obstruction and extracardiac embolization.

The most effective treatment of primary tumors is generally surgical resection with an approximate 2% operative mortality. Recurrence rate in these tumors varies between 3% and 13% but appears to be related to a biologic propensity rather than the surgical technique, as was previously believed. Orthotopic cardiac transplantation has been recommended for unresectable tumors, but the benefit is indeterminate. Although malignant lesions are less common, the surgical risk and outcome for their resection, compared with benign tumor resection, is usually significantly worse, especially in younger patients.

Primary Benign Tumors

Myxoma

Often a diagnostic challenge, myxomas are benign, solitary, and slow-proliferating neoplasms. Microscopically, they often resemble organized thrombi, which may obscure their identity as a primary cardiac tumor. The pedunculated mass is believed to arise from undifferentiated cells in the fossa ovalis and adjoining endocardium, projecting into the left atrium (LA) and the right atrium (RA) 75% and 20% of the time, respectively. However, myxomas appear in other locations of the heart, even occupying more than one chamber. Myxomas predominate in the 30- to 60-year-old age range, but any age group may be affected. More than 75% of the affected patients are women. Although most cases occur sporadically, 7% to 10% of atrial myxomas will occur in a familial pattern with an autosomal dominant transmission pattern known as Carney complex.

Occasionally an incidental finding on echocardiography, myxomas may produce a variety of symptoms. The classic triad includes embolism, intracardiac obstruction, and constitutional symptoms. Approximately 80% of individuals will exhibit one component of the triad. The most common initial symptom, dyspnea on exertion, reflects mitral valve obstruction associated with left atrial myxomas (Fig. 18.1). Because of the pedunculated nature of some myxomas, temporary obstruction of blood flow may cause hemolysis, hypotension, syncope, or sudden death. Other symptoms of mitral obstruction, similar to mitral stenosis, may occur, including hemoptysis, systemic embolization, fever, and weight loss. If the tumor is obstructing the mitral valve, then a *tumor plop* may be heard after the second heart sound on chest auscultation. The persistent sinus rhythm in the presence of such symptoms may help distinguish an atrial myxoma from mitral stenosis. Severe pulmonary hypertension without significant mitral valve involvement suggests recurrent pulmonary emboli, which is known to occur with a myxoma in the RA or right ventricle (RV). Occasionally, right-sided heart tumors may appear as cyanotic congenital heart lesions attributable to intracardiac shunting.

Findings on a chest roentgenogram of a myxoma may be absent in approximately one-third of persons. Calcification on the chest roentgenogram is more diagnostic of right atrial myxoma but may occasionally be present with left atrial myxomas.

IV

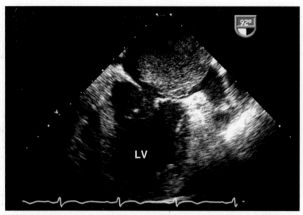

Fig. 18.1 Transesophageal echocardiographic characteristics of a large left atrial myxoma. Midesophageal two-chamber view during systole shows a 5 × 7 cm mass located in the left atrium. *LV,* Left ventricle. (Reproduced with permission from Otto CM, ed. *Practice of Clinical Echocardiography.* 4th ed. Philadelphia: Saunders/Elsevier; 2012.)

Before the availability of echocardiography, angiography was used to identify myxomas; currently, however, angiography is probably only useful to determine coronary anatomy, if considered necessary. CT and MRI can help delineate the extent of a tumor and its relation to surrounding cardiac and thoracic structures. MRI is especially valuable in the diagnosis of myxoma when masses are equivocal or suboptimal with echocardiography or if the tumor is atypical in presentation. Difficulty may arise in differentiating a thrombus from a myxoma, because both are so heterogeneous.

Transthoracic echocardiography (TTE) is excellent for identifying intracavitary tumors, because it is noninvasive, identifies tumor type, and permits complete visualization of each cardiac chamber. TTE is the predominant imaging modality for screening. Transesophageal echocardiography (TEE) allows for better definition of tumor size and location and can be used to identify the site of tumor attachment and the presence of multiple lesions.

When the primary reason for cardiac surgery is the removal of an intracardiac mass, an intraoperative transesophageal echocardiographic evaluation should take place before the surgical incision to ensure that the mass is still present and has not embolized or even dissolved, as in the case of intracardiac thrombus. In the case of myxoma, an intraoperative examination in the presence of the surgeon can aid in finalizing the surgical plan and in detecting previously unseen tumors. After tumor removal, the goal of TEE is to ensure that all visible mass was removed and that no damage occurred to adjacent structures. Specifically, in the case of a myxoma attached to the atrial septum, ensuring that no interatrial shunting has occurred after resection is important. If the tumor was attached on or adjacent to the valvular apparatus, then the examiner must determine whether the valve is competent after removing the tumor.

The first surgical resection of an atrial myxoma was performed in 1954. Subsequently, surgical resection has been recommended even if the myxoma is discovered incidentally, primarily because the risk of embolization to the central nervous system may be 30% to 40%. Surgery is associated with a mortality rate between 0% and 7%. More important, recent studies show that the long-term survival of an individual who has undergone myxoma resection is no different from age- and gender-matched populations.

18

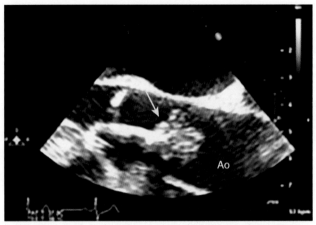

Fig. 18.2 Giant aortic valve papillary fibroelastoma. Transesophageal midesophageal long-axis view of the aortic valve shows the 4.7-cm pedunculated mass attached to the right coronary cusp of the aortic valve *(yellow arrow)*. LV, Left ventricle; Ao, aortic opening. (Reproduced with permission from Fine NM, Foley DA, Breen JF, Maleszewski JJ. Multimodality imaging of a giant aortic valve papillary fibroelastoma. *Case Rep Med.* 2013;2013:705101.)

Papillary Fibroelastoma

Papillomas (papillary fibroelastoma) are rare, benign tumors that tend to affect the cardiac valves. Mostly singular (90%), 1 to 4 cm in size, highly papillary, pedunculated, and avascular, papillomas are covered by a single layer of endothelium containing fine elastic fibrils in a hyaline stroma (Fig. 18.2). They originate most commonly from valvular endocardium, usually involving the ventricular surface of the aortic valve or the atrial surface of the mitral valve, but they only infrequently render the involved valve incompetent. Adults between the ages of 40 and 80 years are primarily affected, with a mean age of 60 years at the time of detection. Many patients are asymptomatic; therefore it is not surprising that 47% of these tumors are discovered incidentally during echocardiography, catheterization, or even cardiac surgery. Echocardiographically they may appear similar to vegetations seen in endocarditis, or they may be confused with Lambl excrescences, which tend to be more nodular in appearance.

Although papillary fibroelastomas were previously believed to be harmless, post-mortem studies have shown a high incidence of embolization to the cerebral and coronary circulations. Not surprisingly, symptoms are often related to stroke or transient ischemic attack and myocardial infarction (MI). Surgical resection is curative but may require valvular repair or replacement in one-third of cases. Recurrence is very rare.

Primary Malignant Tumors

Approximately 25% of primary cardiac tumors are malignant, and 95% of these are sarcomas. They are found infiltrating the RA and causing cavitary obstruction but may have variable clinical presentations based on the location, causing the diagnosis to be elusive. Primary malignant tumors usually occur between the ages of 30 and 50 years and are preceded by vague symptoms such as dyspnea, rapidly progressing to death. Angiosarcomas, the most common sarcoma, are rapidly spreading vascular tumors that arise most often from the RA and appear near the inferior vena cava (IVC) with extension to the mediastinum. Presenting symptoms include chest pain and dyspnea, progressive congestive heart failure (CHF), and bloody pericardial effusion. Treatment is palliative, because the response to chemotherapy and radiation is poor. Resection may be possible, but survival is less than 2 years. Rhabdomyosarcomas are aggressive tumors that have cellular elements that resemble striated muscle. Surgical resection is possible, but distant metastasis reduces the chances of success. Chemotherapy and radiation are ineffective.

In general, malignant primary cardiac tumors may require a combination of surgery, radiation, and chemotherapy to limit cavitary obstruction to blood flow because of rapid growth and metastasis. Local recurrence is more likely to cause death than metastasis. Although still controversial, orthotopic heart transplantation may be considered for unresectable tumors that involve only the heart, but survival is not extended beyond 1 to 2 years. The rate of intraoperative death with malignant tumor resection is seven times that of benign resection, and the morbidity rate is twice as high.

Metastatic Tumors

Although rare in general, secondary or metastatic cardiac tumors are far more common than primary tumors. These tumors may affect primarily the pericardium, the epicardium, the myocardium, or the endocardium. The site of metastasis frequently provides clues to the means of metastasis. Pericardial involvement, for example, often occurs via the direct extension from surrounding intrathoracic structures or from lymphatic spread, whereas endocardial lesions typically reflect hematogenous spread, and epicardial and myocardial lesions tend to arise from lymphatic extension.

Tumors exhibiting high rates of cardiac metastases include mesothelioma (48.4%), melanoma (27.8%), pulmonary adenocarcinoma (21%), undifferentiated lung carcinoma (19.5%), pulmonary squamous cell carcinoma (18.5%), and breast carcinoma (15.5%), although other autopsy series suggest that esophageal carcinoma may also be commonly found in cases of cardiac metastases. When considered by means of extension, direct extension is most likely to occur with tumors of the lung, breast, and esophagus, whereas hematogenous seeding is more likely with melanomas, and lymphatic spread is associated with lymphomas and leukemias. Venous extension, primarily involving right-sided cardiac structures, occurs with tumors of the kidneys (renal cell carcinoma), liver (hepatocellular carcinoma), and uterus (uterine leiomyosarcoma).

Unsurprisingly, the prognosis with a diagnosis of metastatic cardiac disease is poor. In one recent small series, 53.4% of patients diagnosed with metastatic lesions were deceased at 1 year. Although surgical intervention is not typically contemplated, 53.5% of the patients with metastatic disease in that series underwent surgical resection. Of those who underwent resection, 56.5% were alive at 1 year.

Anesthetic Considerations

Anesthetic management of patients with cardiac tumors is likely guided first by the patient's comorbidities and second by tumor location.

In addition to the American Society of Anesthesiologists standard monitors providing continual evaluation of oxygenation, ventilation, circulation, and temperature, anesthesia for resectioning a cardiac tumor will undoubtedly involve placing an arterial line for continuous hemodynamic monitoring and establishing central venous access for vasoactive drug administration, volume infusion, and pressure monitoring. The timing of arterial line placement with respect to anesthetic induction should be guided by the patient's comorbidities and provider experience. Similarly, the choice of catheters and their placement locations for central venous access should be guided by the patient's pathologic condition and the surgical skill of the provider.

18

Anesthetic management is guided by tumor location in addition to patient comorbidity. Left atrial myxomas, for example, will most likely cause mitral valve obstruction, often in conjunction with pulmonary venous hypertension. Anesthetic management will closely resemble that of a patient with mitral stenosis. In contrast, right atrial myxomas may produce signs of right-sided heart failure that correspond to tricuspid valve obstruction. Positioning the patient for surgery must be carefully performed to detect severe restriction of venous return that may often be quickly followed with profound hypotension and arrhythmias. A large tumor may increase the likelihood of hemodynamic instability, whereas small tumors may be associated with increased risk of embolization. Perioperative arrhythmias, especially atrial fibrillation or atrial flutter, may arise in 25% of these patients and may require immediate treatment.

Tumors With Systemic Cardiac Manifestations

Carcinoid Tumors

Carcinoid tumors are metastasizing neuroendocrine tumors that arise primarily from the small bowel, occurring in 1 to 2 per 100,000 people in the population. Upon diagnosis, 20% to 30% of individuals with carcinoid tumors exhibit the symptoms of carcinoid syndrome, characterized by episodic vasomotor symptoms, bronchospasm, hypotension, diarrhea, and right-sided heart disease attributed to the release of serotonin, histamine, bradykinins, and prostaglandins, often in response to manipulation or pharmacologic stimulation. Manifestations of carcinoid syndrome occur primarily in patients with liver metastasis that impairs the ability of the liver to inactivate large amounts of vasoactive substances.

Initially described in 1952, carcinoid heart disease may occur in 20% to 50% of patients with carcinoid syndrome. The prognosis has improved substantially in the last 20 years for individuals with malignant carcinoid tumors and carcinoid heart disease, but it still causes considerable morbidity and mortality. The median life expectancy is 5.9 years without carcinoid heart disease but falls to 2.6 years if it is present.

Carcinoid heart disease characteristically produces tricuspid regurgitation and mixed pulmonic stenosis and regurgitation resulting in severe right-sided heart failure. Tumor growth in the liver permits large amounts of tumor products to reach the RV without the benefit of first-pass hepatic metabolism. Carcinoid plaques composed of myofibroblasts, collagen, and myxoid matrix are deposited primarily on the tricuspid and pulmonary valves, bringing about immobility and thickening of the valve leaflets, causing the distinctive valvular changes. At the time of surgery, 80% of tricuspid valves are observed to be incompetent compared with only 20% with stenosis, whereas the affected pulmonary valves tend to be equally divided between incompetence and stenosis. The exact mechanism that causes valve injury is unknown, but high levels of serotonin are sometimes found in patients with carcinoid heart disease. Fewer than 10% of those with carcinoid heart disease have left-sided heart involvement, possibly attributable to inactivation of serotonin in the lungs, but either the mitral or aortic valve may be affected in the presence of a bronchial carcinoid, a right-to-left intracardiac shunt, or poorly controlled disease with high levels of circulating vasoactive substances.

A careful search for a patent foramen ovale (PFO) should be undertaken, because its presence raises the possibility of left-sided valvular involvement.

Historically, the prognosis of patients with carcinoid syndrome has been poor. In the absence of treatment, median survival was 38 months from the time of development of systemic symptoms. With the development of cardiac involvement and frank

IV

carcinoid heart disease, median survival has dropped to a dismal 11 months. Improvements in medical management and surgical technique, however, have led to improved symptom control and a lower mortality rate. Although the introduction of somatostatin analogs in the mid-1980s was associated with improved symptom control, no evidence suggested that their use was associated with improved survival. Currently, two somatostatin analogs are available for treatment: octreotide and lanreotide.

Treatment of the tumor and the malignant carcinoid syndrome does not result in regression of carcinoid heart disease. The surgical replacement of both the tricuspid and pulmonary valves with either bioprosthetic or mechanical valves is the only viable therapeutic option. The optimal timing of surgical intervention is uncertain but should be considered when signs of right-sided heart failure appear, if not before.

ANESTHETIC CONSIDERATIONS

Patients who have carcinoid heart disease and require cardiac surgical intervention pose an anesthetic challenge. A carcinoid crisis with exuberant vasoactive-mediator release is a life-threatening event that may be precipitated by patient anxiety and fear in anticipation of surgical intervention. A variety of pharmacologic agents, including thiopental, meperidine, morphine, atracurium, and succinylcholine, as well as catecholamines such as epinephrine, norepinephrine, dopamine, and dobutamine, have all been implicated, in crisis precipitation. Furthermore, physical stimulation that may occur with laryngoscopy and endotracheal intubation, vascular access placement and the placement of urinary catheters, and tumor manipulation that may occur during tumor resection may also elicit a brisk release of vasoactive mediators.

Perioperative patient management is facilitated with optimal preoperative symptom control with carefully monitored administration and up-titration of a long-acting somatostatin analog formulation, supplemented preoperatively with additional subcutaneous injections of short-acting medications. Some institutions initiate an octreotide infusion at doses between 50 and 100 μg per hour the night before surgery or the day of surgery in the preoperative holding area, while providing additional intravenous doses of 20 to 100 μg as indicated clinically during anesthetic management. Incidentally, it should be noted that severe hyperglycemia may occur with octreotide because of its inhibition of insulin secretion, especially in combination with steroids.

Because patient anxiety and stress may provoke a carcinoid crisis, consideration should be given to judicious administration of preoperative anxiolytic agents. A variety of strategies have been recommended; however, for a patient whose symptoms are well controlled preoperatively on a regimen of long- and short-acting octreotide or its equivalent, it is likely the case that the drugs used matter less than how they are used and matter less than the vigilance of the anesthesiologist directing the patient's care.

18

Renal Cell Carcinoma

Although renal cell carcinoma may not normally be considered a topic in cardiac anesthesia, cardiac anesthesia team members may increasingly find themselves caring for patients with renal cell carcinoma with significant venous extension. Renal cell cancers represent 2% to 3% of adult malignancies but are the most common and most deadly of renal neoplasms, accounting for approximately 90% of all renal cancers and conferring historic mortality rates between 30% and 40%. Although classically diagnosed by a combination of flank pain, hematuria, and a palpable mass, most renal cell cancers are now found incidentally during radiographic evaluation for other reasons. A small (2–3%) proportion of the cancers may be associated with familial syndromes, such as von Hippel-Lindau disease, although smoking, obesity, and hypertension are considered the three primary modifiable risk factors.

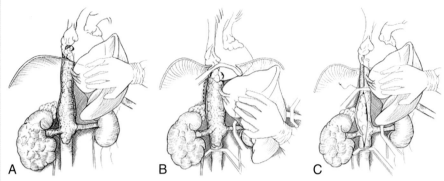

Fig. 18.3 Surgical technique for level IV tumor extraction, avoiding cardiopulmonary bypass. (A) Mobilization of the liver off the retrohepatic inferior vena cava (IVC). (B) Dissection of the IVC and central tendon of the diaphragm off the posterior abdominal wall *(dashed lines)* and clamping of the distal IVC, the right atrium, the left renal vein, and the porta hepatis. (C) Milking the tumor from the supradiaphragmatic IVC, enabling it to be extracted without a sternotomy or the need for cardiopulmonary bypass. (Reproduced with permission from Ciancio G, Shirodkar SP, Soloway MS, et al. Renal carcinoma with supradiaphragmatic tumor thrombus: avoiding sternotomy and cardiopulmonary bypass. *Ann Thorac Surg.* 2010;89:507.)

Historically, surgery for level III and IV tumors has been performed on cardiopulmonary bypass (CPB), often using deep hypothermic circulatory arrest. In an attempt to avoid exposure to extracorporeal circulation, to avoid the neurologic morbidity associated with profound hypothermia and circulatory arrest, and to avoid the ravages of massive transfusion, surgeons have developed strategies for both on-pump resection without hypothermic arrest and off-pump resection, even in the case of lesions extending into the RA (Fig. 18.3).

ANESTHETIC CONSIDERATIONS

Anesthetically, the most important concerns in caring for patients undergoing radical nephrectomy and tumor thrombectomy will be establishing sufficient venous access and performing a thorough intraoperative transesophageal echocardiogram. Placement of a pulmonary artery catheter (PAC) may be unnecessary in patients with normal preoperative biventricular function and may be contraindicated in patients with tumor thrombus extending high into the supradiaphragmatic IVC and RA. Placement of femoral venous catheters for volume use intraoperatively may be of little use, considering the need to interrupt IVC blood flow for surgical resection. For on-pump procedures, consideration should be given to avoiding the use of antifibrinolytic agents, considering a patient's clear hypercoagulable state, although data to guide a rational choice are practically nonexistent.

■ CARDIOMYOPATHY

In 1995 the World Health Organization (WHO) and the International Society of Cardiology (ISC) redefined the cardiomyopathies according to dominant pathophysiologic considerations or, if possible, by "etiological/pathogenetic factors." Cardiomyopathies were then defined as "diseases of the myocardium associated with cardiac dysfunction." The original cardiomyopathies, classified as dilated cardiomyopathy (DCM), restrictive cardiomyopathy (RCM), and hypertrophic cardiomyopathy

IV

(HCM), were preserved, and arrhythmogenic right ventricular cardiomyopathy (ARVC) was added.

Based on the American Heart Association (AHA) definition, cardiomyopathies may be divided into primary and secondary classifications, depending upon the primary organ involvement. Whereas primary cardiomyopathies are confined generally to the myocardium, secondary cardiomyopathies reflect myocardial involvement in the context of a systemic disorder. Primary cardiomyopathies primarily affecting the heart may, in turn, be classified as genetic, mixed, or acquired (Fig. 18.4). Secondary cardiomyopathies, in which cardiac involvement occurs in the context of a systemic disorder, are more numerous (Box 18.1).

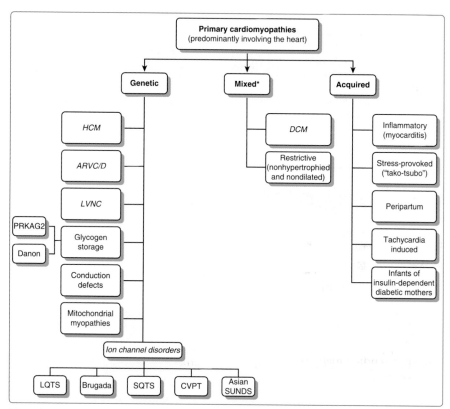

Fig. 18.4 American Heart Association classification of primary cardiomyopathies. Predominantly nongenetic causes, although rare cases of primary cardiomyopathy with a genetic origin, have been reported (see text for details). *ARVC/D,* Arrhythmogenic right ventricular cardiomyopathy/dysplasia; *CVPT,* catecholaminergic polymorphic ventricular tachycardia; *DCM,* dilated cardiomyopathy; *HCM,* hypertrophic cardiomyopathy; *LQTS,* long QT syndrome; *LVNC,* left ventricular noncompaction; *PRKAG2,* adenosine monophosphate–activated protein kinase, subunit gamma-2; *SQTS,* short QT syndrome; *SUNDS,* sudden unexplained nocturnal death. (Reproduced with permission from Maron BJ, Towbin JA, Thiene G, et al; American Heart Association; Council on Clinical Cardiology, Heart Failure and Transplantation Committee; Quality of Care and Outcomes Research and Functional Genomics and Translational Biology Interdisciplinary Working Groups; Council on Epidemiology and Prevention. Contemporary definitions and classification of the cardiomyopathies: an American Heart Association Scientific Statement from the Council on Clinical Cardiology, Heart Failure and Transplantation Committee; Quality of Care and Outcomes Research and Functional Genomics and Translational Biology Interdisciplinary Working Groups; and Council on Epidemiology and Prevention. *Circulation.* 2006;113:181.)

18

As if to confuse the subject further, the European Society of Cardiology Working Group on Myocardial and Pericardial Diseases presented its own classification scheme in 2008. According to the European scheme, cardiomyopathies were divided much as they had been by WHO and the International Society and Federation of Cardiology into hypertrophic, dilated, arrhythmogenic right ventricular, restrictive, and unclassified; and each category, in turn, could be subdivided into familial and genetic or nonfamilial and nongenetic (Fig. 18.5).

With the lack of a consensus on a definition of cardiomyopathy and with its numerous subtypes, it is difficult, if not impossible, to speak of its epidemiologic

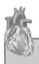

BOX 18.1 *American Heart Association Classification of Secondary Cardiomyopathies*

Infiltrative[a]
    Amyloidosis (primary, familial autosomal dominant,[b] senile, secondary forms)
    Gaucher disease[b]
    Hurler disease[b]
    Hunter disease[b]
Storage[c]
    Hemochromatosis
    Fabry disease[b]
    Glycogen storage disease[b] (type II, Pompe disease)
    Niemann-Pick disease[b]
Toxicity
    Drugs, heavy metals, chemical agents
Endomyocardial
    Endomyocardial fibrosis
    Hypereosinophilic syndrome (Löffler endocarditis)
Inflammatory (granulomatous)
    Sarcoidosis
Endocrine
    Diabetes mellitus[b]
    Hyperthyroidism
    Hypothyroidism
    Hyperparathyroidism
    Pheochromocytoma
    Acromegaly
Cardiofacial
    Noonan syndrome[b]
    Lentiginosis[b]
Neuromuscular and neurologic
    Friedreich ataxia[b]
    Duchenne muscular dystrophy[b]
    Becker muscular dystrophy[b]
    Emery-Dreifuss muscular dystrophy[b]
    Myotonic dystrophy[b]
    Neurofibromatosis[b]
    Tuberous sclerosis[b]
Nutritional deficiencies
    Beriberi (thiamine), pellagra, scurvy, selenium, carnitine, kwashiorkor

IV

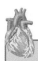

BOX 18.1 *American Heart Association Classification of Secondary Cardiomyopathies—cont'd*

Autoimmune and collagen
    Systemic lupus erythematosus
    Dermatomyositis
    Rheumatoid arthritis
    Scleroderma
    Polyarteritis nodosa
Electrolyte imbalance
Consequence of cancer therapy
    Anthracyclines: doxorubicin (Adriamycin), daunorubicin
    Cyclophosphamide
    Radiation

[a]Extracellular deposition of abnormal substances among myocytes.
[b]Genetic origin.
[c]Extracellular deposition of abnormal substances within myocytes.
Reproduced with permission from Maron BJ, Towbin JA, Thiene G, et al; American Heart Association; Council on Clinical Cardiology, Heart Failure and Transplantation Committee; Quality of Care and Outcomes Research and Functional Genomics and Translational Biology Interdisciplinary Working Groups; Council on Epidemiology and Prevention. Contemporary definitions and classification of the cardiomyopathies: an American Heart Association Scientific Statement from the Council on Clinical Cardiology, Heart Failure and Transplantation Committee; Quality of Care and Outcomes Research and Functional Genomics and Translational Biology Interdisciplinary Working Groups; and Council on Epidemiology and Prevention. *Circulation.* 2006;113:1814.

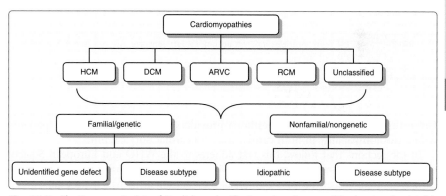

Fig. 18.5 The European Society of Cardiology classification of cardiomyopathies (see text for details). *ARVC,* Arrhythmogenic right ventricular cardiomyopathy; *DCM,* dilated cardiomyopathy; *HCM,* hypertrophic cardiomyopathy; *RCM,* restrictive cardiomyopathy. (Reproduced with permission from Elliott P, Andersson B, Arbustini E, et al. Classification of the cardiomyopathies: a position statement from the European Society of Cardiology Working Group on Myocardial and Pericardial Diseases. *Eur Heart J.* 2008;29:271.)

factors, although likely not uncommon. DCM alone, of whatever cause, has been estimated to have an annual incidence of 5 to 8 cases per 100,000 population and a prevalence in the United States of 36 cases per 100,000 population, leading to approximately 10,000 deaths annually. HCM is even more common, if not the most common inherited cardiomyopathy, with an estimated prevalence between 1:500 and 1:200 and an estimated prevalence of at least 700,000 in the United States alone.

Table 18.2	Characteristics of Cardiomyopathies			
Characteristics	Hypertrophic Cardio-myopathy	Dilated Cardio-myopathy	Arrhythmogenic Right Ventricular Cardiomyopathy	Restrictive Cardiomyopathy
Clinical				
Heart failure	Occasional (LV)	Frequent (LV or BV)	Frequent (RV)	Frequent (BV)
Arrhythmias	Atrial and ventricular arrhythmias	Atrial and ventricular arrhythmias, conduction defects	Ventricular tachycardia (RV), conduction defects	Atrial fibrillation
Sudden death	0.7–11% per year	Frequent (ND)	Frequent (ND)	1–5% per year
Hemodynamically				
Systolic function	Hyperdynamic, outflow tract obstruction (occasionally)	Reduced	Normal-reduced	Near normal
Diastolic function	Reduced	Reduced	Reduced	Severely reduced
Morphologic				
Cavity size				
Ventricle	Reduced (LV)	Enlarged (LV or BA)	Enlarged (RV)	Normal or reduced (BV)
Atrium	Normal-enlarged (LA)	Enlarged (LA or BA)	Enlarged (RV)	Enlarged (BA)
Wall thickness	Enlarged, asymmetric (LV)	Normal-reduced (LV or BV)	Normal-reduced (RV)	Normal (BV)

BA, Both atria; *BV,* both ventricles; *LA,* left atrium; *LV,* left ventricle; *ND,* not determined; *RA,* right atrium; *RV,* right ventricle.
Reproduced with permission from Franz WM, Müller OJ, Katus HA. Cardiomyopathies: from genetics to the prospect of treatment. *Lancet.* 2001;358:1628.

Given this burden of disease, anesthesia providers are likely to encounter patients with a cardiomyopathy in both cardiac and noncardiac surgical units.

In the sections that follow, this text adheres to the WHO and European Society classification, presenting overviews of DCM, HCM, RCM, and ARVC and followed, in turn, by a discussion of the salient points of their anesthetic management (Table 18.2).

Dilated Cardiomyopathy

Formerly referred to as congestive cardiomyopathy or idiopathic cardiomyopathy, DCM is by far the most common of the four cardiomyopathies in adults in the WHO and European Society classification. As developments in molecular biology and genetics have provided better insight into the pathogenesis of DCMs, the term *idiopathic* has become less applicable.

Acknowledging the limitations of any taxonomy, the DCMs run a spectrum from genetic to acquired with an overlap in the middle. The genetics of DCMs and the genetics of familial DCM are complicated and the causes of acquired DCMs are diverse (Box 18.2).

BOX 18.2   *Causes of Dilated Cardiomyopathy*

Idiopathic Causes

- Idiopathic dilated cardiomyopathy
- Idiopathic arrhythmogenic right ventricular dysplasia

Familial (Hereditary) Causes

- Autosomal dominant
- X-chromosomal
- Polymorphism
- Other

Toxic Causes

- Ethanol
- Cocaine
- Adriamycin
- Catecholamine excess
- Phenothiazines, antidepressants
- Cobalt
- Carbon monoxide
- Lead
- Lithium
- Cyclophosphamide
- Methysergide
- Amphetamine
- Pseudoephedrine or ephedrine

Inflammatory: Infectious Causes

- Viral (coxsackievirus, parvovirus, adenovirus, echovirus, influenza virus, human immunodeficiency virus)
- Spirochete (leptospirosis, syphilis)
- Protozoal (Chagas disease, toxoplasmosis, trichinosis)

Inflammatory: Noninfectious Causes

- Collagen vascular disease (scleroderma, lupus erythematosus, dermatomyositis, rheumatoid arthritis, sarcoidosis)
- Kawasaki disease
- Hypersensitivity myocarditis

Causes of Miscellaneous Acquired Cardiomyopathies

- Postpartum cardiomyopathy
- Obesity

Metabolic and Nutritional Causes

- Thiamine
- Kwashiorkor, pellagra
- Scurvy
- Selenium deficiency
- Carnitine deficiency

18

Continued

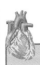

BOX 18.2 *Causes of Dilated Cardiomyopathy—cont'd*

Endocrine Causes

- Diabetes mellitus
- Acromegaly
- Thyrotoxicosis
- Myxedema
- Uremia
- Cushing disease
- Pheochromocytoma

Electrolyte Imbalance

- Hypophosphatemia
- Hypocalcemia

Physiologic Causes

- Tachycardia
- Heat stroke
- Hypothermia
- Radiation

Autoimmune Disorders

- Infiltrative cardiomyopathies (dilated cardiomyopathy usually after progression from restrictive cardiomyopathy; in end-stage)
- Cardiac amyloidosis
- Hemochromatosis

Stress- and Catecholamine-Induced Cardiomyopathies

- Perioperative stress
- Adrenergic stimulation

Reproduced with permission from Bozkurt B. Heart failure as a consequence of dilated cardiomyopathy. In: Mann DL, Felker GM, eds. *Heart Failure: A Companion to Braunwald's Heart Disease*, 3rd ed. Philadelphia: Elsevier; 2016:301.

Phenotypically, the end-stage cardiomyopathies are similar, regardless of the inciting event. There is gross dilatation of all four cardiac chambers, modest thinning of the ventricular walls, and significant hypertrophy of the myocytes and the heart globally, reflecting a myocardium subjected to chronic volume overload. Although valve leaflets may be normal, dilatation of the heart has been associated with regurgitant lesions, secondary to papillary muscle displacement and leaflet malcoaptation, producing the frequently encountered mitral and/or tricuspid regurgitation. Histologic changes are nonspecific and typically shed little insight on the cause. Microscopically, a patchy and diffuse loss of tissue with interstitial fibrosis and scarring is demonstrated. Encroachment on the conduction system produces the bundle branch pattern frequently seen on the electrocardiogram (ECG).

With the DCMs, systolic function is disproportionately impaired, although as systolic function worsens, diastolic function is compromised as well. As contractile function diminishes, stroke volume is initially maintained by augmentation of end-diastolic volume. Ventricular dilatation, combined with valvular regurgitation, compromises the metabolic capabilities of the heart muscle and produces overt

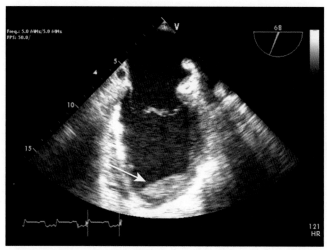

Fig. 18.6 Transesophageal midesophageal two-chamber view shows a thrombus (arrow) at the apex of the left ventricle. (Reproduced with permission from Oliver WC, Mauermann WJ, Nuttall GA. Uncommon cardiac diseases. In: Kaplan JA, Reich DL, Savino JS, eds. *Kaplan's Cardiac Anesthesia: The Echo Era.* 6th ed. Philadelphia: Saunders; 2011:684.)

circulatory failure. Compensatory mechanisms may allow symptoms of myocardial dysfunction to go unnoticed for an extended period.

Echocardiography is extremely useful in the outpatient management of patients with DCM. The characteristic two-dimensional findings are a dilated left ventricle (LV) with globally decreased systolic function. Indeed, all markers of systolic function (ejection fraction, fractional shortening, stroke volume, cardiac output [CO]) are uniformly decreased. Other associated findings may include a dilated mitral annulus with incomplete mitral leaflet coaptation, dilated atria, right ventricular enlargement, and thrombus in the left ventricular apex (Fig. 18.6). In some instances, regional wall motion abnormalities will be present. Well-compensated patients with DCM may have only mild impairment of diastolic function. As the disease progresses and patients become less well compensated, the left ventricular diastolic filling pattern changes to that of restricted filling. Although systolic function may not change in these patients, the increased filling pressures associated with restrictive left ventricular filling will often worsen the symptoms of CHF.

Management of acute decompensated CHF continues to evolve, but the onset of overt CHF is a poor prognostic indicator for persons with DCM. Treatment includes medication regimens and device intervention based on symptom class (Table 18.3).

Patients who are resistant to pharmacologic therapy for CHF have received dual-chamber pacing, cardiomyoplasty, left ventricular assist devices (LVADs), cardiac surgical procedures (nontransplantation), and transplantation in recent years. Cardiac resynchronization therapy with dual ventricular pacing improves the New York Heart Association (NYHA) functional class and ejection fraction 6 months after implantation. Placement of implantable LVADs has enabled end-stage patients to reach transplantation or has become destination therapy for those for whom transplantation is not an option. If mitral regurgitation develops in patients with DCM, then mitral valve repair or replacement is recommended. Surgical intervention in this high-risk population is safe and improves NYHA classification and survival. Transplantation can substantially prolong lives, with current survival at 15 years of 50% if younger than 55 years of age. However, limited organ availability and drug-related morbidity suggest that

18

Table 18.3 Pharmacologic and Device Therapy for Chronic Heart Failure

Indication	ACE Inhibitor	ARB	Diuretic Agent	Beta Blocker	Aldosterone Antagonist	Cardiac Glycosides	CRT	ICD
Asymptomatic LV dysfunction (NYHA class I)	Indicated	If patient is ACE-intolerant	Not indicated	Post-MI Indicated[a]	Recent MI	(1) For rate control with atrial fibrillation or (2) When improved from more severe HF and in sinus rhythm	May be considered[a]	Indicated
Symptomatic HF (NYHA class II)	Indicated	Indicated with or without ACE inhibitor	Indicated if fluid retention is present	Indicated	Indicated	(1) With atrial fibrillation (2) When improved from more severe HF in sinus rhythm	Indicated[b]	
Worsening HF (NYHA classes III–IV)	Indicated	Indicated with or without ACE inhibitor	Combination of diuretic agents indicated	Indicated (under specialist care)	Indicated	Indicated	Indicated[c]	Indicated
End-stage HF (NYHA class IV)	Indicated	Indicated with or without ACE inhibitor	Combination of diuretic agents indicated	Indicated (under specialist care)	Indicated	Indicated	Indicated[c]	Not indicated[d]

[a]May be considered in patients with LVEF 30% or less, of ischemic cause, in sinus rhythm with a QRS of 150 milliseconds or longer, and with morphologic LBBB.
[b]Indicated with QRS of 130 milliseconds or longer with morphologic LBBB or QRS of 150 milliseconds or longer with nonmorphologic LBBB and EF of 30% or less.
[c]Indicated with QRS of 120 milliseconds or more with LBBB or QRS of 150 milliseconds or longer, nonmorphologic LBBB, and EF of 35% or less.
[d]Use of an ICD may be considered in patients with NYHA class IV HF who are undergoing implantation of a CRT device.

ACE, Angiotensin-converting enzyme; ARB, angiotensin-receptor blocker; CRT, cardiac resynchronization therapy; EF, ejection fraction; HF, heart failure; ICD, implantable cardioverter-defibrillator; LBBB, left bundle branch block; LV, left ventricular; LVEF, left ventricular ejection fraction; MI, myocardial infarction; NHYA, New York Heart Association.

Reproduced with permission from Mann DL, Zipes DP, Libby P, et al. *Braunwald's Heart Disease: A Textbook of Cardiovascular Medicine*, 10th ed. Philadelphia: Saunders; 2015:519.

improvements in device therapy, either with LVADs or artificial hearts, may provide the best opportunity for increased survival.

Anesthetic Considerations

The most common cardiac procedures for patients with DCM are correction of mitral and tricuspid regurgitation, placement of an implantable cardioverter-defibrillator (ICD) for refractory ventricular arrhythmias, and device (LVAD, total artificial heart) placement or orthotopic heart transplantation. Anesthetic management is predicated on minimizing further myocardial depression, optimizing preload, and judiciously reducing afterload.

Individuals with DCM may be extremely sensitive to cardiodepressant anesthetic drugs. Historically, high-dose intravenous opioids such as fentanyl (30 µg/kg) were considered to provide excellent analgesia and hemodynamic stability in patients with ejection fractions less than 30%, but opioids will likely contribute to prolonged respiratory depression that may delay extubation. Short-acting narcotics such as remifentanil may be unsuitable for patients undergoing cardiac surgery who have poor left ventricular function attributable to a high incidence of bradycardia and severe hypotension. Although etomidate has been shown to have little effect on the contractility of the cardiac muscle in patients undergoing cardiac transplantation, ketamine has been recommended often for induction in critically ill patients because of its cardiovascular actions attributed primarily to a sympathomimetic effect from the central nervous system. The use of propofol with cardiomyopathy may be a concern, because cardiovascular depression has been observed, possibly attributable to an inhibition of sympathetic activity and a vasodilatory property. However, in a cardiomyopathic hamster model, no direct effect on myocardial contractility was observed with propofol. Caution is prudent with propofol, as it is with any drug, because of its indirect inhibitory effects on the sympathetic activity on which many patients with cardiomyopathy and reduced left ventricular function may depend for hemodynamic stability. As has been stated previously, however, the choice of a particular drug or drug combination is likely less important than how the drugs are used.

Hypertrophic Cardiomyopathy

According to the most recent joint American College of Cardiology (ACC) and AHA guidelines, HCM, the preferred term, is a "disease state characterized by unexplained left ventricular hypertrophy associated with nondilated ventricular chambers in the absence of another cardiac or systemic disease that itself would be capable of producing the magnitude of hypertrophy evident in a given patient." Although the left ventricular hypertrophy, typically quantified with TTE but increasingly assessed with cardiac MRI, may be asymmetric, it need not be nor need it show a preference for the basal septum. Furthermore, although the clinical diagnosis is often made in the context of a left ventricular wall thickness of at least 15 mm in adults, virtually any wall thickness, even measurements within the normal range, may be compatible with the disease. On a microscopic level, HCM is a primary myocardial abnormality with sarcomeric disarray and asymmetric left ventricular hypertrophy. Increased connective tissue, combined with significantly disorganized and hypertrophied myocytes, contributes to the diastolic abnormalities of the disease that exhibit increased chamber stiffness, impaired relaxation, and an unstable electrophysiologic substrate causing complex arrhythmias and sudden death.

HCM is both global and common, perhaps the most common inherited cardiac disease, with a prevalence of at least 1:500 if not closer to 1:200. It is estimated to affect 700,000 Americans if not more. HCM is inherited in autosomal dominant

18

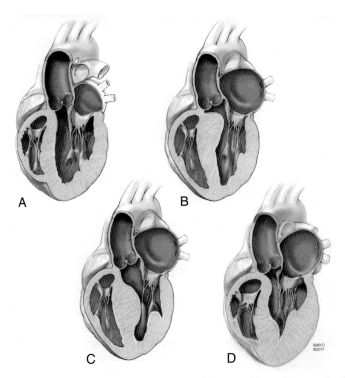

Fig. 18.7 Normal heart and the phenotypic variants of hypertrophic cardiomyopathy. (A) Normal heart. (B) Isolated basal septal hypertrophy. (C) Midventricular septal hypertrophy. (D) Apical hypertrophy. Note that individual patients may have components of more than one type of hypertrophy. (Reproduced with permission from Mayo Foundation for Medical Education and Research. All rights reserved. Illustration No. EBW1078418-001-3.)

fashion, although with variable expressivity and age-related penetrance. It is now known that mutations in at least 11 different genes cause HCM and that these genes encode proteins in both the thick and thin myofilaments, as well as the associated terminal Z-disc.

In the most familiar manifestation of HCM, asymmetric hypertrophy of the basal left ventricular septum produces dynamic left ventricular outflow tract (LVOT) obstruction. More than 50 years of clinical investigation has taught, however, that there are, in fact, multiple patterns of hypertrophy, and the absence of basal hypertrophy, systolic anterior motion (SAM) of the mitral valve, and associated dynamic LVOT obstruction does not exclude the diagnosis of HCM. Other common morphologic types, frequently visualized more clearly with cardiac MRI than with TTE, include a midventricular variant and an apical variant (Fig. 18.7).

Clinically, patients tend to progress along one or more of three pathways: sudden cardiac death, heart failure, and atrial fibrillation with or without cardioembolic stroke (Fig. 18.8).

ICD placement is the only intervention proven to prolong life in patients with HCM. Pharmacologic therapy with β-blockers or calcium channel blockers may offer symptom relief, but it does not improve mortality. Defibrillators are not without complications, however, which occur at an estimated annual rate of 4% to 5% and include inappropriate device discharge, lead fracture or dislodgement, device-related infection, and device-associated bleeding or thrombosis.

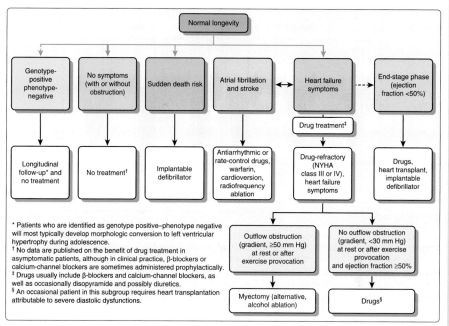

Fig. 18.8 Prognostic pathways and treatment strategies for various presentations of hypertrophic cardiomyopathy. Pathways are not necessarily mutually exclusive. *Colored arrow thickness* represents the proportion of patients affected for every pathway. *NYHA,* New York Heart Association. (Reproduced with permission from Maron BJ, Maron MS. Hypertrophic cardiomyopathy. *Lancet.* 2013;381:247.)

The second pathway along which HCM may progress is that of heart failure, initially diastolic and subsequently systolic. Although many patients with HCM will remain asymptomatic and enjoy a normal life expectancy, others will become symptomatic, complaining of dyspnea on exertion, palpitations, and chest pain. Almost one-half of patients with HCM will develop signs and symptoms of heart failure. Although the symptoms of heart failure frequently reflect dynamic LVOT obstruction and compromise of forward flow, especially under the conditions of hypovolemia, tachycardia, and increased contractility as may occur during exercise or stress, they may occur in the absence of obstruction, reflecting instead an imbalance of myocardial oxygen supply and demand in the context of a grossly hypertrophied heart with an endocardium constantly on the brink of ischemia; impaired left ventricular diastolic function with compromised relaxation and compliance; and the presence often of dynamic mitral regurgitation.

For patients with the classic asymmetric hypertrophy of the basal left ventricular septum, as opposed to those with either the midventricular or apical variant HCM, obstruction occurs as blood ejects from the apex of the LV through the outflow tract and across the aortic valve, passing through a channel of changing caliber created by the hypertrophied basal septum and SAM of the mitral valve apparatus. Hypovolemia, decreased systemic vascular resistance (SVR), tachycardia, and increased contractility, all of which may occur with exercise, stress, and surgical intervention under anesthesia, act in concert to exacerbate outflow tract obstruction. For clinical decision-making purposes, it is the peak (or maximum) instantaneous gradient that influences treatment decisions. A resting gradient 30 mm Hg or greater across the LVOT is consistent with basal obstruction and is an independent predictor of heart failure and death, whereas a gradient 50 mm Hg or greater, either with rest or provocation, is considered sufficient

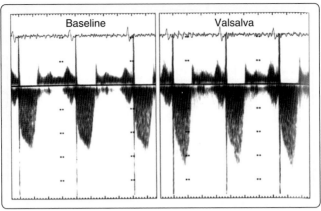

Fig. 18.9 Continuous-wave Doppler spectra obtained from the apex demonstrates dynamic left ventricular (LV) outflow tract obstruction. Note the typical late-peaking configuration resembling a dagger or ski slope *(arrows)*. The baseline *(left)* velocity is 2.8 m/sec, corresponding to the peak LV outflow tract of 31 mm Hg. With the Valsalva maneuver *(right)*, the velocity increases to 3.5 m/sec, corresponding to a gradient of 49 mm Hg. (From Oh JK, Seward JB, Tajik AJ: *The Echo Manual*, ed 3, 2006. Used with permission of Mayo Foundation of Medical Education and Research. All rights reserved.)

to prompt consideration of surgical or percutaneous septal reduction in a severely symptomatic patient.

TTE is the modality of choice for the evaluation of HCM. Continuous-wave Doppler is used to quantify the gradient across the LVOT. The Doppler signal has a unique "dagger-shaped" appearance (Fig. 18.9). With the anterior leaflet likely both pushed and drawn into the outflow tract, the jet of mitral regurgitation is typically directed posteriorly (Fig. 18.10). Although posteriorly directed, mitral regurgitation associated with dynamic LVOT obstruction, even when severe, rarely requires surgical intervention and will largely resolve after the cause is addressed (specifically, LVOT obstruction secondary to basal septal hypertrophy).

For patients with symptoms of heart failure attributable to outflow obstruction, the first-line treatment is pharmacologic therapy with β-blockers with the express purpose of providing symptom relief. For patients unable to tolerate β-blockers, nondihydropyridine calcium channel blockers such as verapamil and diltiazem are second-line agents, although they may exacerbate outflow tract obstruction by lowering mean arterial pressure. For patients who remain symptomatic, despite treatment with either or both β-blockers and calcium channel blockers, both of which may lower exercise-induced but not basal gradients, disopyramide can reduce resting outflow tract gradients and afford a degree of symptom relief.

For patients with persistent symptoms despite pharmacologic therapy, interventional therapy with either alcohol septal ablation or surgical myectomy is the next option. For patients with severe symptoms (NYHA functional class III or IV) and severe resting or provoked LVOT obstruction (≥50 mm Hg), despite maximal medical treatment, surgical septal myectomy is a class I indication. With operative mortality now less than 1%, septal myectomy has the potential to normalize life expectancy for affected individuals.

After the myectomy, TEE is used to assess the degree of residual mitral regurgitation and evidence of continued SAM and LVOT obstruction. The ventricular septum must also be closely evaluated for evidence of shunting via an iatrogenic ventricular septal

IV

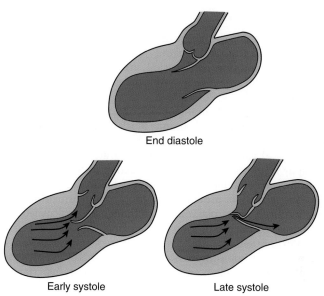

End diastole

Early systole   Late systole

Fig. 18.10 Mechanisms of left ventricular outflow tract (LVOT) obstruction in hypertrophic cardiomyopathy. The systolic anterior motion (SAM) of the anterior leaflet of the mitral valve begins early in systole, often during isovolemic left ventricular contraction (not depicted) when Venturi effects are negligible. As the aortic valve opens and the ejection phase of systole proceeds *(lower left and right images)*, the anterior mitral valve leaflet is both pushed and pulled into the LVOT. In addition, the jet of mitral regurgitation associated with SAM is classically directed posterolaterally (see text for details). (Reproduced with permission from Oliver WC, Mauermann WJ, Nuttall GA. Uncommon cardiac diseases. In: Kaplan JA, Reich DL, Savino JS, eds. *Kaplan's Cardiac Anesthesia: The Echo Era.* 6th ed. Philadelphia: Saunders; 675–736; and from Ommen SR, Shah PM, Tajik AJ. Left ventricular outflow tract obstruction in hypertrophic cardiomyopathy: past, present and future. Heart. 2008;94:1276–1281, 2008.)

defect (VSD). It is common to see small shunts into the area of the LVOT from transection of coronary vessels at the site of the myectomy. It is important that these shunts are not confused with shunting from a VSD. When an iatrogenic VSD occurs, the expected shunt would be from the LV into the RV, as opposed to the flow observed into the LV from transection of septal coronary artery branches. In addition, shunting through a VSD would be expected to occur predominantly during systole, whereas flow into the LV from septal perforators is predominantly during diastole.

For patients with severe symptoms, despite optimal medical management, and those who are poor surgical candidates or show a strong desire to avoid open-heart surgery, alcohol septal ablation is an alternative to septal myectomy. The procedure's objective is to identify a prominent anteroseptal-perforating branch of the left anterior descending coronary artery that is supplying the hypertrophied, culprit portion of the basal septum. Once such a vessel is identified, 1 to 3 mL of ethanol alcohol is infused to create a localized infarction, leading to subsequent necrosis and regression of the area of the basal septum contributing to outflow tract obstruction. Although remodeling takes place over the succeeding months, the injection can affect an immediate decrease in gradient as a result of myocardial stunning. It is associated with a higher risk of need for permanent pacemaker placement; a greater need for repeat procedures, secondary to recurrent or persistent obstruction; and the risk of malignant ventricular arrhythmias attributable to the transmural infarction that is produced.

18

Anesthetic Considerations

The patients most challenging to manage hemodynamically are those with asymmetric hypertrophy of the basal septum and dynamic outflow tract obstruction. The conditions that favor obstruction, and thus hypotension, are the conditions to be avoided and treated quickly should they occur: tachycardia, increased contractility, decreased SVR, and hypovolemia.

After myectomy, a left bundle branch block or a partial left bundle branch block is common. Preoperative right bundle branch block increases the risk of postoperative complete heart block.

Patients with apical variant HCM deserve separate mention. In these patients, apical hypertrophy is not associated with obstruction or SAM but produces a small chamber size, which, in combination with a hypertrophied and stiff myocardium and abnormal diastolic relaxation, produces a significant impairment in diastolic filling and results in abnormally low stroke volumes. Although their calculated left ventricular ejection fraction may be normal or even supranormal, they have a depressed cardiac index in the context of their low stroke volume. It frequently takes very little change in stroke volume to fall from normotensive to uncomfortably hypotensive or to push left-sided filling pressures to the point of pulmonary venous hypertension.

Restrictive Cardiomyopathy

Primary RCM is a rare myocardial disease characterized, in the words of the AHA and in concordance with the European Society of Cardiology, "by normal or decreased volume of both ventricles associated with biatrial enlargement, normal LV wall thickness and AV [atrioventricular] valves, impaired ventricular filling with restrictive physiology, and normal (or near normal) systolic function." Whereas DCM is a morphologic definition, RCM is a pathophysiologic one, characterized by impaired myocardial relaxation and decreased ventricular compliance combining to produce elevated filling pressures (Box 18.3).

Diagnostically, distinguishing RCM from constrictive pericarditis (CP) is important, considering that their treatments are quite different (Table 18.4). In both disorders, filling pressures are elevated; although in restrictive disease, elevated pressures reflect a stiffened myocardium, whereas in constrictive disease, they reflect the constraint of a stiff pericardium. Treatment for RCM should be based on the underlying disease process, if it is known (eg, enzyme-replacement therapy for Gaucher and Fabry diseases, steroids for sarcoidosis); otherwise, pharmacotherapy is tailored toward heart failure symptom relief. With biatrial enlargement, patients with RCM are prone to atrial fibrillation, for which rate therapy and anticoagulation should be used if persistent.

Anesthetic Considerations

Individuals with RCM only infrequently undergo cardiac surgery. One exception, however, is patients with amyloidosis, who may undergo circulatory-assist device placement, orthotopic heart transplantation, or combined heart and liver transplantation.

The choice of induction and maintenance drugs may certainly be based on theoretical concerns related to patient physiologic considerations, but no evidenced-based data exist to support a given pharmacologic regimen clinically. Patients with cardiac amyloid scheduled for transplantation may prove to have particularly labile if not frankly unstable hemodynamics at the time of induction. The combination of severely compromised diastolic function and impaired ventricular filling, likely systolic heart failure, and

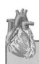

> ## BOX 18.3 *Classification of Types of Restrictive Cardiomyopathy According to Cause*
>
> **Myocardial Causes**
>
> Noninfiltrative
> - Idiopathic cardiomyopathy[a]
> - Familial cardiomyopathy
> - Hypertrophic cardiomyopathy
> - Scleroderma
> - Pseudoxanthoma elasticum
> - Diabetic cardiomyopathy
>
> Infiltrative
> - Amyloidosis[a]
> - Sarcoidosis[a]
> - Gaucher disease
> - Hurler disease
> - Fatty infiltration
>
> Storage diseases
> - Hemochromatosis
> - Fabry disease
> - Glycogen storage disease
>
> **Endomyocardial Causes**
>
> Endomyocardial fibrosis[a]
> Hypereosinophilic syndrome
> Carcinoid heart disease
> Metastatic cancers
> Radiation[a]
> Toxic effects of anthracycline[a]
> Drugs causing fibrous endocarditis (serotonin, methysergide, ergotamine, mercurial agents, busulfan)
>
> [a]Conditions more likely to be encountered in clinical practice.
>
> Reproduced with permission from Oliver WC, Mauermann WJ, Nuttall GA. Uncommon cardiac diseases. In: Kaplan JA, Reich DL, Savino JS, eds. *Kaplan's Cardiac Anesthesia: The Echo Era*, 6th ed. Philadelphia: Saunders; 2011:693.

18

autonomic instability with amyloid infiltration of the nervous system, can conspire to make the effects of even the most judicious doses of drugs unpredictable.

Arrhythmogenic Right Ventricular Cardiomyopathy

Formerly called *arrhythmogenic right ventricular dysplasia*, ARVC is defined by the WHO in 1995 as "progressive fibrofatty replacement of RV myocardium, initially with typical regional and later global RV and some LV involvement, with relative sparing of the septum."

ARVC is familial in 30% to 50% of persons, with primarily autosomal dominant inheritance, variable expressivity, and reduced penetrance. The prevalence of ARVC has been estimated between 1:2000 and 1:5000, with men affected at a ratio of 3:1. Its presentation most commonly begins with the onset of arrhythmias ranging from

Table 18.4 Differentiation of Pericardial Constriction and Myocardial Restriction

Characteristic	Constrictive Pericarditis	Restrictive Cardiomyopathy
Jugular venous waveform	Elevated with less rapid y descent	Elevated with more rapid y descent Large A waves
LAP > RAP	Absent	Almost always
Auscultation	Early S₃ high pitched; no S₄	Late S₃ low pitched; S₄ in some cases
Mitral or tricuspid regurgitation	Frequently absent	Frequently present
Chest roentgenogram	Calcification of pericardium (20–30%)	Pericardial calcification rare
Heart size	Normal to increased	Normal to increased
Electrocardiogram	Conduction abnormalities rare	Conduction abnormalities common
Echocardiogram	Slight enlargement of atria	Major enlargement of atria
Right ventricular pressure waveform	Square-root pattern	Square-root pattern; dip and plateau often less prominent
Right- and left-sided heart diastolic pressures	Within 5 mm Hg of each other in almost all cases	Seldom within 5 mm Hg of each other
Peak right ventricular systolic pressure	Almost always <60 mm Hg, sometimes <40 mm Hg	Usually >40 mm Hg, sometimes >60 mm Hg
Discordant respiratory variation of peak ventricular systolic pressures	Right and left ventricular systolic pressures are out of phase with respiration	In phase with respiration
Paradoxic pulse	Often present	Rare
CT and MRI imaging	Thickened pericardium	Rarely thickened pericardium
Endomyocardial biopsy	Normal or nonspecific changes	Nonspecific abnormalities

CT, Computed tomography; *LAP,* left atrial pressure; *MRI,* magnetic resonance imaging; *RAP,* right atrial pressure.
Reproduced with permission from Hancock EW: Cardiomyopathy: Differential diagnosis of restrictive cardiomyopathy and constrictive pericarditis. *Heart.* 2001;86:343–349; and Chatterjee K, Alpert J. Constrictive pericarditis and restrictive cardiomyopathy: similarities and differences. *Heart Fail Monit.* 2003;3:118–126.
Reproduced with permission from Oliver WC, Mauermann WJ, Nuttall GA. Uncommon cardiac diseases. In: Kaplan JA, Reich DL, Savino JS, eds. *Kaplan's Cardiac Anesthesia: The Echo Era.* 6th ed. Philadelphia: Saunders; 2011:694.

premature ventricular contractions to ventricular fibrillation originating from the RV. The disease is now known to proceed through three phases: (1) concealed phase without symptoms but some electrophysiologic changes that place one at risk for sudden death; (2) overt dysrhythmias; (3) advanced stage with myocardial loss, biventricular involvement, and CHF. Postmortem examination reveals diffuse or segmental loss of the myocardium, primarily in the RV, replaced with fat and fibrous tissue; right ventricular dilation; and thinning of the right ventricular free wall. The replacement of myocardium with fat and fibrous tissue creates an excellent environment for a fatal arrhythmia, possibly the first sign of ARVC. Although a rare disease, ARVC accounts for 20% of sudden death in the young. Diagnosis based on Revised Task Force Criteria graded aberrations (major and minor) include structural alterations (diagnosed by echocardiography, MRI, and/or right ventricular angiography), histologic evaluation, echocardiographic abnormalities, arrhythmias, genetic studies, and family history. Diagnosis may depend on endomyocardial biopsy to reveal the distinctive changes of ARVC, yet be unrewarding if the biopsy is obtained from the septal area of the myocardium known for its lack of characteristic features.

Anesthetic Considerations

During the course of ARVC, arrhythmias of both a supraventricular and ventricular nature may occur. Because arrhythmias are more likely in the perioperative period, noxious stimuli, hypovolemia, hypercarbia, and light anesthesia must be minimized intraoperatively and during recovery. However, general anesthesia, alone, does not appear to be arrhythmogenic. Acidosis may be especially detrimental because of its effect on arrhythmia generation and myocardial function.

▓ MITRAL VALVE PROLAPSE

Mitral valve prolapse (MVP) with severe mitral regurgitation is a common reason for cardiac surgery today. As the most commonly diagnosed cardiac valve abnormality, MVP occurs in adults who are otherwise healthy or in association with many pathologic conditions (Box 18.4) and is equally distributed between men and women. MVP is a degenerative condition with myxoid found on histologic examination that causes thickening, elongation, and a change in the chordae. Currently, MVP is known to be a spectrum of structural and functional valve anomalies affecting 1% to 2% of the population, depending on accepted criteria for diagnosis. In patients with degenerative mitral valve disease, a spectrum of disease is appreciated, ranging from fibroelastic deficiency to Barlow disease (Fig. 18.11). Fibroelastic deficiency was first identified by Carpentier as a form of MVP without billowing or excess valve tissue. The mechanism is impaired connective tissue production attributable to a deficiency of collagens, elastins, and proteoglycans, but the cause is unknown. Unlike Barlow disease, symptoms of fibroelastic deficiency generally arrive with chordal rupture, are frequently observed with advancing age, and include a significantly less pronounced, generalized degeneration of the mitral valve than Barlow disease. Surgical repair is also less complex.

Barlow disease is believed to result from myxomatous degeneration of the mitral valve, elongation and thinning of the chordae tendineae, and the presence of redundant and excessive valve tissue. The mechanism is unknown, but regulation of the extracellular matrix components appears to be a primary issue. Normal mitral valve leaflets may billow slightly with closure, but in MVP, redundant mitral leaflets prolapse into the LA during mid-to-late systole (Fig. 18.12). Superior arching of the mitral leaflets above the level of the atrioventricular ring is diagnostic for MVP. Distortion or malfunction of any of the component structures of the mitral valve may cause prolapse and generate audible clicks or regurgitation associated with a murmur. If the chordae tendineae are lengthened, then the valves may billow even more and progress to prolapse when valve leaflets fail to oppose each other. The degree of these changes will determine the presence of mitral regurgitation. Three-dimensional echocardiography has provided new insight into the characterization of mitral valve disease.

Finally, even histologically, normal mitral valves may prolapse. Normal mitral valve function depends on a number of factors, including the size of the LV and the mitral leaflets. Changes in these components may cause *innocent* MVP.

18

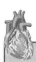
BOX 18.4 *Conditions Associated With Mitral Valve Prolapse*

Connective Tissue Disorders—Genetic

Mitral valve prolapse—isolated
Marfan syndrome
Ehlers-Danlos syndrome—types I, II, and IV
Pseudoxanthoma elasticum
Osteogenesis imperfecta
Polycystic kidney disease

Other Genetic Disorders

Duchenne muscular dystrophy
Myotonic dystrophy
Fragile X syndrome
Mucopolysaccharidoses

Acquired Collagen-Vascular Disorders

Systemic lupus erythematosus
Relapsing polychondritis
Rheumatic endocarditis
Polyarteritis nodosa

Other Associated Disorders

Atrial septal defect—secundum
Hypertrophic obstructive cardiomyopathy
Wolff-Parkinson-White syndrome
Papillary muscle dysfunction
• Ischemic heart disease
• Myocarditis
Cardiac trauma
Post–mitral valve surgery
von Willebrand disease

From Fontana ME, Sparks EA, Boudoulas H, Wooley CF. Mitral valve prolapse and the mitral valve prolapse syndrome. *Curr Probl Cardiol.* 1991;16(5):309–375.

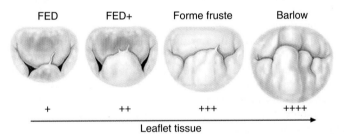

Fig. 18.11 Spectrum of degenerative mitral disease. Degenerative disease spectrum includes: fibroelastic deficiency *(FED)* with thin leaflets and a ruptured chordae *(+)*, long-standing FED leading to myxomatous changes of the prolapsing segment *(++)*, forme fruste with myxomatous disease and excessive tissue in one or more leaflet segments *(+++)*, and Barlow disease with myxomatous changes, excessive leaflet tissue, and large valve size *(++++)*. (Reproduced with permission from Adams DH, Rosenhek R, Falk V. Degenerative mitral valve regurgitation: best practice revolution. *Eur Heart J.* 2010;31:1958–1966.)

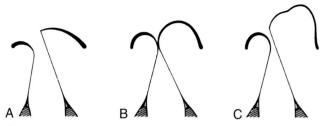

Fig. 18.12 Diagrammatic representation of the pathologic functioning of the mitral valve mechanism. (A) Regurgitation is present with mitral valve prolapse. (B) Billowing mitral valve is demonstrated without prolapse or regurgitation. (C) Billowing and prolapsed mitral leaflets are revealed with regurgitation. (Reproduced with permission of American Heart Association. From Barlow JB, Pocock WA. Mitral valve prolapse enigma—two decades later. *Mod Concepts Cardiovasc Dis.* 1984;53:13.)

No universal criteria for diagnosis of MVP are available. Typical auscultatory features are midsystolic click and late-systolic murmur. Certain maneuvers aid with the auscultatory diagnosis of MVP such as Valsalva, squatting, or leg raises that change the left ventricular end-diastolic volume to move the timing of the click within systole. Currently, MVP is diagnosed more often with two-dimensional echocardiography, because recognition and assessment of the severity is superior. Given the saddle-shaped nature of the mitral annulus, the diagnosis of MVP is typically made from the parasternal long-axis view using TTE. MVP is defined as greater than 2 mm displacement of one or both mitral leaflets into the LA during systole.

Most patients with MVP are asymptomatic; however, controlled studies have reported the presence of palpitations in 50% of patients. Altered autonomic function, catecholamine responsiveness, or possibly a combination of the two may account for complaints of chest pain, fatigue, palpitations, dyspnea, dizziness, syncope, and panic attacks, among others. These symptoms and some clinical findings of thin body type, low blood pressure, and electrocardiographic repolarization abnormalities have been associated with MVP and are termed *MVP syndrome*. Mitral valve regurgitation is the most serious complication associated with MVP. Severe mitral regurgitation develops in approximately 2% to 4% of patients with MVP, two-thirds of whom are male patients. Most patients will have mild-to-moderate mitral regurgitation that does not require surgery. MVP is the most common cause of severe mitral regurgitation, and its onset signals the need for therapeutic intervention. Irrespective of symptoms, the onset of severe mitral regurgitation can result in reduced life expectancy. The posterior leaflet is affected more frequently than the anterior leaflet. Changes are often observed at the site of chordal insertion, leading to rupture of the chordae and a tethering of the valve leaflet. With the development of severe mitral regurgitation, pulmonary hypertension, left atrial enlargement, and atrial fibrillation frequently emerge. Early repair is recommended to preserve left ventricular function and to reduce the likelihood of atrial fibrillation. The management of MVP and mitral regurgitation without symptoms continues to be reconsidered in terms of the timing for cardiac surgical intervention, especially in view of the risk of mitral valve repair and the improved outcomes associated with earlier surgery.

Mitral valve repair is widely recommended for treatment of MVP, compared with replacement. Mitral valve repair confers a significantly improved surgical survival, as well as 5- and 10-year survival, compared with mitral valve replacement. Advantages of mitral valve repair, compared with replacement, include a lower risk of thromboembolism, bleeding, infectious endocarditis, and better ventricular function because the valve structure is preserved. Posterior leaflet prolapse is the most common defect

18

in mitral regurgitation. The posterior leaflet repair is historically low risk, with bileaflet repairs presenting greater technical difficulty. The anterior prolapse repair has a higher rate of reoperation and decreased survival. Recently, endovascular mitral valve repair via MitraClip devices (Abbott Vascular, Santa Clara, CA) has emerged as a viable treatment option for select nonoperable candidates with mitral valve regurgitation.

The association of arrhythmias and sudden death with MVP is a long-held observation. Premature atrial and ventricular beats, atrioventricular block, and supraventricular or ventricular tachyarrhythmias are common during ambulatory monitoring in adults with MVP. The causes of these arrhythmias are multifactorial, probably combining an anatomic substrate with some form of dysautonomia. The occurrence of sudden death with MVP in adults has been debated for years. The risk is low, with an estimated yearly rate of 40 in 10,000, but this number is twice the expected rate in the population. Sudden death does occur within families of patients with MVP. The ECG is abnormal in approximately two-thirds of persons with MVP, but ambulatory electrocardiographic monitoring does not show an excess of atrial or ventricular arrhythmias unless accompanied by severe mitral regurgitation. In general, most low-risk patients do not require treatment for either their symptoms or to prevent sudden death.

Bacterial endocarditis is an infrequent complication of MVP, but its incidence is three to eight times greater in these individuals than in the general population. Current guidelines from the AHA are very specific and do not recommend antibiotic prophylaxis for individuals without a prosthetic cardiac valve, complex congenital heart disease (CHD), postcardiac transplant valvular lesions, or a history of bacterial endocarditis.

Anesthetic Considerations

Understanding the broad nature of the condition called MVP with respect to anesthetic considerations is important. Most individuals with MVP have an uncomplicated general anesthetic, because they have MVP without serious complications, often referred to as MVP syndrome. Anticholinergic preoperative medications are best avoided, despite an increased vagal tone in MVP. A moderate anesthetic depth is desirable to minimize catecholamine levels and potential arrhythmias. Ketamine or drugs that have sympathomimetic effects must be cautiously administered. Hypercapnia, hypoxia, and electrolyte disturbances increase ventricular excitability and should be corrected. If muscle relaxation is desired, then vecuronium is an excellent choice, because it does not cause tachycardia.

Patients with MVP who have mitral regurgitation are at greater risk for complications and warrant a different anesthetic approach compared with those with MVP syndrome. Patients with more severe forms of MVP may rapidly progress to CHF and require cardiac surgery. The severity of mitral regurgitation will strongly influence anesthetic management. Unique aspects of anesthetic management for robotic mitral valve surgery involve peripheral bypass cannulation, single-lung ventilation, and often regional anesthetic techniques (eg, paravertebral block) to facilitate immediate postoperative extubation. Anesthetic management for endovascular mitral valve repair (MitraClip, Abbott Vascular, Santa Clara, CA) typically requires general anesthesia to facilitate frequent transesophageal echocardiographic manipulation for proper device placement.

▣ PATENT FORAMEN OVALE

A PFO is the most common congenital defect involving the atrial septum. Air, thrombus, or fat may travel via PFO from the RA to the LA into the systemic circulation causing a paradoxic embolus that may affect cerebral or coronary circulations. The ability to so readily and safely close a PFO with minimally invasive techniques has created the need to develop guidelines to address the management of PFO.

The foramen ovale is present during fetal circulation to improve the transport of maternal-oxygenated blood from the umbilical veins across the Eustachian valve selectively into the LA. With birth and the onset of respiration, pulmonary vascular resistance decreases, facilitating functional closure of the foramen ovale. If the flaplike covering from the septum primum does not fuse with the septum secundum over a period of a year, then there is anatomic failure of closure forming a PFO (Fig. 18.13). In patients with a PFO, any condition resulting in right atrial pressures exceeding left atrial pressures will facilitate right-to-left shunting. In contrast, left-sided heart conditions that result in left atrial pressures greatly exceeding right atrial pressures will

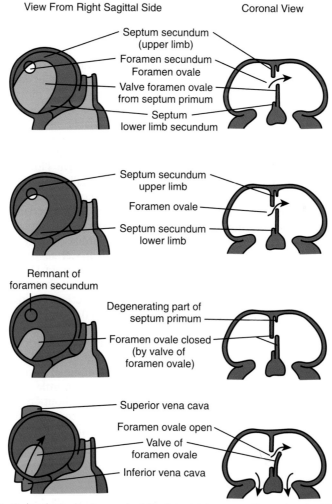

Fig. 18.13 Embryologic development of the interatrial septum. (Reproduced with permission from Hara H, Virmani R, Ladich E, et al. Patent foramen ovale: current pathology, pathophysiology, and clinical status. *J Am Coll Cardiol*. 2005;46:1768–1776.)

cause left-to-right shunting. An individual may remain asymptomatic for years with a PFO, depending on the size of the shunt.

The incidence of PFO in the population has varied, depending on the study and diagnostic technique. TEE has become the gold standard for diagnosing PFO with its higher image resolution than other methods and 100% sensitivity and specificity with autopsy findings. Because TEE is more invasive, additional technical advances in both TTE and transcranial Doppler have improved their sensitivity and, when combined, may be adequate for PFO screening purposes.

The decision to close a PFO will include individual risk factors for stroke or other complications such as migraine headaches and platypnea orthodeoxia syndrome that may occur in the context of a PFO. Paradoxic embolus is more common if an atrial septal aneurysm, a large Eustachian valve, migraines, and an age of 50 years or older are present. Medium-to-large shunts, in combination with coagulation disorders, are highly correlated with paradoxic embolus. To diagnose paradoxic embolus, performing a correct provocative measure to ensure right-to-left movement of air or contrast is essential. Agitated saline directed through an intravenous line with the Valsalva maneuver is most commonly used to confirm the diagnosis. The increased intrathoracic pressure from the Valsalva maneuver will lead to a temporary increased return of venous blood after the maneuver has ended; therefore the right atrial pressure will briefly exceed left atrial pressure to allow contrast administered into the right internal jugular vein to pass to the LA. False-negative results may occur if the left atrial pressure is elevated to such an extent that the provocative measure does not cause right-to-left shunting.

Management of a PFO is dependent on several variables and has been largely debated because of the mixed results of several recent large studies and metaanalyses. Currently, surgically closing an isolated PFO with the safety and availability of percutaneous closure is rare. However, the use of intraoperative TEE during cardiac surgical procedures has increased the number of incidentally diagnosed PFOs. Not only are more PFOs closed as a percentage, but, over time, more surgeons as a percentage are choosing to close them. The cause for these trends is not certain, but a PFO diagnosed incidentally during surgery creates a dilemma for the surgeon.

The decision to close an incidental PFO during cardiac surgery is not always evident, based on short- and long-term risks to the patient. Certain conditions would almost mandate the closure of the PFO, such as the insertion of LVAD that would promote paradoxic embolus or the onset of severe hypoxia attributable to increased right-sided pressures that cause a large right-to-left shunt. Little evidence suggests that incidentally discovered PFOs in patients without respective history increase morbidity or mortality. In fact, one study demonstrated that an alteration in the surgical plan to include the closure of an incidental PFO actually increased the risk of stroke. Certain surgical procedures, such as tricuspid or mitral valve repair or replacement that includes CPB and atriotomy, require minimal deviation from the originally planned procedure to close the PFO and thus incur little risk. In contrast, coronary artery bypass graft (CABG) surgery performed without CPB would entail the risk of going on CPB, aortic cross-clamping, and other complications associated with extracorporeal circulation. The decision to close an incidental PFO in such circumstances must include careful examination of the perceived risk and benefit for each individual patient.

Anesthetic Considerations

Anesthesia management for percutaneous PFO closure typically involves conscious sedation. Intraoperative management for the closure of an incidental PFO during cardiac surgery requires very little deviation from the anesthetic management of the scheduled procedure. However, certain precautions should be undertaken once the PFO has been identified.

Routine care for preventing venous air should be standard for cardiac surgery, including careful injection of medications to remove extraneous air from entering the venous system. Some providers use inline air filters on all intravenous lines once the presence of the PFO has been identified, but such practice is not widespread. Appreciating the potential for paradoxic embolus with any patient requiring mechanical ventilation is important. In situations during which the pulmonary vascular resistance may rise, such as during hypercapnia or with positive end-expiratory pressure (PEEP) greater than 15 mm Hg, the potential for right-to-left shunting increases.

PULMONARY HEMORRHAGE

Pulmonary hemorrhage occurs in approximately 1.5% of patients with hemoptysis; but mortality may reach 85%. The definition of massive hemoptysis varies but is commonly characterized as more than 600 mL of expectorated blood over 24 hours or recurrent bleeding greater than 100 mL per day for several days. Four hundred milliliters of blood in the alveolar space seriously impairs oxygenation. Pulmonary hemorrhage may stabilize, only to worsen again without an obvious explanation, reflecting its unpredictable nature. Notably, death is not attributable to hemodynamic instability with hemorrhage but to excessive blood in the alveoli that causes hypoventilation and refractory hypoxia. Clot formation may lead to occlusion of bronchial segments or even the mainstem bronchus. A delay in initiating treatment because of difficulty in isolating the location of bleeding contributes greatly to the high mortality of pulmonary hemorrhage.

Hemoptysis may occur with various diseases and circumstances (Box 18.5). Massive hemoptysis is usually an emergency, because the underlying pulmonary disorder minimizes the patient's physiologic reserve.

Therapeutic options for bleeding depend on the extent of bleeding. Flexible bronchoscopy may be able to identify the source of bleeding and perform techniques, such as epinephrine flush and cold-saline lavage to minimize hemorrhage and possible balloon bronchial blockers to tamponade any bleeding. Advancements in bronchoscopy have seen success with the use of topically applied agents consisting of oxidized regenerated cellulose mesh injected at the site of bleeding. Additionally, the use of topically applied factor VIIa (FVIIa) has been reported with success in massive hemolysis, secondary to a medical cause, although its use in this manner is off label. Other medications used to reduce bleeding include Premarin, desmopressin, vasopressin, and tranexamic acid. With rapid or persistent bleeding, a double-lumen endotracheal tube (ETT) may be necessary to isolate the bleeding from the unaffected lung.

Continued bleeding after stabilization and conservative therapy necessitates bronchial artery embolization, which is considered first-line therapy for massive hemoptysis. Although success rates of 75% to 98% have been reported, 16% to 20% of patients rebleed within 1 year.

If bleeding persists and/or nonoperative therapies have either failed or are not feasible, then surgical treatment may be required. A localized bleeding site and sufficient lung function are ideally determined before surgical resection, as total pneumonectomy may be required. Postoperative mortality rates vary tremendously from 1% to 50%. Surgery is contraindicated in those with lung carcinoma invading the trachea, mediastinum, heart or great vessels, terminal malignancy, and progressive pulmonary fibrosis.

To reduce the risk for pulmonary artery rupture from PAC, the placement of a PAC distally in the pulmonary artery should be avoided. Advancing the PAC more than 5 cm beyond the pulmonary valve is not advisable. The balloon should not be

18

BOX 18.5 *Causes of Massive Hemoptysis*

Tracheobronchial Disorders

Amyloidosis
Bronchial adenoma
Bronchiectasis[a]
Bronchogenic carcinoma
Broncholithiasis
Bronchovascular fistula
Cystic fibrosis
Foreign body aspiration
Tracheobronchial trauma

Cardiovascular Disorders

Congenital heart disease
Mitral stenosis
Pulmonary arteriovenous fistula
Septic pulmonary emboli
Ruptured thoracic aneurysm
Arteriovenous malformation

Localized Parenchymal Diseases

Amebiasis
Aspergilloma[a]
Atypical mycobacterial infection[a]
Coccidioidomycosis
Lung abscess
Mucormycosis
Pulmonary tuberculosis[a]

Diffuse Parenchymal Diseases

Goodpasture syndrome
Idiopathic pulmonary hemosiderosis
Polyarteritis nodosa
Systemic lupus erythematosus
Wegener granulomatosis

Other Causes

Pulmonary artery rupture from a pulmonary artery catheter
Iatrogenic (eg, bronchoscopy, cardiac catheterization)
Pulmonary hypertension
Pulmonary edema
Pulmonary infarction

[a]Most common causes.
Reproduced with permission from Thompson AB, Teschler H, Rennard SI. Pathogenesis, evaluation, and therapy for massive hemoptysis. *Clin Chest Med.* 1992;13:69.

IV

inflated against increased resistance, particularly if the patient has been given an anticoagulant drug or after separation from CPB. The pulmonary artery waveform should always be carefully observed with inflation and deflation of the balloon. Retracting the PAC into the RV on the initiation of CPB or withdrawing the PAC 5 cm immediately before CPB is advisable.

PERICARDIAL HEART DISEASE

The pericardium is a two-layer sac that encloses the heart and great vessels. The inner layer is a serous membrane (visceral pericardium) covering the surface of the heart. The outer layer is a fibrinous sac (parietal pericardium), which is attached to the great vessels, diaphragm, and sternum. The parietal pericardium is a stiff collagenous membrane that is resistant to acute expansion. The space between the two layers is the pericardial space, normally containing up to 50 mL of clear fluid that is an ultrafiltrate of plasma. It can gradually dilate to accept large volumes of fluid if slowly accumulated; however, rapid fluid accumulation leads to cardiac tamponade. The two layers of the pericardium are joined at the level of the great vessels and at the central tendon of the diaphragm caudally, and a serous layer extends past these junctions to line the inside of the fibrinous sac (parietal pericardium). The lateral course of the phrenic nerve on either side of the heart is an important anatomic relationship because this nerve is encapsulated in the pericardium and thus can easily be damaged during pericardiectomy. The pericardium is not essential for life, and pericardiectomy causes no apparent disability, but it has many subtle functions that are advantageous. Foremost, it acts to minimize torsion of the heart and reduces the friction from surrounding organs.

Acute Pericarditis

Acute pericarditis is common, but the actual incidence is unknown because it often goes unrecognized. It is generally self-limited, with symptoms lasting 6 weeks. Acute pericarditis has many causes (Box 18.6), the most common of which is viral (30–50%). Anesthesiologists encounter patients with acute pericarditis in the context of malignancy,

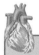

BOX 18.6   *Causes of Acute Pericarditis*

Idiopathic
Infectious
- Viral
- Bacterial
- Fungal
- Parasitic
Immunologic
- Postmyocardial infarction (Dressler syndrome)
- Postcardiotomy syndrome
- Still disease
- Rheumatoid arthritis
- Systemic lupus erythematosus
- Polyarteritis
Neoplastic
Radiation
Traumatic
Renal failure
Drug-induced

Reproduced with permission from Oakley CM. Myocarditis, pericarditis and other pericardial diseases. *Heart*. 2000;84:449–454.

18

Table 18.5	Causes of Constrictive Pericarditis	
Cause		**Percentage**
Idiopathic pericarditis		40
After coronary artery bypass grafting		30
Tuberculosis		10
Radiation-induced		5
Collagen vascular disease		5
Others (malignancy, uremia, purulent)		5

Reproduced with permission from Kabbani SS, LeWinter MM. Diastolic heart failure. Constrictive, restrictive, and pericardial. *Cardiol Clin.* 2000;18:505.

MI, postcardiotomy syndrome, uremia, or infection when surgery is required, because symptoms are incapacitating and medical therapy has failed.

Constrictive Pericarditis

CP is a dense fusion of the parietal and visceral pericardium that limits diastolic filling of the heart, irrespective of the cause. The changes in the pericardium can be due to scarring, induced by a single episode of acute pericarditis, or caused by a prolonged exposure to a recurrent or chronic inflammatory process. Table 18.5 lists some of the causes of chronic CP. Up to 18% of pericardiectomies are attributed to previous cardiac surgeries, which may explain the increase in the number of cases of CP over the last 15 years.

Surgical Considerations for Pericardial Disease

Pericardiectomy is performed for recurrent pericardial effusion and CP refractory to conservative therapies. Pericardial dissection for effusive pericarditis is straightforward; however, pericardiectomy for CP is often a surgical challenge, with an operative mortality of 5.9% to 11.9%. The occurrence of tricuspid regurgitation may occur, similar to CP with signs of right-sided heart failure and volume overload. The presence of tricuspid regurgitation may identify a subset of patients with CP who have more advanced disease.

Persistent low CO immediately after pericardiectomy is a major cause of morbidity and mortality, occurring in 14% to 28% of patients in the immediate postoperative period. These findings are in contrast to the accepted belief that the pericardium is the problem in these patients and the myocardium is normal. Although patients with cardiac tamponade usually improve clinically once the pericardium is opened, improvement is not always apparent immediately after pericardiectomy for patients with CP. Noticeable improvement in cardiac function may take weeks; however, 90% of patients will experience relief of symptoms postoperatively.

Anesthetic Considerations

Anesthetic goals for managing patients with CP for pericardiectomy include minimizing bradycardia, myocardial depression, and decreases in preload and afterload. PAC monitoring is often used because of the risk of low CO syndrome postoperatively.

Low CO syndrome develops in a subset of patients with CP, irrespective of the approach or extent of pericardiectomy. Low CO, hypotension, and arrhythmias (atrial and ventricular) are common during chest dissection. Because of limited and relatively fixed ventricular diastolic filling, CO becomes rate-dependent. If myocardial function or heart rate is depressed, then β-agonists or pacing will improve CO. Catastrophic hemorrhage can occur suddenly if the atrium or ventricle is perforated, necessitating adequate central venous access. Damage to coronary arteries may also occur during dissection; so careful monitoring of the ECG for signs of ischemia is prudent.

Cardiac Tamponade

Tamponade exists when fluid accumulation in the pericardial space dramatically increases intrapericardial pressure and limits filling of the heart. The rate of pericardial fluid accumulation, rather than the absolute fluid volume, is the determinant of tamponade sequelae. The classic Beck triad of acute tamponade, consisting of: (1) decreasing arterial pressure; (2) increasing venous pressure; and (3) a small, quiet heart, is only observed in 10% to 40% of patients. Pulsus paradoxus (Fig. 18.14) may also be observed, which is a fall in systolic blood pressure of more than 10 mm Hg during inspiration, caused by a reduced left ventricular stroke volume that is generated by increased filling of the right-sided heart during inspiration. Pulsus paradoxus is not sensitive or specific for tamponade, because it may be present in those with obstructive pulmonary disease, right ventricular infarction, or CP. Hemodynamic monitoring may aid in the diagnosis of cardiac tamponade. Ultimately, the right atrial pressure, pulmonary artery diastolic pressure, and pulmonary capillary wedge pressure equilibrate. Equilibration of these pressures (within 5 mm Hg of each other) merits immediate action to rule out acute tamponade. Echocardiography is the current method of choice and the most reliable noninvasive method to detect pericardial effusion and exclude tamponade.

Echocardiographic features of tamponade include an exaggerated motion of the heart within the pericardial sac in conjunction with atrial and ventricular collapse.

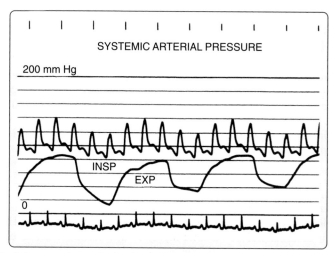

Fig. 18.14 Pulsus paradoxus. During inspiration *(INSP)*, arterial systolic pressure falls by more than 12 mm Hg. *EXP,* Expiration. (Reproduced with permission from Reddy PS, Curtiss EI. Cardiac tamponade. *Cardiol Clin.* 1990;8:628.)

Specific two-dimensional echocardiographic findings that support cardiac tamponade include diastolic collapse of the RV, inversion of the RA during diastole, abnormal ventricular septal motion, and variation of ventricular size with the respiratory cycle. Diastolic collapse of the right-sided chambers occurs because of pericardial pressure exceeding intracardiac pressure during diastole. Right atrial collapse is a specific finding during echocardiographic examination if it is present for more than one-third of the cardiac cycle.

Pericardiocentesis is indicated for life-threatening cardiac tamponade in conjunction with fluid resuscitation to maintain adequate filling pressures. Hemodynamic improvement should ensue after pericardiocentesis. Although pericardiocentesis relieves the symptoms of tamponade, definitive therapy directed at the underlying cause should be pursued. Major complications of pericardiocentesis include coronary artery laceration, cardiac puncture, and pneumothorax. Tamponade attributable to hemorrhage in the patient after cardiac surgery requires immediate mediastinal exploration to determine the source of bleeding and to stabilize hemodynamics.

Anesthetic Considerations

Severe hypotension or cardiac arrest has followed the induction of general anesthesia in patients with tamponade. The causes include myocardial depression, sympatholysis, decreased venous return, and changes in heart rate that often accompany anesthetic medications and positive pressure ventilation. Resuscitation requires immediate drainage of pericardial fluid. Pericardiotomy via a subxiphoid incision with only local anesthetic infiltration or light sedation is an option. If intrapericardial injury is confirmed, then general anesthesia can be induced after decompression of the pericardial space. Ketamine (0.5 mg/kg) and 100% oxygen have been used with local anesthetic infiltration of the preexisting sternotomy to drain severe pericardial tamponade. Spontaneous respirations, instead of positive-pressure ventilation, will support CO more effectively until tamponade is relieved. Correction of metabolic derangements is mandatory. Volume expansion is likely warranted in hypotensive patients. Similar to CP, patients with tamponade have a relatively low and fixed stroke volume and thus rely on heart rate and adequate filling to maintain CO. Catecholamine infusions or pacing may be used to avoid bradycardia.

▣ COMBINED CAROTID AND CORONARY ARTERY DISEASE

The combination of carotid endarterectomy (CEA) and CABG surgery was first proposed by Bernhard and associates in 1972 to reduce morbidity and mortality from coexistent carotid and coronary disease. Renewed interest in this approach now stems from recent controlled trials that demonstrate the benefits of isolated CEA for both symptomatic and asymptomatic severe carotid stenosis. As the population ages, the number of patients with carotid bifurcation stenosis greater than 70% will continue to increase. The result is more patients with combined carotid and coronary disease but with no consensus regarding their treatment.

It is generally accepted that patients with symptomatic carotid disease undergoing CABG surgery are at a significantly increased risk for stroke and merit revascularization of the carotid and coronary disease as a combined or staged procedure. However, the management of unilateral or bilateral *asymptomatic* carotid stenosis continues to evolve. Asymptomatic severe carotid stenosis is a risk for ipsilateral hemispheric stroke with cardiac surgery and CPB, but identifying it in the asymptomatic patient hinders determination of this *true* risk assessment.

Anesthetic Considerations

Beyond the routine monitoring for cardiac surgery, electroencephalography or other modalities to assess neurophysiologic integrity are useful but have a high false-positive rate. For the anesthesiologist, it is helpful to know that the majority of strokes cannot be ascribed to an adverse intraoperative event such as hypotension or low flow. However, it is more difficult to differentiate a *true* stroke from other states of temporary neurologic impairment associated with CABG surgery, such as heavy sedation, residual muscle weakness from a paralyzing agent, or encephalopathy secondary to cerebral edema. By using general anesthesia for CEA, clinical methods to determine neurologic integrity are delayed, as well as a delay in treatment. The use of a local anesthetic for CEA in the combined procedure has proven to be valuable in reducing exposure to anesthesia and reducing shunt-related complications, allowing repair with less risk of damage. The added ability to identify the timing of the neurologic insult may prove valuable, compared with general anesthesia. However, anxiety and pain must be controlled to minimize myocardial ischemia during CEA with local anesthesia. Early extubation is desirable to allow earlier neurologic evaluation in combined cases.

The need for rapid institution of CPB during an awake CEA may prove challenging. Another possibility is the use of general anesthesia for the CEA, followed by a wake-up test, to allow for the evaluation and treatment of any apparent neurologic injury before initiating CPB.

CARDIAC SURGERY DURING PREGNANCY

Heart disease is a major risk factor for maternal and fetal death during pregnancy, with an incidence of 1% to 3%. It is the most common cause of nonobstetric mortality during pregnancy, accounting for 10% to 15% of maternal mortality. Obstetric patients with heart disease are at great risk for serious complications as a result of hemodynamic changes associated with pregnancy and delivery. If cardiac surgery is required during or immediately after pregnancy, then anesthetic management demands an appreciation for the many changes of pregnancy and their effects on the corresponding heart disease and well-being of the fetus.

Certain physiologic changes of pregnancy negatively affect the woman with heart disease. Heart rate and stroke volume are each increased by 25% by the end of the second trimester. Early in the third trimester, intravascular volume has expanded by nearly 50%. These three changes during pregnancy cause a 50% increase in CO that is aggravated by physiologic anemia and aortocaval compression. Labor contractions can rapidly increase the already elevated CO. Such increases in blood volume and CO are especially difficult for a parturient with valvular heart disease. Elevated CO will increase myocardial oxygen demand, exacerbating CHF, and low SVR will worsen coronary perfusion, causing myocardial ischemia.

Mitral valve disease is the most common valvular disorder that requires surgery in pregnancy. Chronic mitral or aortic regurgitation may actually be associated with a small symptomatic improvement, secondary to the normal physiologic changes of pregnancy. In contrast, stenotic valvular lesions tolerate these changes poorly. Aortic and mitral stenosis are common problems that may lead to hemodynamic deterioration, forcing emergency delivery before cardiac surgery. The most frequent indication for emergency cardiac surgery during pregnancy is decompensation from CHF attributable to mitral stenosis. Since the early 1950s, when heart surgery requiring CPB in a pregnant patient was first described, maternal morbidity has fallen from 5% to less than 1%. Fetal mortality remains high, ranging from 16% to 33%. Unfortunately,

18

fetal mortality is related to the use of CPB, duration of the surgery, and hypothermia. The nonphysiologic nature of CPB combines with the changes of pregnancy for an uncertain response and tolerance by both the mother and the fetus. CPB exposes the fetus to many undesirable effects that may have unpredictable consequences. Initiation of CPB activates a whole-body inflammatory response with multiple effects on coagulation, autoregulation, release of vasoactive substances, hemodilution, and other physiologic processes that may adversely affect both the fetus and the mother. Maternal blood pressure may fall immediately after or within 5 minutes of initiating CPB, lowering placental perfusion secondary to low SVR, hemodilution, and the release of vasoactive agents. Fetal heart rate variability is often lost, and fetal bradycardia (<80 bpm) may also occur at this time. Because uterine blood flow is not autoregulated and relies on maternal blood flow, decreases of maternal blood pressure cause fetal hypoxia and bradycardia. Increasing CPB flows (>2.5 L/m^2 per minute) or perfusion pressure (>70 mm Hg) will raise maternal blood flow and usually return the fetal heart rate to 120 bpm. A compensatory catecholamine-driven tachycardia (170 bpm) may ensue that suggests an oxygen debt existed. Nonetheless, increasing CPB flow and mean arterial pressure do not always correct fetal bradycardia, and, if not, then other causes must be considered.

Problems with venous return or other mechanical aspects of extracorporeal circulation may also limit systemic flow, causing reduced placental perfusion. If acidosis persists throughout CPB, then other factors may be responsible for it, rather than low maternal blood pressure such as maternal hypothermia, uterine contractions, or medications that are transferable to the fetus. Monitoring the fetal heart rate is important to assess fetal viability and subsequent therapeutic initiatives. Fetal monitoring reduces mortality partially by early recognition of problems.

Beyond the effect of hypothermia on acid-base status, coagulation, and arrhythmias, it may precipitate uterine contractions that limit placental perfusion and risk fetal ischemia and survival. The explanation for hypothermic-induced contractions may be related to the severe dilution that accompanies CPB and lowers progesterone levels, thus activating uterine contractions. Contractions are more likely to occur the older the gestational age of the fetus. Accordingly, uterine monitoring is strongly recommended if CPB is required during pregnancy. If uterine contractions should begin during CPB, then stopping them is vitally important for fetal survival.

Anesthetic Considerations

Medications for anesthesia must be considered in the context of the maternal heart disease, the influence of CPB, and the effects on the fetus. Maternal safety and optimal fetal outcome must be ensured. Being aware of the safety of the more commonly used drugs in cardiac anesthesia during pregnancy is important. The risk of teratogenesis with a myriad of medications and exposures of the fetus during cardiac surgery and CPB is high, but most infants have successfully avoided the effects. No anesthetic agent has been shown to be teratogenic in humans.

RENAL INSUFFICIENCY AND CARDIAC SURGERY

In recent years, the number of individuals with chronic renal failure (CRF) undergoing cardiac surgery has increased between 2% and 3% of the cardiac surgical population. Patients with CRF may not necessarily be dialysis-dependent before surgery but are more likely to develop worsening renal function after CPB than those with normal preoperative renal function. Because CRF accelerates the development of atherosclerosis, many of these patients will eventually require myocardial revascularization. Irrespective of whether the CRF patient is dialysis-dependent, he or she is an anesthetic challenge, especially in regard to fluid management, electrolyte status, and hemostasis. The ability to avoid dialysis in the nondialysis-dependent patient with CRF is very important to hospital lengths of stay and long-term mortality. A collaborative effort by the cardiac surgeon, anesthesiologist, nephrologist, and cardiologist is instrumental in the care of these patients. Unfortunately, long-term survival is still appreciably diminished, even with minimal perioperative morbidity.

Patients with CRF are more prone to fluid overload, hyponatremia, hyperkalemia, and metabolic acidosis. Optimal hemodynamic and fluid status before surgery is important. Hemodialysis should be strongly considered the day before surgery, especially in those who are strictly dialysis-dependent. Chronic dialysis patients tend to arrive for surgery with worsened left ventricular function, possibly from an inefficient waste and toxin removal. CHF can occur as a result of hypervolemia and poor left ventricular function, manifesting as pulmonary edema and respiratory distress. Dialysis and medical therapy directed at improving cardiac function may be required to optimize the patient preoperatively. Chronic medications should be carefully reviewed to ensure that certain medications, such as antihypertensive agents, are given. The importance of preoperative preparation for patients with CRF is evident by the significantly high mortality rate associated with urgent surgery.

Perioperative mortality of patients with CRF undergoing cardiac surgery is associated with several risk factors. A preoperative creatinine of 2.5 mg/dL is associated with greater mortality even in those patients with nondialysis-dependent CRF. Efforts to find renoprotective agents for patients who are at high risk for renal failure or those with CRF have been unsuccessful. Randomized double-blind prospective trials looking at the use of N-acetylcysteine for patients undergoing CPB with CRF have found mixed results. Fenoldopam, a dopamine-1 receptor agonist, was studied in patients undergoing CPB with preoperative creatinine levels above 1.5 mg/dL. Patients were given a renal dose of dopamine or fenoldopam perioperatively. Postoperative parameters were only improved in those receiving fenoldopam, suggesting a renal protective effect, but additional studies are needed. Mannitol and Lasix may also prevent early oliguric renal failure.

Anesthetic Considerations

CRF affects dosing of medications that have a large volume of distribution. Decreased serum protein concentration diminishes plasma binding, leading to higher levels of free drug to bind with receptors. Many patients with CRF have hypoalbuminemia. In general, anesthetic induction agents and benzodiazepines are safe to use in patients with CRF. Medications that rely totally on renal excretion have a limited role. Fentanyl and sufentanil may be more effective for pain management because excretion is not renally dependent as is the case with morphine sulfate. Currently used volatile anesthetic agents rarely incur any additional renal dysfunction, even with underlying CRF unless severely prolonged duration of anesthesia occurs. Muscle relaxants and agents for antagonism of muscle paralysis have varying degrees of renal excretion.

A rapid-sequence induction is recommended in those with CRF in response to the likelihood of delayed gastric emptying. Significant extracellular volume contraction may also be present before the induction of anesthesia as a result of the 6- to 8-hour fast before surgery and dialysis within 24 hours of surgery that may lead to hypotension on induction. Because fluid requirements are usually high with CPB, a PAC is especially useful to manage fluid administration. TEE may complement fluid management by assessment of left ventricular volume and function. Before the initiation of CPB, fluid administration should be limited, especially if the patient is dialysis-dependent. In the nondialysis-dependent patient, fluid should be given to maintain adequate urine

18

output but to also avoid excessive cardiovascular filling pressures that incite pulmonary edema. Fluids should not be too aggressively restricted, because doing so may cause acute renal failure superimposed on CRF. Low-dose dopamine has been recommended for patients with CRF, but its value is indeterminate.

In general, CRF will worsen after CPB in part because of a combination of non-pulsatile flow, low renal perfusion, and hypothermia. Mean arterial pressure should be kept above 80 mm Hg. The stress of surgery and hypothermia may impair autoregulation so that renal vasoconstriction reduces renal blood flow. The fluid required to initiate CPB may significantly reduce the hemoglobin and oxygen-carrying capacity in view of the preexisting anemia of CRF without the addition of red blood cells (RBCs) to the priming volume or immediately upon initiation of CPB. A hematocrit of 25% should be maintained during CPB. Washed RBCs are recommended for RBC transfusion to lessen excessive potassium and glucose levels intraoperatively. Potassium plasma levels should be checked periodically. Patients with CRF often have glucose intolerance from an abnormal insulin response; therefore more frequent determination of serum glucose levels is advisable.

The anephric patient poorly tolerates post-CPB hypervolemia associated with prolonged duration of CPB. Dialysis can be performed during CPB and is technically easy and effective because small molecules (uremic solutes, electrolytes) are removed. Instead of dialysis during CPB, hemofiltration (ultrafiltration) is more frequently performed effectively, clearing excess water without the hemodynamic instability of dialysis. Circulating blood passes through the hollow fibers of the hemoconcentrators, which have a smaller pore size than albumin (55,000 daltons) that remove water and solutes. Potassium is eliminated, thereby helping reduce excessive potassium concentration commonly associated with cardioplegia administration. Hemofiltration during CPB may not achieve a net reduction in the overall total fluid balance of the patient in part because a minimum volume of fluid must be maintained in the venous reservoir of the extracorporeal circuit.

Excessive bleeding after CPB is not uncommon in those with CRF in part because of preoperative platelet dysfunction. Antifibrinolytic medications are pharmacologic measures used to successfully reduce excessive bleeding and transfusion requirements associated with cardiac surgery. Tranexamic acid, an inexpensive, synthetic antifibrinolytic, is excreted primarily through the kidneys; consequently, a dose reduction will be required, based on the preoperative creatinine level.

Postoperatively, if dialysis is required in patients with end-stage renal disease, then the risk of dialysis dependence is greatly increased. If the patient is dialysis-dependent preoperatively, dialysis is usually resumed within 24 to 48 hours of surgery and then according to the patient's preoperative routine to optimize fluid, electrolyte, and metabolic status. Dialysis may be needed soon after return from the surgical unit if mobilization of fluids into the intravascular space causes CHF. Continuous renal replacement therapy can be instituted intraoperatively and postoperatively to manage acute renal failure with volume overload and metabolic instability with great results in cardiac patients. Continuous renal replacement therapy has become very popular in cardiac surgical patients in the last 10 years because the bedside nurse can direct the degree of fluid pull in response to the patient's changing hemodynamic status.

▨ HEMATOLOGIC PROBLEMS IN PATIENTS UNDERGOING CARDIAC SURGERY

Anesthetic concerns for patients with hematologic problems who undergo cardiac surgery are further complicated by the stress CPB places on coagulation and oxygen-carrying systems. Hemophilia, cold agglutinins (CAs), sickle cell disease (SCD), antithrombin (AT) deficiency, and von Willebrand disease (vWD) are a few of the hematologic disorders that may require special consideration if CPB is used.

Hemophilia

Hemophilia A is the third most common X-linked disorder, occurring in 1 in 5000 male births. Hemophilia B, also known as *Christmas disease*, is also an X-linked disorder with one-fourth the incidence of hemophilia A. FVIII is instrumental for a normally functioning clotting cascade. With a half-life of only 8 to 12 hours, FVIII and FIXa accelerate activation of factor X. Hemophilia is characterized by spontaneous bleeding in the joints and muscles in its severe form. Treatment of hemophilia A and B primarily depends on replacement of FVIII or FIX, respectively.

Mild hemophilia has factor levels between 6% and 30% with occasional symptoms, and represents 30% to 40% of hemophilia cases. Moderate hemophilia has factor levels between 1% and 5%, and represents 10% of hemophilia cases. Severe hemophilia has factor levels below 1%, with easy bleeding that could become severe during surgery if factor activity remains at 1%. Severe hemophilia occurs in approximately 50% of hemophilia cases. Most patients arrive for surgery with an FVIII or FIX activity less than 5%. Although a factor level near 50% of normal is regarded as adequate to achieve noncardiac surgical hemostasis, hemostatic demand and associated coagulation abnormalities with cardiac surgery and CPB will require a higher FVIII level. Preoperatively, FVIII activity should be 80% to 100% for cardiac surgery.

Antibodies to FVIII or FIX may occur in patients with hemophilia who have received replacement therapy. The incidence of FVIII or FIX inhibitors is 18% to 52% and 2% to 16% of the hemophilia population, respectively. The inhibitor titer will characterize the patients as mild or high responders. High responders are at great risk because the anamnestic response may generate very high antibody titers that can render factor replacement therapy totally ineffective hemostatically. The problem with patients who develop inhibitors and require surgery is the inability to predict hemostasis at any point of the hospitalization.

von Willebrand Disease

vWD is the most commonly inherited hemostatic abnormality, with prevalence in the general population of 0.8%. vWD is an autosomal dominant bleeding disorder caused by a deficiency and/or abnormality of von Willebrand factor (vWF). An acquired form of vWD is associated with various disease states and medications. The nomenclature of vWF and FVIII complex have been standardized to resolve past confusion.

Each vWF subunit has a site for a platelet receptor to bind and the extracellular matrix component of the vessel wall to attach. vWF has two major hemostatic functions: (1) a carrier protein and stabilizer for FVIII; and (2) mediation of platelet adhesion to injured sites. It plays a crucial role in mediating platelet adhesion, platelet aggregation, and clotting during high shear conditions. Patients with vWD have an abnormality of both vWF and FVIII. vWD is classified into three major types and four subtypes (Table 18.6). Individuals with type 1 and type 2 make up 70% and 20% of people with vWD, respectively. Type 3 vWD represents only 10% of individuals and is autosomal recessive. Type 3 vWD individuals are severely affected and presentation is similar to individuals with hemophilia who have a very low FVIII activity (1% to 4%).

18

Table 18.6 Classification of von Willebrand Disease

New[a]	Old[a]	Characteristics
1	I platelet normal, I platelet low, 1A, I-1, I-2, I-3	Partial quantitative deficiency of vWF
2A		Qualitative variants with decreased platelet-dependent function that is associated with the absence of high–molecular weight vWF multimers
2B		Qualitative variants with increased affinity for platelet GPIb
2M		Qualitative variants with decreased platelet-dependent function that is not caused by the absence of high–molecular weight vWF multimers
2N		Qualitative variants with significantly decreased affinity for factor VIII
3		Virtually a complete deficiency of vWF

GPIb, Glycoprotein receptor Ib; vWF, von Willebrand factor.
[a]Reproduced with permission from Castaman G, Rodeghiero F. Current management of von Willebrand's disease. Drugs. 1995;50:602.

Correction of vWF deficiency may be accomplished by either facilitating vWF release from in vivo storage sites or administering exogenous components. Each type of vWD requires a specific therapeutic approach. 1-Desamino-8-D-arginine vasopressin (DDAVP) is a synthetic analog of the natural hormone vasopressin without the pressor effect and is the first choice for treatment in vWD; however, not all types of vWD respond to it. DDAVP is effective in type 1 vWD but ill advised in type 2B vWD because thrombocytopenia may result. It is useless in type 3 vWD because there are no stores of vWF to release. DDAVP does not directly cause the release of FVIII/vWF from the endothelial cell but stimulates monocytes to produce a substance that releases vWF. A response to DDAVP should occur in 30 minutes with a threefold to eightfold increase in FVIII and vWF that may persist for 8 to 10 hours. It is readily available, inexpensive, and has minimal risk for patients but may be contraindicated in those with atherosclerosis, CHF, or who require diuretic therapy. Intravenous dosing (0.3 μg/kg) requires 20 to 30 minutes to avoid a decline in mean arterial pressure of 15% to 20%.

Blood products should not be administered to patients with vWD unless another treatment is ineffective or contraindicated. Plasma-derived factor concentrates are the current standard for replacement therapy if the patient is unresponsive to DDAVP. These commercially available concentrates contain large amounts of both vWF and FVIII but differ in their purification and pathogen removal and inactivation techniques. In general, the dosing is 60 to 80 IU/kg for a bolus dose of the factor concentrate to maintain hemostasis. Platelet infusions should be considered in patients with type 3 vWD if bleeding persists after administering replacement concentrates.

Antithrombin

AT and protein C are two primary inhibitors of coagulation. A delicate balance exists between the procoagulant system and the inhibitors of coagulation (Table 18.7). AT is the most abundant and important of the coagulation pathway inhibitors.

Table 18.7 Balance That Normally Exists Between Prothrombotic and Antithrombotic Forces Within the Circulation

Prothrombotic Factors	Antithrombotic Factors
Thrombin	Antithrombin
Factor Xa	Protein C
Factor VIIa	Protein S
Tissue factor	Heparin cofactor II
Activated platelets	Tissue-factor protein inhibitor
Perturbed endothelial cells	Thrombomodulin
Others	Activated protein C cofactor 2
	Others

Reproduced with permission from Blajchman MA. An overview of the mechanism of action of antithrombin and its inherited deficiency states. *Blood Coagul Fibrinolysis*. 1994;5(Suppl 1):S5.

AT deficiency may occur as a congenital or acquired deficiency. Acquired deficiencies are secondary to increased AT consumption, loss of AT from the intravascular compartment (renal failure, nephrotic syndrome) or liver disease (cirrhosis). A normal AT level is 80% to 120%, with activity less than 50% considered clinically important.

In contrast to the rare case of congenital AT deficiency, acquired deficiencies of AT are commonly encountered in cardiac surgical patients. Anticoagulation with heparin for CPB depends on AT to inhibit clotting as heparin, alone, has no effect on coagulation. Heparin catalyzes AT inhibition of thrombin over 1000-fold by binding to a lysine residue on AT and altering its conformation. Thrombin actually attacks AT, disabling it, but in the process attaches AT to thrombin, forming the AT-thrombin complex. This complex has no activity and is rapidly removed. Thirty percent of AT is consumed during this process; consequently, AT levels are reduced temporarily. If AT levels are not restored, then a condition called *heparin resistance* may arise. The many causes of heparin resistance are listed in Box 18.7. Heparin resistance is defined as the failure of a specific heparin dose (300–400 u/kg) to prolong an activated clotting time beyond 480 seconds in preparation for the initiation of CPB. Failure to reach 480 seconds may be considered inadequate anticoagulation with the risk of thrombus formation during CPB.

Heparin resistance was routinely treated with fresh frozen plasma (FFP) for many years. However, a large disparity between AT levels after recombinant AT, compared with FFP, was noted in a prospective, randomized trial of recombinant AT or FFP for patients who were consistently defined as heparin-resistant. More recently, two units of FFP often failed to normalize AT levels in patients who were defined as heparin-resistant. A 75 µg/kg bolus dose of recombinant AT has effectively improved pre-CPB AT levels from 56% to 75% ± 31%. The use of allogeneic blood products to treat AT deficiency should be discouraged.

Cold Agglutinins

CAs are common but rarely clinically important. The incidence rate in cardiac surgical patients varies between 0.8% and 4%. Often associated with lymphoreticular neoplasms, mycoplasma pneumonia, and infectious mononucleosis, they are immunoglobulin M (IgM) class autoantibodies directed against the RBC I-antigen or related antigens.

CAs form a complement antigen-antibody reaction on the surface of the RBC membrane that causes lysis. The degree of hemolysis is related to the circulating titer and thermal amplitude of the CAs. Thermal amplitude, that is, the blood temperature below which the CAs will react, is the key information to assign clinical relevance. The titer and thermal amplitude are determined at a range of temperatures in the serum by an indirect hemagglutination test. Most individuals have cold autoantibodies that react at 4°C but in very low titers. From a pathologic standpoint, thermal amplitude is more important than titer. Pathologic CAs cause RBC clumping and vascular occlusion that injures the myocardium, liver, and kidney. Increasing the temperature will rapidly inactivate CAs.

Blood banks routinely screen for the presence of autoantibodies at 37°C, but cold antibodies, only reactive at lower temperatures, are not detected. The significance of CAs is determined by evaluating agglutination of RBCs in 20°C saline and 30°C albumin. If there is no agglutination, then significant hemolysis is unlikely. Before the initiation of CPB, the titer and thermal amplitude of CAs must be determined to avoid a temperature during CPB that would cause hemolysis. Intraoperatively, low-thermal amplitude CAs can be determined by mixing cold cardioplegia with some of the patient's blood to check for a separation of cells. The occurrence of hemodilution commonly associated with CPB may weaken agglutination and hemolysis in a patient with high reactivity and titer of CAs exposed to hypothermia.

If CAs are suspected or identified preoperatively, then the avoidance of hypothermia is the safest course. Despite normothermic CPB, cold cardioplegia may cause RBC agglutination in small myocardial vessels. If hypothermic CPB is necessary, despite the presence of CAs, then the choices are preoperative plasmapheresis, hemodilution, and maintenance of CPB temperature above the thermal amplitude of the CAs (Fig. 18.15).

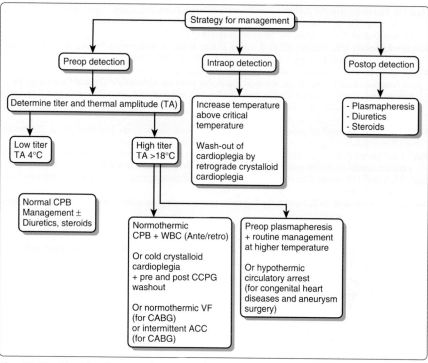

Fig. 18.15 Algorithm illustrates the strategy for the management of cold agglutinin. *ACC,* Aortic cross-clamp; *CABG,* coronary artery bypass grafting; *CCPG,* cold crystalloid cardioplegia; *CPB,* cardiopulmonary bypass; *Intraop,* intraoperative; *Postop,* postoperative; *Preop,* preoperative; *VF,* ventricular fibrillation; *WBC,* warm blood cardioplegia. (Reproduced with permission from Agarwal SK, Ghosh PK, Gupta D. Cardiac surgery and cold-reactive proteins. *Ann Thorac Surg.* 1995;60:1143.)

SUGGESTED READINGS

Abraham WT. Cardiac resynchronization therapy for heart failure: biventricular pacing and beyond. *Curr Opin Cardiol.* 2002;17:346–352.

Anyanwu AC, Adams DH. Etiologic classification of degenerative mitral valve disease: Barlow's disease and fibroelastic deficiency. *Semin Thorac Cardiovasc Surg.* 2007;19:90–96.

Avidan MS, Levy JH, van Aken H, et al. Recombinant human antithrombin III restores heparin responsiveness and decreases activation of coagulation in heparin-resistant patients during cardiopulmonary bypass. *J Thorac Cardiovasc Surg.* 2005;130:107–113.

Barbara DW, Mauermann WJ, Neal JR, et al. Cold agglutinins in patients undergoing cardiac surgery requiring cardiopulmonary bypass. *J Thorac Cardiovasc Surg.* 2013;146:668–680.

Bruce CJ. Cardiac tumors. In: Otto CM, ed. *The Practice of Clinical Echocardiography.* 4th ed. Philadelphia, PA: Elsevier/Saunders; 2012:902–928.

Bruce CJ. Cardiac tumours. Diagnosis and management. *Heart.* 2011;97:151–160.

Castillo JG, Milla F, Adams DH. Surgical management of carcinoid heart valve disease. *Semin Thorac Cardiovasc Surg.* 2012;24:254–260.

Chandrasekhar S, Cook CR, Collard CD. Cardiac surgery in the parturient. *Anesth Analg.* 2009;108:777–785.

Dhoble A, Vedre A, Abdelmoneim SS, et al. Prophylaxis to prevent infective endocarditis: to use or not to use? *Clin Cardiol.* 2009;32:429–433.

Elliott P, Andersson B, Arbustini E, et al. Classification of the cardiomyopathies: a position statement from the European Society of Cardiology Working Group on Myocardial and Pericardial Diseases. *Eur Heart J.* 2008;29:270–276.

Gersh BJ, Maron BJ, Bonow RO, et al. 2011 ACCF/AHA guideline for the diagnosis and treatment of hypertrophic cardiomyopathy: a report of the American College of Cardiology Foundation/American Heart Association Task Force on Practice Guidelines. *Circulation.* 2011;124:e783–e831.

18

Hare JM. The restrictive and infiltrative cardiomyopathies and arrhythmogenic right ventricular dysplasia/cardiomyopathy. In: Mann DL, Felker GM, eds. *Heart Failure: A Companion to Braunwald's Heart Disease*. 3rd ed. Philadelphia, PA: Elsevier; 2016:318–333.

Kandler K, Jensen ME, Nilsson JC, et al. Acute kidney injury is independently associated with higher mortality after cardiac surgery. *J Cardiothorac Vasc Anesth*. 2014;28:1448–1452.

Maron BJ, Towbin JA, Thiene G, et al. Contemporary definitions and classification of the cardiomyopathies: an American Heart Association Scientific Statement from the Council on Clinical Cardiology, Heart Failure and Transplantation Committee; Quality of Care and Outcomes Research and Functional Genomics and Translational Biology Interdisciplinary Working Groups; and Council on Epidemiology and Prevention. *Circulation*. 2006;113:1807–1816.

Naqvi TZ. Restrictive cardiomyopathy: diagnosis and prognostic implications. In: Otto CM, ed. *The Practice of Clinical Echocardiography*. 4th ed. Philadelphia, PA: Saunders; 2012:542–564.

Naylor AR, Mehta Z, Rothwell PM, et al. Carotid artery disease and stroke during coronary artery bypass: a critical review of the literature. *Eur J Vasc Endovasc Surg*. 2002;23:283–294.

Said SM, Schaff HV. Surgical treatment of hypertrophic cardiomyopathy. *Semin Thorac Cardiovasc Surg*. 2013;25:300–309.

Staikou C, Chondrogiannis K, Mani A. Perioperative management of hereditary arrhythmogenic syndromes. *Br J Anaesth*. 2012;108:730–744.

Sukernik MR, Bennett-Guerrero E. The incidental finding of a patent foramen ovale during cardiac surgery: should it always be repaired? A core review. *Anesth Analg*. 2007;105:602–610.

Yawn BP, Buchanan GR, Afenyi-Annan AN, et al. Management of sickle cell disease: summary of the 2014 evidence-based report by expert panel members. *JAMA*. 2014;312:1033–1048.

IV.

Chapter 19

Anesthesia for Heart, Lung, and Heart-Lung Transplantation

Andrew W. Murray, MBChB • Joseph J. Quinlan, MD

Key Points

1. Cardiac denervation is an unavoidable consequence of heart transplantation, and reinnervation is at best partial and incomplete.
2. Drugs acting directly on the heart are the drugs of choice for altering cardiac physiology after heart transplantation.
3. Allograft coronary vasculopathy remains the greatest threat to long-term survival after heart transplantation.
4. Broadening of donor criteria has decreased time to lung transplantation.
5. Air trapping in patients with severe obstructive lung disease may impair hemodynamics and require deliberate hypoventilation.
6. Newly transplanted lungs should be ventilated with a low tidal volume and inspiratory pressure and as low an inspired oxygen concentration as can be tolerated.
7. Reperfusion injury is the most common cause of perioperative death.
8. The frequency of heart-lung transplantation has decreased as the frequency of lung transplantations has increased.

HEART TRANSPLANTATION

The history of heart transplantation spans almost a century. Canine heterotopic cardiac transplantation was first reported in 1905, but such efforts were doomed by ignorance of the workings of the immune system (Box 19.1). Further research in the late 1950s and early 1960s set the stage for the first human cardiac transplant by Barnard in 1966. However, there were few long-term survivors in this era because of continued deficiency in understanding and modulating the human immune system, and the procedure fell into general disfavor. Continued research at selected centers (such as Stanford University) and lessons learned from renal transplantation led to greater understanding of the technical issues and immunology required, and by the early 1980s, cardiac transplantation gained widespread acceptance as a realistic option for patients with end-stage cardiomyopathy.

Heart transplantation experienced explosive growth in the mid-to-late 1980s, but the annual number of heart transplants worldwide plateaued by the early 1990s at approximately 3500 per year. The factor limiting continued growth has been a shortage of suitable donors. As of February 2015, there were slig htly more than 4000 patients on the United Network for Organ Sharing (UNOS) cardiac transplant waiting list (includes all US candidates), an increase of 25% compared with 2004.

473

BOX 19.1   *Heart Transplantation*

Frequency of transplantation remains limited by donor supply
Pathophysiology before transplantation is primarily that of end-stage ventricular failure
Pathophysiology after transplantation reflects the effects of denervation
Allograft coronary vasculopathy is a frequent long-term complication

During that same time period the frequency of heart transplantation also increased (by approximately 17%) but failed to keep pace with the increase in the size of the waiting list. Only 2431 heart transplants were performed in the United States during the 2014 calendar year, slightly above the average of 2290 heart transplants per year over the preceding decade. The median waiting time for a cardiac graft varies widely according to blood type (approximately 52 days for type AB recipients in contrast with 241 days for type O recipients listed for the period 2003–2004, based on Organ Procurement and Transplantation Network [OPTN] data as of February 1, 2015). Of those patients listed for heart transplantation in 2009, 27.5% had spent more than a year waiting for a transplant. Adult patients on the heart transplant waiting list are assigned a status of 1A, 1B, or 2. Status 1A patients require mechanical circulatory support, mechanical ventilation, high-dose or multiple inotropes, with continuous monitoring of left ventricular filling pressure. Status 1B patients require mechanical circulatory support beyond 30 days or inotropic support without continuous monitoring of left ventricular filling pressure. All other patients are classified as Status 2. The most frequent recipient indications for adult heart transplantation remain either idiopathic or ischemic cardiomyopathy. Other less common diagnoses include viral cardiomyopathy, systemic diseases such as amyloidosis, and complex congenital heart disease (CHD).

The 1-year survival rate after heart transplantation has been reported to be 79%, with a subsequent mortality rate of approximately 4%/year. There has been only slight improvement in the survival statistics over the past decade; the OPTN reports that the 1- and 3-year survival rates after heart transplantation for those transplanted in the United States during the period 1997 to 2004 were approximately 87% and 78%, respectively. One-year survival rate after repeat heart transplantation more than 6 months after the original procedure is slightly lower (63%) but substantially worse if performed within 6 months of the original grafting (39%). Risk factors for increased mortality have been associated with recipient factors (prior transplantation, poor human leukocyte antigen matching, ventilator dependence, age, and race), medical center factors (volume of heart transplants performed, ischemic time), and donor factors (race, sex, age), and have remained relatively unchanged over the past two decades. Early deaths most frequently are caused by graft failure, whereas intermediate-term deaths are caused by acute rejection or infection. Late deaths after heart transplantation most frequently are due to allograft vasculopathy, posttransplant lymphoproliferative disease or other malignancy, and chronic rejection.

Recipient Selection

Potential candidates for heart transplantation generally undergo a multidisciplinary evaluation, including a complete history and physical examination, routine hematology, chemistries (to assess renal and hepatic function), viral serology, electrocardiography, chest radiography, pulmonary function tests, and right- and left-heart catheterization. Ambulatory electrocardiography, echocardiography, and nuclear gated scans are performed if necessary. The goals of this evaluation are to confirm a diagnosis of end-stage heart disease that is not amenable to other therapies and that will likely lead to death within 1 to 2 years, as well as to exclude extracardiac organ dysfunction that could lead to death soon after heart transplantation. Patients typically have New York Heart Association (NYHA) class IV symptoms and a left ventricular ejection fraction less than 20%. Although most centers eschew a strict age cutoff, the candidate should have a physiologic age younger than 60. Detecting pulmonary hypertension and determining whether it is due to fixed elevation of pulmonary vascular resistance (PVR) is crucial; early mortality because of graft failure is threefold greater in patients with increased PVR (transpulmonary gradient >15 mm Hg or PVR >5 dynes•sec•cm^{-5}). If increased PVR is detected, a larger donor heart, a heterotopic heart transplant, or a heart-lung transplant (HLT) may be more appropriate. Active infection and recent pulmonary thromboembolism with pulmonary infarction are additional contraindications to heart transplantation. The results of this extensive evaluation should be tabulated and available to the anesthesia team at all times because heart transplantation is an emergency procedure.

Donor Selection and Graft Harvest

Once a brain-dead donor has been identified, the accepting transplant center must further evaluate the suitability of the allograft. Centers generally prefer donors to be free of previous cardiac illness and younger than 35 years because the incidence of coronary artery disease markedly increases at older ages. However, the relative shortage of suitable cardiac donors has forced many transplant centers to consider older donors without risk factors and symptoms of coronary artery disease. If it is necessary and the services are available at the donor hospital, the heart can be further evaluated by echocardiography (for regional wall motion abnormalities) or coronary angiography, to complement standard palpation of the coronaries in the operating room. The absence of sepsis, prolonged cardiac arrest, severe chest trauma, and a high inotrope requirement also are important. The donor is matched to the prospective recipient for ABO blood-type compatibility and size (within 20%, especially if the recipient has high PVR); a crossmatch is performed only if the recipient's preformed antibody screen is positive.

Donors can exhibit major hemodynamic and metabolic derangements that can adversely affect organ retrieval. Most brain-dead donors will be hemodynamically unstable. Reasons for such instability include hypovolemia (secondary to diuretics or diabetes insipidus), myocardial injury (possibly a result of catecholamine storm during periods of increased intracranial pressure), and inadequate sympathetic tone because of brainstem infarction. Donors often also have abnormalities of neuroendocrine function such as low T_3 and T_4 levels.

Donor cardiectomy is performed through a median sternotomy, usually simultaneously with recovery of other organs such as lungs, kidneys, and liver. Just before cardiac harvesting, the donor is heparinized and an intravenous cannula is placed in the ascending aorta for administration of conventional cardioplegia. The superior vena cava (SVC) is ligated and the inferior vena cava (IVC) transected to decompress the heart, simultaneous with the administration of cold hyperkalemic cardioplegia into the aortic root. The aorta is cross-clamped when the heart ceases to eject. The heart also is topically cooled with ice-cold saline. After arrest has been achieved, the pulmonary veins are severed, the SVC is transected, the ascending aorta is divided

19

just proximal to the innominate artery, and the pulmonary artery (PA) is transected at its bifurcation. The heart is then prepared for transport by placing it in a sterile plastic bag that is placed, in turn, in another bag filled with ice-cold saline, all of which are carried in an ice chest. Of all the regimens tested, conventional cardioplegia has proved most effective in maintaining cardiac performance. The upper time limit for ex vivo storage of human hearts appears to be approximately 6 hours.

Surgical Procedures

Orthotopic Heart Transplantation

Orthotopic heart transplantation is carried out via a median sternotomy, and the general approach is similar to that used for coronary revascularization or valve replacement. Frequently, patients will have undergone a prior median sternotomy; repeat sternotomy is cautiously performed using an oscillating saw. The groin should be prepped and draped to provide a rapid route for cannulation for cardiopulmonary bypass (CPB) if necessary. After the pericardium is opened, the aorta is cannulated as distally as possible and the IVC and SVC are individually cannulated via the high right atrium. Manipulation of the heart before institution of CPB is limited if thrombus is detected in the heart with transesophageal echocardiography (TEE). After initiation of CPB and cross-clamping of the aorta, the heart is arrested and excised (Fig. 19.1). The aorta and PA are separated and divided just above the level of their respective valves, and the atria are transected at their grooves. A variant of this classic approach totally excises both atria, mandating bicaval anastomoses. This technique may reduce the incidence of atrial arrhythmias, better preserve atrial function by avoiding tricuspid regurgitation, and enhance cardiac output (CO) after transplantation.

The donor graft then is implanted with every effort to maintain a cold tissue temperature, beginning with the left atrial (LA) anastomosis. If the foramen ovale is patent, it is sutured closed. The donor right atrium is opened by incising it from the IVC to the base of the right atrial (RA) appendage (to preserve the donor sinoatrial node), and the RA anastomosis is constructed. Alternatively, if the bicaval technique is used, individual IVC and SVC anastomoses are sewn. The donor and recipient PAs are then brought together in an end-to-end manner, followed by the anastomosis of the donor to the recipient aorta. After removal of the aortic cross-clamp, the heart is de-aired via a vent in the ascending aorta. Just before weaning from CPB, one of the venous cannulae is withdrawn into the right atrium and the other removed. The patient is then weaned from CPB in the usual manner. After hemostasis is achieved, mediastinal tubes are placed for drainage, the pericardium is left open, and the wound is closed in the standard fashion.

Heterotopic Heart Transplantation

Although orthotopic placement of the cardiac graft is optimal for most patients, certain recipients are not candidates for the orthotopic operation, and instead the graft is placed in the right chest and connected to the circulation in parallel with the recipient heart. The two primary indications for heterotopic placement are significant irreversible pulmonary hypertension and gross size mismatch between the donor and recipient. Heterotopic placement may avoid the development of acute right ventricular (RV) failure in the unconditioned donor heart in the face of acutely increased RV afterload.

Donor harvesting for heterotopic placement is performed in the previously described manner, except that the azygos vein is ligated and divided to increase the length of the donor SVC; the PA is extensively dissected to provide the longest possible main and right PA; and the donor IVC and right pulmonary veins are oversewn, with the

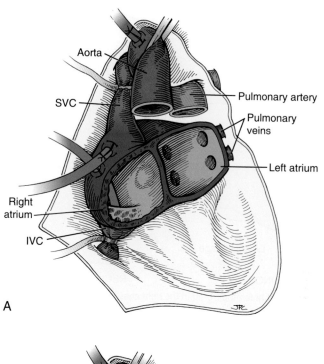

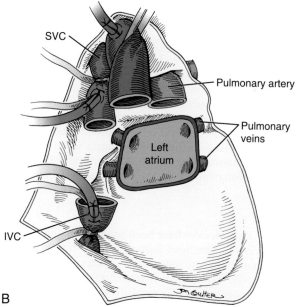

Fig. 19.1 Mediastinum after excision of the heart but before allograft placement. Venous cannulas are present in the superior *(SVC)* and inferior vena cava *(IVC)*, and the arterial cannula is present in the ascending aorta. (A) Classic orthotopic technique. (B) Bicaval anastomotic technique.

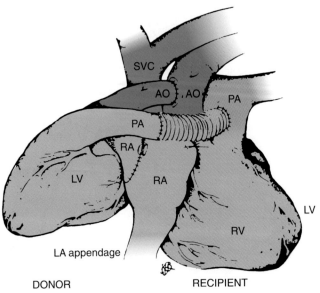

Fig. 19.2 Placement of heterotopic graft in the right chest, with anastomoses to the corresponding native left *(LA)* and right atria *(RA)*, ascending aorta *(AO)*, and an interposition graft to the native pulmonary artery *(PA)*. *LV,* left ventricle; *RV,* right ventricle; *SVC,* superior vena cava. (From Cooper DKC, Lanza LP. *Heart Transplantation: The Present Status of Orthotopic and Heterotopic Heart Transplantation.* Lancaster, United Kingdom: MTP Press; 1984.)

left pulmonary veins incised to create a single large orifice. The operation is performed via a median sternotomy in the recipient, but the right pleura is entered and excised. The recipient SVC is cannulated via the RA appendage, and the IVC via the lower right atrium. After arresting the recipient heart, the LA anastomosis is constructed by incising the recipient left atrium near the right superior pulmonary vein and extending this incision inferiorly and then anastomosing the respective left atria. The recipient RA-SVC is then incised and anastomosed to the donor RA-SVC, after which the donor aorta is joined to the recipient aorta in an end-to-side manner. Finally, the donor PA is anastomosed to the recipient main PA in an end-to-side manner if it is sufficiently long; otherwise, they are joined via an interposed vascular graft (Fig. 19.2).

Special Situations

Mechanical ventricular assist devices have been used successfully to bridge patients who would otherwise die of acute heart failure awaiting transplantation. Although ventricular assist devices may improve the survival of patients awaiting transplantation, complications associated with their use may negatively impact survival after transplantation. The technique of transplantation is virtually identical in such patients to that for ordinary orthotopic transplantation. However, repeat sternotomy is obligatory, and repeat sternotomy is associated with higher morbidity and mortality, as well as higher intraoperative blood use, postoperative length of intensive care unit (ICU) and hospital stays, and frequency of reoperation for bleeding after subsequent heart transplantation.

Rarely, patients will present for cardiac transplantation combined with transplantation of the liver. The cardiac allograft usually is implanted first to better enable the patient to survive potential hemodynamic instability associated with reperfusion of the hepatic allograft. Large-bore intravenous access is mandatory. Conventional full heparinization protocols or low-dose heparin with heparin-bonded circuits may be used. A venous cannula can be left in the right atrium at the completion of the heart transplant procedure to serve as a return site for subsequent venovenous bypass during liver transplantation.

Pathophysiology Before Transplantation

The pathophysiology of heart transplant candidates is predominantly end-stage cardiomyopathy. Normally, such patients will have both systolic dysfunction (character-ized by decreased stroke volume and increased end-diastolic volume) and diastolic dysfunction, characterized by an increased intracardiac diastolic pressure. As compensa-tory mechanisms to maintain CO fail, the increased left ventricular (LV) pressures lead to increases in pulmonary venous pressures and development of pulmonary vascular congestion and edema. A similar process occurs if RV failure also occurs. Autonomic sympathetic tone is increased in patients with heart failure, leading to generalized vasoconstriction, as well as salt and water retention. Vasoconstriction and ventricular dilation combine to substantially increase myocardial wall tension. Over time, the high levels of catecholamines lead to a decrease in the sensitivity of the heart and vasculature to these agents via a decrease in receptor density (ie, downregula-tion) and a decrease in myocardial norepinephrine stores.

Therapy of heart failure seeks to reverse or antagonize these processes. Almost all candidates will be maintained on diuretics; hypokalemia and hypomagnesemia second-ary to urinary losses are likely, and the anesthesiologist must be alert to the possibility that a patient is hypovolemic from excessive diuresis. Another mainstay of therapy is vasodilators (such as nitrates, hydralazine, and angiotensin-converting enzyme inhibitors), which decrease the impedance to LV emptying and improve cardiac function and survival in patients with end-stage heart failure. Paradoxically, slow incremental β-blockade with agents such as the β_1-antagonist metoprolol also can improve hemodynamics and exercise tolerance in some patients awaiting heart transplantation. Patients who are symptomatic despite these measures often will require inotropic therapy. Digoxin is an effective but weak inotrope, and its use is limited by toxic side effects. Phosphodiesterase inhibitors such as amrinone, milrinone, and enoximone are efficacious, but chronic therapy is restricted by concerns about increased mortality in those receiving these agents. Therefore inotrope-dependent patients often are treated with intravenous infusions of β-adrenergic agonists such as dopamine or dobutamine. Patients refractory to even these measures may be supported with intraaortic balloon counterpulsation, but its use is fraught with significant vascular complications and essentially immobilizes the patient. Many patients with low CO are maintained on anticoagulants such as warfarin to prevent pulmonary or systemic embolization, especially if they have atrial fibrillation.

Pathophysiology After Transplantation

The physiology of patients after heart transplantation is of interest not only to anesthesiologists in cardiac transplant centers but to the anesthesiology community at large because a substantial portion of these patients return for subsequent surgical procedures.

Cardiac denervation is an unavoidable consequence of heart transplantation. Many long-term studies indicate that reinnervation is absent, or at best partial or incomplete,

19

in humans. Denervation does not significantly change baseline cardiac function, but it does substantially alter the cardiac response to demands for increased CO. Normally, increases in heart rate can rapidly increase CO, but this mechanism is not available to the transplanted heart. Heart rate increases only gradually with exercise, and this effect is mediated by circulating catecholamines. Increases in CO in response to exercise are instead mostly mediated via an increase in stroke volume. Therefore maintenance of adequate preload in cardiac transplant recipients is crucial. Lack of parasympathetic innervation probably is responsible for the gradual decrease in heart rate after exercise seen in transplant recipients, rather than the usual sharp decline.

Denervation has important implications in the choice of pharmacologic agents used after cardiac transplantation. Drugs that act indirectly on the heart via either the sympathetic (ephedrine) or parasympathetic (atropine, pancuronium, edrophonium) nervous systems generally will be ineffective. Drugs with a mixture of direct and indirect effects will exhibit only their direct effects (leading to the absence of the normal increase in refractory period of the atrioventricular node with digoxin, tachycardia with norepinephrine infusion, and bradycardia with neostigmine). Thus agents with direct cardiac effects (such as epinephrine or isoproterenol) are the drugs of choice for altering cardiac physiology after transplantation. However, the chronically high catecholamine levels found in cardiac transplant recipients may blunt the effect of α-adrenergic agents, as opposed to normal responses to β-adrenergic agents.

Allograft coronary vasculopathy remains the greatest threat to long-term survival after heart transplantation. Allografts are prone to the accelerated development of an unusual form of coronary atherosclerosis that is characterized by circumferential, diffuse involvement of entire coronary arterial segments, as opposed to the conventional form of coronary atherosclerosis with focal plaques often found in eccentric positions in proximal coronary arteries. The pathophysiologic basis of this process remains elusive, but it is likely due to an immune cell-mediated activation of vascular endothelial cells to upregulate the production of smooth muscle cell growth factors. More than half of all heart transplant recipients have evidence of concentric atherosclerosis 3 years after transplant, and more than 80% at 5 years. Because afferent cardiac rein-nervation is rare, a substantial portion of recipients with accelerated vasculopathy will have silent ischemia. Noninvasive methods of detecting coronary atherosclerosis are insensitive for detecting allograft vasculopathy. Furthermore, coronary angiography often underestimates the severity of allograft atherosclerosis; other diagnostic regimens such as intravascular ultrasound and dobutamine stress echocardiography may detect morphologic abnormalities or functional ischemia, respectively, in the absence of angiographically significant lesions. Therefore the anesthesiologist should assume that there is a substantial risk for coronary vasculopathy in any heart transplant recipient beyond the first 2 years, regardless of symptoms, the results of noninvasive testing, and even angiography.

Anesthetic Management

Preoperative Evaluation and Preparation

The preoperative period often is marked by severe time constraints because of the impending arrival of the donor heart. Nevertheless, a rapid history should screen for last oral intake, recent anticoagulant use, intercurrent deterioration of ventricular function, or change in anginal pattern; a physical examination should evaluate present volume status, and a laboratory review (if available) and a chest radiograph should detect the presence of renal, hepatic, or pulmonary dysfunction. Many hospitalized patients will be supported with inotropic infusions and/or an intraaortic balloon pump, and the infusion rates and timing of the latter should be reviewed.

Equipment and drugs similar to those usually used for routine cases requiring CPB should be prepared. A β-agonist such as epinephrine should be readily available both in bolus form and as an infusion to treat ventricular failure rapidly, and an α-agonist such as phenylephrine or norepinephrine is useful to compensate for the vasodilatory effects of anesthetics because even small decreases in preload and afterload can lead to catastrophic changes in CO and coronary perfusion in these patients.

Placement of invasive monitoring before induction will facilitate rapid and accurate response to hemodynamic events during induction. In addition to standard noninvasive monitoring, an arterial catheter and a PA catheter (PAC, with a long sterile sheath to allow partial removal during graft implantation) are placed after judicious use of sedation and local anesthetics. Placing the PAC in a central site rather than the radial artery will avoid the discrepancy between radial and central arterial pressure often seen after CPB, but it also may be necessary to cannulate a femoral artery for arterial inflow for CPB if there has been a prior sternotomy. Floating the PAC into correct position may be difficult because of cardiac chamber dilation and severe tricuspid regurgitation. Large-bore intravenous access is mandatory, especially if a sternotomy has been previously performed, in which case external defibrillator/pacing patches also may be useful. The overall hemodynamic picture should be evaluated and optimized insofar as possible just before induction. If the hemodynamics seem tenuous, then starting or increasing an inotrope infusion may be advisable.

Induction

Most patients presenting for heart transplantation will not be in a fasting state and should be considered to have a full stomach. Therefore the induction technique should aim to rapidly achieve control of the airway to prevent aspiration while avoiding myocardial depression. A regimen combining a short-acting hypnotic with minimal myocardial depression (etomidate, 0.3 mg/kg), a moderate dose of narcotic to blunt the tachycardic response to laryngoscopy and intubation (fentanyl, 10 µg/kg), and succinylcholine (1.5 mg/kg) is popular; high-dose narcotic techniques with or without benzodiazepines also have been advocated. Vasodilation should be countered with an α-agonist. Anesthesia can be maintained with additional narcotic and sedatives (benzodiazepines or scopolamine).

Intraoperative Management

After induction, the stomach can be decompressed with an orogastric tube and a TEE probe introduced while the bladder is catheterized. A complete TEE examination often will reveal useful information not immediately available from other sources, such as the presence of cardiac thrombi, ventricular volume and contractility, and atherosclerosis of the ascending aorta and aortic arch. Crossmatched blood should be immediately available once surgery commences, especially if the patient has had a previous sternotomy; patients not previously exposed to cytomegalovirus should receive blood from donors who are likewise cytomegalovirus negative. Sternotomy and cannulation for CPB are performed as indicated earlier. The period before CPB often is uneventful, apart from arrhythmias and slow recovery of coronary perfusion because of manipulation of the heart during dissection and cannulation. The PAC should be withdrawn from the right heart before completion of bicaval cannulation.

Once CPB is initiated, ventilation is discontinued and the absence of a thrill in the carotid arteries is documented. Most patients will have an excess of intravascular volume, and administration of a diuretic and/or the use of hemofiltration via the pump may be beneficial by increasing the hemoglobin concentration. A dose of glucocorticoid (methylprednisolone, 500 mg) is administered as the last anastomosis is being completed before release of the aortic cross-clamp to attenuate any hyperacute immune response. During the period of reperfusion, an infusion of an inotrope is begun for both inotropy and chronotropy. TEE is used to monitor whether the cardiac chambers are adequately de-aired before weaning from CPB.

Weaning from bypass begins after ventilation is resumed and the cannula in the SVC is removed. The donor heart should be paced if bradycardia is present despite the inotropic infusion. Once the patient is separated from CPB, the PAC can be advanced into position. Patients with increased PVR are at risk for acute RV failure and may benefit from a pulmonary vasodilator such as prostaglandin E_1 (0.05–0.15 µg/kg/min). Rarely, such patients will require support with a RV assist device. TEE often will provide additional useful information about right- and left-heart function and volume, and document normal flow dynamics through the anastomoses. Unless a bicaval anastomosis was created, a ridge of redundant tissue will be evident in the left atrium and should not cause alarm.

Protamine then is given to reverse the effect of heparin after satisfactory weaning from CPB. Continued coagulopathy despite adequate protamine is common after heart transplantation, especially if there has been a prior sternotomy. Treatment is similar to that used for other postbypass coagulopathies: meticulous attention to surgical hemostasis, empiric administration of platelets, and subsequent addition of fresh-frozen plasma and cryoprecipitate guided by subsequent coagulation studies. After adequate hemostasis is achieved, the wound is closed in standard fashion and the patient transported to the ICU.

Postoperative Management and Complications

Management in the ICU after the conclusion of the procedure essentially is a continuation of the anesthetic management after CPB. The electrocardiogram; arterial, central venous, and/or PA pressures; and arterial oxygen saturation are monitored continuously. Cardiac recipients will continue to require β-adrenergic infusions for chronotropy and inotropy for up to 3 to 4 days. Vasodilators may be necessary to control arterial hypertension and decrease impedance to LV ejection. Patients can be weaned from ventilatory support and extubated when the hemodynamics are stable and hemorrhage has ceased. The immunosuppressive regimen of choice (typically consisting of cyclosporine, azathioprine, and prednisone, or tacrolimus and prednisone) should be started after arrival in the ICU. Invasive monitoring can be withdrawn as the inotropic support is weaned, and mediastinal tubes removed after drainage subsides (usually after 24 hours). Patients usually can be discharged from the ICU after 2 or 3 days.

Early complications after heart transplantation include acute and hyperacute rejection, cardiac failure, systemic and pulmonary hypertension, cardiac arrhythmias, renal failure, and infection. Hyperacute rejection is an extremely rare but devastating syndrome mediated by preformed recipient cytotoxic antibodies against donor heart antigens. The donor heart immediately becomes cyanotic from microvascular thrombosis and ultimately ceases to contract. This syndrome is lethal unless the patient can be supported mechanically until a suitable heart is found. Acute rejection is a constant threat in the early postoperative period and may present in many forms (eg, low CO, arrhythmias). Acute rejection occurs most frequently during the initial 6 months after transplantation, so its presence is monitored by serial endomyocardial biopsies, with additional biopsies to evaluate any acute changes in clinical status. Detection of rejection mandates an aggressive increase in the level of immunosuppression, usually including pulses of glucocorticoid or a change from cyclosporine to tacrolimus. Low CO after transplantation may reflect a number of causative factors: hypovolemia, inadequate adrenergic stimulation, myocardial injury during harvesting, acute rejection, tamponade, or sepsis. Therapy should be guided by invasive monitoring, TEE, and endomyocardial biopsy. Systemic hypertension may be caused by pain, so adequate analgesia should be obtained before treating blood pressure with a vasodilator. Because fixed pulmonary hypertension will have been excluded during the recipient evaluation, pulmonary hypertension after heart transplantation usually will be transient and responsive to vasodilators such as prostaglandin E_1, nitrates, or hydralazine after either orthotopic or heterotopic placement. Atrial and ventricular tachyarrhythmias are common after heart transplantation; once rejection has been ruled out as a cause, antiarrhythmics are used for conversion or control (except those acting via indirect mechanisms such as digoxin, or those with negative inotropic properties such as β-blockers and calcium channel blockers). Almost all recipients will require either β-adrenergic agonists or pacing to increase heart rate in the immediate perioperative period, but 10% to 25% of recipients also will require permanent pacing. Renal function often improves immediately after transplantation, but immunosuppressives such as cyclosporine and tacrolimus may impair renal function. Finally, infection is a constant threat to immunosuppressed recipients. Bacterial pneumonia is frequent early in the postoperative period, with opportunistic viral and fungal infections becoming more common after the first several weeks.

LUNG TRANSPLANTATION

History and Epidemiology

Although the first human lung transplant was performed in 1963, surgical technical problems and inadequate preservation and immunosuppression regimens prevented widespread acceptance of this procedure until the mid-1980s (Box 19.2). Advances in these areas have since made lung transplantation a viable option for many patients with end-stage lung disease. According to data collected by UNOS between 2000 and 2002, the annual frequency of lung transplantation has remained stagnant, with the total number still averaging in the vicinity of 1000. Further growth in lung transplantation was feared to be constrained by a shortage of donor organs, with demand for organs still vastly exceeding supply. This was expected to be potentially exacerbated by data that were published in 2009, revealing that double-lung transplant afforded fewer hospitalizations and potentially better long-term survival. Despite these data, since 2003 the number of double-lung transplants has increased significantly in the United States, whereas the number of single-lung transplants has remained stagnant. The greatest growth in double-lung transplant occurred in the population with chronic obstructive pulmonary disease without alpha-1 antitrypsin deficiency and interstitial lung disease.

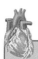

BOX 19.2 *Lung Transplantation*

Broader donor criteria have decreased the time from listing to transplantation
Nitric oxide minimizes reperfusion injury
Donor lungs should be ventilated with a protective strategy (low inspired oxygen, low tidal volume/inspired pressure) after transplantation

19

It is estimated that more than one million individuals with end-stage lung disease are potential recipients of lung transplants. The OPTN has 1643 patients listed as candidates for lung transplantation in the United States. This number does not accurately reflect the number of organs required because some patients will require bilateral lung transplantation. Average time to transplant increased to as high as 451 days in 1999; however, most recently, that time has declined to 325 days. After stagnating from 2001 to 2003 at slightly more than 1000 transplants annually, the number of transplants in the United States has grown steadily since 2010 to between 1700 and 1900 annually. Currently, about one-fourth of patients undergo transplant within 251 days. Most of this improvement has been seen with recipients who are 50 years and older. One explanation for this may be increasing leniency in organ-selection criteria. The use of expanded criteria does not appear to have been associated with an increase in mortality. Mortality for patients on the waiting list also has continued to decline, from a 2001 high of about 500 to approximately 198 in 2014. Although some of this improvement may be ascribed to better medical management of patients on the waiting list, it is also likely due to broadened criteria for acceptance for transplantation and the corresponding increase in the number of transplants performed per year.

Data from 1990 to 2012 have shown a median survival of about 5.7 years. Double-lung transplant recipients did better than single-lung transplants, with median survival being 7.0 years as compared with 4.5 years for single-lung transplants. Better survival data have been reported from centers with extensive experience with these procedures (1-year survival rates of 82% for double-lung recipients and 90% for single-lung recipients). Infection is the most frequent cause of death in the first year after transplant, but this is superseded in later years by bronchiolitis obliterans (BO). Additional causes for mortality are primary graft failure, technical problems with the procedure, and cardiovascular causes. In patients who have longer survival, the causes shift more toward BO, chronic rejection, and malignancy.

Some of the most challenging patients are those with cystic fibrosis. The 1-year survival rate of 79% and 5-year survival rate of 57% after lung transplantation have shown that, despite the high incidence of poor nutrition and the almost ubiquitous colonization by multidrug-resistant organisms, these patients can still successfully undergo lung transplantation with acceptable outcomes data.

It is a sign of the maturity of lung transplantation procedures that survival data for redo lung transplantation also are becoming available. Retransplantation has very high early mortality and a median survival rate of only 2.5 years. Infection and multiorgan failure before repeat transplant are associated with an almost uniformly fatal outcome. Subsequent data from UNOS, however, have shown an improvement, with the 1-year survival rate at 66.3% in the retransplant patients as compared with 83.8% in the primary transplant population. This is, however, significantly worse at 3 years, with repeat survival rate at 38.8% compared with 63.2% (Box 19.3).

Recipient Selection

Because donor lungs are scarce, it is important to select those most likely to benefit from lung transplantation as recipients. In general, candidates should be terminally ill with end-stage lung disease (NYHA class III or IV, with a life expectancy of approximately 2 years), be psychologically stable, and be devoid of serious medical illness (especially extrapulmonary infection) compromising other organ systems. Patients already requiring mechanical ventilation are poor candidates, although lung transplantation can be successful in such a setting. Other factors, such as advanced age, previous thoracic surgery or deformity, and steroid dependence, may be regarded as relative

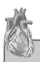

BOX 19.3 *Risk Factors for Increased Mortality*

Smaller transplant center: 30 transplants per year
Greater donor-to-recipient height mismatch
Older recipient: older than 55
Higher bilirubin
Higher supplemental oxygen therapy
Lower cardiac output
Lower forced vital capacity
Higher creatinine

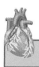

BOX 19.4 *Absolute Contraindications for Lung Transplantation*

Malignancy within 2 years (preferably 5 years)
Untreatable significant disease in another organ system
Atherosclerotic disease not corrected
Acute medical instability: hepatic failure
Bleeding diathesis that is not correctable
Mycobacterium tuberculosis infection
Highly virulent or resistant microbial infections
Chest wall deformity
Obesity
Medical noncompliance
Psychiatric disease leading to noncooperation in management plan
Absent social support system
Substance abuse/addiction
Severely impaired functional status

19

contraindications by individual transplant centers. Hepatic disease solely caused by right-heart dysfunction should not preclude candidacy (Boxes 19.4 and 19.5).

Potential recipients undergo a multidisciplinary assessment of their suitability, including pulmonary spirometry, radiography (plain film and chest CT scan), and echocardiography or multigated image acquisition scan. Patients older than 40 years and those with pulmonary hypertension usually undergo left-heart catheterization to exclude significant coronary atherosclerosis or an intracardiac shunt. TEE may yield data (eg, unanticipated atrial septal defect) that will alter subsequent surgical approach in approximately one-quarter of patients with severe pulmonary hypertension. Candidates who are accepted often are placed on a physical conditioning regimen to reverse muscle atrophy and debilitation and kept within 20% of their ideal body weight. Because lung transplantation is an emergency procedure (limited by a lung preservation time of 6–8 hours), results of this comprehensive evaluation should be readily available to the anesthesiology team at all times.

Donor Selection and Graft Harvest

The ongoing shortage of suitable donor organs has led to a liberalization of selection criteria. Prospective lung donors who were cigarette smokers are no longer rejected

BOX 19.5 *Relative Contraindications for Lung Transplantation*

Age >65 years with limited functional reserve
Obesity
Malnutrition
Severe osteoporosis
Prior lung resection surgery
Mechanical ventilation or extracorporeal life support
Highly resistant bacterial colonization
Hepatitis B and C
HIV infection with detectable viral load
Burkholderia and *Mycobacterium abscessus* infection in which good control is not expected

simply based on a pack-year history. Computed tomography has been used to assess the structural integrity of the lung, particularly in donors who have suffered traumatic chest injury. Lungs that have contusion limited to less than 30% of a single lobe can be considered adequate. Greater use also has been made of organs from older but otherwise healthy donors (55 to 60 years old), especially when the ischemic period will be short. A clear chest radiograph, normal blood gas results, unremarkable findings on bronchoscopy, sputum stain, and direct intraoperative bronchoscopic and gross evaluation confirm satisfactory lung condition. The lungs are matched to the recipient for ABO blood type and size (oversized lungs can result in severe atelectasis and compromise of venous return in the recipient, especially after double-lung transplantation). Donor serology and tracheal cultures will guide subsequent antibacterial and antiviral therapy in the recipient.

Most lung grafts are recovered during a multivisceral donor harvest procedure. The heart is removed as described for heart transplantation, using inflow occlusion and cardioplegic arrest, with division of the IVC and SVC, the aorta, and the main PA. Immediately after cross-clamping, the pulmonary vasculature is flushed with ice-cold extracellular preservative solution, which often contains prostaglandin E_1. This is believed to promote pulmonary vasodilation, which aids homogeneous distribution of the preserving solution. Other additives that have been included are nitroglycerin and low-potassium 5% dextran. The left atrium is divided to leave an adequate LA cuff for both the heart graft and lung graft(s) with the pulmonary veins. After explantation, the lung also may be flushed to clear all pulmonary veins of any clots. After the lung is inflated, the trachea (or bronchus for an isolated lung) is clamped, divided, and stapled closed. Inflating the lung has been shown to increase cold ischemia tolerance of the donor organ. The lung graft is removed, bagged, and immersed in ice-cold saline for transport. The use of extracellular preservation fluid has been shown to be beneficial in protecting the lungs from ischemia/reperfusion injury. However, the most important factor to consider when determining resistance to ischemia/reperfusion is the duration of the ischemia itself. When the ischemia time exceeds 330 minutes, the risk of mortality rapidly increases.

Surgical Procedures

Because of the relative shortage of lung donors and the finding that recipients can gain significant exercise tolerance even with only one transplanted lung, single-lung transplantation used to be the procedure of choice for all lung transplant candidates. Subsequently, however, the published data have indicated better outcomes for those patients receiving double-lung transplant. Certain situations exist in which it is, practically speaking, better to transplant both lungs. For example, the presence of lung disease associated with chronic infection (cystic fibrosis and severe bronchiectasis) mandates double-lung transplantation to prevent the recipient lung from acting as a reservoir of infection and subsequently cross-contaminating the allograft. Patients with severe air trapping may require double-lung transplantation if uncontrollable ventilation/perfusion mismatching will be likely after transplantation.

Single-Lung Transplant

The choice of which lung to transplant is usually based on multiple factors, including avoidance of a prior operative site, preference for removing the native lung with the worst ventilation/perfusion ratio, and donor lung availability. The recipient is positioned for a posterolateral thoracotomy, with the ipsilateral groin prepped and exposed in case CPB becomes necessary. With the lung isolated, a pneumonectomy is performed, with special care to preserve as long a PA segment as possible. After removal of the diseased native lung, the allograft is positioned in the chest, with particular attention taken to maintaining its cold tissue temperature. The bronchial anastomosis is performed first. A telescoping anastomosis is used if there is significant discrepancy in size between the donor and the recipient. The object of the technique is to minimize the chance of dehiscence. Although it was once common to wrap bronchial anastomoses with omentum, wrapping produces no added benefit when a telescoping anastomosis is performed. The PA is anastomosed next, and finally, the left atrial cuff on the allograft containing the pulmonary venous orifices is anastomosed to the native left atrium. The pulmonary circuit is then flushed with blood and de-aired. The initial flush solution is usually cold (4°C) but is followed by a warm (37°C) flush. The warm flush usually is performed during final completion of the vascular anastomoses. The administration of pulmonoplegia aims to achieve a controlled reperfusion. The contents of this solution are listed in Box 19.6.

After glucocorticoid administration, the vascular clamps are removed and reperfusion is begun. The vascular anastomoses are inspected for any areas of hemorrhage, and then the lung is reinflated with a series of ventilations to full functional residual capacity. After achieving adequate hemostasis and satisfactory blood gases, chest tubes are placed, the wound is closed, and the patient is transported to the ICU.

BOX 19.6 *Warm Pulmonoplegia*

Hematocrit 18 to 20, leukocyte-depleted
L-Glutamate
L-Aspartate
Adenosine
Lidocaine
Nitroglycerin
Verapamil
Dextrose
Insulin

Double-Lung Transplant

Early attempts at double-lung transplantation using an en bloc technique via a median sternotomy were plagued by frequent postoperative airway dehiscence because of poor vascular supply of the tracheal anastomosis, by hemorrhage caused by extensive mediastinal dissection (which also resulted in cardiac denervation), by the requirement for complete CPB and cardioplegic arrest (to facilitate pulmonary arterial and venous anastomoses), and by poor access to the posterior mediastinum. The subsequent development of the bilateral sequential lung transplant technique via a "clamshell" thoracosternotomy (essentially, two single-lung transplants performed in sequence) has avoided many of the problems inherent in the en bloc technique. An alternative to using a clamshell incision in slender patients is an approach through two individual anterolateral thoracotomies. This can result in a particularly pleasing cosmetic result in female patients because the scar can be hidden in the breast crease. Use of CPB is optional, but it does result in better exposure of the posterior mediastinum, thus improving hemostasis, and cardiac denervation usually can be avoided. Pleural scarring usually is extensive in patients with cystic fibrosis, and postoperative hemorrhage and coagulopathy are common and potentially exacerbated if CPB is required.

Transplantation of both lungs is performed in the supine position. The groin is prepped and exposed in case CPB is required. If a clamshell incision is used, the arms are padded and suspended over the head on an ether screen. In the slender patient whose anteroposterior chest dimensions are normal, the arms may be tucked at the patient's sides. Recipient pneumonectomy and implantation of the donor lung are performed sequentially on both sides in essentially the same manner as described earlier for a single-lung transplant. The native lung with the worst function should be transplanted first. In patients whose indication for transplantation is suppurative disease, the pleural cavity is pulse-lavaged with antibiotic-containing solution that has been tailored to that patient's antimicrobial sensitivity profile, although it is unclear if this has any effect on subsequent infection. In addition to this, the anesthesiologist irrigates the trachea and bronchi with diluted iodophor solution before the donor lung is brought onto the surgical field.

Pathophysiology Before Transplantation

Patients with highly compliant lungs and obstruction of expiratory airflow cannot completely exhale the delivered tidal volume, resulting in positive intrapleural pressure throughout the respiratory cycle (auto-PEEP [positive end-expiratory pressure] or intrinsic PEEP), which decreases venous return and causes hypotension. The presence of auto-PEEP is highly negatively correlated with forced expiratory volume in 1 second (FEV_1; percentage predicted) and highly positively correlated with pulmonary flow resistance and resting hypercarbia. Hyperinflation is a frequent complication of single-lung ventilation during lung transplantation in patients with obstructive lung disease. Hyperinflation-induced hemodynamic instability can be confirmed by disconnecting the patient from the ventilator for 30 seconds and opening the breathing circuit to the atmosphere. If the blood pressure returns to its baseline value, hyperinflation is most likely the underlying cause. Hyperinflation can be ameliorated with deliberate hypoventilation (decreasing both the tidal volume and rate). Although this may result in profound hypercarbia, high carbon dioxide tensions are often well tolerated in the absence of hypoxemia. PEEP also may decrease air trapping because it decreases expiratory resistance during controlled mechanical ventilation. However, the application of PEEP requires close monitoring because, if the level of extrinsic PEEP applied exceeds the level of auto-PEEP, further air trapping may result.

RV failure frequently is encountered in lung-transplant recipients with pulmonary hypertension because of chronically increased RV afterload. The response of the right ventricle to a chronic increase in afterload is to hypertrophy, but eventually this adaptive response is insufficient. As a result, RV stroke volume decreases and chamber dilation results. The combination of increasing afterload for the right ventricle coupled with decreased stroke volume (and subsequent decrease in the LV stroke volume) creates an unfavorable supply-and-demand situation that makes the right ventricle more prone for failure. The following should be kept in mind when caring for patients with severe dysfunction (Box 19.7). First, increases in intrathoracic pressure may markedly increase PVR, leading to frank RV failure in patients with chronic RV dysfunction. Changes in RV function may occur immediately after adding PEEP, increasing tidal volume, or decreasing expiratory time, and can have devastating consequences. In addition, although intravascular volume expansion in the presence of normal PVR increases CO, overzealous infusion in patients with increased PVR will increase RV end-diastolic pressure and RV wall stress, decreasing CO. Inotropes with vasodilating properties (such as dobutamine or milrinone) often are a better choice than volume for augmenting CO in the setting of increased PVR. Furthermore, the right ventricle has a greater metabolic demand yet a lower coronary perfusion pressure than normal. RV performance can be augmented by improving RV coronary perfusion pressure with α-adrenergic agents, provided these vasoconstrictors do not disproportionately increase PVR. Vasopressin is a good choice to achieve this result. This can sometimes be a better choice than augmenting the perfusion pressure with β-adrenergic agents because the oxygen supply is increased without a large increase in oxygen demand. Additionally, the use of norepinephrine has also been shown to improve the ratio of systemic to pulmonary pressures. Finally, vasodilators such as nitroprusside or prostaglandin E_1 may be effective in decreasing PVR and improving RV dysfunction early in the disease process, when only mild-to-moderate pulmonary hypertension is present. However, they are of notably limited value in the presence of severe, end-stage pulmonary hypertension. Systemic vasodilation and exacerbation of shunting often limit their use. Inhaled nitric oxide activates guanylate cyclase and raises the level of cyclic guanosine monophosphate that results in local vasodilation; it has shown promise as a means of acutely decreasing PVR without altering systemic hemodynamics before and during the explantation phase, as well as after lung transplantation. Nitric oxide decreases both PA pressure and intrapulmonary shunting.

19

BOX 19.7 *Treatment of Intraoperative Right Ventricular Failure*

- Avoid large increases in intrathoracic pressure from:
  - Positive end-expiratory pressure (PEEP)
  - Large tidal volumes
  - Inadequate expiratory time
- Intravascular volume
  - Increase preload if pulmonary vascular resistance is normal
  - Rely on inotropes (dobutamine) if pulmonary vascular resistance is increased
- Maintain right ventricular coronary perfusion pressure with α-adrenergic agonists
- Cautious administration of pulmonary vasodilators (avoid systemic and gas exchange effects)
  - Prostaglandin E_1 (0.05–0.15 µg/kg per min)
  - Inhaled nitric oxide (20–40 ppm)

Further, the combination of inhaled nitric oxide and aerosolized prostacyclin had a synergistic effect, without causing deleterious effects on the systemic perfusion pressure. The use of nitric oxide with or without inhaled prostacyclin may be helpful in avoiding CPB in patients having lung transplantation. In addition to the medications just mentioned, patients with pulmonary hypertension may also have been started on phosphodiesterase-5 inhibitors, soluble guanylate cyclase, and endothelin receptor antagonists. Patients may also be on a prostaglandin infusion preoperatively, which should be kept running during the transplant procedure.

Pathophysiology After Lung Transplantation

The implantation of the donor lung(s) causes marked alterations in recipient respiratory physiology. In single-lung recipients, the pattern of ventilation/perfusion matching depends on the original disease process. For example, with pulmonary fibrosis, blood flow and ventilation gradually divert to the transplanted lung, whereas in patients transplanted for diseases associated with pulmonary hypertension, blood flow is almost exclusively diverted to the transplanted lung, which still receives only half of the total ventilation. In such patients the native lung represents mostly dead-space ventilation. Transplantation results in obligatory sympathetic and parasympathetic denervation of the donor lung and therefore alters the physiologic responses of airway smooth muscle. Exaggerated bronchoconstrictive responses to the muscarinic agonist metha-choline have been noted in some (but not all) studies of denervated lung recipients. The mechanism of hyperresponsiveness may involve cholinergic synapses, inasmuch as they are the main mediators of bronchoconstriction. For example, electrical stimula-tion of transplanted bronchi (which activates cholinergic nerves) produces a hyper-contractile response. This suggests either enhanced release of acetylcholine from cholinergic nerve endings because of an increased responsiveness of parasympathetic nerves or else a loss of inhibitory innervation. Such effects are unlikely to be postsynaptic in origin because the number and affinity of muscarinic cholinergic receptors on transplanted human bronchi are similar to controls. Reinnervation during subsequent weeks to months has been demonstrated in several animal models, but there was no definitive evidence concerning reinnervation of transplanted human lungs until a small study was published in 2008 that showed return of cough reflex to noxious stimuli (distal to the anastomosis) within 12 months. Mucociliary function is transiently severely impaired after lung transplantation and remains depressed for up to a year after the procedure. Thus transplant recipients require particularly aggressive endo-tracheal suctioning to remove airway secretions.

Lung transplantation also profoundly alters the vascular system. The ischemia and reperfusion that are an obligatory part of the transplantation process damages endothelium. Cold ischemia alone decreases β-adrenergic cyclic adenosine monophosphate–mediated vascular relaxation by approximately 40%, and subsequent reperfusion produces even greater decreases in both cyclic guanosine monophosphate–mediated and β-adrenergic cyclic adenosine monophosphate–mediated pulmonary vascular smooth muscle relaxation. Endothelial damage in the pulmonary allograft also results in leaky alveolar capillaries and the development of pulmonary edema. Pulmonary endothelial permeability is approximately three times greater in donor lungs than in healthy volunteers. Regulation of pulmonary vasomotor tone solely by circulating humoral factors is another side effect of denervation. Changes in either the levels of circulating mediators or in the responsiveness of the pulmonary vasculature to such mediators may result in dramatic effects on the pulmonary vasculature. An example of the former is the finding that the potent vasoconstrictor endothelin is present at markedly increased levels (two to three times normal) immediately after transplantation and remains increased for up to a week thereafter. Alterations in the response of denervated pulmonary vasculature to α_1-adrenergic agents and prostaglandin E_1, as well as a reduction in nitric oxide activity, also have been demonstrated in acutely denervated lung. Dysfunctional responses to mediators may be exaggerated if CPB is required. PVR can be substantially decreased with the administration of inhaled nitric oxide after reperfusion. It remains unclear whether nitric oxide also ameliorates reperfusion injury. Several studies suggest that nitric oxide prevents or modulates reperfusion injury as measured by decreased lung water, lipid peroxidase activity, and neutrophil aggregation in the graft. However, a number of studies suggest that, although nitric oxide has an effect on pulmonary hemodynamics, it does not ameliorate reperfusion injury.

Aerosolized inhaled prostacyclin also decreases PVR after reperfusion and improves oxygenation without the added theoretic risk for worsening reperfusion injury. Inhaled prostacyclin has approximately the same effectiveness as nitric oxide in treating lungs damaged by reperfusion injury and offers the added benefit of being less expensive.

Given these pathophysiologic derangements, it is not surprising that PVR increases in the transplanted lung. However, what the clinician observes in the lung-transplant patient will depend on the severity of pulmonary vascular dysfunction present before surgery. PA pressures decrease dramatically during lung transplantation in patients who had pulmonary hypertension before transplantation, and pressures remain decreased for weeks to months thereafter. Concomitant with the decrease in PA pressure, there is an immediate decrease in RV size after lung transplantation in those patients with preexisting pulmonary hypertension, as well as a return to a more normal geometry of the interventricular septum. Both of these effects are sustained over several weeks to months. Although echocardiographic indices of RV function (RV fractional area change) have not shown a consistent improvement in the immediate posttransplant period, several other studies have documented improvement in RV function during the first several months after lung transplantation. One striking finding was that persistent depression of RV function (defined as baseline RV fractional area change of less than 30% with failure to increase after transplant by either at least 5% or by 20% of baseline) was statistically associated with death in the immediate perioperative period.

Anesthetic Management

Preoperative Evaluation and Preparation

Immediate pretransplant reevaluation pertinent to intraoperative management includes a history and physical examination to screen for intercurrent deterioration or additional abnormalities that affect anesthetic management. Particular attention should be given to recent physical status, especially when the transplant evaluation was performed more than 9 to 12 months previously. A decrease in the maximal level of physical activity from that at the time of initial evaluation can be a sign of progressive pulmonary disease or worsening RV function. Most patients are maintained on supplemental nasal oxygen yet are mildly hypoxemic. Patients who are bedridden or those who must pause between phrases or words while speaking possess little functional reserve and are likely to exhibit hemodynamic instability during induction. The time and nature of the last oral intake should be determined to aid in deciding the appropriate method of securing the airway. The physical examination should focus on evaluation of the airway for ease of laryngoscopy and intubation, on the presence of any reversible pulmonary dysfunction such as bronchospasm, and on signs of cardiac failure. Patients with scleroderma can present difficulty in that they often have a small mouth opening, and in some cases, they can have restricted cervical range of motion. New laboratory data often are not available before the beginning of anesthesia care, but special attention should be directed to evaluation of the chest radiograph for signs of pneumothorax, effusion, or hyperinflation because they may affect subsequent management.

Equipment necessary for this procedure is analogous to that used in any procedure in which CPB and cardiac arrest are real possibilities. Special mandatory pieces of equipment include some method to isolate the ventilation to each lung; although bronchial blockers have their advocates, double-lumen endobronchial tubes offer the advantages of easy switching of the ventilated lung, suctioning of the nonventilated lung, and facile independent lung ventilation after surgery. A left-sided double-lumen endobronchial tube is suitable for virtually all lung transplant cases (even left-lung transplants). Regardless of whether a bronchial blocker or double-lumen tube is used, a fiberoptic bronchoscope is absolutely required to rapidly and unambiguously verify correct tube positioning, evaluate bronchial anastomoses, and clear airway secretions. An adult-sized bronchoscope offers better field of vision and superior suctioning capability but can be used only with 41 or 39 French double-lumen tubes. A ventilator with low internal compliance is necessary to adequately ventilate the noncompliant lungs of recipients with restrictive lung disease or donor lungs suffering from reperfusion injury. The added capability of the ventilator to deliver pressure-controlled ventilation also is important, especially for the patients who have pulmonary fibrotic disease or reperfusion injury. Single-lung recipients with highly compliant lungs may require independent lung ventilation with a second ventilator after transplantation. A PAC capable of estimating right ventricular ejection fraction (RVEF) can be useful in diagnosing RV failure and its response to inotropes and vasodilators, as well as the response of the right ventricle to clamping of the PA. However, RVEF catheters are not accurate in the presence of significant tricuspid regurgitation or when malpositioned. Continuous mixed venous oximetry is beneficial in evaluating tissue oxygen delivery in patients subject to sudden, severe cardiac decompensation in the course of the operation, as well as the responses to therapy. A rapid-infusion system can be lifesaving in cases in which major hemorrhage occurs because of anastomotic leaks, inadequate surgical ligation of mediastinal collateral vessels, chest wall adhesions, or coagulopathy after CPB.

Induction of Anesthesia

Patients presenting for lung transplantation frequently arrive in the operating room area without premedication. Indeed, many will be admitted directly to the operating room from home. Because of the nature of the procedure planned, and many months on the transplant waiting list, these patients are often extremely anxious. Considering the risk for respiratory depression from sedatives in patients who are chronically hypoxic or hypercapnic, or both, only the most judicious use of intravenous benzo-diazepines or narcotics is warranted. Assiduous administration of adequate local anesthesia during placement of invasive monitoring will also considerably improve conditions for both the patient and anesthesiologist. The standard noninvasive monitoring typical of cardiovascular procedures is used (ie, two electrocardiogram leads, including a precordial lead, blood pressure cuff, pulse oximetry, capnography, and temperature measurement). Intravenous access sufficient to administer large volumes of fluid rapidly is required. Generally, two large-bore (16- or, preferably, 14-gauge catheters, or a 9 French introducer sheath) intravenous catheters are placed. Patients for bilateral sequential lung transplantation who will receive a clamshell thoracosternotomy should have intravenous catheters placed in the internal or external jugular veins, because peripherally placed intravenous catheters often are unreliable when the arms are bent at the elbow and suspended from the ether screen. An intraarterial catheter is an absolute requirement for blood pressure monitoring and for obtaining specimens for arterial blood gases. Continuous monitoring via a fiberoptic electrode placed in the arterial catheter occasionally may be useful if this technology is available. One femoral artery should be left free of vascular access to allow for cannulation access for CPB or extracorporeal membrane oxygenation (ECMO). Although the radial or brachial artery may be used in single-lung transplantation patients, these sites are not optimal in those who will require CPB (eg, en bloc double-lung transplants or patients with severe pulmonary hypertension) because the transduced pressure may inaccurately reflect central aortic pressure during and after CPB, as well as in patients undergoing a clamshell thoracosternotomy, because of the positioning of the arms. An axillary arterial catheter may also be useful in the latter situations because it provides a more accurate measure of central aortic pressure and allows sampling blood closer to that perfusing the brain. This may be important if partial CPB with a femoral arterial cannula is used because differential perfusion of the upper and lower half of the body may result. A PAC is inserted via the internal or external jugular veins. A TEE probe is placed after the airway is secured. PA pressure monitoring is most useful in patients who have preexisting pulmonary hypertension, especially during induction and during initial one-lung ventilation (OLV) and PA clamping. Position of the PAC must be verified by TEE to ensure that it is residing in the main PA.

If the procedure is planned without CPB, care should be taken to ensure that the patient is kept at ideal physiologic temperature to minimize coagulopathy and increases in the oxygen consumption. This can be achieved with a warming blanket on the bed, on the patient's head and arms, and on the legs below the knees. A fluid warmer is also useful in this regard.

Three main principles should guide the formulation of a plan for induction: (1) protection of the airway; (2) avoidance of myocardial depression and increases in RV afterload in patients with RV dysfunction; and (3) avoidance and recognition of lung hyperinflation in patients with increased lung compliance and expiratory airflow obstruction (Box 19.8). All lung transplants are done on an emergency basis, and the majority of patients will have recently had oral intake and must be considered to have full stomachs. Because aspiration during induction would be catastrophic, every measure must be taken to protect the airway. Patients with known or suspected abnormalities of airway anatomy should be intubated awake after topical anesthesia is applied to the airway. Although a conventional rapid-sequence intravenous induction with a short-acting hypnotic (such as etomidate, 0.2–0.3 mg/kg), a small amount of narcotic (eg, up to 10 µg/kg of fentanyl) and succinylcholine usually will be tolerated, patients with severe RV dysfunction may exhibit profound hemodynamic instability

19

BOX 19.8 *Key Principles of Anesthetic Induction for Lung Transplantation*

Secure the airway
Intravenous rapid sequence induction versus gradual narcotic induction with continuous cricoid pressure
Avoid myocardial depression and increases in right ventricular afterload
Avoid lung hyperinflation

in response to this induction regimen. For such patients, a more gradual induction is recommended, with greater reliance on high doses of narcotics and ventilation with continuous application of cricoid pressure. Consideration should also be given to possibly starting an inotrope or indicator before induction to allow for support of the right ventricle. Patients with bullous disease or fibrotic lungs requiring high inflation pressures may develop a pneumothorax during initiation of positive-pressure ventilation. Acute reductions in SaO_2 accompanied by difficulty in ventilating the lungs and refractory hypotension should generate strong suspicions that a tension pneumothorax has developed. RV function can be impaired during induction by drug-induced myocardial depression, increases in afterload, or by ischemia secondary to acute RV dilation. Agents that act as myocardial depressants should be avoided in such patients. Increases in RV afterload can result from inadequate anesthesia, exacerbation of chronic hypoxemia and hypercarbia and metabolic acidosis, as well as increases in intrathoracic pressure because of positive-pressure ventilation. Systemic hypotension is poorly tolerated because increased RV end-diastolic pressure will diminish net RV coronary perfusion pressure. In addition, chronic increase of RV afterload increases the metabolic requirements of RV myocardium. Once the trachea is intubated and positive-pressure ventilation initiated, the avoidance of hyperinflation in patients with increased pulmonary compliance or bullous disease is crucial. Small tidal volumes, low respiratory rates, and inspiratory/expiratory (I:E) ratios should be used even if this allows increased end tidal carbon dioxide (permissive hypercapnia), although attention should be paid to the effect of this action on the pulmonary artery pressure. If hemodynamic instability does occur with positive-pressure ventilation, the ventilator should be disconnected from the patient. If hyperinflation is the cause of hypotension, blood pressure will increase within 10 to 30 seconds of the onset of apnea. Ventilation then can be resumed at a tidal volume and/or rate compatible with hemodynamic stability.

Anesthesia can be maintained using a variety of techniques. A moderate dose of narcotic (5–15 μg/kg of fentanyl or the equivalent), combined with low doses of a potent inhalation anesthetic, offers the advantages of stable hemodynamics, a high inspired oxygen concentration, a rapidly titratable depth of anesthesia, and the possibility of extubation in the early postoperative period. Patients with severe RV dysfunction who cannot tolerate even low concentrations of inhalation anesthetics may require a pure narcotic technique. Nitrous oxide generally is not used because of the requirement for a high inspired oxygen concentration throughout the procedure and its possible deleterious effects if gaseous emboli or an occult pneumothorax is present.

Intraoperative Management

Institution of OLV occurs before hilar dissection and may compromise hemodynamics or gas exchange, or both (Box 19.9). Patients with diminished lung compliance often can tolerate OLV with normal tidal volumes and little change in hemodynamics. In contrast, patients with increased lung compliance and airway obstruction often will exhibit marked hemodynamic instability, unless the tidal volume is decreased and the expiratory time is increased. The magnitude of hypoxemia generally peaks about 20 minutes after beginning OLV. Hypoxemia during OLV may be treated with continuous positive airway pressure applied to the nonventilated lung, PEEP to the ventilated lung, or both. Continuous positive airway pressure attempts to oxygenate the shunt fraction but may interfere with surgical exposure. PEEP attempts to minimize atelectasis in the ventilated lung, but may concomitantly increase shunt through the nonventilated lung. Definitive treatment of shunt in the nonventilated lung is provided by rapid isolation and clamping of the PA of the nonventilated lung. Pneumothorax on the nonoperative side may result during OLV if a large tidal volume is used.

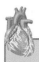

BOX 19.9 *Management Principles for One-Lung Ventilation During Lung Transplantation*

- Tidal volume and respiratory rate
  - Maintain in patients with normal or decreased lung compliance (ie, primary pulmonary hypertension, fibrosis)
  - Decrease both tidal volume and rate in patients with increased compliance (eg, obstructive lung disease) to avoid hyperinflation (permissive hypercapnia)
- Maintain oxygenation by:
  - 100% inspired oxygen
  - Applying continuous positive airway pressure (5–10 cm H_2O) to nonventilated lung
  - Adding positive end-expiratory pressure (5–10 cm H_2O) to ventilated lung
  - Intermittent lung reinflation if necessary
  - Surgical ligation of the pulmonary artery of the nonventilated lung
- Be alert for development of pneumothorax on nonoperative side
  - Sharp decline in oxygen saturation, end-tidal carbon dioxide
  - Sharp increase in peak airway pressures
  - Increased risk with bullous lung disease
- Therapy
  - Relieve tension
  - Resume ventilation
  - Emergency cardiopulmonary bypass

BOX 19.10 *Indications for Cardiopulmonary Bypass During Lung Transplantation*

Cardiac index	<2 L/min/m²
Svo_2	<60%
Mean arterial pressure	<50 to 60 mm Hg
Sao_2	<85% to 90%
pH	<7.00

19

PA clamping usually is well tolerated, except in the face of pulmonary hypertension with diminished RV reserve. If the degree of RV compromise is uncertain, a 5- to 10-minute trial of PA clamping is attempted; then the right ventricle is evaluated by serial COs and RVEF measurements and inspection by TEE. A significant decrease in CO may predict patients who will require extracorporeal support. Other indications for CPB in lung transplantation are listed in Box 19.10.

Patients with severe pulmonary hypertension (greater than two-thirds of systemic pressure) generally will be placed on CPB before PA clamping. The intraoperative use of nitric oxide (20 to 40 parts per million [ppm]) may allow some procedures to proceed without the use of CPB.

Lung transplantation usually can be performed without the aid of CPB; even during bilateral sequential lung transplantation, experienced teams use CPB for only about one-quarter of patients. Although CPB may provide stable hemodynamics, it is associated with an increased transfusion requirement. In addition, graft function (as reflected by alveolar-arterial oxygen gradient) may be compromised, endothelium-dependent cyclic guanosine monophosphate–mediated and β-adrenergic cyclic adenosine monophosphate–mediated pulmonary vascular relaxation may be impaired to a greater degree, and a longer period of mechanical ventilation may be necessary. Several exceptional circumstances require CPB: the presence of severe pulmonary hypertension because clamping of the PA will likely result in acute RV failure and flooding of the nonclamped lung, the repair of associated cardiac anomalies (eg, patent foramen ovale, atrial or ventricular septal defects), treatment of severe hemodynamic or gas exchange instabilities, and living-related lobar transplantation. Hypercarbia generally is well tolerated and should not be considered a requirement for CPB per se. Thus the frequency of CPB will depend on recipient population factors such as prevalence of end-stage pulmonary vascular disease and associated cardiac anomalies.

The use of femoral venous and arterial cannulae for CPB during lung transplantation may lead to poor venous drainage and/or differential perfusion of the lower and upper body. Moreover, native pulmonary blood flow continues and may act as an intrapulmonary shunt during what will be partial CPB. In this case, the cerebral vessels receive this desaturated blood, whereas the lower body is perfused with fully oxygenated blood from the CPB circuit. This effect is detectable by blood gas analysis of samples drawn from suitable arteries or by appropriately located pulse oximeter probes. Treatment includes conventional measures to increase venous return and augment bypass flow, or placing a venous cannula in the right atrium if this is feasible. The anesthesiologist also should maximize the inspired oxygen concentration and add PEEP to decrease intrapulmonary shunt. If all other measures fail, ventricular fibrillation can be induced using alternating current, although this is exceedingly rare.

ECMO also has been suggested as an alternative method of CPB during lung transplantation. It has been suggested that the use of ECMO with heparin-bonded circuits might improve the outcome of both single- and double-lung transplants by lessening the amount of pulmonary edema. An added benefit of this technique is that it clears the operative field of bypass cannulae, making left-sided transplant as unimpeded as right-sided transplant. Another added benefit of using ECMO in situ is that reperfusion of the lungs can be more easily controlled because the CO transiting the newly transplanted lung can be precisely controlled. This is especially the case for patients with advanced pulmonary hypertension.

If CPB is used, weaning from circulatory support occurs when the graft anastomoses are complete. Ventilation is resumed with a lung protection strategy similar to that used in the ARDSnet (Acute Respiratory Distress Syndrome Network) trial. This demonstrated that patients with decreased compliance related to acute respiratory distress syndrome had a 22% decrease in mortality rate when applying tidal volumes of 6 mL/kg and a plateau pressure less than 30 cm H_2O. Minimizing the inspired fraction of oxygen may help prevent generation of oxygen free radicals and modulate reperfusion injury. FiO_2 can be decreased to the minimum necessary to maintain the SpO_2 greater than 90%. Special attention should be directed to assessing and supporting RV function during this period, inasmuch as RV failure is the most frequent reason for failure to wean. Although the right ventricle often can be seen in the surgical field, TEE is more valuable for visualizing this structure's functional properties at this juncture. TEE also allows the evaluation of PA and pulmonary vein anastomoses. The PA diameter should be greater than 1 cm. Interrogating the pulmonary veins should demonstrate a two-dimensional diameter that is at least 0.5 cm with the presence of flow as measured by color-flow Doppler. In addition, pulse wave Doppler interrogation should yield flow rates less than 100 cm/second to indicate adequacy of anastomosis. Care should be taken to measure these flow rates with both lungs being perfused because the measurements could be erroneous if measured with one PA clamped. Inotropic support with dobutamine or epinephrine, as well as pulmonary vasodilation with nitroglycerin, nitroprusside, milrinone, or nitric oxide, may be necessary if RV dysfunction is evident. Milrinone has the advantage of providing both inotropic and vasodilatory effects; however, its administration can be complicated by significant systemic hypotension.

Coagulopathy after weaning from CPB is common. The severity of coagulopathy may be worse after double- than single-lung transplantation, probably because of the more extensive dissection, presence of collaterals and scarring, and the longer duration of CPB. Factors under the anesthesiologist's control include incomplete reversal of heparin's effects, which should be assayed by the activated coagulation time. Similarly, preexisting deliberate anticoagulation (eg, caused by warfarin) should be aggressively corrected with fresh-frozen plasma. Because platelet dysfunction is common after CPB, empiric administration is justified if coagulopathy persists. The thrombotic and fibrinolytic systems are activated during lung transplantation, especially if CPB is used, and, although aprotinin can reduce this activation and perhaps reduce perioperative hemorrhage, it has been withdrawn from production. The utility of epsilon-aminocaproic acid, tranexamic acid, and desmopressin (DDAVP) in replacing aprotinin in this setting remains unknown, although some preliminary data suggest that tranexamic acid may be similar in efficacy to aprotinin.

Reperfusion without CPB often is accompanied by a mild-to-moderate decrease in systemic blood pressure and occasionally is complicated by severe hypotension. This is usually the result of profound systemic vasodilation. The causative factor is unknown but may be caused by ionic loads such as potassium or additives such as prostaglandin E_1 in preservation solutions or by vasoactive substances generated during ischemia and reperfusion. This hypotension generally responds well to large doses of α-adrenergic agents and fortunately is short-lived. Agents of greatest use in this setting are norepinephrine and vasopressin. Ventilation is resumed with a lung protection strategy identical to that used when weaning from CPB.

Patients with preexisting increased lung compliance, as found in chronic obstructive pulmonary disease, can manifest great disparity in lung compliance after single-lung transplant. The donor lung usually will exhibit normal to decreased compliance, depending on the presence of reperfusion injury. This will result in relative hyperinflation of the native lung and underinflation with loss of functional residual capacity in the donor lung. Hyperinflation of the native lung may cause hemodynamic instability because of mediastinal shift, especially if PEEP is applied. Therefore patients exhibiting signs of hyperinflation during OLV, which improves with deliberate hypoventilation, should be treated with independent lung ventilation after reperfusion. To accomplish this, the patient's postoperative ventilator is brought to the operating room while the donor lung is being implanted. When all anastomoses are completed, the donor lung is ventilated with a normal tidal volume (8 to 10 mL/kg) and rate, with PEEP initially applied at 10 cm H_2O. These settings can be adjusted according to blood gas analysis. Most gas exchange will take place in the transplanted lung. The native lung is ventilated with a low tidal volume (2 to 3 mL/kg) and a low rate (2 to 4/min) without PEEP. The objective is to prevent this lung from overinflating or developing a large shunt. Carbon dioxide exchange occurs predominantly in the donor lung.

Although some degree of pulmonary edema commonly is detected by chest radiograph after surgery, it is uncommon to encounter severe pulmonary edema in the operating room immediately after reperfusion of the graft. However, when it does occur, postreperfusion pulmonary edema can be dramatic and life-threatening. Copious pink frothy secretions may require almost constant suctioning to maintain a patent airway and may be accompanied by severe gas exchange and compliance abnormalities. Treatment includes high levels of PEEP using selective lung ventilation, diuresis, and volume restriction. Occasionally, patients may require support with

19

ECMO for several days until reperfusion injury resolves; a high percentage of patients so treated ultimately survive.

Adequate analgesia is crucial for these patients to facilitate the earliest possible extubation, ambulation, and participation in spirometric exercises to enhance or preserve pulmonary function. Lumbar or thoracic epidural narcotic analgesia provides excellent analgesia while minimizing sedation. Placement of an epidural catheter in cases in which a high expectation exists for the necessity of CPB remains a controversial topic.

Postoperative Management and Complications

Routine postoperative management of the lung transplant recipient continues many of the monitoring modes and therapies begun in the operating room. Positive-pressure ventilation is continued for at least several hours; if differential lung ventilation was used intraoperatively, this is continued in the early postoperative period. Because the lung graft is prone to the development of pulmonary edema because of preservation/ reperfusion and the loss of lymphatic drainage, fluid administration is minimized and diuresis encouraged when appropriate. When hemorrhage has ceased, the chest radiograph is clear, and the patient meets conventional extubation criteria, the endotracheal tube can be removed. Prophylactic antibacterial, antifungal, and antiviral therapies, as well as the immunosuppressive regimen of choice, are begun after arrival in the ICU.

Surgical technical complications are uncommon immediately after lung transplantation but may be associated with high morbidity. Pulmonary venous obstruction usually presents as acute, persistent pulmonary edema of the transplanted lung. Color-flow and Doppler TEE will show narrowed pulmonary venous orifices with turbulent, high-velocity flow and loss of the normal phasic waveform. PA anastomotic obstruction should be suspected if PA pressures fail to decrease after reperfusion of the lung graft. If the right PA is obstructed, this usually is evident on a TEE examination in the same way as for pulmonary venous obstruction; it is usually much more difficult to inspect the left PA anastomosis adequately with TEE, although some centers have reported a high success rate. The diagnosis can be definitively made by measuring the pressure gradient across the anastomosis either by inserting needles on both sides of the anastomosis to transduce the respective pressures or by advancing the PAC across it. However, care should be taken not to measure this gradient while the contralateral PA is clamped, because the shunting of the entire CO through one lung will exaggerate the gradient present. Angiography and perfusion scanning also are useful for making this diagnosis but are not immediately available in the operating room. Bronchial dehiscence or obstruction is extremely rare in the immediate perioperative period and can be evaluated by fiberoptic bronchoscopy.

Pneumothorax must be a constant concern for the anesthesiologist, especially involving the nonoperative side. Diagnosis of pneumothorax on the nonoperative side during a thoracotomy is extremely difficult. A sudden increase in inflation pressures with deterioration of gas exchange and possibly hypotension are characteristic. However, these same findings are possible with hyperinflation, mucous plugging, or malpositioning of the endobronchial tube. Transient cessation of ventilation and immediate fiberoptic bronchoscopy may rule out the former explanations, and the observation of an upward shift of the mediastinum in the surgical field may be observed in the presence of tension pneumothorax. If this diagnosis is strongly suspected, needle thoracostomy on the field may be lifesaving. Alternatively, the surgeon may be able to dissect across the mediastinum directly and decompress the nonoperative thorax, facilitating reinflation.

Tension pneumopericardium and postoperative hemothorax with complete ventilation/perfusion mismatch are other rare complications that have been reported after lung transplantation. Patients with pulmonary hypertension and RV hypertrophy occasionally may develop dynamic RV outflow obstruction when transplantation acutely decreases RV afterload; the diagnosis can be confirmed using TEE. Hyperacute rejection of a kind similar to that seen with heart transplantation has not been noted with lung transplantation.

The most common cause of death in the immediate perioperative period is graft dysfunction from reperfusion injury, which usually presents with hypoxemia, pulmonary infiltrates, poor lung compliance, pulmonary hypertension, and RV failure. If there are no technical reasons to account for pulmonary hypertension and RV failure, then graft dysfunction must be suspected. Unfortunately, few treatments will specifically ameliorate graft dysfunction and therapy is largely supportive. Vasodilator therapy to directly decrease PVR and, therefore, RV afterload may improve hemodynamics and, in some cases, may improve gas exchange. Both prostaglandin E_1 and nitrates can reverse severe hypoxemia and pulmonary hypertension after lung transplantation, and the latter attenuate the increase in transcription of vasoconstrictor genes (such as for endothelin and platelet-derived growth factor) induced by hypoxia. Indeed, a prophylactic low-dose infusion of prostaglandin E_1 has been reported to preserve arterial oxygen tension without altering pulmonary hemodynamics. and improvement in pulmonary hemodynamics and gas exchange in patients with graft dysfunction also have been reported with the administration of nitric oxide. Compared with historic control patients who developed graft dysfunction before the advent of nitric oxide, inhalation of nitric oxide decreased the duration of mechanical ventilation, frequency of airway complications, and mortality. Improved hemodynamics and gas exchange may reflect the ability of nitric oxide to compensate for the decrease in endothelium-derived relaxant factor activity after transplantation. If nitric oxide has been used to control pulmonary hypertension after surgery, it should be weaned gradually to avoid any rebound pulmonary vasoconstriction. Finally, ECMO may be used to support the patient until there is adequate recovery of pulmonary function.

Infection is a constant threat in these immunosuppressed patients. Prophylactic antibiotic coverage is aimed at agents commonly causing nosocomial and aspiration pneumonias because these are common in donors. Coverage can be modified once culture results from the donor trachea are available. Patients with cystic fibrosis should receive antibiotics targeted at bacteria found in the native lungs before transplantation. Infection should be suspected as the cause of any infiltrate found on chest radiograph, especially if fever or leukocytosis develops, but distinguishing infection from reperfusion injury and rejection may be difficult. Diagnostic bronchoscopy and bronchoalveolar lavage are useful in defining therapy and differentiating infection from rejection, but open-lung biopsy occasionally is necessary for definitive diagnosis. Patients who are seronegative to viral agents to which the donor was seropositive (eg, cytomegalovirus) will require prophylactic antiviral therapy. Rejection episodes are common and may occur as early as several days after transplantation. Rejection often presents as new infiltrates on chest radiograph in the setting of deteriorating gas exchange. Bronchoscopy with transbronchial biopsy helps to rule out other causes of deterioration and document acute changes consistent with rejection. Therapy for acute lung rejection consists of large pulses of steroids such as methylprednisolone or changing the immunosuppressive agents (cyclosporine to tacrolimus or vice versa). Expired nitric oxide has been shown to be an indicator of chronic rejection in post–lung-transplant patients. Measurements of expired nitric oxide have been shown to decrease with the switch of cyclosporine to tacrolimus, reflecting a decrease in the inflammation in the pulmonary mucosa. Expired nitric oxide may be a useful tool to observe patients for the presence or change in chronic graft rejection.

19

One of the most serious complications of lung transplantation occurs late. BO is a syndrome characterized by alloimmune injury leading to obstruction of small airways with fibrous scar. Patients with BO present with cough, progressive dyspnea, obstruction on flow spirometry, and interstitial infiltrates on chest radiograph. Therapy for this syndrome includes augmentation of immunosuppression, cytolytic agents (which have been used with varying degrees of success), or retransplantation in refractory cases.

Living-Related Lung Transplantation

The scarcity of suitable donor lungs has resulted in waiting times on transplant lists in excess of 2 years, during which time up to 30% of candidates succumb to their illness. Living-related lung transplantation programs have developed to address the needs of lung transplant candidates with acute deterioration expected to preclude survival. Successful grafting of a single lobe for children with bronchopulmonary dysplasia or Eisenmenger syndrome, or two lobes for children and young adults with cystic fibrosis, has encouraged several centers to consider such procedures. The anesthetic management issues related to such undertakings have been reviewed. Donor candidates will have undergone a rigorous evaluation to ensure that there are no contraindications to lobe donation and that the donation is not being coerced. Donor lobectomy is performed via a standard posterolateral thoracotomy. Of special note to the anesthesiologist during such procedures is the requirement for OLV to optimize surgical exposure, the continuous infusion of prostaglandin E_1 to promote pulmonary vasodilation, and the administration of heparin and steroids just before lobe harvest. Anesthetic management of the recipient is identical to that for a standard lung transplant, except that the use of CPB is mandatory for bilateral lobar transplant.

▓ HEART-LUNG TRANSPLANTATION

History and Epidemiology

The diminished frequency of heart-lung transplantation since 1990 reflects that it is being supplanted by lung transplantation. The number of HLTs worldwide peaked at 241 in 1989, and there has been a continual decline in subsequent years to approximately half that number. Only 173 HLT candidates were registered with UNOS as of early March 2005, less than 5% of the number on the lung transplant list. The most common recipient indications remain primary pulmonary hypertension, CHD (including Eisenmenger syndrome), and cystic fibrosis.

One-year survival rate after heart-lung transplantation is 60%, significantly less than that for isolated heart or lung transplantation. Mortality in subsequent years is approximately 4% per year, similar to that for heart transplantation. Risk factors for increased mortality after HLT are recipient ventilator dependence, male recipient sex, and a donor age older than 40 years. Early deaths are most often due to graft failure or hemorrhage, whereas midterm and late deaths primarily are due to infection and BO, respectively. Repeat HLT is a rare procedure and is likely to remain so because the 1-year survival rate after repeat HLT is dismal (28%).

Recipient Selection

As more patients with pulmonary hypertension and cystic fibrosis are treated with isolated lung transplantation, it is likely that the indications for heart-lung transplantation will be limited to CHD with irreversible pulmonary hypertension that is not amenable to repair during simultaneous lung transplantation or diseases with both pulmonary hypertension and concomitant severe left ventricular dysfunction.

Donor Selection and Graft Harvest

Potential heart-lung donors must meet not only the criteria for heart donors but also those for lung donation, both described earlier in this chapter. Graft harvesting is carried out in a manner similar to that previously described for heart transplantation. After mobilization of the major vessels and trachea, cardiac arrest is induced with inflow occlusion and infusion of cold cardioplegia into the aortic root. After arrest, the PA is flushed with a cold preservative solution often containing prostaglandin E_1. The ascending aorta, SVC, and trachea are transected, and the heart-lung bloc removed after it is dissected free of the esophagus. The trachea is clamped and the graft immersed in cold solution before being bagged for transport.

Surgical Procedures

The operation generally is performed through a median sternotomy, but a clamshell thoracosternotomy also is an acceptable approach. Both pleurae are incised. Any pulmonary adhesions are taken down before anticoagulation for bypass. Cannulae for CPB are placed in a manner similar to that for heart transplantation. After the aorta is cross-clamped, the heart is excised in a manner similar to that for orthotopic heart transplant. Each lung is then individually removed, including its pulmonary veins. The airways are divided at the level of the respective main bronchi for bibronchial anastomoses. For a tracheal anastomosis, the trachea is freed to the level of the carina without stripping its blood supply and an anastomosis is constructed just above the level of the carina. The atrial anastomosis is performed in a manner similar to that for orthotopic heart transplantation, and finally, the aorta is joined to the recipient aorta. After de-airing and reperfusion, the patient is weaned from CPB, hemostasis is achieved, and the wound is closed.

Pathophysiology Before Transplantation

The pathophysiology of HLT recipients combines the elements discussed earlier in this chapter. Patients usually will have end-stage biventricular failure with severe pulmonary hypertension. The cardiac anatomy may be characterized by complex congenital malformations. If obstruction of pulmonary airflow is present, there is a danger of hyperinflation after application of positive-pressure ventilation.

Pathophysiology After Transplantation

As with isolated heart recipients, the physiology of HLT recipients is characterized by cardiac denervation, transient cardiac ischemic insult during graft harvest, transport, and implantation, and long-term susceptibility to accelerated allograft vasculopathy and rejection. As is the case for lung recipients, heart-lung recipients have denervated pulmonary vascular and airway smooth muscle responses, transient pulmonary ischemic insult, altered pulmonary lymphatic drainage, and impaired mucociliary clearance.

Anesthetic Management

The anesthetic management of heart-lung transplantation more closely resembles that of heart than lung transplantation because the use of CPB is mandatory. After placement of invasive and noninvasive monitoring similar to that used for heart transplantation, anesthesia can be induced with any of the techniques previously described for heart and lung transplantation. As with lung transplantation, avoidance of myocardial depression and protection and control of the airway are paramount. Although a double-lumen endotracheal tube is not mandatory, it will aid in exposure of the posterior mediastinum for hemostasis after weaning from CPB. Otherwise, anesthetic management before CPB is similar to that for heart transplantation.

A bolus of glucocorticoid (eg, methylprednisolone, 500 mg) is given when the aortic cross-clamp is removed. After a period of reperfusion, an inotrope infusion is started and the heart is inspected with TEE for adequate de-airing. Ventilation is resumed with normal tidal volume and rate, along with the addition of PEEP (5–10 cm) before weaning from CPB. After successful weaning from CPB, the PAC can be advanced into the PA again. Protamine then is administered to reverse heparin-induced anti-coagulation. The inspired oxygen concentration often can be decreased to less toxic levels based on blood gas analysis.

Problems encountered after weaning from CPB are similar to those encountered after isolated heart or lung transplantation. Lung reperfusion injury and dysfunction may compromise gas exchange, so administration of crystalloid should be minimized. Occasionally, postreperfusion pulmonary edema may require support with high levels of PEEP and inspired oxygen in the operating room. Ventricular failure usually responds to an increase in β-adrenergic support. Unlike isolated heart or lung transplantation, frank RV failure is uncommon immediately after heart-lung transplantation unless lung preservation was grossly inadequate. Coagulopathy often is present after HLT and should be aggressively treated with additional protamine (if indicated), platelets, and fresh-frozen plasma.

Postoperative Management and Complications

The principles of the immediate postoperative care of HLT recipients are a combination of those of isolated heart and lung recipients. Invasive and noninvasive monitoring done in the operating room is continued. Inotropic support is continued in a manner similar to that for heart transplantation. Ventilatory support is similar to that after lung transplantation; the lowest acceptable inspired oxygen concentration is used to avoid oxygen toxicity, and the patient is weaned from the ventilator after hemodynamics have been stable for several hours, hemorrhage has ceased, and satisfactory gas exchange is present. Diuresis is encouraged. Finally, the immunosuppressive regimen of choice is begun.

Infection is a more frequent and serious complication in heart-lung recipients than in isolated heart recipients. Bacterial and fungal infections are especially common in the first month after transplantation, with viral and other pathogens (*Pneumocystis carinii* and *Nocardia*) occurring in subsequent months.

Similar to isolated heart or lung transplants, rejection episodes are common early after heart-lung transplantation. Rejection may occur independently in either the heart or lung. Therapy is similar to that for rejection of isolated heart or lung grafts.

Heart grafts in heart-lung blocs are prone to accelerated coronary vasculopathy in a manner similar to those of isolated heart grafts. As with lung transplantation, a feared late complication of heart-lung transplantation is BO. Approximately one-third of heart-lung recipients develop this process. Anecdotal reports indicate that most affected patients also have accelerated coronary vasculopathy.

SUGGESTED READINGS

Atluri P, Gaffey A, Howard J, et al. Combined heart and liver transplantation can be safely performed with excellent short- and long-term results. *Ann Thorac Surg.* 2014;98:858.

Awad M, Czer LS, Mirocha J, et al. Prior sternotomy increases the mortality and morbidity of adult heart transplantation. *Transplant Proc.* 2015;47:485.

Canter CE, Shaddy RE, Bernstein D, et al. Indications for heart transplantation in pediatric heart disease: a scientific statement from the American Heart Association Council on Cardiovascular Disease in the Young; the Councils on Clinical Cardiology, Cardiovascular Nursing, and Cardiovascular Surgery and Anesthesia; and the Quality of Care and Outcomes Research Interdisciplinary Working Group. *Circulation.* 2007;115:658.

Chetham P. Anesthesia for heart or single or double lung transplantation. *J Card Surg.* 2000;15:167–174.

Dipchand AI, Kirk R, Edwards LB, et al. The Registry of the International Society for Heart and Lung Transplantation: Sixteenth Official Pediatric Heart Transplantation Report—2013; focus theme: age. *J Heart Lung Transplant.* 2013;32:979.

Gabbay E, Walters EH, Orsida B, et al. Post-lung transplant bronchiolitis obliterans syndrome (BOS) is characterized by increased exhaled nitric oxide levels and epithelial inducible nitric oxide synthetase. *Am J Respir Crit Care Med.* 2000;162:2182–2187.

Gilbert S, Dauber J, Hattler B, et al. Lung and heart-lung transplantation at the University of Pittsburgh 1982–2002. *Clin Transpl.* 2002;16:253–261.

Hoskote A, Carter C, Rees P, et al. Acute right ventricular failure after pediatric cardiac transplant: predictors and long-term outcome in the current era of transplantation medicine. *J Thorac Cardiovasc Surg.* 2010;139:146.

Itescu S, Burke E, Lietz K, et al. Intravenous pulse administration of cyclophosphamide is an effective and safe treatment for sensitized cardiac allograft recipients. *Circulation.* 2002;105:1214.

Ko WJ, Chen YS, Lee YC. Replacing cardiopulmonary bypass with extracorporeal membrane oxygenation in lung transplantation operations. *Artif Organs.* 2001;25:607–612.

Kwak YL, Lee CS. The effect of phenylephrine and norepinephrine in patients with chronic pulmonary hypertension. *Anesthesia.* 2002;57:9.

Lang JD Jr, Leill W. Pro: Inhaled nitric oxide should be used routinely in patients undergoing lung transplantation. *J Cardiothorac Vasc Anesth.* 2001;15:785–789.

McIlroy DR, Pilcher DV, Snell GI. Does anaesthetic management affect early outcomes after lung transplant? An exploratory analysis. *Br J Anesth.* 2009;102:506–514.

Quader MA, Wolfe LG, Kasirajan V. Heart transplantation outcomes in patients with continuous-flow left ventricular assist device-related complications. *J Heart Lung Transplant.* 2014;34:75.

Tallaj JA, Pamboukian SV, George JF, et al. Have risk factors for mortality after heart transplantation changed over time? Insights from 19 years of Cardiac Transplant Research Database study. *J Heart Lung Transplant.* 2014;33:1304.

Thabut G, Mal H, Cerrina J, et al. Graft ischemic time and outcome of lung transplantation: a multicenter analysis. *Am J Respir Crit Care Med.* 2005;171:786. American Thoracic Society.

Trivedi JR, Cheng A, Singh R. Survival on the heart transplant waiting list: impact of continuous flow left ventricular assist device as bridge to transplant. *Ann Thorac Surg.* 2014;98:830.

Voeller RK, Epstein DJ, Guthrie TJ, et al. Trends in the indications and survival in pediatric heart transplants: a 24-year single-center experience in 307 patients. *Ann Thorac Surg.* 2012;94:807.

Weiss ES, Allen JG, Merlo CA, et al. Factors indicative of long-term survival after lung transplantation: a review of 836 10 year survivors. *J Heart Lung Transplant.* 2010;29:240–246.

Whitson BA, Lehman A, Wehr A, et al. To induce or not to induce: a 21st century evaluation of lung transplant immunosuppression's effect on survival. *Clin Transplant.* 2014;28:450.

19

Chapter 20

Pulmonary Thromboendarterectomy for Chronic Thromboembolic Pulmonary Hypertension

Dalia A. Banks, MD, FASE • William R. Auger, MD • Michael M. Madani, MD

Key Points

1. The incidence of thromboembolic disease is difficult to estimate because of the nonspecific nature of presenting symptoms and a lack of awareness of the disorder.
2. Chronic thromboembolic pulmonary hypertension (CTEPH) results from incomplete resolution of a pulmonary embolus (PE) or from recurrent PE.
3. The cause of CTEPH after acute PE is not fully understood. Proposed mechanisms include abnormalities in fibrinolytic enzymes or resistance of the thrombus to fibrinolysis.
4. Pulmonary thromboendarterectomy (PTE) is the most effective treatment for patients with CTEPH.
5. Patients typically present with progressive exertional dyspnea and exercise intolerance because of increased pulmonary vascular resistance (PVR), decreased cardiac output, and increased minute ventilation requirements secondary to increased alveolar dead space.
6. Right-sided heart catheterization defines the severity of pulmonary hypertension and the degree of cardiac dysfunction.
7. Patients with preoperative PVR greater than 1000 dynes·s·cm^{-5} have a greater operative mortality rate, but a markedly increased preoperative PVR does not contraindicate surgical treatment.
8. Postsurgical complications include: reperfusion pulmonary edema and persistent pulmonary hypertension.
9. Riociguat is the first medication approved by the US Food and Drug Administration for treating certain patients with CTEPH.
10. Balloon pulmonary angioplasty is an alternative approach to PTE in patients believed to have surgically inaccessible chronic thromboembolic disease.
11. Reperfusion pulmonary edema and airway bleeding are two of the most difficult complications of PTE to manage.

Chronic thromboembolic pulmonary hypertension (CTEPH) is a form of pulmonary hypertension (PH) that is characterized by complete or partial obstruction of the pulmonary vascular bed as a result of a recurrent or residual intraluminal organized fibrotic clot leading to increased pulmonary vascular resistance (PVR), severe PH, and eventually right-sided heart failure. Its incidence is difficult to estimate because of the uncertainty regarding the frequency of acute pulmonary embolism (PE) and the percentage of patients in whom emboli fail to resolve. The incidence reflects a wide range, from less than 1% to as high as 9% of patients with acute PE.

Screening for CTEPH in patients with PH or unexplained dyspnea is of paramount importance because this form of PH is potentially curable with pulmonary thromboendarterectomy (PTE), also known as pulmonary endarterectomy. The success of the operation centers on endarterectomy of the organized fibrous thrombus in the intima and part of the medial layers of the pulmonary vascular tree. Lung transplantation is another potential option, but it is usually not a choice for patients with CTEPH because of the risk of death while on the waiting list, a shortage of organ supply, the expense, the risk of immunosuppressive agents, infection, and rejection.

CLASSIFICATION OF PULMONARY HYPERTENSION

Classifications of PH began in 1973 at the World Health Organization (WHO) conference and have since undergone multiple revisions as the appreciation of the disease and treatment of PH has evolved. Currently PH is divided into five distinct subgroups of patients sharing specific features (Box 20.1).

Further classification of PH defines the presence of precapillary (groups I, III, IV, and V) or postcapillary (group II) patterns. CTEPH is precapillary PH, as assessed by right-sided heart catheterization characterized by a mean pulmonary artery pressure (mPAP) greater than 25 mm Hg with normal pulmonary capillary wedge pressure lower than 15 mm Hg and an elevated PVR greater than 300 dynes·s·cm^{-5}. Postcapillary PH secondary to left-sided heart disease is the most frequent form of PH, and it is characterized by mPAP greater than 25 mm Hg and pulmonary capillary wedge pressure greater than 15 mm Hg with normal PVR. Differentiating pulmonary arterial hypertension (PAH) from pulmonary venous hypertension in group II is important given the high prevalence of left-sided heart disease. Echocardiography is an essential tool for initial screening and assessment for PH (Table 20.1).

20

BOX 20.1 *Revised World Health Organization Classification of Pulmonary Hypertension*

Group I: Pulmonary arterial hypertension (PAH) and other subtypes of PAH
Group II: Left-sided heart disease
Group III: Respiratory disease and hypoxemia
Group IV: Chronic thromboembolic pulmonary hypertension
Group V: Miscellaneous causes

Adapted from McLaughlin V, Langer A, Tan M, et al. Contemporary trends in the diagnosis and management of pulmonary arterial hypertension. *Chest.* 2013;143:324–332.

Table 20.1	Echocardiography in the Initial Screening and Assessment for Pulmonary Hypertension	
Completed?	Action Item	Notes
☐	Record estimated PASP	• Underestimated when Doppler beam alignment is poor or when TR jet is minimal • Overestimated in patients with significant anemia or in some cases of agitated saline-enhanced TR jet on continuous wave Doppler (from feathering) • Assumes absence of pulmonic stenosis • Echocardiographic PASP does not equal mean PA pressure (definition of PH per guidelines is on the basis of invasive hemodynamics: mean PA pressure ≥ 25 mm Hg)
☐	Evaluate RV size and function	• Signs of RV enlargement (apical four-chamber view): right ventricle shares apex with left ventricle, right ventricle larger than left ventricle, RV basal diameter >4.2 cm • RV hypertrophy (subcostal view): RV end-diastolic wall thickness >5 mm • RV systolic dysfunction: RV fractional area change <35%, TAPSE <1.6 cm, RV tissue Doppler s´ velocity <10 cm/s at base of the RV free wall (tricuspid annulus) • Septal flattening: in systole = RV pressure overload and in diastole = RV volume overload
☐	Evaluate for signs of elevated PVR	• RVOT notching on pulse-wave Doppler profile is a sign of elevated PVR • Peak TR velocity (m/s)/RVOT VTI (cm) <0.18: unlikely PVR is elevated
☐	Estimate volume status	• Use size and collapsibility of IVC (during sniff maneuver) to determine RA pressure • Hepatic vein flow: systolic flow reversal can be a sign of severe TR, RV overload, and/or increased RV stiffness • Signs of RA overload or enlargement: RA area >18 cm², interatrial septum bowing from right to left
☐	Evaluate severity of TR	• Features suggestive of severe TR: dense TR jet on continuous-wave Doppler, V-wave cutoff sign, and systolic flow reversal on hepatic vein pulse-wave Doppler imaging
☐	Evaluate for pericardial effusion	• In patients with PAH, the presence of a pericardial effusion = poor prognostic sign
☐	Evaluate for causes of PH (left-sided heart disease, shunt lesions)	• Left-sided heart disease: look for overt LV systolic dysfunction, grade 2 or worse diastolic dysfunction, severe aortic or mitral valvular disease, and less common abnormalities of the left side of the heart (eg, hypertrophic cardiomyopathy, cor triatriatum) • Shunt lesions: perform agitated saline bubble study

Table 20.1	Echocardiography in the Initial Screening and Assessment for Pulmonary Hypertension—cont'd	
Completed?	**Action Item**	**Notes**
☐	Differentiate PAH from PVH	• Signs favoring PVH: LA enlargement (LA size >RA size), interatrial septum bows from left to right, E/A ratio >1.2; *E/e'* (lateral) >11; lateral e" <8 cm/s • In patients with significantly elevated PASP at rest: grade 1 diastolic dysfunction pattern (E/A ratio <0.8) favors PAH diagnosis because of underfilled LA and decreased LV compliance secondary to RV-LV interaction (extrinsic compression of left ventricle by right ventricle)

E/A ratio, Ratio of early to late (atrial) mitral inflow velocities; *IVC*, inferior vena cava; *LA*, left atrial; *LV*, left ventricular; *PA*, pulmonary artery; *PAH*, pulmonary arterial hypertension; *PASP*, pulmonary artery systolic pressure; *PH*, pulmonary hypertension; *PVH*, pulmonary vascular hypertension; *PVR*, pulmonary vascular resistance; *RA*, right atrial; *RV*, right ventricular; *RVOT*, right ventricular outflow tract; *TAPSE*, tricuspid annular-plane systolic excursion; *TR*, tricuspid regurgitation; *VTI*, velocity-time integral.

Reprinted with permission from McLaughlin V, Shah S, Souza R, et al. Management of pulmonary arterial hypertension. *J Am Coll Cardiol.* 2015;65;1976–1997.

■ PATHOPHYSIOLOGY

Acute or recurrent PE is thought to be the inciting event in the development of CTEPH. Incomplete resolution of the embolus followed by thrombus organization and fibrosis leads to partial or complete vessel obstruction. In addition, vascular remodeling in the distal pulmonary arteries (pulmonary arteriopathy) also may contribute to the increased PVR, and it is the cause of residual PH seen in some patients after otherwise successful PTE. Unresolved PE in the proximal pulmonary arterial tree causes vascular obstruction in two ways: canalization of the clot leading to multiple small endothelized channels separated by bands and webs or fibrin clot organization or absent canalization leading to dense fibrous connective tissue that completely occludes the arterial lumen. This fibrous plug is firm and adherent to the arterial wall, and the surgical challenge is to remove enough of the fibrous plug as one unit to reduce the vascular resistance without disrupting the arterial wall.

The natural history of PE in most patients is complete resolution of the thromboembolic event with restoration of normal blood flow and hemodynamics. However, in some patients embolic resolution is incomplete, resulting in the development of CTEPH. The mechanism by which thromboembolic material remains unresolved is not fully understood. A variety of factors may play a role. The volume of the embolic substance may simply overwhelm the lytic system, with total occlusion of a major arterial branch preventing the lytic material from reaching and dissolving the embolus completely. The emboli may be made of substances such as well-organized fibrous thrombus that cannot be dissolved by normal mechanisms. Some patients may have tendencies to thrombus formation, a hypercoagulable state, or abnormal lytic mechanisms. Larger perfusion defects at diagnosis, idiopathic thromboembolic disease, high PA pressure (PAP) at the time of presentation, and a history of multiple PEs are risk factors for development of CTEPH after an acute PE.

Other identified risk factors include: ventriculoatrial shunts, infected pacemakers, splenectomy, previous venous thromboembolism, recurrent venous thromboembolism, blood group other than O, lupus anticoagulant or antiphospholipid antibodies, thyroid replacement therapy, or a history of malignant disease. Despite being a risk factor for venous thromboembolism, the prevalence of hereditary thrombophilic states (deficiencies of antithrombin III, protein C, and protein S, and factor II and factor V Leiden mutations) is similar to that in normal control subjects or in patients with idiopathic PH. In contrast, lupus anticoagulant or antiphospholipid antibodies can be found in up to 21% of patients with CTEPH, and increased levels of factor VIII were identified in 41% of patients with CTEPH. Finally, small, preliminary studies suggest the possibility of structural and functional abnormalities of fibrinogen in patients with CTEPH that perhaps confer resistance to fibrinolysis.

CLINICAL MANIFESTATIONS

A history of a previous acute thromboembolic event is not present in 25% to 30% of patients diagnosed with CTEPH. Thus a high index of suspicion is important for the diagnosis of CTEPH in any patient presenting with exertional dyspnea and exercise intolerance, even without evidence of previous PE. Early in the disease process, patients may go through a "honeymoon period" in which signs and symptoms of PH are not obvious. Symptoms appear when the right ventricle is unable to increase contractility sufficiently to augment left ventricular (LV) preload and cardiac output (CO) during exercise. Progressive exertional dyspnea is often the initial symptom of CTEPH, and, unfortunately, it is often attributed to more common medical conditions such as obstructive lung disease, obesity, or deconditioning. Exertional dyspnea results from increased PVR limiting CO and increased breathing requirements because of increased alveolar dead space.

As the disease progresses and the right side of the heart fails, patients may develop ascites, early satiety, epigastric or right upper quadrant fullness, edema, chest pain, and presyncope or syncope. Other symptoms may include nonproductive cough, hemoptysis, and palpitations. Left vocal cord dysfunction and hoarseness may arise from compression of the left recurrent laryngeal nerve between the aorta and an enlarged left main PA. Early in the disease process the physical examination may be normal or may reveal an accentuated pulmonic component of the second heart sound. Pulmonary flow murmurs or bruits heard over the lung fields are caused by turbulent blood flow through partially occluded or recanalized thrombi. These flow murmurs are heard in 30% of patients with CTEPH and are not found in idiopathic PH.

Late in the disease process, patients experience exertion-related syncope and resting dyspnea. The physical signs are far from uniform, and the physical examination may be surprisingly unrewarding if right ventricular (RV) failure is not yet present, even in patients with severe dyspnea. Physical findings of RV failure such as jugular venous distension, RV lift, fixed splitting of the second heart sound, murmur of tricuspid regurgitation (TR), RV gallop, hepatomegaly, ascites, and edema may appear in later stages of the disease. Most patients are hypoxic, with room-air arterial oxygen tension in the range of 65 mm Hg. This hypoxia is a result of ventilation/perfusion ($\dot{V}/\dot{Q}$) mismatch and low mixed venous oxygen saturation. Marked hypoxemia at rest implies severe RV dysfunction or the presence of a considerable right-to-left shunt, typically through a patent foramen ovale (PFO). Carbon dioxide tension is slightly reduced with metabolic compensation (reduced bicarbonate). Dead-space ventilation is increased, along with $\dot{V}/\dot{Q}$ mismatch, although these features correlate poorly with the degree of pulmonary vascular obstruction.

🔲 DIAGNOSTIC EVALUATION

Pulmonary Function Studies

Basic pulmonary function studies do not provide specific clues to the diagnosis of CTEPH, and these tests are most useful in evaluating patients for coexisting parenchymal lung disease or airflow obstruction. Twenty percent of patients with CTEPH exhibit a mild-to-moderate restrictive defect, often a result of parenchymal scarring from previous lung infarction. Similarly, a modest reduction in single-breath diffusing capacity of the lung for carbon monoxide (DLCO) may be present in some patients with CTEPH. A normal value does not exclude the diagnosis, and severe reduction in DLCO indicates that the distal pulmonary vascular bed is significantly compromised, thus making an alternative diagnosis likely.

Chest Radiography

The chest radiograph may be unremarkable in the early stages of CTEPH. However, as the disease progresses with the development of PH, the proximal pulmonary vascular bed enlarges. In some patients with chronic thromboembolic disease of the main or lobar PAs, this central PA enlargement can be asymmetric. This is not a radiographic finding in those patients with PH resulting from small-vessel disease. As the right ventricle adapts to the rise in PVR, radiographic signs of chamber enlargement such as obliteration of the retrosternal space and prominence of the right heart border can be observed. Relatively avascular lung regions can be appreciated if an organized thrombus has compromised blood flow to that area. In these poorly perfused lung regions, peripheral alveolar opacities, linear scarlike lesions, and pleural thickening may be found as a result of parenchymal injury and infarction.

Transthoracic Echocardiography

Transthoracic echocardiography (TTE) is a frequently used screening modality in patients with suspected PH. It often provides the first objective indication of the presence of elevated PAPs or RV compromise. Current technology allows for estimates of systolic PAP (using Doppler analysis of the velocity of TR), along with CO and RV performance. Enlargement of the right heart chambers and the resultant TR, flattening or paradoxical motion of the interventricular septum, and encroachment of an enlarged right ventricle on the LV cavity resulting in impaired LV filling are findings in patients with significant PH. Contrast echocardiography using intravenous agitated saline may show the presence of an intracardiac shunt, as a result of a PFO or another previously undetected septal defect. The echocardiogram is also useful in excluding LV dysfunction, valvular disease, or congenital heart disease, which may cause PH. In some patients with suspected CTEPH, TTE showing normal or minimally elevated PAPs at rest can sometimes demonstrate a substantial rise in PAP or dilatation of the right ventricle with exertion.

Ventilation/Perfusion Scintigraphy

The next step in the evaluation of patients for CTEPH is the acquisition of a V̇/Q̇ scan. For those patients with diagnosed PH, and for patients with dyspnea of unclear origin and suspected pulmonary vascular disease, the V̇/Q̇ scan is the recommended screening test for CTEPH. In CTEPH, at least one, and more commonly several, segmental or larger mismatched perfusion defects are present (Fig. 20.1). In

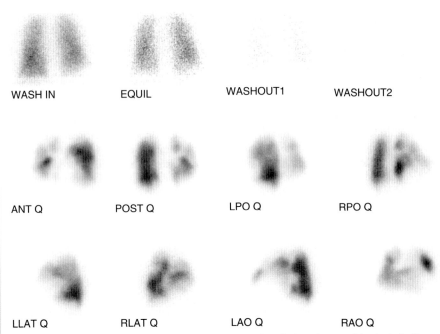

WASH IN   EQUIL   WASHOUT1   WASHOUT2

ANT Q   POST Q   LPO Q   RPO Q

LLAT Q   RLAT Q   LAO Q   RAO Q

Fig. 20.1 Lung ventilation-perfusion scan. Unmatched perfusion abnormalities include "hypo-perfused" left upper lobe, with scattered segmental perfusion defects in the lingula and throughout the right lung. *ANT,* Anterior; *EQUIL,* equilibrium; *LAO,* left anterior oblique; *LLAT,* left lateral; *LPO,* left posterior oblique; *POST,* posterior; *Q,* perfusion; *RAO,* right anterior oblique; *RLAT,* right lateral; *RPO,* right posterior oblique.

those patients with small-vessel pulmonary vascular disease, perfusion scan results either are normal or exhibit a "mottled" appearance characterized by nonsegmental defects. The greatest value of a $\dot{V}/\dot{Q}$ scan as a screening study is that a relatively normal perfusion pattern excludes the diagnosis of surgical CTEPH. Investigators have also observed that the magnitude of perfusion defects exhibited by patients with CTEPH with operable disease may understate the degree of pulmonary vascular obstruction determined by angiography. Therefore CTEPH should be considered, and an evaluation for operable disease is warranted, even if the $\dot{V}/\dot{Q}$ scan demonstrates a limited number of mismatched perfusion defects or regions of relative hypoperfusion ("gray zones").

Although an abnormal perfusion scan finding is observed in patients with CTEPH, this finding lacks specificity. Several other disorders affecting the proximal pulmonary vessels may result in scan findings similar to those in CTEPH, and, as such, further diagnostic imaging is necessary. Depending on imaging modality availability, and interpretive expertise, conventional catheter-based angiography—computed tomography pulmonary angiography (CTPA)—and magnetic resonance imaging (MRI) are most valuable methods for defining large-vessel, pulmonary vascular anatomy and providing the necessary diagnostic information for the confirmation of CTEPH.

Catheter-Based Pulmonary Angiography

Catheter-based pulmonary angiography has traditionally been considered the gold standard for confirming the diagnosis of CTEPH and assessing the proximal extent of chronic thromboembolic disease in evaluating patients for PTE. In most

IV

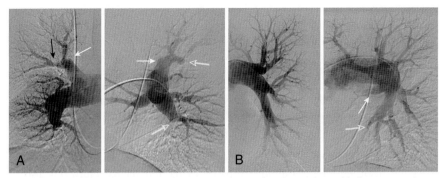

Fig. 20.2 (A) The accompanying pulmonary angiogram showing angiographic features consistent with chronic thromboembolic disease: "web" narrowing *(black arrow);* proximal vessel occlusion, anterior right upper lobe *(solid white arrows);* and rounded "pouch" lesions of the posterior right upper lobe artery and right descending pulmonary artery *(open white arrow).* (B) The left pulmonary angiogram demonstrates nearly complete occlusion of the proximal lingula *(solid white arrow)* and segmental narrowing of the anterior left lower lobe, best seen on the lateral view *(open white arrow).*

circumstances, a properly performed pulmonary angiogram, including lateral projections, provides sufficient information on which to base a decision regarding chronic thrombus location and surgical accessibility. The angiographic appearance of CTEPH is distinct from the well-defined, intraluminal filling defects of acute PE. The angiographic patterns encountered in CTEPH reflect the complex patterns of organization and recanalization that occur following an acute thromboembolic event. Several angiographic patterns have been described in CTEPH, including "pouch defects," PA webs or bands, intimal irregularities, abrupt and frequently angular narrowing of the major PAs, and complete obstruction of main, lobar, or segmental vessels at their point of origin. In most patients with CTEPH, two or more of these angiographic findings are present, typically involving both lungs (Fig. 20.2).

Computed Tomography of the Chest

With advances in technology, CTPA of the chest has played an increasing role in the evaluation for CTEPH. Certain vascular and parenchymal computed tomography (CT) findings are seen in patients with chronic thromboembolic disease. These include "mosaic perfusion" of the lung parenchyma, enlargement of the central PAs and right heart chambers, variability in the size of lobar and segmental-level vessels with a reduction in vessel caliber of those involved with chronic thrombi, and peripheral, scarlike lesions in poorly perfused lung regions. With contrast enhancement of the pulmonary vasculature during CT imaging, organized thrombus can be seen to line the pulmonary vessels, often in an eccentric manner. Associated narrowing of PAs, web strictures or bands, poststenotic vessel dilatation, and other irregularities of the intima may also be appreciated. These radiologic signs are distinct from the isolated finding of intraluminal filling defects observed with acute thromboemboli. With appropriate timing of the intravenous contrast bolus for CTPA, opacification of both the pulmonary and systemic circulation is possible. This type of imaging allows examination of both the pulmonary vascular bed and several cardiac features, including cardiac chamber size, the position and shape of the interventricular septum (deviated toward the left ventricle in the setting of significant RV pressure overload), the presence of congenital cardiac abnormalities, anomalous pulmonary venous drainage, and the size and distribution of collateral vessels arising from the systemic

20

arterial circulation, such as bronchial arteries off the aorta and collateral vessels arising from coronary vessels.

What remains incompletely evaluated is the utility of CTPA in determining operability in certain subgroups of patients with CTEPH. This has become particularly relevant because operative techniques allow for resection of chronic thromboembolic material at the segmental vessel level. Clinical experience has demonstrated that the absence of lining thrombus or thickened intima of the central vessels on CTPA does not exclude the diagnosis of CTEPH or the possibility of surgical resection. Studies directly comparing CTPA with conventional pulmonary angiography are limited.

Supplemental information provided by CT is of considerable value, not only in detecting disorders of the pulmonary parenchyma and mediastinum but also in differentiating CTEPH from "radiologic mimics." In patients with CTEPH and coexisting interstitial lung disease or emphysema, CT can define the extent and location of the parenchymal lung process. An attempted PTE leading to diseased lung parenchyma risks an undesirable postoperative outcome; such circumstances therefore should exclude a patient from surgical consideration. When a $\dot{V}/\dot{Q}$ scan demonstrates absence or nearly complete absence of perfusion to an entire lung, CT is an essential study to rule out extrinsic pulmonary vascular compression from mediastinal adenopathy, fibrosis, or neoplasm. CTEPH "mimics" such as primary sarcomas of the proximal pulmonary vessels, arteritis of medium to large pulmonary vessels (eg, Takayasu arteritis or sarcoidosis), and mediastinal fibrosis involving the proximal PAs or pulmonary veins are often revealed with CT.

Magnetic Resonance Imaging

At some CTEPH specialty centers, MRI and magnetic resonance angiography (MRA) to visualize the pulmonary vascular bed have been shown to be reliable methods for diagnosing CTEPH and for determining surgical candidacy. In a study of 34 patients with CTEPH, wall-adherent thromboembolic material involving the central PAs down to the segmental level could be seen. Intraluminal webs and bands, as well as abnormal vessel tapering and cutoffs, were also detected. Investigators have also shown that MRA was superior to digital subtraction angiography (DSA) in determining the proximal location of resectable chronic thromboembolic material.

Additional features of MRI that can be useful in the evaluation of patients with CTEPH include cine imaging, which allows an assessment of RV and LV function and provides data on end-systolic and end-diastolic volumes, ejection fraction, and muscle mass. Furthermore, phase-contrast imaging may be used to measure CO, along with pulmonary and systemic arterial flow.

Evaluation of the Patient With Chronic Thromboembolic Pulmonary Hypertension for Pulmonary Thromboendarterectomy

The evaluation of a patient with suspected CTEPH has the objectives of establishing the diagnosis, determining whether PTE is feasible, and, after careful assessment of comorbidities, risks, and anticipated benefits, whether surgical treatment should be pursued. Once the diagnosis of CTEPH has been confirmed, the next consideration in establishing the surgical candidacy of any patient is the determination of surgical accessibility of the chronic thrombotic lesions and, as such, "operability" (Box 20.2). Despite advances in diagnostics and an expanding surgical experience, this assessment

BOX 20.2 *Patient Selection Criteria for Pulmonary Thromboendarterectomy*

- Presence of surgically resectable chronic thromboembolic disease
- Symptomatic chronic thromboembolic disease, with or without pulmonary hypertension and right-sided heart dysfunction at rest
- Absence of concurrent illnesses representing an immediate threat to life
- Patient's desire for surgical treatment based on dissatisfaction with poor cardiorespiratory function or prognosis
- Patient's willingness to accept the mortality risk of the pulmonary thromboendarterectomy surgical procedure

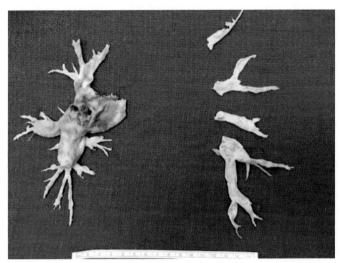

Fig. 20.3 Material removed at the time of pulmonary thromboendarterectomy that shows organized thrombus accompanied by semiorganized clot beginning in the right main pulmonary artery, whereas on the left, segmental level thrombus was endarterectomized. Preoperative pulmonary hemodynamics: mean atrial right pressure, 10; pulmonary artery pressure, 88/33 (55 mean); cardiac index, 2.09 L/min/m². Postoperative hemodynamics: central venous pressure, 9; pulmonary artery pressure, 43/15 (24 mean); cardiac index, 4.8 L/min/m² per minute.

remains subjective. Experience with interpretation of the diagnostic studies outlined in the previous sections and knowledge of the capabilities of the surgical team at a specialized center for PTE dictate which chronic thromboembolic lesions can be removed. As surgical experience is gained, it becomes possible to resect not only main PA and lobar level disease, but also more distal, segmental chronic thromboembolic lesions (Fig. 20.3). Although early experience with PTE procedures focused on the treatment of patients with PH and RV failure, the indications for surgical intervention have expanded to include those patients with symptomatic chronic thromboembolic disease without PH at rest. A report of 42 patients with symptomatic chronic thromboembolic disease and a baseline mPAP lower than 25 mm Hg concluded that PTE resulted in a significant improvement in functional status and quality of life. Thromboendarterectomy and reperfusion of lung regions before the development of

20

significant PH may prevent the development of the small-vessel arteriopathy in this patient group.

Equally essential in defining surgical candidacy is the assessment of perioperative risks. Properly performed right-sided heart catheterization enables a clinician accurately to determine the severity of PH and the degree of RV dysfunction in patients with CTEPH undergoing surgical evaluation. Early observations indicated that patients with severe PH, as defined by a PVR greater than 1000 dynes·s·cm^{-5}, bear a greater perioperative mortality risk. Although worldwide perioperative mortality rates have declined, patients with more severe PH and those with decompensated RV failure from CTEPH remain at greater risk. Madani and colleagues reported a declining overall operative mortality risk of 2.2% following PTE in 500 patients operated on between 2006 and 2010; in this same group, those patients with a preoperative PVR greater than 1000 dynes·s·cm^{-5} had a mortality rate of 4.1% compared with 1.6% in those patients with a PVR lower than 1000 dynes·s·cm^{-5}.

Finally, one should anticipate PTE will result in a meaningful outcome for the patient undergoing this complex and technically challenging procedure. Patients with significant comorbid conditions such as severe emphysema or those with a life-limiting malignant disease are not only at considerable perioperative risk but also are unlikely to realize the functional status benefit from PTE. Although the operation would possibly be technically feasible, such an aggressive intervention could be ill advised. Furthermore, when the degree of PH appears out of proportion to the extent of accessible chronic thromboembolic disease apparent by angiography, and surgical resection is not expected to result in a substantive improvement in pulmonary hemodynamics, surgical treatment should not be undertaken. Unfortunately, this assessment continues to be subjective. In previous attempts to establish objective criteria whereby small-vessel disease could be contributing to the PVR in patients with CTEPH, PA occlusion waveform analysis was used to "partition" the proximal versus distal components of vascular resistance. Although specialized equipment is required and obtaining adequate occlusion waveforms may be difficult in this patient population, the available data from this technique underscore the heterogeneity of pulmonary vascular lesions present in CTEPH; those patients with operable disease had a greater degree of upstream resistance.

OPERATION

Historical Background

Chronic thromboembolic disease was not recognized as a distinct diagnostic entity until the late 1920s. The first surgical attempt to remove the adherent thrombus from the PA wall was reported in 1958. This landmark operation distinguished endarterectomy, rather than embolectomy, as the surgical procedure of choice for chronic thromboembolic disease. In 1961 and 1962, systemic hypothermia with cardiopulmonary bypass (CPB) was used to perform two successful endarterectomies. Since the progressive modifications to the surgical technique have been made, these improvements have led to a reduction in mortality rates to 1% to 2%.

Pulmonary Thromboendarterectomy Procedure

PTE is the only curative treatment for CTEPH, with periprocedural mortality rates lower than 2% to 5% in experienced centers, nearly normalized hemodynamics, and substantial improvement in clinical symptoms in the majority of patients. Treatment decisions in CTEPH should be made by a CTEPH team and based on interdisciplinary discussions among internists, radiologists, and expert surgeons. A patient's condition should not be considered inoperable unless at least two independent experienced PTE surgeons have evaluated the patient. Detailed preoperative patient evaluation and selection, surgical and anesthetic technique, and meticulous postoperative management are essential for surgical success. Following complete endarterectomy, a significant decrease in PVR can be expected with near normalization of pulmonary hemodynamics. The procedure follows four basic but important principles:

1. The endarterectomy must be bilateral; therefore the approach is through a median sternotomy.
2. Identification of the correct dissection plane is crucial, and the plane must be identified in each of the segmental and subsegmental branches.
3. Perfect visualization is essential, and thorough distal endarterectomy cannot be performed without the use of circulatory arrest. Circulatory arrest is usually limited to 20 minutes at a time and is supported by cooling to 18°C.
4. Complete endarterectomy all the way to the distal ends of the smallest vessels is essential.

The endarterectomy must be bilateral because bilateral thromboembolic disease is present in almost all patients with CTEPH, and PH is a bilateral phenomenon. Historically, many reports described unilateral operations, and, occasionally these are still performed by lateral thoracotomy in inexperienced centers. However, the unilateral approach ignores the disease on the contralateral side, subjects the patient to hemodynamic jeopardy during clamping of the PA, does not allow adequate visibility because of the continued presence of bronchial blood flow, and exposes the patient to a repeat operation on the contralateral side. In addition, collateral channels develop in CTEPH not only through the bronchial arteries, but also from diaphragmatic, intercostal, and pleural vessels. Dissection of the lung in the pleural space through a thoracotomy incision can therefore be extremely bloody. The median sternotomy, apart from providing bilateral access, avoids entry into the pleural cavities and allows the ready institution of CPB.

CPB is essential to ensure cardiovascular stability when the operation is performed and to cool the patient to allow circulatory arrest. Excellent visibility is required, in a bloodless field, to define an adequate endarterectomy plane and to then follow the PTE specimen deep into the subsegmental vessels. Because of the copious bronchial blood flow usually present in these cases, periods of circulatory arrest are necessary to ensure perfect visibility. However, sporadic reports have described the performance of this operation without circulatory arrest. The circulatory arrest periods are limited to 20 minutes, with restoration of blood flow between each arrest. With experience, the endarterectomy usually can be performed with a single period of circulatory arrest on each side. A true endarterectomy in the plane of the media must be accomplished. It is essential to appreciate that the removal of visible thrombus is largely incidental to this operation.

When CPB is initiated, surface cooling with both a head-wrap jacket and a body cooling blanket is begun, and the blood is cooled with the pump oxygenator. During cooling, no more than a 10°C gradient between arterial blood and bladder or rectal temperature is maintained. Cooling generally takes 45 to 60 minutes. When ventricular fibrillation occurs, an additional vent is placed in the left atrium through the right superior pulmonary vein. This vent prevents left atrial (LA) and LV distension from the large amount of bronchial blood flow.

20

> **BOX 20.3   University of California San Diego Chronic Thromboemboli Classification**
>
> Level I: Chronic thromboembolic disease in the main pulmonary arteries
> Level IC: Complete occlusion of one main pulmonary artery with chronic thromboembolic disease
> Level II: Chronic thromboembolic disease starting at the level of the lobar arteries or in the main descending pulmonary arteries
> Level III: Chronic thromboembolic disease starting at the level of the segmental arteries
> Level IV: Chronic thromboembolic disease starting at the level of the subsegmental arteries
> Level 0: No evidence of chronic thromboembolic disease in either lung
>
> From Madani MM, Jamieson SW, Pretorius V, et al. Subsegmental pulmonary endarterectomy: time for new surgical classification. Abstract presented at the International CTEPH Conference, Paris, 2014.

Five categories of pulmonary occlusive disease related to thrombus can be appreciated. The University of California San Diego (UCSD) classification system describes the different levels of the thromboembolic specimen and corresponds to the degree of difficulty of the endarterectomy (Box 20.3). Level 0 is no evidence of chronic thromboembolic disease present. In other words, a misdiagnosis has occurred, or perhaps one lung is completely unaffected by thromboembolic disease; both situations are rare. This entity is characterized by intrinsic small-vessel disease, although secondary thrombus may occur as a result of stasis. Small-vessel disease may be unrelated to thromboembolic events ("primary" PH) or may occur in relation to thromboembolic hypertension as a result of a high-flow or high-pressure state in previously unaffected vessels similar to the generation of Eisenmenger syndrome. Investigators believe that sympathetic "cross-talk" from the affected contralateral side or stenotic areas in the same lung may also be present.

Level I disease refers to the condition in which thromboembolic material is present and readily visible on the opening of the main left and right PAs. A subset of level I disease, level Ic is complete occlusion of either the left or right PA and nonperfusion of that lung. Complete occlusion may represent an entirely different disease, especially when it is unilateral and on the left side. This group of patients, typically young women with complete occlusion of the left PA, may not have reperfusion of their affected lung despite a complete endarterectomy, thus indicating a different intrinsic pulmonary vascular disease unrelated to thromboembolic disease.

In level II, the disease starts at the lobar or intermediate-level arteries, and the main PA is unaffected. Level III disease is limited to thromboembolic disease originating in the segmental vessels only. Level IV is disease of the subsegmental vessels, with no other disease appreciated at more proximal levels. Level III disease and level IV disease present the most challenging surgical situations. The disease is very distal and is confined to the segmental and subsegmental branches. These levels are most often associated with presumed repetitive thrombi from upper extremity sources, long-term indwelling catheters, pacemaker leads, or ventriculoatrial shunts.

After completion of the endarterectomies, CPB is reinstituted and warming is commenced. Methylprednisolone (500 mg, intravenously) and mannitol (12.5 g, intravenously) are administered, and during warming no more than a 10°C temperature gradient is maintained between the perfusate and body temperature, with a maximum perfusate temperature of 37°C. If the systemic vascular resistance (SVR) is high, nitroprusside is administered to promote vasodilatation and warming.

When the left pulmonary arteriotomy has been repaired, the PA vent is replaced into the left PA. If the intraoperative transesophageal echocardiogram (TEE) showed evidence of a septal defect, the right atrium is opened and examined. Any intraatrial communication is closed. Although TR is invariable in these patients and is often severe, tricuspid valve repair is not performed unless an independent structural abnormality of the tricuspid valve is present. If the tricuspid valve morphology is normal, tricuspid valve competence returns with RV remodeling over the course of a few days postoperatively. If other cardiac procedures are required, such as coronary artery or mitral or aortic valve operations, these are performed during the systemic rewarming period. Myocardial cooling is discontinued once all cardiac procedures have been concluded. The LA vent is removed, and the vent site is repaired. All air is removed from the heart, and the aortic cross-clamp is removed. When the patient has rewarmed, CPB is discontinued. Despite the duration of CPB, hemostasis is readily achieved, and blood products are generally unnecessary. Wound closure is routine. Vigorous diuresis is usual for the first few hours after CPB.

ANESTHETIC MANAGEMENT OF PATIENTS UNDERGOING PULMONARY THROMBOENDARTERECTOMY

Hemodynamic Considerations and Anesthetic Induction

On the day of the operation, a large-bore peripheral intravenous catheter and a radial arterial catheter are placed in the preoperative area. Benzodiazepines occasionally are administered for sedation but with extreme caution, with full monitoring, and preferably in the operating room. Sedation should be administered on a case-by-case basis, noting that anxiety and pain can increase PVR, whereas excessive sedation can cause hypercarbia and hypoxia, leading to acidosis that exacerbates high PVR. A PA catheter (PAC) may be placed preoperatively but usually is placed after anesthetic induction.

CTEPH, according to its classification as precapillary PH, is characterized by normal LV systolic function and abnormal right-sided hemodynamics. Thus induction and decision making are centered on RV function. The right ventricle typically is hypertrophied and dilated and is associated with a dilated right atrium. Patients undergoing PTE have a fixed PVR and concomitant RV dysfunction; therefore any significant decrease in mean arterial pressure during induction may compromise RV perfusion and cause cardiovascular collapse. Maintenance of adequate SVR, an adequate inotropic state, and a normal sinus rhythm serves to preserve systemic hemodynamics, as well as RV coronary perfusion. Attempts to reduce PVR pharmacologically by using nitroglycerin or nitroprusside should be avoided because these agents have minimal efficacy in treating the relatively fixed PVR, and they result in SVR reduction that compromises RV coronary perfusion and RV function, thus rapidly leading to hypotension and cardiovascular collapse. Inhaled nitric oxide (NO) is safe to use, but some patients are not responsive to NO, and it is rarely required on induction. Administration of vasopressors, such as phenylephrine or vasopressin, is vital in treating hypotension and promoting adequate RV perfusion. Despite a relatively fixed PVR, attempts should be made to minimize conditions that increase PVR further, such as episodes of hypoxia and hypercarbia.

20

> ### BOX 20.4 *Signs of Impending Collapse*
>
> - Right ventricular end-diastolic pressure >15 mm Hg
> - Severe tricuspid regurgitation
> - Pulmonary vascular resistance >1000 dynes·s·cm^{-5}

The choice of anesthetic induction drugs depends on the degree of hemodynamic instability. Etomidate frequently is used because it maintains sympathetic tone and does not have a significant direct myocardial depressant effect. Succinylcholine or rocuronium can be used to achieve a rapid intubation environment and control of the airway. It is recommended that titration of narcotics to blunt the response to intubation takes place after control of ventilation to avoid rigidity and hypoventilation. Inotropic support with an infusion of a catecholamine is used in patients who are at high risk for cardiovascular collapse (Box 20.4).

A PAC is routinely placed after induction rather than before because the right-sided heart catheterization data are usually available for review preoperatively. The TEE can be very useful to guide PAC placement and confirm the position of the PAC in the PA. Patients undergoing PTE tend to have a dilated right atrium and right ventricle, thereby potentially making placement of the PAC difficult. A PAC is vital to assess the impact of surgical intervention on pulmonary vascular reactivity. Patients with advanced disease may be unable to lie supine or in the Trendelenburg position, which sometimes can lead to cardiorespiratory collapse. If the preoperative TTE reveals evidence of right atrial (RA), RV, or main PA thrombi, TEE is performed immediately after induction and before placement of the PAC. In this instance, PAC placement is guided with TEE, and the PAC is left in the superior vena cava (at 20 cm) until completion of the surgical procedure. Because all patients undergoing PTE also undergo prolonged CPB and circulatory arrest, a femoral arterial catheter is placed after induction to monitor arterial pressure after CPB because a radial artery catheter significantly underestimates systemic arterial pressure with a gradient of as much as 20 mm Hg.

SEDLine brain-function monitoring (Hospira, Lake Forest, IL) is used to monitor the electroencephalogram. This four-channel processed electroencephalograph provides confirmation of cerebral isoelectricity and thus minimal use of oxygen by the brain before circulatory arrest. It also serves as a monitor for the level of consciousness during the procedure. Cerebral near-infrared spectroscopy is used to monitor the patient's cerebral oxygen saturation status within tissues of the frontal lobe during the procedure and circulatory arrest. The device is a noninvasive method of estimating jugular bulb venous oxygen saturation ($SjvO_2$) and therefore global cerebral oxygen balance in the clinical setting. Patients with a cerebral oxygen saturation of less than 40% for longer than 10 minutes have had an increased incidence of neurocognitive dysfunction.

Temperature monitoring is achieved in several ways during all PTE procedures to allow accurate quantification of thermal gradients and to ensure even cooling and rewarming. Bladder temperature and rectal probes are used for core temperature estimation. A tympanic membrane probe is used for brain temperature estimation, and the PAC measures blood temperature.

Acute normovolemic hemodilution often is used in the setting of an increased starting hematocrit without the presence of any concomitant cardiac disease. Typically, 1 to 2 units of whole blood is harvested after anesthetic induction, depending on the starting hematocrit, and it is replaced with colloid if needed to maintain hemodynamic stability. Acute normovolemic hemodilution has added benefits for deep hypothermic circulatory arrest because it will help decrease blood viscosity, optimize capillary blood flow, and promote uniform cooling. This autologous harvested whole blood is reinfused after protamine administration, thus providing platelets and factors and replacing the diluted clotting factors resulting from the pump prime. Antifibrinolytic agents are not used routinely with PTE because patients are often inherently hypercoagulable.

TEE is used routinely in patients undergoing PTE to monitor hemodynamics, evaluate RV and LV function, identify intracardiac thrombus or valvular disease, and evaluate RV function and de-airing after bypass. A thorough intraatrial septal evaluation is performed to rule out a PFO, which has an incidence of 35% in the PTE population. All patients are evaluated with two methods: color-flow Doppler and agitated echocardiographic contrast. Agitated echocardiographic contrast imaging is particularly useful if results of color-flow Doppler imaging are inconclusive. Positive pressure at 30 cm H_2O is applied for 10 seconds, and with release of the Valsalva maneuver, the agitated echocardiographic contrast (agitated blood or 5% albumin without adding any air) is injected. The echocardiographic contrast study is preferably performed after the patient is prepared and draped because instances of hemodynamic collapse have occurred following contrast injection. Most PFOs are repaired intraoperatively. An algorithm for PFO study assessment is shown in Fig. 20.4. In rare instances when results of the operation are not favorable, and high right-sided pressures are expected, the PFO is left open as a "pop-off" to improve RV function and increase CO at the expense of some hypoxemia. In this instance, closure of a PFO can be detrimental to clinical status by reducing LV filling and increasing filling of the noncompliant right ventricle.

The patient's head is wrapped in a cooling blanket because all PTE-treated patients undergo circulatory arrest. The head-wrap system is composed of two items: the Polar Care 500 cooling device (cooling bucket, pump, pump bracket, and AC power transformer), which is reusable, and the actual wrap, which is a single-use item. In a series of 55 patients who used this device during circulatory arrest, the mean tympanic

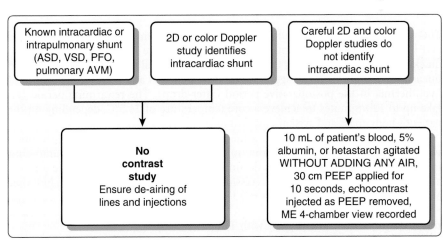

Fig. 20.4 Algorithm for performance of intraoperative echocardiographic contrast study for pulmonary thromboendarterectomy procedures. *ASD,* Atrial septal defect; *AVM,* arteriovenous malformation; *ME,* midesophageal; *PEEP,* positive end-expiratory pressure; *PFO,* patent foramen ovale; *VSD,* ventricular septal defect; *2D,* two-dimensional.

membrane temperature was 15.1°C. The head wrap provides sufficient cooling to the brain, wraps the whole head, and is much easier to use than ice bags.

Cardiopulmonary Bypass Prime, Cooling, and Hypothermic Circulatory Arrest

The prebypass time is typically short unless concomitant coronary artery bypass grafting is planned. The bypass system is primed with 1000 mL of Plasma-Lyte A (Baxter, Deerfield, IL), 100 mL of 25% albumin, 5 to 12 mL (100 units/kg) of heparin, 12.5 g mannitol, and 8.4% 50 mL sodium bicarbonate. For circulatory arrest, 30 mg/kg of methylprednisolone to a maximum dose of 3 g is added to the prime, and an additional 500 mg is added at rewarming. The steroid theoretically functions as a cell membrane stabilizer and antiinflammatory agent. Phenytoin (15 mg/kg) is administered by the perfusionist for postoperative seizure prophylaxis, after initiation of bypass.

Cooling begins immediately after initiation of bypass, by using CPB temperature adjustment and the cooling blankets present under the patient, together with the head wrap. Allowing appropriate time to cool and warm the patient in each direction using rectal, bladder, tympanic, PA, and perfusate temperatures with appropriate thermal gradients ensures even and thorough cooling and warming, respectively. Propofol, 2.5 mg/kg, is administered immediately before initiation of deep hypothermic circulatory arrest to ensure complete isoelectricity. SEDLine brain-function monitoring is used for this purpose because brain cooling may be uneven or incomplete, and cerebral emboli may occur, given that PTE is an open procedure; in case of sparse electroencephalographic activity, it will monitor for any residual activity.

The following must be confirmed before circulatory arrest: the electroencephalogram is isoelectric, the tympanic membrane temperature is lower than 18°C, bladder and rectal temperatures are lower than 20°C, and all monitoring catheters to the patient are turned off, to decrease the risk for entraining air into the vasculature during exsanguination.

Rewarming Phase and Separation From Bypass

The rewarming perfusate should not exceed 37°C, and the gradient between blood and bladder or rectal temperatures should not be more than 10°C. Warming too quickly promotes systemic gas bubble formation, cerebral oxygen desaturation, and uneven warming, which can aggravate cerebral ischemia and increase the chance of hypothermia in the postoperative period (after-drop). The rewarming period can take up to 120 minutes to achieve a core temperature of 36.5°C, depending on the patient's body mass and systemic perfusion.

Separation from CPB follows the same process as in most other cardiac operations, with a few minor exceptions. Communication with the surgeon is of paramount importance because surgical classification of the thromboembolic disease and the amount of organized clot that was successfully removed will dictate how much inotropic and vasopressor support (if any) is needed to separate from bypass. With successful endarterectomy, substantial reduction in PVR and improved RV function occur, as revealed immediately after bypass with TEE (Fig. 20.5).

If residual PH is observed, the patient may need aggressive inotropic support (eg, dopamine, 3–7 µg/kg per minute; or epinephrine, 0.03–0.15 µg/kg per minute), together with pulmonary vasodilators, such as milrinone, and inhaled prostacyclin or NO. Inhaled NO is preferred because it acts on the pulmonary vasculature with minimal

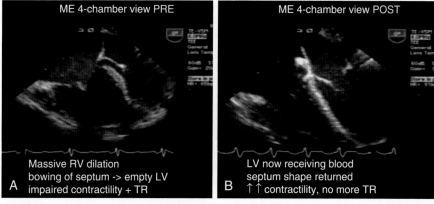

ME 4-chamber view PRE	ME 4-chamber view POST
Massive RV dilation bowing of septum -> empty LV **A** impaired contractility + TR	LV now receiving blood septum shape returned **B** ↑↑ contractility, no more TR

Fig. 20.5 (A) Midesophageal *(ME)* four-chamber view in a patient with chronic thromboembolic pulmonary hypertension before pulmonary thromboendarterectomy (PTE). Note the severely dilated right atrium, right ventricle, and the interatrial and intraventricular septum bulging toward the left atrium and left ventricle *(LV)*. (B) After successful PTE, note the improvement in the right atrial and right ventricular *(RV)* size. *TR,* Tricuspid regurgitation.

systemic effects. The right atrium is routinely paced at a rate of 90 to 100 beats/min with temporary epicardial pacing electrodes to ensure incomplete RV filling reducing wall tension. Ventricular epicardial electrodes are placed as well, but they are used only if atrioventricular conduction is impaired. End-tidal carbon dioxide is a poor measure of ventilation adequacy and does not represent the true arterial carbon dioxide in these patients both before and after CPB because dead-space ventilation is an integral part of the disease process. The arterial end-tidal carbon dioxide gradient usually improves after successful surgical treatment, but the response and time course vary. Higher minute ventilation is often required to compensate for metabolic acidosis that develops from CPB, circulatory arrest, and hypothermia. Before separation from CPB, intracardiac air and RV and LV function are assessed with TEE and PAC. With successful operative results, immediate improvements of RV function and resolution of the interventricular septal distortion and flattening are seen on intraoperative TEE. With the dramatic resolution of PH following PTE, transmitral diastolic flow improves in a predictable manner. Not surprisingly, this change correlates with improvements in the CO and cardiac index (CI).

To standardize ventilation and maintain hyperventilation postoperatively, a portable transport ventilator is used to transport patients to the intensive care unit after PTE. If postoperative care is uneventful, most patients are discharged from the unit on the second or third postoperative day, with subsequent hospital discharge approximately 1 to 2 weeks after the operation.

Management of Airway Bleeding

Reperfusion pulmonary edema and airway bleeding are two of the most dreaded complications of PTE. Anesthesiologists must therefore be prepared to provide diagnostic and therapeutic maneuvers for these rare complications and routinely check the endotracheal tube during the rewarming phase before separation from CPB to inspect for bleeding or frothy fluid in the endotracheal tube.

Most cases of bleeding are spontaneous and are discovered only after resuming cardiac ejection. However, the surgeon may anticipate bleeding if an adventitial injury is suspected during PTE and will help in promptly identifying the bronchial side that needs to be isolated. If dark frank blood is seen in the endotracheal tube after separation from CPB, it usually indicates a surgical violation of the blood-airway barrier in one of the PA branches. In contrast, pink frothy blood usually indicates early and severe reperfusion injury and is suspected when the PTE increased blood flow to a previously occluded vessel. Management of airway bleeding centers on prevention of exsanguination and maintenance of adequate gas exchange. Conservative management consists of positive end-expiratory pressure, lung isolation of the segment bleeding with a bronchial blocker, reversal of heparin, and correction of coagulopathies. These maneuvers often reduce minor bleeding and reperfusion injury. If bleeding is recognized before separation from CPB, the surgeon should allow the heart to eject briefly with the bleeding area under direct visualization with fiberoptic bronchoscopy to establish the location of bleeding. An attempt is made to isolate the affected segment by using bronchial blockade to prevent spilling blood into other segments and causing further impaired air flow and gas exchange. Therefore, immediately before separation from CPB, special attention should be paid to optimizing oxygenation and ventilation. In addition, while the patient is undergoing CPB and with the PA vent on suction, an attempt may be made to exchange the endotracheal tube with a larger (9–10 mm) endotracheal tube. This allows the use of a large bronchoscope together with a 9-Fr Uniblocker (LMA North America, San Diego, CA). We recommend the use of an airway exchange catheter because of the high incidence of poor direct visualization resulting from bleeding, edema, and suboptimal conditions. Use of the Uniblocker is good for isolation of a lung or lobe, and the Arndt blocker (Cook Medical, Bloomington, IN) is more appropriate for isolation of a specific segment. The use of a double-lumen tube is not recommended because it presents a challenge when using a large bronchoscope that has superior suction and diagnostic capabilities. In cases of minor adventitial injuries, the blocker balloon can be deflated under direct visualization, and normal ventilation can be resumed; however, if persistent hemorrhage is noted, continued lung isolation is needed.

In severe circumstances in which inadequate oxygenation, ventilation, and hemodynamics persist, various forms of extracorporeal life support should be considered. Three options exist:

1. With biventricular dysfunction, venoarterial extracorporeal membrane oxygenation (ECMO) can be used with anticoagulation.
2. With RV dysfunction and persevered LV function, ECMO with RA inflow and PA outflow cannula bypassing and unloading the right ventricle aids in gas exchange and supports RV function.
3. With preserved RV and LV function, venovenous ECMO using a heparin-bonded circuit, without systemic anticoagulation, improves oxygenation but does not provide ventricular support.

An algorithm for management of post-CPB hemorrhage is presented in Fig. 20.6. The Avalon Elite Bicaval Dual-Lumen Catheter (Maquet, Rastatt, Germany) typically is inserted via the Seldinger technique into the right internal jugular vein with ultrasound and TEE guidance. A bicaval view using color-flow Doppler is used to ensure that the outflow jet is toward the tricuspid valve. This technique is efficient, requires no anticoagulants, and maintains appropriate gas exchange with preservation of pulsatile pulmonary and systemic flow while allowing natural hemostatic processes to repair the affected PA or capillary bed. The natural repair is usually complete after 24 to 48 hours, thus allowing weaning from ECMO. The third most common cause of perioperative death in patients undergoing PTE is massive pulmonary hemorrhage after PTE, with residual PH and reperfusion pulmonary edema as the leading two causes.

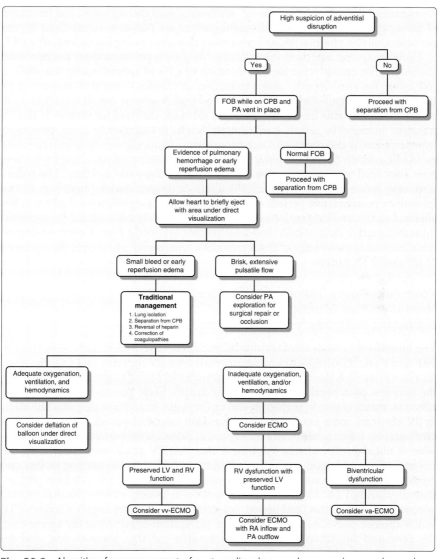

Fig. 20.6 Algorithm for management of post–cardiopulmonary bypass pulmonary hemorrhage for the pulmonary thromboendarterectomy procedure. *CPB,* Cardiopulmonary bypass; *FOB,* fiberoptic bronchoscopy; *ECMO,* extracorporeal membrane oxygenation; *LV,* left ventricular; *PA,* pulmonary artery; *RA,* right atrial; *RV,* right ventricular; *va,* venoarterial; *vv,* venovenous. (Reprinted with permission from Cronin B, Maus T, Pretorius V, et al. Case 13—2014: management of pulmonary hemorrhage after pulmonary endarterectomy with venovenous extracorporeal membrane oxygenation without systemic anticoagulation. *J Cardiothorac Vasc Anesth.* 2014;28(6):1667–1676.)

▣ MANAGEMENT OF THE POSTOPERATIVE PATIENT

In many respects the principles of postoperative management of patients undergoing PTE are similar to those following other procedures requiring sternotomy and CPB. The desire to minimize the time of mechanical ventilation, the use of vasoactive medications for inotropic and hemodynamic support, wound care, mediastinal chest tube management, the use of "prophylactic" antibiotics, pain management, and treatment of postoperative arrhythmias and coagulopathies are common issues faced by the physicians, nurses, pharmacists, and respiratory therapists caring for patients after PTE.

However, several aspects of this operation frequently present unique postoperative challenges. For example, the median duration of CPB of approximately 4 hours is a risk factor for coagulopathy and a reduction in platelet count that may result in transient, albeit significant, mediastinal blood loss. A modest rise in creatinine level postoperatively is also frequently observed, although the need for dialysis is rare. A transient increase in serum transaminase levels, presumptively from prolonged hypoperfusion, is also observed. Deep hypothermia frequently results in postoperative metabolic acidosis during the rewarming phase, and prolonged circulatory arrest has been associated with postoperative mental status changes and delirium. The endarterectomy procedure itself dramatically alters cardiopulmonary physiology in the immediate postoperative period. After successful PTE, a significant reduction in RV afterload occurs, and lung regions supplied by vessels previously occluded by organized thrombus receive dramatically increased pulmonary blood flow. Understanding of these immediate physiologic changes provides a rationale for the unique management of the post-PTE patient.

Post–Pulmonary Thromboendarterectomy Hemodynamic Management and Persistent Pulmonary Hypertension

The immediate hemodynamic results following effective PTE include reductions in PAP and PVR (RV afterload) and improvements in RV function and CO. However, transient sinus node dysfunction often requiring atrial pacing frequently occurs during the first few postoperative days. This dysfunction likely results from the residual effects of intraoperative hypothermia and cardioplegia. In addition, despite a reduction in RV afterload, some persistent RV dysfunction can be observed. As seen on echocardiography, a degree of RV strain can persist, although the pattern is different from what is noted preoperatively. We believe that this RV strain may result from the residual effects of hypothermia (including the use of a cardiac cooling jacket) and cardioplegia, as a response to poor pulmonary vascular compliance, or from pericardiotomy during PTE. Modest inotropic support is usually effective in maintaining adequate CO during this brief period. Sometimes a persistently low SVR follows PTE in the absence of evidence of infection or medication effect. As in the earlier case, the profound hypothermia may be responsible for this phenomenon, and an α-adrenergic agonist is generally effective in supporting blood pressure. On rare occasions, adrenal insufficiency may be the basis for this hypotension, and cortisol levels (after administration of adrenocorticotropic hormone) should be assessed to verify this diagnosis. Some patients do not achieve normal PAPs and RV function following PTE; the incidence is between 5% and 35% of operated patients. Plausible explanations include residual chronic thromboembolic disease that could not be surgically resected or a significant amount of coexisting small-vessel arteriopathy.

Long-term information on the level of residual PH that negatively affects functional status and survivorship is lacking. In the immediate postoperative period, significant RV dysfunction greatly complicates the clinical course. Attention to oxygenation status and careful volume management, correction of acid-base imbalance, inotropic support, and at times the use of PH-targeted medical therapy with parenteral prostanoid administration may be necessary to support patients through this tenuous postoperative period. In extreme circumstances, ECMO support has been used when other measures fail, particularly when concurrent hypoxic respiratory failure is present. Success with this approach presupposes a reversal component to the cardiopulmonary instability, and sometimes this aggressive management can be viewed as a bridge to organ transplantation in the acute setting.

Other Pulmonary Considerations and Management of Hypoxemia

After successful PTE, lung perfusion shifts, with blood flow preferentially going to regions supplied by PAs that have been opened. This shift is accompanied by a reduction in perfusion in lung regions uninvolved with chronic thrombotic material, a phenomenon termed *perfusion steal*. Although this reperfusion of previously nonperfused lung parenchyma is the basis for the reduction in RV afterload, the postoperative perfusion shifts are responsible for $\dot{V}/\dot{Q}$ mismatch, an important contributor to the development of acute reperfusion lung injury. This form of acute lung injury occurs in the endarterectomized lung region, is associated with varying degrees of hypoxemia (ratio of arterial oxygen partial pressure to fractional inspired oxygen [P/F ratio] <300), begins within 72 hours of operation, and occurs in the absence of an alternative clinical explanation for the pulmonary infiltrates on chest radiograph. The pathophysiologic basis is incompletely understood, although initial observations suggested a high-permeability, inflammatory-mediated mechanism. Such observations were supported by anecdotal experience with high-dose corticosteroids resulting in reductions in both the incidence and the severity of the reperfusion response. Furthermore, a randomized, placebo-controlled clinical trial examining the use of a selectin analog to block neutrophil adhesion and migration was shown to reduce the relative risk of lung injury by 50% in patients undergoing PTE. However, well-designed follow-up studies investigating the perioperative use of high-dose corticosteroids failed to show effectiveness, and the declining incidence over the years of this postoperative complication without evident cause, or change in surgical or anesthetic management, brings the "inflammatory" response as the sole physiologic basis for this lung injury into question. Furthermore, reports that a higher preoperative PVR is associated with a higher incidence of lung injury after PTE, and more observations that postcapillary microvascular disease can be observed in patients with CTEPH, suggest that a hemodynamic component contributes to reperfusion lung injury after PTE.

The approach to patients with reperfusion lung injury is primarily supportive, and the intensity of intervention depends on the degree of hypoxemia. The difficulties in management of this patient population are augmented by the shift in pulmonary blood flow that occurs as noted previously: the normal compensatory mechanism of hypoxic pulmonary vasoconstriction is blunted in injured lung regions receiving a large percentage of blood flow, thus resulting in regions that are edematous, poorly ventilated, and noncompliant. In the mildest forms, diuresis to decrease lung edema and supplemental oxygen may be the only treatment required. For more severe lung injury, aggressive diuresis, lung-protective ventilator strategies, and prompt treatment of concurrent lung infection (if present) are mainstays of therapy. For severe lung injury, when other measures have failed, ECMO support has been used with success. The use of inhaled NO to correct $\dot{V}/\dot{Q}$ mismatch can be associated with an improvement in oxygenation in some patients, at least initially. However, this approach was not consistently effective in a small trial of patients with other forms of lung injury. Similarly, the use of a low-lung-volume ventilation strategy during the immediate post-PTE period, as an independent factor, is unlikely to prevent reperfusion lung injury.

Hypoxemia during the immediate postoperative period may also simply be secondary to atelectasis in a region of newly reperfused lung. Ventilator adjustments using slightly higher tidal volumes, positive end-expiratory pressure, and lung recruitment maneuvers

20

525

can be effective in improving $\dot{V}/\dot{Q}$ matching in this setting. For extubated patients, mobilization and aggressive lung recruitment maneuvers to diminish atelectasis usually improve oxygenation.

Low $\dot{V}/\dot{Q}$ and resultant hypoxemia can be observed following PTE operations in the absence of evident lung injury. These findings may be the result of a high perfusion state in relatively small lung regions after endarterectomy of segmental and subsegmental vessels. Other than supportive measures and oxygen supplementation, no specific treatment exists for this condition. This perfusion shift improves over time.

Postoperative Thrombosis Prophylaxis and Anticoagulation

Once hemostasis has been achieved in the early hours following PTE, thrombosis prophylaxis is typically initiated with subcutaneous heparin and the use of pneumatic compression devices. Experience has suggested that patients with a history of antiphospholipid syndrome, those patients with CTEPH who have undergone level 1C resection, and those with evidence of a recent thromboembolic event are at greater risk for postoperative thrombosis, including within the pulmonary vessels. For these patients, therapeutic-level anticoagulation is attempted early postoperatively as long as significant hemorrhage does not occur.

Lifelong anticoagulation is strongly advised in patients who have undergone PTE. Once epicardial pacing wires are removed, and further invasive procedures are unlikely, warfarin is begun with a target international normalized ratio (INR) of 2.5 to 3.5. Although data are lacking on the ideal level of anticoagulation over time, thromboembolic recurrence is rare in patients who have been maintained on long-term anticoagulation. Individualization of the care plan is emphasized. For example, in patients with antiphospholipid syndrome who have considerable thrombophilia, INR targets are frequently higher. For older patients and for those patients concurrently taking antiplatelet agents, targeting an INR between 2.0 and 3.0 is common practice. The use of the newer oral anticoagulants, targeting thrombin or factor Xa, has yet to be examined in this patient population.

▓ NONSURGICAL APPROACH TO CHRONIC THROMBOEMBOLIC DISEASE

Pulmonary Hypertension–Targeted Medical Therapy

PTE is the preferred treatment option for patients with CTEPH. However, patient subgroups in whom PH-targeted medical therapy was examined in randomized, placebo-controlled trials include patients deemed to have inoperable CTEPH and patients with residual PH following PTE. PH-targeted medical therapy is also sometimes beneficial as a bridge to PTE in preoperative patients with severe PH and RV dysfunction (Box 20.5).

Existing data have not justified the routine use of PH-targeted medical therapy in patients with operable CTEPH as a bridge to surgical treatment, although logic dictates that a subgroup of patients with CTEPH with severe PH and RV failure may benefit from hemodynamic stabilization before undergoing anesthetic induction and the cardiopulmonary stress of operation. Despite the uncertainties surrounding medical therapy, increasing numbers of patients with CTEPH with surgical disease are given medical treatment preoperatively.

BOX 20.5 *Patient Groups With Chronic Thromboembolic Pulmonary Hypertension to Consider for Targeted Medical Therapy for Pulmonary Hypertension*

- Patients with inoperable chronic thromboembolic pulmonary hypertension
- Patients with residual pulmonary hypertension after a pulmonary thromboendarterectomy surgical procedure
- Patients with chronic thromboembolic pulmonary hypertension in whom comorbidities are so significant that surgical treatment is contraindicated
- Patients who have severe pulmonary hypertension and right-sided heart failure, in whom targeted medical therapy for pulmonary hypertension may be a "clinically stabilizing bridge" to surgical treatment

Percutaneous Balloon Pulmonary Angioplasty

The use of balloon pulmonary angioplasty (BPA) in the management of selected patients with chronic thromboembolic disease has grown. Application of this technique in a patient with CTEPH was first reported in 1988. In 2001 BPA was described as an alternative to PTE in patients believed to have surgically inaccessible CTEPH or in patients whose comorbidities precluded surgical consideration.

Specialized centers in Japan have reported the greatest experience with BPA. In a prospective study of 12 patients deemed to have nonsurgical CTEPH and "stabilized" with pulmonary vasodilators (including two patients with residual PH after PTE), Sugimura and associates performed multiple angioplasty sessions until the mPAP was less than 30 mm Hg. Not only did this approach result in an overall improvement in pulmonary hemodynamics and functional status, but also, when compared with historical controls, showed an improvement in survivorship. Mild-to-moderate hemoptysis was observed in 50% of patients following this procedure. In 68 patients, Mizoguchi and colleagues reported a refinement of the angioplasty procedure in which the selection of appropriate balloon size was made using intravascular ultrasound; the hypothesis was that this technique could reduce the incidence of postprocedure reperfusion lung injury. Although 60% of patients developed a degree of reperfusion injury (including the development of "hemosputum"), improvements in mPAP (45.4 ± 9.6 to 24.0 ± 6.4 mm Hg) and functional status were reported. One patient died of RV failure 28 days following the procedure. The ultimate role of BPA in the treatment of patients with CTEPH requires ongoing assessment. Appropriate patient selection, the optimal procedural technique to avoid reperfusion lung injury or pulmonary vascular injury, the appropriate timing of repeated BPAs, hemodynamic benefits, and functional improvement must be determined.

INTRAOPERATIVE ECHOCARDIOGRAPHY IN PATIENTS WITH CHRONIC THROMBOEMBOLIC PULMONARY HYPERTENSION

CTEPH results in myriad changes leading to functional and morphologic alterations of both right and left ventricles. Echocardiographic evaluation of patients with CTEPH

20

includes a complete examination of all cardiac structures. This examination encompasses evaluation of RV anatomy and function, including dilation and hypertrophy, with attention to leftward ventricular septal motion. Therefore the midesophageal (ME) four-chamber, ME ascending aortic short-axis, RV inflow-outflow, and bicaval views are essential.

The *ME four-chamber* view is the first view used for assessment of RV dilation and hypertrophy, RA size, and tricuspid valve function. The right ventricle exhibits several changes in response to chronic pressure and volume overload to that ventricle. The response seen as a result of chronic increased afterload includes volume-adapting dilatory changes, as well as pressure-related changes such as RV enlargement, hypertrophy, and paradoxical septal motion that eventually lead to RV systolic failure.

The normal right ventricle typically occupies two-thirds, in cross-sectional area, of the LV area. With RV enlargement, its size becomes greater than two-thirds, sharing the cardiac apex; whereas with severe enlargement, the right ventricle becomes larger than the left ventricle, thus forming the cardiac apex. An effective way to assess the right ventricle rapidly is by looking at the makeup of the cardiac apex in the ME four-chamber view.

RV hypertrophy is the compensatory mechanism for the right ventricle to maintain stroke volume in the presence of increased PVR. Normally, RV free wall thickness at end-diastole is 5 mm in diameter. With long-standing severe chronic PH, RV hypertrophy can exceed 10 mm in thickness, and a prominent moderator band may be noted. This measurement may be obtained in the ME four-chamber, ME RV inflow-outflow, or transgastric midpapillary views, often aided by the use of M-mode echocardiography.

The right ventricle is normally adapted to eject against a low-pressure pulmonary circuit. With acute or chronic elevation in PAP, RV systolic dysfunction ensues. The right ventricle has a characteristic "peristaltic-like" movement beginning with contraction at the inflow portion, followed by the apex, and ending with contraction of the outflow infundibulum. Several modalities have been suggested for evaluating RV systolic function.

Tricuspid annular plane systolic excursion is a measure of global RV systolic function and a prognostic indicator in PH. This excursion is the amount of shortening of the base of the tricuspid valve annulus toward the apex at peak systole, thus measuring the excursion between end-diastole and end-systole. The normal value is more than 16 mm; a value of less than 15 mm is associated with mortality risk.

Interventricular septal motion is seen with RV overload, and it results in flattening of the septum and loss of the natural crescent shape of the RV, thus leading to the characteristic "D-shaped" sign most noticeable in the transgastric midpapillary short-axis view (Fig. 20.7). The right and left ventricles share the interventricular septum, which is usually concave toward the right ventricle during the entire cardiac cycle. Evaluation of the nature and timing of septal flattening relative to diastole versus systole can help differentiate between RV volume overload and RV pressure overload. In conditions characterized by RV volume overload, the septum is flattened at end-diastole, whereas in pressure overload, the septum is flattened at end-systole. With severe CTEPH and pressure overload, right-sided pressures exceed left-sided pressures in both systole and diastole, so the septum may remain deformed throughout the cardiac cycle, a condition that may eventually lead to impaired LV filling and decreased CO. The *eccentricity index* (*EI*) is the ratio of the anteroposterior to septolateral diameter of the left ventricle in the transgastric mid–short-axis view. In normal values, the EI has a value of 1 in both systole and diastole. In cases with pressure overload, the EI value is greater than 1 during end-systole, whereas in volume overload it is greater than 1 during end-diastole.

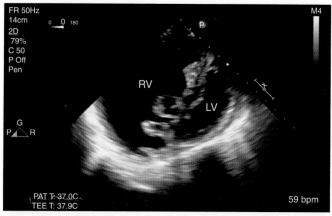

Fig. 20.7 Transgastric midpapillary short-axis view showing flattening of the interventricular septum as a result of right ventricular pressure or volume overload leading to the characteristic D-shaped sign. *LV*, Left ventricle; *RV*, right ventricle.

Pulsed-wave Doppler tissue imaging allows evaluation of the peak systolic velocity (S′) of the basal RV free wall in the ME four-chamber view. A peak systolic velocity of less than 10 cm/s suggests abnormal RV function. Peak systolic velocity has correlated well with RV ejection fraction using cardiac MRI.

The *RV myocardial performance index (RV MPI)*, also known as the Tei index, is another global assessment of RV systolic and diastolic cardiac performance that combines both systolic and diastolic time intervals. The RV MPI is easily derived using two methods:

1. Pulsed Doppler method from two separate cardiac cycles is used.
2. Tissue Doppler method from a single cardiac cycle. The RV MPI greater than 0.4 by pulsed-wave Doppler and greater than 0.55 by tissue Doppler signifies impaired RV function. The Tei index is simple, noninvasive, and easy to estimate.

Interatrial septum position and motion serve as a surrogate of RV function. In the setting of CTEPH and a failing right ventricle, high right-sided pressure is transmitted to the right atrium, thus leading to dilatation, increasing RA pressure, and shifting the interatrial septum toward the left atrium (Fig. 20.8). In the setting of long-standing PH and overt RV failure, decreased CO leads to increased right-sided volume and diastolic pressure that, when transmitted to the right atrium, causes RA dilatation. Patients with CTEPH often present with pericardial effusions correlating with increased RA pressure. Marked elevations in RV and RA pressures may lead to impaired lymphatic and venous drainage from the pericardium that results in pericardial effusions. Similarly, elevated RA pressure and severe TR may impair coronary sinus drainage and lead to a dilated coronary sinus, best visualized in the deep ME four-chamber view.

Patients with CTEPH with long-standing elevated RA pressure exhibit a higher incidence of PFO than the estimated 25% seen in the adult population. The ME four-chamber, ME RV inflow-outflow, and ME bicaval views are all used to evaluate for PFO, with the aid of color-flow Doppler or agitated saline injection.

The *ME RV inflow-outflow* view is often used to assess RV free wall hypertrophy and function, as well as to evaluate peak regurgitation velocity. Systolic PAP can be easily estimated using peak TR velocity (V_{TR}) with continuous-wave Doppler and

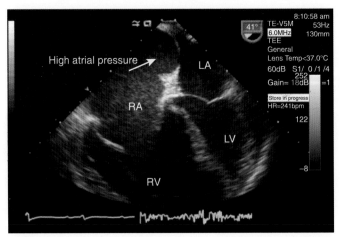

Fig. 20.8 Midesophageal four-chamber view showing a dilated right ventricle *(RV)*, right atrium *(RA)* with increased right atrial pressure *(arrow)*, and an underfilled left ventricle *(LV)*. HR, Heart rate; *LA,* left atrium.

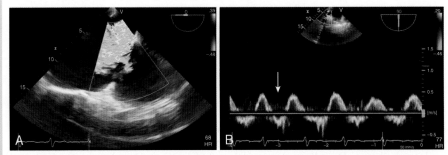

Fig. 20.9 (A) Midesophageal four-chamber view showing a dilated right ventricle with severe tricuspid regurgitation. (B) Hepatic vein reversal, with S-wave reversal *(arrow)*. HR, Heart rate.

applying the modified Bernoulli equation ($\Delta P = 4v^2$) with the addition of central venous pressure.

It is not uncommon to encounter difficulty in floating the PAC because of severe TR, as well as a dilated right atrium and right ventricle. TEE is routinely used to float the PAC by using the bicaval and ME RV inflow-outflow views.

RA pressure can be approximated by imaging the inferior vena cava (IVC) by echocardiography. The IVC diameter should not exceed 1.7 cm and should collapse by at least 50% during spontaneous inspiration in healthy persons. The presence of a dilated IVC and the lack of more than 50% inspiratory collapse implies elevation of RA pressure in the range of 10 to 14 mm Hg. In more severe cases, in which RA pressure is greater than 20 mm Hg, the IVC diameter does not collapse at all with ventilation.

RV failure ultimately leads to RV dilation, with a dilated tricuspid valve annulus together with chordal traction resulting in significant TR. This condition is confirmed by a *vena contracta* greater than 0.7 cm and systolic reversal of hepatic vein flow (Fig. 20.9). Notably, TR does not correlate directly with the degree of PH, but rather with the degree of RV enlargement and alterations in RV geometry. Echocardiography helps appraise the degree of TR before and after surgical treatment.

The *ME ascending aortic short-axis* and upper esophageal aortic arch short-axis views frequently are used to evaluate the pulmonary vasculature for the presence of clots. Therefore a thorough evaluation throughout the venous system, right side of the heart, and pulmonary vasculature is required. Indirect clues to thrombus formation include a dilated right atrium and right ventricle, intracardiac devices, or the presence of spontaneous echocardiographic contrast. Dilated main PA and right PA are also common in CTEPH.

Mitral valve prolapse (MVP) has been described in patients with CTEPH as "pseudo-MVP." The phenomenon is thought to result from pressure deformation of the left ventricle by the right ventricle, thereby leading to distortion of the mitral valve annulus. The EI was greater for patients with MVP and deformation of the left ventricle compared with patients with no MVP without deformation. Reduction of PH after PTE reversed this deformation and allowed for resolution of "pseudo-MVP."

Impaired LV relaxation seen in patients with CTEPH is largely the result of low LV volume and relative underfilling and is not solely caused by LV chamber distortion secondary to the geometric effects of RV enlargement. LV diastolic filling patterns improve with the resolution of PH after successful PTE. The transmitral E (peak early filling [E wave]) velocity increases, and pulmonary venous S (systolic forward flow [S wave]) and D (diastolic forward flow wave [D wave]) velocity increase significantly, suggesting higher preload with improvement in the CO. TEE is critical in the intraoperative management of patients with CTEPH for assessment of the right ventricle, tricuspid valve, right atrium, and intracardiac thrombus or other cardiac disease. It also allows for postbypass cardiovascular evaluation and assessment of de-airing of the cardiac chambers, as well as changes affecting the right ventricle.

◼ OUTCOME AND FUTURE OF CHRONIC THROMBOEMBOLIC PULMONARY HYPERTENSION

With increased awareness of CTEPH and with several major cardiovascular centers around the world performing the procedure, progress in surgical and medical management has improved outcomes.

The reported world literature on this operation (exclusive of UCSD) is more than 3000 cases. The mortality rate at UCSD has declined significantly, from 16% in the 1980s to 1.3% by 2012, and, despite a patient population at higher risk, the mortality rate declined to 1% to 2% (Fig. 20.10). This change likely reflects the evolution and refinements in all aspects of patient care: correct preoperative diagnosis, meticulous preparation for operation, advances in surgical and anesthetic technique, and improved postoperative management. The secret to the success of this procedure is the close collaboration of multiple medical teams, including pulmonary medicine, anesthesiology, perfusion, and cardiac surgery.

Efforts from the international community have put forth a prospective registry for long-term follow-up and continued awareness of CTEPH. PTE has revolutionized the treatment of CTEPH by providing significant and permanent lifestyle improvements. With increased awareness of the disease, excellent surgical outcomes in specialized centers, and innovations in medical therapy, treatment of severe PH resulting from CTEPH is now within reach of many patients around the world. However, many questions remain to be answered through future studies and innovations.

20

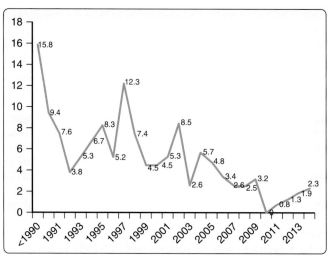

Fig. 20.10 Perioperative mortality rates: University of California San Diego.

SUGGESTED READINGS

Adams A, Fedullo PF. Postoperative management of the patient undergoing pulmonary endarterectomy. *Semin Thorac Cardiovasc Surg.* 2006;18:250–256.

Auger WR, Kerr KM, Kim NH, et al. Evaluation of patients with chronic thromboembolic pulmonary hypertension for pulmonary endarterectomy. *Pulm Circ.* 2012;2:155–162.

Bermudez CA, Rocha RV, Sappington PL, et al. Initial experience with single cannulation for venovenous extracorporeal oxygenation in adults. *Ann Thorac Surg.* 2010;90:991–995.

Bossone E, D'Andrea A, D'Alto M, et al. Echocardiography in pulmonary arterial hypertension: from diagnosis to prognosis. *J Am Soc Echocardiogr.* 2013;26:1–14.

Cronin B, Maus T, Pretorius V, et al. Management of pulmonary hemorrhage after pulmonary endarterectomy with venovenous extracorporeal membrane oxygenation without systemic anticoagulation. *J Cardiothorac Vasc Anesth.* 2014;28(6):1667–1676.

D'Armini AM, Morsolini M, Mattiucci G, et al. Pulmonary endarterectomy for distal chronic thromboembolic pulmonary hypertension. *J Thorac Cardiovasc Surg.* 2014;148(3):1005–1011.

Fedullo PF, Auger WR, Kerr KM, et al. Chronic thromboembolic pulmonary hypertension. *N Engl J Med.* 2001;345:1465.

Ikeda K, MacLeod DB, Grocott HP, et al. The accuracy of a near-infrared spectroscopy cerebral oximetry device and its potential value for estimating jugular venous oxygen saturation. *Anesth Analg.* 2014;119(6):1381–1392.

Jamieson SW, Kapelanski DP, Sakakibara N, et al. Pulmonary endarterectomy; experience and lessons learned in 1,500 cases. *Ann Thorac Surg.* 2003;76:1457.

Kerr KM. Pulmonary artery sarcoma masquerading as chronic thromboembolic pulmonary hypertension. *Nat Clin Pract Cardiovasc Med.* 2005;2:108–112.

Kreitner K-F, Ley S, Kauczor H-U, et al. Chronic thromboembolic pulmonary hypertension: pre- and postoperative assessment with breath-hold magnetic resonance techniques. *Radiology.* 2004;32:535–543.

Madani MM, Auger WR, Pretorius V, et al. Pulmonary endarterectomy: recent changes in a single institution's experience of more than 2,700 patients. *Ann Thorac Surg.* 2012;94:97–103.

McLaughlin V, Langer A, Tan M, et al. Contemporary trends in the diagnosis and management of pulmonary arterial hypertension. *Chest.* 2013;143(2):324–332.

Mizoguchi H, Ogawa A, Munemasa M, et al. Refined balloon pulmonary angioplasty for inoperable patients with chronic thromboembolic pulmonary hypertension. *Circ Cardiovasc Interv.* 2012;5:748–755.

Pengo V, Lensing AW, Prins MH, et al; Thromboembolic Pulmonary Hypertension Study Group. Incidence of chronic thromboembolic pulmonary hypertension after pulmonary embolism. *N Engl J Med.* 2004;350:2257–2264.

Raisinghani A, Ben-Yehuda O. Echocardiography in chronic thromboembolic pulmonary hypertension. *Semin Thorac Cardiovasc Surg*. 2006;18:230–235.

Simonneau D, Gatzoulis M, Adatia I, et al. Updated clinical classification of pulmonary hypertension. *J Am Coll Cardiol*. 2013;62(suppl):D34–D41.

Sugimura K, Fukumoto Y, Satoh K, et al. Percutaneous transluminal pulmonary angioplasty markedly improves pulmonary hemodynamics and long-term prognosis in patients with chronic thromboembolic pulmonary hypertension. *Circ J*. 2012;76:485–488.

Svyatets M, Tolani K, Zhang M, et al. Perioperative management of deep hypothermic circulatory arrest. *J Cardiothorac Vasc Anesth*. 2010;24(4):644–655.

Thistlethwaite PA, Kemp A, Du L, et al. Outcomes of pulmonary thromboendarterectomy for treatment of extreme thromboembolic pulmonary hypertension. *J Thorac Cardiovasc Surg*. 2006;131:307–313.

Willemink MJ, van Es HW, Koobs L, et al. CT evaluation of chronic thromboembolic pulmonary hypertension. *Clin Radiol*. 2012;67:277–285.

Wolf M, Boyer-Neumann C, Parent F, et al. Thrombotic risk factors in pulmonary hypertension. *Eur Respir J*. 2000;116:503.

20

Chapter 21

Procedures in the Hybrid Operating Room

Waseem Zakaria Aziz Zakhary, MD • Joerg Karl Ender, MD

Key Points

1. A hybrid operating room combines advanced imaging capabilities with a fully functioning operating suite.
2. Transcatheter aortic valve replacement (TAVR) is recommended for patients with severe symptomatic aortic stenosis who are inoperable or at high risk for needing surgical aortic valve replacement and have a predicted post-TAVR survival of more than 12 months.
3. Vascular complications are the most common complications with the transfemoral approach.
4. The concept of multimodal imaging plays an important role in preprocedural assessment.
5. The presence of a heart team is a prerequisite for establishing a TAVR program.
6. Catheter-based mitral valve repair techniques are primarily guided by transesophageal echocardiography.

Hybrid operating rooms (ORs) were conceived two decades ago. They were first designed to combine percutaneous coronary interventions (PCIs) and stent implantations with minimally invasive coronary artery bypass grafting (CABG) procedures. However, widespread building of hybrid ORs started only after the development of transcatheter valve replacements. After the first report of successful percutaneous balloon valvuloplasty in patients with severe aortic stenosis (AS) in 1983, the first human transcatheter aortic valve replacement (TAVR) was performed in 2002. Despite high costs and structural complexity, there has been a steady increase in new hybrid ORs as a result of the development of more and more percutaneous interventions, which require a facility that combines the capabilities of the angiographic catheterization laboratory with the cardiac surgical OR. Typical procedures performed in the hybrid ORs include TAVR, percutaneous mitral valve repair, thoracic endovascular aortic repair (TEVAR), percutaneous pulmonary valve implantation, implantable pacemaker and cardioverter-defibrillator lead explantations, and combined coronary and valve procedures.

TECHNICAL CONSIDERATIONS

Definition of a Hybrid Operating Room

A hybrid OR combines advanced imaging capabilities with a fully functioning operating suite. This means that angiographic, fluoroscopic, and other imaging capabilities (eg, computed tomography [CT], echocardiography) are integrated into a cardiac OR.

Equipment and Layout

In addition to components of a surgical suite, the following features should be available:

1. High-quality fluoroscopy (generally with flat-panel imaging) in a lead-lined room.
2. Integration of other modalities, such as a biplane system, C-arm CT, integrated ultrasound, and electromagnetic navigation systems (optional).
3. A control area for radiologic technicians either inside or outside of the hybrid OR with a direct view to the surgical field.
4. A radiolucent, thin, nonmetallic carbon fiber operating table that can accommodate both angiography and open operations. It must also be integrated to the imaging system to avoid collisions. Because of a lack of metal parts, some operating table functions are lost, such as isolated movement of upper or lower parts of the patient's body. Nevertheless, a floating tabletop with multidirectional tilt function is needed for accurate catheter maneuvering.
5. Adequate room size (800 square feet [74.3 m^2] to 1000 square feet or more) to accommodate the equipment required by cardiac or vascular surgeons and interventional cardiologists, as well as the anesthesia team, nursing team, perfusionist, and radiologic technicians. Careful equipment positioning is required to allow fast conversion to conventional surgery if needed.
6. Ceiling-mounted monitors placed in positions that allow all team members (surgeons, anesthesiologists, and interventionists) to visualize the images simultaneously. Images from angiography, echocardiography, and hemodynamic monitoring need to be displayed.
7. Circulating heating, ventilation, and laminar air flow to provide a smooth undisturbed air flow suitable for conventional surgical operations.
8. Adequate high-output lighting for surgical interventions.
9. Other inevitable requirements such as adequate number of power receptacles, gas and suction outlets for both the anesthesia machine and the cardiopulmonary bypass (CPB) system, and hot and cold water outlets for the CPB.
10. Equipment: high-definition displays and monitors, oxygen (O_2) analyzer, suction, O_2 supply, defibrillator/resuscitation cart, echocardiographic equipment, sonographers, anesthesia equipment, CPB equipment, syringe pumps, radiation protection (along with the imaging system), blood warmers and blood bank access, point-of-care laboratory monitoring for blood gases and coagulation parameters, and so on. Because of the life-threatening complications that may be encountered during the procedure, ready-made crash carts consisting of any equipment necessary in an emergency must be available.
11. A complete sterile environment.

▣ IMAGING SYSTEMS

Fluoroscopy

Fluoroscopy may be portable or fixed. In general, fixed systems enable higher imaging quality and less radiation exposure compared with portable systems. The fixed C-arm may be mounted on the ceiling or the floor. Ceiling-mounted systems do not occupy OR floor space, but they need higher ceilings, which affects lighting, monitor placement, and laminar air flow. While these disadvantages can be avoided using floor-mounted systems, this comes at the cost of the available floor space. The fluoroscopy operating system generates a considerable amount of heat and noise, and it is suitable to put it outside the hybrid OR.

Digital Subtraction Angiography

This technique is used to visualize the blood vessels and identify any abnormalities without interference from background structures. In TAVR, it is used for identification of the coronary arteries immediately before valve implantation.

Echocardiography

Transesophageal echocardiography (TEE) is used during TAVR preprocedure, intraprocedure, and postprocedure for diagnosis of the disease and complications. Real-time 3D TEE can be a helpful tool that facilitates maneuvering of the delivery system and proper positioning of the aortic prosthesis. Transthoracic echocardiography (TTE) may be used in interventions performed under monitored anesthetic care (MAC) in which TEE is not possible.

▣ RADIATION SAFETY

The most important aspect of radiation safety is education. The whole team must understand how to reduce the radiation dosage and exposure. Certain safety measures should be available during procedures. Hybrid ORs must have lead-lined walls and doors. Both portable and built-in shielding for personnel must be considered during design of a hybrid OR. Moreover, lead aprons must be attached to the table. Enough lead aprons must be hung in a dedicated space outside the hybrid OR for all personnel. Finally, the radiation exposure should be measured regularly for all personnel.

▣ TRANSCATHETER AORTIC VALVE REPLACEMENT

Patient Selection and Indications

Currently, TAVR is recommended for patients with severe symptomatic AS who are inoperable or at high risk for needing surgical AVR and have a predicted post-TAVR survival of more than 12 months. High-risk patients are generally defined as those with a Society of Thoracic Surgeons (STS) score of 10% or European System for Cardiac Operative Risk Evaluation (EuroSCORE) of 20%. According to the American Heart Association (AHA) and the American College of Cardiology (ACC), high risk is defined as an STS predicted risk of mortality (PROM) of 8% or higher; or two or more indices of frailty (moderate to severe); or up to two major organ systems compromised, not to be improved postoperatively; or possible procedure-specific impediment.

The approach to patient selection for TAVR is optimal with a multidisciplinary team (MDT) that includes a primary cardiologist, cardiac surgeon, interventional cardiologist, echocardiographer, imaging specialists (CT or cardiac magnetic resonance [CMR]), heart failure and valve disease specialist, cardiac anesthesiologist, nurse practitioner, and cardiac rehabilitation specialists. At minimum, cardiologists, cardiac surgeons, cardiac anesthesiologists, and an imaging specialist should be involved in daily clinical practice.

IV

The following issues must be discussed during the patient selection process:

1. Indication for aortic valve replacement (AVR), either surgical or TAVR.
2. Risk assessment and indication for TAVR.
3. Feasibility of the procedure for specific patient and choice of most proper access (eg, severe peripheral arterial disease).
4. Selection of specific valve type and size for the individual patient.

Other factors that may affect the decision-making process include availability, experience, and institutional commitment to managing very high-risk patients, technical skills, local results, referral patterns, and patient preference.

Indication for Aortic Valve Replacement: Surgical or Transcatheter

Diagnosis of AS should not differ according to whether or not a minimally invasive technique is chosen but should be made according to established guidelines. Echocardiography and, to some extent, cardiac catheterization are the main diagnostic tools for AS. The echocardiographic criteria to define severe AS include decreased systolic opening of a calcified or congenital stenotic valve with an aortic valve area (AVA) of 1.0 cm^2 or less, indexed AVA 0.6 cm^2/m^2 or less, aortic velocity 4.0 m/s or higher, and/or a mean transvalvular pressure gradient of 40 mm Hg or higher. Symptomatic patients may have heart failure, syncope, exertional dyspnea, angina, or presyncope by history or on exercise testing. AVR is recommended for asymptomatic patients provided that left ventricular ejection fraction (LVEF) is 50% or less. Stress echocardiography may be useful during the assessment of low-flow/low-gradient AS. If stress results in increases in stroke volume and AVA larger than 0.2 cm^2 with little change in pressure gradient, it is not severe AS; with true severe AS, patients have a fixed valve area with increases in stroke volume and pressure gradient during a stress state.

Risk Assessment and Indication for TAVR

The two most commonly used scores for risk assessment are the STS risk score and the EuroSCORE and the related logistic EuroSCORE. Five risk factors have special importance, either because of their impact on outcome or because they are not presented in risk models in spite of their prevalence. These factors are chronic kidney disease, coronary artery disease, chronic lung disease, mitral valve disease, and systolic dysfunction. Some patients are generally eligible for surgical AVR, but because of local disease abnormalities they may be scheduled for TAVR (eg, severe calcification of ascending aorta, porcelain aorta, friable aortic atheroma, and previous radiation therapy to the mediastinum). Two other factors that may affect the decision on surgery are (1) very elderly with associated comorbidities, and (2) frailty and futility.

The inclusion and exclusion criteria have been subjected to many modifications as a result of advances in technology and the specifications of next generation valves. Other clinical and anatomic contraindications also must be considered, such as valve endocarditis, elevated risk of coronary ostium obstruction (asymmetric valve calcification, short distance between annulus and coronary ostium, small aortic sinuses), and untreated coronary artery disease requiring revascularization (Box 21.1).

Feasibility of the Procedure for Specific Patients and Choice of Access

Access routes for TAVR include transfemoral, transapical, transaortic (via left anterior minithoracotomy or ministenotomy), suprasternal (aortic/innominate), transcarotid, or axillary and subclavian. Caval-aortic access also has been described for TAVR,

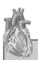

BOX 21.1 *Inclusion Criteria and Contraindications for TAVR*

Inclusion Criteria

- Calcific aortic valve stenosis
- Echocardiography: mean gradient >40 mm Hg or jet velocity >4.0 m/s and AVA <0.8 cm^2 or indexed EOA <0.5 cm^2/m^2
- High risk for conventional AVR assessed by one cardiac interventionist and two experienced cardiothoracic surgeons
- Symptomatic

Contraindications (Candidates Will Be Excluded If Any of the Following Conditions Are Present)

- Absolute
  - Absence of a heart team and no cardiac surgery on the site
  - Appropriateness of TAVR, as an alternative to AVR, not confirmed by a heart team
- Clinical
  - Estimated life expectancy <1 year
  - Improvement of quality of life by TAVR unlikely because of comorbidities
  - Severe primary associated disease of other valves with major contribution to the patient's symptoms, which can be treated only by surgery
- Anatomic
  - Inadequate annulus size (<18 mm, >29 mm) (when using the current devices)
  - Thrombus in the left ventricle
  - Active endocarditis
  - Elevated risk of coronary ostium obstruction (asymmetric valve calcification, short distance between annulus and coronary ostium, small aortic sinuses)
  - Plaques with mobile thrombi in the ascending aorta or arch
  - For transfemoral/subclavian approach: inadequate vascular access (vessel size, calcification, tortuosity)
- Relative
  - Bicuspid or noncalcified valves
  - Untreated coronary artery disease requiring revascularization
  - Hemodynamic instability
  - LVEF <20%
  - For transapical approach: severe pulmonary disease, LV apex not accessible
  - Mixed aortic valve disease (aortic stenosis and aortic regurgitation with predominant aortic regurgitation >3+)
  - Hypertrophic cardiomyopathy
  - Severe incapacitating dementia
  - Renal insufficiency (creatinine >3.0 mg/dL) and/or end-stage renal disease requiring chronic dialysis
  - Severe pulmonary hypertension and RV dysfunction

AVA, Aortic valve area; *AVR,* aortic valve replacement; *EOA,* effective orifice area; *LV,* left ventricular; *LVEF,* left ventricular ejection fraction; *RV,* Right ventricle; *TAVR,* transcatheter aortic valve replacement.

wherein percutaneous entry is obtained into the abdominal aorta from the femoral vein through the adjoining inferior vena cava. All of these routes are retrograde except for transapical and transseptal approaches, which are antegrade. The most common approaches are transfemoral and transapical.

The primary access route is transfemoral as long as the diameter of the femoral vessels is 6 to 8 mm or larger and the degree of atherosclerosis allows. Vascular complications are the most common complications with the transfemoral approach and are due to large-caliber devices and the atherosclerotic disease of the patients. Peripheral vascular diseases with related vascular calcification, narrow arterial diameter, tortuosity and intramural thrombus or dissection are the most important factors. Planning access requires assessment of the luminal size and the degree of vessel calcification and tortuosity. The high-quality thin-slice CT scan with contrast that extends from the femoral artery to the subclavian artery is considered the key study in this context. Angiography and intravascular ultrasound may be adjuvants. Limitations of the transfemoral approach will be fewer with the use of the newer generation lower-profile valves and reduction in the size of the delivery sheath. Subclavian access is an alternative approach for TAVR, with less reported vascular injury, but rare brachial plexus neuropathies have been reported. Left subclavian artery access could be an unsuitable choice for patients who have undergone a previous CABG with left internal mammary anastomosis, because of the risk of myocardial ischemia during temporary occlusion of the artery.

The transapical and direct aortic approaches are comparable. Both have the disadvantage of being a surgical technique that violates the chest wall and the advantage of avoiding the aortic arch with a theoretical reduction of stroke incidence. Moreover, because the distance from the entry point to implantation is short, implantation is easier and more accurate.

The transapical approach has the risk of ventricular rupture and life-threatening bleeding. The concept of multimodal imaging plays an important role in preprocedural assessment, not only in helping determine the feasibility of the procedure but also in evaluating the access size and the size of the aortic annulus. This includes angiography and cardiac catheterization, echocardiography, multidetector computed tomography (MDCT), and magnetic resonance imaging (MRI). Some relative or absolute contraindications may be discovered during imaging, such as a bicuspid valve, left ventricular (LV) thrombus, significant mitral regurgitation with mitral annulus calcifications, a substantially high anatomic risk for coronary ostial obstruction (<10 mm), and infective endocarditis.

Selection of Specific Valve Type and Size for the Patient

Because of the variety of the valves present on the market now, many cardiologists use the concept of "anatomy-dependent" valve selection. The close proximity to the coronary ostia, the width and height of the sinuses, the membranous ventricular septum with the His bundle, and the anterior leaflet of the mitral valve are important anatomic considerations.

Imaging techniques play a major role in:

- Identifying suitable prosthesis size.
- Measuring the distance of the coronary ostia from the aortic annulus to avoid occlusion by the valve stent (>11 mm).
- The diameter of the tubular aorta 45 mm from the aortic valve annulus in case of CoreValve use, which is designed to have a frame with hooks deployed in the supraannular aorta. This diameter must be less than 40 to 45 mm according to valve size.
- Presence of atheroma in the thoracic aorta.
- Other valve dysfunctions, especially mitral regurgitation.
- Left ventricular outflow tract (LVOT) and septal hypertrophy.
- Diameter of the femoral vessels.

Prosthesis size: Slight oversizing is required for prevention of dislocation of these sutureless valves. Undersizing may lead to paravalvular regurgitation (PVR) or valve

21

embolization, whereas oversizing may lead to incomplete valve deployment or annular rupture. Contrast CT measurement is the ideal technique for aortic annulus sizing before TAVR; the annulus is larger than that measured by TEE by 1.5 ± 1.6 mm.

Three-dimensional TEE measurements are superior to 2D TEE measurements and correlate closely with those from MDCT. TTE underestimates the annulus size by up to 15% or 1.36 mm. The 3D TEE is also very accurate in measuring the true aortic annulus diameter via proper alignment of the short and long axes of the aortic valve. It should be used whenever CT is not available. Sizing using cardiac MRI also may be an alternative to CT. Operator experience is the main factor in valve selection.

In the absence of severe atherosclerosis and severe vascular tortuosity, femoral artery size is considered the main limiting factor in determining the most suitable route for TAVR. Sheaths allow access to the vessel without loss of blood when a hemostatic valve is used. Sheath diameter has decreased over time from 25-Fr in the first generation to 18-Fr in the third generation (or even 14-Fr in expandable sheaths [Edwards Lifesciences, Irvine, Calif]). Vessel diameter less than 6 mm (measured by angiography, ultrasound, or CT) presently is considered nonsuitable for the smallest sheath. The Edwards SAPIEN valve consists of a trileaflet bovine pericardium valve, pretreated to decrease calcification, mounted in a balloon-expandable stainless steel stent that can be implanted transfemorally or transapically. The CoreValve (now produced commercially by Medtronic, Irvine, Calif) has an auto-expandable nitinol stent containing a porcine pericardial valve. This valve has only been used by a retrograde approach, either via transfemoral, subclavian, or direct aortic access. Several newer transcatheter valves are in various stages of evaluation.

Logistical Considerations

The presence of a heart team is a prerequisite for establishing a TAVR program. The presence of on-site cardiac surgery, anesthesiologist, and CPB is essential regardless of the location in the OR, cardiac catheterization laboratory (CCL), or hybrid OR. During a TAVR procedure, patients may require conversion to emergency cardiac surgery if a complication occurs that cannot be managed conservatively. Although many patients having TAVR are not candidates for conventional aortic valve replacements, rescue CPB should be instituted to allow the correction of reversible complications. Further measures in case of major complications should be discussed with the patient before the procedure. These decisions must be documented in the medical notes and discussed with the whole medical team involved in the procedure.

Some complications (eg, coronary obstruction, vessel injury) do not require open surgery but instead a lot of support for the interventionist from other team members such as anesthesiologists and radiologists. It is obvious that these complicated procedures need the MDT approach and a hybrid OR that provides an environment suitable for the team to ensure the safety and efficacy of the procedure and to manage complications that may arise.

Multidisciplinary Team

Two important issues must be highlighted when evolving a TAVR program: First, it is not a solo procedure that can be done only by a group of physicians away from other team members. This team approach, which is known also as an MDT approach, is essential for a successful procedure. While the importance of full collaboration between interventional cardiologist and cardiac surgeon is obvious, it is even more critical to incorporate other key providers from other physician groups (eg, anesthesiology, radiology, noninvasive cardiology, intensive care) into the process. Second, it is

IV

important to emphasize that TAVR therapy program is a process that starts outside the OR with patient evaluation and selection of suitability for this procedure and does not stop after the procedure, but continues in the postoperative period.

Responsibilities for the different heart team members must be assigned before starting the procedure:

- Normally, instrumentation of the patient as well as anesthetic management belongs to the anesthesiologist.
- The intervention itself is performed by cardiologists, cardiac surgeons, or (ideally) both.
- Temporary transvenous pacemaker implantation can be done by the anesthesiologist from the jugular vein or by the interventionist from the femoral vein.
- Rapid pacing can be induced by the anesthesiologist or by the interventionist. No matter who is responsible, clear communication is mandatory.
- Echocardiographic imaging is done by the anesthesiologist or an echocardiographer.

Anesthetic Management

Anesthetic Technique

The decision whether the patient receives general anesthesia (GA) or local anesthesia (LA) of the access site with or without sedation or MAC depends on the route of access, institutional practice, and the patient's comorbidities. GA remains the mainstay in management of patients undergoing TAVR. In many institutions (especially in Europe), transfemoral TAVR is done under MAC with satisfying results. The transapical TAVR is done under GA or, in rare cases, using thoracic epidural. Otherwise, other access approaches are done under GA mostly because of lack of experience and familiarity to such procedures.

Advantages to using a MAC technique include avoidance of the circulatory depressant effects of GA, decreased use of vasoactive drugs, easy intraoperative central nervous system monitoring in case of embolic stroke, reduced procedural time, faster patient recovery, need for a lower level of postoperative care, and shorter hospital stay duration. Even when LA or MAC is used, the anesthesiologist has to be prepared to switch to GA in emergency situations.

On the other hand, GA has its own advantages. The airway is secured, avoiding emergency airway intervention in case of an unfavorable hemodynamic situation. The use of TEE under GA is of particular importance in diagnosis and management intraoperatively. No anesthetic drug is superior to another. In general, short-acting anesthetics with less hemodynamic effects are preferred to ensure early extubation after the procedure. Etomidate, propofol, remifentanil, sevoflurane, and desflurane are the most frequently used anesthetics.

Procedure-Related Anesthetic Considerations

MONITORING

In addition to standard monitoring (ie, electrocardiography [ECG], pulse oximetry, end-tidal CO_2, anesthetic gas concentration, and noninvasive blood pressure), invasive monitoring is mandatory because of the complicated nature of the procedure, the patient's comorbidities, intraoperative cardiovascular compromise (especially with rapid pacing), and the possibility of life-threatening complications. Both arterial and central venous catheters should be inserted under LA or GA. Although a pulmonary artery catheter has been recommended, there is still debate about whether it is needed in every patient. It may be useful in patients with moderate-to-severe pulmonary hypertension, because pulmonary hypertension per se is an independent risk for mortality in patients undergoing TAVR. In these patients, the use of elective femorofemoral CPB also may be considered. At least one large-bore venous access catheter should be inserted for volume resuscitation. Urinary output and temperature monitoring are helpful.

RAPID VENTRICULAR PACING

Rapid ventricular pacing is a special and important issue during the procedure. It is essential to have no ejection with a cardiac arrest during balloon aortic valvuloplasty and during deployment of a balloon-expandable valve such as the SAPIEN valve. On the other hand, the longer profile of the CoreValve, which extends from the aortic annulus to the supracoronary aorta, allows its gradual release without need of rapid pacing. The rapid pacing phase is usually brief, and the heart recovers in seconds after stopping rapid pacing. Communication during this period is essential. A clear command "rapid pacing on" has to be followed by the clear reaction that rapid pacing has been started and the heart does not eject anymore. At the end of the maneuver the command "rapid pacing off" has to be followed by the reaction "rapid pacing is off" and the state of the circulation (ie, blood pressure and heart rate recovery).

Transesophageal Echocardiography

TEE is one of the two most important intraoperative imaging modalities used during TAVR. It stands side-by-side with fluoroscopy for a successful TAVR process. The radiation exposure to the patient and to the personnel is the major problem with fluoroscopy. In spite of that, it is used extensively because of its ability to better assess the guidewire and catheter locations and the valve stent position. On the other hand, TEE, in spite of being very useful in this context, is used intraoperatively only with patients under GA.

The aortic valve has special anatomy that increases the imaging assessment difficulties, and it is important for the echocardiographer to have a good understanding of what is called the functional aortic annulus for good TAVR guidance. The functional aortic annulus contains the following components: the aortic annulus, the sinus segment with the sinuses of Valsalva and the origins of the coronary arteries, and the sinotubular junction where the sinus segment joins the tubular ascending aorta. The definition of *aortic annulus* varies significantly among operators. The aortic annulus has at least three definitions. It is either the ring formed by the anatomic ventriculoarterial junction, the ring formed by the hinge point at the attachment of the valve leaflet to the myocardium, or the ring formed at the top of the valve leaflets at the sinotubular junction (Fig. 21.1). Actually, the most commonly used "hinge points" ring is a virtual

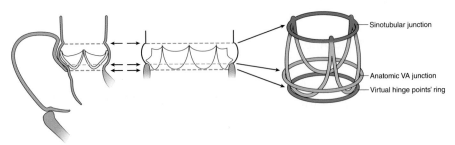

Sinotubular junction

Anatomic VA junction

Virtual hinge points' ring

Fig. 21.1 The various rings associated with the aortic annulus. VA, Ventriculoarterial. (Modified from Piazza N, de Jaegere P, Schultz C, et al. Anatomy of the aortic valvar complex and its implications for transcatheter implantation of the aortic valve. *Circ Cardiovasc Interv.* 2008;1:74–81.)

ring, as there is no anatomic plane for this ring. Anatomically, it is located in the upper part of the LVOT, below the other two rings. It was found that the functional aortic annulus is not a spherical but an elliptical structure, with both major and minor diameters, which makes the measurements more difficult, with need for a multiplane, rather than one-plane (2D), assessment. Three-dimensional imaging either by TEE or MDCT plays a major role to overcome this problem.

TEE should be used before, during, and after TAVR procedures to assess various factors.

PREPROCEDURAL ASSESSMENTS

- The severity of AS and associated aortic regurgitation if present.
- Aortic valve system (cusps, annulus, root) morphology and abnormalities.
- Aortic annulus size: the anterior-posterior aortic annulus diameter in systole at the hinge point of the cusps, either in the 2D long-axis view or 3D in the long-axis and the short-axis views using multiplanar reconstruction mode.
- LV size and function.
- The aortic annulus to coronary ostia distance, which must be greater than 11 mm to avoid inadvertent coronary occlusion during implantation. Both 2D and 3D modes are used. For left coronary ostium, 3D multiplanar reconstruction must be used, while the right coronary ostium can be measured also in a 2D long-axis view.
- Diameter of tubular aorta (a diameter >45 mm is a contraindication for CoreValve implantation).
- Presence of atheroma in thoracic aorta.
- Other valve dysfunctions, especially mitral valve regurgitation.
- LVOT and septal hypertrophy.

INTRAPROCEDURAL ASSESSMENTS

- The ventricular puncture site in the transapical approach using the midesophageal two-chamber view.
- The proper position of the wires, balloon, and valve delivery systems during and after the implantation. During the transapical approach it is important to ensure that the guidewire is not stuck in the mitral valve apparatus. The mitral valve chordae and the degree of mitral regurgitation must always be reevaluated as catheter advancement in these circumstances risks mitral valve injury and acute mitral regurgitation. Real-time 3D echo is superior in mitral valve apparatus visualization.
- The severity and the location (and sometimes the cause) of transvalvular and PVR. Semiquantitative methods of PVR assessment include the diastolic flow reversal in the descending aorta and the percentage circumferential extent of PVR.
- The valve after implantation concerning the pressure gradients, valve area and the dimensionless velocity index when applicable.
- Global and regional LV and right ventricular (RV) function, especially after the rapid pacing phases.
- Possible complications (ie, new regional wall motion abnormalities, mitral regurgitation, pericardial effusion/tamponade, aortic dissection or trauma, and coronary occlusion of the circumflex artery).

POSTPROCEDURAL ASSESSMENTS

- The aortic valve prosthesis function and position.
- LV function and mitral regurgitation.
- Any possible complication (eg, pericardial tamponade)
- To follow up a paraprosthetic regurgitation, if present.

21

Intraoperative Fluoroscopy

Valve positioning is currently based on fluoroscopy with or without (in patients receiving only MAC/LA) TEE guidance. Originally, the operator depends on the aortic calcifications that appear in the 2D view of the fluoroscopy for valve positioning.

Digital Subtraction Angiography

Digital subtraction angiography (DSA) is used mainly to visualize the blood vessels and identify any abnormality without interference from background structures. An advanced visualization of the entire DSA flow (iflow) with color coding is another advancement in this field that allows the operator to visualize the entire vascular tree in just one image.

Multidetector Computed Tomography

MDCT is the "gold standard" method in assessment of complex aortic valve geometry. It can give almost all the information needed for TAVR. It is used in the assessment of the annular size and shape, degree of calcification, the distance between annulus and coronary ostia, and in planning for the precise coaxial alignment of the stent-valve along the centerline of the aortic valve and aortic root. In addition, the atherosclerosis of the iliofemoral and the thoracoabdominal aorta can be easily assessed.

Three-dimensional reconstruction of the heart is a very helpful realistic method that can be used at the desired phase of the cardiac cycle (eg, 30–40% of the systole) for valve area and annular assessment. Four-dimensional reconstruction of the heart for the whole cardiac cycle can be done, but at the expense of a high radiation dose. Another risk that must be considered is the low-osmolar iodinated contrast agent causing contrast nephropathy. The noncontrast scan is not optimal, but the assessment of the vessel's size, calcification, and tortuosity is feasible.

The elliptical shape of the aortic annulus gives the 3D CT reconstruction special importance, as it allows the measurement of both annular minimal and maximal diameters, which can be measured also by 3D TEE but not with 2D TEE. A difference of 2 mm or more between the maximum aortic annulus and nominal prosthesis diameters by MDCT is considered as an independent risk factor for postoperative moderate-to-severe PVR.

Complications

In some patients who have required relatively long rapid pacing because of multiple adjustments to balloon or valve positions before inflation, heart stunning has occurred and has not recovered without medical or mechanical support. Usually a small bolus of metaraminol (0.5–1 mg), phenylephrine (0.1–0.5 mg), or norepinephrine (10–20 μg) is sufficient for recovery. Epinephrine (10–20 μg) sometimes is necessary and can be injected through the central venous catheter or directly into the aortic root pigtail catheter used for contrast administration. This direct injection into the aorta is more effective, especially with a noncontracting heart. External cardiac massage must be initiated, without any delay, to obtain an acceptable cardiac output and coronary perfusion pressure. Failure of these measures must lead the team to move forward to mechanical circulatory support using emergency CPB. Institution of CPB must not take much time and the arterial and venous cannulas are inserted over the femoral guidewires already in situ for emergency situations. During this time, the situation must be assessed to discover any possible complication that led to the condition. Sometimes the only rescue maneuver is conversion to an open surgical operation through a sternotomy. Such a decision must be discussed with the patient before the operation takes place. Patients under LA usually have unpleasant feelings and nausea during the phase of rapid pacing and hypotension, which is distressing when this phase is prolonged. This can require changing to GA and rapidly securing the airway with an endotracheal tube, adding a major burden to the anesthesiologist during this critical situation. Additionally, the anesthesiologist must help to find the reason for the circulatory failure using TEE; however, this must not come before patient care and management. The possible causes of severe acute hemodynamic collapse during the procedure that can be discovered by TEE include valve embolization, severe aortic regurgitation, severe mitral regurgitation, aortic rupture or dissection, LV or RV perforation, and hypovolemia. Ventricular fibrillation is another rare complication that may arise after rapid ventricular pacing that mandates rapid defibrillation. External defibrillator pads should be attached to every patient before the procedure. Electrolytes levels, especially potassium, must be measured and corrected.

The two most common (rare, ≈1% of cases) complications that cause conversion to open surgery are valve embolization into the left ventricle and procedure-related aortic injury, including annular rupture, aortic dissection, and perforation. In spite of active management of such complications, including the surgical team's using CPB, the mortality rate is still very high, ranging from 46% to 67%. While it is highest in patients with aortic dissection or perforation (80%), it is about 33% following severe aortic regurgitation. For annular rupture, myocardial perforation, and prosthesis embolization, mortality rates are 67%, 50%, and 40%, respectively.

Coronary artery obstruction, which occurs in about 0.7% of cases, affects mainly the left main artery and requires emergency coronary intervention with a success rate of 82% and a 30-day mortality of 41%. Another relatively common complication is vascular injuries; occurrences range from 1.9% to 17.3% of patients and mortality is increased by 2.4- to 8.5-fold. These complications may require surgery, advanced endovascular stenting, ballooning, or intravascular ultrasound.

The common complications of TAVR are major bleeding, vascular injury, heart block, acute kidney injury, paravalvular leak, stroke, and postprocedural myocardial infarction.

Vascular Injury

As mentioned earlier, vascular complications (eg, rupture, perforation, dissection, hematoma, and pseudoaneurysm) were common (up to 27%) at the beginning of the era of TAVR, especially with the transfemoral approach because of relatively large valve delivery systems, lack of experience, and inadequate preoperative vascular system assessment tools. These complications have negative effects on morbidity and mortality. Over the past few years, the size of the valve delivery systems has been reduced and the precise assessment of the whole vascular system has become available.

Vascular injury must be considered if there is hemodynamic instability or a decrease in hemoglobin concentration at the end of the procedure. Good communication with the operator is essential in this situation.

Pericardial Hemorrhage

This life-threatening complication may arise at any time of the procedure. It occurs either by annular rupture or by wire perforation. The annular rupture and the ventricular or aortic wire perforation are very serious and usually require sternotomy and surgical repair. Venous bleeding by the guidewire or by the pacemaker wire can be managed by pericardial drainage and close observation.

Conduction System Abnormalities and Arrhythmias

As the atrioventricular node and bundle of His pass superficially through the interventricular septum, they are liable to be injured during aortic valve surgical procedures

21

by mechanical trauma, tissue edema, or local inflammation. This dysfunction may be temporary or permanent, for which a permanent pacemaker must be implanted. The same problems occur during TAVR, especially with long valve stents that extend into the LVOT as with the CoreValve, low implantation of the valve, or oversizing. The incidence for a permanent pacemaker after implantation of a CoreValve ranges from 23.4% to 39%, whereas it is only 4.9% to 6% for the SAPIEN valve.

Valve Malpositioning

This includes either low (in LVOT) or high (in aortic root) valve implantation or valve embolization in the worst-case scenario. Low valve deployment in the LVOT may impinge on the anterior mitral leaflet, in addition to the high risk for postoperative heart block. On the other hand, high valve implantation in the aortic root carries the risk of coronary ostial obstruction leading to myocardial ischemia and potential cardiovascular collapse. To avoid delay in stenting for high-risk patients, either a prophylactic stent insertion or at least a wire in the left coronary artery before valve deployment can be used.

Paraprosthetic aortic regurgitation can occur as a result of valve malpositioning, undersizing, extensive valve calcifications, or incomplete expansion of the valve. Mild regurgitation is found in about 70% of patients after TAVR. Moderate-to-severe regurgitation occurs in 11.7% of the patients and is an independent predictor of mid- to long-term mortality. Management options for moderate and severe regurgitation include a second balloon dilation, snares, and valve-in-valve implantation. Second balloon dilation must be done carefully as it risks valve leaflet disruption.

The rapid pacing technique is very important during valve deployment as any cardiac ejection during this phase may lead to valve malpositioning. Therefore, the temporary pacer must be adjusted to a nonsensing fixed mode with maximum output to minimize ventricular ejection risk.

Embolization of the valve into the left ventricle or into the aorta is a complication that usually needs surgical intervention. It also has been managed by implanting a second device and leaving the dislocated valve safely in the descending aorta.

Stroke

At the beginning of the TAVR era, neurologic complications were cumbersome. Recently, the incidence of stroke has declined from 7.8% to between 2.1% and 2.8%, but is still higher than in surgical AVR. Stroke in TAVR has many causes, including atherotic material from the ascending aorta or arch, calcific material from the native aortic valve, thromboembolism from the catheters used in the procedure, air micro-embolism during LV cannulation, prolonged hypotension, or dissection of brachio-cephalic vessels. Manipulation of the aortic root and valve by guidewires and catheters, and during implantation of the prosthesis, are the critical phases in which embolism mostly occurs.

Renal Dysfunction

Acute renal injury occurs in 12% to 21% (8.3–57% in other studies) of patients and is mostly reversible. Diabetes mellitus, peripheral vascular disease, chronic renal failure, and the need for blood transfusions increase its incidence.

Future Perspectives for TAVR

TAVR technology continues to improve the process and overcome the already known problems, as well as to find new applications for the procedure. The trend to smaller introducer systems has reduced vascular complications. New valve sizes are being produced to fit larger patients. Valve-in-valve TAVR, TAVR in bicuspid aortic valve, TAVR in medium- and low-risk surgical groups and in younger patients, and TAVR for aortic valve regurgitation are under clinical investigation. Moreover, new access routes have been used with patients for whom none of the known access routes are feasible.

▣ TRANSCATHETER MITRAL VALVE REPAIR: MITRACLIP

Different transcatheter mitral valve repair techniques have been developed over the past few years addressing the leaflets, the mitral annulus, or the left ventricle. These techniques usually mimic well-known surgical techniques. The MitraClip (Abbott Laboratories, Abbott Park, IL) is the most commonly used catheter-based mitral valve repair technique. It mimics the surgical edge-to edge technique first described by Alfieri and coworkers and creates a double orifice mitral valve (Fig. 21.2).

Patient Selection and Indications

The MitraClip procedure should be considered in patients with chronic severe structural mitral regurgitation (Carpentier classification type II) or chronic severe secondary or functional mitral regurgitation in patients who are severely symptomatic (New York Heart Association functional class III or IV) with a prohibitive risk for surgery or judged inoperable, favorable anatomy for a repair procedure, and a reasonable life expectancy (>1 year).

Routinely used risk scores like the logistic EuroSCORE, EuroSCORE II, or STS-PROM overestimate the predicted mortality in these patients. The procedure has been found to have a low rate of complications and in-hospital mortality.

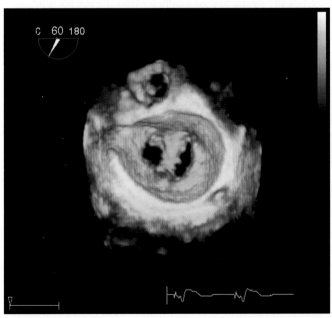

Fig. 21.2 Three-dimensional zoom double-orifice mitral valve after successful MitraClip implantation.

Access Routes

The procedure is performed via the left femoral vein. First, a steerable guide is placed through a transseptal puncture into the left atrium. Then, a clip delivery system together with the MitraClip device is introduced via the guide. After capturing both leaflets, the MitraClip is fixed to create the typical double orifice mitral valve.

Anesthetic Management

Usually this procedure is performed under GA to create optimal conditions for the interventionist and the echocardiographer, although there have been some attempts to do this procedure in sedated patients. Owing to the patients' high-risk profile, invasive blood pressure and central venous catheters are mandatory, whereas the use of a pulmonary artery catheter is not recommended. Early extubation right after the procedure can be achieved in most patients. The procedure can be done in the CCL or in the hybrid OR.

Complications

Complications such as atrial perforation with pericardial effusion or tamponade are extremely rare and can be treated without the use of CPB.

Imaging Techniques and Guidance

In contrast to TAVR, this procedure is primarily echo-guided. Angiography can be used for transseptal puncture and for visualization of the groin vessels. However, the guidance of the MitraClip system is performed by TEE. The main steps are:

- Transseptal puncture
- Introduction of the steerable guide catheter into the left atrium
- Advancement of the clip delivery system into the left atrium
- Steering and positioning of the MitraClip above the mitral valve
- Alignment of the clip
- Advancing of the MitraClip into the left ventricle
- Grasping the leaflets and assessment of proper leaflet insertion (Fig. 21.3)
- Control of leaflet insertion
- Functional control of the result (ie, residual mitral regurgitation, new mitral stenosis)
- Assessment of iatrogenic residual atrial septal defect after withdrawing of the steerable guide catheter.

For most of the main steps, real-time 3D TEE either in the wide sector zoom mode or in the X-plane mode is preferred over 2D TEE.

TRANSCATHETER PULMONARY VALVE REPLACEMENT (MELODY VALVE)

The right ventricular outflow tract (RVOT) and the pulmonary valve and artery are subjected to many abnormalities of either congenital origin (ie, tetralogy of Fallot with pulmonary atresia and truncus arteriosus) or acquired origin (ie, Ross operation). These patients are often treated with surgical placement of a right ventricular–to–pulmonary artery (RV-PA) conduit. RVOT conduits develop stenosis, insufficiency,

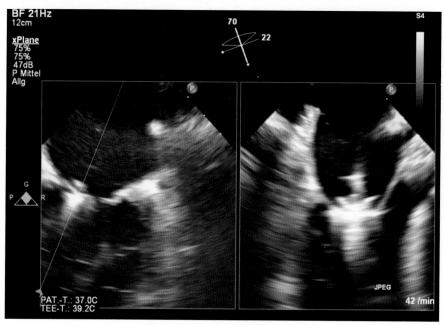

Fig. 21.3 Grasping the leaflets.

or both, over time owing to the development of calcification, intimal proliferation, and graft degeneration; consequently, RV dysfunction by volume and/or pressure overload occurs. Such patients are subjected to multiple RVOT conduit reoperations. Bare metal stenting of stenotic conduits decreases RV pressures and is associated with immediate hemodynamic improvement and potentially prolonged conduit life span. Nevertheless, this treatment option comes at the expense of significant pulmonary regurgitation. Transcatheter pulmonary valve replacement provides a good option to treat such cases without the risk of reoperation.

The Melody transcatheter pulmonary valve (Medtronic, Minneapolis, MN) has been used to treat RVOT conduit dysfunction for more than 10 years, with procedural success, excellent short-term function, and low reintervention and reoperation rates at 1 year.

The Melody valve is composed of a bovine jugular venous valve and a balloon-expandable stent. The valved stent is crimped on a balloon-in-balloon front-loading delivery system (Ensemble, Medtronic). For implantation, the inner balloon is inflated first, followed by inflation of the outer balloon. The utility of a balloon-in-balloon system increases stability of the stent on the balloon during the implantation. The device is available only in one size, while the delivery system comes in three sizes.

21

SUGGESTED READINGS

Agarwal S, Tuzcu EM, Krishnaswamy A, et al. Transcatheter aortic valve replacement: current perspectives and future implications. *Heart.* 2015;101:169–177.

Armstrong AK, Balzer DT, Cabalka AK, et al. One-year follow-up of the Melody transcatheter pulmonary valve multicenter post-approval study. *JACC Cardiovasc Interv.* 2014;7:1254–1262.

Arnold SV, Reynolds MR, Lei Y, et al. Predictors of poor outcomes after transcatheter aortic valve replacement: results from the PARTNER (Placement of Aortic Transcatheter Valve) trial. *Circulation.* 2014;129:2682–2690.

Costopoulos C, Latib A, Maisano F, et al. Comparison of results of transcatheter aortic valve implantation in patients with severely stenotic bicuspid versus tricuspid or nonbicuspid valves. *Am J Cardiol.* 2014;113:1390–1393.

Frohlich GM, Lansky AJ, Webb J, et al. Local versus general anesthesia for transcatheter aortic valve implantation (TAVR)–systematic review and meta-analysis. *BMC Med.* 2014;12:41.

Guarracino F, Baldassarri R, Ferro B, et al. Transesophageal echocardiography during MitraClip(R) procedure. *Anesth Analg.* 2014;118:1188–1196.

Holmes DR Jr, Mack MJ, Kaul S, et al. 2012 ACCF/AATS/SCAI/STS expert consensus document on transcatheter aortic valve replacement: developed in collaboration with the American Heart Association, American Society of Echocardiography, European Association for Cardio-Thoracic Surgery, Heart Failure Society of America, Mended Hearts, Society of Cardiovascular Anesthesiologists, Society of Cardiovascular Computed Tomography, and Society for Cardiovascular Magnetic Resonance. *J Thorac Cardiovasc Surg.* 2012;144:e29–e84.

Jilaihawi H, Chakravarty T, Weiss RE, et al. Meta-analysis of complications in aortic valve replacement: comparison of Medtronic-Corevalve, Edwards-Sapien and surgical aortic valve replacement in 8,536 patients. *Catheter Cardiovasv Interv.* 2012;80:128–138.

Jilaihawi H, Doctor N, Kashif M, et al. Aortic annular sizing for transcatheter aortic valve replacement using cross-sectional 3-dimensional transesophageal echocardiography. *J Am Coll Cardiol.* 2013;61:908–916.

Kaneko T, Davidson MJ. Use of the hybrid operating room in cardiovascular medicine. *Circulation.* 2014;130:910–917.

Klein AA, Skubas NJ, Ender J. Controversies and complications in the perioperative management of transcatheter aortic valve replacement. *Anesth Analg.* 2014;119:784–798.

Miller DC, Blackstone EH, Mack MJ, et al. Transcatheter (TAVR) versus surgical (AVR) aortic valve replacement: occurrence, hazard, risk factors, and consequences of neurologic events in the PARTNER trial. *J Thorac Cardiovasc Surg.* 2012;143:832–843 e13.

Nishimura RA, Otto CM, Bonow RO, et al. 2014 AHA/ACC guideline for the management of patients with valvular heart disease: a report of the American College of Cardiology/American Heart Association Task Force on Practice Guidelines. *J Am Coll Cardiol.* 2014;63:e57–e185.

Patel PA, Ackermann AM, Augoustides JGT, et al. Anesthetic evolution in transcatheter aortic valve replacement: expert perspectives from high-volume academic centers in Europe and the United States. *J Cardiothorac Vasc Anesth.* 2017;31:777–790.

Patel PA, Gutsche JT, Vernick WJ, et al. The functional aortic annulus in the 3D era: focus on transcatheter aortic valve replacement for the perioperative echocardiographer. *J Cardiothorac Vasc Anesth.* 2015;29:240–245.

Piazza N, De Jaegere P, Schultz C, et al. Anatomy of the aortic valvar complex and its implications for transcatheter implantation of the aortic valve. *Circ Cardiovasc Interv.* 2008;1:74–81.

Roy DA, Schaefer U, Guetta V, et al. Transcatheter aortic valve implantation for pure severe native aortic valve regurgitation. *J Am Coll Cardiol.* 2013;61:1577–1584.

Sintek M, Zajarias A. Patient evaluation and selection for transcatheter aortic valve replacement: the heart team approach. *Prog Cardiovasc Dis.* 2014;56:572–582.

Smith CR, Leon MB, Mack MJ, et al. Transcatheter versus surgical aortic-valve replacement in high-risk patients. *N Engl J Med.* 2011;364:2187–2198.

Sürder D, Pedrazzini G, Gaemperli O, et al. Predictors for efficacy of percutaneous mitral valve repair using the MitraClip system: the results of the MitraSwiss registry. *Heart.* 2013;99:1034–1040.

Tang GH, Lansman SL, Cohen M, et al. Transcatheter aortic valve replacement: current developments, ongoing issues, future outlook. *Cardiol Rev.* 2013;21:55–76.

Vahanian A, Alfieri O, Andreotti F, et al. Guidelines on the management of valvular heart disease (version 2012): The Joint Task Force on the Management of Valvular Heart Disease of the European Society of Cardiology (ESC) and the European Association for Cardio-Thoracic Surgery (EACTS). *Eur J Cardiothorac Surg.* 2012;42:S1–S44.

Willson A, Toggweiler S, Webb JG. Transfemoral aortic valve replacement with the SAPIEN XT valve: step-by-step. *Semin Thorac Cardiovasc Surg.* 2011;23:51–54.

550

Chapter 22

Mechanical Assist Devices for Heart Failure

Marc E. Stone, MD • Joseph Hinchey, MD, PhD

Key Points

1. Mechanical circulatory support (MCS) for the failing heart has become a mainstay of the modern management of patients with both acute and chronic heart failure refractory to pharmacologic and other usual interventions.
2. Outcomes with MCS have improved so dramatically that the main focus of this arena has now shifted away from simple survival and toward mitigation of risk and minimization of adverse events.
3. Data taken from experience gained with the first generation of pulsatile devices may no longer be applicable in the current era of nonpulsatile support, but the valuable lessons learned continue to help shape management and clinical decision making.
4. In addition to the traditional indications for MCS (eg, short-term bridge to recovery and long-term bridge to transplantation), MCS is currently employed for a variety of both short- and long-term modern indications.
5. Patient status at the time of implementation of rescue MCS is a key factor determining outcome. Deterioration from delayed implementation is associated with worse outcome.
6. The timing of implantation of a durable left ventricular assist device (LVAD) (eg, as a bridge to transplantation and/or as destination therapy) and perioperative optimization of the patient's nutritional status are key factors determining outcome.
7. Nonpulsatile support devices have supplanted the first generation of pulsatile ventricular assist devices worldwide, and outcomes have improved dramatically with the technology now available.
8. Extracorporeal membrane oxygenation is being incorporated more and more often into modern extracorporeal life support algorithms.
9. The implantable total artificial heart has undergone a resurgence of interest as a bridge to transplantation for patients with biventricular failure and in other scenarios where an LVAD alone would not be ideal.

▨ THE CURRENT ERA OF MECHANICAL CIRCULATORY SUPPORT

Mechanical circulatory support (MCS) for the failing heart has become a mainstay of current management of patients with both acute and chronic heart failure refractory to pharmacologic and other usual interventions. In fact, the successes realized to date have been so significant that the main focus of this arena has now shifted away from simple survival and toward mitigation of risk and minimization of adverse events. Undeniably, continued advances in device technology have made this possible, but when coupled with analyses of the enlarging patient management experience, we now have better understandings regarding optimal patient selection and timing of intervention, the expectation of significant improvement in multiorgan function during ventricular assist device (VAD) support, and the ways in which preexisting and demographic risk factors may result in complications.

Although some of the data taken from the experience with the first generation of pulsatile devices may no longer be applicable in the modern era of nonpulsatile support, the valuable lessons learned help shape management and clinical decision making. All of these factors have now resulted in more widespread acceptance of VADs by physicians and patients as a management strategy, as well as an earlier use of VADs in the course of a patient's cardiac deterioration. As such, in addition to the traditional indications for MCS (eg, short-term bridge to recovery and long-term bridge to transplantation), MCS is currently employed for a variety of both short- and long-term indications, including rescue of patients from acute low cardiac output situations (bridge to immediate survival), prevention of further myocardial damage following an ischemic event, prevention of deterioration in multisystem organ function, as a temporizing measure to buy time for recovery, as a bridge to the next step of management, as a bridge to improved candidacy (for transplantation) and, increasingly, as a final management strategy for end-stage heart failure (destination therapy).

Equally important to the advances in MCS technology has been the formal sharing of outcomes data from centers nationwide through the Interagency Registry for Mechanically Assisted Circulatory Support (INTERMACS), a North American registry database sponsored by the National Heart, Lung, and Blood Institute; the US Food and Drug Administration (FDA); and the Centers for Medicare and Medicaid Services. INTERMACS was established in 2005 for adult patients receiving long-term MCS device therapy to treat advanced heart failure. A similar European-based database called EuroMACS exists in Europe. Additional databases collect pediatric MCS data (PEDIMACS) and data about adult heart failure patients with higher (less sick) INTERMACS levels (discussed later) still being medically managed (MEDAMACS).

INTERMACS collects clinical data about patients implanted with durable MCS devices at 1 week, 1 month, 3 months, 6 months, and every 6 months thereafter. Major outcomes after implant (eg, death, explant, rehospitalization, and adverse events) are updated frequently and also as part of the defined follow-up intervals. Additional end points include patients' level of function and quality of life, and the reported improvements in both of these areas have been compelling. These data have proven invaluable to appropriate risk stratification and patient selection, and as new devices are introduced, documentation of functional outcomes beyond simple survival assist in differentiating the value of MCS devices.

The sixth INTERMACS annual report, released in 2014, summarizes the enrollment and outcomes of more than 12,300 patients implanted with left ventricular assist devices (LVADs) between 2006 and 2013. This latest INTERMACS report reveals the dynamic and expanding landscape of modern MCS:

- Patient accrual now exceeds 2000 VAD implants per year in the United States alone, and the number of implanting centers in the United States has grown to 158.
- At 1 year, overall survival with a durable MCS device now approaches 80%. This is a marked improvement over the 52% 1-year survival rate demonstrated with the pulsatile HeartMate VE in the REMATCH trial reported in 2001 and is a major advance when compared to the medically managed patients in that trial that demonstrated only a 25% 1-year survival rate.

- Overall survival rate at 2 years with a durable MCS device now approaches 70%, 3-year survival rate now approaches 60%, and 4-year survival rate now approaches 50%. Survival rate after destination therapy is now higher than 75% at 1 year and higher than 50% at 3 years.

Survival has improved dramatically in recent years, but this has also been influenced by the earlier implantation in the course of a patient's cardiac deterioration. Classification in this regard is denoted by INTERMACS level, a scale of clinical condition ranging from 1 to 7. An INTERMACS 7 patient is simply in the advanced stages of heart failure, with the clinical condition of the patient worsening as the INTERMACS profile number gets lower. An INTERMACS 4 has symptoms at rest, an INTERMACS 3 is hemodynamically stable but inotrope-dependent, an INTERMACS 2 is clinically deteriorating with signs of end-organ dysfunction despite the use of inotropes, and an INTERMACS 1 is in cardiogenic shock.

Based on the collective outcome data in the INTERMACS registry, guidelines for device implantation have developed. For early elective implantation of a durable LVAD, at numerically higher INTERMACS levels (5–7), the risks of adverse events may outweigh the benefits. Conversely, waiting until the patient is at too low an INTERMACS level (1 or 2) with multisystem organ failure is associated with a low probability of ultimate rescue and poor survival. Consequently, at least in the United States, elective LVAD patients are being implanted with durable LVADs when at an INTERMACS level 3 (and in some cases 4), because this seems to be the best timing to balance the risks and benefits and to achieve the best outcomes.

Until 2009, MCS was used most often as a bridge to transplantation. Since 2010, use of destination therapy has grown exponentially, once the HeartMate II received approval as a destination therapy device. INTERMACS data show that destination therapy is now the most common utilization of MCS in the United States, accounting for 41.6% of all LVAD implants in the time period 2011–2013 (compared with 14.7% in 2006–2007). Bridge to candidacy (for transplantation) is now the second most common indication for VADs. The percentage of patients listed for transplantation at the time of VAD implantation has decreased to 21.7% in 2011–2013, compared to 42.4% in 2006–2007. Bridge to recovery and bridge to next decision with short-term VADs and/or extracorporeal membrane oxygenation (ECMO) currently constitutes only a very small percentage of the usage of this technology, compared with the long-term indications.

MECHANICAL CIRCULATORY SUPPORT: THEORY AND PRACTICE

Cardiogenic shock may be defined as the inability of the heart to deliver sufficient blood flow to meet the metabolic requirements of the body, despite the presence of adequate intravascular volume. Generally, cardiogenic shock entails sustained hypotension (systolic blood pressure [SBP] <90 mm Hg or 30 mm Hg below baseline), low cardiac output with high central filling pressures (eg, cardiac index <2.2 L/min/m^2 with pulmonary capillary wedge pressure (PCWP) >12 mm Hg) and signs of diminished tissue perfusion.

What distinguishes cardiogenic shock from the other forms of shock is the mechanical impairment of pump function. Once a patient develops mechanical pump failure and the intracardiac volumes and pressures begin to rise, the vicious cycles (Fig. 22.1) can result in an imbalance of myocardial oxygen supply and demand, worsening

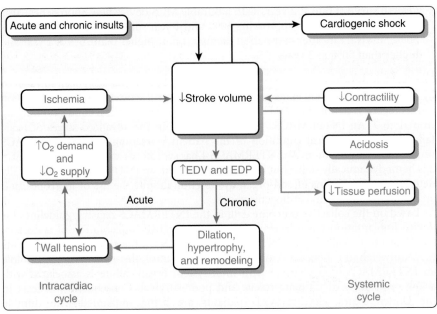

Fig. 22.1 Vicious cycles leading to cardiogenic shock. *EDP,* End-diastolic pressure; *EDV,* end-diastolic volume.

ischemia and resulting in further decreases in ventricular function. Cardiogenic shock may ultimately result if the cycle is not broken.

Manipulations and optimization of preload, afterload, heart rate, and contractility are generally the first-line treatments for acute heart failure. Facilitating recovery requires maintaining adequate myocardial oxygen supply, with the lowest feasible myocardial oxygen demand.

Pharmacologic therapies can potentially improve hemodynamics and stabilize the patient with mild or perhaps moderate cardiac failure. In severe failure, however, pharmacologic management with inotropes and vasopressors comes at the cost of increased myocardial oxygen demand and decreased perfusion to the peripheral and splanchnic circulations during attempts to attain acceptable central hemodynamics. For the myocardium, β-adrenergic stimulation may improve contractility of areas that are well perfused, but it will greatly increase myocardial oxygen demand, feeding into and fueling the vicious cycle.

Vasoconstriction may improve coronary and systemic perfusion pressures but, depending on which vasoconstrictor is used, α-adrenergic stimulation will increase both systemic and pulmonary vascular resistances, making it harder for failing ventricles to eject. This is especially problematic when there is right ventricular (RV) failure, because this will increase the workload of the already struggling right ventricle. Furthermore, intentional vasoconstriction often leaves the peripheral and splanchnic beds underperfused.

Afterload reduction with vasodilators is a common strategy to assist the failing heart because the physiologic principle of ventriculoarterial coupling holds that, regardless of the poor intrinsic systolic mechanics of the failing ventricle, its overall function as a pump can be improved by decreasing the afterload against which it must pump. However, decreased afterload in the setting of developing cardiogenic shock results in hypotension and poor tissue perfusion that predisposes the patient to multisystem organ failure and a poor outcome.

This is where mechanical circulatory assistance can play an important role, effectively breaking the cycle and improving the balance between myocardial supply and demand as well as systemic perfusion. By decompressing the failing ventricle, the increased wall tension that is adversely affecting the supply-to-demand ratio is addressed, which potentially sets the stage for myocardial recovery. Concurrently, effective perfusion is resumed to the heart and the rest of the body, which can stave off multisystem organ failure.

Thus, by using a mechanical device to take over the pumping function of the failing ventricle, the ravages of cardiogenic shock can often be addressed with the one intervention, albeit an extremely invasive one, with potential advantages and disadvantages. Thus, the implementation of mechanical assistance is often approached in a stepwise fashion.

The Role of the Intraaortic Balloon Pump

The first step that specifically targets the problem is implementation of intraaortic balloon pump (IABP) counterpulsation. Despite the fact that it was introduced in 1968, the IABP still remains a very commonly used VAD (especially in the United States) because counterpulsation with a properly timed IABP simultaneously increases myocardial oxygen supply and decreases oxygen demand, and is often an effective treatment for left ventricular (LV) failure.

Fig. 22.2 demonstrates a deployed IABP. The device has been inserted percutaneously into the femoral artery and then advanced retrograde up the aorta to its correct position that is just distal to the left subclavian artery. Balloon inflation during diastole occludes the aorta and displaces arterial blood, abruptly increasing the aortic root pressure. This increases coronary perfusion pressure, which increases myocardial oxygen supply (assuming the patient has an adequate level of saturated hemoglobin). Abrupt deflation just before the next systolic ejection decreases the pressure in the aorta in a sudden fashion, facilitating forward ejection from the heart by decreasing impedance to opening of the aortic valve. This results in increased stroke volume and decreased myocardial work and therefore less oxygen demand on the struggling left ventricle. It has been reported that a properly timed, optimally functioning balloon pump can increase cardiac output by 20% or perhaps 30% and decrease afterload by as much as 15%. Of the two, it is generally believed that it is the decrease in oxygen demand that most benefits the failing ventricle supported by this device. In the setting of acute myocardial stunning (eg, as a result of an acute myocardial infarction [AMI]), such a decrease in oxygen demand can help to set the stage for myocardial recovery. In the setting of an acute deterioration of a chronically failing ventricle, the IABP may be used to stabilize hemodynamics as a bridge to intervention. Additional reported benefits of IABP counterpulsation include reduction in systemic acidosis and improvements in cerebral and renal microcirculatory perfusion. However, although a balloon pump is well known to improve cardiac function and overall hemodynamics, as mentioned earlier, it augments forward cardiac output by only 25% to 30% at maximum, and it will not augment anything if there is a complete absence of LV output. As a sole intervention, the IABP cannot be expected to rescue a patient from catastrophic myocardial failure.

Appropriate timing of balloon inflation and deflation is key to realizing the hemodynamic benefits of the device. The usual trigger for balloon inflation is the R wave of the patient's electrocardiogram (ECG); however, an arterial pressure tracing

22

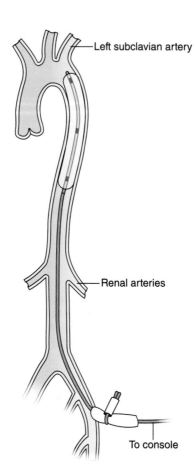

Left subclavian artery

Renal arteries

To console

Fig. 22.2 The intraaortic balloon pump.

and pacing spikes can also be used. Regardless of the trigger used, as illustrated in Fig. 22.3, inflation should always coincide with the dicrotic notch of the arterial tracing and should continue throughout diastole. Deflation should always occur just at end-diastole, immediately before the next systolic ejection. Inflation and deflation at any other point in the cardiac cycle must be manually corrected by adjustments in balloon timing. Fig. 22.4 shows and discusses potential timing errors. Helium is used as the inflation gas in the IABP because of its low viscosity and inert nature. Depending on the level of assistance required, the balloon can be triggered with each cardiac cycle (so-called 1:1 assistance), every other cycle (1:2), every third cycle (1:3), and so forth. Ratios of 1:2 or 1:3 are ideal for optimizing the timing of inflation and deflation.

Contraindications to the use of the IABP include clinically significant aortic insufficiency, aortic aneurysms, and significant friable atherosclerotic plaques in the aorta. However, the widespread availability of echocardiography to assess patients with cardiac problems, as well as the nearly routine use of transesophageal echocardiography (TEE) during IABP placement in the operative setting, can detect significant atherosclerotic disease in the arch and descending aorta and may help identify patients at

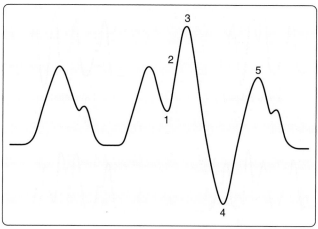

Fig. 22.3 A well-timed intraaortic balloon pump (IABP) inflation. The figure demonstrates an arterial pressure tracing taken from a patient with an IABP. The first pulse seen on the left is the familiar waveform of an arterial pulse. An IABP is triggered to inflate during the second pulse, generating a typical sinusoidal balloon inflation-deflation waveform. The third pulse represents an assisted ejection due to the action of the IABP. Characteristics of the typical balloon waveform include the following. *1,* The balloon inflation point coinciding with the location of the patient's dicrotic notch (representing aortic valve closure at the end of systole). *2,* A steep slope of increasing pressure indicating rapid balloon inflation. This creates a rapid rise in aortic root pressure to reach point 3. *3,* The assisted diastolic peak pressure perfusing the coronary arteries while the IABP is inflated. This increase in coronary perfusion pressure creates the increased myocardial oxygen supply associated with IABP action. *4,* A steep slope of pressure decline indicates a rapid balloon deflation, resulting in a decrease in end-diastolic aortic root pressure. This localized decreased afterload decreases impedance to opening of the aortic valve at the beginning of systole, and creates the decreased myocardial oxygen demand associated with IABP action. *5,* The assisted systolic peak pressure of the next beat perfusing the body. The systolic pressure attained by this ejection was accomplished with less myocardial work thanks to the IABP. Depending on the level of assistance required, the balloon can be triggered with each cardiac cycle (so-called 1:1 assistance), every other cycle (1:2), every third cycle (1:3), and so forth.

high risk. While an ascending aortic dissection still contraindicates IABP use, a descending aortic dissection may no longer constitute an absolute contraindication to IABP use, because, in this era of echocardiography, TEE can be used to ensure the device comes to rest in the true lumen of the aorta.

Indications for the IABP have not changed, but routine IABP usage has recently become somewhat controversial, especially in Europe. It is estimated that 5% to 10% of patients will develop cardiogenic shock following an AMI, and early survival rates for these patients have always been reportedly of the order of 5% to 21%. However, 75% of such patients who were unresponsive to pharmacologic interventions were well known to exhibit hemodynamic improvement with IABP therapy alone, and early survival rates in these patients were reported to approach 93% when treated with IABP counterpulsation. Although decades of nonrandomized studies and clinical observational trials reported such benefit of IABP use, until recently, limited data were available from randomized trials regarding the outcomes of patients with AMI cardiogenic shock in whom IABP counterpulsation was employed.

In the era of thrombolysis as a primary management of AMI, the IABP enjoyed a class I recommendation in international guidelines. However, in current international guidelines (Box 22.1), in the era of percutaneous coronary interventions (PCIs), the

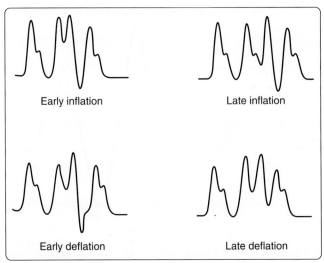

Fig. 22.4 Intraaortic balloon pump (IABP) timing errors. *Early inflation,* before the dicrotic notch (ie, before systolic ejection is completed) immediately forces the aortic valve closed, resulting in prematurely terminated systolic ejection. This results in decreased stroke volume for that cardiac cycle and increased preload for the next cardiac cycle. Not only does this reduce an already impaired cardiac output, but acutely increased end-diastolic volumes stress the failing ventricle by increasing wall tension, which can increase myocardial oxygen demand, impair perfusion, and lead to ischemia. Thus early inflation must be corrected because it increases myocardial oxygen demand and decreases myocardial oxygen supply. *Late inflation,* after the dicrotic notch, fails to augment coronary perfusion pressure optimally. Thus myocardial oxygen supply is not maximally enhanced. *Early deflation* allows time for aortic root pressure to return to baseline before systolic ejection and therefore fails to decrease impedance to opening the aortic valve. Thus myocardial oxygen demand is not decreased. Recall that it is the decrease in myocardial oxygen demand that most benefits the failing ventricle and allows for increased stroke volume with less myocardial work. *Late deflation* can be identified by a failure of the pressure to fall back to baseline or, ideally, below baseline, before the next systolic ejection. Late deflation impedes systolic ejection like an aortic cross clamp. The ventricle is forced to develop such a high pressure to open the aortic valve that ventricular wall tension is significantly increased, which increases myocardial oxygen demand, impairs perfusion, and can lead to ischemia.

IV

recommendation for routine IABP use in the setting of AMI cardiogenic shock has now been downgraded from class I to class IIa in the 2013 American Heart Association (AHA) guidelines and to a class IIb recommendation in European guidelines, on the basis of registry data and a small number of retrospective meta-analyses and randomized trials that failed to demonstrate a mortality benefit from use of the device. However, a number of serious concerns and criticisms (eg, regarding patient selection and timing of intervention) have been raised about the methodologies and protocols used in these trials (and thus in trials analyzed in the meta-analyses), and their negative conclusions have been questioned at the international level because several modern-era trials and analyses have demonstrated outcome benefits from IABP use in the AMI cardiogenic shock population.

A summary of available published data at the time of this writing regarding the routine use of the IABP to treat patients with AMI cardiogenic shock is as follows:

1. There are no strong data to support the routine use of the IABP in the management of AMI with or without cardiogenic shock, certainly when the device is deployed after PCI.

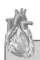

BOX 22.1 *2013 ACCF/AHA STEMI Guidelines for the Use of IABP and VADs*

Class I

1. Emergency revascularization with either PCI or CABG is recommended in suitable patients with cardiogenic shock due to pump failure after STEMI irrespective of the time delay from MI onset. (Level of evidence: B)
2. In the absence of contraindications, fibrinolytic therapy should be administered to patients with STEMI and cardiogenic shock who are unsuitable candidates for either PCI or CABG. (Level of evidence: B)

Class IIa

1. The use of IABP counterpulsation can be useful for patients with cardiogenic shock after STEMI who do not quickly stabilize with pharmacologic therapy. (Level of evidence: B)

Class IIb

1. Alternative LVADs for circulatory support may be considered in patients with refractory cardiogenic shock. (Level of evidence: C)

ACCF, American College of Cardiology Foundation; *AHA,* American Heart Association; *CABG,* coronary artery bypass graft; *IABP,* intraaortic balloon pump; *LVADs,* left-ventricular assist devices; *MI,* myocardial infarction; *PCI,* percutaneous coronary intervention; *STEMI,* ST-segment elevation myocardial infarction; *VAD,* ventricular assist device.
From O'Gara PT, Kushner FG, Ascheim DD, et al. 2013 ACCF/AHA guideline for the management of ST-elevation myocardial infarction: executive summary: a report of the American College of Cardiology Foundation/American Heart Association Task Force on Practice Guidelines: developed in collaboration with the American College of Emergency Physicians and Society for Cardiovascular Angiography and Interventions. *Catheter Cardiovasc Interv.* 2013;82(1):E1–E27.

2. Conversely, no strong data support the avoidance of the use of an IABP in a timely manner in appropriately selected patients who might benefit from the hemodynamic optimization it can provide. Overall, minimal harm has been demonstrated from its use, specifically regarding the incidence of stroke, bleeding, peripheral ischemic complications, and sepsis.
3. There are data suggesting that the routine inclusion of an IABP before high-risk PCI decreases the number of procedural complications and the need for rescue.
4. There are data suggesting that long-term mortality is improved by timely inclusion of an IABP when placed before PCI to ameliorate myocardial ischemia, decompress the ischemic left ventricle, and assist forward flow.

Clearly, the IABP remains useful for stabilizing and improving the hemodynamics of selected patients with low cardiac output. It cannot, however, substantially augment forward cardiac output in patients with severe LV failure. This is where more formal MCS comes into play. Despite the absence of strong data and only a class IIb recommendation in current American College of Cardiology (ACC)/AHA guidelines regarding MCS for acute situations (see Box 22.1), the immediate survival of acute cardiogenic shock of any origin will be minimal if nothing is done and is disappointingly low (<20%) if medical management alone is instituted.

22

Implementation of Mechanical Circulatory Support

When the patient with a failing ventricle has failed to improve substantially following all the usual attempts to optimize and maximize, including an IABP, signs that the patient likely needs formal MCS include the following:

- Hypotension (mean arterial pressure [MAP] <60 mm Hg or SBP <90 mm Hg)
- Cardiac index <2 liters per minute [LPM]/m²
- PCWP or right atrial pressure (RAP) >20 mm Hg
- Systemic vascular resistance (SVR) >2000 dyne-sec/cm
- Oliguria, low mixed venous oxygen saturation, and rising lactate.

It cannot be overemphasized that fixing numbers will not inevitably improve outcome. Even if somewhat acceptable central hemodynamics can be created pharmacologically, it is very important to consider evidence of poor organ and peripheral perfusion, such as oliguria, low mixed venous oxygen saturation, and rising serum lactate as indications of the need to support the circulation in a more formal way.

Moreover, it is critically important that the failure of the usual maneuvers to adequately stabilize the patient be promptly recognized, because experience of the past few decades has shown that the timing of implementation of MCS is the most important factor in patient outcome.

One cannot wait to initiate support until there is profound cardiogenic shock with deterioration in major organ function. Some recovery may be possible with restoration of adequate perfusion, but it is very difficult to predict, and study after study has shown that patient status at the time of implantation is the primary determinant of outcome. *The longer one waits, the worse the outcome.*

To provide formal MCS, the heart and great vessels must be cannulated and connected to a pump. Fig. 22.5 shows the classic cannulation strategies in the heart and

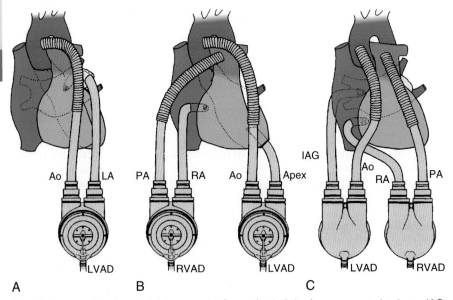

Fig. 22.5 (A–C) Classic cannulation strategies for mechanical circulatory support. *Ao,* Aorta; *IAG,* interatrial groove; *LA,* left atrium; *LVAD,* left ventricular assist device; *PA,* pulmonary artery; *RA,* right atrium; *RVAD,* right ventricular assist device.

great vessels that, until recently, were the only options, regardless of which manufacturer's device was selected to provide the support.

While diversion of blood to the pump provides the stroke volume that is ejected, it also facilitates decompression of the failing ventricle, which is critical, because decreased ventricular wall tension dramatically reduces myocardial oxygen demand, interrupting the cycle of worsening ventricular failure. It should also be noted that currently available VADs do not provide any oxygenation or removal of waste from the blood but simply act as pumps that can promote perfusion of the arterial circulation downstream from the failing ventricle. It is possible with some devices, however, to introduce an in-line membrane oxygenator and extracorporeal carbon dioxide (CO_2) removal system for patients with concomitant respiratory failure.

Once the decision to provide MCS has been made, an appropriate device is selected. A number of different devices may be available, and the device selected for a given patient depends primarily on the following factors:

1. The anticipated duration of support required (different devices have different intended durations of use rooted in their engineering, and there are also considerations of FDA approval of the various devices).
2. Whether univentricular or biventricular support is required (some devices are intended to support just the left ventricle, although some can be configured to support either, or both simultaneously).
3. The degree of pulmonary dysfunction such that ECMO is required.
4. The urgency of the situation (some devices can be deployed rapidly, perhaps even at the bedside, whereas others require transfer to the operating room for sternotomy and cardiopulmonary bypass [CPB]).
5. The availability of the device.

As patient management experience in the field has grown and the outcomes have improved with more advanced devices, there has been an interesting shift away from the question, who needs a VAD? to the more pertinent question, who probably should not receive one? The only absolute contraindications to even temporary VAD use are prognostic factors that would preclude survival even with the restoration of perfusion to the vital organs and peripheral tissues. Thus, the potential for recovery is the paramount consideration. On many occasions, however, the myocardial insult is at least initially the primary problem, and more relative contraindications to VAD support will need to be considered.

Box 22.2 lists a number of commonly encountered considerations and relative contraindications to VAD support that include a variety of anatomic issues and other patient factors that create management issues, make VAD placement or use difficult, make complications more likely, or make meaningful recovery unlikely. Although the advent of modern devices and management strategies has rendered some of these relative contraindications essentially moot, all must be considered and addressed.

SHORT-TERM SUPPORT

INTERMACS data reveal that short-term MCS support constitutes a relative minority of the usage of this technology, but the use of a VAD as a bridge to recovery remains critical to the survival of patients with acute, refractory, severe cardiac failure. However, the traditional conception of short-term use of a VAD only as a bridge to recovery has now been expanded to include concepts such as a bridge to immediate survival,

BOX 22.2 *Conditions or Comorbidities That Make Ventricular Assist Device Placement or Use Difficult, Make the Patient More Likely to Have Major Complications, or Make Meaningful Recovery Unlikely*

Absolute Contraindication

- The patient will not survive regardless of the restoration of adequate systemic perfusion

Relative Contraindications or Issues That Need to Be Addressed

- Patient is not a transplant candidate (unless destination therapy or bridging to improved candidacy is the intention and a durable LVAD is being implanted)
- In situ prosthetic valves
- Clinically significant aortic insufficiency
- Clinically significant tricuspid insufficiency
- Mitral or tricuspid stenosis
- Congenital heart disease
- Intracardiac shunts
- Previous cardiac surgery
- Poor nutritional status
- Extremes of body surface area
- Advanced systemic disease (severe COPD, malignancy, ESLD, ESRD, sepsis, progressive neurologic disorder, etc.)

COPD, Chronic obstructive pulmonary disease; *ESLD,* end-stage liver disease; *ESRD,* end-stage renal disease; *LVAD,* left ventricular assist device.

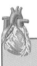

BOX 22.3 *Common Clinical Scenarios in Which Short-Term Mechanical Circulatory Support May Be Indicated*

Stunned myocardium following open heart surgery
Acute myocardial infarction
Following a failed heart transplantation
Cardiogenic shock due to acute myocarditis
Stress-induced cardiomyopathy
Following a cardiac catheterization lab misadventure
In the setting of right ventricular failure in the patient already supported by left ventricular assist device

bridge to next decision, bridge to a bridge, and bridge to surgery (sometimes at another center). It is common for MCS to be implemented to allow for patient transport to a transplant center.

Thus, as listed in Box 22.3, common scenarios in which temporary VAD insertion may be indicated include ventricular failure due to stunned myocardium following open heart surgery, AMI, following a failed heart transplantation, cardiogenic shock due to acute myocarditis, stress-induced cardiomyopathy, following a cardiac catheterization laboratory complication, and in the setting of RV failure in the patient already supported by an LVAD.

Available Devices for Short-Term Support

Before 1992, when the Abiomed BVS 5000 became clinically available, standard centrifugal pumps were used to provide either univentricular or biventricular short-term mechanical circulatory assistance. Currently, this type of very basic device would be used for pediatric applications (with small-caliber cannulas to limit flow) or for ECMO; clinicians are beginning to incorporate ECMO more frequently into resuscitative efforts as a bridge to next decision. Such a strategy has been termed *extracorporeal life support*, in which a patient with refractory cardiogenic shock with uncertain outcome is placed on ECMO for a few days. In this fashion, a less expensive centrifugal device is used to determine if there is reasonable likelihood of survival, before committing the patient to a more formal (and much more expensive) VAD. As experience grows, ECMO utilization is likely to increase in these circumstances, concurrent with the availability of more advanced devices that are replacing standard centrifugal pump head technology.

CentriMag

The CentriMag (Thoratec Corporation, Pleasanton, CA; Fig. 22.6) is a small centrifugal pump with a magnetically levitated impeller that is now being used widely in the United States, in Europe, and in other parts of the world to provide short-term support for almost any modern indication. As with other short-term devices, the pump head itself remains paracorporeal during support, connected to cannulas in the heart and great vessels, so it can be used for left-sided, right-sided, or biventricular support.

Earlier short-term support devices were usually pulsatile and made of polyurethane and other suboptimal materials; they included artificial valves and had a high rate of thrombosis. In contrast, the CentriMag produces nonpulsatile continuous flow, and its design has demonstrable advantages. The impeller of the CentriMag is magnetically levitated and hydrodynamically suspended in the patient's blood; there is no central bearing and, without a bearing, less heat is produced. As a result, there is less hemolysis and therefore less inflammatory response, less peripheral vasoconstriction, and less microvascular occlusion related to plasma free hemoglobin. There may also be a lower incidence of thromboembolic events, and the derangement of liver function tests generally seen after a few days with a standard centrifugal pump head are reportedly not seen to nearly the same extent with the CentriMag.

Despite its small size, the pump itself can provide flow rates of up to 9.9 LPM and can pump through a membrane oxygenator if ECMO is desired. This versatility coupled with its superior performance profile has made the CentriMag the device of choice for short-term support in many experienced institutions.

At the time of this writing, the CentriMag is FDA cleared for 30 days as a right ventricular assist device (RVAD), but only for 6 hours as an LVAD. It should be understood, however, that the off-label use of the CentriMag as an LVAD for periods longer than 6 hours is common. A smaller version called the PediVAS is approved for 6 hours of use as either an LVAD or an RVAD. Recent publications of experiences using the CentriMag for biventricular support as a bridge to next decision report 30-day survival in the range of 44% to 73%.

Bridge to Immediate Survival: Concepts and Devices

A key determinant of the overall success of bridge to recovery is the rapidity with which the failing ventricle can be decompressed and resumption of adequate systemic perfusion

22

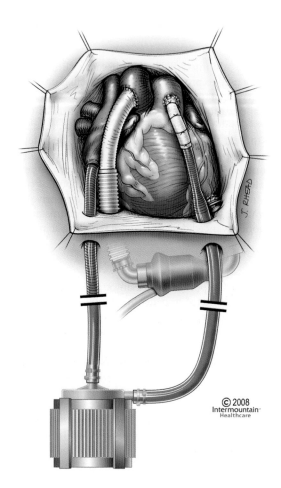

Fig. 22.6 The Thoratec CentriMag. (*Courtesy of Thoratec Corporation, Pleasanton, CA*)

IV

ensured. One of the recognized limitations of currently available devices as a bridge to recovery following an acute myocardial insult is that they must be implanted in a cardiac operating room, often utilizing CPB. Even assuming the immediate availability of the operating room, the device, and the necessary surgical, anesthesia, perfusion, and nursing personnel, delays are inevitable. Poor patient selection aside, it is conceivable that a factor contributing to the low rates of successful bridge to recovery seen in the past was delay in treatment due to operating room and personnel availability. During this interval, the failing ventricle was invariably pressure- and volume-overloaded, while the splanchnic beds and peripheral tissues were underperfused.

Deploying a rescue device rapidly at the first recognition of refractory ventricular insufficiency (whether acute, or acute on chronic) in the emergency room, the cardiac catheterization laboratory, or an intensive care unit without the need for sternotomy and CPB is theoretically a superior option. Additionally, commonly encountered complications of CPB, such as perioperative bleeding, and the sequelae of the systemic inflammatory response would be minimized. Once immediate survival is ensured, such a strategy/device can conceivably be switched to another that is capable of providing a longer period of support. Considerations such as these led to the development of innovative short-term assist devices and continue to drive the use of time-honored strategies in new ways.

Extracorporeal Membrane Oxygenation

ECMO can be rapidly deployed in experienced centers as a lifesaving intervention to provide temporary cardiopulmonary support as a bridge to immediate survival, a bridge to recovery, and/or as a bridge to support by a longer term support device. Developed from CPB technology in the 1970s, a simple ECMO circuit generally uses only a centrifugal pump head, a membrane oxygenator, and a heat exchanger. Survival to hospital discharge has always been the best for full-term neonatal patients with respiratory failure, but experience suggests that appropriately selected adults can also benefit. Clearly, similar considerations govern patient selection for ECMO as for acute implementation of MCS in general, with a high likelihood of recovery being the key consideration prior to initiating the therapy. Patients with poor clinical prognosis beyond their respiratory or cardio-pulmonary failure, those with multisystem organ failure, and those who have already been intubated and mechanically ventilated for several days at the time of proposed intervention are not likely to demonstrate optimal outcomes from ECMO.

Where respiratory failure is the principal issue and the heart is able to provide adequate output to potentially meet circulatory needs, venovenous (VV) ECMO can provide the necessary oxygenation and ventilation of the blood. In this strategy, venous blood is drained from a caval cannula (introduced through either the femoral or the jugular route), pumped through a membrane oxygenator, and returned to the venous circulation (usually at the level of the right atrium).

Patients with both respiratory and cardiac pump failure are best supported by venoarterial (VA) ECMO, in which venous blood is oxygenated, ventilated, and pumped back into the arterial circulation. Such a strategy is essentially providing CPB. Although cannulations for VA ECMO can be peripheral (eg, femoral vein to femoral artery) or central (eg, right atrium to aorta), central venous cannulation generally provides optimal decompression of the cardiac chambers, which is important for myocardial recovery.

Thus, both VV and VA ECMO provide respiratory support, but only VA ECMO provides MCS. Potential complications of ECMO include all of those inherent to extracorporeal circulation, including bleeding (due to the requisite anticoagulation during support) and limb ischemia distal to peripherally inserted cannulas.

Echocardiography plays an important role in determining the type of ECMO needed (VV vs VA) to ensure proper positioning of cannulas, to assess the extent of ventricular decompression, to monitor potential myocardial recovery, and to aid in subsequent decision making.

Current AHA guidelines for cardiopulmonary resuscitation give ECMO a class IIb recommendation (may be considered, benefit may outweigh risk) for clinical scenarios where recovery is possible. A position article, published in 2011 by the European Extracorporeal Life Support (ECLS) Working Group, outlines the indications, contraindications, and various aspects of patient management regarding ECMO.

Impella and TandemHeart

The Impella (Abiomed, Danvers, MA; Fig. 22.7) and the TandemHeart (CardiacAssist, Pittsburgh, PA; Fig. 22.8) percutaneous VADs (pVADs) represent potential bridge-to-immediate-survival devices. Both are designed to support the failing left ventricle, and both are rapidly deployable percutaneously at the time of diagnosis of acute ventricular insufficiency in the emergency room, cardiac catheterization laboratory,

22

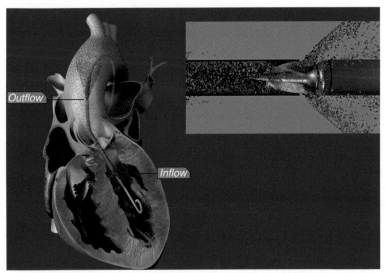

Fig. 22.7 The Impella support device. (*Courtesy of Abiomed Inc., Danvers, MA*)

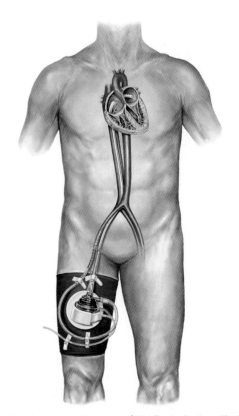

Fig. 22.8 TandemHeart. (*Courtesy of CardiacAssist Inc., Pittsburgh, PA*)

or intensive care unit. There is no need for sternotomy and CPB, which has clear potential advantages (as discussed earlier).

Despite the enormous potential of these devices when employed early as a lifesaving intervention, the most frequent use of both devices has been in the catheterization and electrophysiology labs as an extra margin of safety for high-risk patients undergoing high-risk percutaneous interventions and hemodynamically challenging electrophysiologic interventions (eg, ablation of ventricular tachycardia or fibrillation pathways); the least frequent use has been as a bridge to immediate survival or recovery.

Unfortunately, similar to the initial experience with VADs themselves, when such devices first became available, they were implemented for rescue only as a last resort, once patients had already developed profound cardiogenic shock and organ dysfunction refractory to pharmacology and IABP counterpulsation. Not surprisingly, this led initially to suboptimal results. Outcomes, however, are reportedly improving, and such devices may ultimately demonstrate benefit over ECMO or long-term VADs in the setting of isolated LV or RV failure without pulmonary dysfunction, major valvular abnormality, or biventricular failure. Accordingly, clinical experiences with these devices for acute rescue now appear in the peer-reviewed, published literature. There seems to be an advantage of these devices over the IABP in terms of the level of support provided and the output they can generate, but with a higher risk of bleeding, and the clinical situations in which they might be optimally employed are still being elucidated.

IMPELLA

The Impella pump system is a family of microaxial continuous flow support devices that can be used to support the left, right, or both ventricles. Clinical trials intended to establish the efficacy and optimal utilization of each Impella device are ongoing.

Percutaneously deployable members of the Impella family include the LP 2.5 (provides 2.5 LPM of flow as an LVAD), the LP 5.0 (provides 5 LPM of flow as an LVAD) and the recently approved RP (provides 4 LPM of flow as an RVAD). Other members of the Impella family include directly implantable versions for both left and right ventricular support (LD and RD). All of these devices are FDA-cleared, and theoretically all hold the international class IIb recommendation for VAD use in the AMI cardiogenic shock population.

As illustrated in Fig. 22.7, the percutaneous Impella LVAD devices can be inserted from the femoral or subclavian arterial approach retrograde across the aortic valve into the left ventricle to pump blood into the ascending aorta, actively unloading the left ventricle. Relative contraindications to this approach include significant aortic valvular disease or significant atherosclerotic burden in the aorta (eg, mobile plaques or vascular stenosis). The Impella RP is inserted via the femoral vein through the right atrium and into the pulmonary artery, unloading the failing right ventricle and ensuring pulmonary blood flow as an RVAD.

Although reasonably easy to deploy with fluoroscopy or TEE guidance, the majority of use of the LP 2.5 has been in the cardiac catheterization lab or electrophysiology lab as an extra margin of safety for high-risk patients undergoing PCIs and arrhythmia ablations. This is because 2.5 LPM of flow is generally insufficient to rescue by accommodating the circulatory needs of a full grown adult with cardiogenic shock. Since the mid-1990s, it has been understood that patient status at the time of implementation of MCS is the primary determinant of outcome. Early and sufficient MCS leads to the best possible outcomes. Cardiologists and emergency physicians are the providers who must make the decision to employ MCS when patients present with acute symptoms, typically in the emergency department setting. Cause of the cardiogenic shock and appropriate patient selection are critical factors as well. The outcome of a young person with acute

22

myocarditis cannot be compared to an older person with coronary artery disease, long-standing heart failure, and varying levels of multisystem deterioration. Furthermore, it is also important to consider that simply preventing imminent death is not the same thing as prolonging a high quality of life. Goals of care are important to these decisions.

By comparison to the LP 2.5, the Impella 5.0 can produce a physiologically relevant amount of forward flow, and there is a rapidly growing experience with the use of that device as a bridge to immediate survival, a bridge to recovery, and a bridge to surgery. In contrast to the experience with the LP 2.5 in the setting of AMI cardiogenic shock, a 2013 publication reported the results of a multicenter assessment of the Impella 5.0 as a rescue device for postcardiotomy LV failure. Survival rates were very encouraging, with 30-day, 3-month, and 1-year survival rates of 94%, 81%, and 75%, respectively. It is important to consider that in MCS for postcardiotomy, LV failure is associated with superior outcomes when compared with MCS for AMI cardiogenic shock. This is likely related to shorter intervals separating diagnosis and active management. A recent publication also reported the utility of the Impella 5.0 as a bridge to improved candidacy for transplantation with a durable long-term LVAD.

THE TANDEMHEART

The TandemHeart pVAD (CardiacAssist, Pittsburgh, PA) uses a full-sized centrifugal pump and a percutaneous cannulation strategy that results in reasonable decompression of the failing left ventricle and rapid resumption of systemic perfusion. As illustrated in Fig. 22.8, with this device, a long percutaneous venous inflow cannula is advanced retrograde from the femoral vein through the right atrium and across the interatrial septum into the left atrium. Up to 5 LPM of continuous, nonpulsatile outflow from the centrifugal device (strapped to the patient's leg) is directed into the femoral artery to maintain systemic perfusion.

The TandemHeart holds a CE mark in Europe and is FDA-cleared in the United States for up to 6 hours of use as an LVAD. In current guidelines, the TandemHeart holds a class IIb recommendation for the management of AMI cardiogenic shock. Although this device was envisioned to be a comparatively rapidly deployable bridge to immediate survival device, the need for a transseptal puncture guided by fluoroscopy and/or echcardiography may limit the ease of implantation, and it would be impossible to implement this device during cardiopulmonary resuscitation.

The superiority of the TandemHeart to provide MCS when compared to a balloon pump was reported in a number of studies, but there is a paucity of published data regarding outcomes with the TandemHeart LVAD by itself. The main complications with the TandemHeart appear to be bleeding at the cannulation sites and limb ischemia. Cannula dislodgement is also a potential issue. The TandemHeart is currently the subject of a multicenter pivotal trial called TRIS (TandemHeart to Reduce Infarct Size) looking at myocardial salvage in patients with AMI, and experience with the use of the TandemHeart as an RVAD is growing.

A 2013 study compared outcomes of 79 patients in acute cardiogenic shock supported by the TandemHeart, the Impella 5.0, and conventional VA ECMO. Overall, in-hospital mortality, rates of successful weaning, rates of successful bridging to a bridge with a longer-term device and incidence of limb complications did not differ between the devices. Younger age was the only predictor for improved in-hospital survival, and cost considerations favored ECMO.

Fig. 22.9 depicts a logical decision-making algorithm for MCS in the setting of severe refractory cardiogenic shock, but what works well in one institution may not be generalizable to another. Thus, each institution should ideally develop its own algorithm, taking available devices, resources, and experiences into account.

IV

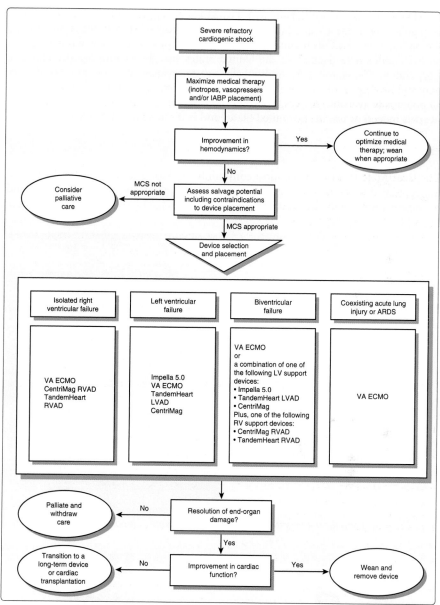

Fig. 22.9 A logical decision-making algorithm for mechanical circulatory support *(MCS)* in the setting of severe refractory cardiac shock. *ARDS,* Acute respiratory distress syndrome; *IABP,* intraaortic balloon pump; *LVAD,* left ventricular assist device; *RVAD,* right ventricular assist device; *VA ECMO,* venoarterial extracorporeal membrane oxygenation.

LONG-TERM SUPPORT

As revealed by the INTERMACS data, long-term, durable devices are being implanted in thousands of people each year who otherwise would succumb to heart failure. A number of long-term VADs are available at the time of this writing, but only the HeartMate II (Thoratec Corporation, Pleasanton, CA; Fig. 22.10) and the HeartWare

HVAD (HeartWare, Framingham, MA; Fig. 22.11) are approved for use and currently in regular use in the United States. Efficacious devices exist in other countries (eg, the Berlin Heart INCOR, Berlin Heart, Berlin, Germany). Several new durable devices are still under investigation in the United States (eg, the HeartMate III, Thoratec Corporation, Pleasanton, CA). Additionally, some previously used or approved devices may still be employed infrequently in specific centers, but a complete discussion of all potentially available devices is beyond the scope of this chapter. The total artificial heart is indeed in use in the United States and is discussed in detail later.

HeartMate II

The HeartMate II is by far the most commonly used long-term LVAD in the United States at the time of this writing. Approved as a bridge to transplantation in 2008 and for destination therapy in 2010, the device is a small axial flow pump, about the size

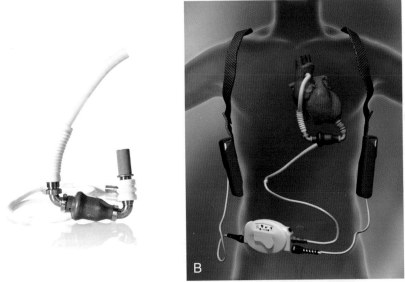

A   B

Fig. 22.10 (A) and (B) The HeartMate II. (*Courtesy of Thoratec Corporation, Pleasanton, CA*)

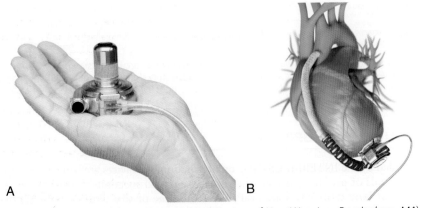

A   B

Fig. 22.11 (A) and (B) HeartWare HVAD. (*Courtesy of HeartWare Inc., Framingham, MA*)

of a D-battery, with a rotating impeller shaped like an Archimedes screw. It has an internal volume of 63 mL and a maximum output of 10 LPM against a mean pressure of 100 mm Hg. This is a continuous flow device that initially results in a mostly nonpulsatile circulation, but pulsatility returns in most patients once the ventricle starts to recover. According to the manufacturer, more than 16,000 patients worldwide have been implanted with the HeartMate II, with the longest duration of support greater than 8 years. Out of all the patients implanted with this device for the purpose of bridge to transplantation, 87% have received a heart transplantation.

Fig. 22.10 shows how the device is configured internally. The only visible external component is a driveline that exits the skin of the abdomen, usually on the right somewhere convenient between the upper and lower quadrants. The device draws blood from the LV apex and pumps the blood continuously into the ascending aorta. This does not prevent the left ventricle from ejecting through the aortic valve, and the amount of support provided by the device depends on several factors, including intrinsic myocardial function, preload, and afterload

HeartWare HVAD

The HeartWare ventricular assist device (HVAD) is a small intrapericardially positioned continuous flow centrifugal pump, with a bearingless, hydrodynamically suspended, magnetically driven impeller. Technically, the HVAD is a third-generation device because it is bearingless. Typical for a centrifugal pump, rotational speeds of 2000 to 3000 rpm can produce upward of 10 LPM of flow. There are the usual external system controller and power supply that are connected to the device by a tunneled driveline. The configuration of the HVAD is depicted in Fig. 22.11.

The HVAD was CE marked for clinical use in Europe in 2009, was approved by the Australian Therapeutic Goods Administration (TGA) in 2011, and received FDA approval as a bridge to transplantation in the United States in November 2012 following its demonstration as noninferior to other implantable devices in the ADVANCE trial. In this trial, 140 patients implanted with the HVAD were followed for 180 days or until transplantation or death, and their outcomes compared with 544 patients implanted with other commercially available devices. Of the 140 in the investigational group, at 180 days, 62% were still supported by their original device, 29% had been transplanted, 5% had required device exchange (2% for pump thrombosis), and 4% had died. Overall the 1-year survival rate was 85%.

The HVAD, because of its small size, has also been used as an implantable RVAD. Experience with the use of the HVAD for RV support (while limited at this time) is steadily increasing. The HVAD is already approved as a device for use in destination therapy in Ontario (since 2012), and it is anticipated that data from the ENDURANCE trial and the ENDURANCE supplemental trial, which began enrolling patients in late 2013, will establish the HVAD as a device for this use in the United States.

A recent analysis of real-world experience with the HeartWare HVAD over 4 years in the UK revealed a 75% survival rate at 1 year and 66% at 2 years. It should be noted, however, that European patients are generally implanted at lower INTERMACS levels (higher acuity) than in the United States, which may account for the lower rate of survival when compared to the ADVANCE trial conducted in the United States.

COMPLICATIONS OF MECHANICAL CIRCULATORY SUPPORT

As outcomes have improved, simple survival of mechanically supported patients has become less of an issue, and the primary focus of MCS research has shifted toward

22

optimizing outcomes through limiting adverse events. Unfortunately, no single risk-stratification method or scoring system has yet been devised to predict the various adverse events inherent to the MCS population. For example, although the preimplant Sequential Organ Failure Assessment (SOFA) score was recently reported to predict survival reliably after 6, 9, 12, 24, and 36 months of support, the SOFA score did not predict other long-term adverse events (eg, stroke, bleeding, infection, need for pump replacement). It is also important to understand that, because of the distinct mechanical underpinnings, materials, and functional specifications of modern devices, all data, predictive indices, and risk-stratification scores generated during the era of first-generation pulsatile devices cannot be extrapolated to the current generation of nonpulsatile devices.

Overall, there has been a major decrease in the rates of specific adverse events with the continuous flow devices compared to the first generation of pulsatile devices, according to INTERMACS and other data sources. Conversely, only minor decreases in the total burden of adverse events have been reported in the current era compared to the previous era. Although the rates of some classic problems have decreased significantly (eg, mediastinal bleeding, RV failure, perhaps stroke), the rates of some important ones (eg, renal failure and respiratory failure) have not changed. Moreover, new complications have appeared that did not exist with the first generation of pulsatile devices, such as arteriovenous malformations in the gastrointestinal tract, von Willebrand syndrome resulting in gastrointestinal and intracerebral bleeding, and pump thrombosis, among others.

New information is rapidly emerging, and certain modern complications of VAD support have now been linked with certain preexisting factors and/or aspects of modern MCS technology.

- Gastrointestinal arteriovenous malformations are now understood to result from the nonpulsatile flow produced by modern MCS devices, much as they are known to form in patients with severe aortic stenosis (Heyde syndrome).
- Acquired von Willebrand syndrome (from the loss of high-molecular-weight von Willebrand monomers) is now understood to result from the shear stresses imposed by the continuous flow devices.
- Pump thrombosis has been seen with surprisingly high frequency with both the HeartMate II and the HVAD. Starting in approximately 2011, the rate of confirmed HeartMate II pump thromboses at 3 months after implantation rose from approximately 2.2% to 8.4% by 2013. This was alarming, because previously the median time from implantation to identification of any significant incidence of pump thrombosis had been 18.6 months. To date, any single reason for this increase remains elusive. In all likelihood, this is a multifactorial problem. In addition to design changes to the HeartMate II introduced in 2010 (a new gelatin sealing of the grafts), as reviewed by Lindenfeld and Keebler, additional potential causes of the increased rate and number of HeartMate II thromboses may have included inadequate anticoagulation and/or antiplatelet therapy during VAD support, overestimation of the actual level of anticoagulation present, the use and dosage of erythropoiesis stimulating agents, abnormal angulation of the inflow and/or outflow cannula, strategically decreased rates of flow, heat production by the bearing, infection, atrial fibrillation, and RV failure. For the HVAD, the addition of titanium sintering to the inflow conduit (which should encourage the ingrowth of a nonthrombogenic neointima, as was present in the first-generation, pulsatile HeartMate I) in 2011 appears to have decreased the incidence of HVAD thrombosis seen during early clinical experience with the device.

Hemolysis and increasing lactate dehydrogenase levels are now recognized as premonitory signs of thrombosis. These can be monitored, and pharmacologic strategies may be employed in many cases as alternatives to device exchange or transplantation.

Additionally, new associations are being established between adverse events and potentially modifiable risk factors. For example, stroke has recently been linked to vitamin D deficiency and also to elevated SBP during support.

■ TOTAL ARTIFICIAL HEARTS

From the original pneumatically driven devices with their massive external control consoles to the totally implantable computer-controlled AbioCor implantable replacement heart (Abiomed, Danvers, MA), a mechanical total artificial heart (TAH) that could permanently replace the failing human heart has been the subject of intensive research and development for decades.

The first TAH was a pneumatically driven biventricular pump developed by Dr. Domingo Liotta and colleagues in the 1960s. This device (the Liotta TAH) was first implanted in a 47-year-old patient with severe heart failure by Dr. Denton Cooley, and was used for 64 hours as a bridge to heart transplantation. The patient died of *Pseudomonas* pneumonia 32 hours after his transplantation, but the Liotta heart proved that a mechanical device could be successfully used clinically to sustain a patient, and, in fact, the original intention of such a device was the permanent replacement of the failing heart. The second human implantation, the Akutsu III TAH, was successfully used for 55 hours as bridge to transplantation in a 36-year-old patient with end-stage heart failure. The Jarvik-7 TAH was first implanted as a permanent replacement heart (destination device) in August 1985 in a 61-year-old man with primary cardiomyopathy and chronic obstructive pulmonary disease. Although the patient survived only 112 days, the duration of his survival was encouraging.

The SynCardia Temporary Total Artificial Heart

From 1991, the Jarvik-7 was known as the CardioWest TAH. Now known as the SynCardia temporary TAH (TAH-t; SynCardia Systems Inc., Tucson, AZ), the current incarnation of this device is in use today as a bridge to transplantation in more than 100 centers in North America, Europe, Asia, and Australia/New Zealand.

The TAH-t is a pneumatically driven, orthotopically placed, biventricular pump weighing less than 0.5 pounds that can produce in excess of 9 LPM of pulsatile flow. Metal tilting-disk prosthetic valves within the device mandate anticoagulation during support. FDA approval of this TAH as a bridge to transplantation came in 2004, and a CE mark was granted for its use in Europe in 2006.

This device has seen a major resurgence of interest in the past few years as an implantable support device for patients with end-stage biventricular failure (instead of biventricular support with paracorporeal VADs), as a bridge to retransplantation in patients experiencing rejection and failure of a transplanted heart (instead of reimplanting an LVAD), and when there is LVAD failure (in lieu of device exchange).

According to the manufacturer, more than 1400 implantations have now been performed, with the longest duration of support at approximately 4 years. The rate of successful bridge to transplantation with this device has been reported at approximately 75% to 80% for over a decade, but it remains to be seen if such success will continue to be manifested as the number of implants grows beyond the confines of

22

clinical trials. As with other devices used to provide MCS, stroke and infection are encountered, but data regarding rates of these complications are not currently available from the INTERMACS database. A recent update publication in the *Texas Heart Institute Journal* reported that "most" (4%) of the strokes associated with the TAH-t occur essentially in the perioperative period, and the rate of fatal infections with this device is approximately 2%. As it produces pulsatile flow, acquired von Willebrand syndrome and bleeding complications from arteriovenous malformations (now commonly observed with continuous flow VADs) may not be seen with the TAH-t.

Originally powered and controlled by a massive control console ("Big Blue"), the availability of a small, wearable controller weighing less than 15 pounds (the Freedom portable driver) now allows for easy ambulation and hospital discharge. An even smaller controller will soon be available, as will a smaller version of the TAH itself (with 50-mL ventricles), for use in small adults and children. Ironically, although it was originally conceived of and used as a destination device, the TAH-t is only now currently the subject of a formal destination therapy trial.

AbioCor Implantable Replacement Heart

The AbioCor implantable replacement heart (Abiomed, Danvers, MA; Fig. 22.12) potentially represents a major advance in artificial heart technology because it is truly totally implantable; there are no percutaneous cables, conduits, or wires. The device is motor-driven, so a source of compressed air to drive the pumping action is not required, allowing patients complete mobility without the need for even a portable or wearable controller. The device itself weighs approximately 2 pounds and is orthotopically implanted.

The AbioCor is indicated for patients not eligible for transplant who are younger than 75 years old and have end-stage, biventricular failure. Transcutaneous energy transfer is used (in lieu of a percutaneous cable) to supply the motor-driven hydraulic

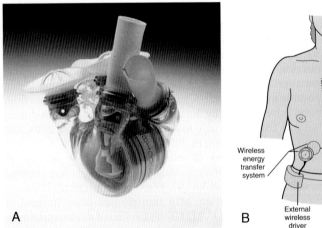

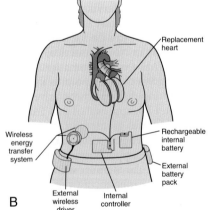

A

B

Fig. 22.12 (A) The AbioCor implantable replacement heart. (B) Orthotopic implantation of the AbioCor implantable replacement heart. The native failed heart is removed, and the AbioCor is implanted orthotopically, anastomosed to cuffs of native atria and the great vessels. Transcutaneous energy transfer technology eliminates the need for percutaneous wires. (*Courtesy of Abiomed, Inc., Danvers, MA*)

pumping of the artificial ventricles with power and system control. Artificial unidirectional valves within the device mandate anticoagulation during support.

A relatively small number (14) of implantations of this device at the University of Louisville and three other centers in the early 2000s demonstrated a moderate amount of success (survival of over 1 year was achieved, but there were high rates of stroke and infection and a few device failures).

The FDA initially denied application for approval of this device in 2005, citing "quality of life vs quantity of life" issues, but the AbioCor eventually received FDA approval in 2006 under the Humanitarian Device Exemption Program, largely as a result of the testimony of patients and families of those supported regarding the ability of the supported patients to be present to "share significant life events" with their families. A very small number of implants apparently followed as part of a postmarket study, but there have been no recent publications about this device, and it is essentially no longer available.

▨ PERIOPERATIVE ANESTHETIC CONSIDERATIONS FOR VAD SUPPORT

The anesthetic approach to the patient requiring VAD implantation depends entirely on the urgency of the situation. Patients requiring emergent VAD support are in extremis and health professionals can do little but provide supportive care until the patient can be placed on CPB. In contrast, patients presenting for elective VAD implantation as a bridge to transplantation or as destination therapy have end-stage heart failure and, when medically optimized, can appear remarkably well despite significantly depressed cardiac function. Some patients presenting for elective LVAD insertion have suffered an acute decompensation of long-standing heart failure and will have been admitted preoperatively to an intensive care unit with pharmacologic therapy (eg, milrinone, nesiritide, dobutamine) and intraaortic balloon counterpulsation therapy in an attempt to stabilize and optimize hemodynamics.

Regardless of their outward appearance, all patients requiring VAD support decompensate easily from even the most transient of hemodynamic aberrations (eg, tachycardia, bradycardia, hypercarbia, loss of sinus rhythm, sudden alterations in volume status, hypotension) and thus must be approached with caution.

Patients Presenting for Elective LVAD Implantation

Severely depressed cardiac function is the key consideration in the management of all patients presenting for LVAD insertion. The majority will have a dilated cardiomyopathy that is accompanied by mitral regurgitation, diastolic dysfunction, a dilated tricuspid annulus with functional tricuspid regurgitation, and varying degrees of pulmonary hypertension. Renal insufficiency, cerebral vascular disease, and mild coagulopathy owing to hepatic congestion are not uncommon. As coronary artery disease has become one of the most common causes of heart failure (31.8% of all patients currently listed for heart transplantation), ongoing ischemia is a potential concern. Many of these patients will have undergone previous cardiac surgery (eg, coronary artery bypass grafting, valve repair/replacement, ventricular reshaping, correction of congenital heart disease), adding the attendant risks of repeat sternotomy to the anesthetic concerns. Finally, it is common for this population to have a pacemaker and/or implantable cardioverter-defibrillator that must be managed perioperatively.

22

Issues Related to Outpatient Medications

Patients presenting for elective LVAD implantation have generally been managed with medications that reduce afterload, promote diuresis, prevent arrhythmias, control heart rate and antagonize the adverse myocardial remodeling that accompanies chronic, progressive heart failure. Typically employed agents include angiotensin-converting enzyme (ACE) inhibitors, angiotensin receptor blockers, aldosterone antagonists, amiodarone, β-blockers, diuretics, and digoxin. While effective for the preoperative optimization of this population, agents with long elimination half-lives, such as ACE inhibitors and amiodarone, result in significant vasodilation that will need to be addressed and countered pharmacologically in the period after bypass. Where feasible, it is generally recommended to withhold diuretics in the immediate preoperative period in an attempt to lessen the relative hypovolemia and electrolyte depletion seen with these commonly used agents. There is currently no consensus about whether or not to withhold ACE inhibitors preoperatively.

Preoperative Nutritional Optimization

It is widely understood that preoperative malnutrition predisposes the general surgical population to an array of postoperative complications, including delayed wound healing and increased risk of infection. Nutritional status has also been established as an important determinant of survival in patients with heart failure, and in patients with a VAD there is growing evidence that nutrition, as measured by traditional surrogates, such as serum albumin and body mass index, is a critical determinant of postimplantation survival. In a study by Lietz and colleagues, poor preoperative nutrition status was identified as one of several predictors of poor postimplantation outcomes as part of a risk-stratification score. More recently, preoperative hypoalbuminemia was reported as an independent risk factor of mortality in a large cohort of patients with nonpulsatile devices. Interestingly, postoperative correction of albumin levels also correlated with a significant survival advantage in this study.

Postoperative indicators of suboptimal nutritional status, such as low prealbumin levels, have also been shown to correlate with increased mortality in this population. Based on these findings, aggressive optimization of nutritional status has become an important component of patient management before and after operations. In patients refractory to conventional approaches to nutritional augmentation, enteral and/or parenteral feeding should be considered. Of note, parenteral nutrition, despite its traditional association with increased risk of infection, has been shown to be a safe and effective alternative to enteral nutrition preoperatively for patients with a VAD and may prove in the future to be a standard component of perioperative nutritional optimization in patients refractory to other methods.

The Immediate Preoperative Period

It is prudent to provide supplemental oxygen (via nasal cannula or face mask) and monitor vital signs during the preoperative period, especially if anxiolytic medications are given. The potential for hypoventilation always exists with sedation, and this population will not generally tolerate sudden decreases in sympathetic tone, hypoxemia, and the potentially increased pulmonary vascular resistance that may accompany a sudden respiratory acidosis. Preinduction insertion of an intraarterial catheter for blood pressure monitoring is of critical importance for patients with severely depressed cardiac function.

Induction and Maintenance

The anesthetic plan must take into account the severe degree of cardiac dysfunction and potential preexisting organ insufficiency. The failing heart is at least partially compensated by a heightened adrenergic state, and anesthetic induction agents that markedly blunt sympathetic tone should be avoided as they may result in rapid cardiovascular decompensation or collapse. Additionally, management goals for patients with heart failure should also include the avoidance of anesthetic agent–induced depression of cardiac function and of hemodynamic conditions that increase myocardial demand, such as tachycardia and increased ventricular afterload. In summary, the induction strategy should aim to strike a balance between adequate depth of anesthesia and maintenance of stable hemodynamics.

Etomidate (0.2 mg/kg IV) is an ideal induction agent for patients with heart failure because it does not cause a significant reduction in SVR nor does it decrease myocardial contractility. An induction technique based on a high-dose opioid (eg, fentanyl 50–100 μg/kg) and a neuromuscular blocking agent will likely result in several hours of hemodynamic stability. The resultant bradycardia with high doses of opioids, however, could result in further decreases in cardiac output. Additionally, amnesia is usually inadequate with narcotics alone, and ventilatory support will be required for several hours after the procedure has ended. Thus, high-dose opioid techniques are less frequently used currently.

Ketamine remains an extremely useful alternative agent in patients with severely decreased ventricular function. A ketamine induction (1–2.5 mg/kg IV or 2.5–5 mg/kg IM) followed by a maintenance infusion (50–100 μg/kg/min) will usually provide excellent hemodynamic stability while ensuring adequate analgesia and amnesia. Before administering ketamine, a small dose of midazolam (eg, 1–2 mg IV) is often given to theoretically lessen the potential postemergence psychomimetic side effects that may occur in some patients, and an antisialagogue (eg, glycopyrrolate 0.2 mg IV) is generally employed, which is ordinarily balanced by its indirect sympathomimetic properties. In the setting of advanced heart failure, where partial compensation is achieved through chronic activation of the adrenergic system and downregulation of myocardial β-adrenergic receptors, there is a theoretical risk of unmasking and seeing primarily the direct depressant effects of ketamine on the heart with doses adequate for induction.

Thus, a standard balanced technique consisting of small doses of midazolam, etomidate as the induction agent, moderate doses of opioid (eg, total fentanyl dose 10–20 μg/kg), a neuromuscular blocking agent, and potent volatile inhaled agents as tolerated is often used in well-optimized patients. As a general rule, however, high doses of all the potent inhaled volatile agents are poorly tolerated in this population because they all interfere with calcium handling and cyclic nucleotide secondary messengers in the myocardium. By comparison with the other currently available agents, sevoflurane appears to cause less myocardial depression and decrease in SVR, although low concentrations of isoflurane are commonly used without difficulty. In addition to direct myocardial depression and vasodilation, the inhaled anesthetic agents may also adversely affect myocardial automaticity, impulse conduction, and refractoriness, potentially resulting in reentry phenomena and dysrhythmias. Dysrhythmias are especially likely when the delivered concentration of an agent is abruptly increased.

As perioperative bleeding is a common problem following VAD implantation, an antifibrinolytic agent (eg, ε-aminocaproic acid or tranexamic acid) is used during these cases.

Monitoring

In addition to standard American Society of Anesthesiologists monitors (eg, ECG, end-tidal CO_2, temperature, pulse oximetry, and blood pressure), an intraarterial catheter, a pulmonary artery catheter, and TEE are routinely employed during LVAD implantation.

Before LVAD implantation, TEE is used to detect anatomic pathologies that will:

- Impede optimal LVAD filling (eg, mitral stenosis, severe tricuspid regurgitation, severe RV dysfunction)
- Decrease the potential for optimal LV decompression (eg, aortic regurgitation) and
- Cause complications once the LVAD is functioning (eg, patent foramen ovale, atrial septal defect, intracardiac thrombus, ascending aortic atherosclerosis, mobile ascending aortic plaques).

During LVAD implantation, TEE is used to:

- Ensure proper inflow cannula position (in the center of the left ventricle, pointing toward the mitral valve; often the midesophageal two-chamber view at a 90-degree angle best reveals the cannula position, but three-dimensional imaging can also be helpful), and
- Ensure adequate de-airing of the device (and the heart) before and after engagement of support.

The Postimplantation Period

Hemodynamics can initially be quite labile once LVAD support is engaged until intravascular volume is restored, vasomotor tone is reestablished in both the systemic circuit and the pulmonary beds, and RV function is optimized. Thus, despite a properly functioning device, inotropic and vasoactive agents are often required to enable separation from CPB. Certain management strategies appear to be more advantageous than others, and an understanding of the physiology of the LVAD-supported state greatly aids in decision making.

POTENTIAL EFFECTS OF LVAD SUPPORT ON RIGHT VENTRICULAR FUNCTION

Data from the era of the pulsatile VADs consistently reported the response of the right ventricle to LV unloading by an LVAD to include an increased RV preload, increased RV compliance, decreased RV afterload, and overall decreased RV contractility. It has also been established that preexisting or perioperative RV disorders (eg, regional ischemia, poorly compensated chronic ventricular failure, inflammatory insults) can predispose the patient to profound deterioration of RV function when LVAD support is engaged.

To understand RV decompensation in the post-LVAD implantation setting, several key physiologic principles must be appreciated; namely, ventricular interdependence,

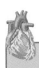

BOX 22.4 *Key Physiologic Principles in Ventricular Assist Devices*

Ventricular interdependence
Series circulatory effects
Ventriculoarterial coupling

series circulatory effects, and ventriculoarterial coupling (Box 22.4). First, the concept of *ventricular interdependence* centers on the continuous nature of the muscle fibers between the free wall of the right ventricle and the left ventricle and the presence of a common interventricular septum (IVS), which results in anatomic and mechanical coupling of the ventricles. Second, the concept of *series circulatory effects* holds that it is the output of the right ventricle that fills the LVAD and that the LVAD output in turn becomes the preload of the right ventricle. Third, the concept of *ventriculoarterial coupling* holds that no matter how impaired the intrinsic systolic mechanics of the ventricle are, the chamber can always function better as a pump if one reduces the afterload against which it must pump. Additionally, one must appreciate the unique anatomic and physiologic properties of the right ventricle as they relate to pump function.

Ejection of blood from the right ventricle is accomplished by two separate simultaneous actions: (1) compression of the chamber caused by contraction of the single layer of transverse fibers that make up the free RV wall, and (2) a twisting caused by sequential contraction of the two layers of obliquely oriented septal fibers.

In the absence of normal septal twisting, RV ejection must be produced only by contraction of the basal wall that contains a single layer of predominantly transverse fibers. This compression may not always provide enough contractile force to ensure adequate cardiac output, especially if pulmonary vascular resistance is increased. It has long been known that normal septal function can compensate for loss of the RV free wall with respect to overall RV systolic performance, but the RV free wall cannot always compensate for loss of septal function, and RV failure appears to be a problem primarily when the septum becomes dysfunctional.

Perhaps the most obvious effect of LV decompression by an LVAD is the potential shift of the IVS to the left, but bowing of the IVS to the left creates what has been called an *architectural septal disadvantage* because the distortion of the normal architecture of the IVS results in the otherwise obliquely oriented septal muscle layers assuming a more transverse orientation with respect to one another, with subsequent loss of normal septal twisting. Numerous investigators have demonstrated the critical contribution of the IVS to RV pump function, and it has long been demonstrated that, as long as septal function is unimpaired, contraction of the RV free wall is of little consequence where overall RV pressure development and volume outflow are concerned.

Another consequence of deforming the septum is dysfunction of the electrical conduction system owing to stretching of the conducting pathways. Intraventricular conduction delays resulting in dyssynchronous contraction of the ventricle lead to a decrease in overall systolic function. Additionally, it is clear that stunning of the IVS is common following prolonged CPB despite the best of myocardial protective efforts, and there can be residual adverse electrophysiologic effects of cardioplegia that can persist through the early period after bypass. One or both of these factors can act to

22

increase the degree of septal dysfunction. Thus, decompression of the left ventricle plays a big role in the baseline predisposition to RV failure, because it causes septal shift leftward, which can result in septal dysfunction, but this is not the only factor predisposing to RV failure during LVAD support.

The LVAD and right ventricle exist in series, as codependent pumps in a circuit. Given that the right ventricle may be mechanically disadvantaged because of septal dysfunction of various causes when LVAD support is engaged, it may not tolerate even modestly increased preload. Potential sources of increased RV preload during LVAD support include high LVAD outputs, requisite perioperative transfusions of blood and blood products, and the potential for increased tricuspid regurgitation if the level of LV decompression results in septal displacement. Potential causes of increased tricuspid regurgitation include: (1) deformation of the tricuspid annulus; and (2) distraction of the subvalvular apparatus attached to the IVS, resulting in failure of apposition of the leaflets.

Despite the predisposition to RV dysfunction based on ventricular interdependence and the potential problems that may come from the series circulatory effects, it appears that the beneficial effect of decreased RV afterload due to LVAD action still tends to outweigh any impairment of intrinsic RV systolic mechanics. An overall improvement in RV pump function is generally seen during LVAD support in patients with normal pulmonary vascular resistance. This illustrates the principle of *ventriculoarterial coupling,* in which a conceptual separation of RV systolic mechanics from overall RV pump function reveals the critical importance of RV afterload.

As discussed in detail earlier, and as might be surmised from the success of Fontan physiology, RV pumping function is probably dispensable in the LVAD-supported patient, so long as the pulmonary vascular resistance is normal. Pulmonary vascular resistance, however, is not always normal after LVAD implantation. In many patients, pulmonary vascular resistance rises owing to pulmonary vascular endothelial injury from inflammatory mediators resulting from prolonged exposure to extracorporeal circulation, as well as from perioperative blood and platelet transfusions. Other causes include the routine ones that are encountered in the care of critically ill patients, such as hypoxemia, hypercarbia, acidosis, hypothermia, large tidal volumes, pain, and catecholamine infusions. Fig. 22.13 demonstrates the potential consequences of increased RV afterload.

Furthermore, the potential roles of perioperative events and management cannot be discounted in the etiology of potential RV failure during LVAD support. Numerous factors potentially influence the outcome of the patient, including the timing of LVAD insertion in the course of the patient's heart failure, surgical misadventures, stunning of the right coronary artery distribution during CPB, and hypotension in the post-CPB period compromising coronary perfusion. While ischemic insults or other injuries to the RV free wall do not appear to have great influence on the development of RV failure when LVAD support is engaged, ischemic insults to the septum will likely have profoundly negative consequences.

The quality of perioperative care is also a major determinant of success in LVAD implantation, and it is imperative that staff caring for patients immediately after LVAD implantation be well versed in the relevant physiology and associated risks. While relative hypovolemia is a common issue in the LVAD-supported patient, large rapid volume loads are a potential problem for a right ventricle that is already mechanically disadvantaged, and fluid management must be approached judiciously. Perhaps the biggest concern is increased pulmonary vascular resistance. As described earlier, once the septum becomes deformed from LV decompression, the transversely oriented fibers can only generate enough pressure to eject into a low resistance pulmonary vascular bed. Thus, between the physiology of the LVAD-supported state and potential

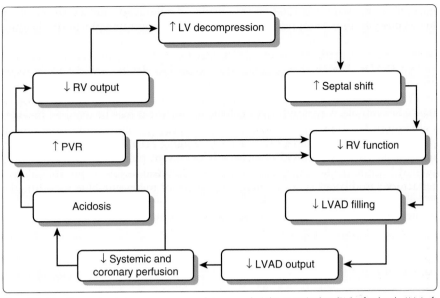

Fig. 22.13 The potential consequences of increased right ventricular *(RV)* afterload. *LV,* Left ventricular; *LVAD,* left ventricular assist device; *PVR,* pulmonary vascular resistance.

perioperative events and requisite postoperative care, there are many reasons why the right ventricle is at increased risk of failure during LVAD support.

Intravascular Volume Status

LVADs are dependent on adequate volume in the LV chamber. Most elective LVAD patients will have started out volume-overloaded and with a massively dilated left ventricle. With the nonpulsatile devices, if the amount of blood removed from the ventricle by continuous VAD action exceeds the amount of blood present in the left ventricle, *suckdown* occurs; that is, the continuous flow VAD sucks the ventricle empty, which results in decreased output and hypotension. Thus, the goal for perioperative fluid management is to maintain a euvolemic, if not slightly hypervolemic, state (which may help minimize vasopressor requirements), assuming the unsupported and potentially dysfunctional right ventricle is able to handle the volume load. An empty left ventricle also shifts the IVS to the left, changing the geometry of the right ventricle, which decreases its function (septal architectural disadvantage discussed earlier), and decreased RV function is another important reason for an inadequate preload to an LVAD. Furthermore, the effect of surgical positioning and/or retractors must be monitored so as not to obstruct venous return to the right ventricle, and high intrathoracic pressures (eg, from excessively large tidal volumes) should be avoided once the chest is closed for the same reason. Overall, LVADs generally function well as long as there is sufficient intravascular volume (and RV function) to fill the pump, but management must be individualized.

Afterload and Contractility

In general, the profound vasodilatation that often follows LVAD implantation requires administration of vasoconstrictors to maintain adequate perfusion pressures. A major goal following LVAD implantation is to maintain pulmonary vascular resistance as low as possible; thus, vasopressin may have advantages over norepinephrine because of vasopressin's lack of pulmonary vasoconstrictive effects. Physicians must be cautious, however, because markedly increased SVR may sometimes impair forward flow from certain LVADs. The current generation of axial flow devices are not likely to be affected, but the output from the new miniaturized centrifugal devices can be sensitive to afterload. Inotropic agents are also typically required to support the function of the right ventricle. A typical pharmacologic regimen that may be required includes milrinone (0.3–0.75 µg/kg per minute), vasopressin (2.5–5 units/h), nitric oxide (20–40 parts per million) and epinephrine (0.05–0.25 µg/kg per minute). As noted earlier, norepinephrine may be disadvantageous if significant pulmonary hypertension is present because of the imperative to keep RV afterload as low as possible. Where refractory vasodilatory shock is manifest, a bolus of methylene blue (0.5–2 mg/kg IV) may be of help in restoring vasomotor tone. In severe cases, a continuous infusion of methylene blue (0.5 mg/kg per hour) may be required.

Bleeding

Anecdotally, and for a number of potential reasons, intraoperative or postoperative bleeding does not seem to be as severe with the modern devices as it once may have been with the large pulsatile devices, but coagulopathy following VAD implantation remains common despite the routine use of antifibrinolytic agents, and the transfusion of platelets, cryoprecipitate, and fresh frozen plasma (FFP) is often necessary to restore hemostatic competence. However, practitioners must be cautious, because rapid infusion of large volumes can precipitate RV failure. Moreover, significant risk of transfusion-associated lung injury (TRALI) exists with the transfusion of platelets and FFP. Where available, thromboelastography can be extremely useful to help guide the judicious transfusion of blood products. Factor concentrates such as prothrombin complex concentrates (PCC) represent a compelling alternative to FFP, both from the perspective of avoiding volume overload and TRALI. When compared to FFP, PCCs have been shown to restore target factors and reverse factor-dependent coagulopathy more rapidly, with negligible additional volume, and lower risk of TRALI.

Another source of coagulopathy uniquely associated with LVAD implantation involves the dysfunction of von Willebrand factor (vWF). Sheer forces generated by some VAD devices promote cleavage of vWF multimers by the metalloprotease ADAMTS13, leading to an acquired vWF deficiency and increased tendency for gastrointestinal bleeding, wound site bleeding, and epistaxis. Recent data from a population of nearly 1000 HeartMate II patients demonstrated an overall 38% incidence and prevalence of bleeding, with gastrointestinal bleeding in 29% of those implanted as destination therapy and 13% of those implanted as bridge to transplantation. Thus, strategies to control bleeding in these patients should ideally include the use of vWF-containing concentrates, factor VIII concentrates, antifibrinolytics, and desmopressin (DDAVP).

The Postimplantation Role of Transesophageal Echocardiography

After LVAD placement, TEE is used to:

- Ensure adequate LV decompression (but not complete obliteration of the LV cavity).
- Ensure RV function does not deteriorate (may need RVAD as well).
- Ensure tricuspid regurgitation does not worsen (may need annuloplasty).

IV

- Reevaluate for patent foramen ovale (must be closed if detected).
- Assist with diagnosis of new patient problems that arise in the postoperative period (eg, hypovolemia, tamponade, cannula misalignment or obstruction).

SUGGESTED READINGS

Aaronson KD, Slaughter MS, Miller LW, et al. Use of an intrapericardial, continuous-flow, centrifugal pump in patients awaiting heart transplantation. *Circulation.* 2012;125(25):3191–3200.

Beckmann A, Benk C, Beyersdorf F, et al. Position article for the use of extracorporeal life support in adult patients. *Eur J Cardiothorac Surg.* 2011;40:676–681.

Chamogeorgakis T, Rafael A, Shafii AE, et al. Which is better: a miniaturized percutaneous ventricular assist device or extracorporeal membrane oxygenation for patients with cardiogenic shock? *ASAIO J.* 2013;59(6):607–611.

Copeland JG, Smith RG, Arabia FA, et al. Cardiac replacement with a total artificial heart as a bridge to transplantation. *N Engl J Med.* 2004;351:859–867.

Geisen U, Heilmann C, Beyersdorf F, et al. Non-surgical bleeding in patients with ventricular assist devices could be explained by acquired von Willebrand disease. *Eur J Cardiothorac Surg.* 2008;33:679–684.

Hanke AA, Joch C, Gorlinger K. Long-term safety and efficacy of a pasteurized nanofiltrated prothrombin complex concentrate (Beriplex P/N): a pharmacovigilance study. *Br J Anaesth.* 2013;110:764–772.

John R, Long JW, Massey HT, et al. Outcomes of a multicenter trial of the Levitronix CentriMag ventricular assist system for short-term circulatory support. *J Thorac Cardiovasc Surg.* 2011;141:932–939.

Kato TS, Kitada S, Yang J, et al. Relation of preoperative serum albumin levels to survival in patients undergoing left ventricular assist device implantation. *Am J Cardiol.* 2013;112(9):1484–1488.

Kirklin JK, Naftel DC, Pagani FD, et al. Sixth INTERMACS annual report: a 10,000-patient database. *J Heart Lung Transplant.* 2014;33(6):555–564.

Landis ZC, Soleimani B, Stephenson ER, et al. Severity of end-organ damage as a predictor of outcomes after implantation of left ventricular assist device. *ASAIO J.* 2015;61(2):127–132.

Lietz K, Long JW, Kfoury AG, et al. Outcomes of left ventricular assist device implantation as destination therapy in the post-REMATCH era: implications for patient selection. *Circulation.* 2007;116:497–505.

Lindenfeld J, Keebler ME. Left ventricular assist device thrombosis: another piece of the puzzle? *JACC Heart Fail.* 2015;3(2):154–158.

O'Gara PT, Kushner FG, Ascheim DD, et al. 2013 ACCF/AHA guideline for the management of ST-elevation myocardial infarction: a report of the American College of Cardiology Foundation/American Heart Association Task Force on Practice Guidelines. *Circulation.* 2013;127(4):e362–e425.

Patel MR, Smalling RW, Thiele H, et al. Intra-aortic balloon counterpulsation and infarct size in patients with acute anterior myocardial infarction without shock. The CRISP AMI randomized trial. *JAMA.* 2011;306(12):1329–1337.

Rose EA, Gelijns AC, Moskowitz AJ, et al. Long-term use of a left ventricular assist device for end-stage heart failure. *N Engl J Med.* 2001;345(20):1435–1443.

Saleh S, Liakopoulos OJ, Buckberg GD. The septal motor of biventricular function. *Eur J Cardiothorac Surg.* 2006;29S:S126–S138.

Sarkar J, Golden PJ, Kajiura LN, et al. Vasopressin decreases pulmonary-to-systemic vascular resistance ratio in a porcine model of severe hemorrhagic shock. *Shock.* 2015;43:475–482.

Stainback RF, Estep JD, Agler DA, et al. Echocardiography in the Management of Patients with Left Ventricular Assist Devices: Recommendations from the American Society of Echocardiography. *J Am Soc Echocardiogr.* 2015;28:853–909, 245.

Starling RC, Moazami N, Silvestry SC, et al. Unexpected abrupt increase in left ventricular assist device thrombosis. *N Engl J Med.* 2014;370(1):33–40.

Stern DR, Kazam J, Edwards P, et al. Increased incidence of gastrointestinal bleeding following implantation of the HeartMate II LVAD. *J Card Surg.* 2010;25:352–356.

Thiele H, Zeymer U, Neumann FJ, et al. Intraaortic balloon support for myocardial infarction with cardiogenic shock. *N Engl J Med.* 2012;367:1287–1296.

22

Chapter 23

Reoperative Cardiac Surgery

Amanda J. Rhee, MD • Joanna Chikwe, MD

Key Points

1. Reoperative cardiac surgery presents greater risk than first-time surgery because patients are usually older, have more comorbidity, and have more advanced cardiovascular disease. Also, resternotomy can be hazardous due to adhesions of cardiac structures to the sternum. Bypass conduits may not be available owing to prior use, and the frequency of valve replacement versus valve repair is higher.
2. A thorough history, clinical evaluation, and review of imaging must be performed—with particular thought to weighing the risk of surgery against the possibility of medical management with multidisciplinary expertise—before making the decision to proceed.
3. Preinduction anesthestic preparations include placement of defibrillator pads, pacemaker or defibrillator adjustments, and placement of invasive monitoring in the setting of the possibility of peripheral cannulation strategies and alternative cardiopulmonary bypass techniques such as cooling before sternotomy.
4. Emergency reexploration is a high-risk situation in which expedited surgical intervention is required, usually in the setting of bleeding with pericardial tamponade. Transfusion should be anticipated, hemodynamics supported, and heparin ready to administer in anticipation of possible cardiopulmonary bypass.

In contemporary practice, 3% to 4% of coronary artery bypass graft (CABG) operations and approximately 10% of valve surgery procedures are reoperations. Reoperative cardiac surgery carries an incremental risk of mortality and major morbidity compared with first-time or primary cardiac surgery because patients are usually older, with additional comorbidity and more advanced cardiac disease, and because of specific technical challenges presented by prior cardiac surgery. The surgical approach to incision and cannulation in coronary and valve surgery reoperations often differs significantly from the approach used in primary cases, and adverse intraoperative events that require immediate changes to the planned strategy are common and often predictable. Preoperative assessment and planning with the surgical team is therefore particularly important because optimal patient care may require the modification of several aspects of standardized cardiac anesthetic approaches. The incidence of emergency reexploration ranges from 1% to 5% after cardiac surgery, and the primary challenges relate to effectively managing major cardiopulmonary instability and ensuring safe and efficient surgery, either in the operating room or outside the operating room setting.

Indications for Reoperative Cardiac Surgery

The indications for reoperative cardiac surgery are based on the same principles as for primary cardiac surgery. However, the incremental hazard of resternotomy, the lack of bypass conduits, the greater age and comorbidity of this patient group, and the likelihood of valve replacement rather than repair are additional considerations. Consequently, the threshold for recommending surgery rather than medical or transcatheter approaches is higher for reoperative patients. Most patients with symptomatic coronary artery or graft stenoses after CABG surgery are most effectively treated by percutaneous coronary intervention (PCI). Very symptomatic patients with significant lesions to a left anterior descending graft are generally considered to gain symptomatic and prognostic benefit from reoperative coronary artery surgery. The main indications for reoperative valve surgery include prosthetic valve dysfunction (for which the results of transcatheter valve-in-valve implantation are still preliminary) and endocarditis, which is a contraindication to transcatheter valve replacement. Paravalvular leaks are increasingly addressed by percutaneous placement of occluder devices. Late reoperation for isolated severe tricuspid regurgitation is associated with particularly high mortality and major morbidity because of the high prevalence of preoperative moderate-to-severe right ventricular dysfunction, pulmonary arterial hypertension, and multiorgan dysfunction in this population.

Preoperative Assessment

History

Patients undergoing reoperative cardiac surgery are generally older, have more comorbidity, and more advanced cardiovascular disease than patients undergoing first-time surgery. The decision to operate usually depends on correlating a precise account of the nature, timing, and severity of symptoms with the findings from diagnostic studies and balancing the benefits of intervention against the incremental risk of mortality and morbidity posed by reoperation. Additionally, the medical history should establish details of all prior cardiovascular procedures, including date and type of PCI; any previous cardiac surgery, including incisions; history of difficult intubation or adverse reaction to anesthesia, respiratory failure, or tracheostomy; coagulopathy and blood transfusions; and postoperative sepsis and organ dysfunction. Although the balance of risks generally favors continuing antiplatelet medication until surgery in non-reoperative patients, this may not be the case in patients scheduled for reoperative surgery, who will be at greater risk of postoperative coagulopathy and bleeding. It may be appropriate to admit patients preoperatively to discontinue oral anticoagulation and transition to a shorter-acting regimen, such as a heparin infusion.

Clinical Examination

One of the most important risk factors for poor outcomes is frailty. Although this is not well defined, and consequently is not included in most risk models, it is a relatively easy, albeit subjective, judgment often made by looking at a patient. Physical examination of all patients referred for cardiac surgery includes a careful inspection of the entire chest and abdomen. Patients may omit to mention distant cardiac and thoracic surgery procedures, and these may become evident only from incisions, which can be inframammary, posterior thoracotomy, or axillary. All incisions, including conduit harvest sites,

23

pacemaker or defibrillator insertion sites, and potential sites of peripheral cannulation for cardiopulmonary bypass (CPB) in upper and lower extremities, should be assessed for signs of distant or recent infection, poor healing, and vascular complications such as stenosis or aneurysm formation. Evaluation of the airway includes inspection of the suprasternal notch and trachea for evidence of prior tracheostomy.

Imaging

With the exception of young adult patients without risk factors for acquired or congenital coronary artery disease, all patients should have recent cardiac catheterization, including coronary angiography, to assess the patency and anatomy of native vessels and any CABG. In young patients, computed tomographic (CT) coronary angiography usually provides sufficient information about coronary anatomy. Coronary angiograms should be reviewed to determine whether grafts are close or even adherent to the sternum.

Noncontrast computed tomography provides helpful visualization of calcification and aneurysmal segments along the entire arterial tree from aortic root to femoral vessels that may dictate choice of cannulation site. The presence of large amounts of prosthetic material indicates potentially severe adhesions. Intravenous contrast may be employed in CT angiography to demonstrate the course of bypass grafts more clearly; contrast is required to assess patency, and it provides detailed information on the presence of peripheral vascular disease, which is particularly relevant if peripheral arterial cannulation is planned or the patient is likely to need an intraaortic balloon pump.

Echocardiography is necessary to quantify right and left ventricular function, the presence of pulmonary hypertension, and the nature and grade of any valvular dysfunction. Transesophageal echocardiography (TEE) is particularly valuable in the detailed assessment of prosthetic valve endocarditis and failed valve repair or if transthoracic echocardiographic windows are poor.

Before Induction

Days Before Induction

Reoperative patients require the same laboratory tests as patients undergoing first-time surgery. The presence of renal or hepatic dysfunction at baseline means that particular attention must be paid to maintenance of adequate systemic flows, perfusion pressure, and venous drainage on CPB. Patients with preoperative anemia and thrombocytopenia, particularly if they have low body surface areas, are more likely to require blood products than if they were undergoing first-time surgery. In reoperative patients, the hemostatic benefits of stopping antiplatelet drugs (particularly dual antiplatelet therapy) before surgery outweigh the risks of acute coronary ischemia. In patients with or at high risk of acute coronary syndromes, short-acting antiplatelet drugs can be used as a bridge to surgery. Intravenous heparin should be stopped 4 to 6 hours before the planned surgery time and eptifibatide (Integrilin) infusions at least 12 to 24 hours beforehand. Withholding long-acting vasodilators, particularly angiotensin-converting enzyme inhibitors, for 48 hours before surgery may reduce the risk of postoperative vasoplegia.

Immediately Before Induction

Adhesive external defibrillator pads must be attached to the patient before induction. The external defibrillator pads are retained throughout the case for several reasons: internal paddles usually cannot be used because of dense adhesions; electrocautery of adhesions close to myocardium may directly induce ventricular fibrillation; and damage to patent bypass grafts during mediastinal dissection can cause severe myocardial ischemia leading to ventricular fibrillation.

A significant proportion of reoperative patients have cardiovascular implantable electronic devices that should be checked preoperatively by an individual familiar with the device to ascertain its functionality and to devise a plan for intraoperative management. The defibrillator function mode of an implantable cardioverter-defibrillator should be disabled for the duration of surgery. Otherwise, defibrillation shocks (which can precipitate asystole or ventricular fibrillation) may be triggered by electrocautery. The devices should be interrogated again and appropriate defibrillator and pacing settings restored postoperatively, before the removal of temporary epicardial pacing wires. The external defibrillator pads should remain in place for the entire period that the permanent devices are disabled.

In reoperative cases in which CPB times may be prolonged, with associated vasoplegia or low cardiac output states, arterial pressure tracings from distal arteries are often damped and may be unreliable. The presence of two arterial catheters is particularly valuable in reoperative patients. The plan should be discussed with the surgical team because cannulation and the operative strategy will dictate the available location and utility of these catheters.

Anesthesia

Balanced and high-dose narcotic techniques can be used in the reoperative setting. Particular attention must be paid to patients who are at high risk of cardiovascular collapse during induction, such as those with unprotected critical left main (or left main equivalent) coronary artery stenosis, severe aortic stenosis, or cardiac tamponade. Emergency sternotomy, internal cardiac massage, and institution of central CPB are usually not possible because of adhesions that prevent safe, rapid access to the mediastinum. Therefore, in selected reoperative patients thought to be at particularly high risk of cardiovascular decompensation during induction of anesthesia, it may be appropriate to place arterial and central lines in the awake patient and then perform preparation and draping for sternotomy and/or rapid femoral cannulation with the surgeon scrubbed before anesthesia is induced.

Before Incision

The strategy and order of sternotomy, heparinization, cannulation, and institution of bypass may be very different in a reoperation because the safest sequence of these steps is dictated by the risk posed by resternotomy (Table 23.1). Cross-matched blood should be checked and made immediately available before incision. The CPB circuit should be fully primed, and the bypass lines should be brought up to the field before sternotomy, during which time the perfusionist, attending anesthesiologist, and circulating nurse must be present.

Incision

The sternal skin incision is usually made in the standard fashion, and then the sternal wires are untwisted, cut, and either bent to the sides or removed entirely. This can theoretically result in laceration of vascular structures in close proximity underneath, including the right ventricle. Some surgeons elect routinely to perform an initial dissection under the sternum using thoracoscopic guidance. In cases in which an aneurysmal aorta is thought to be densely adherent to the posterior sternal table, a small transverse incision may be made in the second or third left intercostal space to allow the aorta to be dissected free before median sternotomy.

23

Table 23.1	Risk Stratification of Low-, Medium-, High-, and Very-High-Risk Sternotomies, With a Summary of Operative Strategy Tailored to Address Risks	
Preoperative Assessment of Risk		**Intraoperative Strategy**
Increasing risk of major injury	Low-risk resternotomy: • Prior cardiac surgery without patent coronary bypass grafts • Aorta and mediastinal structures a safe distance from the sternum	• Resternotomy, dissection of adhesions, standard aortocaval cannulation; initiate bypass; proceed with residual adhesiolysis and cardiac surgical procedure • Optional: expose peripheral cannulation sites before stenotomy
	Moderate-risk resternotomy: • Patent coronary bypass grafts that lie >1 cm from the sternum, including patent left internal mammary artery (IMA) to left anterior descending coronary artery routed lateral to the sternum	• As above • Optional: peripheral arterial cannulation, with 5000 units of heparin given and arterial line flushed intermittently by perfusion; resternotomy and division of adhesions as above • If major vascular injury occurs, venous cannulation can be performed peripherally, and centrally and after full heparinization cardiopulmonary bypass (CPB) is commenced
	High-risk resternotomy: • Patent left IMA graft crossing midline close to sternum, right ventricle adherent to sternum, normal aorta in close proximity to sternum • Third- or fourth-time resternotomy	• Peripheral and arterial cannulation with full heparinization before resternotomy • Optional: institute CPB, stop ventilation, and drain venous return into pump reservoir to decompress right side of heart
	Very-high-risk resternotomy: • Patent left IMA graft crossing midline adherent to sternum and large area of myocardium at risk, aortic tube graft or aneurysm adherent to sternum	• Peripheral and arterial cannulation with full heparinization, institution of CPB, cooling before resternotomy • Optional: circulatory arrest under moderate hypothermia during sternotomy

Adapted from Akujuo A, Fischer GW, Chikwe J. Current concepts in reoperative cardiac surgery. *Semin Cardiothorac Vasc Anesth*. 2009;13:206–214.

The anterior sternal table is divided with an oscillating saw. Under an optional period of apnea, the posterior table is then divided along its entire length with either the oscillating saw or a heavy blunt-tipped scissors. This part of the sternotomy poses the most risk to underlying structures. Injury to these structures is particularly problematic because hemorrhage and hemodynamic instability may prevent completion of the sternotomy—in which case the surgeon will have insufficient surgical access to address the injury effectively. To minimize the risk of this scenario, surgeons commonly try to decompress the mediastinal structures by asking the anesthesiologist to hold ventilation and, in the case of patients who have been cannulated and heparinized, asking the perfusionist to exsanguinate the patient into the pump temporarily. On rare occasions, the safest option is to commence CPB using peripheral cannulation, cool the patient, and arrest the circulation before skin incision and sternotomy (see Table 23.1). Electrocautery is used to dissect the heart away from the left sternal edge and then the right sternal edge. Excessive retraction of the sternum before this dissection is fully completed can result in right ventricular rupture. Other possible complications during this initial dissection are ventricular arrhythmias, including fibrillation as a result of electrocautery in proximity to the myocardium and injury to a patent left internal mammary artery (IMA) graft resulting in myocardial ischemia and a high likelihood of ventricular dysfunction and/or ventricular fibrillation.

Subsequent mediastinal dissection is targeted at obtaining access to central cannulation and aortic cross-clamp sites, specifically the aorta and the right atrium. A "no touch" technique is used for bypass grafts to avoid distal embolization and myocardial ischemia. The most common injuries during this phase of dissection are to the right atrium, which is frequently thin walled and densely adherent at sites of prior cannulation and atriotomy. Such injuries can usually be addressed with primary suture closure, but occasionally institution of CPB is mandated to effect a repair.

For patients undergoing a mitral, a tricuspid, or (occasionally) an aortic valve procedure, a right thoracotomy may be less hazardous than a median sternotomy. This technique is used to reduce the risk of injury to structures lying adjacent to the sternum. The disadvantage with a right thoracotomy approach is that access to the lateral border of the heart, the ascending aorta, and the aortic valve is limited.

Cannulation

Arterial and/or venous cannulation for CPB can be peripheral, central, or a combination of both. The choice depends on the risks posed by sternal reentry and the presence of peripheral arterial disease, as well as the presence of multiple sites of previous surgery on the aorta and right atrium, which may limit the room available for central cannulation. For example, the presence of multiple patent graft anastomoses to the aorta may favor peripheral arterial cannulation. For patients who are at high risk of catastrophic injury to mediastinal structures, arterial (and in certain cases venous) cannulation may be carried out peripherally before sternotomy. The choice of cannulas should take into account the patient's body surface area: if the venous cannula is too small, the perfusionist will be unable to drain the venous return adequately, and if the arterial cannula is too small, the perfusionist will be unable to provide adequate arterial flow without excessive line pressures. Should the peripheral vessels be too small to permit adequately sized cannulas, it is usually possible to add additional cannulas centrally subsequently, if needed, to improve the adequacy of systemic perfusion.

The right or left axillary artery and vein may be exposed by a 5-cm incision in the deltopectoral groove. Use of the axillary artery for arterial cannulation offers less risk of limb ischemia and cerebrovascular events than use of the femoral artery, which is less well collateralized and provides retrograde arterial flow. The most common complication of axillary artery cannulation involves trauma to the branches of the brachial plexus that are intimately involved with the artery. Injury to the artery itself, causing ischemia, dissection, and hyperperfusion, is also possible. The risks of ischemia and dissection are minimized by cannulating a T-graft sewn to the axillary artery rather than cannulating the artery directly. Institution of CPB via the T-graft may be associated with hyperperfusion of the ipsilateral arm. If arterial cannulation alone is carried out peripherally, it is unnecessary to fully heparinize the patient initially. A single dose of 5000 units of heparin will be sufficient to keep the line free of thrombus if the perfusionist flushes the cannula intermittently before institution of CPB. Full heparinization to an activated coagulation time greater than 480 seconds is usually required before venous cannulation, use of pump (cardiotomy) suction, or institution of CPB, although policies may vary from institution to institution.

The main indication for peripheral venous cannulation (which mandates full heparinization) before sternotomy is the surgeon's decision to institute CPB before sternotomy. The axillary vein is sometimes used, but the larger femoral vein, which has a straighter course to the right atrium, provides the most reliable access and venous drainage. A major complication of femoral venous and arterial cannulation, which may not manifest until later in the case, is retroperitoneal hemorrhage caused by perforation of the femoral or iliac vessel or retrograde dissection of the aorta. A significant retroperitoneal bleed or dissection on CPB is characterized by low flows, low systemic pressures, poor venous drainage owing to loss of circulating volume and, eventually, abdominal distension from accumulating hematoma and venous stasis.

Cardiopulmonary Bypass

The patient can be placed on CPB before resternotomy, if indicated. Safe institution of CPB should be confirmed by the anesthesiologist, perfusionist, and surgeon. This is even more important if the patient has been placed on bypass emergently because cannula choice and placement may not be optimal.

If proximity of right-sided heart structures to the sternum is a concern (particularly the right ventricle in patients with severe pulmonary hypertension), some surgeons take the precaution of temporarily draining the circulating volume into the venous reservoir of the CPB circuit before sternotomy. This has the theoretical advantage of decompressing the right side of the heart, which may reduce the risk of injury from the sternal saw. After the sternotomy is completed, the remainder of the mediastinal dissection can be carried out with the patient on or off CPB, depending on the challenges presented by adhesions and pathology. Although starting CPB early increases bypass time, it likely reduces the risk of injury to important structures and does not appear to increase morbidity, mortality, or postoperative bleeding. The main reason this is not done routinely is that the patient is fully heparinized while lysis of adhesions is carried out, potentially leading to increased transfusion requirements during the procedure; red cell salvaging may minimize transfusions.

Myocardial Protection

Whereas the approach to myocardial protection for reoperative cardiac surgery follows the same basic principles as for first-time surgery (ie, decompression of the heart, usually in cold diastolic arrest to minimize myocardial oxygen demand), there are several additional factors that commonly impact the myocardial protection strategy. Patients undergoing reoperative cardiac surgery typically have worse myocardial function and more advanced coronary and valvular heart disease than patients having first-time surgery. In most reoperations, technical challenges increase the cross-clamp time significantly. If one or more patent IMA grafts are present, they will perfuse the coronary circulation with systemic blood flow after the aorta is cross-clamped. The subsequent washing out of cardioplegic solution from the myocardium with systemic blood, which is usually warmer and normokalemic, will cause the heart to resume electrical activity. If this is not addressed, the areas of myocardium not perfused by the IMA may become ischemic. If there is any more than mild aortic insufficiency, fibrillatory arrest will result in ventricular distension unless the left ventricle is vented, and retrograde blood flow from the aorta can make mitral valve surgery very challenging in this scenario.

Retrograde cardioplegia is a useful adjunct, but correct placement of a coronary sinus catheter is more challenging in reoperative patients because manual palpation is usually prevented by diaphragmatic adhesions. Consequently, the surgeon is more reliant on TEE to assess coronary sinus placement, and it is crucial to monitor the coronary sinus pressure continuously during cardioplegia to confirm an appropriate pressure response. Additionally, if the aorta is open, the surgeon should see cardioplegia effluent from the left and right main coronary ostia.

Coagulation Management

Because of the large surface area of dissection (particularly in a fully heparinized patient) and prolonged CPB time, coagulopathy is common in reoperative patients. Point-of-care testing, including platelet function assays and thrombelastography, and transfusion algorithms are useful to guide therapy toward restoration of hemostasis and minimizing transfusion requirements.

Intraoperative Emergency Scenarios

Intraoperative adverse events occur in 3% to 10% of reoperative cardiac procedures, with a quarter occurring before or during sternotomy and most of the remainder occurring during mediastinal dissection before institution of CPB. Potentially life-threatening injuries related to sternotomy include trauma to patent bypass grafts (which are the most frequently injured structures) and injury to the aorta. Additionally, injuries to the right atrium, right ventricle, and innominate vein are common and challenging to address, especially in patients with right-sided heart failure. Rapid volume replacement via large peripheral or central venous catheters or via the arterial cannula may be required. Major injury to arterial structures is immediately life-threatening, either from hemorrhage or from myocardial ischemia, and usually mandates immediate heparinization, cannulation, and institution of CPB.

In the event of major hemodynamic instability that is likely to necessitate CPB (including major bleeding), the anesthesiologist should administer a dose of heparin sufficient to institute CPB (300–400 units/kg or an in vitro titration dose calculated to exceed 2.5–3.0 units/mL of blood). Assuming no access to central cannulation sites, extrathoracic sites should be cannulated emergently and CPB initiated. When the patient is fully heparinized and an arterial cannula is in place, "suction bypass" may be initiated to allow for partial temporary CPB. In this scenario, all venous return to the CPB circuit comes from cardiotomy suction ("coronary suckers") placed into the mediastinum and/or lacerated cardiac structures until venous cannulation can be established. The patient should still be ventilated because the left side of the heart is likely to be ejecting blood returning from the pulmonary veins. The period of cardiotomy suction bypass should be as short as possible; extensive hemolysis results from the turbulent flow and mixture with air in the cardiotomy tubing.

If there is a major injury to the aorta, institution of CPB alone will not be sufficient to control the problem. The primary goal is to obtain some degree of control of the bleeding by direct compression or occlusion sufficient to allow effective CPB for several minutes. Restoration of aortic continuity often requires institution of systemic hypothermia so that the aorta may be assessed and repaired during a period of moderate hypothermic circulatory arrest.

If a patent CABG is inadvertently lacerated or transected, it is possible to reduce the risk of resultant myocardial ischemia and ventricular fibrillation by inserting an

23

intracoronary shunt to restore flow across the injured portion. It is frequently necessary to rapidly institute CPB, however. This is clearly the case if significant ST-segment elevation, bradycardia, or ventricular fibrillation is associated with arterial bleeding in this setting. The primary aim initially is decompression of the left ventricle and restoration of adequate systemic circulation. The eventual goal is restoration of coronary perfusion by repair of the injury or replacement of the graft.

▨ EMERGENCY REEXPLORATION

Indications

Emergency reexploration is needed in approximately 1% to 3% of patients in the first few hours to days after cardiac surgery. Emergency resternotomy is indicated for definitive management of cardiac tamponade and acute massive mediastinal hemorrhage. Emergency resternotomy permits internal cardiac massage (which has been shown to increase the cardiac index to 1.3 L/min per m^2 from 0.6 L/min per m^2 in the closed chest), placement of epicardial pacing wires, relief of tension pneumothorax, internal defibrillation, and management of excess mediastinal bleeding. Consequently, the other main indication for emergency reexploration is cardiac arrest that does not respond satisfactorily to a few minutes of cardiopulmonary resuscitation and is likely to have a cause that can be addressed by emergency resternotomy. After cardiac surgery, 20% to 50% of cardiac arrests result in emergency sternotomy.

With the exception of catastrophic surgical bleeding or acute cardiac tamponade, the timing of intervention for excess mediastinal bleeding is almost always subject to some debate. When the surgical team has specific concerns about surgical bleeding sites, the threshold for surgical reexploration may be low. It may be much higher in the setting of significant coagulopathy, particularly if an extended effort was made to secure hemostasis in the operating room. In general, indications that the patient may require reexploration for bleeding include (1) greater than 400 mL bleeding in 1 hour; (2) greater than 200 mL/hour for more than 2 hours; (3) greater than 2 L of blood loss in 24 hours; (4) increasing rate of bleeding, particularly in the absence of coagulopathy; and (5) bleeding associated with hypotension, low cardiac output, or tamponade.

General Considerations

Anesthetic and surgical considerations in patients undergoing emergency reexploration differ from those in patients undergoing reoperative cardiac surgery, including surgical revision of bypass grafts or other cardiac procedures in the early postoperative setting. In the setting of emergency reexploration, patients are characteristically hemodynamically unstable and often undergoing cardiopulmonary resuscitation with external cardiac massage. The trigger for emergency resternotomy may have been preceded by several hours of a low cardiac output state, with profound metabolic disturbances. In the case of persistent hemorrhage, the patient may be coagulopathic and may have already received massive transfusions. Emergency reexploration often takes place in the intensive care unit if the patient is too unstable to be transferred to the operating room. Advanced preparation in the form of practice drills and team protocol development is important to help overcome the disadvantages of reduced access to operating room personnel, equipment, and space that can be major obstacles to the safe and effective resuscitation of these patients. Additionally, the longer the time between the index cardiac surgery procedure and cardiac arrest, the less likely it is that the cause of cardiac arrest can be effectively addressed by emergency resternotomy.

Akujuo A, Fischer GW, Chikwe J. Current concepts in reoperative cardiac surgery. *Semin Cardiothorac Vasc Anesth.* 2009;13:206–214.

Braunwald E, Antman EM, Beasley JW. ACC/AHA guideline update for the management of patients with unstable angina and non–ST-segment elevation myocardial infarction—2002: summary article. *Circulation.* 2002;106:1893–1900.

Breglio A, Anyanwu A, Itagaki S, et al. Does prior coronary bypass surgery present a unique risk for reoperative valve surgery? *Ann Thorac Surg.* 2013;95:1603–1608.

Chikwe J, Adams DH. Frailty: the missing element in predicting operative mortality. *Semin Thorac Cardiovasc Surg.* 2010;22:109–110.

Crooke GA, Schwartz CF, Ribakove GH, et al. Retrograde arterial perfusion, not incision location, significantly increases the risk of stroke in reoperative mitral valve procedures. *Ann Thorac Surg.* 2010;89:723–729.

Dunning J, Fabbri A, Kolh PH, et al. Guideline for resuscitation in cardiac arrest after cardiac surgery. *Eur J Cardiothorac Surg.* 2009;36:3–28.

Etz CD, Plestis KA, Kari FA, et al. Axillary cannulation significantly improves survival and neurologic outcome after atherosclerotic aneurysm repair of the aortic root and ascending aorta. *Ann Thorac Surg.* 2008;86:441–446, discussion 446–447.

Ferraris VA, Saha SP, Oestreich JH, et al. 2012 Update to The Society of Thoracic Surgeons guideline on use of antiplatelet drugs in patients having cardiac and noncardiac operations. *Ann Thorac Surg.* 2012;94:1761–1781.

Ghanta RK, Kaneko T, Gammie JS, et al. Evolving trends of reoperative coronary artery bypass grafting: an analysis of The Society of Thoracic Surgeons Adult Cardiac Surgery Database. *J Thorac Cardiovasc Surg.* 2013;145:364–372.

Roselli EE, Pettersson GB, Blackstone EH, et al. Adverse events during reoperative cardiac surgery: frequency, characterization, and rescue. *J Thorac Cardiovasc Surg.* 2008;135:316–323.

Shore-Lesserson L, Manspeizer HE, DePario M, et al. Thromboelastography-guided transfusion algorithm reduces transfusions in complex cardiac surgery. *Anesth Analg.* 1999;88:312–319.

The Society of Thoracic Surgeons Task Force on Resuscitation After Cardiac Surgery. The Society of Thoracic Surgeons expert consensus for the resuscitation of patients who arrest after cardiac surgery. *Ann Thorac Surg.* 2017;103:1005–1020.

Thourani VH, Suri RM, Gunter R, et al. Contemporary real-world outcomes of surgical aortic valve replacement in 141,905 low-risk, intermediate-risk and high-risk patients. *Ann Thorac Surg.* 2015;99:55–61.

Yusuf S, Zhao F, Mehta SR, et al. Effects of clopidogrel in addition to aspirin in patients with acute coronary syndromes without ST-segment elevation. *N Engl J Med.* 2001;345:494–502.

23

Chapter 24

Patient Safety in the Cardiac Operating Room

Joyce A. Wahr, MD, FAHA • T. Andrew Bowdle, MD, PhD, FASE • Nancy A. Nussmeier, MD, FAHA

Key Points

1. Cardiac surgical patients are at significant risk from preventable adverse events. These events occur through human error, by either faulty decision making (diagnosis, decision for treatment) or faulty actions (failure to implement the plan correctly).
2. Human error is ubiquitous and cannot be prevented or eliminated by trying harder or by eliminating the one who errs. Reduction in human error requires system changes that prevent errors from occurring or prevent errors from reaching the patient.
3. Sleep deprivation and fatigue can render a person more likely to make an error. Although residents' hours are limited, those of other physicians in the United States are not, unlike in other countries.
4. Nontechnical skills such as leadership, communication, cooperation, and situational awareness are critical to patient safety, but they are rarely taught. Distractions, disruptions, noise, and alarms contribute to technical errors and increase mortality rates in cardiac surgery.
5. Communication is the leading root cause of sentinel events, whether through missing information or through misunderstanding. Use of structured communication protocols reduces errors. Handoffs performed without a protocol involve significant numbers of omitted items.
6. Team training reduces surgical mortality rates, but it must be done with careful preparation and with regular retraining.
7. Surgical briefings that use a checklist significantly reduce surgical mortality rates. Debriefings allow teams to identify hazards and formulate improvements.
8. Simulation is an effective means to teach both technical and nontechnical skills and to allow teams to train for rare but dangerous events.
9. Cognitive aids should be available in every operating room to provide direction during rare crisis events (eg, malignant hyperthermia, pulseless electrical activity).
10. Medication errors occur approximately in 1 in every 150 to 200 anesthetic cases. The Anesthesia Patient Safety Foundation published a set of recommendations to reduce medication errors, including standardization, use of technology such as bar codes and smart infusion pumps, having pharmacy involvement in every step of the medication process, and building a culture of safety.

Cardiac surgical patients each year become ill and die because of preventable adverse events, and they are more likely to have adverse events than other surgical patients (12.2% vs 3%), with 54% of these events considered to be preventable. These numbers may underestimate the true rate of adverse events. Despite significant attention and discussion, eradication of these preventable medical events has proved difficult, largely because medical education remains focused on technical rather than nontechnical aspects of medicine. Far more time is spent teaching anesthesia residents how to cannulate the internal jugular vein than how to communicate clearly and without error or how to understand the complexities of human error.

Patient safety involves both doing the right thing (ie, applying best practice to every situation) and doing the right thing the right way (ie, avoiding human error). Whereas most of this textbook is devoted to discussion of the right thing to do in a given circumstance, this chapter discusses both requirements for safe practice: (1) formulation of the correct plan for patient care (implementing evidence-based best practices); and (2) flawlessly carrying out the plan (preventing or correcting human error.)

THE SCIENCE OF SAFETY

Rigorous patient safety science has improved the understanding of how errors occur and how to design safe practices, test them for efficacy, implement changes effectively, and measure the effectiveness of interventions, thus ensuring improvements.

One such comprehensive observational study of the hazards in the cardiac operating room (OR) was undertaken in the Locating Errors Through Networked Surveillance (LENS) group as part of the FOCUS (Flawless Operative Cardiac Unified Systems) project. This collaborative study involved the Society of Cardiovascular Anesthesiologists, and consisted of observations of 20 cardiac operations by a team of trained observers, including human factors engineers, anesthesiologists, and organizational psychologists. The analysis identified a myriad of hazards in the cardiac OR and detailed the complex interaction of organizational structure (lack of policies), teamwork behaviors (poor communication), system shortcomings (inadequate support requiring multiple workarounds), equipment and technologies (poorly designed and integrated), and individual failings (situational awareness). The complexity of interactions among systems, providers, and processes highlights the truth that a simple solution to patient safety is not feasible. Experts from a variety of disciplines will be required to examine every aspect of perioperative cardiac surgical care and to integrate proposed solutions.

24

HUMAN ERROR

Theory of Human Error

The universality of human error is well known and is accepted in virtually every walk of life, except perhaps medicine. Here it is expected that physicians and providers will be perfect, that the natural cognitive slips and trips and biases inherent in daily life will be overcome by the importance of the work being done and the fact that lives hang in the balance.

The elegant exploration of human error and system accidents have made it clear that patient safety in the cardiac OR will not come about by identifying and eliminating error-prone individual clinicians. In general, if the system is designed such that one

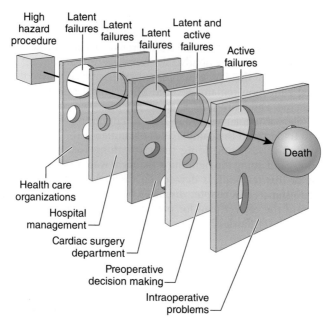

Fig. 24.1 Accident model. Active and latent failures in health care organizations, hospital management, and individual human error can all contribute to adverse events during high-risk procedures. (From Carthey J, de Leval MR, Reason JT. The human factor in cardiac surgery: errors and near misses in a high technology medical domain. *Ann Thorac Surg.* 2001;72:300–305.)

person can make a given error, it is virtually guaranteed that another human will as well. For example, despite a Joint Commission Sentinel Alert in 2006 to caution care providers of the dangerous errors made possible by the use of universal connectors (Luer), hundreds of patients have died since then because intravenous fluids, pressure lines, or enteral feedings were erroneously connected to epidural catheters or arterial lines and vice versa. The appropriate system change is now being implemented, with unique connectors for intravenous, arterial, enteral feeding, and pressure tubing and neuraxial catheters established by the International Standards Organization.

Highly complex systems such as health care or the nuclear power industry are far more vulnerable, even though many of the worst events begin with a trivial misstep (eg, O-ring not tested in low temperatures in the space shuttle rocket). Even when the initiating event is a human error, correcting or preventing adverse outcomes nearly always requires a system change. Reason's Swiss cheese model is now well accepted to demonstrate how system defenses must be in place to prevent or at least detect human errors before harm is done to patients (Fig. 24.1).

Personal Readiness (Fatigue, Stress)

It has been concluded that working for more than 16 consecutive hours is unsafe for both trainees (marked increased risk of an accident while driving home) and for their patients (attention failure, serious errors, and diagnostic mistakes). After 24 hours of being awake, impairment of reaction time is comparable to that produced by a blood alcohol concentration of 0.10 g/dL. Sleep-deprived persons have a poor capacity to recognize their fatigue, thus reducing their capacity to work safely. A survey of resident physicians suggested that fatigue-related errors resulting in death or injury of a patient are not uncommon.

Fatigue has been implicated as a contributor to impaired performance, critical incidents, and errors in anesthesia. The work hours and schedules of anesthesiologists expose them to circadian disruption, with both acute and chronic sleep deprivation causing fatigue. Anesthesiologists may be more susceptible to even mild sleep deprivation compared with other medical specialties because of the vigilance required to provide safe anesthesia care.

In a well-designed, realistic, simulation-based trial, in both a sleep-deprived state and a rested state, 12 residents anesthetized a simulated patient for 4 hours. The sleep-deprived group had a trend to poorer vigilance with slower response times. The sleep-deprived group took numerically longer to detect and correct abnormal clinical events, and during the simulated anesthetic regimen, nearly one-third of the sleep-deprived group fell asleep at some stage. Similarly, when surveyed, 50% of perfusionists reported that they had performed CPB after 36 hours of being awake; 15% of surveyed perfusionists reported episodes of microsleep while performing CPB. Two-thirds reported fatigue-related errors, and 6.7% reported serious perfusion accidents related to fatigue.

Vigilance While Performing Transesophageal Echocardiograms

The introduction and subsequent widespread use of transesophageal echocardiography (TEE) brought about a major advance in cardiac surgery and anesthesia for both diagnosis and intraoperative monitoring. Anecdotally, we have noticed times when all attention in the OR is focused on the TEE machine rather than on the patient, especially with trainees. This seems to be more noticeable during the phase of learning TEE than with clinicians who are more experienced.

This area needs further investigation, but consideration should be given to where the TEE machine is placed in relation to the patient and the other monitors. The anesthesiologist working alone may be more vulnerable, given that attention can be focused on only one place at a time. Although all cardiac anesthesiologists recognize the poor ergonomics of machines and monitors, no studies define best practices.

TEAMWORK AND COMMUNICATION

24

As noted earlier, preventable adverse events or human errors in the cardiac OR often are related not to technical skill or knowledge base but to cognitive, teamwork, or system failures. Skills such as communication, cooperation, and leadership are recognized to be critical components of teamwork, and deficiencies in these skills have been associated with adverse outcomes.

Communication failures, human factors, and leadership deficiencies have been found to be the top three causes underlying sentinel events in every review from The Joint Commission since 2004. In a review of litigated surgical outcomes, a communication failure among caregivers was responsible for the adverse outcome in 87% of cases. Clearly, teamwork behaviors and communication are critical to patient safety.

Disruptions, Distractions, Major and Minor Events

The cardiac OR is a highly complex setting where professionals from multiple disciplines interact with complicated and often poorly designed equipment to complete hazardous interventions—typically under significant time constraints—in patients with challenging cardiac disease and other comorbidities. Despite the apparent need for quiet concentration, distractions and disruptions rule the day. In cardiac surgical cases, door openings average 19.2/hour, 22.8/hour if prosthetic devices are involved. OR traffic, door openings, conversations, alarms, and even music can result in an excessive noise level. It is no wonder that failures of teamwork resulting in surgical flow disruptions occurred at a rate of 11.7/hour.

Team members perceive disruptions and distractions, as well as team behaviors, in discipline-specific ways. Surgeons tend to downplay disruptions and report them as having a lesser effect on performance than do nurses or trained observers. All too often, significant disruptions and distractions simply are treated as annoyances and part of the daily work. Data show, however, that technical errors and adverse patient outcomes increase as disruptions accumulate.

Equipment and Alarms

The quantity and complexity of the equipment required for cardiac operations are significant. Equipment-related problems are responsible for 10% to 12% of flow disruptions. Even though ergonomic design is known to be an important factor in patient safety, it has been suboptimal, both for OR room design and layout and for equipment design. ORs built years or decades ago are now necessarily cluttered with equipment, each device requiring electrical cords and communication tethers.

In a study of disruptions observed in 10 cardiac operations, 33% of flow disruptions were related to OR design and physical layout. A literature review regarding hazards associated with cardiac surgery identified four ways in which equipment harms the patient: (1) poor design and ergonomics; (2) poor training or negligence with use; (3) poor maintenance and upkeep; and (4) risk inherent in use of the device (eg, the risk that a TEE probe will cause esophageal injury). Medical devices and equipment typically are designed by engineers who spend little time in the environment in which the devices will be used. Even rarer is the participation of human factors engineers in the prepurchase evaluation of equipment for device-specific form and function, as well as for integration of the equipment into the existing physical layout of a typical OR. As a result, the interaction between people and technologies in the OR is suboptimal. Perhaps the most distressing single contribution to OR noise is the frequency of alarms. Alarms clearly are designed to alert to parameters outside the norm, but a typical cardiac OR has some 18 alarms, each with manufacturer-chosen visual and audio alerts. Unfortunately, the volume or tonality of the alarm has no rhyme or reason. A "not ventilating" alarm can be quiet and nearly undetectable, whereas a circuit humidifier alarm can be hair-raising. It was reported that 359 alarms occurred per cardiac operation, at a rate of 1.2/*minute*. In one study, 90% of alarms were found to be false-positive events, often resulting in alarms being turned off or ignored. In a study of 731 alarm warnings, only 7% were found to be useful, and 13% were triggered by a planned intervention. As concerning as the noise and disruption are, even more concerning is the tendency to tune out the alarms or even turn off the alarms when they become too annoying, potentially resulting in a serious preventable adverse event. The Joint Commission made alarm management a goal in 2012, but true correction will require a comprehensive national (or international) approach to standardize the volume and tonality of alarms by system (eg, ventilation, cardiac) and by urgency and then to require all manufacturers to meet these standards.

Teamwork

In the highly complex world of cardiac surgery, teamwork and communication are critical to outcome. Team members (especially physicians) are poor at assessing their

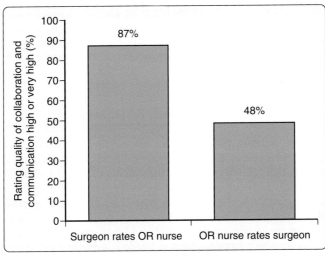

Fig. 24.2 Differences in perceptions of teamwork between surgeons and operating room (OR) nurses. (From Makary MA, Sexton JB, Freischlag JA, et al. Operating room teamwork among physicians and nurses: teamwork in the eye of the beholder. *J Am Coll Surg.* 2006;202:746–752.)

own teamwork and communication skill level. In multiple studies, surgeons' and anesthesiologists' teamwork and communication skills were rated much more highly by themselves than by nurses and perfusion staff members. In one study, surgeons rated the quality of other surgeons' teamwork as high or very high 85% of the time, whereas nurses rated the collaboration with surgeons as high or very high only 48% of the time (Fig. 24.2).

Communication

One very specific aspect of communication is that required during a transition of care from one provider to another (relief during surgical procedures) or between teams (OR to intensive care unit [ICU]), termed "the handoff" (also known as the handover). A handoff is essentially a contemporaneous process of passing patient-specific information from one caregiver to another to ensure continuity and safety of patient care. Standardized handoff communication was a safety goal of The Joint Commission for 2006. Handoffs occur multiple times during surgical procedures as staff members are relieved, and multiple handoffs occur among teams: from cardiology to cardiac surgery, from the preoperative team to the intraoperative team, even from anesthesia to perfusion at the initiation of bypass, from the OR to the ICU, from the ICU to the ward, and, finally, from the hospital back to the primary care provider or cardiologist. One group reviewed 258 surgical malpractice cases in which error led to injury of a patient; 60 cases involved communication failures. Forty-three percent of the failures occurred during a handoff, and 19% occurred across departments. Most of the communication failures (92%) were verbal, involved a single transmitter and receiver, and were equally the result of omission of critical information (49%) and misinterpretation (44%).

These errors are understandable, given the complexity of cardiac surgical procedures, the nuances of patients' physiology (often understood as much at a subconscious level as at a conscious one), and the frequent distractions that arise during patient care. Handoffs rarely occur in a quiet setting, and distractions are common. Occasionally,

24

no handoff occurs at all. A review of the literature portrays handoffs as being highly variable, unstructured, and performed under pressure from competing tasks. In one study of pediatric cardiac surgical handoffs, important content items were reported only 53% of the time, and distractions occurred at a rate of 2.3/minute of reporting.

INTERVENTIONS TO IMPROVE PATIENT SAFETY

It is clear from the preceding discussion that nontechnical aspects of cardiac surgical procedures play a vital role in patient outcomes. Efforts to improve these aspects of cardiac operations are required to decrease the number of patients who suffer preventable harm. Key areas of focus include the following: standardizing care as much as possible, including implementing evidence-based best practices; undertaking formal training and practice in teamwork behaviors and skills; implementing presurgery briefings, and the use of cognitive aids such as checklists; using regular debriefings to identify areas in which improvement is needed; strengthening structured communication protocols both during surgical procedures and during transitions of care; and using simulation to provide directed practice both for nontechnical skills and for the technical aspects of crisis management.

Although these interventions have been shown to increase patient and staff satisfaction and to reduce mortality rates, interventions are often met with ambivalence at best and hostility at worst. As noted, this response can have several causes: overestimation of skill level; discounting of the effects of stress, fatigue, and disruptions; and a view that imposition of external guidelines limits individualized patient care or is insulting to staff members' intelligence and dedication.

Teamwork Training

The evidence presented earlier (ie, that poor teamwork skill is directly linked to technical errors and adverse patient outcomes) indicates that specific teamwork training should improve outcomes. Many investigators and experts have pointed to the aviation industry's use of Crew Resource Management (CRM) to achieve excellent teamwork and reduce errors and accidents, and have suggested that medical teams adopt CRM. Key components of effective teamwork are similar between aviation and medicine: leadership and management, situational awareness, shared decision making, cooperation, and coordination. However, the effect of teaching CRM to surgical teams has been mixed. When pilots were brought in to teach surgical staff how to perform effective briefings, no change in safety attitudes occurred among faculty physicians, and only a modest change occurred among junior physicians.

Checklists and Briefings

Checklists are simple cognitive aids that can improve performance of simple tasks (shopping) or complex endeavors (landing a fighter plane on an aircraft carrier deck), and they serve as reminders of routine tasks that may otherwise be missed. Checklists successfully have been used to ensure completion of critical steps in a variety of surgical procedures, as well as in preparation for anesthesia.

Checklists can help drive implementation of best practices, often by reducing voluminous guidelines to a simple set of the most critical evidence-based best practices. The Keystone Project implemented a list of five key evidence-based elements to prevent central line–associated bloodstream infections (CLABSI). In the 108 ICUs participating, the median rate of CLABSI fell from 2.7 per 1000 catheter-days to 0 at 3 months, and the mean rate decreased from 7.7 per 1000 catheter-days to 1.4 at 18 months. Similar evidence-based checklists have reduced ventilator-associated pneumonia and mortality rates. Briefings are reviews of the salient points of the plan, and they allow teams to develop a closely shared mental model of the operation to be performed. In aviation, even training runs that have been performed countless times before by the same team begin with an extensive brief. During a brief, all members of the team assume equal hierarchy in terms of raising concerns and identifying vulnerabilities. In surgery, as was common in aviation before implementation of CRM, strict hierarchies inhibit trainees and low-status staff from raising concerns or questioning the plan. Many OR personnel report that they would have trouble speaking up, even if they believed that patient safety was compromised. Without formal intervention or team training, few, if any, briefings are performed, and poor agreement exists about what constitutes a briefing. The SURPASS is a checklist that covers the entire continuum of surgery and includes a presurgical briefing as well as a postsurgical debriefing. Implementation of the SURPASS tool reduced the complication rate from 27.3% to 16.7% and decreased the mortality rate from 1.5% to 0.8% in one series. A closed claim review of adverse events that occurred before implementation found that some 40% of the events would have been prevented with use of the SURPASS tool.

Briefings enhance team performance and require little time. In an analysis of 37,133 briefings, it was found that briefings averaged 2.9 minutes and debriefings averaged 2.5 minutes. Implementing briefings reduced the number of nonroutine events in cardiac surgical procedures by 25%, and it increased the perception that wrong-site operations would be prevented. After briefings were instituted at 16 cardiac surgical centers, surgical flow disruptions decreased from 5.4 per case to 2.8, disruptions resulting from inadequate procedural knowledge decreased from 4.1 to 2.2, and miscommunication events fell from 2.5 per case to 1.2. Briefings improved communication; they reduced the number of communication failures per case from 3.95 to 1.31 and identified new problems or knowledge gaps.

Debriefings and Learning From Defects

Regular team debriefings at the end of surgical procedures can serve as a means to identify hazards and formulate improvements. Although debriefings are often discussed in conjunction with briefings and occur in the same context as briefings, they differ in timing, content, purpose, and practice. Debriefings should occur at the end of each surgical procedure and provide an opportunity for the team to reflect on the procedure and verbalize lessons learned or deficiencies identified. It can be as simple as asking, "Did everything go as well as we wanted it to (or as we expected) today?" Debriefings allow the team to come together to rectify problems and to find ways to improve performance in the next case. They give the teams a chance to identify latent hazards and vulnerabilities, develop and implement system improvements, address areas of teamwork weakness, and formulate future plans.

▨ MEDICATION SAFETY

Drug Errors

Substantial evidence indicates that drug administration errors are common in anesthetic practice. The incidence of drug administration errors in an academic practice in the

24

Table 24.1	Types of Drug Errors
Error Type	**Definition**
Incorrect dose	Wrong dose of an intended drug
Substitution	Incorrect drug instead of the desired drug; a syringe or vial swap
Omission	Intended drug not given (eg, missed antibiotic redosing)
Repetition	Extra dose of an intended drug
Incorrect route	Intended drug erroneously given by an unintended route
Other	Drug administered when contraindicated; rapid infusion of drug intended to be given slowly; antibiotic administered prior to collection of microbial cultures

Modified from Webster CS, Merry AF, Larsson L, et al. The frequency and nature of drug administration error during anaesthesia. *Anaesth Intensive Care.* 2001;29:494–500 and reproduced with the kind permission of the Australian Society of Anaesthetists.

United States appears to be similar to that reported from elsewhere in the world. In a self-reporting study performed in a single center in the United States, a rate of error of 0.40% (35 in 8777, or 1 in 203 anesthetic cases) and a rate of pre-error of 0.19% (17 in 8777) was found. More recently, an observational study found that a medication error or adverse drug reaction occurred in 1 in 5 operations.

The majority of reported drug errors can be classified (Table 24.1). In one study, nearly 50% of the errors were syringe and drug preparation errors, with 18.9% being swaps of correctly labeled syringes and 20.8% caused by selection of the wrong ampoule or vial, thus resulting in an incorrectly labeled syringe. Equipment misuse or failure accounted for 26%, incorrect route for 14%, and communication error for 4%. Administration of a drug in the OR is a complex procedure, with up to 41 steps involved in the first-time administration of a drug. Human factors experts classify 36 of these steps as automatic behavior, whereas 5 steps require conscious attention, decision, and judgment. Traditionally, the anesthesiologist performs all the steps alone, eliminating the opportunity for a double-check that is common elsewhere in medicine, in which a pharmacist checks the physician's prescription and a nurse checks both.

In addition, cardiac surgical procedures requiring CPB present the relatively unusual situation in which the anesthesiologist and the perfusionists may be administering drugs intravenously. Perfusionists frequently administer anesthetic drugs during CPB, and they may administer a variety of other drugs as well. Rarely, the perfusionist also may be an anesthesiologist, but whether the anesthesiologist supervises the perfusionist in the administration of drugs varies depending on the particular practice setting. Infusion pumps have become increasingly prevalent in the cardiac OR, and they offer significant advantages, including the ability to deliver very small volumes of fluids or drugs at precisely programmed rates. They are not, however, a panacea for medication errors. From 2005 through 2009, the US Food and Drug Administration (FDA) received approximately 56,000 reports of adverse events associated with the use of infusion pumps, including numerous injuries and deaths. Adverse events were related to hardware issues (battery failures, sparking, and fires), as well as software issues (error messages, double recording a single key strike such that 10 becomes 100). However, as any anesthesiologist can attest, many were related to poor user interface design or human factors issues. In addition to issues with the pumps, user error is common. Compliance with the drug library is critical for prevention of error, but a systematic review found numerous studies showing high rates of user override of soft alerts, as well as a variable compliance rate with drug library use.

Prevention of Drug Administration Errors

In 2010, the Anesthesia Patient Safety Foundation convened a consensus conference of more than 100 participants to develop strategies to improve medication safety in the OR. The consensus statements focused on four key areas: standardization, technology, pharmacy involvement, and culture (Box 24.1). Standardization focused primarily on having a single concentration of a drug available in the OR, but it also involved using standardized drug trays across all anesthetizing locations and having a single concentration of infusions that are administered by infusion devices with drug libraries. Pharmacy involvement was believed to be critical to reducing errors, from educational duties to managing the entire dispensing process, from ordering of drugs to providing them to the anesthesiologists. Bar code reading devices represent an underused technology, and bar coding drugs at the point of care to verify the correctness of the drug and the dose is widely regarded as a technologic solution that could improve

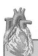

> **BOX 24.1** *Anesthesia Patient Safety Foundation Consensus Recommendations for Improving Medication Safety in the Operating Room*
>
> **Standardization**
>
> 1. High-alert drugs (eg, phenylephrine and epinephrine) should be available in standardized concentrations or diluents prepared by the pharmacy in a ready-to-use (bolus or infusion) form that is appropriate for both adult and pediatric patients. Infusions should be delivered by an electronically controlled smart device containing a drug library.
> 2. Ready-to-use syringes and infusions should have standardized, fully compliant, machine-readable labels.
> 3. *Additional ideas*
>   a. Interdisciplinary and uniform curriculum for medication administration safety to be available to all training programs and facilities
>   b. No concentrated versions of any potentially lethal agents in the operating room
>   c. Required read-back in an environment for extremely high-alert drugs such as heparin
>   d. Standardized placement of drugs within all anesthesia workstations in an institution
>   e. Convenient required method to save all used syringes and drug containers until the case is concluded
>   f. Standardized infusion libraries and protocols throughout an institution
>   g. Standardized route-specific connectors for tubing (intravenous, arterial, epidural, enteral).
>
> **Technology**
>
> 1. Every anesthetizing location should have a mechanism to identify medications before drawing up or administering them (bar code reader) and a mechanism to provide feedback, decision support, and documentation (automated information system).
> 2. *Additional ideas*
>   a. Technology training and device education for all users, possibly requiring formal certification
>   b. Improved and standardized user interfaces on infusion pumps
>   c. Mandatory safety checklists incorporated into all operating room systems.

24

> **BOX 24.1** *Anesthesia Patient Safety Foundation Consensus Recommendations for Improving Medication Safety in the Operating Room—cont'd*
>
> **Pharmacy/Prefilled/Premixed**
>
> 1. Routine provider-prepared medications should be discontinued whenever possible.
> 2. Clinical pharmacists should be part of the perioperative and operating room team.
> 3. Standardized preprepared medication kits by case type should be used whenever possible.
> 4. *Additional ideas*
>   a. Interdisciplinary and uniform curriculum for medication administration safety for all anesthesia professionals and pharmacists
>   b. Enhanced training of operating room pharmacists specifically as perioperative consultants
>   c. Deployment of ubiquitous automated dispensing machines in the operating room suite (with communication to central pharmacy and its information management system).
>
> **Culture**
>
> 1. Establish a "just culture" for reporting errors (including near misses) and discussion of lessons learned.
> 2. Establish a culture of education, understanding, and accountability through a required curriculum and continuing medical education and through dissemination of dramatic stories in the *APSF Newsletter* and educational videos.
> 3. Establish a culture of cooperation and recognition of the benefits of the STPC (standardization, technology, pharmacy/prefilled/premixed, and culture) paradigm within and among institutions, professional organizations, and accreditation agencies.
>
> Reprinted from Eichhorn JH. APSF hosts medication safety conference: consensus group defines challenges and opportunities for improved practice. *APSF Newslett.* 2010;25:1–8.

the accuracy of drug administration. The FDA issued a rule in February 2004 (updated in April 2014) that requires bar codes on most prescription drugs, certain over-the-counter drugs, and blood products. The FDA believes that effective bar code use could result in a 50% reduction in medication errors, thereby preventing 500,000 adverse events and transfusion errors while saving $93 billion over 20 years.

Some infusion pumps use drug libraries with predefined dosing limits and warn the practitioner if the dosing parameters entered will result in a dose that is outside the predefined dosing limits. Smart infusion pumps, although not perfect, repeatedly have been shown to intercept and prevent errors, primarily wrong rate and dose. A smart pump can potentially intercept errors during multiple steps in the medication delivery process. Most intercepted errors represented a low level of harm, but some studies included examples of many-fold errors of high-alert drugs (100 times the intended dose of norepinephrine) or more than 100-fold underdoses.

REDUCING SYSTEM VULNERABILITY

The preceding section focused on individual interventions designed to improve teamwork and communication and to avoid certain common errors in the cardiac

OR. However, most quality improvement initiatives in cardiac surgery represent comprehensive, multidisciplinary, and multiunit approaches.

The Geisinger Health System in Danville, Pennsylvania, asked surgeons to develop a care bundle for patients undergoing coronary artery bypass graft that would be evidence based and hard-wired into the care processes. A continual improvement approach was used to improve the implementation of the bundle. Significant improvements were seen in ICU readmissions, hospital readmissions, blood product use, and overall costs. Developed in 2006, this program has grown into a true "pay-for-performance" program, in which surgeons receive a base salary with incentives that are based on benchmarks of patient satisfaction and outcomes.

Multicenter collaboratives in cardiac surgery have been developed for the purpose of sharing site-specific and physician-specific data, as well as identifying best practices; these collaboratives have improved quality and safety over the past two decades. The first collaborative model began in 1987 with the formation of the Northern New England Cardiovascular Disease Study Group. Five hospitals in New England agreed to share patients' demographic, process, and outcome data, and developed risk-adjusted methods to create predictive models. Variability in actual versus predicted mortality rates led to round-robin site visits and frequent face-to-face meetings to understand how differences in practices affected outcomes. The teams met to share practices and to develop, test, and implement standardized protocols. This model of shared learning led to reductions in overall mortality rates, lower mortality rates in women undergoing cardiac operations, reduced rates of reexploration for significant bleeding, and more appropriate use of aspirin in patients undergoing coronary artery bypass graft.

SUGGESTED READINGS

Arriaga AF, Bader AM, Wong JM, et al. Simulation-based trial of surgical-crisis checklists. *N Engl J Med.* 2013;368:246–253.

Barbeito A, Lau WT, Weitzel N, et al. FOCUS: the Society of Cardiovascular Anesthesiologists' initiative to improve quality and safety in the cardiovascular operating room. *Anesth Analg.* 2014;119:777–783.

Catchpole K, Mishra A, Handa A, et al. Teamwork and error in the operating room—analysis of skills and roles. *Ann Surg.* 2008;247:699–706.

Catchpole K, Wiegmann D. Understanding safety and performance in the cardiac operating room: from 'sharp end' to 'blunt end'. *BMJ Qual Saf.* 2012;21:807–809.

Craig R, Moxey L, Young D, et al. Strengthening handover communication in pediatric cardiac intensive care. *Paediatr Anaesth.* 2012;22:393–399.

Culig MH, Kunkle RF, Frndak DC, et al. Improving patient care in cardiac surgery using Toyota production system based methodology. *Ann Thorac Surg.* 2011;91:394–399.

ElBardissi AW, Duclos A, Rawn JD, et al. Cumulative team experience matters more than individual surgeon experience in cardiac surgery. *J Thorac Cardiovasc Surg.* 2013;145:328–333.

ElBardissi AW, Wiegmann DA, Henrickson S, et al. Identifying methods to improve heart surgery: an operative approach and strategy for implementation on an organizational level. *Eur J Cardiothorac Surg.* 2008;34:1027–1033.

Hudson CC, McDonald B, Hudson JK, et al. Impact of anesthetic handover on mortality and morbidity in cardiac surgery: a cohort study. *J Cardiothorac Vasc Anesth.* 2015;29:11–16.

Manser T, Foster S. Effective handover communication: an overview of research and improvement efforts. *Best Pract Res Clin Anaesthesiol.* 2011;25:181–191.

Martinez EA, Marsteller JA, Thompson DA, et al. The Society of Cardiovascular Anesthesiologists' FOCUS initiative: Locating Errors Through Networked Surveillance (LENS) project vision. *Anesth Analg.* 2010;110:307–311.

Martinez EA, Thompson DA, Errett NA, et al. Review article: high stakes and high risk: a focused qualitative review of hazards during cardiac surgery. *Anesth Analg.* 2011;112:1061–1074.

Nagpal K, Abboudi M, Fischler L, et al. Evaluation of postoperative handover using a tool to assess information transfer and teamwork. *Ann Surg.* 2011;253:831–837.

Palmer G 2nd, Abernathy JH 3rd, Swinton G, et al. Realizing improved patient care through human-centered operating room design: a human factors methodology for observing flow disruptions in the cardiothoracic operating room. *Anesthesiology.* 2013;119:1066–1077.

24

Rothschild JM, Keohane CA, Rogers S, et al. Risks of complications by attending physicians after performing nighttime procedures. *JAMA*. 2009;302:1565–1572.

Schmid F, Goepfert MS, Kuhnt D, et al. The wolf is crying in the operating room: patient monitor and anesthesia workstation alarming patterns during cardiac surgery. *Anesth Analg*. 2011;112:78–83.

Spiess BD, Rotruck J, McCarthy H, et al. Human factors analysis of a near-miss event: oxygen supply failure during cardiopulmonary bypass. *J Cardiothorac Vasc Anesth*. 2015;29:204–209.

Thompson DA, Marsteller JA, Pronovost PJ, et al. Locating Errors Through Networked Surveillance: a multimethod approach to peer assessment, hazard identification, and prioritization of patient safety efforts in cardiac surgery. *J Patient Saf*. 2015;11:143–151.

Trew A, Searles B, Smith T, et al. Fatigue and extended work hours among cardiovascular perfusionists: 2010 survey. *Perfusion*. 2011;26:361–370.

Wadhera RK, Parker SH, Burkhart HM, et al. Is the "sterile cockpit" concept applicable to cardiovascular surgery critical intervals or critical events? The impact of protocol-driven communication during cardiopulmonary bypass. *J Thorac Cardiovasc Surg*. 2010;139:312–319.

IV

Section V

Extracorporeal Circulation

Chapter 25

Cardiopulmonary Bypass Management and Organ Protection

Hilary P. Grocott, MD, FRCPC, FASE •
Mark Stafford-Smith, MD, CM, FRCPC, FASE •
Christina T. Mora-Mangano, MD

Key Points

1. Cardiopulmonary bypass (CPB) is associated with a number of profound physiologic perturbations. The central nervous system, kidneys, gut, and heart are especially vulnerable to ischemic events associated with extracorporeal circulation.
2. Advanced age is the most important risk factor for stroke and neurocognitive dysfunction after CPB.
3. Acute renal injury from CPB can contribute directly to poor outcomes.
4. Drugs such as dopamine and diuretics do not prevent renal failure after CPB.
5. Myocardial stunning represents injury caused by short periods of myocardial ischemia that can occur during CPB.
6. Gastrointestinal complications after CPB include pancreatitis, gastrointestinal bleeding, bowel infarction, and cholecystitis.
7. Pulmonary complications such as atelectasis and pleural effusions are common after cardiac surgery with CPB.
8. Embolization, hypoperfusion, and inflammatory processes are common central pathophysiologic mechanisms responsible for organ dysfunction after CPB.
9. Controversy regarding the optimal management of blood flow, pressure, and temperature during CPB remains. Perfusion should be adequate to support ongoing oxygen requirements; mean arterial pressures of more than 70 mm Hg may benefit patients with cerebral and/or diffuse atherosclerosis. Arterial blood temperatures should never exceed 37.5°C.
10. Organ dysfunction cannot definitively be prevented during cardiac surgery with off-pump techniques.

The American Society of Anesthesiologists (ASA) states that the absence of anesthesia personnel during the conduct of a general anesthetic violates the first of the ASA Standards for Basic Anesthetic Monitoring. The absence of a member of the anesthesia care team during cardiopulmonary bypass (CPB) is below the accepted standard of care. At a minimum, the anesthesiologist's role during CPB is to maintain the anesthetic state—a more challenging task than the usual case when the patient's blood pressure, heart rate, and movement provide information regarding the depth of anesthesia. The complexities of CPB and the necessary integration of risk factors with the nuances of cardiac surgery warrant constant thinking and rethinking of how the conduct of CPB and surgery modulates the risks and what protective strategies need implementation.

GOALS AND MECHANICS OF CARDIOPULMONARY BYPASS

The CPB circuit is designed to perform four major functions: oxygenation and carbon dioxide elimination, circulation of blood, systemic cooling and rewarming, and diversion of blood from the heart to provide a bloodless surgical field. Typically, venous blood is drained by gravity from the right side of the heart into a reservoir that serves as a large mixing chamber for all blood return, additional fluids, and drugs. Because (in most instances) negative pressure is not employed, the amount of venous drainage is determined by the central venous pressure (CVP), the column height between the patient and reservoir, and resistance to flow in the venous circuitry. Negative pressure will enhance venous drainage and is used in some bypass approaches, including port-access CPB. Venous return may be decreased deliberately (as is done when restoring the patient's blood volume before coming off bypass) by application of a venous clamp. From the reservoir, blood is pumped to an oxygenator and heat exchanger unit before passing through an arterial filter and returning to the patient. Additional components of the circuit generally include pumps and tubing for cardiotomy suction, venting, and cardioplegia delivery and recirculation, as well as in-line blood gas monitors, bubble detectors, pressure monitors, and blood sampling ports. A schematic representation of a typical bypass circuit is depicted in Fig. 25.1.

The cannulation sites and type of CPB circuit used are dependent on the type of operation planned. Most cardiac procedures use full CPB, in which the blood is drained from the right side of the heart and returned to the systemic circulation through the aorta. The CPB circuit performs the function of the heart and lungs. Aorto-atriocaval cannulation is the preferred method of cannulation for CPB, although femoral arteriovenous cannulation may be the technique of choice for emergency access, "redo" sternotomy, and other clinical settings in which aortic or atrial cannulation is not feasible. Procedures involving the thoracic aorta are often performed using partial bypass in which a portion of oxygenated blood is removed from the left side of the heart and returned to the femoral artery. Perfusion of the head and upper extremity vessels is performed by the beating heart, and distal perfusion is provided below the level of the cross-clamp by retrograde flow by the femoral artery. All blood passes through the pulmonary circulation, eliminating the need for an oxygenator.

PHYSIOLOGIC PARAMETERS OF CARDIOPULMONARY BYPASS

The primary objective of CPB is maintenance of systemic perfusion and respiration. Controversy arises with the question of whether systemic oxygenation and perfusion should be "optimal or maximal" or "adequate or sufficient." Remarkably, after more than 60 years of CPB, there is continued disagreement regarding many fundamental management issues of extracorporeal circulation. Clinicians and investigators disagree on what the best strategies are for arterial blood pressure goals, pump flow, hematocrit,

25

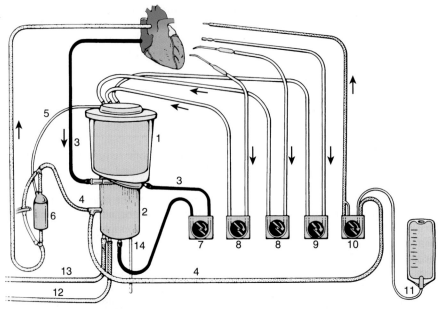

Fig. 25.1 Components of the extracorporeal circuit. *1*, Integral cardiotomy reservoir; *2*, membrane oxygenator bundle; *3*, venous blood line; *4*, arterial blood line; *5*, arterial filter purge line; *6*, arterial line filter; *7*, venous blood pump (also called the arterial pump head; this pump forces venous blood through the membrane oxygenator and arterialized blood to the patient's aortic root); *8*, cardiotomy suction pump; *9*, ventricular vent pump; *10*, cardioplegia pump; *11*, crystalloid cardioplegia; *12*, water inlet line; *13*, water outlet line; and *14*, gas inlet line. (From Davis RB, Kauffman JN, Cobbs TL, Mick SL. *Cardiopulmonary Bypass*. New York: Springer-Verlag; 1995:239.)

temperature, blood gas management, or mode of perfusion (pulsatile vs nonpulsatile). Whereas each of these physiologic parameters used to be taken into account individually, the application of each has organ-specific effects.

END-ORGAN EFFECTS OF CARDIOPULMONARY BYPASS

Modern cardiac surgery continues to be challenged by the risk of organ dysfunction and the morbidity and mortality that accompany it. A number of injurious common pathways may account for the organ dysfunction typically associated with cardiac surgery. CPB itself initiates a whole-body inflammatory response with the release of various injurious inflammatory mediators. Add to this the various preexisting patient comorbidities and the potential for organ ischemic injury caused by embolization and hypoperfusion, and it becomes clear why organ injury can occur. Most cardiac surgery, because of its very nature, causes some degree of myocardial injury. Other body systems can be affected by the perioperative insults associated with cardiac surgery (particularly CPB), including the kidneys, lungs, gastrointestinal (GI) tract, and central nervous system.

The following section describes the various organ dysfunction syndromes that can occur in patients undergoing cardiac surgical procedures, with particular emphasis directed at strategies for reducing these injuries.

Incidence and Significance of Injury

Central nervous system dysfunction after CPB represents a spectrum of clinical entities ranging from neurocognitive deficits, occurring in approximately 25% to 80% of patients, to overt stroke, occurring in 1% to 5% of patients. The significant disparity among studies in the incidence of these adverse cerebral outcomes relates in part to their definition and to numerous methodologic differences in the determination of neurologic and neurocognitive outcomes. Retrospective versus prospective assessments of neurologic deficits account for a significant portion of this inconsistency, as do the experience and expertise of the examiner. The timing of postoperative testing also affects determinations of outcome. For example, the rate of cognitive deficits can be as high as 80% for patients at discharge, between 10% and 35% at approximately 6 weeks after coronary artery bypass grafting (CABG), and 10% to 15% more than a year after surgery. Higher rates of cognitive deficits have been reported 5 years after surgery, when as many as 43% of patients have documented deficits.

Although the incidence of these deficits varies greatly, the significance of these injuries cannot be overemphasized. Cerebral injury is a most disturbing outcome of cardiac surgery. To have a patient's heart successfully treated by the planned operation but discover that the patient no longer functions as well cognitively or is immobilized from a stroke can be devastating. There are enormous personal, family, and financial consequences of extending a patient's life with surgery, only to have the quality of the life significantly diminished. Death after CABG, although having reached relatively low levels in the past decade (generally less than 1% overall), is increasingly attributable to cerebral injury.

Risk Factors for Central Nervous System Injury

Successful strategies for perioperative cerebral and other organ protection begin with a thorough understanding of the risk factors and pathophysiology involved. Risk factors for central nervous system injury can be considered from several different perspectives. Most studies outlining risk factors take into account only stroke. Few describe risk factors for neurocognitive dysfunction. Although it is often assumed that their respective risk factors are similar, few studies have consistently reported the preoperative risks of cognitive loss after cardiac surgery. Factors such as a poor baseline (preoperative) cognitive state, years of education (ie, more advanced education is protective), age, diabetes, and CPB time are frequently described.

Stroke is better characterized with respect to risk factors. Although studies differ somewhat as to all the risk factors, certain patient characteristics consistently correlate with an increased risk for cardiac surgery–associated neurologic injury. In a study conducted by the Multicenter Study of Perioperative Ischemia of 2108 patients from 24 centers, incidence of adverse cerebral outcome after CABG surgery was determined, and the risk factors were analyzed. Two types of adverse cerebral outcomes were defined. Type I included nonfatal stroke, transient ischemic attack, stupor or coma at time of discharge, and death caused by stroke or hypoxic encephalopathy. Type II included new deterioration in intellectual function, confusion, agitation, disorientation, and memory deficit without evidence of focal injury. A total of 129 (6.1%) of the 2108 patients had an adverse cerebral outcome in the perioperative period. Type I outcomes occurred in 66 (3.1%) of 2108 patients, with type II outcomes occurring in 63 (3.0%) of 2108 patients. Stepwise logistic regression analysis identified eight independent predictors of type I outcomes and seven independent predictors of type II outcomes (Table 25.1).

In a subsequent analysis of the same study database, a stroke risk index using preoperative factors was developed (Fig. 25.2). This risk index allowed for the preoperative calculation of the stroke risk based on the weighted combination of the preoperative factors, including age, unstable angina, diabetes mellitus, neurologic disease, previous coronary artery or other cardiac surgery, vascular disease, and pulmonary disease. Of all the factors in the Multicenter Study of Perioperative Ischemia analysis and in multiple other analyses, age appears to be the most overwhelmingly robust predictor of stroke and of neurocognitive dysfunction after cardiac surgery. Tuman and colleagues described that age has a greater impact on neurologic outcome than it does on perioperative myocardial infarction (MI) or low cardiac output states (LCOSs) after cardiac surgery (Fig. 25.3).

The influence of gender on adverse perioperative cerebral outcomes after cardiac surgery has been evaluated. Women appear to be at higher risk for stroke after cardiac surgery than men.

Another consistent risk factor for stroke after cardiac surgery is the presence of cerebrovascular disease and atheromatous disease of the aorta. With respect to cerebrovascular disease, patients who have had a prior stroke or transient ischemic attack are more likely to suffer a perioperative stroke. Even in the absence of symptomatic cerebrovascular disease, such as the presence of a carotid bruit, the risk of stroke increases with the severity of the carotid disease.

Although the presence of cerebrovascular disease is a risk factor for perioperative stroke, it does not always correlate well with the presence of significant aortic atherosclerosis. Atheromatous disease of the ascending aorta, aortic arch, and descending thoracic aorta has been consistently implicated as a risk factor for stroke in cardiac surgical patients. The widespread use of transesophageal echocardiography (TEE)

Table 25.1 Risk Factors for Adverse Cerebral Outcomes After Cardiac Surgery

Risk Factor	Type I Outcomes	Type II Outcomes
Proximal aortic atherosclerosis	4.52 (2.52–8.09)[a]	
History of neurologic disease	3.19 (1.65–6.15)	
Use of IABP	2.60 (1.21–5.58)	
Diabetes mellitus	2.59 (1.46–4.60)	
History of hypertension	2.31 (1.20–4.47)	
History of pulmonary disease	2.09 (1.14–3.85)	2.37 (1.34–4.18)
History of unstable angina	1.83 (1.03–3.27)	
Age (per additional decade)	1.75 (1.27–2.43)	2.20 (1.60–3.02)
Admission systolic BP >180 mm Hg		3.47 (1.41–8.55)
History of excessive alcohol intake		2.64 (1.27–5.47)
History of CABG		2.18 (1.14–4.17)
Arrhythmia on day of surgery		1.97 (1.12–3.46)
Antihypertensive therapy		1.78 (1.02–3.10)

[a]Adjusted odds ratio (95% confidence intervals) for type I and type II cerebral outcomes associated with selected risk factors from the Multicenter Study of Perioperative Ischemia.
BP, Blood pressure; CABG, coronary artery bypass graft surgery; IABP, intraaortic balloon pump.
From Arrowsmith JE, Grocott HP, Reves JG, Newman MF. Central nervous system complications of cardiac surgery. Br J Anaesth 2000;84:378–393.

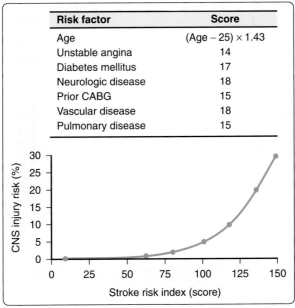

Risk factor	Score
Age	(Age − 25) × 1.43
Unstable angina	14
Diabetes mellitus	17
Neurologic disease	18
Prior CABG	15
Vascular disease	18
Pulmonary disease	15

Fig. 25.2 Preoperative stroke risk for patients undergoing CABG surgery. The individual patient's stroke risk can be determined from the corresponding cumulative risk index score in the nomogram. *CABG*, Coronary artery bypass graft; *CNS*, central nervous system. (Modified from Arrowsmith JE, Grocott HP, Reves JG, Newman MF. Central nervous system complications of cardiac surgery. *Br J Anaesth*. 2000;84:378–393.)

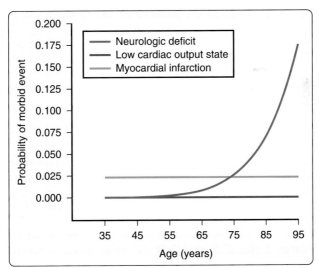

Fig. 25.3 The relative effect of age on the predicted probability of neurologic and cardiac morbidity after cardiac surgery. (Modified from Tuman KJ, McCarthy RJ, Najafi H, Ivankovich AD. Differential effects of advanced age on neurologic and cardiac risks of coronary artery operations. *J Thorac Cardiovasc Surg*. 1992;104:1510–1517.)

25

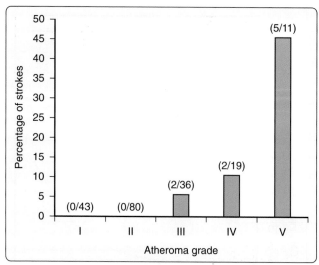

Fig. 25.4 Stroke rate 1 week after cardiac surgery as a function of atheroma severity. Atheroma was graded by transesophageal echocardiography as follows: I, normal; II, intimal thickening; III, plaque <5 mm thick; IV, plaque >5 mm thick; V, any plaque with a mobile segment. (From Hartman GS, Yao FS, Bruefach M 3rd, et al. Severity of aortic atheromatous disease diagnosed by transesophageal echocardiography predicts stroke and other outcomes associated with coronary artery surgery: a prospective study. *Anesth Analg.* 1996;83:701–708.)

and epiaortic ultrasonography has added new dimensions to the detection of aortic atheromatous disease and the understanding of its relation to stroke risk. These imaging modalities have allowed the diagnosis of atheromatous disease to be made in a more sensitive and detailed manner, contributing greatly to the information regarding potential stroke risk. The risk of cerebral embolism from aortic atheroma was described early in the history of cardiac surgery and has been described repeatedly and in detail since then. Studies have consistently reported higher stroke rates for patients with increasing atheromatous aortic involvement (particularly the ascending and arch segments). This relationship is outlined in Fig. 25.4.

Causes of Perioperative Central Nervous System Injury

Because central nervous system dysfunction represents a wide range of injuries, differentiating the individual causes of these various types of injuries becomes somewhat difficult (Box 25.1). They are frequently grouped together and superficially discussed as representing different severities on a continuum of brain injury. This likely misrepresents the different causes of these injuries. The following section addresses stroke and cognitive injury (Table 25.2), and their respective causes are differentiated when appropriate.

Cerebral Embolization

Macroemboli (eg, atheromatous plaque) and microemboli (ie, gaseous and particulate) are generated during CPB, and many emboli find their way to the cerebral vasculature. Macroemboli are responsible for stroke, with microemboli being implicated in the development of less severe encephalopathies. Sources for the microemboli are numerous and include those generated de novo from the interactions of blood within the CPB

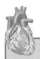

Potential Contributors to Central Nervous System Complications After Cardiopulmonary Bypass

Cerebral emboli
Global hypoperfusion
Inflammation
Cerebral hyperthermia
Cerebral edema
Blood-brain barrier dysfunction
Genetics

Table 25.2 Potential Contributors to Causes of Cognitive Dysfunction After Cardiac Surgery

Cause	Possible Settings
Cerebral microemboli	Generated during cardiopulmonary bypass (CPB); mobilization of atheromatous material or entrainment of air from the operative field; gas injections into the venous reservoir of the CPB apparatus
Global cerebral hypoperfusion	Hypotension, occlusion by an atheromatous embolus leading to stroke
Inflammation (systemic and cerebral)	Injurious effects of CPB, such as blood interacting with the foreign surfaces of pump-oxygenator; upregulation of proinflammatory cyclooxygenase mRNA
Cerebral hyperthermia	Hypothermia during CPB; hyperthermia during and after cardiac surgery, such as aggressive rewarming
Cerebral edema	Edema from global cerebral hypoperfusion or increased cerebral venous pressure from cannula misplacement
Blood-brain barrier dysfunction	Diffuse cerebral inflammation; ischemia from cerebral microembolization
Genetic influences	Effects of single nucleotide polymorphisms on risk for neurologic injury or impaired recovery from injury

25

apparatus (eg, platelet-fibrin aggregates) and those generated within the body by the production and mobilization of atheromatous material or entrainment of air from the operative field. Other sources for emboli include lipid-laden debris that can be added by cardiotomy suction. Other gaseous emboli may be generated through injections into the venous reservoir of the CPB apparatus itself.

Global Cerebral Hypoperfusion

The concept that global cerebral hypoperfusion during CPB may lead to neurologic and neurocognitive complications originates from the earliest days of cardiac surgery, when significant (in degree and duration) systemic hypotension was a relatively common event. Although this concept (ie, that hypotension would lead to global cerebral hypoperfusion) makes intuitive sense, studies that have examined the relationship between mean arterial pressure (MAP) and cognitive decline after cardiac surgery have generally failed to show any significant relationship.

This is not the case for stroke, for which a link between hypotension and the presence of a significantly atheromatous aorta with an increased risk of stroke has been demonstrated. This is not a clear relationship, however, and likely represents an interaction between macroembolism and global cerebral hypoperfusion. It is likely, for example, that if an area of the brain that is being perfused by a cerebral vessel becomes occluded by an atheromatous embolus, it may be more susceptible to hypoperfusion if collateral perfusion is compromised by concomitant systemic hypotension.

Temperature-Related Factors

During rewarming from hypothermic CPB, there can be an overshoot in cerebral temperature due to aggressive rewarming generally aimed at decreasing time on CPB and overall operating room time. This cerebral hyperthermia may well be responsible for some of the injury that occurs in the brain. The postoperative period is also a critical time in which hyperthermia can contribute to brain injury. It is not clear whether this hyperthermia causes de novo injury or exacerbates injury that has already occurred (eg, injury that might be induced by cerebral microembolization or global cerebral hypoperfusion). It is assumed that the brain is injured during CPB, and because experimental brain injury is known to cause hyperthermia (resulting from hypothalamic injury), the hyperthermia that is demonstrated in the postoperative period may be caused by the occurrence or extent of brain injury. However, if hyperthermia results from the inflammatory response to CPB, the hyperthermia itself may induce or exacerbate cerebral injury.

Inflammation

Although it is well known that blood interacts with the foreign surfaces of the pump-oxygenator to stimulate a profound inflammatory response, the systemic end-organ effects of this inflammatory response are less clearly defined. In settings other than cardiac surgery, inflammation has been demonstrated to injure the brain directly (eg, sepsis-mediated encephalopathy), but it is also known to result as a response to various cerebral injuries (eg, ischemic stroke). There is no direct evidence that inflammation causes cardiac surgery–associated adverse cerebral outcome; however, there is some supportive indirect evidence. There is increasing genetic evidence linking inflammation to adverse cerebral outcomes, both stroke and cognitive loss.

Cerebral Edema

Cerebral edema after CPB has been reported in several studies. The explanation for why cerebral edema may occur early in the period after bypass is not clear. It may be caused by cytotoxic edema resulting from global cerebral hypoperfusion or possibly by hyponatremia-induced cerebral edema. Generalized cerebral edema due to increases in cerebral venous pressure caused by cannula misplacement, which frequently occurs during CPB, is another reason. Specifically, use of a dual-stage venous cannula can often lead to cerebral venous congestion during the vertical displacement of the heart during access to the lateral and posterior epicardial coronary arteries. It is not clear from these studies whether the edema results because of injury that occurs during CPB, leading to cognitive decline, or whether the edema itself directly causes the injury by consequent increases in intracranial pressure with global or regional decreases in cerebral blood flow (CBF) and resulting ischemia.

Blood-Brain Barrier Dysfunction

The function of the blood-brain barrier (BBB) is to aid in maintaining the homeostasis of the extracellular cerebral milieu protecting the brain against fluctuations in various ion concentrations, neurotransmitters, and growth factors that are present in the serum. The impact of CPB on the function and integrity of the BBB is not clearly known.

It is difficult to determine whether the changes in BBB integrity, if present at all, are a primary cause of brain dysfunction or simply a result of other initiating events such as ischemia (ie, from cerebral microembolization) or a diffuse cerebral inflammatory event. Changes in the BBB could cause some of the cerebral edema that has been demonstrated, or could result from cerebral edema if the edema resulted in ischemic injury (from increases in intracranial pressure).

Neuroprotective Strategies

Emboli Reduction

There are multiple sources of particulate and gaseous emboli during cardiac surgery. Within the CPB circuit itself, particulate emboli in the form of platelet-fibrin aggregates and other debris are generated. Gaseous emboli can be created in the circuit or augmented if already present by factors such as turbulence-related cavitation and potentially even by vacuum-assisted venous drainage. Air in the venous return tubing is variably handled by the bypass circuit (ie, reservoir, oxygenator, and arterial filters). The ability of the circuit to prevent the transit of gaseous emboli through the oxygenator varies considerably between manufacturers and remains a significant source of emboli. The impact of perfusionist interventions on cerebral embolic load has also been confirmed.

Significant quantities of air can be entrained from the surgical field into the heart itself; flooding the field with carbon dioxide has been proposed as being effective in reducing this embolic source. Its ability to specifically reduce cerebral injury has not been rigorously evaluated, although it has been demonstrated to reduce the amount of TEE-detectable bubbles in the heart after cardiac surgery significantly. Even with the use of carbon dioxide in the surgical field, significant amounts of entrained air can be present. Although the oxygenator-venous reservoir design attempts to purge this air before reaching the inflow cannula, the arterial line filter handles a great deal of what is left. The capacity of the arterial filter to remove all sources of emboli (gaseous or particulate) has significant limitations, and, despite its use, emboli can easily pass through and on into the aortic root.

The aortic cannula may be very important to reduce cerebral emboli production. Placement of the cannula into an area of the aorta with a large atheroma burden may cause the direct generation of emboli from the "sandblasting" of atherosclerotic material in the aorta. The use of a long aortic cannula, where the tip of the cannula lies beyond the origin of the cerebral vessels, has been found to reduce emboli load. The type of cannula itself may be an important factor. Various designs have allowed the reduction of various sandblasting-type jets emanating from the aortic cannula. Blood that is returned from the surgical field though the use of the cardiotomy suction may significantly contribute to the particulate load in the CPB circuit and subsequently in the brain. The use of cell-salvage devices to process shed blood before returning it to the venous reservoir may minimize the amount of particulate- or lipid-laden material that contributes to embolization. Most of this material is small enough or so significantly deformable (because of its high lipid content) that it can pass through standard 20- to 40-μm arterial filters. There are several issues with the cell saver, however. One is the cost that is incurred with its use, and the other is its side effects of reducing platelet and coagulation factors through its intrinsic washing processes. Modest use of cell salvage up to a certain, although as yet undefined, volume of blood is likely prudent. Despite this rationale, the results from studies examining neurologic outcome have shown variable effects of cell-saver use on cognitive outcome.

25

Management of Aortic Atherosclerosis

The widespread use of TEE and complementary (and preferably routine) epiaortic scanning has contributed greatly to the understanding of the risks involved in managing patients with a severely atheromatous aorta. There is indisputable evidence linking stroke to atheroma. However, the strength of association between atheroma and cognitive decline seen after cardiac surgery is less clear. Regardless of whether atheroma causes cognitive dysfunction, its contribution to cardiac surgery–associated stroke is enough to warrant specific strategies for management.

One of the difficulties in interpreting studies that have evaluated atheroma avoidance strategies is the absence of any form of blinding of the investigators. For the most part, a strategy is chosen based on the presence of known atheroma, and the results of these patients are compared with historic controls. What constitutes the best strategy is unclear. Multiple techniques can be used to minimize atheromatous material liberated from the aortic wall from getting into the cerebral circulation. These range from optimizing placement of the aortic cannula in the aorta to an area relatively devoid of plaque to the use of specialized cannulas that reduce the sandblasting of the aortic wall. The avoidance of partial occlusion clamping for proximal vein graft placement by performing all of the anastomoses in a single application of an aortic cross-clamp has demonstrated a benefit. Specialized cannulas that contain filtering technologies and other means to deflect emboli to more distal sites have been developed and studied. Technology is advancing rapidly, and proximal (and distal) coronary artery anastomotic devices are becoming increasingly available and focus on minimizing manipulation of the ascending aorta. None of these aortic manipulations has yet yielded significant neuroprotective results in large, prospective, randomized trials, but their potential holds promise.

Pulsatile Perfusion

A large body of literature has accumulated comparing the physiology of pulsatile with nonpulsatile perfusion. Nevertheless, it remains uncertain whether pulsatile CPB has shown substantive clinical improvement in any outcome measure compared with standard, nonpulsatile CPB. Claims of advantages to pulsatile flow are effectively offset by conflicting studies of similar design.

Nonpulsatile CPB is the most commonly practiced form of artificial perfusion. As intuitive as it may seem that this type of nonphysiologic, nonpulsatile pump flow could be injurious, there is an overall lack of data to suggest that using pulsatile flow during clinical CPB has a neurologic benefit. A significant limitation to most pulsatility studies is that, because of technical limitations, true "physiologic" pulsatility is almost never accomplished. Instead, variations of sinusoidal pulse waveforms are produced that do not replicate the kinetics and hydrodynamics of normal physiologic pulsation. A fundamental difference between pulsatile and nonpulsatile flow is that additional hydraulic energy is required and applied to move blood when pulsatile flow is used. This extra kinetic energy is known to improve red blood cell transit, capillary perfusion, and lymphatic function. CPB may influence many of the properties of the blood (viscosity) and the vasculature itself (arterial tone, size, and geometry) as a result of hemodilution, hypothermia, alteration of red blood cell deformability, and redistribution of flow. As a result of these changes, generation of what appears to be a normal pulsatile *pressure* waveform may not result in a normal pulsatile *flow* waveform. Simply reproducing pulsatile pressure is not sufficient to ensure reproduction of pulsatile flow, nor does it allow quantification of energetics.

Newer pulsatile technologies may better reproduce the normal biologic state of cardiac pulsatility. Computer technologies that allow creating a more physiologic pulsatile perfusion pattern have demonstrated, at least experimentally, preservation of cerebral oxygenation. However, most studies do not present convincing evidence to suggest that routine pulsatile flow during CPB, as can be achieved by widely available technology, is warranted.

Acid-Base Management: Alpha-Stat Versus pH-Stat

Optimal acid-base management during CPB has long been debated. Theoretically, alpha-stat management maintains normal CBF autoregulation with the coupling of cerebral metabolism ($CMRO_2$) to CBF, allowing adequate oxygen delivery while minimizing the potential for emboli. Although early studies were unable to document a difference in neurologic or neuropsychologic outcome between the two techniques, later studies showed reductions in cognitive performance when pH-stat management was used, particularly in cases with prolonged CPB times. pH-Stat management (ie, CO_2 is added to the oxygenator fresh gas flow) results in a higher CBF than is needed for the brain's metabolic requirements. This luxury perfusion risks excessive delivery of emboli to the brain. Except for congenital heart surgery, for which most outcome data support the use of pH-stat management because of its improvement in homogenous brain cooling before circulatory arrest, adult outcome data support the use of only alpha-stat management.

Temperature and Rewarming Strategies

The use of some hypothermia remains a mainstay of perioperative management in the cardiac surgical patient. Its widespread use relates to its putative, although not definitively proved, global organ protective effects. Although hypothermia has a measurable effect on suppressing cerebral metabolism (approximately 6% to 7% decline per 1°C), it is likely that its other neuroprotective effects may be mediated by nonmetabolic actions. In the ischemic brain, for example, moderate hypothermia has multimodal effects. Although experimental demonstrations of this are abundant, clinical examples of hypothermia neuroprotection have been elusive.

Just as hypothermia has some likely protective effects on the brain, hyperthermia, in an opposite and disproportionate fashion, has some injurious effects. Although the studies referred to previously demonstrated no neuroprotective effect, there is emerging evidence that, if some degree of neuroprotection is afforded by hypothermia, it may be negated by the obligatory rewarming period that must ensue. Although there are numerous sites for monitoring temperature during cardiac surgery, several warrant special consideration. One of the lessons learned from the three warm versus cold trials, as well as from other information regarding temperature gradients between the CPB circuit, nasopharynx, and brain, is that it is important to monitor (and use as a target) a temperature site relevant to the organ of interest. If it is the body, a core temperature measured in the bladder, rectum, pulmonary artery, or esophagus is appropriate. However, if the temperature of the brain is desired, it is important to look at surrogates of brain temperature. These include nasopharyngeal temperature and tympanic membrane temperature. Testing these different temperature sites has demonstrated that vast temperature gradients appear across the body and across the brain. It is likely that during periods of rapid flux (eg, during rewarming), these temperature gradients are maximal.

Mean Arterial Pressure Management During Cardiopulmonary Bypass

The relationship between blood pressure during CPB and CBF is pertinent to understanding whether MAP can be optimized to reduce neurologic injury. Clinically, the available data suggest that, in an otherwise normal patient, CBF during nonpulsatile hypothermic CPB using alpha-stat blood gas management is largely independent of MAP as long as that MAP is within or near the autoregulatory range for the patient (ie, 50–100 mm Hg). Underlying essential hypertension as a comorbidity, however, likely includes a rightward shift in the autoregulatory curve. The degree to which this rightward shift occurs is not clear, but it would be reasonable to expect that it is at least 10 mm Hg, suggesting that the lower range of autoregulatory blood flow is more likely to be 60-70 than 50 mm Hg. In addition, diabetes may lead to autoregulatory disturbances that make CBF more pressure passive than in patients without diabetes.

Although the data relating MAP to neurologic and neurocognitive outcome after CABG surgery are inconclusive, most data suggest that MAP during CPB is not the primary predictor of cognitive decline or stroke after cardiac surgery. However, with increasing age, MAP during CPB may play a role in improving cerebral collateral perfusion to regions embolized, improving neurologic and cognitive outcome. Some experimental data in the noncardiac surgical setting suggest that collateral perfusion to penumbral areas of brain suffering from ischemic injury are relatively protected by higher perfusion pressure. Overall, it appears that MAP (in the normal range) has little effect on cognitive outcome, but in those with significant aortic atheroma, it may be prudent to increase blood pressure modestly.

Rather than choosing a specific or fixed (and arguably arbitrary) blood pressure threshold based on the conflicting preceding data, a more prudent approach may be to individualize the blood pressure targets based on the emerging concept of cerebral oximetry–based real-time physiologic feedback. Technologies such as near-infrared spectroscopy-based cerebral oximetry have played an important role in guiding this approach. This may allow for the determination of individual autoregulatory-driven blood pressure targets.

Glucose Management

Hyperglycemia is a common occurrence during the course of cardiac surgery. Administration of cardioplegia containing glucose and stress response–induced alterations in insulin secretion and resistance increase the potential for significant hyperglycemia. Hyperglycemia has been repeatedly demonstrated to impair neurologic outcome after experimental focal and global cerebral ischemia. The explanation for this adverse effect likely relates to the effects that hyperglycemia has on anaerobic conversion of glucose to lactate, which ultimately causes intracellular acidosis and impairs intracellular homeostasis and metabolism. A second injurious mechanism relates to an increase in the release of excitotoxic amino acids in response to hyperglycemia in the setting of cerebral ischemia. If hyperglycemia is injurious to the brain, the threshold for making injuries worse appears to be 180 to 200 mg/dL.

The appropriate type of perioperative serum glucose management and whether it adversely affects neurologic outcome in patients undergoing CPB remain unclear. The major difficulty in hyperglycemia treatment is the relative ineffectiveness of insulin therapy. Using excessive amounts of insulin during hypothermic periods may lead to rebound hypoglycemia after CPB. Studies that have attempted to maintain normoglycemia during cardiac surgery with the use of an insulin protocol have shown that, even with aggressive insulin treatment, hyperglycemia is often resistant and may actually predispose patients to postoperative hypoglycemia. This concern over potentially increasing adverse effects by exerting tight glycemic controls has reportedly been supported. Attempting to mediate injury may predispose patients to additional injury.

Off-Pump Cardiac Surgery

Off-pump coronary artery bypass (OPCAB) surgery is frequently used for the operative treatment of coronary artery disease. The impact on adverse cerebral outcomes after cardiac surgery has been variably reported. Although early data suggested less cognitive decline after OPCAB procedures, most studies have not seen it eliminated altogether. The reasons for this are unclear but likely reflect the complex pathophysiology involved. For example, if inflammatory processes play a role in initiating or propagating cerebral injury, OPCAB, with its continued use of sternotomy, heparin administration, and wide hemodynamic swings, all of which may contribute to a stress and inflammatory response, may be a significant reason why cognitive dysfunction is still seen. Ascending aortic manipulation, with its ensuing particulate embolization, is also still commonly used.

Pharmacologic Neuroprotection

No pharmacologic therapies have been approved by the US Food and Drug Administration or foreign regulatory agencies for the prevention or treatment of cardiac surgery–associated cerebral injury, despite numerous previous investigations of specific pharmacologic agents in this setting (Table 25.3). The failure to discern any single compound that might protect the brain is not unique to cardiac surgery. With the exception of thrombolysis, there are no other therapies in the general medical field either.

THIOPENTAL

Thiopental was one of the first agents investigated as a potential neuroprotective agent for patients undergoing cardiac surgery. The proposed mechanism related to the suppressive effects of barbiturates on cerebral metabolism. This mechanism, along with experimental data reporting the beneficial effects of the barbiturates, made it a logical choice for cardiac surgery. However, results of additional investigations of the use of thiopental were not as positive. These negative trials and the side effects of prolonged sedation with barbiturates served to quell the optimism for barbiturates. The beneficial effects of the thiopental might not be related to a direct neuroprotective effect but to an indirect effect on reducing emboli. The well-known cerebral vaso-constricting effects of thiopental (matching CBF with a barbiturate-induced reduction in $CMRO_2$) may result in a reduction in embolic load to the brain during CPB and, as a result, a beneficial effect on neurologic outcome. It has subsequently been shown that isoelectricity itself is not necessary to incur a neuroprotective benefit from barbiturates.

25

Table 25.3	Agents Studied as Pharmacologic Neuroprotectants During Cardiac Surgery	
Agent	**Agent**
Thiopental	Lidocaine
Propofol	β-Blockers
Acadesine	Pegorgotein
Aprotinin	C5 complement inhibitor (pexelizumab)
Nimodipine	Lexiphant (platelet-activating factor antagonist)
GM_1 ganglioside	Clomethiazole
Dextromethorphan	Ketamine
Remacemide	

PROPOFOL

Propofol has effects similar to those of thiopental on $CMRO_2$ and CBF and has some antioxidant and calcium channel antagonist properties. Along with supportive data from experimental cerebral ischemia studies, propofol has been evaluated as a neuroprotectant in the setting of cardiac surgery. In a randomized trial ($N = 215$) of burst-suppression doses of propofol, there was no beneficial effect on cognitive outcome at 2 months. The investigators concluded that electroencephalogram (EEG) burst-suppression doses of propofol provided no neuroprotection during valvular cardiac surgery. No other studies in nonvalve cardiac surgery have assessed the effects of propofol on the brain.

APROTININ

In a large, multicenter trial of aprotinin for primary or redo CABG and valvular surgery evaluating its blood loss–reducing effects, the high-dose aprotinin group also had a lower stroke rate compared with placebo ($P = .032$). There has been considerable investigation of the potential mechanism for aprotinin-derived neuroprotection. Initial enthusiasm focused on its antiinflammatory effects potentially preventing some of the adverse inflammatory sequelae of cerebral ischemia. However, aprotinin may have beneficial effects independent of any direct neuroprotective effect through an indirect effect of modulating cerebral emboli. If a drug reduces the amount of particulate-containing blood returning from the operative field to the cardiotomy reservoir (by decreasing overall blood loss), cerebral emboli and the resulting neurologic consequences may also be decreased.

More recently, the potential adverse effects of aprotinin were reported by Mangano and coworkers in their observational study of 4374 patients. In that study, patients having received aprotinin had a significantly higher rate of cerebrovascular complications ($P < .001$). The Blood Conservation Using Antifibrinolytics: A Randomized Trial (BART) reported a significant reduction in bleeding but an overall mortality risk with aprotinin compared with other antifibrinolytics. Although the Mangano study and the BART trial contributed to the market withdrawal of aprotinin, the relevance of the potential neurologic effects of kallikrein inhibition remains.

NIMODIPINE

Calcium plays a central role in propagating cerebral ischemic injury. For this reason, as well as a demonstrated beneficial effect of the calcium channel blocker nimodipine in subarachnoid hemorrhage and experimental cerebral ischemia, a randomized, double-blind, placebo-controlled, single-center trial was undertaken to assess the effect of nimodipine on outcomes after valvular surgery. The trial was not completed after safety concerns regarding an increased bleeding and death rate in the nimodipine group prompted an external review board to suspend the study. There was also no neuropsychologic deficit difference between the placebo or nimodipine groups at this interim review. As a result, the true effect of this drug or similar calcium trial blockers may never be fully known in this setting.

LIDOCAINE

Intravenous lidocaine, because of its properties as a sodium channel blocking agent and potential antiinflammatory effects, has been investigated as a neuroprotectant in cardiac surgery. Lidocaine cannot be recommended at this time as a clinical neuroprotective agent in cardiac surgery, but it continues to be investigated.

β-BLOCKERS

Although the use of β-blockers in patients with cardiac disease has been predominantly directed toward the prevention of adverse myocardial events, in a study of neurologic outcomes after cardiac surgery, β-blockers have been demonstrated to have mixed effects in neurologic outcomes. Support for a potential neuroprotective effect from β-blockers has come from a study of carvedilol, which is known to have mixed adrenergic antagonist effects, as well as acting as an antioxidant and inhibitor of apoptosis. Any potential benefit to β-blocker therapy needs to be tempered by recent data in the non–cardiac surgery population that demonstrated neurologic harm. The POISE trial, although demonstrating a reduction in MI, demonstrated an increase in stroke rate in patients randomized to receive metoprolol perioperatively. It is unclear how this information pertains to the cardiac surgical population.

STEROIDS

Corticosteroids have long been considered as potential cerebroprotective agents, in part because of their ability to reduce the inflammatory response. Inflammation is considered an important factor in propagating ischemia-mediated brain injury. However, with the exception of spinal cord injury, steroids have never been demonstrated to possess any significant clinical neuroprotective properties. Part of their lack of effect may result from the hyperglycemia that generally follows their administration. Hyperglycemia in animal models and several human studies of cerebral injury has been associated with worsened neurologic outcome. In the largest-ever trial of a potentially neuroprotective agent in cardiac surgery, they were unable to show any beneficial effort in stroke, cognitive outcome, or delirium. The administration of steroids with the intent of conferring some degree of neuroprotection during cardiac surgery cannot be recommended.

KETAMINE

The neuroprotective effects of S(+D)-ketamine, a frequently used anesthetic that is also an N-methyl-D-aspartate (NMDA)-receptor antagonist, was evaluated in a small ($N = 106$) study enrolling cardiac surgery patients. The incidence of neurocognitive dysfunction 10 weeks after surgery trended toward being lower in the ketamine group (20% for ketamine vs 25% for controls; $P = .54$), but, because the study was underpowered, it was not a significant change. There has been renewed interest in ketamine for its potential to reduce the incidence of delirium. This drug awaits further large trials to determine its potential benefit. Although there is some experimental evidence supporting its role as a neuroprotectant, there is insufficient clinical evidence to support its use for this specific indication.

◼ ACUTE KIDNEY INJURY

Despite concern for almost half a century over the seriousness of renal dysfunction as a complication after cardiac surgery, acute kidney injury (AKI) persists as a prevalent and important predictor of early death. Even during procedures where there is no evidence of AKI based on serum creatinine levels, more subtle markers often demonstrate renal tubular injury. Increasing degrees of AKI after cardiac surgery are associated with poorer outcome, greater costs, and more short- and long-term resource utilization. The degree of AKI also predicts poorer long-term survival in patients returning home. While some of the harm associated with AKI simply reflects its accompaniment of other serious complications as an "epiphenomenon" (eg, sepsis), there is also compelling evidence that AKI itself contributes to adverse outcome. Accumulation of "uremic toxins" beyond creatinine has widespread adverse effects on most organ systems, and, where it is best studied in chronic renal disease, inadequate clearance of uremic toxins adversely affects survival.

Even when postoperative dialysis is avoided, the strong relationship of AKI with adverse outcome continues to fuel the search for therapies to protect the kidney. Although practicing avoidance of the numerous recognized renal insults is a well-established approach to reducing AKI rates, the search for renoprotective strategies has otherwise been extremely disappointing.

Clinical Course, Incidence, and Significance

The specific surgical procedure is important when considering postoperative AKI. The incidence varies widely by operation, each cardiac surgery having its own characteristic renal insult and pattern of serum creatinine change. For example, creatinine often drops immediately after CABG surgery (presumably as a result of hemodilution), but then rises, typically peaking on postoperative day 2, then returning toward or even below baseline values in subsequent days. Up to 30% of patients having CABG sustain sufficient insult to meet threshold AKI criteria (eg, RIFLE–injury/AKIN criteria: a creatinine rise >0.3 mg/dL or 50% within the first 48 hours). The reported incidence thus varies according to the definition of kidney injury, as well as by the institution reporting their results.

Of the 1% to 3% of patients sustaining AKI severe enough to require dialysis following CABG, up to 60% will die before being discharged from the hospital, and many of the survivors will require continuing dialysis or be left with chronic kidney disease. The rate of "renal recovery" after AKI is also difficult to predict, but emerging evidence suggests it is highly associated with outcome and apparently independent of AKI.

Risk Factors and Surgery-Related Acute Kidney Injury Pathophysiology

Numerous studies have characterized risk factors for nephropathy after cardiac surgery (Fig. 25.5). Despite an increasing understanding of perioperative renal dysfunction, known risk factors account for only one-third of the observed variability in creatinine rise after cardiac surgery. Procedure-related risk factors include emergent and redo operations, valvular procedures, and operations requiring a period of circulatory arrest or extended durations of CPB. Infection and sepsis, atrial fibrillation, and indicators of LCOS, including need for inotropic agents and insertion of an intraaortic balloon pump (IABP) during surgery, also have been associated with renal impairment.

Preoperative demographic risk factors identified include advanced age, increased body weight, African American ethnicity, hypertension and wide pulse pressure, baseline anemia, peripheral or carotid atherosclerotic disease, diabetes, preoperative hyperglycemia, and/or elevated hemoglobin A1c in nondiabetics, reduced left ventricular (LV) function, and obstructive pulmonary disease. Interestingly, baseline chronic kidney disease is not a risk factor for AKI, but since even small amounts of additional renal impairment may lead to dialysis when severe renal disease is present at baseline, these individuals are at greatest risk for dialysis. A genetic predisposition to AKI exists and explains more variation in AKI after cardiac surgery than conventional clinical risk factors alone.

Using intraoperative epiaortic scanning, ascending aortic atheroma burden has been shown to correlate with AKI. Similarly, postoperative AKI has been correlated with arterial emboli load. Other emboli sources may be relevant to AKI in some circumstances. Fat droplets, particulates, and bubbles are common during cardiac surgery. Renal embolic infarcts from any source are wedge-shaped and involve adjacent

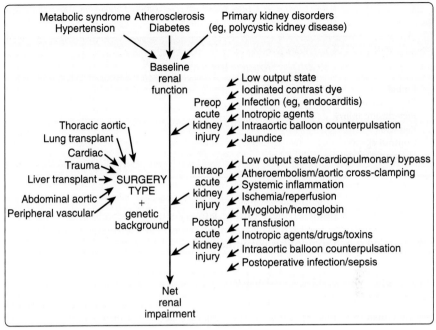

Fig. 25.5 Numerous sources of kidney insult play a variably important role for each patient during the perioperative period. (Used with permission and modified from Stafford-Smith M, Patel UD, Phillips-Bute BG, et al. Acute kidney injury and chronic kidney disease after cardiac surgery. *Adv Chronic Kidney Dis.* 2008;15:257–277.)

cortex and medulla, highlighting the vascular arrangement and lack of redundancy of kidney perfusion.

Many elements of cardiac surgery contribute to the risk of hypoperfusion and ischemia-reperfusion–mediated AKI. Embolism, LCOS, and exogenous catecholamines can all contribute, leading to cellular high-energy phosphate depletion, calcium accumulation, oxygen free radical generation, local leukocyte activation, and nuclear factor-κB (NF-κB) activation. Femoral artery cannulation can be complicated by leg ischemia and has been blamed for myoglobinuric AKI. Myoglobin and hemoglobin avidly bind nitric oxide and are believed to cause AKI through vasoconstrictor effects but also direct cytotoxicity and frank tubular obstruction.

Withdrawal of the antifibrinolytic agent aprotinin from the market eliminates one concern of perioperative renal toxicity for cardiac surgery patients. In contrast, the lysine analogue antifibrinolytics, ε-aminocaproic acid and tranexamic acid, can raise concern because of their renal effects of small protein spillage into the urine (tubular proteinuria). While tubular proteinuria often heralds tubular injury, with lysine analogue antifibrinolytics this is completely resolved within 15 minutes after the agent is discontinued. Other perioperative nephrotoxins include some antibiotics, α-adrenergic agonist agents, cyclosporine, and nonsteroidal antiinflammatory agents. However, the net effect on post–cardiac surgery AKI of α_1-mediated vasoconstriction and dopaminergic and α_2-mediated renal vasodilation with hemodynamic compromise is unknown.

Considerable evidence has emerged with respect to the potential for colloid solutions, particularly hydroxyethyl starches, to contribute to AKI in a number of settings (Box 25.2). Cardiac surgery is no different, and several studies have provided evidence suggesting that hydroxyethyl starches are one of the factors associated with renal

25

dysfunction. As a result of these cardiac surgery studies, as well as the mounting evidence against the use of starches in other critical care settings, the avoidance of hydroxyethyl starch solutions is recommended.

Strategies for Renal Protection

The sluggish serum creatinine rise consequent to sudden drops in glomerular filtration is now considered inadequate to be the signal for acute renoprotection, much as Q waves are too late to be useful for cardioprotection. When serum creatinine is employed, the obligatory delay in AKI recognition has even been suggested to explain some of the disappointing results from past renoprotection studies. Developing and validating tools for more prompt AKI diagnosis has become a priority. The hope is that early AKI biomarkers can be identified that can play a role in renal protection, much like myocardial creatine kinase isoenzyme (CK-MB) and troponin currently serve for myocardial protection.

Nonetheless, despite its limitations as an early biomarker, serum creatinine remains an important clinical tool because of its many other uses. Indisputably, creatinine accumulation serves as a prognostic gold standard heralding AKI that is highly predictive of other major adverse outcomes, including death. Validation for even the most promising of newer early AKI biomarkers is very limited or lacking in comparison. In addition to injury, serum creatinine characterizes renal recovery, unlike most AKI biomarkers. Renal recovery as reflected by declining creatinine levels is highly predictive of short- and long-term outcomes beyond the magnitude of kidney insult. Finally, the generalizability across studies and settings of creatinine-based consensus definitions for AKI, such as RIFLE and AKIN, are gaining popularity.

Early Acute Kidney Injury Biomarkers

Beyond serum creatinine, the race is on to identify one or more "early biomarkers" for AKI. As a condition whose treatment paradigm demands prompt intervention, AKI currently has no equivalents to CK-MB, troponin, and the ST segment for the heart.

While only a few new early biomarker candidates involve a substitute "ideal" creatinine, most involve one of three other early consequences of AKI: tubular cell damage, tubular cell dysfunction, and the adaptive stress response of the kidney. For example, damaged renal cells leak contents directly into urine; this strategy underpins tubular enzymuria AKI biomarkers, including β-N-acetyl-β-D-glucosaminidase and at least eight other candidates. Monitoring markers of the kidney's stress response provides another strategy for AKI recognition, including some frontrunners; these include neutrophil gelatinase-associated lipocalcin, urinary IL-18, and at least three other candidates. Simple urinary partial pressure of oxygen (PO_2) monitoring correlates with changes in renal medullary oxygen levels and predicts subsequent AKI in cardiac surgery patients.

Several large prospective observational studies are currently under way that may help identify the winner(s) of the early AKI biomarker race. It will be important for surgical and anesthesia advocates to highlight AKI biomarker issues unique to cardiac surgery lest these be overlooked in the broader pursuit of consensus AKI definitions.

Cardiopulmonary Bypass Management and the Kidney

Basic issues in the management of CPB that relate to the kidney involve the balance between oxygen supply and oxygen demand, particularly to the renal medulla. Perfusion pressure (ie, MAP during CPB) and oxygen-carrying capacity (as related to hemodilution and transfusion) address the supply issues, with the use of hypothermia being directed at modulating renal oxygen demand.

Profound hypothermia is a highly effective component of the protective strategy used during renal transplantation. Mild hypothermia during CPB would, therefore, seem to be a logical component of a perioperative renal protective strategy. However, three separate studies have not found any protective benefit of mild hypothermia during CPB.

Low CPB blood pressure is typically not associated with the hypoperfusion characteristic of hypovolemic shock and LCOS, conditions that are highly associated with AKI. Studies addressing the role of perfusion pressure have not shown an association with AKI. Interestingly, some data are emerging on the interrelationship between cerebral autoregulatory limits (ie, defining individual blood pressure targets) and AKI after cardiac surgery.

Moderate hemodilution is thought to reduce the risk of kidney injury during cardiac surgery through blood viscosity–related improvement in regional blood flow. However, the practice of extreme hemodilution (hematocrit <20%) during CPB has been linked to adverse renal outcome after cardiac surgery. Studies suggest that profound hematocrit change (eg, >50% drop) may be even less well tolerated, highlighting the importance of a clinical strategy including transfusion only after all measures of hemodilution avoidance have been taken.

Glycemic control during CPB has been identified as a potential opportunity to attenuate AKI. Despite widespread adoption of intensive insulin protocols, numerous subsequent studies have failed to reproduce Van den Berghe's findings of benefit. In a study combining Van den Berghe–like postoperative management of 400 cardiac surgery patients randomized to intensive intraoperative insulin therapy (target 80–100 mg/dL) versus usual management, Gandhi and associates found no benefit and similar dialysis rates (6/199 vs 4/201; $P = .54$), even noting an unexpected increase in 30-day mortality and stroke with tight control.

Pharmacologic Intervention

There is very little in terms of interventions available to the clinician to prevent or treat established perioperative AKI pharmacologically. Proposed changes to improve the likelihood of success in finding renoprotective strategies have included increasing the size of studies designed to see benefit should it be present and, as outlined earlier, improving timely AKI detection to allow earlier intervention.

Unfortunately, because of the limitations of current research tools, most potential renoprotective therapies have not been subjected to the rigor of a large randomized trial or even meta-analysis, and none has been given the opportunity to be used

25

immediately after the onset of AKI. Additional data, including rationale and existing studies for a number of these therapies, is outlined next.

DOPAMINE

Mesenteric dopamine$_1$ (D_1) receptor agonists increase renal blood flow, decrease renal vascular resistance, and enhance natriuresis and diuresis. Despite the absence of clinical evidence of renoprotection, this rationale has been used to justify the use of low-dose ("renal-dose") dopamine (<5 µg/kg per min) for decades. However, numerous double-blind, randomized studies in several surgical and nonsurgical settings have failed to demonstrate any renal benefits. Despite the lack of benefit and accumulating concerns regarding the use of low-dose dopamine, many centers continue to use this agent for renoprotection.

FENOLDOPAM

Fenoldopam mesylate, a derivative of benzazepine, is a selective D_1-receptor agonist. Although first approved as an antihypertensive agent, fenoldopam has shown promise in the prevention of contrast-induced nephropathy. There is, however, very little in the way of randomized, controlled studies to evaluate the agent as a therapy for postoperative renal dysfunction.

DIURETIC AGENTS

Diuretics increase urine generation by reducing reuptake of tubular contents. This can be achieved by numerous mechanisms, including inhibiting active mechanisms that lead to solute reuptake (eg, loop diuretics), altering the osmotic gradient in the tubular contents to favor solute remaining in the tubule (eg, mannitol), or hormonal influences that affect the balance of activities of the tubule to increase urine generation (eg, atrial natriuretic peptide). The general renoprotective principle of diuretic agents is that increasing tubular solute flow through injured renal tubules will maintain tubular patency, avoiding some of the adverse consequences of tubular obstruction, including oliguria or anuria and possibly the need for dialysis. Other agent-specific properties (eg, antioxidant effects, reduced active transport) have also been proposed to have beneficial effects in the setting of ischemic renal injury.

Loop diuretics, such as furosemide, produce renal cortical vasodilation and inhibit reabsorptive transport in the medullary thick ascending limb, causing more solute to remain in the renal tubule and increasing urine generation. In contrast to evidence from animal experiments, several clinical studies have shown no benefit and possibly even harm from perioperative diuretic therapy in cardiac surgery patients. Although they may facilitate avoidance of dialysis in responsive patients by maintaining fluid balance, there is insufficient evidence to support the routine use of loop diuretics as specific renoprotective agents. However, in situations of severe hemoglobinuria, they may facilitate urine production and tubular clearance of this nephrotoxin.

Mannitol, an osmotic diuretic, has been evaluated in several studies of cardiac surgical patients. Although an increased diuresis has been documented, very few studies have carefully assessed postoperative renal dysfunction in these patients. In addition to the lack of beneficial effect on the kidney, several studies have identified a nephrotoxic potential of high-dose mannitol, especially in patients with preexisting renal insufficiency.

N-ACETYLCYSTEINE

N-Acetylcysteine is an antioxidant that enhances the endogenous glutathione scavenging system and has shown promise as a renoprotective agent by attenuating intravenous contrast-induced nephropathy. The weight of evidence, including four meta-analyses, suggests that potential benefits that may exist with contrast nephropathy are not pertinent to perioperative patients.

ADRENERGIC AGONISTS

The α_1- and α_2-adrenergic receptors in the kidney modulate vasoconstrictor and vasodilatory effects, respectively. Agents that attenuate renal vasoconstriction may have potential as renoprotective drugs because vasoconstriction most likely contributes to the pathophysiology of AKI. Clonidine, an α_2-agonist, has been shown experimentally to inhibit renin release and cause diuresis, and it has been evaluated in an experimental AKI model confirming its potential as a renoprotective agent. Despite being positively supported, clonidine has not gained popular acceptance as a renoprotective agent. Notably, decreased afferent α_1-adrenergic receptor–mediated vasoconstriction has been suggested as an explanation for the renal protective benefit of thoracic epidural blockade in cardiac surgery patients.

CALCIUM CHANNEL BLOCKERS

Diltiazem is the calcium channel blocker that has been most evaluated as a renoprotective agent in cardiac surgery, with its ability to antagonize vasoconstricting signals and reports of beneficial effects in experimental models of toxic and ischemic acute renal failure. However, in humans, numerous small randomized trials and a retrospective study combine to provide a confusing picture, including evidence suggesting diltiazem therapy in cardiac surgery patients may have minor renal benefits, no benefit, or even potential harm.

SODIUM BICARBONATE

The perioperative infusion of sodium bicarbonate has recently attracted attention because of reduced AKI compared to a placebo saline infusion in 100 post–cardiac surgery patients. Despite evidence that sodium bicarbonate–based hydration appears to be of benefit in other settings such as contrast-induced nephropathy, the considerable additional fluid and sodium load required with this therapy has raised concern with some clinicians.

ANGIOTENSIN-CONVERTING ENZYME INHIBITOR AND ANGIOTENSIN I RECEPTOR BLOCKERS

The renin-angiotensin-aldosterone system mediates vasoconstriction and is important in the paracrine regulation of the renal microcirculation. Angiotensin-converting enzyme (ACE) inhibitor and angiotensin I receptor blocker agents act by inhibiting steps in activation of the renin-angiotensin-aldosterone system. Although ACE inhibitor and angiotensin receptor blocker agents have demonstrated effects at slowing the progression of most chronic renal diseases, their role in AKI has not been well studied.

MYOCARDIAL INJURY

From the earliest days of modern cardiac surgery, perioperative myocardial dysfunction, with its associated morbidity and mortality, has been reported. Evidence, including substantial subendocardial cellular necrosis, led to the conclusion that this injury resulted from an inadequate substrate supply to the metabolically active myocardium. Optimizing myocardial protection during cardiac surgery involves several compromises inherent in allowing surgery to be performed in a relatively immobile, bloodless field, while preserving postoperative myocardial function. The fundamental tenets of this protection center on the judicious use of hypothermia along with the induction and

25

maintenance of chemically induced electromechanical diastolic cardiac arrest. Despite continued efforts directed at myocardial protection, it is clear that myocardial injury, although reduced, still remains a problem, and with it, the representative phenotype of postoperative myocardial dysfunction.

Incidence and Significance of Myocardial Dysfunction After Cardiopulmonary Bypass

Unlike other organs at risk of damage during cardiac surgery, it is assumed, because of the very nature of the target of the operation being performed, that all patients having cardiac surgery will suffer some degree of myocardial injury. Although the injury can be subclinical, represented only by otherwise asymptomatic elevations in cardiac enzymes, it frequently manifests more overtly. The degree to which these enzymes are released by injured myocardium, frequently to levels sufficiently high to satisfy criteria for MI, have been related to perioperative outcome after cardiac surgery.

Risk Factors for Myocardial Injury

With an increasingly sicker cohort of patients presenting for cardiac surgery, many with acute ischemic syndromes or significant LV dysfunction, the need has never been greater for optimizing myocardial protection to minimize the myocardial dysfunction consequent to aortic cross-clamping and cardioplegia. The continued increase in cardiac transplantation and other complex surgeries in the patient with heart failure has served to fuel the search for better myocardial protection strategies.

Pathophysiology of Myocardial Injury

Myocardial stunning represents the myocardial dysfunction that follows a brief ischemic event. It is differentiated from the reversible dysfunction associated with chronic ischemia, which is called hibernation. Myocardial stunning typically resolves over the 48 to 72 hours after the ischemic event and is frequently observed after aortic cross-clamping with cardioplegic arrest. Important factors that contribute to stunning include not only the metabolic consequences of oxygen deprivation but also the premorbid condition of the myocardium, reperfusion injury, acute alterations in signal transduction systems, and the effects of circulating inflammatory mediators.

The metabolic consequences of oxygen deprivation become apparent within seconds of coronary artery occlusion. With the rapid depletion of high-energy phosphates, accumulation of lactate and intracellular acidosis in the myocytes soon follows, with the subsequent development of contractile dysfunction. When myocyte adenosine triphosphate (ATP) levels decline to a critical level, the subsequent inability to maintain electrolyte gradients requiring active transport (eg, Na^+, K^+, Ca^{2+}) leads to cellular edema, intracellular Ca^{2+} overload, and loss of membrane integrity.

Predictably with the release of the aortic cross-clamp and the restoration of blood flow, myocardial reperfusion occurs. With reperfusion the paradox, represented by the balance of substrate delivery restoration needed for normal metabolism that also can serve as the substrate for injurious free radical production, becomes a significant issue for consideration. Reperfusion causes a rapid increase in free radical production within minutes, and it plays a major role in initiating myocardial stunning.

In addition to free radical upregulation, myocardial reperfusion associated with acute myocardial ischemic injury induces inflammation mediated by neutrophils and an array of humoral inflammatory components. Prostaglandins are also generated during reperfusion, and their adverse effects appear to be synergistic with increases in intracellular calcium.

A potential additional mechanism for myocardial dysfunction specific to the setting of CPB relates to proposed acute alterations in β-adrenergic signal transduction. Acute desensitization and downregulation of myocardial β-adrenergic receptors during CPB has been demonstrated after cardiac surgery. Although the role of the large elevations in circulating catecholamines seen with CPB on β-adrenergic malfunction is unclear, it has been proposed that an increased incidence of post-CPB LCOS and reduced responsiveness to inotropic agents may be attributed in part to this effect.

Myocardial Protection During Cardiac Surgery: Cardioplegia

Optimizing the metabolic state of the myocardium is fundamental to preserving its integrity. The major effects of temperature and functional activity (ie, contractile and electrical work) on the metabolic rate of the myocardium have been extensively described. With the institution of CPB, the emptying of the heart significantly reduces contractile work and myocardial oxygen consumption (Mvo_2). Nullifying this cardiac work reduces the Mvo_2 by 30% to 60%. With subsequent reductions in temperature, the Mvo_2 further decreases, and with induction of cardiac arrest and hypothermia, 90% of the metabolic requirements of the heart can be reduced. Temperature reductions diminish metabolic rate for all electromechanical states (ie, beating or fibrillating) of the myocardium.

Although cardiac surgery on the empty beating heart or under conditions of hypothermic fibrillation (both with the support of CPB) is sometimes performed, aortic cross-clamping with cardioplegic arrest remains the most prevalent method of myocardial preservation. Based on the principle of reducing metabolic requirements, the introduction of selective myocardial hypothermia and cardioplegia (ie, diastolic arrest) marked a major clinical advance in myocardial protection. With the various additives in cardioplegia solutions (designed to optimize the myocardium during arrest and attenuate reperfusion injury) and the use of warm cardioplegia, the idea of delivering metabolic substrates (as opposed to solely reducing metabolic requirements) is also commonplace. Several effective approaches to chemical cardioplegia are employed. The clinical success of a cardioplegia strategy may be judged by its ability to achieve and maintain prompt continuous arrest in all regions of the myocardium, early return of function after cross-clamp removal, and minimal inotropic requirements for successful separation from CPB. Composition, temperature, and route of delivery constitute the fundamentals of cardioplegia-derived myocardial protection.

Composition of Cardioplegia Solutions

The composition of the various cardioplegia solutions used during cardiac surgery varies as much between institutions as it does between individual surgeons. In very general terms, cardioplegia can be classified into blood-containing and non–blood-containing (ie, crystalloid) solutions. Whereas crystalloid cardioplegia has fallen out of favor, blood cardioplegia in various combinations of temperatures and routes of delivery is the most used solution. However, even within the category of blood cardioplegia, the individual chemical constituents of the solution vary considerably with respect to the addition of numerous additives. Table 25.4 outlines the various additives to cardioplegia solutions along with their corresponding rationale for use. Although

Table 25.4 **Strategies for the Reduction of Ischemic Injury With Cardioplegia**

Principle	Mechanism	Component
Reduce O_2 demand	Hypothermia Perfusion Topical/lavage	Blood, crystalloid, ice slush, lavage
	Asystole	KCl, adenosine (?), hyperpolarizing agents
Substrate supply and use	Oxygen	Blood, perfluorocarbons, crystalloid (?)
	Glucose	Blood, glucose, citrate-phosphate-dextrose
	Amino acids	Glutamate, aspartate
	Buffer acidosis	Hypothermia (Rosenthal factor), intermittent infusions
	Buffers	Blood, tromethamine, histidine, bicarbonate, phosphate
	Optimize metabolism	Warm induction (37°C), warm reperfusion
Reduce Ca^{2+} overload	Hypocalcemia	Citrate, Ca^{2+} channel blockers, K channel openers (?)
Reduce edema	Hyperosmolarity	Glucose, KCl, mannitol
	Moderate infusion pressure	50 mm Hg

From Vinten-Johansen J, Thourani VH. Myocardial protection: an overview. *J Extra Corpor Technol.* 2000;32:38–48.

all cardioplegia solutions contain higher-than-physiologic levels of potassium, solutions used for the induction of diastolic arrest contain the highest concentrations of potassium as opposed to solutions used for the maintenance of cardioplegia. In addition to adjustment of electrolytes, manipulation of buffers (eg, bicarbonate, tromethamine), osmotic agents (eg, glucose, mannitol, potassium), and metabolic substrates (eg, glucose, glutamate, and aspartate) constitute the most common variations in cardioplegia content. Oxygenation of crystalloid cardioplegia before infusion is aimed at increasing aerobic metabolism, but the limited oxygen-carrying capacity of crystalloid makes a rapid decline in metabolic rate through immediate and sustained diastolic arrest critical to effective cardioprotection with this technique.

Blood cardioplegia has the potential advantage of delivering sufficient oxygen to ischemic myocardium to sustain basal metabolism or even augment high-energy phosphate stores, as well as possessing free radical scavenging properties. Although low-risk cardiac surgical patients appear to do equally well with crystalloid or blood cardioplegic protection, evidence is compelling that more critically ill patients, including those with "energy-depleted" hearts, have improved outcomes using blood cardioplegia.

Infusion of a single, warm (37°C) reperfusion dose of cardioplegia (so-called hot shot) containing metabolic substrates (ie, glucose, glutamate, and aspartate) just before aortic cross-clamp removal is preferred by some clinicians. The rationale for this is evidence that normothermia maximally enhances myocardial aerobic metabolism and recovery after an ischemic period.

Cardioplegia Temperature

The composition of cardioplegia solutions varies considerably; in contrast, myocardial temperature during cardioplegia is almost uniformly reduced to between 10°C and

12°C or less by the infusion of refrigerated cardioplegia and external topical cooling with ice slush. However, the introduction of warm cardioplegia has challenged this once universally considered necessity of hypothermia for successful myocardial protection. Although hypothermic cardioplegia is the most commonly used temperature, numerous investigations have examined tepid (27–30°C) and warm (37–38°C) temperature ranges for the administration of cardioplegia. Much of the work aimed at determining the optimum temperature of the cardioplegia solution centered on the fact that, although hypothermia clearly offered some advantages to the myocardium in suppressing metabolism (particularly when intermittent cardioplegia was delivered), it may have some detrimental effects.

The deleterious effects of hypothermia include the increased risk of myocardial edema (through ion pump activity inhibition) and the impaired function of various membrane receptors on which some pharmacologic therapy depends (such as the various additives to the cardioplegia solutions). The other disadvantages of hypothermic cardioplegia, in addition to the production of the metabolic inhibition in the myocardium, are an increase in plasma viscosity and a decrease in red blood cell deformability. As a result, investigations aimed at using warmer cardioplegia temperatures have been explored.

Cardioplegia Delivery Routes

If using tepid or warm cardioplegia administration, the continuous administration of this cardioplegia needs to be ensured. Retrograde cardioplegia, where a cardioplegia catheter is introduced into the coronary sinus, allows for almost continuous cardioplegia administration. Retrograde delivery is also useful in settings where antegrade cardioplegia is problematic, such as with severe aortic insufficiency or during aortic root or aortic valve (and, frequently, mitral) surgery (Box 25.3). It also allows the distribution of cardioplegia to areas of myocardium supplied by significantly stenosed coronary vessels. The acceptable perfusion pressure to limit perivascular edema and hemorrhage needs to be limited to less than 40 mm Hg.

Retrograde cardioplegia does have some limitations. Although the retrograde approach has been shown to effectively deliver cardioplegia adequately to the left ventricle, because of shunting and blood flowing into the atrium and ventricles by the thebesian veins and various arteriosinusoidal connections, the right ventricle and septum frequently receive inadequate delivery of cardioplegia. Difficulties with retrograde delivery can also occur if the coronary sinus catheter is placed beyond the great cardiac vein, or if anatomic variants occur that communicate with systemic veins, such as a persistent left superior vena cava (SVC). Because retrograde cardioplegia is inefficient in producing arrest of the beating heart, induction of arrest with this technique must be achieved by a single antegrade infusion of cardioplegia before its institution.

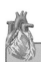

BOX 25.3   Uses for Retrograde Cardioplegia

Along with anterograde cardioplegia
In the presence of aortic insufficiency
For aortic (and mitral) valve surgery
To perfuse severely diseased coronary arteries

▧ GASTROINTESTINAL COMPLICATIONS

Incidence and Significance

GI complications after cardiac surgery, although occurring relatively infrequently (0.5–5.5%), portend a significantly increased risk of overall adverse patient outcome. The variability in the reported incidence of GI complications is partly a reflection of how they are defined as well as the variable patient and operative risk factors in the studied cohorts. As devastating as they are, because of the relative low incidence, studies of GI complications are few. Although the most commonly considered GI complications include pancreatitis, GI bleeding, cholecystitis, and bowel perforation or infarction, hyperbilirubinemia (total bilirubinemia >3.0 mL/dL) has also been described as an important complication after cardiac surgery.

In addition to their association with other morbid events, adverse GI complications are significantly associated with increased mortality after cardiac surgery. The average mortality rate among subtypes of GI complications in the study by McSweeney was 19.6%, and in other reports, the mortality rate ranges from 13% to 87%, with an overall average mortality rate of 33%. Even the seemingly insignificant complication of having an increased laboratory measurement of total bilirubin was associated with a 6.6 odds ratio of death in the McSweeney study, compared with a death odds ratio of 8.4 for all adverse GI outcomes combined. Apart from the significant effect on mortality, the occurrence of an adverse GI outcome also significantly increases the incidence of perioperative MI, renal failure, and stroke, as well as significantly prolonging intensive care unit (ICU) and hospital lengths of stay.

Risk Factors

A long list of preoperative, intraoperative, and postoperative risk factors for GI complications has been identified in a number of studies. As many factors are associated with one another, it is only when these risk factors are examined in multivariable analyses that a more accurate understanding of what the most significant risk factors for visceral complications after cardiac surgery are. Preoperatively, age (>75 years), history of congestive heart failure, presence of hyperbilirubinemia (>1.2 mg/dL), combined cardiac procedures (eg, CABG plus valve), repeat cardiac operation, preoperative ejection fraction less than 40%, preoperative elevations in partial thromboplastin time, emergency operations; intraoperatively, prolonged CPB, use of TEE, and blood transfusion; and postoperatively, requirements for prolonged inotropic or vasopressor support, IABP use for the treatment of LCOS; and prolonged ventilatory support are all risk factors. These factors identify patients at high risk, and they lend some credence to the overall pathophysiology and suspected causes of these adverse events. If there is a common link among all these risks, it is that many of these factors would be associated with impairment in oxygen delivery to the splanchnic bed.

Pathophysiology and Causative Factors

Impairments in splanchnic perfusion commonly occur during even the normal conduct of cardiac surgery. When this is superimposed on an already depressed preoperative cardiac output (CO) or is associated with prolonged postoperative LCOS, the impairment in splanchnic blood flow is further perpetuated. The systemic inflammatory response to CPB itself can be initiated by splanchnic hypoperfusion by means of translocation of endotoxin from the gut into the circulation. De novo splanchnic

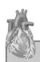

> **BOX 25.4** *Protecting the Gastrointestinal Tract During Cardiopulmonary Bypass*
>
> Avoiding high doses of vasopressors
> Maintaining a high perfusion flow
> Reducing emboli-producing maneuvers

hypoperfusion can be a result of the humoral vasoactive substances that are released by inflammation remote from the gut. Another causative factor for GI complications directly related to splanchnic hypoperfusion is atheroembolism. Prolonged ventilator support is another causative factor for GI complications, with several lines of investigation having described a relationship between prolonged ventilation and GI adverse events; this likely results from a direct effect of positive pressure ventilation impairing CO and subsequently splanchnic perfusion.

Protecting the Gastrointestinal Tract During Cardiac Surgery

As with other aspects of organ protection, critical causative factors need to be addressed with specific targeted therapies (Box 25.4). Unfortunately, as with most other organ-protective strategies, the major limitation in making definitive recommendations is an overall lack of large, well-controlled, prospectively randomized studies to provide supportive data for any one particular technique.

Cardiopulmonary Bypass Management

Because CPB itself has been shown to impair splanchnic blood flow, modifications in how it is conducted may have some salutary effects on GI tract integrity. Several studies have focused on the issue of the relative importance of pressure versus flow during CPB, demonstrating that it is likely more beneficial to maintain an adequate bypass flow rate than only maintaining pressure during bypass. The addition of significant vasoconstrictors to maintain an adequate MAP artificially in the presence of inadequate flow on CPB may lead to further compromise of splanchnic blood flow. The optimal CPB temperature to protect the gut is also unknown. Just as aggressive rewarming can be injurious to the brain, there is some evidence that rewarming can cause increases in visceral metabolism, making any overshoot in temperature suspect by adversely altering the balance of gut oxygen consumption and delivery.

Emboli Reduction

Whereas microembolization and macroembolization to the splanchnic bed clearly occur during CPB and possibly even during the period after bypass, there are few data to determine whether emboli reduction strategies can alter GI outcome. It remains prudent to avoid maneuvers (ie, aortic cannulation and cross-clamping) in areas of high atheroma burden, which is an overall tenet of cardiac surgery for the prevention of all complications.

Drugs

Various vasoactive drugs have been used to enhance splanchnic blood flow during CPB. It is likely that most of these drugs, such as the phosphodiesterase III inhibitors,

25

dobutamine, and other inotropic agents, maintain or enhance splanchnic blood flow, not because of a direct effect on the vasculature but by the inherent enhancement in CO. An increasingly common drug in the setting of cardiac surgery is vasopressin. Although vasopressin can clearly augment systemic MAP, it does so at the cost of severe impairments to splanchnic blood flow. Although there are always trade-offs when choosing which vasoactive agent to use, if having a very low MAP is going to be detrimental to other organ systems, the choice to use vasopressin should at least be made with the knowledge that it can have an adverse effect on splanchnic blood flow.

Off-Pump Cardiac Surgery

There is little evidence that the use of off-pump cardiac surgery is in any way beneficial to the GI tract. One reason for this lack of apparent difference between on-pump and off-pump cardiac surgery may again be related to the common denominator of splanchnic perfusion. OPCAB surgery is fraught with hemodynamic compromise that may lead to prolonged periods of splanchnic hypoperfusion by itself or as a result of the concurrent administration of vasopressors to maintain normal hemo-dynamics during the frequent manipulations of the heart.

LUNG INJURY DURING CARDIAC SURGERY

Incidence and Significance

Pulmonary dysfunction was one of the earliest recognized complications of cardiac surgery employing CPB. However, as improvements in operative technique and CPB perfusion technologies occurred, the overall frequency and severity of this complication decreased. Juxtaposed to the improvements in cardiac surgery, which led to an overall reduction in complications, is an evolving patient population that now comprises a higher-risk group with a higher degree of pulmonary comorbidities, increasing their risks of postoperative pulmonary dysfunction. With the advent of fast-track techniques, even minor degrees of pulmonary dysfunction have reemerged as significant contributors to patient morbidity and the potential need for extended postoperative ventilation. As with most postoperative organ dysfunction, there is a range of dysfunction severity. Arguably, some degree of pulmonary dysfunction occurs in most patients after cardiac surgery; however, it manifests clinically only when the degree of dysfunction is particularly severe or the pulmonary reserve is significantly impaired. As a result, even minor CPB-related pulmonary dysfunction can cause significant problems in some patients.

The full range of reported pulmonary complications includes simple atelectasis, pleural effusions, pneumonia, cardiogenic pulmonary edema, pulmonary embolism, and various degrees of acute lung injury ranging from the mild to the most severe (ie, acute respiratory distress syndrome [ARDS]). Although the final common pathway in all of these forms of pulmonary dysfunction complications is the occurrence of hypoxemia, these complications vary widely in their incidence, cause, and clinical significance. Atelectasis and pleural effusions are the most common pulmonary abnormalities seen after cardiac surgery, presenting in more than 60% of patients. Atelectasis is commonly attributed to a number of intraoperative and postoperative events. With the induction of general anesthesia, physical compression of the left lower lobe to aid exposure of the heart and facilitate in the dissection of the internal mammary artery, as well as the apnea occurring during the conduct of CPB, have all been implicated. Postoperative causes include the poor respiratory efforts by patients with impaired coughing, lack of deep inspirations, and pleural effusions. Despite a high incidence of these radiographically recognized complications, the clinical significance is relatively low.

Similar to atelectasis, pleural effusions, despite occurring commonly after cardiac surgery (40–50%), rarely cause significant perioperative morbidity. More common in the left thorax, likely as a consequence of the bleeding from the dissection of the internal mammary artery, other causes of pleural effusions relate to continued postoperative bleeding, pulmonary edema from cardiogenic and noncardiogenic causes, and pneumonia. Pneumonia after cardiac surgery also has a variable incidence but a much higher significance to overall patient outcome. Reported rates of pneumonia range widely from 2% to 22%. Pneumonia occurring early after cardiac surgery portends a very poor outcome, illustrated in one study by a mortality rate of 27%. Factors that increase the risk for postoperative pneumonia include smoking, the presence of chronic obstructive pulmonary disease, other pulmonary complications requiring prolonged intubation, significant heart failure, and the transfusion of large volumes of blood products.

Pathophysiology and Causative Factors

Studies have demonstrated CPB-induced changes in the mechanical properties (ie, elastance or compliance and resistance) of the pulmonary apparatus (particularly the lung as opposed to the chest wall) and changes in pulmonary capillary permeability. Impairment in gas exchange has been demonstrated to be a result of atelectasis with concomitant overall loss of lung volume. Most research has focused on the development of increases in pulmonary vascular permeability (leading to various degrees of pulmonary edema) as the principal cause of the impaired gas exchange that occurs during cardiac surgery and results in a high alveolar-arterial (A-a) gradient.

The cause of pulmonary dysfunction and ARDS after cardiac surgery is complex, but largely revolves around the CPB-induced systemic inflammatory response with its associated increase in pulmonary endothelial permeability. A central causative theme is a significant upregulation in the inflammation induced because of the interaction between the blood and foreign surfaces of the heart-lung machine or the inflammation related to the consequences of splanchnic hypoperfusion with the subsequent translocation of significant amounts of endotoxin into the circulation. Endotoxin is proinflammatory, and it has direct effects on the pulmonary vasculature. In addition to CPB-mediated inflammation, inflammation mediated by endotoxemia has been reported. Several studies have identified transfusion of packed red blood cells (>4 units) as a risk factor for ARDS in cardiac surgical patients.

Pulmonary Thromboembolism

Although not an injury to the lungs occurring as a direct result of CPB itself, deep vein thrombosis (DVT) and pulmonary embolism occur with regular frequency in the cardiac surgical population. The incidence of pulmonary embolism after cardiac surgery ranges from 0.3% to 9.5%, with a mortality rate approaching 20%. The incidence of pulmonary embolism appears to be lower after valve surgery compared with CABG, which may be due to the anticoagulation that is started soon after valve surgery.

The incidence of DVT is 17% to 46%, with most cases being asymptomatic. The higher incidences were reported from series that used lower extremity ultrasound to examine populations more comprehensively. DVT has been reported for the leg from

BOX 25.5 *Strategies to Protect the Lungs*

Reduced fraction of inspired oxygen (FIO_2) during bypass
Low postoperative tidal volume
Vital capacity breath before bypass separation

which the saphenous vein grafts were harvested and from the contralateral leg. The recommendations for DVT prophylaxis in cardiac surgery are aspirin and elastic gradient compression stockings in patients who ambulate within 2 to 3 days after surgery and low-molecular-weight heparin and sequential compression stockings in nonambulatory patients.

Pulmonary Protection

Ventilatory Strategies

Several studies have examined the use of continuous positive airway pressure (CPAP) during CPB as a means to minimize the decrement in the A-a gradient that can occur after surgery. Overall, it is unlikely that CPAP plays any major role in preventing or treating the pulmonary dysfunction that occurs in the setting of cardiac surgery.

The inspired oxygen content of the gases that the lungs see during the period of apnea during CPB may have an effect on the A-a gradient, probably because of the enhanced effect of higher FIO_2 on the ability of atelectasis (so-called absorption atelectasis) on these gradients. With these findings in mind, it would be prudent to reduce the FIO_2 to room air levels during CPB. Several simple therapies can be introduced before separation from CPB, including adequate tracheobronchial toilet and the delivery of several vital capacity breaths that may reduce the amount of atelectasis that has occurred during bypass (Box 25.5).

Pharmacologic Pulmonary Protection

STEROIDS

Antiinflammatory therapies may play a role in moderating the effects of the more significant forms of pulmonary dysfunction that occur after cardiac surgery and that have inflammation as a central causative factor. However, with the exception of corticosteroids, few antiinflammatory therapies are available for routine use. Corticosteroid use can reduce the amount of systemic inflammation as measured by circulating cytokines. However, this has not been coupled with a reduction in pulmonary dysfunction.

MANAGEMENT OF BYPASS

The Prebypass Period

An important objective of this phase is to prepare the patient for CPB (Box 25.6). This phase invariably involves two key steps: anticoagulation and vascular cannulation. With rare exceptions, heparin is still the anticoagulant clinically used for CPB. Dose, method of administration, and opinions as to what constitutes adequate anticoagulation

BOX 25.6 *Management Before Cardiopulmonary Bypass*

Anticoagulation
Cannulation of the heart
Careful monitoring to minimize organ dysfunction
Protection of the heart
Preparation for cardiopulmonary bypass

vary. Heparin must be administered before cannulation for CPB, even if cannulation must be done emergently. Failure to do so is to risk thrombosis in both the patient and extracorporeal circuit. After heparin has been administered, a period of at least 3 minutes is customarily allowed for systemic circulation and onset of effect; an activated coagulation time or heparin concentration measurement demonstrating actual achievement of adequate anticoagulation is then performed.

Vascular Cannulation

The next major step in the prebypass phase is vascular cannulation. The goal of vascular cannulation is to provide access whereby the CPB pump may divert all systemic venous blood to the pump-oxygenator at the lowest possible venous pressures and deliver oxygenated blood to the arterial circulation at pressure and flow sufficient to maintain systemic homeostasis.

Arterial Cannulation

Arterial cannulation is generally established before venous cannulation to allow volume resuscitation of the patient, should it be necessary. The ascending aorta is the preferred site for aortic cannulation because it is easily accessible, does not require an additional incision, accommodates a larger cannula to provide greater flow at a reduced pressure, and carries a lower risk of aortic dissection compared with other arterial cannulation sites (femoral or iliac arteries). Because hypertension increases the risk of aortic dissection during cannulation, the aortic pressure may be temporarily lowered (MAP <70 mm Hg) during aortotomy and cannula insertion. Several potential complications are associated with aortic cannulation, including embolization of air or atheromatous debris, inadvertent cannulation of aortic arch vessels, aortic dissection, and other vessel wall injury.

Reviews and clinical reports emphasize the importance of embolization as the major mechanism of focal cerebral injury in cardiac surgery patients. Intraoperative use of two-dimensional epiaortic ultrasound imaging as a guide to selection of cross-clamping and cannulation site is increasing. A femoral or axillary artery, rather than the ascending aorta, can be cannulated for systemic perfusion. These alternate sites can be used when ascending aortic cannulation is considered relatively contraindicated, as in severe aortic atherosclerosis, aortic aneurysm or dissection, or known cystic medical necrosis. Historically, the anesthesiologist sought evidence of cannula malposition by looking for unilateral blanching of the face, gently palpating carotid pulses and checking for new unilateral diminution, and by measuring blood pressure in both arms and to check for new asymmetries. However, robust assessments of CBF symmetry can more reliably be made with the use of near-infrared spectroscopy cerebral oximetry.

25

Venous Cannulation

Venous cannulation can be achieved using a single atrial cannula that is inserted into the right atrium and directed inferiorly (Fig. 25.6). Drainage holes in this multistage cannula are located in the inferior vena cava (IVC) and right atrium to drain blood returning from the lower extremities and the SVC and coronary sinus, respectively. This technique has the advantage of being simpler, faster, and requiring only one incision; however, the quality of drainage can be easily compromised when the heart is lifted for surgical exposure. The bicaval cannulation technique, required in cases in which right atrial access is needed, involves separately cannulating the SVC and IVC (Fig. 25.7). Loops placed around the vessels can be tightened to divert all caval blood flow away from the heart. Blood returning to the right atrium from the coronary sinus will not be drained using this technique, so an additional vent or atriotomy is necessary.

During CPB, blood will continue to return to the left ventricle from a variety of sources, including the bronchial and thebesian veins, as well as blood that traverses the pulmonary circulation. Abnormal sources of venous blood include a persistent left SVC, systemic-to-pulmonary shunts, and aortic regurgitation. It is important to avoid LV filling and distension during CPB to prevent myocardial rewarming, minimize

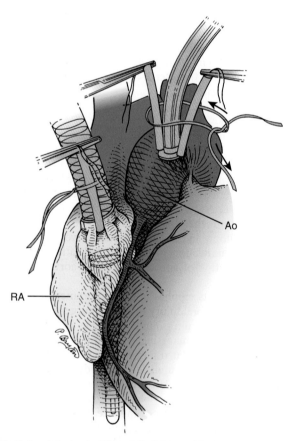

Fig. 25.6 Aortic *(Ao)* and single, double-staged, right atrial *(RA)* cannulation. Notice the drainage holes of venous cannula in right atrium and inferior vena cava. (From Connolly MW. *Cardiopulmonary Bypass.* New York: Springer-Verlag; 1995:59.)

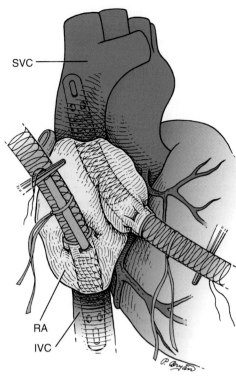

Fig. 25.7 Position of two-vessel cannulation of right atrium *(RA)* with placement of drainage holes into superior vena cava *(SVC)* and inferior vena cava *(IVC)*. The aortic cannula is not shown. (From Connolly MW. *Cardiopulmonary Bypass*. New York: Springer-Verlag; 1995:59.)

LV wall tension, and limit myocardial oxygen demand. This can be accomplished with the use of a vent placed in the left ventricle via the left superior pulmonary vein. Alternate sites include the pulmonary artery, the aortic root, or directly in the left ventricle via the ventricular apex.

Venous cannulas, using a multistage or bicaval cannula, are large and can impair venous return from the IVC or SVC. Superior vena caval obstruction is detected by venous engorgement of the head and neck, conjunctival edema, and elevated SVC pressure. Inferior vena caval obstruction is far more insidious, presenting only as decreased filling pressures because of lowered venous return.

Femoral venous cannulation is sometimes used for CPB without, or before, sternotomy or right atrial cannulation (eg, redos, ascending aortic aneurysms). Because of the femoral venous cannula's comparatively small size and long length, venous return can be impaired but is optimized when the tip of the cannula is advanced (under TEE guidance) until it is placed at the level of the SVC–right atrium junction. Kinetic or vacuum-assisted negative pressure can be applied to further enhance drainage.

Other Preparations

Once anticoagulation and cannulation are complete, CPB can be instituted. Because there usually is redundant pulmonary artery catheter length in the right ventricle, and the heart is manipulated during CPB, there is a tendency for distal migration of

25

the catheter into pulmonary artery branches. This distal migration of the catheter increases the risks of "overwedging" and pulmonary artery damage. During the prebypass phase it is advisable to withdraw the pulmonary artery catheter 3 to 5 cm to decrease the likelihood of these untoward events. It is also advisable to check the integrity of all vascular access and monitoring devices. A pulmonary artery catheter placed through an external jugular or subclavian vein can become kinked or occluded on full opening of the sternal retractor. If TEE is being used, the probe should be placed in the "freeze" mode and the tip of the scope placed in the neutral and unlocked position. Leaving the electronic scanning emitter turned on during hypothermic CPB adds heat (in some TEE models) to the esophagus and posterior wall of the ventricle.

Before initiating CPB, the anesthesiologist should assess the depth of anesthesia and adequacy of muscle relaxation. It is important to maintain paralysis to prevent patient movement that could result in dislodgement of bypass-circuit cannulas and prevent shivering as hypothermia is induced (with the attendant increases in oxygen consumption). It is often difficult to determine the depth of anesthesia during the various stages of CPB. Because blood pressure, heart rate, pupil diameter, and the autonomic nervous system are profoundly affected by extracorporeal circulation (eg, the heart is asystolic, blood pressure is greatly influenced by circuit blood flow, and sweating occurs with rewarming), these variables do not reliably reflect the anesthetic state. Although hypothermia decreases anesthetic requirements, it is necessary to provide analgesia, hypnosis, and muscle relaxation during CPB. Useful adjuncts to assessing depth of anesthesia are available in the form of processed electroencephalographic devices. For example, the bispectral index has proven useful in preventing awareness during cardiac surgery. With the initiation of CPB and hemodilution, blood levels of anesthetics and muscle relaxants acutely decrease. However, plasma protein concentrations also decrease, which increases the free-fraction and active drug concentrations. Every drug has a specific kinetic profile during CPB, and kinetics and pharmacodynamics during CPB vary greatly among patients. Many clinicians administer additional muscle relaxants and opioids at the initiation of CPB. A vaporizer for potent inhalation drugs may be included in the bypass circuit. A final inspection of the head and neck for color, symmetry, adequacy of venous drainage (neck vein and conjunctiva engorgement), and pupil equality is reasonable to serve as a baseline for the anesthetic state. A summary of preparatory steps to be accomplished during the prebypass phase is given in Box 25.7.

INITIATION AND DISCONTINUATION OF BYPASS SUPPORT: AN OVERVIEW

Initiation of Cardiopulmonary Bypass

Uncomplicated Initiation

Once all preparatory steps have been taken, the perfusionist progressively increases delivery of oxygenated blood to the patient's arterial system, as systemic venous blood is diverted from the patient's right side of the heart, maintaining the pump's venous reservoir volume. After full flow is achieved, all systemic venous blood is (ideally) draining from the patient to the pump reservoir. An on-bypass checklist of issues to address shortly after initiation of bypass can serve as a valuable safety tool (Box 25.8). The CVP and pulmonary arterial pressure should decrease to near zero (2–5 mm

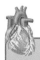

BOX 25.7 *Bypass Preparation Checklist*

1. Anticoagulation
   a. Heparin administered
   b. Desired level of anticoagulation achieved
2. Arterial cannulation
   a. Absence of bubbles in arterial line
   b. Evidence of dissection or malposition?
3. Venous cannulation
   a. Evidence of superior vena cava obstruction?
   b. Evidence of inferior vena cava obstruction?
4. Pulmonary artery catheter (if used) pulled back
5. Are all monitoring and/or access catheters functional?
6. Transesophageal echocardiograph (if used)
   a. In "freeze" mode
   b. Scope in neutral or unlocked position
7. Supplemental medications
   a. Neuromuscular blockers
   b. Anesthetics, analgesics, amnestics
8. Inspection of head and neck
   a. Color
   b. Symmetry
   c. Venous drainage
   d. Pupils

Hg), whereas systemic flow, arterial pressure, and oxygenation are maintained at desired values.

Hypotension With Onset of Bypass

Systemic arterial hypotension (MAP, 30–40 mm Hg) is relatively common on initiation of CPB. Much of this can be explained by the acute reduction of blood viscosity that results from hemodilution with nonblood priming solutions. MAP increases with initiation of hypothermia-induced vasoconstriction, along with levels of endogenous catecholamines and angiotensin. The hemodilution also results in the loss of nitric oxide binding by hemoglobin; the excess free nitric oxide can lead to further vasodilation. Treatment with α-agonists is *usually* not necessary if the hypotension is brief (<60 s). Of concern is the potential for myocardial and cerebral ischemia because hypothermia has not yet been achieved.

Until the aortic cross-clamp is applied, the coronary arteries are perfused with hemodiluted, nonpulsatile blood. If placement of the aortic cross-clamp is delayed, MAP should be maintained in the range of 60 to 80 mm Hg to support myocardial perfusion, especially in the presence of known coronary stenosis or ventricular hypertrophy. This arterial pressure is likely adequate to maintain CBF until hypothermia is induced.

Unless pulsatile perfusion is used, once at full flow, the arterial pressure waveform should be nonpulsatile except for small (5–10 mm Hg) sinusoidal deflections created by the roller pump heads. Continued pulsatile arterial pressure indicates that the left ventricle is receiving blood from some source.

25

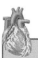

BOX 25.8 *Bypass Procedure Checklist*

1. Assess arterial inflow
   a. Is arterial perfusate oxygenated?
   b. Is direction of arterial inflow appropriate?
   c. Evidence of arterial dissection?
   d. Patient's arterial pressure persistently low?
   e. Inflow line pressure high?
   f. Pump/oxygenator reservoir level falling?
   g. Evidence of atrial cannula malposition?
   h. Patient's arterial pressure persistently high or low?
   i. Unilateral facial swelling, discoloration?
   j. Symmetrical cerebral oximetry?
2. Assess venous outflow
   a. Is blood draining to the pump/oxygenator's venous reservoir?
   b. Evidence of SVC obstruction?
   c. Facial venous engorgement or congestion, CVP elevated?
3. Is bypass complete?
   a. High CVP/low PA pressure?
   b. Impaired venous drainage?
   c. Low CVP/high PA pressure?
   d. Large bronchial venous blood flow?
   e. Aortic insufficiency?
   f. Arterial and PA pressure nonpulsatile?
   g. Desired pump flow established?
4. Discontinue drug and fluid administration
5. Discontinue ventilation and inhalation drugs to patient's lungs

CVP, Central venous pressure; *PA,* pulmonary artery; *SVC,* superior vena cava.

Pump Flow and Pressure During Bypass

Pump flow during CPB represents a careful balance between the conflicting demands of surgical visualization and adequate oxygen delivery. Two theoretical approaches exist. The first is to maintain oxygen delivery during CPB at normal levels for a given core temperature. Although this may limit hypoperfusion, it increases the delivered embolic load. The second approach is to use the lowest flows that do not result in end-organ injury. This approach offers the potential advantage of less embolic delivery as well as potential improved myocardial protection and surgical visualization. However, some of these advantages are not seen when the left ventricle is vented during CPB.

During CPB, pump flow and pressure are related through overall arterial impedance, a product of hemodilution, temperature, and arterial cross-sectional area. This is important because the first two factors, hemodilution and temperature, are critical determinants of pump flow requirements. Pump flows of 1.2 L/min per m^2 perfuse most of the microcirculation when the hematocrit is near 22% and hypothermic CPB is being employed. However, at lower hematocrits or periods of higher oxygen consumption, these flows become inadequate. Because of changes in oxygen demand with temperature and the plateauing of oxygen consumption with increasing flow, a series of nomograms has been developed for pump flow selection (Fig. 25.8).

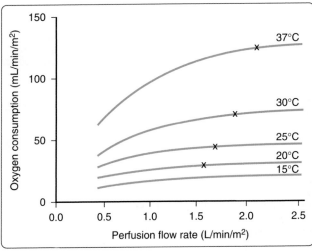

Fig. 25.8 Nomogram depicting the relationship of oxygen consumption (VO_2) to perfusion flow rate and temperature. The *x* on the curves represents common clinically used flow rates at the various temperatures. (From Kirklin JW, Barratt-Boyes BG. *Cardiac Surgery*. New York: Wiley; 1986:35.)

In addition to use of these nomograms, most perfusion teams also monitor mixed venous oxygen saturation, targeting levels of 70% or greater. Unfortunately, this level does not guarantee adequate perfusion of all tissue beds, because some (muscle, subcutaneous fat) may be functionally removed from the circulation during CPB. Hypothermic venous saturation may overestimate end-organ reserves.

Preparation for Separation

Before discontinuation of CPB, conditions that optimize cardiac and pulmonary function must be restored. To a great extent this is achieved by reversing the processes and techniques used to initiate and maintain CPB (Box 25.9).

Potential for Patient Awareness

It is not uncommon for patients to sweat during rewarming. This is almost certainly caused by perfusion of the hypothalamus (ie, the thermoregulatory site) with blood that is warmer than the latter organ's set-point (37°C). The brain is a high-flow organ and can be assumed to equilibrate fairly quickly (10 to 15 minutes) with cerebral perfusate temperature (ie, nasopharyngeal temperature). A less likely, but more disturbing, possibility is that restoration of brain normothermia with decreased anesthetic concentration may result in an inadequate depth of anesthesia and the potential for awareness. It is estimated that awareness occurs during cardiac surgery in up to 0.1% of patients.

Patient movement before discontinuation of CPB is, at the least, extremely disruptive and may be genuinely life-threatening if it results in cannula dislodgement or disruption of the procedure. Additional muscle relaxant should be administered. If awareness is suspected, supplemental amnestics or anesthetics should be administered during rewarming. Because sweating stops almost immediately on discontinuation of CPB, continued sweating after emergence from CPB may be a sign of awareness. Neurologic monitors such as the bispectral index can be used to help judge the depth of anesthesia during and after weaning from CPB.

25

BOX 25.9 *Preparation for Separation From Bypass Checklist*

1. Air clearance maneuvers completed
2. Rewarming completed
   a. Nasopharyngeal temperature 36–37°C
   b. Rectal/bladder temperature ≥35°C, but ≤37°C
3. Address issue of adequacy of anesthesia and muscle relaxation
4. Obtain stable cardiac rate and rhythm (use pacing if necessary)
5. Pump flow and systemic arterial pressure
   a. Pump flow to maintain mixed venous saturation ≥70%
   b. Systemic pressure restored to normothermic levels
6. Metabolic parameters
   a. Arterial pH, PO_2, PCO_2 within normal limits
   b. Hct: 20–25%
   c. K^+: 4.0–5.0 mEq/L
   d. Possibly ionized calcium
7. Ensuring all monitoring/access catheters are functional
   a. Transducers re-zeroed
   b. TEE (if used) out of freeze mode
8. Respiratory management
   a. Atelectasis cleared/lungs re-expanded
   b. Evidence of pneumothorax?
   c. Residual fluid in thoracic cavities drained
   d. Ventilation reinstituted
9. Intravenous fluids restarted
10. Inotropes/vasopressors/vasodilators prepared

Hct, Hematocrit; *TEE,* transesophageal echocardiography.

Rewarming

When systemic hypothermia is used, body temperature is restored to normothermia by gradually increasing perfusate temperature with the heat exchanger. Time required for rewarming (ie, heat transfer) varies with arterial perfusate temperature, patient temperature, and systemic flow. Excessive perfusate heating is not advisable for at least three key reasons: possible denaturation of plasma proteins, possible cerebral hyperthermia, and the fact that dissolved gas can come out of solution and coalesce into bubbles if the temperature gradient is too great. Because small increases (0.5°C) in cerebral temperature exacerbate ischemic injury in the brain, it is critical to perfuse the patient with blood temperatures at or below 37°C. Although this will increase the duration of rewarming, the risk of hyperthermic brain injury is greatly increased with hyperthermic blood temperatures. Most centers now employ mild hypothermia (ie, systemic temperature 32–35°C) instead of moderate hypothermia (26–28°C), reducing the amount of heat transfer required to achieve normothermia during rewarming.

Rewarming may be enhanced by increasing pump flow, which thereby increases heat input. At levels of hypothermia routinely used (25–30°C), the patient behaves as if vasoconstricted (calculated SVR is relatively high). Increasing pump flow in this setting may result in unacceptable hypertension. There are two approaches to this problem: wait out the vasoconstriction or pharmacologically induce patient vasodilation. When rectal or bladder temperature approaches 30–32°C, patients appear to vasodilate

V

rapidly. This is probably the result of decreasing blood viscosity or relaxation of cold-induced vasoconstriction with warming. Increasing pump flow at this point serves several purposes: increased heat transfer, support of systemic arterial pressure, and increased oxygen delivery in the face of increasing oxygen consumption. Often, waiting for the patient to spontaneously vasodilate is sufficient, and with subsequent increased pump flows, rewarming will be adequate at separation from CPB support. Circumstances in which more aggressive rewarming may be needed include profound hypothermia with a large hypoperfused "heat sink" and late initiation of warming by accident or design.

Skeletal muscle and subcutaneous fat are relatively hypoperfused during CPB. These tissues cool slowly and are also slow to warm. Temperatures at high-flow regions (eg, esophagus, nasopharynx) do not reflect the temperature of these tissues. Pharmacologic vasodilation allows an earlier increase in pump flow and delivery of warmed arterial blood to low-flow beds, making the rewarming process more uniform. Arteriolar vasodilators (eg, nicardipine, sodium nitroprusside) are much more likely to be effective in this process than venodilators (eg, nitroglycerin). Other aids to warming during or after CPB are sterile forced-air rewarming devices and servoregulated systems, as well as heating blankets, warmed fluids, heated humidified gases, and increased room temperature. The issue of afterdrop is less of a concern during routine cardiac surgery but manifests frequently in patients following deep hypothermic circulatory arrest (DHCA).

Restoration of Systemic Arterial Pressure to Normothermic Value

After aortic cross-clamp release, the heart is again perfused through the native coronary arteries. Until the proximal anastomoses are made, myocardial perfusion may be compromised in the presence of a low MAP. Consequently, it is advisable to increase MAP gradually during rewarming to levels of approximately 70 to 80 mm Hg.

With discontinuation of CPB, a marked discrepancy often exists between blood pressure readings measured from the radial artery and the central aorta. Radial arterial catheters may underestimate central aortic systolic pressures by 10 to 40 mm Hg. Discrepancies in MAP tend to be of a lesser magnitude (5–15 mm Hg). Such a discrepancy is not present before CPB, nor is it present after CPB in all patients. Mechanisms are undefined, but evidence supports vasodilatory and arteriovenous shunting phenomena in the forearm and hand. It is unknown at what point during CPB that radial artery–central aortic blood pressure discrepancies develop, but most investigators report their resolution 20 to 90 minutes after discontinuation of CPB. If measured radial arterial pressure is suspected to be low in relation to central aortic pressure, several actions can be taken. The surgeon can estimate central aortic pressure by palpation of the ascending aorta, place a small needle in the aortic lumen, use an aortic cannula to allow temporary monitoring of aortic pressure, or place a femoral arterial catheter.

Removal of Intracardiac Air

At the end of the procedure, intracardiac air is present in virtually all cases that require opening the heart (ie, valve repair or replacement, aneurysmectomy, septal defect repair, repair of congenital lesions). In such cases, it is important to remove as much air as possible before resumption of ejection. Surgical techniques differ. With the aortic cross-clamp still applied, the surgeon or perfusionist can partially limit venous return and LV vent flow, causing the left atrium and left ventricle to fill with blood. Through a transventricular approach, the left ventricle can then be aspirated. The left atrium and left ventricle are balloted to dislodge bubbles, and the cycle is repeated. The operating table can be rotated from side to side and the lungs ventilated to

25

promote clearance of air from the pulmonary veins. Rather than using transventricular aspiration, some surgeons vent air through the cardioplegia cannula or a needle vent in the ascending aorta. Before removal of the aortic cross-clamp, the patient is placed head down, so that bubbles will float away from the dependent carotid arteries. Some surgeons favor temporary manual carotid occlusion before cross-clamp removal, but safety and efficacy of this potentially dangerous maneuver are undocumented. A venting cannula is often left in the aorta at a location that should allow air pickup after resumption of ejection.

TEE has shown that routine air clearance techniques are not completely effective. Transcranial Doppler studies document a high incidence of intracranial gas emboli on release of the aortic cross-clamp or resumption of ejection. Three essential elements of air removal are: mobilization of air by positive chamber filling, stretching of the atrial wall, and repeated chamber ballottement; removal of mobilized air by continuous ascending aortic venting; and proof of elimination by TEE. Carbon dioxide gas insufflated by gravity into open cardiac chambers during CPB helps replace nitrogen in the bubbles with a more soluble gas. Accordingly, the persistence of gas bubbles observed by TEE after release of the aortic cross-clamp was lower in patients exposed to CO_2 in the chest. However, CO_2 insufflation should be used in addition to, rather than instead of, other de-airing maneuvers.

Intracardiac air may be present in 10% to 30% of closed cardiac cases as well (eg, CABG). During aortic cross-clamping, air may enter the aorta and left ventricle retrograde through native coronary arteries opened in the course of CABG surgery, particularly when suction is applied to vent the left side of the heart or aortic root. Efforts to expel air from the left ventricle and aortic root should be routine before unclamping the aorta. It is unclear to what extent gas emboli originating from the heart and aorta contribute to neurologic injury. However, microembolic load correlates with magnitude of cognitive dysfunction. Other studies report that air ejected from the left ventricle can also travel to the coronary arteries, resulting in sudden and sometimes extreme myocardial ischemia and failure after separation from bypass.

Defibrillation

Before discontinuation of CPB, the heart must have an organized rhythm that is spontaneous or pacer-induced. Ventricular fibrillation, common after cross-clamp release and warming, will often spontaneously convert to some other rhythm. Prolonged ventricular fibrillation is undesirable during rewarming for at least three reasons: subendocardial perfusion is compromised in the presence of normothermic ventricular fibrillation; myocardial oxygen consumption is greater with ventricular fibrillation compared with a beating heart at normothermia; and, if the left ventricle receives a large amount of blood (aortic insufficiency or bronchial return) in the absence of mechanical contraction, the left ventricle may distend. LV distension increases wall tension and further compromises subendocardial perfusion. On the other hand, early resumption of mechanical contraction may make some surgical procedures difficult (eg, modification of distal anastomoses).

Defibrillation, when necessary, is accomplished with internal paddles at much lower energies than would be used for external cardioversion. In the adult, starting energies of 5 to 10 J are routine. Defibrillation is less effective when the heart has not fully rewarmed, and it is rarely successful if myocardial (perfusate) temperature is less than 30°C. Repeated attempts at defibrillation, particularly with escalating energy levels, can lead to myocardial injury. If defibrillation is not successful after two to four attempts, options include further warming, correction of blood gas and electrolyte abnormalities if present (high PO_2 and high normal serum potassium [K^+] seem favorable), increased MAP, and antiarrhythmic therapy. Bolus administration of 100 mg of lidocaine before the release of the cross-clamp significantly lowers the incidence of reperfusion ventricular fibrillation. Increasing coronary perfusion by increased MAP is believed to result in myocardial reperfusion and recovery of the energy state.

Restoration of Ventilation

Before discontinuation of CPB, the lungs must be reinflated. Positive pressure (20–40 cm H_2O) is repeatedly applied until all areas of atelectasis are visually reinflated. Attention is specifically directed at the left lower lobe, which seems more difficult to reexpand. Fluid that has collected in the thoracic cavities during CPB is removed by the surgeon, and if the pleural cavity has not been opened, evidence of pneumothorax is also sought. The ventilatory rate can be increased 10% to 20% above prebypass values to compensate for increased V_d/V_t if present. Ventilation is resumed with 100% oxygen and subsequent adjustments in F_{IO_2} are made based on arterial blood gas analysis and pulse oximetry.

Correction of Metabolic Abnormalities and Arterial Oxygen Saturation

When rewarming is nearly complete and separation from CPB is anticipated to occur in 10 to 15 minutes, an arterial blood sample is taken and analyzed for acid-base status, P_{O_2}, partial pressure of carbon dioxide (P_{CO_2}), hemoglobin or hematocrit, potassium, and ionized calcium.

OXYGEN-CARRYING CAPACITY

Generally, a hematocrit of approximately 25% is sought before bypass is discontinued. The primary compensatory mechanism to ensure adequate systemic oxygen delivery in the presence of normovolemic anemia is increased CO. Increased CO results in an increased myocardial oxygen need, which is met by increased coronary oxygen delivery by coronary vasodilation. The lower limit of the hematocrit, below which increased CO can no longer support systemic oxygen needs, is reported to be 17% to 20% in dogs with completely healthy hearts. With increases in systemic V_{O_2}, such as occur with exercise, fever, or shivering, higher values of the hematocrit are required. Patients with good ventricular function and good coronary reserve (or good revascularization) might be expected to tolerate hematocrit values in the 20s. When ventricular function is impaired or revascularization is incomplete, hematocrit above 25% may aid in support of the systemic circulation and concomitantly lower myocardial oxygen requirements on discontinuation of bypass. When pump or oxygenator reservoir volume is in excess, the hematocrit can be increased by use of hemofiltration.

ARTERIAL PH

Considerable debate has centered on the extent to which acidemia affects myocardial performance and whether correction of arterial pH with sodium bicarbonate is advantageous or deleterious to the heart. Studies have challenged long-held beliefs that acidemia impairs myocardial performance. Nevertheless, most in vivo and clinical studies have found metabolic acidosis impairs contractility and alters responses to exogenous catecholamines. Hemodynamic deterioration is usually mild above pH 7.2 because of compensatory increases in sympathetic nervous system activity. Attenuation of sympathetic nervous system responses by β-blockade or ganglionic blockade increases the detrimental effect of acidosis. The ischemic myocardium has been found to be particularly vulnerable to detrimental effects of acidosis. Patients with poor contractile function or reduction of myocardial sympathetic responsiveness (eg, chronic LV failure), those treated with β-blockers, or those with myocardial ischemia are

25

especially susceptible to the adverse effects of acidosis. For these reasons arterial pH is corrected to near-normal levels before discontinuation of CPB, using sodium bicarbonate. Concerns regarding carbon dioxide generation and acidification of the intracellular space can be obviated by slow administration and appropriate adjustment of ventilation, both of which are easily achieved during CPB.

ELECTROLYTES

Electrolytes most commonly of concern before discontinuation of CPB are potassium and calcium. Serum potassium concentration may be acutely low because of hemodilution with nonpotassium priming solutions, large-volume diuresis during CPB, or the use of insulin to treat hyperglycemia. More commonly, potassium concentration is elevated as a result of systemic uptake of potassium-containing cardioplegic solution; values exceeding 6 mEq/L are not uncommon. Other potential causes of hyperkalemia that must be considered are hemolysis, tissue ischemia or necrosis, and acidemia. Hypokalemia can be rapidly corrected during CPB with relative safety because the heart and systemic circulation are supported. Increments of 5 to 10 mEq of KCl over 1- to 2-minute intervals can be given directly into the oxygenator by the perfusionist, and potassium subsequently is rechecked. Depending on severity and urgency of correction, elevated potassium can be treated or reduced by any of several standard means: alkali therapy, diuresis, calcium administration, or insulin and glucose. Alternatively, hemofiltration can be used to lower serum potassium. While the patient is still on CPB, potassium-containing extracellular fluid is removed and replaced with fluid not containing potassium.

Ionized calcium is involved in the maintenance of normal excitation-contraction coupling and therefore in maintaining cardiac contractility and peripheral vascular tone. Low concentrations of ionized calcium lead to impaired cardiac contractility and lowered vascular tone. Concerns have been raised about the contribution of calcium administration to myocardial reperfusion injury and to the action of various inotropes. Some investigators argue in favor of measuring ionized calcium before discontinuation of CPB and to administer calcium in patients with low concentrations to optimize cardiac performance. Although they routinely measure ionized calcium before discontinuation of bypass, calcium salts are not routinely administered. When confronted with poor myocardial or peripheral vascular responsiveness to inotropes or vasopressors after bypass in the presence of a low level of ionized calcium, calcium salts should be administered to restore ionized calcium to normal (not elevated) levels in the hope of restoring responsiveness. The same strategy can be used for measuring and administering magnesium.

Other Final Preparations

Before the patient is separated from CPB, all monitoring and access catheters should be checked and calibrated. The zero-pressure calibration points of the pressure transducers are routinely checked. Not uncommonly, finger pulse oximeter probes do not have a good signal after CPB. In those cases, a nasal or ear probe is placed to obtain reliable oximetry. Intravenous infusions are restarted before separation from CPB, and their flow characteristics are assessed for evidence of obstruction or disconnection.

During warming and preparation for separation, an assessment should be made of the functional status of the heart and peripheral vasculature based on visual inspection, hemodynamic indices, and metabolic parameters. Based on this assessment, inotropes, vasodilators, and vasopressors thought likely to be necessary for successful separation from CPB should be prepared and readied for administration.

Separation From Bypass

After all preparatory steps are taken, CPB can be discontinued. Venous outflow to the pump or oxygenator is impeded by slowly clamping the venous line, and the patient's intravascular volume and ventricular loading conditions are restored by transfusion of perfusate through the aortic inflow line. When loading conditions are optimal, the aortic inflow line is clamped, and the patient is separated from CPB.

At this juncture it must be determined whether oxygenation, ventilation, and, more commonly, myocardial performance (systemic perfusion) are adequate. Should separation fail for any reason, CPB can simply be reinstituted by unclamping the venous outflow and arterial inflow lines and restoring pump flow. This allows for support of systemic oxygenation and perfusion while steps are taken to diagnose and treat those problems that precluded successful separation.

▦ PERFUSION EMERGENCIES

Accidents or mishaps occurring during CPB can quickly evolve into life-threatening emergencies (Box 25.10). Many of the necessary conditions of CPB (cardiac arrest, hypothermia, volume depletion) preclude the ability to resume normal cardiorespiratory function if an accident threatens the integrity of the extracorporeal circuit. Fortunately, major perfusion accidents occur infrequently and are rarely associated with permanent injury or death. However, all members of the cardiac surgery team must be able to respond to perfusion emergencies to limit the likelihood of perfusion-related disasters. Some of the most common emergencies are discussed in the subsequent sections.

Arterial Cannula Malposition

Ascending aortic cannulas can be malpositioned such that the outflow jet is directed primarily into the innominate artery, the left common carotid artery (rare), or the left subclavian artery (rare). The latter two can occur with the use of long arch-type cannulas. In the first two circumstances, unilateral cerebral *hyperperfusion*, usually with systemic hypoperfusion, occurs, whereas flow directed to the subclavian artery results in global cerebral *hypoperfusion*. Despite the fact that not all combinations of arterial pressure monitoring site and cannula malposition produce systemic hypotension, it is commonly regarded as a cardinal sign of cannula malposition. For example, right arm blood pressure monitoring and innominate artery cannulation, or left arm monitoring and left subclavian artery cannulation, may result in *high* arterial pressure on initiation of bypass. With other positioning and monitoring combinations, investigators report persistently low systemic arterial pressure (MAP, 25–35 mm Hg), which is poorly responsive to increasing pump flow or vasoconstrictors. Over time (minutes), signs of systemic hypoperfusion (eg, acidemia, oliguria) develop. Because

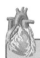

BOX 25.10   *Perfusion Emergencies*

Arterial cannula malposition
Aortic dissection
Massive air embolism
Venous air lock
Reversed cannulation

a variable period of systemic hypotension with CPB initiation is nearly always seen with hemodilution, hypotension alone is not significant evidence to establish a diagnosis of arterial cannula malposition. On initiation of CPB and periodically thereafter, it is advisable to inspect the face for color change and edema, rhinorrhea, or otorrhea, and to palpate the neck with onset of cooling for temperature asymmetry. Electroencephalographic monitoring was first advocated as a method of detecting cannula malposition. However, transcranial Doppler, and more commonly available cerebral oximetry, is the monitor of choice to detect malperfusion secondary to cannula complications.

Two other arterial cannula malpositions are possible: abutment of the cannula tip against the aortic intima, which results in high line pressure, poor perfusion, or even acute dissection when CPB is initiated, and the cannula tip directed caudally toward the aortic valve. This may result in acute aortic insufficiency, with sudden LV distension and systemic hypoperfusion on bypass. If the aortic inflow cannula is soft, aortic cross-clamping will occlude the arterial perfusion line, which can rupture the aortic inflow line. Suspicion of any cannula malposition must immediately be brought to the attention of the surgeon.

Aortic or Arterial Dissection

Signs of arterial dissection, often similar to those of cannula malposition, must also be sought continuously, especially on initiation of CPB. Dissection may originate at the cannulation site, aortic cross-clamp site, proximal vein graft anastomotic site, or partial occlusion (side-biting) clamp site. Dissections are due to intimal disruption or, more distally, to fracture of atherosclerotic plaque. In either case, some systemic arterial blood flow becomes extraluminal, being forced into the arterial wall. The dissection propagates mostly but not exclusively in the direction of the systemic flow. Extraluminal blood compresses the luminal origins (take-offs) of major arterial branches such that vital organs (heart, brain, kidney, intestinal tract, spinal cord) may become ischemic. Because systemic perfusion may be low, and origins of the innominate and subclavian arteries may be compressed, probably the best sign of arterial dissection is persistently low systemic arterial pressure. Venous drainage to the pump decreases (blood is sequestered), and arterial inflow "line pressure" is usually inappropriately high. The surgeon may see the dissection if it involves the anterior or lateral ascending aorta (bluish discoloration), or both. It is possible the surgeon may *not* see any sign of dissection, because the dissection is out of view (eg, posterior ascending aorta, aortic arch, descending aorta). A careful TEE examination at this time may show the dissection and its extent. Dissection can occur at any time before, during, or after CPB. As with cannula malposition, a suspicion of arterial dissection must be brought to the attention of the surgeon. The anesthesiologist must not assume that something is suddenly wrong with the arterial pressure transducer but should "think dissection."

After a dissection of the ascending aorta is diagnosed, immediate steps to minimize propagation must be taken. If it has occurred before CPB, the anesthesiologist should take steps to reduce MAP and the rate of rise of aortic pressure (dP/dt). If it occurs during CPB, pump flow and MAP are reduced to the lowest acceptable levels. Arterial perfusate is frequently cooled to profound levels (14–19°C) as rapidly as possible to decrease metabolic demand and protect vital organs. A different arterial cannulation site is prepared (eg, the femoral artery is cannulated or the true aortic lumen is cannulated at a site more distal on the aortic arch). Arterial inflow is shifted to that new site with the intent that perfusing the true aortic lumen will reperfuse vital organs. The ascending aorta is cross-clamped just below the innominate artery, and cardioplegia is administered (into the coronary ostia or coronary sinus). The aorta is opened to expose the site of disruption, which is then resected and replaced. Reimplantation of the coronary arteries or aortic valve replacement, or both, may be necessary. The false lumina at both ends of the aorta are obliterated with Teflon buttresses, and the graft is inserted by end-to-end suture. With small dissections it is sometimes possible to avoid open repair by application of a partial occlusion clamp with plication of the dissection and exclusion of the intimal disruption.

Arterial dissections originating from femoral cannulation also necessitate reductions in arterial pressure, systemic flow, and temperature. If the operation is near completion, the heart may be transfused and CPB discontinued; otherwise, the aortic arch must be cannulated and adequate systemic perfusion restored to allow completion of the operation.

Massive Arterial Gas Embolus

Macroscopic gas embolus is a rare but disastrous CPB complication. Two independent studies in 1980 reported incidences of recognized massive arterial gas embolism of 0.1% to 0.2%. The current incidence is probably lower because of the widespread use of reservoir-level alarms and other bubble detection devices. Between 20% and 30% of affected patients died immediately, with another 30% having transient or nondebilitating neurologic deficits, or both. Circumstances that most commonly contributed to these events were inattention to oxygenator blood level, reversal of LV vent flow, or unexpected resumption of cardiac ejection in a previously opened heart. Rupture of a pulsatile assist device or IABP may also introduce large volumes of gas into the arterial circulation.

The pathophysiology of cerebral gas embolism (macroscopic and microscopic) is not well understood. Tissue damage after gas embolization is initiated from simple mechanical blockage of blood vessels by bubbles. Although gas emboli may be absorbed or pass through the circulation within 1 to 5 minutes, the local reaction of platelets and proteins to the blood gas interface or endothelial damage is thought to potentiate microvascular stasis, prolonging cerebral ischemia to the point of infarction. Areas of marginal perfusion, such as arterial boundary zones, do not clear gas emboli as rapidly as well-perfused zones, producing patterns of ischemia or infarction difficult to distinguish from those due to hypotension or particulate emboli.

Recommended treatment for massive arterial gas embolism includes immediate cessation of CPB with aspiration of as much gas as possible from the aorta and heart, assumption of steep Trendelenburg position, and clearance of air from the arterial perfusion line. After resumption of CPB, treatment continues with implementation or deepening of hypothermia (18–27°C) during completion of the operation and clearance of gas from the coronary circulation before emergence from CPB. In many reports of patients suffering massive arterial gas embolus, seizures occurred postoperatively and were treated with anticonvulsants. Because seizures after ischemic insults are associated with poor outcomes, perhaps because of hypermetabolic effects, prophylactic phenytoin seems reasonable. Hypotension has been shown to lengthen the residence time of cerebral air emboli and worsen the severity of resulting ischemia. Maintenance of moderate hypertension therefore is reasonable and clinically attainable to hasten clearance of emboli from the circulation and, hopefully, improve neurologic outcome.

Many clinicians have reported dramatic neurologic recovery when hyperbaric therapy was used for arterial gas embolism, even if delayed up to 26 hours after the event. Spontaneous recovery from air emboli has also been reported, and no prospective study of hyperbaric therapy in the cardiac surgery setting has been performed. Few

25

institutions that do cardiac surgery have an appropriately equipped and staffed hyperbaric chamber to allow expeditious and safe initiation of hyperbaric therapy. Nonetheless, immediate transfer by air is often possible and should seriously be considered. It seems reasonable to expect that institutions that perform cardiac surgery should have policies regarding catastrophic air embolism.

Venoarterial perfusion as an alternative to hyperbaric therapy has also been suggested, with the goal of flushing air from the cerebral arterial circulation. None of the patients so treated had evidence of neurologic injury. Other reports using this technique have followed. The timing of the embolism is also a major consideration. For example, if massive air embolism occurs during connection, serious consideration should be given to abandoning the procedure to allow immediate therapy and awakening the patient to assess neurologic status. Air embolism and its subsequent cerebral ischemia are likely worsened by the nonphysiologic nature of CPB as well as its inherent inflammatory processes.

Venous Air Lock

Air entering the venous outflow line can result in complete cessation of flow to the venous reservoir, and this is called *air lock*. Loss of venous outflow necessitates immediate slowing, even cessation of pump flow, to prevent emptying the reservoir and subsequent delivery of air to the patient's arterial circulation. After an air lock is recognized, a search for the source of venous outflow line air must be undertaken (eg, loose atrial purse-string suture, atrial tear, open intravenous access) and repaired before reestablishing full bypass.

Reversed Cannulation

In reversed cannulation, the venous outflow limb of the CPB circuit is incorrectly connected to the arterial inflow cannula, and the arterial perfusion limb of the circuit is attached to the venous cannula. On initiation of CPB, blood is removed from the arterial circulation and returned to the venous circulation at high pressure. Arterial pressure is found to be extremely low by palpation and arterial pressure monitoring. Very low arterial pressures can also (more commonly) be due to dissection in the arterial tree. In the latter case, the perfusionist will rapidly lose volume, whereas with reversed cannulation, the perfusionist will have an immediate gross excess of volume. If high pump flow is established, venous or atrial rupture may occur. The CVP will be dramatically elevated, with evidence of facial venous engorgement.

Line pressure is the pressure in the arterial limb of the CPB circuit. Because arterial cannulas are much smaller than the aorta, there is always a pressure drop across the aortic cannula. Arterial inflow line pressure will always be considerably higher than systemic (patient) arterial pressure. The magnitude of the pressure drop depends on cannula size and systemic flow; small cannulas and higher flows result in greater gradients. The CPB pump must generate a pressure that overcomes this gradient to provide adequate systemic arterial pressure. For a typical adult (ie, MAP of about 60 mm Hg, systemic flow of about 2.4 L/min/m^2, and a 24-Fr aortic cannula), line pressure in an uncomplicated case usually ranges from 150 to 250 mm Hg. The fittings on the arterial inflow line are plastic; the fittings and the line itself can rupture. Perfusionists typically do not want a line pressure in excess of 300 mm Hg.

CPB must be discontinued and the cannula disconnected and inspected for air. If air is found in the arterial circulation, an air embolus protocol is initiated. Once arterial air is cleared, the circuit is correctly reconnected and CPB restarted. In adults, the venous outflow limb of the CPB circuit is a larger-diameter tubing than the arterial inflow tubing, precisely to eliminate reversed cannulation. This is why reversed cannulation is rare in adults—but it has happened. In pediatric cases, the arterial inflow and venous outflow limbs of the CPB circuit are close or equal in size.

SPECIAL PATIENT POPULATIONS

Care of the Gravid Patient During Bypass

Studies assessing the effects of cardiac surgery and CPB on obstetric physiology and fetal well-being are lacking. However, several reviews and many case reports describe individual experience in caring for the gravid patient and fetus during cardiac surgery and extracorporeal circulation. These surveys and anecdotal reports, along with an understanding of the well-documented physiology of pregnancy and the effects of cardiac therapeutics on fetal physiology, can serve as a basis for a rational approach to care for the pregnant patient and fetus during cardiac surgery (Box 25.11). The reported experience on maternal and fetal outcomes after cardiac procedures with CPB suggests that cardiac surgery is well tolerated by the mother, but poses a significant risk to the fetus.

Considerations Before Bypass

PREMEDICATION AND PATIENT POSITIONING

Premedication should be appropriate for the specific cardiac lesion and physical status of the patient. Teratogenic drugs should be avoided, especially in the first trimester of pregnancy. After the 34th week of gestation, stomach emptying is delayed and patients are at increased risk for pulmonary aspiration. Although it is not possible to ensure gastric emptying before anesthesia induction, sodium citrate and an H_2-receptor antagonist may provide some protection against aspiration pneumonia. The gravid uterus obstructs aortic flow and IVC blood return to the heart. Gravid patients should never be supine; they must be positioned with left uterine displacement throughout the perioperative period.

MATERNAL AND FETAL MONITOR INFORMATION

The pregnant patient undergoing cardiac surgery requires the usual monitors employed during cardiac surgery, as well as monitors that can assess fetal well-being. Monitors that help assess the adequacy of maternal cardiovascular performance and oxygen delivery to the fetus are of paramount importance. Little is known about the effects of cardiovascular drugs and other therapeutic measures on the pregnant cardiac

25

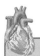

BOX 25.11   *Special Patients Who May Need Cardiopulmonary Bypass*

Pregnant women
Accidental hypothermia victims
Neurosurgical patient with an intracranial aneurysm

patient undergoing CPB. Appropriate monitors permit the assessment of an individual therapy on maternal and fetal oxygen delivery.

Uterine activity should be monitored with a tocodynamometer applied to the maternal abdomen. This monitor transduces the tightening of the abdomen during uterine contractions. As is the case with other types of major surgery, the tocodynamometer should not interfere with the conduct of cardiac surgery; if necessary, the monitor may be intermittently displaced by the operating surgeon. The use of an intraamniotic catheter to monitor uterine activity and pressure may be inadvisable in a patient who is fully heparinized. Intraoperative uterine contractions may have a deleterious effect on fetal oxygen delivery (by causing an increase in uterine venous pressure and decrease in uterine blood flow) and signal the onset of preterm labor. Use of the tocodynamometer is imperative, as it provides important information about the state of the uterus and allows intervention if necessary. Various reports have documented the common occurrence of uterine contractions during cardiac surgery and CPB. Uterine contractions may appear at any time during the perioperative period but occur most frequently immediately after the discontinuation of CPB and in the early ICU period. It is therefore important to leave the tocodynamometer in place after the completion of surgery. Although uterine contractions occur frequently in the perioperative course, they usually are effectively treated with magnesium sulfate, ritodrine, or ethanol infusions, and they do not result in preterm labor or fetal demise.

Fetal heart rate (FHR) monitors should be used in all gravid patients after 20 weeks' gestation because one of the primary perioperative goals is to avoid fetal loss. Use of an FHR monitor permits recognition of fetal distress and allows the clinician to institute measures to improve fetal oxygen delivery. The FHR monitor recognizes and records the FHR, FHR variability, and uterine contractions. A spinal electrode placed on the fetal scalp gives the most reliable fetal electrocardiogram (ECG) and therefore the best FHR information. However, this method may be undesirable in the presence of maternal anticoagulation. External FHR monitoring—using ultrasound, phonocardiography, or external abdominal ECG—is less exact but preferable in this clinical setting.

The cardiac surgeon, perfusionist, and cardiac anesthesiologist may not be familiar with uterine and FHR monitors. As a result, having a perinatologist or an obstetrician present during cardiac surgery is desirable to assess for preoperative fetal distress and the anticipated need for emergency cesarean section during cardiac surgery.

FHR is usually normal in the prebypass period, but decreases precipitously with the initiation of CPB and remains below normal for the entire bypass period. There are many potential causes of this observed decrease in FHR. Persistent fetal bradycardia is a classic sign of acute fetal hypoxia. However, in the CPB setting, especially when hypothermia is employed, it is difficult to ascribe fetal bradycardia to hypoxia or to decreased fetal oxygen demand. Fetal tachycardia typically occurs after the discontinuation of CPB. This tachycardia may represent a compensatory mechanism for the oxygen debt incurred during CPB. The FHR usually returns to normal by the end of the operative period.

Interventions optimizing maternal blood oxygen content, correcting any acid-base imbalance, and replenishing fetal glycogen stores may alleviate signs of fetal hypoxia. Some clinicians recommend an increase in CPB pump flow to improve fetal oxygen delivery.

Conducting the Bypass Procedure

The conditions of extracorporeal circulation—nonpulsatile blood flow, hypothermia, anemia, and anticoagulation—will likely have a negative impact on fetal well-being during CPB. There are no studies that recommend a particular CPB management

Table 25.5   Recommendations for the Conduct of Extracorporeal Circulation in the Gravid Patient

Variable	Recommended Value/Characteristic	Rationale
Blood flow	3.0 L/min/m^2	Cardiac index normally is increased during pregnancy
Blood pressure (MAP)	60–70 mm Hg	Uterine blood flow depends on maternal MAP
Temperature	32–34°C	Mild hypothermia decreases fetal oxygen requirements and is less likely to cause fetal arrhythmia
Oxygenator type	Membrane	Membrane oxygenators are associated with fewer embolic phenomena than bubblers
Hematocrit	25–27%	The quantity of oxygen carried in maternal blood (and therefore the oxygen available to the fetus) greatly depends on hemoglobin concentration
Duration of perfusion	Minimized	The duration of bypass is dictated by the complexity of the operative procedure
Cardioplegia	?	No data
Pulsatile perfusion	?	No data

MAP, Mean arterial pressure.

strategy in gravid patients. Recommendations are summarized (Table 25.5) for the management of CPB in pregnant patients, based on the survey and anecdotal reports in the literature.

BLOOD FLOW

Optimal CPB blood flow in the gravid patient is unknown. However, the increase in CO associated with pregnancy is well defined, and it might be argued that high blood flows during CPB are more physiologic in the gravid patient. It has been suggested that flow during CPB in the pregnant patient be maintained at a minimum of 3.0 L/min per m^2. A few reports demonstrate that increasing CPB circuit blood flow improves FHR, suggesting improvement in fetal oxygen delivery.

BLOOD PRESSURE

Under normal conditions, uterine blood flow is determined solely by maternal blood pressure, as the placental vasculature is maximally dilated. However, it is not known what factors determine uterine blood flow during the very abnormal condition of CPB. For example, catecholamine levels increase by several times during CPB; therefore, uterine vascular resistance may increase during extracorporeal circulation in response to increased levels of norepinephrine and epinephrine. However, regardless of the state of uterine vascular resistance during CPB, maternal blood pressure will be an important determinant of uterine blood flow and fetal oxygen delivery. Moderately high pressure (MAP ≥65 mm Hg) should be employed during perfusion in the gravid patient.

In theory, the use of short-acting vasodilators, such as nitroglycerin or sodium nitroprusside, may counteract the effects of CPB and norepinephrine- or epinephrine-induced increases in uterine vasculature resistance. If maternal blood pressure is maintained by increasing extracorporeal circuit pump flow, uterine blood flow and fetal oxygen delivery may be increased with vasodilators. Monitoring should be conducted to assess the effect of a given therapeutic on fetal oxygen delivery during CPB.

TEMPERATURE

Controversy exists regarding temperature management during CPB in the nongravid patient, although most perfusions are conducted under hypothermic conditions. Similarly, there are few data and no consensus regarding temperature management in the gravid patient undergoing CPB.

There are theoretical advantages and disadvantages for normothermic and hypothermic CPB in the gravid patient. Hypothermia can cause fetal bradycardia and may lead to fetal ventricular arrhythmias, resulting in fetal wastage. Rewarming after hypothermic CPB may precipitate uterine contractions and preterm labor. However, others reported the onset of uterine contractions at the time of discontinuation of CPB in spite of normothermic perfusion. Uterine contractions also occur at various times in the postbypass and postoperative periods. The association of uterine contractions with rewarming after hypothermic bypass is unclear.

Hypothermia may be protective to the fetus during extracorporeal circulation by decreasing fetal oxygen requirements. Perfusion temperatures of 25°C to 37°C have been used in gravid patients undergoing CPB. However, the optimal gravida temperature during CPB has not been established. There are no data that suggest hypothermia is harmful to the mother or fetus undergoing bypass.

Accidental Hypothermia

Patient Selection

Clinicians lack consensus regarding the absolute indications or contraindications for the use of CPB in the treatment of accidental deep hypothermia. However, there are theoretical considerations and some data to help guide the decision-making process regarding the rewarming of accidental hypothermia patients. Phenomena that greatly limit the likelihood of successful resuscitation include the presence of asphyxia before the initiation of hypothermia, as occurs commonly in avalanche and drowning victims. Similarly, patients with severe traumatic injury, or extremely elevated potassium levels (≥10 mmol/L) are unlikely to benefit from resuscitative efforts.

Caring for the Accidental Hypothermia Victim

After the decision is made to resuscitate an accidental hypothermia victim, the patient should be maintained at the hypothermic temperature and rapidly transferred to a facility that can provide extracorporeal rewarming. In the operating room, various vascular sites may be cannulated to initiate rewarming. Femoral vessels or mediastinal vasculature may serve as conduits for rewarming. Because the ventricle is noncompliant at temperatures below 32°C, sternotomy or thoracotomy may be preferable to facilitate direct cardiac massage and defibrillation. Although hypothermia reduces anesthetic requirements, the prudent use of anesthetics, analgesics, sedative-hypnotics, and volatile drugs is recommended. These agents should be administered through the extracorporeal circuit.

To treat an asystolic patient, the extracorporeal circuit must include a pump, oxygenator, and heat exchange water bath. At flow rates of 2 to 3 L/min, with the water bath at 37°C, the patient's core temperature can increase by as much as 1 to

2°C every 3 to 5 minutes. Slowly, the flow rate can be increased as determined by venous return. Given the data regarding the adverse effects of mildly hyperthermic blood on ischemic cerebral damage, the accidental hypothermia patient should not be perfused with blood warmed to temperatures in excess of 37°C. If the victim has a perfusing cardiac rhythm, venovenous rewarming may be used. Indeed, strong arguments can be made for limiting the rewarming to only 32°C to 33°C and then adhering to cardiac arrest protocols that use prolonged mild hypothermia to optimize cerebral outcomes.

Intracranial Aneurysm Surgery

Surgery for intracranial aneurysm represents a major challenge for the surgeon and anesthesiologist. For a small number of these cases, DHCA has been applied to improve surgical access and cerebral protection. Like many areas, significant evolution in technique and application has occurred over time. Initial enthusiasm for DHCA in intracranial aneurysm surgery was tempered by the unfortunate occurrence of coagulopathies. Its use was further restricted by advances in neurosurgical microscopic techniques (aneurysm wrapping, parent vessel ligation, and use of temporary clips). Improvements in perioperative monitoring and neuroanesthesia have reserved a use for DHCA in the approach to giant aneurysms that might otherwise be inoperable.

Given that the overall numbers involved are small, it is very difficult to develop precise estimates for morbidity and mortality rates. However, given that DHCA in intracranial aneurysm surgery has been reserved for only the most difficult cases, the results seen are encouraging. As in most areas of cardiac surgery, continued developments have led to an evolution in neurosurgery as well and in how these intracranial aneurysms are being addressed. For example, many more are now being addressed with neurovascular radiologic coiling than are being treated open under DHCA. It is likely that this will be a continuing trend in the declining use of DHCA to treat intracranial aneurysms.

▨ MINIMALLY INVASIVE SURGERY AND CARDIOPULMONARY BYPASS

25

Port-Access Bypass Circuit

The port-access system consists of a series of catheters that are introduced through various puncture sites, including the femoral artery and vein, and threaded through the aorta and venous system to the heart. The perfusion is usually set up from the femoral vein to the oxygenator and then returned via the femoral artery. An inflatable balloon on the end of an endoaortic clamp (EAC) catheter can be used to arrest the blood flow in the aorta, and other catheters help drain and reroute the blood flow to the heart-lung machine. Through two of the catheters, cardioplegia solution can be administered to the heart (Fig. 25.9).

The EAC is an occlusion balloon that functions as an aortic cross-clamp and permits antegrade cardioplegia infusion into the aortic root and coronary arteries. The lumen used to administer cardioplegia can also function as an aortic root–venting catheter. Some surgeons prefer to use a direct modified aortic cross-clamp inserted through a port in the right side of the chest instead of using the EAC; they depend on administration of cardioplegia in a retrograde fashion via the coronary sinus. Retrograde cardioplegia can be delivered through an endocoronary sinus catheter (ECSC) that is placed with a percutaneous approach.

V

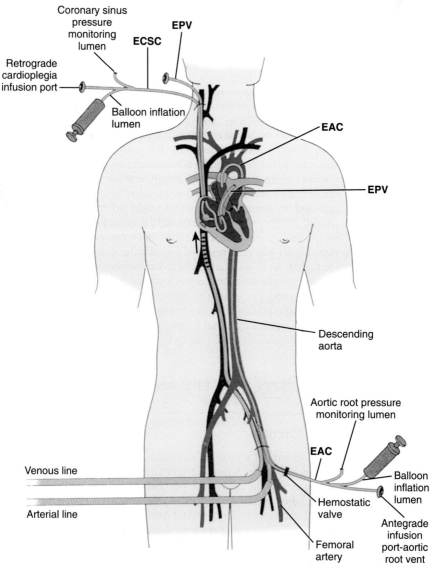

Fig. 25.9 Positioning of endovascular catheters. The femoral venous drainage catheter tip is positioned at the right atrium–superior vena cava junction by fluoroscopy and transesophageal echocardiography. *EAC,* Endoaortic clamp; *ECSC,* endocoronary sinus catheter; *EPV,* endopulmonary vent. (From Toomasian JM, Peters SP, Siegel LC, Stevens JH. Extracorporeal circulation for port-access cardiac surgery. *Perfusion.* 1997;12:83–91.)

Blood returns to the CPB through the femoral venous catheter that is advanced to the level of the IVC–right atrium junction. Because extrathoracic gravity drainage is usually insufficient in providing adequate blood flow for complete CPB support, kinetic-assisted venous drainage, with controlled suction, is used to augment the drainage of blood to the heart-lung machine.

Port-access CPB demands an expanded role of the anesthesiologist during CPB. The anesthesiologist is responsible for inserting the ECSC (and even the endopulmonary vent [EPV]) through introducer sheaths placed in the right internal jugular vein. The ECSC should be placed first with the assistance of both fluoroscopy and TEE. TEE guidance is used for engaging the coronary sinus and fluoroscopy for advancing the catheter in the coronary sinus. Proper placement is judged by attaining a pressure in the coronary sinus greater than 30 mm Hg during cardioplegia administration at a rate of 150 to 200 mL/min. Failure can occur for a number of reasons, but the most common reason is displacement of the catheter from the coronary sinus during surgical manipulations. Complications, including perforation and dissections, have been reported in a small percentage of patients.

Monitoring for Endovascular Clamp Bypass

The aorta catheter with the EAC should be positioned in the ascending aorta 2 to 4 cm distal to the aortic valve. Because cephalad migration of the endovascular aortic root clamp may compromise CBF, it is imperative to monitor endovascular clamp position continuously. There are several proposed methods to achieve this essential goal (Table 25.6). TEE and color-flow Doppler aid in visualizing the placement of the EAC balloon in the ascending aorta and in detecting any leakage of blood around the balloon. Right radial artery pressure will decrease acutely if the EAC migrates and obstructs the brachiocephalic artery. Some clinicians choose to measure blood pressure in the left and right radial arteries. The occurrence of acute difference in radial artery pressures may indicate cephalad migration of the EAC. Pulse-wave Doppler of the right carotid artery can verify cerebral perfusion but is frequently difficult to assess under the conditions of nonpulsatile blood flow. The ability of transcranial Doppler monitoring of the middle cerebral artery and cerebral oximetry techniques to determine the adequacy of CBF requires further evaluation. The TEE probe may be useful in visualizing the ascending aorta and location of the balloon; however, many clinicians report the inadequacy of this technique.

Port-Access Cardiac Surgery Outcome Data

Early advocates of port-access cardiac surgery (PACS) hoped that this new approach would provide the benefits of minimally invasive surgery with the advantage of extracorporeal support and myocardial preservation during procedures on the heart. A relatively slow learning curve exists, and multiple, unexpected complications have been reported (eg, inadequate de-airing of the ventricle before discontinuation of CPB support, aortic or femoral artery dissection, malposition of the endovascular clamp). Coronary artery surgery can be done using PACS, but it has not become a popular technique compared with OPCAB and other minimally invasive revascularization procedures. The use of robotic assistance for mitral valve repairs performed via a thoracotomy using PACS has gained popularity in some centers; results have shown good success rates, less transfusion need, and shorter hospital stays.

661

Table 25.6 Potential Strategies to Monitor Cerebral Blood Flow During Port-Access Bypass

Monitor	Limitations	Observation With Cephalad Migration of Endoaortic Clamp[a]
Fluoroscopy	Must interrupt surgery to use monitor	EAC occluding great vessels
Transesophageal echocardiography	May be difficult to visualize EAC position during cardiopulmonary bypass	EAC in area of great vessels
Carotid ultrasound	Difficult to monitor signal continuously—depends on index of suspicion Difficult to obtain signal with nonpulsatile blood flow	Sudden loss of blood flow signal
Transcranial Doppler	Difficult to monitor MCA blood flow continuously—depends on index of suspicion Difficult to insonate MCA during nonpulsatile blood flow Poor sensitivity/specificity	Loss of MCA blood flow velocity signal Change in ratio of RMCA vs LMCA blood flow velocity Change in RMCA or LMCA blood flow direction
Cerebral oximetry (R vs L signal)	Sensitivity/specificity?	Decrease in cerebral venous blood oxygen saturation; change in R vs L signal[b]
Electroencephalography	Hypothermia, anesthetics, and roller pump artifacts limit interpretation of EEG signals	EEG slowing/change in right vs left EEG signal
Right and left radial arterial pressures	Requires cannulation of both radial arteries; increased risk for hand ischemia Left radial arterial free graft conduit not possible	Change in the ratio of right and left radial arteries measured MAP

EAC, Endoaortic clamp; *EEG,* electroencephalographic; *L,* left; *MAP,* mean arterial pressure; *MCA,* middle cerebral artery; *R,* right.
[a]Hypothetical observation; the sensitivity and specificity of these monitors in this clinical setting have not been evaluated.
[b]The rate and magnitude of change depend on many factors, including the patient's cerebral temperature, magnitude of obstruction, and collateral blood flow.

SUGGESTED READINGS

Arrowsmith JE, Grocott HP, Reves JG, et al. Central nervous system complications of cardiac surgery. *Br J Anaesth.* 2000;84:378–393.

Bainbridge D, Martin J, Cheng D. Off pump coronary artery bypass graft surgery versus conventional coronary artery bypass graft surgery: a systematic review of the literature. *Semin Cardiothorac Vasc Anesth.* 2005;9:105–111.

Duebener LF, Hagino I, Sakamoto T, et al. Effects of pH management during deep hypothermic bypass on cerebral microcirculation: alpha-stat versus pH-stat. *Circulation.* 2002;106:I103–I108.

Duncan AE, Abd-Elsayed A, Maheshwari A, et al. Role of intraoperative and postoperative blood glucose concentrations in predicting outcomes after cardiac surgery. *Anesthesiology*. 2010;112:860–871.

Engelman R, Baker RA, Likosky DS, et al. The society of thoracic surgeons, the society of cardiovascular anesthesiologists, and the American society of ExtraCorporeal technology: clinical practice guidelines for cardiopulmonary bypass-temperature management during cardiopulmonary bypass. *Ann Thorac Surg*. 2015;100:748–757.

Gandhi GY, Nuttall GA, Abel MD, et al. Intraoperative hyperglycemia and perioperative outcomes in cardiac surgery patients. *Mayo Clin Proc*. 2005;80:862–866.

Grigore AM, Grocott HP, Mathew JP, et al. The rewarming rate and increased peak temperature alter neurocognitive outcome after cardiac surgery. *Anesth Analg*. 2002;94:4–10.

Grigore AM, Mathew J, Grocott HP, et al. Prospective randomized trial of normothermic versus hypothermic cardiopulmonary bypass on cognitive function after coronary artery bypass graft surgery. *Anesthesiology*. 2001;95:1110–1119.

Hudetz JA, Pagel PS. Neuroprotection by ketamine: a review of the experimental and clinical evidence. *J Cardiothorac Vasc Anesth*. 2010;24:131–142.

Laffey JG, Boylan JF, Cheng DC. The systemic inflammatory response to cardiac surgery: implications for the anesthesiologist. *Anesthesiology*. 2002;97:215–252.

Lebon JS, Couture P, Rochon AG, et al. The endovascular coronary sinus catheter in minimally invasive mitral and tricuspid valve surgery: a case series. *J Cardiothorac Vasc Anesth*. 2010;24:746–751.

Lennon MJ, Gibbs NM, Weightman WM, et al. Transesophageal echocardiography-related gastrointestinal complications in cardiac surgical patients. *J Cardiothorac Vasc Anesth*. 2005;19:141–145.

Mangano DT, Tudor IC, Dietzel C. The risk associated with aprotinin in cardiac surgery. *N Engl J Med*. 2006;354:353–365.

Mathew JP, Grocott HP, Podgoreanu MV, et al. Inflammatory and prothrombotic genetic polymorphisms are associated with cognitive decline after CABG surgery. *Anesthesiology*. 2004;101:A274.

McSweeney ME, Garwood S, Levin J, et al. Adverse gastrointestinal complications after cardiopulmonary bypass: can outcome be predicted from preoperative risk factors? *Anesth Analg*. 2004;98:1610–1617.

Mehta RL, Kellum JA, Shah SV, et al. Acute Kidney Injury Network: report of an initiative to improve outcomes in acute kidney injury. *Crit Care*. 2007;11:R31.

Newman MF, Kirchner JL, Phillips-Bute B, et al. Longitudinal assessment of neurocognitive function after coronary-artery bypass surgery. *N Engl J Med*. 2001;344:395–402.

Ono M, Brady K, Easley RB, et al. Duration and magnitude of blood pressure below cerebral autoregulation threshold during cardiopulmonary bypass is associated with major morbidity and operative mortality. *J Thorac Cardiovasc Surg*. 2014;147:483–489.

Rubens FD, Boodhwani M, Mesana T, et al. The cardiotomy trial: a randomized, double-blind study to assess the effect of processing of shed blood during cardiopulmonary bypass on transfusion and neurocognitive function. *Circulation*. 2007;116:I89–I97.

Swaminathan M, Grocott HP, Mackensen GB, et al. The "sandblasting" effect of aortic cannula on arch atheroma during cardiopulmonary bypass. *Anesth Analg*. 2007;104:1350–1351.

van den Berghe G, Wouters P, Weekers F, et al. Intensive insulin therapy in critically ill patients. *N Engl J Med*. 2001;345:1359–1367.

Zacharias M, Conlon NP, Herbison GP, et al. Interventions for protecting renal function in the perioperative period. *Cochrane Database Syst Rev*. 2008;(9):CD003590.

Zarychanski R, Abou-Setta AM, Turgeon AF, et al. Association of hydroxyethyl starch administration with mortality and acute kidney injury in critically ill patients requiring volume resuscitation: a systematic review and meta-analysis. *JAMA*. 2013;309:678–688.

25

Chapter 26

Extracorporeal Devices Including Extracorporeal Membrane Oxygenation

Robert C. Groom, MS, CCP, FPP •
David Fitzgerald, MPH, CCP • Jacob T. Gutsche, MD •
Harish Ramakrishna, MD, FASE, FACC

Key Points

1. Two predominant methods of blood propulsion are used: positive displacement roller pumps and constrained vortex centrifugal-type pumps.
2. Modern heart-lung machines are equipped with a number of alarm systems and redundant backup systems to overcome primary system failures.
3. Blood gas exchange devices have improved over time in terms of reduced blood-surface interface, improved efficiency, and improved blood device-related inflammatory response.
4. Gaseous and particulate microemboli enter the cardiopulmonary bypass (CPB) circuit from entrainment in the venous inflow to the circuit and also through the cardiotomy suction system. None of the currently available CPB systems remove all of the emboli.
5. Cardioplegia must be delivered accurately to prevent myocardial damage, and new pump delivery systems provide a better operator-interface for effective delivery.
6. Blood conservation is paramount, and an effective system involves proper equipment selection for the size of the patient, careful coagulation management, and the use of advanced techniques such as acute normovolemic hemodilution, retrograde and antegrade priming, ultrafiltration, and autotransfusion.
7. Extracorporeal membrane oxygenation (ECMO) has had a profound resurgence as therapy for acute cardiopulmonary failure.
8. Advancements in equipment and improvements in techniques and management have led to better outcomes for patients undergoing ECMO.
9. Venoarterial (VA) ECMO should be considered for patients with acute cardiac or combined cardiac and respiratory failure.
10. Venovenous (VV) ECMO is indicated for patients with adequate cardiac function in the setting of severe acute respiratory failure refractory to standard management.

Since the 1950s, cardiopulmonary bypass (CPB) has undergone a dramatic metamorphosis from a lifesaving, yet life-threatening, technique to a procedure practiced nearly 1 million times a year throughout the world. It is uncommon in today's medical environment to encounter such an invasive procedure, with such significant risk and inherent morbidity, being practiced as routine. The goal of all techniques of CPB has always been to design an integrated system that could provide nutritive solutions with appropriate hemodynamic driving force to maintain whole-body homeostasis, without causing inherent injury.

MECHANICAL DEVICES

Blood Pumps

All extracorporeal flow occurs through processes that incorporate a transfer of energy from mechanical forces to a perfusate and, ultimately, to the tissue. Most extracorporeal pumps fall into one of the following categories: positive displacement (PD) roller pumps or constrained vortex (centrifugal).

Positive Displacement Pumps

The PD pump operates by occluding tubing between a stationary raceway and rotating roller pumps (Fig. 26.1). The pumping mechanism is also referred to as the *pump*

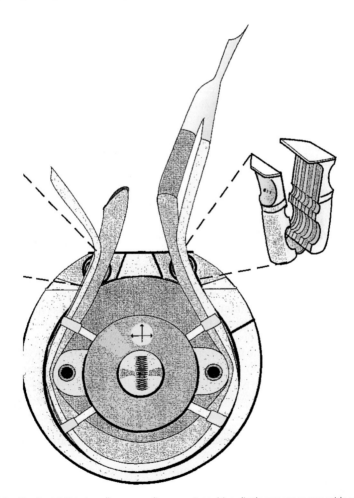

Fig. 26.1 Stockert S-3 twin roller pump diagram. A positive displacement pump with a stationary raceway and rotating twin roller pumps. (Courtesy Sorin Group, Arvada, CO.)

26

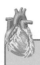
> **BOX 26.1   *Roller Pumps***
>
> Composed of twin rollers
> Deliver flow using positive displacement of the fluid in the tubing
> Blood flow is calculated using tubing stroke volume and pump revolutions per minute
> An underocclusive roller pump or an open shunt in the circuit may result in retrograde
> flow in the patient and in the cardiopulmonary bypass circuit
> An overocclusive roller pump may increase hemolysis and produce spallation of the
> perfusion tubing

head, and the tubing that traverses the raceway is referred to as the *pump header.* In a PD pump, fluid is displaced in a progressive fashion from suction to discharge, with the capacity of the displacement dependent both on the volume of the tubing occluded by the rollers and on the number of revolutions per minute (rpm) of the roller. All PD roller pumps (RPs) use the volume in the pump header, which is referred to as a *flow constant* and is specific to each size of tubing referred to by the internal diameter of tubing, for calculating the flow of the pump. This is displayed on a digital readout and is referred to as the *output* (flow) of the pump. It is measured in liters per minute (Box 26.1).

A modern heart-lung machine consists of between four and five of these RPs positioned on a base console (Figs. 26.2 and 26.3). Most machines are modular in design, permitting the rapid change-out of a defective unit in the case of single-pump failure. Each pump is independently controlled by a rheostat that functions to regulate the rpm of the rollers. Each pump is calibrated according to specific flow constants that are calculated from the internal diameter of tubing, as well as the tubing length, placed in the pump raceway. Periodically, PD pumps are calibrated by performing a timed collection of pumped fluid to verify that after proper calibration the pump delivers the volume indicated on the pump flow display. Most of the hemolysis generated during a routine CPB procedure is not related to the occlusiveness of the arterial pump head but rather to the air-surface interface interaction occurring with the use of suction and "vent" line components of the circuit.

Centrifugal Pumps

The second type of extracorporeal pump is a resistance-dependent pump termed a centrifugal pump (CP) or constrained vortex pump. The CP conducts fluid movement by the addition of kinetic energy to a fluid through the forced centrifugal rotation of an impeller or cone in a constrained housing (Box 26.2). The greatest force, highest energy, is found at a point most distal to the center axis of rotation. CPs operate as pressure-sensitive pumps, with blood flow directly related to downstream resistance. Blood flow is, therefore, related to both the rpm of the cones or impellers and the total resistance.

The acceptance of these devices in routine CPB has increased tremendously since first being introduced into clinical practice in 1969, and it is the pump of choice during emergency bypass procedures. The CP also has been used as a temporary ventricular assist device (VAD) because of its inherent safety features and pressure sensitivity, as well as relatively low cost.

Electromagnetic and Doppler ultrasonic flow meters are the two methods of measuring CP flow, as compared with the calculated flow display of the PD pumps, which is the product of a flow constant and the rpms. Some have argued that separate flow meters should be used with PD pumps to measure the flow directly to avoid

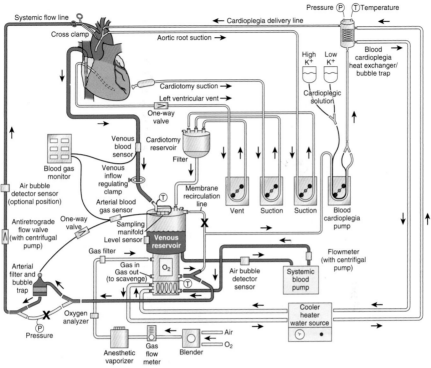

Fig. 26.2 Schematic diagram of cardiopulmonary bypass circuit, including four roller pumps (one vent pump, two suction pumps, and a cardioplegia deliver pump). A centrifugal blood pump for systemic blood propulsion is shown on the lower right. (From Hensley FA, Martin DE, Gravlee GP. *A Practical Approach to Cardiac Anesthesia,* 4th ed. Philadelphia: Lippincott Williams & Wilkins; 2008: Fig. 18.1.)

BOX 26.2 *Centrifugal Pumps*

Operate on the constrained vortex principle
Blood flow is inversely related to downstream resistance
Flow rate is determined using an ultrasonic flow meter
Increase in centrifugal pump revolutions per minute may result in heat generation and
  hemolysis
If the centrifugal pump is stopped, the line must be clamped to prevent
  retrograde flow

26

errors that may occur related to an unocclusive roller head, open shunts in the circuit, or selection of the wrong flow constant.

Safety Mechanisms for Extracorporeal Flow

Some of the most recent advances in pump design have been a result of a heightened awareness of increasing safety associated with complex operating systems. The PD

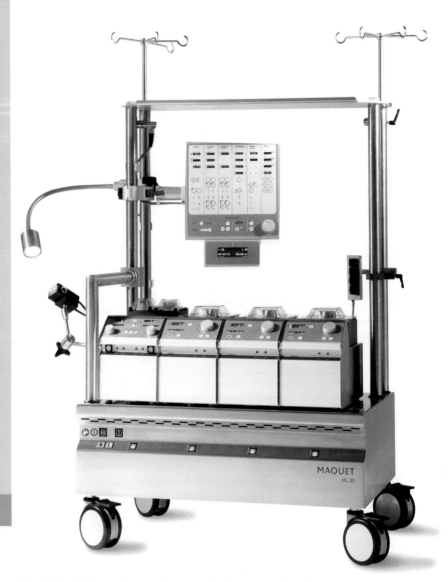

Fig. 26.3 HL20 heart-lung machine console. (Reproduced from Maquet Cardiopulmonary GmbH, with permission.)

pumps are pressure-independent, which means they will continue to pump regardless of downstream resistance. In a CPB circuit, the summation of resistances against which a pump must function includes the total tubing length, the oxygenator, the heat exchanger, the arterial line filter, the cannula, and the patient's systemic vascular resistance (SVR). Additional factors that influence SVR include the viscosity of the perfusate, related to the total formed element concentration, which primarily is dependent on the formed elements of blood and the temperature of the solution. Perfusionists routinely monitor the summation of all resistances and record this value as the arterial line, or system, pressure. Any acute change in resistance, such as unexpected clamping or kinking of the arterial line, results in an abrupt increase in arterial line pressure, which can lead to catastrophic line separation or circuit fracture anywhere on the high-pressure side of the circuit. A life-threatening event could occur on the initiation of CPB if the tip of the arterial cannula lodges against the wall of the aorta, undermining the intima of the vessel. Under these conditions, aortic dissection can occur as the vessel intima separates from the media, directing blood flow into a newly created false lumen. This dissection can extend throughout the entire length of the aorta. For this reason, perfusionists routinely check the line pressure after cannulation before the onset of CPB to ensure the presence of a pulsatile waveform, indicating proper cannula placement in the central lumen of the aorta. Either the absence of pulsatile pressure in the outflow portion of the perfusion circuit or an extremely high line pressure (>400 mm Hg when CPB is initiated) should immediately be investigated.

All heart-lung machines include a microprocessor-controlled safety interface with their pump consoles. These systems monitor and control pump function and serve as the primary mechanical safety control system for regulating extracorporeal flow. Pressure limits are set by the perfusionist and are determined by patient characteristics and the type of intervention performed. These units consist of early-warning alarms that alert the user to abrupt changes in pressure and will automatically turn off a pump when preset limits are exceeded. These safety devices have been used in both the main arterial pump and the cardioplegia pump; the latter become more important with the utilization of retrograde cardioplegia administration into the coronary sinus.

Electrical failure in the operating room (OR) can be especially catastrophic in the conduct of extracorporeal circulation (ECC) when the native heart and lungs are unable to function. When such an event occurs during CPB, it is imperative that instantaneous actions be instituted to minimize the risk for whole-body hypoperfusion. The perfusionist should be mindful of the power limitations of the electrical outlet used in the cardiac OR and also be aware of the location of the circuit breaker panel for the room and the specific number of the breaker in the panel for the outlet used for the heart-lung machine and other support equipment. Methods to ensure the safe conduct of CPB involve the incorporation of an emergency power source in the extracorporeal circuit that provides a secondary power source in the event of electrical interruption. Electrical failure during CPB was reported by 42.3% of respondents in a survey on perfusion accidents. Although hospitals are equipped with emergency generators for such events, their availability may be limited to certain electrical circuits within the operating suite. Furthermore, these emergency power systems require a brief interruption in power before a generator or backup source of power is initiated. Most heart-lung machines are equipped with uninterrupted backup power, sometimes referred to as the *uninterrupted power source* (UPS), whereby there is a seamless transfer from the wall power source to an internal battery within the pump should the wall power fail. Thus with this system, there is no loss of flow from the pumps that could result in retrograde flow and entrainment of air or disruption of settings and timers.

26

EXTRACORPOREAL CIRCUITRY

Blood Gas Exchange Devices

The ECC of blood incorporating total heart-lung bypass could not be accomplished were it not for the development of devices that could replace the function of the lungs in pulmonary gas exchange. The technology of pumps to replace the mechanical action of the heart was developed well before their incorporation in ECC. Therefore the limiting factor hindering the progression of CPB was the development of an

BOX 26.3 *Membrane Oxygenators*

Hollow-fiber membrane oxygenators are commonly used for cardiopulmonary bypass
An oxygen gas mixture flows through microporous polypropylene hollow fibers
Blood flow is directed over the microporous hollow fibers
Recently nonporous polymethylpentene (PMP) hollow fibers have been developed
PMP fibers provided a more durable surface for prolonged oxygenation such as
   extracorporeal membrane oxygenation
PMP fibers do not permit the passage of volatile anesthetics such as isoflurane

artificial lung, or blood gas exchange device (BGED), commonly referred to as a *membrane oxygenator* (Box 26.3). The term *membrane* denotes the separation of blood and gas phases by a semipermeable barrier, whereas *oxygenator* refers to the change in oxygen partial pressure that occurs by the arterialization of venous blood. However, "oxygenator" is a misrepresentation of the functional ability of these systems to perform ventilatory control of carbon dioxide. Numerous engineering challenges hindered the development of BGEDs, but two of the most pressing were the design of high-capacity units for gas exchange with low rates of bioreactivity. The latter requirement, also termed *biocompatibility*, was imperative to reduce both red blood cell (RBC) trauma and activation of the formed elements of blood.

Membrane oxygenators are made of three distinct compartments: gas, blood, and water. The latter phase is also termed the *heat exchange compartment* and is used for temperature control. Gas and blood are partitioned into separate compartments with either a limited or absent gas-blood interface. Microporous membrane oxygenators have a blood-gas interface that is formed when the inner blood contact surface has been exposed to plasma; and a protein layer is deposited, acting as a diffusible barrier to gas exchange. The most common material in use today in membrane oxygenators is microporous polypropylene, which has excellent capacity for gas exchange and good biocompatibility. Despite the improvements made to extracorporeal devices over the past several decades, once blood is exposed to synthetic surfaces, hematologic changes result. Initially, complement is activated mainly through alternative pathways, resulting in the liberation of toxic mediators such as C3a and C5a. Both platelets and leukocytes that elicit a complex series of inflammatory and hemostatic reactions that ultimately increase the risk for postoperative complications are activated.

Gas transfer in membrane oxygenators is a function of several factors, including surface area, the partial pressures of venous oxygen and carbon dioxide, blood flow, ventilation flow (called *sweep rate*), and gas flow composition. Membrane devices independently control arterial oxygen and carbon dioxide tensions (PaO_2 and $PaCO_2$). PaO_2 is a function of the FIO_2, whereas $PaCO_2$ is determined by the sweep rate of the ventilating gas. This independent control of ventilating gas results in arterial blood gas values more closely resembling normal physiologic blood gas status. However, it is common for perfusionists to maintain PaO_2 levels in the 150- to 250-mm Hg range during CPB because of the limited reserve capacity of membrane oxygenators.

Venous and Cardiotomy Reservoirs

There are two general categories for venous reservoirs: open and closed systems (Box 26.4). Open systems have a hard polycarbonate venous reservoir and usually

BOX 26.4   *Venous Reservoirs*

Open Systems

- Open systems have polycarbonate hard-shell reservoirs and are usually equipped with an integrated cardiotomy reservoir
- With open systems, venous return may be improved by applying regulated suction to the reservoir (vacuum-assisted venous drainage)
- With open systems, buoyant air bubbles escape to the atmosphere at the top of the reservoir

Closed Systems

- Closed systems consist of collapsible polyvinylchloride bags
- Closed systems require a separate cardiotomy reservoir
- Buoyant air from the venous line accumulates in the bag and must be actively aspirated
- Closed systems have a reduced contact surface of the blood with air or plastic
- A separate centrifugal pump may be used to increase venous return (kinetic-assisted venous drainage)

incorporate a cardiotomy reservoir and defoaming compartment (see Fig. 26.2). Closed systems are collapsible polyvinylchloride bags that have a minimal surface area and often a thin single-layer screen filter, and they require a separate external cardiotomy reservoir for cardiotomy suction. The use of an open system offers several distinct advantages. Unlike collapsible reservoirs, it is not necessary to aspirate air actively, which may be entrained in the venous line during CPB. The large buoyant air migrates to the top of the reservoir and escapes through strategically placed vents on the reservoir cover.

Heat Exchangers

Patients who are exposed to ECC will become hypothermic in the absence of an external source of heat to regulate body temperature. Most CPB systems use some form of heat exchanger in the circuit to warm and/or cool the patient's blood. All oxygenators contain integrated heat exchangers through which blood passes before undergoing gas exchange.

Heat exchangers can be placed in the circuit in a variety of locations, although the most common location is on the proximal side of the oxygenator. It is hypothesized that with proximal, or venous-side, heat exchange, there is less chance of "outgassing of solution" caused by rapid rewarming of blood after hypothermic CPB, which could generate large gas bubbles.

Arterial Line Filters

Arterial line filters significantly reduce the load of gaseous and particulate emboli and should be used in CPB circuits. Some studies suggest that 20-μm screen filtration is superior to 40-μm filtration in the reduction of cerebral embolic counts. Some studies have demonstrated a protective effect of arterial line filtration on neurologic outcomes.

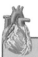

Screen filters are the predominant type in current use. They trap particulate and gaseous emboli that are of larger diameter than their effective pore size. The filter material is accordion-pleated to provide a larger surface area within a lower prime housing (Box 26.5).

Cannulae and Tubing

The major devices of CPB are those that replace the systems from which the heart-lung machine has derived its name. However, as with most technologic advances, it is the combination of all component parts that function to ensure success. Besides the pump and oxygenator, a seamless array of tubing is required to connect the patient to the heart-lung machine.

The majority of cardiac procedures using CPB through a median sternotomy are performed with venous cannulation of the right atrium (RA) and arterial return into the ascending aorta.

Although cannulation of the ascending aorta is preferred for most procedures, femoral arterial cannulation often is selected for reoperations or minimally invasive surgical procedures. The axillary or subclavian artery often is selected for arterial return for patients with severe atherosclerosis of the ascending aorta. This site offers the advantage of providing antegrade flow to the arch vessels, protection of the arm and hand, and avoidance of inadvertent cannulation of the false lumen in cases in which type A aortic dissection has occurred. The axillary artery is accessed through a subclavicular incision.

Blood flows out of the RA cannula and into the venous reservoir when CPB is initiated. The venous line connects the cannula to the venous reservoir. Mixed venous oxygen saturation is measured by optical or chemical fluorescence by flow through cells placed in the venous line. A stopcock manifold is placed in the venous line to facilitate the delivery of medications and for venous sampling. Blood then enters the venous reservoir, which serves as a volume chamber for settling and acts as a safety feature, providing additional response time to the perfusionist.

From the venous reservoir, blood is pumped into the heat exchanger of a membrane oxygenator by the actions of the arterial pump. The heat exchanger is connected to an external water source that maintains the perfusate temperature according to the temperature of the water pumped from the cooler/heater. Blood then passes directly to the oxygenator, where gas exchange occurs in accordance with the operation of a gas blender that controls the FIO_2 by mixing oxygen with medical-grade air, along with a flow meter that regulates the ventilation rate. The gas blender is attached to the inlet gas port of the oxygenator via a section of 1/4-inch tubing and a bacteriostatic (0.2-μm) filter. Gas exchange across the blood and gas phases of the fiber occurs through the process of simple diffusion. Levels of high gas molecule concentration

V

are permitted to diffuse through tiny slit pores of the oxygenator fiber strands to lower levels of gas concentration. During CPB support, this typically results in the addition of O_2 to the blood phase and the uptake of CO_2 to the gas phase. Many circuits also have a vaporizer for the delivery of volatile, inhaled anesthetic gases placed in-line between the gas blender and the oxygenator.

CARDIOPLEGIA DELIVERY

During aortic cross-clamping, the heart is rendered globally ischemic by the cessation of coronary blood flow. Some myocardial perfusion undoubtedly occurs through the involvement of noncoronary collateral circulation from mediastinal sources and the bronchial circulation. There are numerous methods of achieving mechanical arrest, and the combination of these techniques is referred to as *myocardial preservation.* Myocardial preservation encompasses both the pharmacologic manipulation of the solutions (cardioplegia) used to protect the heart and methods of mechanical delivery. Potassium-containing solutions arrest the cardiac muscle in a depolarized state by disruption of the myocardial action potential.

Adjunct means of cooling and protecting the myocardium during aortic cross-clamping include the use of topical application of cold solutions to prevent early transmural myocardial rewarming. A common method for cooling the myocardium is achieved by the surgeon creating a "pericardial well" in the chest by suspending the pericardium with stay sutures to the chest retractor. Cold (4°C) topical saline solution is then applied to the pericardium, bathing the heart in cold solution while a sucker line is placed in the well to evacuate the saline solution. Topical saline has been shown to cool the epicardium and diminish transmural gradients, but it also has resulted in phrenic nerve paresis and myocardial damage. An alternate technique involves a topical cooling device, which consists of a coolant flow pad in which cold (4°C) saline flows, separated from the body by a metal skeleton and polyurethane insulator, which protects the posterior mediastinum and phrenic nerve from hypothermic injury. The benefits of a topical cooling device over topical cold saline include a reduction in total hemodilution, procurement of a drier operative field, reduced blood loss in waste suction, and more uniform distribution of cooling. However, these devices are costly, require a separate RP for delivery, and may not be applicable for all procedures in which the heart will be lifted and elevated away from the posterior pericardium.

There are two major disposable circuit configurations for cardioplegia delivery: a recirculating system with a heat exchanger for asanguineous delivery and a single-pass cardioplegia system for nonrecirculating delivery. In recirculating systems, crystalloid cardioplegic solution is kept constantly recirculating throughout the cardioplegia circuit and is delivered to the patient by the movement of a clamp, directing flow away from the recirculation line and into the infusion line. Another type of cardioplegia delivery system is termed a *blood cardioplegia system,* which involves the shunting of arterialized blood from the oxygenator into the cardioplegia circuit, where it is mixed with a crystalloid base solution, usually of high potassium concentration, before it is delivered into the coronary circulation. Most sanguineous cardioplegia systems are nonrecirculating and only make a single pass through a heat exchanger before passing to the heart. For this reason, these systems must have a high efficiency rating for caloric exchange between the cardioplegic solution and the cooling, or warming, source. These devices can deliver varying ratios of blood-to-crystalloid base, ranging from a 1:1 to a 1:20 ratio of crystalloid to blood. Most are equipped with temperature monitoring ports and pressure-measuring sites to monitor delivery pressures.

26

◼ THE HEART-LUNG MACHINE PRIMING SOLUTIONS

Before ECC can be attempted, the patient must be connected to the CPB machine, necessitating the creation of a fluid-filled circuit to ensure continuity with the patient. Not only is it important that the circuit be "primed," but it also must be completely devoid of any gaseous bubbles or particulate matter that potentially could embolize. For this reason, perfusionists often perform painstaking maneuvers to rid the circuit of bubbles before bypass.

When nonhemic primes are used during CPB, a concomitant reduction in SVR occurs at the onset of ECC as a result of the reduced viscosity of the blood. Although the oxygen-carrying capacity of the pump perfusate is reduced by hemodilution, overall oxygen delivery may not be significantly affected because the reduced viscosity enhances perfusion. Safe levels of hemodilution are dependent on multiple factors that include the patient's metabolic rate, cardiovascular function and reserve, degree of atherosclerotic disease and resultant tissue perfusion, and core temperature. Although an absolute value for the degree of hemodilution tolerated will vary among individual patients, studies supported a minimal hematocrit value of 20% to ensure oxygen delivery and tissue extraction. More recently, several large retrospective studies have described a trend toward increased morbidity and mortality with nadir hematocrits less than 23%.

Priming of the CPB circuit with crystalloid solutions alone reduces colloid oncotic pressure, and this reduction is directly related to the total volume of prime solution and the overall level of hemodilution. Hypo-oncotic primes promote tissue edema through interstitial expansion with plasma water. A significant decline in plasma albumin occurs after CPB in patients who have been exposed to crystalloid-only primes. Albumin and various high-molecular-weight colloid solutions are added by some groups to the prime to offset these changes, although the benefits associated with each practice remain controversial.

Further important considerations in choosing a priming solution for CPB circuits include alterations induced by changes in electrolyte activity. Balanced electrolyte solutions are the first-choice base solutions of most prime solution "cocktails" used by perfusionists. Lactated Ringer's solution, Normosol-A, and Plasmalyte are used frequently because of their electrolyte compositions and isotonicity. Calcium concentration varies depending on the type of prime constituents, as well as the presence of citrate in allogeneic blood products.

Perioperative Salvage and Autotransfusion

Cardiotomy Suction

Shed blood from the surgical field and blood vented from the left atrium, left ventricle, pulmonary artery, or the aorta is collected and reinfused into the CPB circuit through the cardiotomy suction system. Cardiotomy suction blood contains fat, bone, lipids, and other debris from the surgical field. This blood is also exposed to air, shear forces, and artificial surfaces that cause exacerbation of the systemic inflammatory response and result in microcirculatory dysfunction. These substances may traverse the CPB circuit, enter into the arterial line, and ultimately obstruct the microcapillary circulation of the patient. Cardiotomy suction blood has been identified as a major source of lipid emboli in several studies. For this reason, some have advocated eliminating the use of cardiotomy suction, which is returned directly to the ECC.

Cell Salvaging Through Centrifugation and Washing Techniques

One of the simplest forms of autotransfusion is the use of a cell-salvaging system that uses aspiration and anticoagulation to collect shed blood and return it to the patient. Another form of autotransfusion uses specific machines that salvage and process shed blood and include a cell-washing step. The term *cell saving* has come to denote the process of autotransfusion that involves centrifugation of collected operative blood and processing with a wash solution, 0.9% NaCl, and reinfusing the product back to the patient. The basic operating principles found in autotransfusion include aspiration, anticoagulation, centrifugation, washing, and reinfusion.

Several large systematic reviews and metaanalyses have demonstrated the efficacy of routine autotransfusion usage in CPB surgery. Cost-effectiveness always has been a concern, with the prevailing belief that autotransfusion should be considered only when anticipated blood loss would result in a reinfusion of 1 to 2 units of processed RBCs. However, the active interest in minimizing patient exposure, combined with the use of smaller-volume centrifuge bowls, has prompted increased use of autotransfusion during cardiac surgery. In addition to aspirating shed blood from cardiac patients, the autotransfusion device can be used to concentrate the pump perfusate at the termination of CPB. Although this process is known to reduce the protein concentration of the perfusate when compared with reinfusion of the unprocessed pump contents, this method significantly reduces allogeneic banked blood exposure. Many centers will infuse the blood contained in the CPB circuit at the termination of bypass. The blood in the CPB circuit is displaced with a balanced electrolyte solution so that the pump remains primed should it be necessary to return to bypass. Sometimes vasodilators are administered to the patient to increase capacitance and allow this blood to be reinfused.

Monitoring During Cardiopulmonary Bypass

After ensuring that an appropriate level of anticoagulation has been achieved, the perfusionist initiates CPB. Undoubtedly, the most important assessment of CPB after initiation of perfusion is the function of the oxygenator. Without the proper delivery of oxygen to the venous blood and the removal of carbon dioxide, the arterial pump serves no purpose. Traditionally, isolated blood analysis was performed at a distant site from the OR and provided the clinician with a historic marker of oxygenator and patient performance. Unfortunately, this event is only a "snapshot" of one point during CPB. For this reason, the use of in-line blood gas monitoring is imperative and should not be considered a "luxury" because of its added cost. Indeed, in this litigious society, it is questionable not to use readily available technologies that may reduce unnecessary patient risk.

Optical fluorescence technology has made reliable in-line blood gas and electrolyte monitoring a reality, providing minute-to-minute accurate surveillance of these parameters during CPB. In-line blood gas monitoring allows for real-time monitoring of the "adequacy of perfusion," and one device currently available for use in CPB is the CDI500 (Terumo Cardiovascular Group, Ann Arbor, MI; Figs. 26.4 and 26.5). The CDI500 provides continuous real-time blood gas and electrolyte measurements for PO_2, PCO_2, pH, HCO_3^-, and K^+. The enhanced safety conferred by the use of this technology has been documented.

Arterial blood oxygen saturation always should be maintained at greater than 99%, with PO_2 tensions between 150 and 250 mm Hg. Arterial PCO_2 levels will vary depending on whether alpha-stat or pH-stat blood gas management is used.

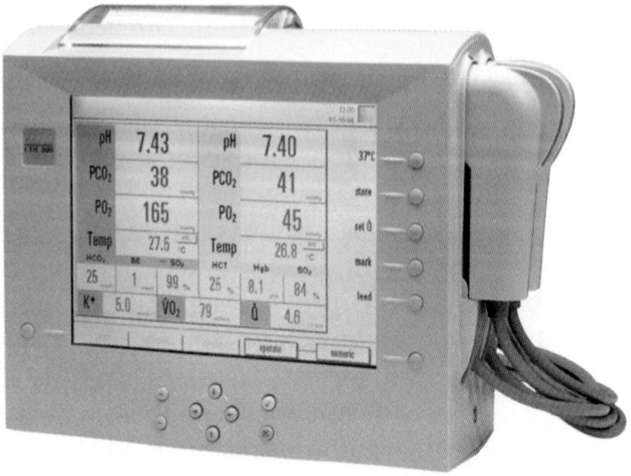

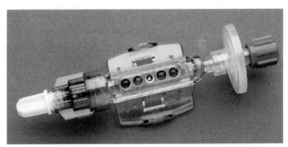

Fig. 26.4 CDI500 continuous blood gas and saturation monitor. Measures arterial and venous pH, P_{CO_2}, P_{O_2}, potassium, hemoglobin saturation, hematocrit, and hemoglobin. (Courtesy Terumo Cardiovascular Group, Ann Arbor, MI.)

Fig. 26.5 CDI500 sensor. Blood flows through the sensor so that continuous monitoring may be accomplished. (Courtesy Terumo Cardiovascular Group, Ann Arbor, MI.)

V

During alpha-stat management, the rule of thumb for controlling carbon dioxide is to maintain P_{CO_2} levels equal to the temperature of arterial blood. For pH-stat management, the P_{CO_2} is kept constant at 40 mm Hg, and the pH at 7.4 at all temperatures. The venous oxygen saturation (S_{VO_2}) will vary during the operative procedure depending on the metabolic state of the patient but is generally maintained above 70%.

The benefits of venous blood gas monitoring have been well accepted in cardiovascular medicine, and the information gained from such assessment has been used to guide therapeutic interventions in numerous clinical situations. Changes in both venous P_{CO_2} and P_{O_2} levels have been shown to correlate well with changes in global tissue perfusion. During CPB, the importance of mixed venous oxygen saturation monitoring cannot be overemphasized. This parameter has global utility and is the one parameter universally monitored during most extracorporeal procedures. The mixed venous oxygen saturation is used to calculate whole-body oxygen consumption when, according to the Fick equation, perfusion flow and the oxygen content of arterial blood are also known.

HISTORY, EVOLUTION, AND CURRENT STATUS OF EXTRACORPOREAL MEMBRANE OXYGENATION

There are two basic types of modern ECMO: venoarterial (VA) ECMO, which supports the heart and lungs, and venovenous (VV) ECMO, which supports the lungs only. VV ECMO can be easily converted to venovenous arterial VVA if left ventricular support is subsequently required. ECMO can temporarily support cardiopulmonary function as the patient recovers or serve as a bridge to a permanent solution such as a ventricular support device or transplantation. Although ECMO is challenging to manage and is associated with relatively high morbidity and mortality rates, increased experience and the durability of ECMO circuits have allowed care teams to support patients for several weeks.

Interest in ECMO for respiratory support has dramatically increased in the past decade and has been aided by advancements in extracorporeal technology, publication of key randomized trials, and the resurgence of viral infections causing respiratory failure (particularly the H1N1 influenza pandemic in 2009).

The steep increase in the use of ECMO worldwide in the past 5 years (Fig. 26.6) can be attributed to two important events. The first was publication of the results of the Conventional Ventilatory Support Versus Extracorporeal Membrane Oxygenation for Severe Adult Respiratory Failure (CESAR) trial in 2009, which randomized patients with severe respiratory failure to conventional medical therapy in general hospitals or ECMO support in specialized medical centers.

The second event that promoted ECMO was the 2009 influenza A (H1N1) pandemic, which dramatically increased VV ECMO use worldwide as emergent salvage therapy for patients with severe viral pneumonia or acute respiratory distress syndrome (ARDS) unresponsive to mechanical ventilation.

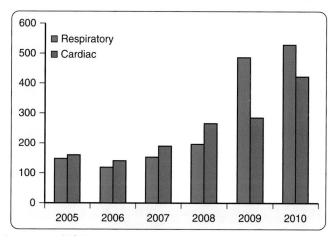

Fig. 26.6 Extracorporeal Life Support Organization registry data for venoarterial (VA) and venovenous (VV) extracorporeal membranous oxygenation (ECMO). VA ECMO is indicated for patients with acute cardiac or cardiopulmonary failure. VV ECMO is indicated for those with adequate cardiac function but acute respiratory failure refractory to standard management. (Data from Extracorporeal Life Support Organization. *ECLS registry report: international summary.* July 2015. *http:www.elso.org.*)

26

The trend has continued, as demonstrated in a 2014 study that reported a significant (433%) increase in ECMO use in adults in the United States from 2006 to 2011.

Survival rates have improved significantly for both types of ECMO, with respiratory ECMO survivors having a clear survival advantage over cardiac ECMO patients. Survival rates for ECMO-treated adults after cardiac arrest increased from 30% in 1990 to 59% in 2007.

EXTRACORPOREAL MEMBRANE OXYGENATION PHYSIOLOGY AND GAS EXCHANGE

A basic ECMO circuit consists of inflow and outflow cannulas, tubing, a pump, and a membrane oxygenator with heat exchanger (Fig. 26.7). The oxygen and CO_2 levels

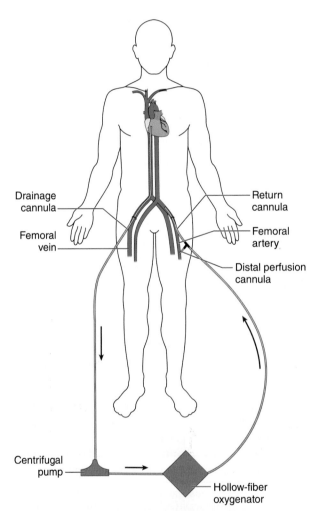

Fig. 26.7 Standard ECMO circuit. (From Sidebotham D, McGeorge A, McGuinness S, et al. Extracorporeal membrane oxygenation for treating severe cardiac and respiratory failure in adults. Part 2: technical considerations. *J Cardiothorac Vasc Anesth.* 2010;24:164–172.)

in the blood pumped through the ECMO circuit are controlled by altering the oxygen content and the flow rate (ie, sweep) of gas through the membrane oxygenator.

MANAGEMENT OF VENOARTERIAL EXTRACORPOREAL MEMBRANE OXYGENATION

Extracorporeal Membrane Oxygenation for Hemodynamic Support

VA ECMO may be used to provide circulatory support or a combination of pulmonary and circulatory support. The VA ECMO circuit consists of venous drainage to a CP in series with a membrane oxygenator and return of oxygenated blood to the arterial circulation to maintain end-organ perfusion.

There are numerous acute and subacute indications for VA ECMO (Box 26.6), but most can be classified as severe cardiac insufficiency causing end-organ ischemia. Practitioners determining the need for VA ECMO or VV ECMO in cases of pulmonary insufficiency must evaluate right and left ventricular function. Although no established standards exist for the minimal ventricular function that should trigger the use of VA ECMO, patients with severe ventricular dysfunction do not benefit from VV ECMO. VA ECMO may be used as a means of support during recovery of native cardiac function or in patients with little hope of cardiac recovery as a bridge to a mechanical VAD or heart transplantation.

Initiation of Venoarterial Extracorporeal Membrane Oxygenation

After cannulation, the ECMO circuit flows are increased to the target range, which should be based on clinical parameters, including arterial blood pressure, oxygen saturation of the venous return to the circuit, and measures of global ischemia such as serum lactate (Box 26.7). Initial settings should be standardized based on patient size (estimated at 50–60 mL/kg per minute). Additional determinants of arterial blood pressure include arterial blood flow and arterial vascular tone.

The volume of arterial blood flow is supplied by the combination of native heart function and the ECMO circuit. Patients with an adequate volume of blood flow who

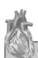

BOX 26.6 *Indications for Venoarterial ECMO*

Pulmonary embolism
Myocardial infarction
Myocarditis
Postcardiotomy cardiac failure
Heart transplantation
Acute-on-chronic heart failure
Cardiac arrest
Acute respiratory distress syndrome with severe cardiac dysfunction
Refractory ventricular arrhythmia
Cardiac trauma
Acute anaphylaxis
Cardiac support for percutaneous cardiac procedures

BOX 26.7 *Initial Settings and Goals After Implementation of Venoarterial ECMO*

Circuit flow	≥2 L/min per 1 m²
Sweep gas flow	Equal to blood flow
Fraction of inspired oxygen (sweep gas)	100%
Inlet pressure (centrifugal pump)	≥ −100 mm Hg
Oxygen saturation (outflow cannula)	100%
Oxygen saturation (inflow cannula)	>65%
Arterial oxygen saturation	>95%
Mixed venous oxygen saturation	>65%
Arterial carbon dioxide tension	35–45 mm Hg
pH	7.35–7.45
Mean arterial pressure	60–90 mm Hg
Hematocrit	30–40%
Activated partial thromboplastin time	1.5–2.0 times normal
Platelet count	>100,000/mm³
Lactate level	<2 mmol/L

Adapted from Sidebotham D, McGeorge A, McGuinness S, et al. Extracorporeal membrane oxygenation for treating severe cardiac and respiratory failure in adults. Part 2: technical considerations. *J Cardiothorac Vasc Anesth.* 2010;24:164–172.

have persistent hypotension need vasopressors to maintain sufficient vascular resistance and preserve adequate blood pressure. Sweep flows should initially be set to match arterial flow and then adjusted based on system arterial partial pressure of carbon dioxide ($PaCO_2$) and pH. Regardless of the indication for ECMO, the ventilator should be managed with lung-protective strategies.

Weaning From Venoarterial Extracorporeal Membrane Oxygenation

Daily clinical, hemodynamic, and echocardiographic evaluation of cardiac function should guide the strategy and timing of weaning from ECMO. Weaning is not commenced until after cardiac rest for at least 24 to 48 hours to facilitate recovery. After successful cardiac rest and recovery, the arterial monitor should demonstrate pulsatility on low doses of an inotrope and a mean arterial pressure of at least 60 mm Hg. Metabolic disturbances should be corrected, and lung function should be adequate to increase the chance of successful weaning. If cardiac function has recovered but lung function remains compromised, conversion to VV ECMO should be considered.

Pump flows are systematically decreased over a period of hours under echocardiographic and hemodynamic guidance. As circuit flows decrease in increments of 0.5 to 1 L/min, preload increases and afterload decreases, facilitating cardiac ejection. If hemodynamic parameters are met and organ and limb perfusion are satisfactory, the patient is evaluated on a 1-L/min flow for up to 1 hour before decannulation. Serial echocardiographic assessment, a left ventricular ejection fraction of at least 20% to 25%, and a multidisciplinary approach are important to maximize successful liberation from VA EMCO support.

▧ MANAGEMENT OF VENOVENOUS EXTRACORPOREAL MEMBRANE OXYGENATION

Indications for Venovenous Extracorporeal Membrane Oxygenation

The most rapidly growing aspect remains VV ECMO, spurred on by the CESAR trial results and the 2009–2010 H1N1 pandemic. In the key data published, ECMO duration averaged 9 to 10 days, and it was initiated within the first 7 days of mechanical ventilation; mortality rates ranged from 21% to 37%. VV ECMO is considered in patients with life-threatening but potentially reversible respiratory failure.

The Murray score played a key role in determining the need for ECMO support in the CESAR trial. The score is based on the assessed severity of respiratory failure. It uses four criteria (Table 26.1): PaO_2/FIO_2 ratio, positive end-expiratory pressure (PEEP), dynamic lung compliance, and the number of quadrants infiltrated on the chest radiograph. In this trial, a Murray score greater than 3.0 was the key criterion for patient enrollment in addition to uncompensated hypercapnia with a pH lower than 7.20.

As described in the 2013 Extracorporeal Life Support Organization (ELSO) guidelines, VV ECMO recommendations are based on the impending mortality risk. For patients with a 50% risk of death (ie, PaO_2/FIO_2 <150 on FIO_2 >90% and/or Murray score of 2–3), ECMO should be considered. When the anticipated risk of death approaches 80% (PaO_2/FIO_2 <100 on FIO_2 >90% and/or Murray score 3–4 despite optimal care for ≥6 hours), VV ECMO is indicated.

In addition to ARDS, the ELSO guidelines also recommend VV ECMO for severe air leak syndromes, for CO_2 retention in mechanically ventilated patients despite a high (>30 cm H_2O) plateau pressure (Pplat), and for miscellaneous patient conditions such as airway support in a patient listed for lung transplantation and a patient with acute respiratory failure unresponsive to optimal care.

26

Table 26.1	**Murray Lung Injury Score for Grading Acute Respiratory Distress Syndrome Severity**				
	ARDS Severity				
Parameter	*0*	*1*	*2*	*3*	*4*
Consolidation on chest radiograph (no. of quadrants)	0	1	2	3	4
PEEP (cm H_2O)	≤5	6–8	9–11	12–14	≥15
PaO_2/FIO_2	≥300	225–299	175–224	100–174	<100
Compliance (mL/cm H_2O)	≥80	60–79	40–59	20–39	≤19

ARDS, Acute respiratory distress syndrome; *FIO₂*, fraction of inspired oxygen; *PaO₂*, arterial partial pressure of oxygen; *PEEP*, positive end-expiratory pressure.
Modified from Murray JF, Matthay MA, Luce JM, Flick MR. An expanded definition of the adult respiratory distress syndrome. *Am Rev Respir Dis.* 1988;138:720–723.

Care of Patients on Venovenous Extracorporeal Membrane Oxygenation

The standard of care requires intravenous administration of 5000 U of heparin when the guidewires are in place during percutaneous insertion, and the dose should be titrated to an activated coagulation time greater than 180 seconds. Activated partial thromboplastin time (PTT) has been shown to correlate closely with blood heparin level and is commonly monitored every 6 hours during ECMO. Most patients requiring ECMO are intubated, deeply sedated, and mechanically ventilated at this point, but they may require additional neuromuscular blockade and opiates.

Initial Venovenous Extracorporeal Membrane Oxygenation Management

After cannulation has been performed, ECMO is commenced by unclamping the circuit and slowly increasing flows to the target range. For VV ECMO, key parameters used to determine pump flows are Sao_2 and Sdo_2 (ie, oxygen saturation of blood in the VV ECMO drainage cannula). The European Consensus Conference data suggest that, for ideal oxygenation in VV ECMO, the pump blood flow should be 60% or greater of the calculated cardiac output, with an arterial saturation goal of 88% or greater and a sweep gas rate that produces a $Paco_2$ between 30 and 40 mm Hg. The 2013 ELSO guidelines for VV ECMO also recommended a sweep gas flow titrated to maintain $Paco_2$ at 40 mm Hg. Unlike VA ECMO, VV ECMO does not provide added hemodynamic support. The need for pressors, inotropes, vasodilators, and volume replacement does not change.

Ventilator settings for VV ECMO can vary based on clinical pathophysiology. Current ELSO guidelines recommend rest settings, with Fio_2 as low as possible (<40%) and the avoidance of plateau pressures greater than 25 mm Hg. Typical rest settings consist of pressure-controlled ventilation with low respiratory rates, very low tidal volumes, low Fio_2, peak inspiratory pressure no higher than 25 cm H_2O, and PEEP of 10 to 15 cm H_2O.

A progressive, tapered sedation plan should be instituted for all VV ECMO patients, with moderate to heavy sedation for the first 24 hours. The goal is minimal to no sedation to accompany a plan to extubate or perform tracheotomy within 3 to 5 days of VV ECMO commencement. Most ECMO centers have protocols for management of temperature, blood volume, and nutrition; infection prevention; patient positioning; and management of bleeding.

Analogous to CPB, ECMO creates significant alterations in drug pharmacokinetics that require dose adjustments, particularly in the intensive care unit setting. With additional multisystem organ dysfunction, systemic inflammatory response, hemodilution from the circuit and acute renal failure that is associated with critically ill patients, drug responses can be difficult to predict, and possibilities range from drug toxicity to lack of effect. The increased volumes of distribution, decreased drug elimination, and sequestration of drugs in the ECMO circuit contribute to altered pharmacokinetics.

Weaning From Venovenous Extracorporeal Membrane Oxygenation

Weaning from ECMO is a complex process. The question of when a patient on VV ECMO should be weaned should be posed daily with each clinical assessment. For most patients, recovery can take 1 to 3 weeks. Possibilities for recovery or

> **BOX 26.8   Venovenous Complications of Extracorporeal Membrane Oxygenation**
>
> | | |
> |---|---|
> | Oxygenator failure | 10.2% |
> | Cannula site bleeding | 13.9% |
> | Gastrointestinal hemorrhage | 6.0% |
> | Hemolysis | 5.6% |
> | Disseminated intravascular coagulation | 3.1% |
> | CNS infarct | 2.0% |
> | CNS hemorrhage | 3.8% |
> | Pulmonary hemorrhage | 6.5% |
> | Renal failure requiring dialysis | 10.4% |
>
> *CNS*, Central nervous system.
> Data from the Extracorporeal Life Support Organization. *ECLS Registry Report: International summary.* http://www.elso.org.

discontinuation due to futility should be explained to the family before ECMO institution. Patients should be carefully watched for signs of potential irreversibility, such as fluid overload refractory to aggressive diuresis and progressively worsening pulmonary hypertension. Right ventricular failure in conjunction with a mean pulmonary artery pressure that is more than two-thirds of systemic pressure usually indicates irreversibility.

VV ECMO weaning durations are not established. Weaning trials can be 1 to 6 hours or longer. Key monitoring issues include hemodynamic stability (ie, standard parameters, including transesophageal echocardiography to monitor cardiac function with or without inotropes and vasopressors), serial arterial blood gas measurements, and assessment of respiratory mechanics, particularly if the patient is on spontaneous assisted ventilation. If the patient meets all criteria, circuit flows are reduced to zero, the cannulas are clamped, and decannulation takes place.

Complications of Venovenous Extracorporeal Membrane Oxygenation

ECMO is used to treat critically ill neonates, infants, and adults worldwide, with a trend toward earlier use in high-risk patients. Despite the high-risk population, overall outcomes suggest that almost 50% of patients who have received ECMO survive to discharge from the hospital. Improvements in pump circuitry allow longer periods of extracorporeal circulatory support.

Complications from ECMO can be devastating, and troubleshooting circuit issues can be challenging in an unstable patient. ECMO complications can arise from the circuit or be patient-related (Box 26.8).

SUGGESTED READINGS

Atallah S, Liebl M, Fitousis K, et al. Evaluation of the activated clotting time and activated partial thromboplastin time for the monitoring of heparin in adult extracorporeal membrane oxygenation patients. *Perfusion.* 2014;29:456–461.

Australia and New Zealand Extracorporeal Membrane Oxygenation (ANZ ECMO) Influenza Investigators, Davies A, Jones D, et al. Extracorporeal membrane oxygenation for 2009 influenza A(H1N1) acute respiratory distress syndrome. *JAMA*. 2009;302:1888–1895.

Barry AE, Chaney MA, London MJ. Anesthetic management during cardiopulmonary bypass: a systematic review. *Anesth Analg*. 2015;120:749–769.

Beck JR, Fung K, Lopez IIH, et al. Real-time data acquisition and alerts may reduce reaction time and improve perfusionist performance during cardiopulmonary bypass. *Perfusion*. 2015;30(1):41–44.

de Jong A, Popa BA, Stelian E, et al. Perfusion techniques for minimally invasive valve procedures. *Perfusion*. 2015;30(4):270–276.

de Somer F. Impact of oxygenator characteristics on its capability to remove gaseous microemboli. *J Extra Corpor Technol*. 2007;39:271–273.

Ferraris VA, Brown JR, Despotis GJ, et al. Perioperative blood transfusion and blood conservation in cardiac surgery: The Society of Thoracic Surgeons and The Society of Cardiovascular Anesthesiologists clinical practice guideline. *Ann Thorac Surg*. 2011;91:944–982.

Lazar HL, McDonnell M, Chipkin SR, et al. The Society of Thoracic Surgeons practice guideline series: blood glucose management during adult cardiac surgery. *Ann Thorac Surg*. 2009;87(2):663–669.

MacLaren G, Combes A, Bartlett RH. Contemporary extracorporeal membrane oxygenation for adult respiratory failure: life support in the new era. *Intensive Care Med*. 2012;38:210–220.

Mehta RH, Castelvecchio S, Ballotta A, et al. Association of gender and lowest hematocrit on cardiopulmonary bypass with acute kidney injury and operative mortality in patients undergoing cardiac surgery. *Ann Thorac Surg*. 2013;96(1):133–140.

Menkis AH, Martin J, Cheng DC, et al. Drug, devices, technologies, and techniques for blood management in minimally invasive and conventional cardiothoracic surgery: a consensus statement from the International Society for Minimally Invasive Cardiothoracic Surgery (ISMICS) 2011. *Innovations*. 2012;7(4):229–241.

Peek GJ, Mugford M, Tiruvoipati R, et al. Efficacy and economic assessment of conventional ventilatory support versus extracorporeal membrane oxygenation for severe adult respiratory failure (CESAR): a multicentre randomised controlled trial. *Lancet*. 2009;374:1351–1363.

Rex S, Brose S, Metzelder S, et al. Normothermic beating heart surgery with assistance of miniaturized bypass systems: the effects on intraoperative hemodynamics and inflammatory response. *Anesth Analg*. 2006;102:352–362.

Saczkowski R, Maklin M, Mesana T, et al. Centrifugal pump and roller pump in adult cardiac surgery: a meta-analysis of randomized controlled trials. *Artif Organs*. 2012;36(8):668–676.

Sauer CM, Yuh DD, Bonde P. Extracorporeal membrane oxygenation use has increased by 433% in adults in the United States from 2006 to 2011. *ASAIO J*. 2015;61:31–36.

Saur CM, Yuh DD, Bonde P. Extracorporeal membrane oxygenation use has increased by 433% in adults in the United States from 2006–2011. *ASAIO J*. 2015;61:31–36.

Scott DA, Silbert BS, Doyle TJ, et al. Centrifugal versus roller head pumps for cardiopulmonary bypass: effect on early neuropsychologic outcomes after coronary artery surgery. *J Cardiothorac Vasc Anesth*. 2002;16:715–722.

Shann KG, Likosky DS, Murkin JA, et al. An evidence-based review of the practice of cardiopulmonary bypass in adults: a focus on neurologic injury, glycemic control, hemodilution, and the inflammatory response. *J Thorac Cardiovasc Surg*. 2006;132:283–290.

Sidebotham D, McGeorge A, McGuinness S, et al. Extracorporeal membrane oxygenation for treating severe cardiac and respiratory failure in adults. Part 2: technical considerations. *J Cardiothorac Vasc Anesth*. 2010;24:164–172.

Soar J, Perkins GD, Abbas G, et al. European Resuscitation Council Guidelines for Resuscitation 2010. Section 8. Cardiac arrest in special circumstances: electrolyte abnormalities, poisoning, drowning, accidental hypothermia, hyperthermia, asthma, anaphylaxis, cardiac surgery, trauma, pregnancy, electrocution. *Resuscitation*. 2010;81:1400–1433.

Wiesenack C, Wiesner G, Keyl C, et al. In vivo uptake and elimination of isoflurane by different membrane oxygenators during cardiopulmonary bypass. *Anesthesiology*. 2002;97:133–138.

Chapter 27

Transfusion Medicine and Coagulation Disorders

Bruce D. Spiess, MD, FAHA • Sarah Armour, MD •
Jay Horrow, MD, FAHA • Joel A. Kaplan, MD, CPE, FACC •
Colleen G. Koch, MD, MS, MBA •
Keyvan Karkouti, MD, FRCPC, MSc • Simon C. Body, MD

Key Points

1. It is easiest to think of coagulation as a wave of biologic activity occurring at the site of tissue injury, consisting of initiation, acceleration, control, and lysis.
2. Hemostasis is part of a larger body system: inflammation. The protein reactions in coagulation have important roles in signaling inflammation.
3. Thrombin is the most important coagulation modulator, interacting with multiple coagulation factors, platelets, tissue plasminogen activator, prostacyclin, nitric oxide, and various white blood cells.
4. The serine proteases that compose the coagulation pathway are balanced by serine protease inhibitors, termed *serpins*. Antithrombin is the most important inhibitor of blood coagulation, but others include heparin cofactor II and alpha 1 antitrypsin.
5. Platelets are the most complex part of the coagulation process, and antiplatelet drugs are important therapeutic agents.
6. Heparin requires antithrombin to anticoagulate blood and is not an ideal anticoagulant for cardiopulmonary bypass. Newer anticoagulants are actively being sought to replace heparin.
7. Protamine can have many adverse effects. Ideally, a new anticoagulant will not require reversal with a toxic substance such as protamine.
8. Antifibrinolytic drugs are often given during cardiac surgery; these drugs include ε-aminocaproic acid and tranexamic acid.
9. Recombinant factor VIIa is an off-label "rescue agent" to stop bleeding during cardiac surgery, but it can also be prothrombotic, which is an off-label use of the drug.
10. Every effort should be made to avoid transfusion of banked blood products during routine cardiac surgery. In fact, bloodless surgery is a reality in many cases. Patient blood management, including techniques to reduce coagulation precursors, has been shown to be cost effective and to have better outcomes than routine surgery.
11. The evolving risks of transfusion have shifted from viral transmission to transfusion-related acute lung injury and immunosuppression. Those patients who receive allogeneic blood have a measurable increased rate of perioperative serious infection (approximately 16% increase per unit transfused).
12. Cardiac centers that have adopted multidisciplinary blood management strategies have improved patient outcomes and decreased costs. The careful application of these strategies in use of coagulation drugs and products is very beneficial.
13. New purified human protein adjuncts are replacing fresh-frozen plasma and cryoprecipitate with four-agent prothrombin complex concentrate and human lyophilized fibrinogen.

Coagulation and bleeding assume particular importance when surgery is performed on the heart and great vessels using extracorporeal circulation. This chapter provides an understanding of the depth and breadth of hemostasis relating to cardiac procedures, beginning with coagulation pathophysiology. The pharmacology of heparin and protamine follows. This background is then applied to treatment of the bleeding patient.

■ OVERVIEW OF HEMOSTASIS

Proper hemostasis requires the participation of innumerable biologic elements (Box 27.1). This section groups them into four topics to facilitate understanding: coagulation factors, platelet function, the endothelium, and fibrinolysis. The reader must realize this is for simplicity of learning, and that, in biology, the activation creates many reactions (perhaps >800) and control mechanisms, all interacting simultaneously. The interaction of the platelets, endothelial cells, and proteins either to activate or to deactivate coagulation is a highly buffered and controlled process. It is perhaps easiest to think of coagulation as a wave of biologic activity occurring at the site of tissue injury (Fig. 27.1). Although there are subcomponents to coagulation itself, the injury/control leading to hemostasis is a four-part event: initiation,

BOX 27.1 *Components of Hemostasis*

Coagulation factor activation
Platelet function
Vascular endothelium
Fibrinolysis and modulators of coagulation

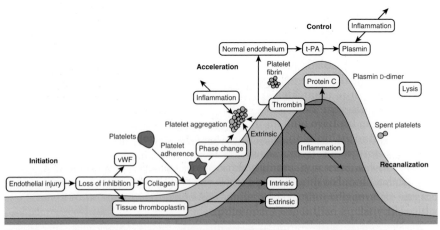

Fig. 27.1 Coagulation is a sine wave of activity at the site of tissue injury. It goes through four stages: initiation, acceleration, control, and lysis/recanalization. *t-PA,* Tissue plasminogen activator; *vWF,* von Willebrand factor. (Redrawn from Spiess BD. Coagulation function and monitoring. In: Lichtor JL, ed. *Atlas of Clinical Anesthesia.* Philadelphia: Current Medicine; 1996.)

acceleration, control, and lysis (recanalization/fibrinolysis). The initiation phase begins with tissue damage, which really is begun with endothelial cell destruction or dysfunction. This initiation phase leads to binding of platelets, as well as protein activations; both happen nearly simultaneously, and each has feedbacks into the other. Platelets adhere, creating an activation or acceleration phase that gathers many cells to the site of injury. From that adhesion a large number of events of cellular/protein messaging cascade. As the activation phase ramps up into an explosive set of reactions, counter-reactions are spun off, leading to control proteins damping the reactions. It is easiest, conceptually, to think of these control mechanisms as analogous to a nuclear reactor. The activation phase would continue to grow and overcome the whole organism unless control rods were inserted (eg, thrombomodulin, proteins C and S, and tissue plasminogen activator [t-PA]) to stop the spread of the reaction. The surrounding normal endothelium acts quite differently from the disturbed (ischemic) endothelium. Eventually, the control reactions overpower the acceleration reactions and lysis comes into play. A key concept is that hemostasis is part of a larger body system: inflammation. Most, if not all, of the protein reactions of coagulation control have importance in signaling inflammation leading to other healing mechanisms. It is no wonder that cardiopulmonary bypass (CPB) has such profound inflammatory effects when it is considered that each of the activated coagulation proteins and cell lines then feeds into upregulation of inflammation.

Protein Coagulation Activations

Coagulation Pathways

The coagulation factors participate in a series of activating and feedback inhibition reactions, ending with the formation of an insoluble clot. A *clot* is the sum total of platelet-to-platelet interactions, leading to the formation of a platelet plug (initial stoppage of bleeding). The cross-linking of platelets to each other by way of the final insoluble fibrin leads to a stable clot. Clot is not simply the activation of proteins leading to more protein deposition.

With few exceptions, the coagulation factors are glycoproteins (GPs) synthesized in the liver, which circulate as inactive molecules termed *zymogens*. Factor activation proceeds sequentially, each factor serving as substrate in an enzymatic reaction catalyzed by the previous factor in the sequence. Hence this reaction sequence classically has been termed a *cascade* or *waterfall*. Cleavage of a polypeptide fragment changes an inactive zymogen to an active enzyme often by creating a conformational change of the protein, exposing an active site. The active form is termed a *serine protease* because the active site for its protein-splitting activity is a serine amino acid residue. Many reactions require the presence of calcium ion (Ca^{2+}) and a phospholipid surface (platelet phosphatidylserine). The phospholipids occur most often either on the surface of an activated platelet or endothelial cell and occasionally on the surface of white cells. So anchored, their proximity to one another permits reaction rates profoundly accelerated (up to 300,000-fold) from those measured when the enzymes remain in solution. The factors form four interrelated *arbitrary* groups (Fig. 27.2): the contact activation, intrinsic, extrinsic, and common pathways.

CONTACT ACTIVATION

Factor XII, high-molecular-weight kininogen (HMWK), prekallikrein (PK), and factor XI form the contact or surface activation group. Because factor XII autoactivates by undergoing a shape change in the presence of a negative charge, in vitro coagulation tests use glass, silica, kaolin, and other compounds with negative surface charge. One potential in vivo mechanism for factor XII activation is disruption of the endothelial

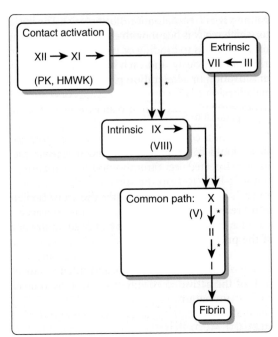

Fig. 27.2 Depiction of coagulation protein activation sequence. *Asterisks* denote participation of calcium ion. *HMWK*, High-molecular-weight kininogen; *PK*, prekallikrein.

cell layer, which exposes the underlying negatively charged collagen matrix. Activated platelets also provide negative charges on their membrane surfaces. HMWK anchors the other surface activation molecules, PK and factor XI, to damaged endothelium or activated platelets. Factor XIIa cleaves both factor XI, to form factor XIa, and PK, to form kallikrein.

INTRINSIC SYSTEM

Intrinsic activation forms factor XIa from the products of surface activation. Factor XIa splits factor IX to form factor IXa, with Ca^{2+} required for this process. Then factor IXa activates factor X with help from Ca^{2+}, a phospholipid surface (platelet-phosphatidylserine), and a GP cofactor, factor VIIIa.

EXTRINSIC SYSTEM

Activation of factor X can proceed independently of factor XII by substances classically thought to be extrinsic to the vasculature. Any number of endothelial cell insults can lead to the production of tissue factor by the endothelial cell. At rest, the endothelial cell is quite antithrombotic. However, with ischemia, reperfusion, sepsis, or cytokines (particularly interleukin [IL]-6), the endothelial cell will stimulate its production of intracellular nuclear factor-κB and send messages for the production of messenger RNA for tissue factor production. This can happen quickly and the resting endothelial cell can turn out large amounts of tissue factor. It is widely held today that the activation of tissue factor is what drives many of the abnormalities of coagulation after cardiac surgery, rather than contact activation. Thromboplastin, also known as tissue factor, released from tissues into the vasculature, acts as a cofactor for initial activation of factor X by factor VII. Factors VII and X then activate one another with the help of

V

platelet phospholipid and Ca^{2+}, thus rapidly generating factor Xa. (Factor VIIa also activates factor IX, thus linking the extrinsic and intrinsic paths.)

COMMON PATHWAY

Factor Xa splits prothrombin (factor II) to thrombin (factor IIa). The combination of factors Xa, Va, and Ca^{2+} is termed the *prothrombinase complex*—a critical step. Factor Xa anchors to the membrane surface (of platelets) via Ca^{2+}. Factor Va, assembling next to it, initiates a rearrangement of the complex, vastly accelerating binding of the substrate, prothrombin. Most likely, the factor Xa formed from the previous reaction is channeled along the membrane to this next reaction step without detaching from the membrane.

Thrombin cleaves the fibrinogen molecule to form soluble fibrin monomer and polypeptide fragments termed *fibrinopeptides A and B*. Fibrin monomers associate to form a soluble fibrin matrix. Factor XIII, activated by thrombin, cross-links these fibrin strands to form an insoluble clot. Patients with lower levels of factor XIII have been found to have more bleeding after cardiac surgery.

VITAMIN K

Those factors that require calcium (II, VII, IX, X) depend on vitamin K to add between 9 and 12 γ-carboxyl groups to glutamic acid residues near their amino terminal. Calcium tethers the negatively charged carboxyl groups to the phospholipid surface (platelets), thus facilitating molecular interactions. Some inhibitory proteins also depend on vitamin K (proteins C and S) for their functional completion.

Modulators of the Coagulation Pathway

Thrombin, the most important coagulation modulator, exerts a pervasive influence throughout the coagulation factor pathways. It activates factors V, VIII, and XIII; cleaves fibrinogen to fibrin; stimulates platelet recruitment, creates chemotaxis of leukocytes and monocytes; releases t-PA, prostacyclin, and nitric oxide from endothelial cells; releases IL-1 from macrophages; and with thrombomodulin, activates protein C, a substance that then inactivates factors Va and VIIIa. Note the negative feedback aspect of this last action. Coagulation function truly centers on the effects of thrombin as far-reaching accelerant. The platelets, tissue factor, and contact activation all are interactive and activated by a rent in the surface of the endothelium or through the loss of endothelial coagulation control. Platelets adhere to a site of injury and, in turn, are activated, leading to sequestration of other platelets. It is the interaction of all of those factors together that eventually creates a critical mass of reacting cells and proteins, which, in turn, leads to clot formation. Once enough platelets are interacting together, with their attached surface concomitant serine protease reactions, then a thrombin burst is created. Only when enough thrombin activation has been encountered in a critical time point is a threshold exceeded, and the reactions become massive—much larger than the sum of the parts. It is thought that the concentration and ability of platelets to react fully affect the ability to have a critical thrombin burst. CPB may affect the ability to get that full thrombin burst because it reduces platelet number, decreases platelet-to-platelet interactions, and decreases the concentration of protein substrates.

The many serine proteases that compose the coagulation pathways are balanced by serine protease inhibitors, termed *serpins*. Thus a biologic yin and yang leads to an excellent buffering capacity. It is only when the platelet-driven thrombin burst so overwhelms the body's localized anticoagulation or inhibitors that clot proceeds forward. Serpins include α_1-antitrypsin, α_2-macroglobulin, heparin cofactor II, α_2-antiplasmin, antithrombin (AT; also termed *antithrombin III* [AT III]), and others.

AT III constitutes the most potent and widely distributed inhibitor of blood coagulation. It binds to the active site (serine) of thrombin, thus inhibiting action of thrombin. It also inhibits, to a much lesser extent, the activity of factors XIIa, XIa, IXa, and Xa; kallikrein; and the fibrinolytic molecule, plasmin. Thrombin bound to fibrin is protected from the action of AT, thus partially explaining the poor efficacy of heparin in treating established thrombosis. AT III is a relatively inactive zymogen. To be most effective, AT must bind to a unique pentasaccharide sequence contained on the wall of endothelial cells in the glycosaminoglycan surface known as heparan; the same active sequence is present in the drug heparin.

An important point is that activated AT III is active only against free thrombin (fibrin-bound thrombin cannot be seen by AT III). Prothrombin circulates in the plasma but is not affected by heparin-AT III complexes; it is only thrombin, and thrombin does not circulate freely. Most thrombin in its active form is either bound to GP binding sites of platelets or in fibrin matrices. When blood is put into a test tube and clot begins to form (such as in an activated coagulation time [ACT]), 96% of thrombin production is yet to come. Most thrombin generation is on the surface of platelets and on clot-held fibrinogen. Platelets, through their GP binding sites and phospholipid folds, protect activated thrombin from attack by AT III. Therefore the biologic role of AT III is to create an anticoagulant surface on endothelial cells. It is not present biologically to sit and wait for a dose of heparin before CPB.

Another serpin, *protein C,* degrades factors Va and VIIIa. Like other vitamin K–dependent factors, it requires Ca^{2+} to bind to phospholipid. Its cofactor, termed *protein S,* also exhibits vitamin K dependence. Genetic variants of protein C are less active and lead to increased risk for deep vein thrombosis and pulmonary embolism. When endothelial cells release thrombomodulin, thrombin then accelerates by 20,000-fold its activation of protein C. Activated protein C also promotes fibrinolysis through a feedback loop to the endothelial cells to release t-PA.

Regulation of the extrinsic limb of the coagulation pathway occurs via tissue factor pathway inhibitor (TFPI), a glycosylated protein that associates with lipoproteins in plasma. TFPI is not a serpin. It impairs the catalytic properties of the factor VIIa–tissue factor complex on factor X activation. Both vascular endothelium and platelets appear to produce TFPI. Heparin releases TFPI from endothelium, increasing TFPI plasma concentrations by as much as sixfold. *von Willebrand factor* (vWF), a massive molecule composed of disulfide-linked glycosylated peptides, associates with factor VIII in plasma, protecting it from proteolytic enzymes. It circulates in the plasma in its coiled inactive form. Disruption of the endothelium either allows for binding of vWF from the plasma or allows for expression of vWF from tissue and from endothelial cells. Once bound, vWF uncoils to its full length and exposes a hitherto cryptic domain in the molecule. This A-1 domain has a very high affinity for platelet GPs. Initially, vWF attaches to the glycoprotein Iα (GPIα) platelet receptor, which slows the platelet forward movements against the shear forces of blood flow. Shear forces are activators of platelets. As the platelet's forward movement along the endothelial brush border is slowed (because of vWF attachment), shear forces actually increase; thus the binding of vWF to GPI acts to provide a feedback loop for individual platelets, further activating them. The activation of vWF and its attachment to the platelet are not enough to bind the platelet to the endothelium, but it creates a membrane signal that allows for early shape change and expression of other GPs, GPIb, and GPIIb/IIIa. Then secondary GPIb binding connects to other vWF nearby, binding the platelet and beginning the activation sequence. It bridges normal platelets to damaged subendothelium by attaching to the GPIb platelet receptor. An ensuing platelet shape change then releases thromboxane, β-thromboglobulin, and serotonin, and exposes GPIIb/IIIa, which binds fibrinogen. Table 27.1 summarizes the coagulation factors, their activation sequences, and vehicles for factor replacement when deficient.

Table 27.1 The Coagulation Pathway Proteins, Minimal Amounts Needed for Surgery, and Replacement Sources

Factor	Activated By	Acts On	Minimal Amount Needed	Replacement Source	Alternate Name and Comments
XIII	IIa	Fibrin	<5%	FFP, CRYO	Fibrin-stabilizing factor; not a serine protease, but an enzyme
XII	Endothelium	XI	None	Not needed	Hageman factor; activation enhanced by XIIa
XI	XIIa	IX	15%–25%	FFP	Plasma thromboplastin antecedent
X	VIIa or IXa	II	10%–20%	FFP, 9C	Stuart-Prower factor; vitamin K–dependent
IX	VIIa or XIa	X	25%–30%	FFP, 9C, PCC	Christmas factor; vitamin K–dependent
VIII	IIa	X	>30%	CRYO, 8C, FFP	Antihemophilic factor; a cofactor; RES synthesis
VII	Xa	X	10%–20%	FFP, PCC	Serum prothrombin conversion accelerator; vitamin K–dependent
V	IIa	II	<25%	FFP	Proaccelerin; a cofactor; RES and liver synthesis
IV	—	—	—	—	Calcium ion; binds II, VII, IX, X to phospholipid
III	—	X	—	—	Thromboplastin/tissue factor; a cofactor
II	Xa	—	20%–40%	FFP, PCC	Prothrombin; vitamin K–dependent
I	IIa	—	1 g/L	CRYO, FFP, FC	Fibrinogen; activated product is soluble fibrin
vWF	—	VIII	See VIII	CRYO, FFP	von Willebrand factor; endothelial cell synthesis

Unless otherwise specified, all coagulation proteins are synthesized in the liver. Note that there is no factor VI. For von Willebrand factor, cryoprecipitate or fresh-frozen plasma (*FFP*) is administered to obtain a factor VIII coagulant activity >30%. *8C*, Factor VIII concentrate; *9C*, purified factor IX complex concentrate; *CRYO*, cryoprecipitate; *FC*, fibrinogen concentrate; *PCC*, prothrombin complex concentrate; *RES*, reticuloendothelial system.

Platelet Function

Most clinicians think first of the coagulation proteins when considering hemostasis. Although no one element of the many that participate in hemostasis assumes dominance, platelets may be the most complex. Without platelets, there is no coagulation and no hemostasis. Without the proteins, there is hemostasis, but it lasts only about 10 to 15 minutes because the platelet plug is inherently unstable and breaks apart under the shear stress of the vasculature. Platelets provide phospholipid for coagulation factor reactions; contain their own microskeletal system and release coagulation factors; secrete active substances affecting themselves, other platelets, the endothelium, and other coagulation factors; and alter shape (through active actin-myosin contraction) to expose membrane GPs essential to hemostasis. The initial response to vascular injury is formation of a platelet plug. Good hemostatic response depends on proper functioning of platelet adhesion, activation, and aggregation.

Platelet Adhesion

Capillary blood exhibits laminar flow, which maximizes the likelihood of interaction of platelets with the vessel wall. Red cells and white cells stream near the center of the vessels and marginate platelets. However, turbulence causes reactions in endothelium that lead to the secretion of vWF, adhesive molecules, and tissue factor. Shear stress is high as fast-moving platelets interact with the endothelium. When the vascular endothelium becomes denuded or injured, the platelet has the opportunity to contact vWF, which is bound to the exposed collagen of the subendothelium. A platelet membrane component, GPIb, attaches to vWF, thus anchoring the platelet to the vessel wall. Independently, platelet membrane GPIa and GPIIa and IX may attach directly to exposed collagen, furthering the adhesion stage.

The integrin GPs form diverse types of membrane receptors from combinations of 20 α and 8 β subunits. One such combination is GPIIb/IIIa, a platelet membrane component that initially participates in platelet adhesion. Platelet activation causes a conformational change in GPIIb/IIIa, which results in its aggregator activity.

Platelet adhesion begins rapidly—within 1 minute of endothelial injury—and completely covers exposed subendothelium within 20 minutes. It begins with decreased platelet velocity when GPIb/IX and vWF mediate adhesion, followed by platelet activation, GPIIb/IIIa conformational change, then vWF binding and platelet arrest on the endothelium at these vWF ligand sites.

Platelet Activation and Aggregation

Platelet activation results after contact with collagen, when adenosine diphosphate (ADP), thrombin, or thromboxane A_2 binds to membrane receptors, or from certain platelet-to-platelet interactions. Platelets then release the contents of their dense (δ) granules and α granules. Dense granules contain serotonin, ADP, and Ca^{2+}; α granules contain platelet factor V (previously termed platelet factor 1), β-thromboglobulin, platelet factor 4 (PF4), P-selectin, and various integrin proteins (vWF, fibrinogen, vitronectin, and fibronectin). Simultaneously, platelets use their microskeletal system to change shape from a disk to a sphere, which changes platelet membrane GPIIb/IIIa exposure. Released ADP recruits additional platelets to the site of injury and stimulates platelet G protein, which, in turn, activates membrane phospholipase. This results in the formation of arachidonate, which platelet cyclooxygenase converts to thromboxane A_2. Other platelet agonists besides ADP and collagen include serotonin, a weak agonist, and thrombin and thromboxane A_2, both potent agonists. Thrombin is by far the most potent platelet agonist, and it can overcome all other platelet antagonists, as well as inhibitors. In total, more than 70 agonists can produce platelet activation and aggregation.

V

Agonists induce a graded platelet shape change (the amount based on the relative amount of stimulation), increase platelet intracellular Ca^{2+} concentration, and stimulate platelet G protein. In addition, serotonin and thromboxane A_2 are potent vasoconstrictors (particularly in the pulmonary vasculature). The presence of sufficient agonist material results in platelet aggregation. Aggregation occurs when the integrin proteins (mostly fibrinogen) released from α granules form molecular bridges between the GPIIb/IIIa receptors of adjacent platelets (the final common platelet pathway).

Prostaglandins and Aspirin

Endothelial cell cyclooxygenase synthesizes prostacyclin, which inhibits aggregation and dilates vessels. Platelet cyclooxygenase forms thromboxane A_2, a potent aggregating agent and vasoconstrictor. Aspirin irreversibly acetylates cyclooxygenase, rendering it inactive. Low doses of aspirin, 80 to 100 mg, easily overcome the finite amount of cyclooxygenase available in the nucleus-free platelets. However, endothelial cells can synthesize new cyclooxygenase. Thus with low doses of aspirin, prostacyclin synthesis continues, whereas thromboxane synthesis ceases, decreasing platelet activation and aggregation. High doses of aspirin inhibit the enzyme at both cyclooxygenase sites.

In many centers, a majority of the patients presenting for coronary artery bypass grafting (CABG) will have received aspirin within 7 days of surgery in hopes of preventing coronary thrombosis. Platelets have a life span of approximately 9 days, so the idea of taking somebody off aspirin for 5 to 7 days seems reasonable in that the majority of platelets circulating will not have cyclooxygenase poisoned by aspirin. Aspirin is a drug for which an increased risk for bleeding often has been demonstrated. Today, it probably is more likely that, in some patients, a mild-to-moderate increased risk for bleeding is possible.

Drug-Induced Platelet Abnormalities

Many other agents inhibit platelet function. β-Lactam antibiotics coat the platelet membrane, whereas the cephalosporins are rather profound but short-term platelet inhibitors. Many cardiac surgeons may not realize that their standard drug regimen for antibiotics may be far more of a bleeding risk than aspirin. Hundreds of drugs can inhibit platelet function. Calcium channel blockers, nitrates, and β-blockers are ones commonly used in cardiac surgery. Nitrates are effective antiplatelet agents, and that may be part of why they are of such benefit in angina, not only for their vasorelaxing effect on large blood vessels. Nonsteroidal antiinflammatory drugs reversibly inhibit both endothelial cell and platelet cyclooxygenase.

In addition to the partial inhibitory effects of aspirin and the other drugs mentioned earlier, new therapies that inhibit platelet function in a more specific manner have been developed. These drugs include platelet adhesion inhibitor agents, platelet-ADP-receptor antagonists, and GPIIb/IIIa receptor inhibitors (Table 27.2).

ADENOSINE DIPHOSPHATE RECEPTOR ANTAGONISTS

Clopidogrel (Plavix), and prasugrel (Effient), are thienopyridine derivatives that inhibit the ADP receptor pathway to platelet activation. They have a slow onset of action because they must be converted to active drugs, and their potent effects last the lifetime of the platelets affected (5–10 days). Clopidogrel and prasugrel are the preferred drugs. They are administered orally once daily to inhibit platelet function and are quite effective in decreasing myocardial infarctions (MIs) after percutaneous coronary interventions (PCIs). The combination of aspirin and clopidogrel has led to increased bleeding, but is used in an effort to keep vessels and stents open. Recently,

27

Table 27.2 Antiplatelet Therapy

Drug Type	Composition	Mechanism	Indications	Route	Half-Life	Metabolism
Aspirin	Acetylsalicylic acid	Irreversible COX inhibition	CAD, AMI, PVD, PCI, ACS	Oral	10 days	Liver, kidney
NSAIDs	Multiple	Reversible COX inhibition	Pain	Oral	2 days	Liver, kidney
Adhesion inhibitors (eg, dipyridamole)	Multiple	Block adhesion to vessels	VHD, PVD	Oral	12 hours	Liver
ADP Receptor Antagonists						
—Clopidogrel (Plavix), prasugrel (Effient)	Thienopyridines	Irreversible	AMI, CVA, PVD, ACS, PCI	Oral	5 days	Liver
—Ticagrelor (Brilinta)	Nonthienopyridine	Reversible	AMI, CVA, PVD, ACS, PCI	Oral	3–5 days	Liver
—Cangrelor (Kengreal)	Nonthienopyridine	Reversible	AMI, CVA, PVD, ACS, PCI	IV	3–10 min	Blood
PAR-1 Inhibitors						
—Vorapaxar (Zontivity)	PAR-1 antagonist	Irreversible—inhibits thrombin-induced platelet activation	AMI, PVD	Oral	20 hr–4 wk	Liver
GPIIb/IIIa Receptor Inhibitors						
—Abciximab (ReoPro)	Monoclonal antibody	Nonspecific—binds to other receptors	PCI, ACS	IV	12–18 hours	Plasma proteinase
—Eptifibatide (Integrilin)	Peptide	Reversible—specific to GPIIb/IIIa	PCI, ACS	IV	2–4 hours	Kidney
—Tirofiban (Aggrastat)	Nonpeptide-tyrosine derivative	Reversible—specific to GPIIb/IIIa	PCI, ACS, AMI, PVD	IV	2–4 hours	Kidney

ACS, Acute coronary syndrome; AMI, acute myocardial infarction; CAD, coronary artery disease; COX, cyclooxygenase; CVA, cerebrovascular disease; IV, intravenous; NSAID, nonsteroidal antiinflammatory drug; PAR-1, protease-activated receptor; PCI, percutaneous coronary intervention; PVD, peripheral vascular disease; VHD, valvular heart disease.

two new nonthienopyridine ADP P_2Y_{12} inhibitors have become available. Ticagrelor is a direct-acting oral drug, and cangrelor is a short-acting intravenous agent. The latter drug may be a very valuable bridging drug for use in the PCI laboratory and perioperative period.

GLYCOPROTEIN IIB/IIIA RECEPTOR INHIBITORS

These are the most potent (>90% platelet inhibition) because they act at the final common pathway of platelet aggregation with fibrinogen, no matter which agonist began the process. All of the drugs mentioned earlier work at earlier phases of activation of platelet function. These drugs are all administered by intravenous infusion, and they do not work orally. The GPIIb/IIIa inhibitors often are used in patients taking aspirin because they do not block thromboxane A_2 production. The dose of heparin usually is reduced when used with these drugs (ie, PCI to avoid bleeding at the vascular puncture sites). Platelet activity can be monitored to determine the extent of blockade. Excessive bleeding requires allowing the short-acting drugs to wear off, while possibly administering platelets to patients receiving the long-acting drug abciximab. Most studies have found increased bleeding in patients receiving these drugs who required emergency CABG.

Fibrinolysis

Fibrin breakdown, a normal hematologic activity, is localized to the vicinity of a clot. It remodels formed clot and removes thrombus when endothelium heals. Like clot formation, clot breakdown may occur by intrinsic and extrinsic pathways. As with clot formation, the extrinsic pathway plays the dominant role in clot breakdown. Each pathway activates plasminogen, a serine protease synthesized by the liver, which circulates in zymogen form. Cleavage of plasminogen by the proper serine protease forms plasmin. Plasmin splits fibrinogen or fibrin at specific sites. Plasmin is the principal enzyme of fibrinolysis, just as thrombin is principal to clot formation. Plasma normally contains no circulating plasmin because a scavenging protein, α_2-antiplasmin, quickly consumes any plasmin formed from localized fibrinolysis. Thus localized fibrinolysis, not systemic fibrinogenolysis, accompanies normal hemostasis.

Extrinsic Fibrinolysis

Endothelial cells synthesize and release t-PA. Both t-PA and a related substance, urokinase plasminogen activator, are serine proteases that split plasminogen to form plasmin. The activity of t-PA magnifies on binding to fibrin. In this manner, also, plasmin formation remains localized to sites of clot formation. Epinephrine, bradykinin, thrombin, and factor Xa cause endothelium to release t-PA, as do venous occlusion and CPB.

Intrinsic Fibrinolysis

Factor XIIa, formed during the contact phase of coagulation, cleaves plasminogen to plasmin. The plasmin so formed then facilitates additional cleavage of plasminogen by factor XIIa, forming a positive feedback loop.

Exogenous Activators

Streptokinase (made by bacteria) and urokinase (found in human urine) both cleave plasminogen to plasmin but do so with low fibrin affinity. Thus systemic plasminemia

27

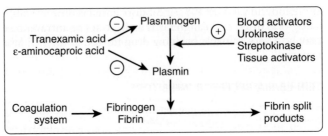

Fig. 27.3 The fibrinolytic pathway. Antifibrinolytic drugs inhibit fibrinolysis by binding to both plasminogen and plasmin. Intrinsic blood activators (factor XIIa), extrinsic tissue activators (tissue plasminogen activator, urokinase plasminogen activator), and exogenous activators (streptokinase, acetylated streptokinase plasminogen activator complex) split plasminogen to form plasmin. (From Horrow JC, Hlavacek J, Strong MD, et al. Prophylactic tranexamic acid decreases bleeding after cardiac operations. *J Thorac Cardiovasc Surg.* 1990;99:70.)

and fibrinogenolysis, as well as fibrinolysis, ensue. Acetylated streptokinase plasminogen activator complex provides an active site, which is not available until deacetylation occurs in blood. Its systemic lytic activity lies intermediate to those of t-PA and streptokinase. Recombinant t-PA (Alteplase) is a second-generation agent that is made by recombinant DNA technology and is relatively fibrin-specific.

Clinical Applications

Fig. 27.3 illustrates the fibrinolytic pathway, with activators and inhibitors. Streptokinase, acetylated streptokinase plasminogen activator complex, and t-PA find application in the lysis of thrombi associated with MI. These intravenous agents "dissolve" clots that form on atheromatous plaque. Clinically significant bleeding may result from administration of any of these exogenous activators or streptokinase.

Fibrinolysis also accompanies CPB. This undesirable breakdown of clot after surgery may contribute to postoperative hemorrhage and the need to administer allogeneic blood products. Regardless of how they are formed, the breakdown products of fibrin intercalate into sheets of normally forming fibrin monomers, thus preventing cross-linking. In this way, extensive fibrinolysis exerts an antihemostatic action. Factor XIII is an underappreciated coagulation protein. It circulates and, when activated, cross-links fibrin strands and protects fibrin from the lytic actions of plasmin. It has been known for some time that low levels of factor XIII are associated with increased hemorrhage after CPB. Factor XIII levels are reduced by hemodilution, but it also appears that there is active destruction in some patients with CPB.

HEPARIN

The *N*-sulfated-D-glucosamine and L-iduronic acid residues of heparin alternate in copolymer fashion to form chains of varying length. As a linear anionic polyelectrolyte, the negative charges being supplied by sulfate groups, heparin demonstrates a wide spectrum of activity with enzymes, hormones, biogenic amines, and plasma proteins. A pentasaccharide segment binds to AT. Heparin is a heterogenous compound; the carbohydrates vary in both length and side-chain composition, yielding a range of molecular weights from 5000 to 30,000, with most chains between 12,000 and 19,000. Today, the standard heparin is called *unfractionated heparin (UFH)*.

Most commercial preparations of heparin now use pig intestine, 40,000 pounds of which yield 5 kg heparin. Heparin potency is determined by comparing the test specimen against a known standard's ability to prolong coagulation. Current United States Pharmacopeia (USP) and British Pharmacopoeia (BP) assays use a PT-like method on pooled sheep's plasma obtained from slaughterhouses.

UFH dose should not be specified by weight (milligrams) because of the diversity of anticoagulant activity expected from so heterogenous a compound. One USP unit of heparin activity is the quantity that prevents 1.0 mL of citrated sheep's plasma from clotting for 1 hour after addition of calcium. Units cannot be cross-compared among heparins of different sources, such as mucosal versus lung, or low-molecular-weight heparin (LMWH) versus UFH, or even lot to lot, because the assay used may or may not reflect actual differences in biologic activity. None of these measures has anything to do with the effect of a unit on anticoagulation effect for human cardiac surgery.

Pharmacokinetics and Pharmacodynamics

The heterogeneity of UFH molecules produces variability in the relation of dose administered to plasma level of drug. In addition, the relation of plasma level to biologic effect varies with the test system. A three-compartment model describes heparin kinetics in healthy humans: rapid initial disappearance, saturable clearance observed in the lower dose range, and exponential first-order decay at greater doses. The rapid initial disappearance may arise from endothelial cell uptake. The reticuloendothelial system, with its endoglycosidases and endosulfatases, and uptake into monocytes, may represent the saturable phase of heparin kinetics. Finally, renal clearance via active tubular secretion of heparin, much of it desulfated, explains heparin's exponential clearance.

Loading doses for CPB (200–400 U/kg) are substantially greater than those used to treat venous thrombosis (70–150 U/kg). Plasma heparin levels, determined fluorometrically, vary widely (2–4 units/mL) after doses of heparin administered to patients about to undergo CPB. The ACT response to these doses of heparin displays even greater dispersion. However, the clinical response to heparin administered to various patients is more consistent than suggested by in vitro measurements.

Actions and Interactions

Heparin exerts its anticoagulant activity via AT III, one of the many circulating serine protein inhibitors (serpins), which counter the effects of circulating proteases. The major inhibitor of thrombin and factors IXa and Xa is AT III; that of the contact activation factors XIIa and XIa is α_1-proteinase inhibitor; kallikrein inhibition arises mostly from C1 inhibitor. AT activity is greatly decreased at a site of vascular damage, underscoring its primary role as a scavenger for clotting enzymes that escape into the general circulation.

AT inhibits serine proteases even without heparin. The extent to which heparin accelerates AT inhibition depends on the substrate enzyme; UFH accelerates the formation of the thrombin-AT complex by 2000-fold but accelerates formation of the factor Xa-AT complex by only 1200-fold. In contrast, LMWH fragments preferentially inhibit factor Xa. Enzyme inhibition proceeds by formation of a ternary complex consisting of heparin, AT, and the proteinase to be inhibited (eg, thrombin, factor Xa). For UFH, inhibition of thrombin occurs only on simultaneous binding to both AT and thrombin. This condition requires a heparin fragment of at least 18 residues. A pentasaccharide sequence binds to AT. LMWHs, consisting of chains 8 to 16 units long, preferentially inhibit factor Xa. In this case, the heparin fragment activates AT, which then sequentially inactivates factor Xa; heparin and factor Xa do not directly interact.

Several investigators have demonstrated continued formation of fibrinopeptides A and B, as well as prothrombin fragment F1.2 and thrombin-AT complexes, despite clearly acceptable anticoagulation for CPB by many criteria. These substances indicate thrombin activity. The clinical significance of this ongoing thrombin activity has had limited study. The ACT must be more prolonged to prevent fibrin formation during cardiac surgery compared with during extracorporeal circulation without surgery because surgery itself incites coagulation. UFH in conjunction with AT appears to work in plasma only on free thrombin. When considering what is known today about thrombin burst and thrombin activity, heparin appears to be relatively inefficient because there is not much free thrombin. Thrombin is held on the surface of activated platelets at various GP binding sites, including the GPIIb/IIIa site. Most thrombin is fibrin-bound, and heparin-AT complexes do not bind at all to this thrombin unless the level of heparin is pushed far above what is used routinely for CPB.

Heparin Resistance

Patients receiving UFH infusions exhibit a much-diminished ACT response to full anticoagulating doses of UFH for CPB (200–400 U/kg). With widespread use of heparin infusions to treat myocardial ischemia and infarction, heparin resistance or, more appropriately, "altered heparin responsiveness" has become more problematic during cardiac surgery (Box 27.2).

Hemodilution accompanying CPB decreases AT levels to about 66% or even half of normal levels. There are, however, outlier patients who have profoundly low AT levels. It is possible to see AT III levels as low as 20% of normal, and these levels correspond to levels seen in septic shock and diffuse intravascular coagulation. However, supplemental AT may not prolong the ACT, which means that the heparin available has been bound to sufficient or available AT. The only way that the ACT would be prolonged is if there is excess heparin beyond available AT. Reports of heparin resistance for CPB ascribe its occurrence variously to the use of autotransfusion, previous heparin therapy, infection, and ventricular aneurysm with thrombus. The individual anticoagulant response to heparin varies tremendously. Some presumed cases of heparin resistance may represent nothing more than this normal variation. Regardless of cause, measurement of each individual's anticoagulant response to heparin therapy for CPB is warranted. Heparin resistance helps focus the debate regarding whether

BOX 27.2 *Problems With Heparin as an Anticoagulant for Cardiopulmonary Bypass*

Heparin resistance
Heparin-induced thrombocytopenia
Heparin rebound
Heparin's heterogeneity and variable potency
AT III decrease

AT III, Antithrombin.

anticoagulation monitoring should measure heparin concentrations or heparin effect; the goal of anticoagulation is not to achieve heparin presence in plasma but to inhibit the action of thrombin on fibrinogen, platelets, and endothelial cells. Therefore the effect of heparin usually is measured.

Most commonly, additional heparin prolongs the ACT sufficiently for the conduct of CPB. Amounts up to 800 U/kg may be necessary to obtain an ACT of 400 to 480 seconds or longer. Although administration of fresh-frozen plasma (FFP), which contains AT, should correct AT depletion and suitably prolong the ACT, such exposure to transfusion-borne infectious diseases should be avoided whenever possible.

AT concentrate specifically addresses AT deficiency. Two products are available for utilization. One is a recombinant DNA engineered product made from goat's milk and the other is a purified human plasma harvest derivative.

Heparin Rebound

Several hours after protamine neutralization for cardiac surgery, some patients experience development of clinical bleeding associated with prolongation of coagulation times. This phenomenon is often attributed to reappearance of circulating heparin. Theories accounting for "heparin rebound" include late release of heparin sequestered in tissues, delayed return of heparin to the circulation from the extracellular space via lymphatics, clearance of an unrecognized endogenous heparin antagonist, and more rapid clearance of protamine in relation to heparin. Studies demonstrating uptake of heparin into endothelial cells suggest that these cells may slowly release the drug into the circulation once plasma levels decline with protamine neutralization. It is questionable how much heparin rebound contributes to actual bleeding.

Although still debated by a few, most clinicians accept heparin rebound as a real phenomenon. However, clinical bleeding does not always accompany heparin rebound. When it does, administration of supplemental protamine will neutralize the remaining heparin (Box 27.3).

Heparin-Induced Thrombocytopenia

Heparin normally binds to platelet membranes at GPIb and other sites and aggregates normal platelets by releasing ADP. A moderate, reversible heparin-induced thrombocytopenia (HIT), now termed *type I,* has been known for half a century. The fact that heparin actually triggers an acute decline in platelet count should be considered a biologic event, because heparin, even in trace amounts, triggers the expression of many different platelet GPs. This has been termed *activation of platelets,* but it is not total activation. Heparin's prolongation of the bleeding time probably is related to activation of the platelets, as well as heparin binding to the GPIb surface.

27

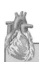

BOX 27.3 *Considerations in Determining the Proper Dose of Protamine to Reverse Heparin*

The proper dose is broad and difficult to determine exactly
The dose should be determined by a measurement of coagulation
The dose should be administered over at least 10 minutes
Excess protamine is a mild antithrombin agent; it may well lead to bleeding itself

   In contrast with these predictable effects of heparin, occasionally patients experience development of progressive and severe thrombocytopenia (<100,000/mm³), sometimes accompanied by a debilitating or fatal thrombosis (HIT with thrombosis [HITT]). This syndrome is termed *type II HIT (HIT II)*. A platelet count in excess of 100,000/mm³ does not mean that HIT II is not present. A decline in platelet count in excess of 30% to 50% over several days in a patient who is receiving or who has just finished receiving heparin is probably caused by HIT II.

Mechanism

These patients with HIT demonstrate a heparin-dependent antibody, usually IgG, although others are described, which aggregates platelets in the presence of heparin. During heparin therapy, measured antibody titers remain low because of antibody binding to platelets. Titers rise after heparin therapy ceases; but paradoxically, antibody may be undetectable a few months later. Two other features are unexpected: first, the antibody does not aggregate platelets in the presence of excess heparin; and second, not all reexposed patients experience development of thrombocytopenia.

   The platelet surface contains complexes of heparin and platelet factor 4 (PF4). Affected patients have an antibody to this complex. Antibody binding activates platelets via their FcγII receptors and activates endothelium (Fig. 27.4). The activation of the

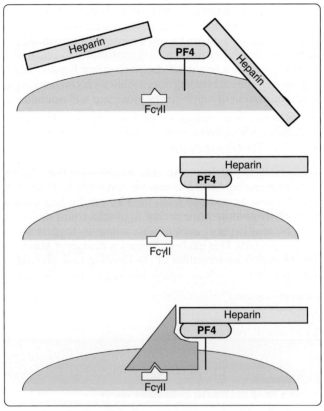

Fig. 27.4 Presumed mechanism of the interaction among heparin, platelets, and antibody in heparin-induced thrombocytopenia. *Top,* Platelet factor 4 (*PF4*) released from platelet granules is bound to the platelet surface. *Middle,* Heparin and PF4 complexes form. *Bottom,* The antibody binds to the PF4-heparin complex and activates platelet FcγII receptors.

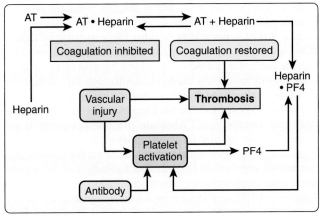

Fig. 27.5 Mechanism of thrombosis accompanying heparin-induced thrombocytopenia. Normally, heparin and antithrombin (*AT*) form a complex that inhibits coagulation. Platelet factor 4 (*PF4*), released from platelets on activation, binds heparin and drives the dissociation reaction of the AT-heparin complex to the right, restoring coagulation locally. Restored coagulation mechanisms and activated platelets form thrombus in the presence of vascular injury. (Adapted from Parmet JL, Horrow JC. Hematologic diseases. In: Benumof J, ed. *Anesthesia and Uncommon Diseases.* 3rd ed. Philadelphia: WB Saunders Company; 1997.)

platelet surface triggers a secondary thrombin release. Platelets can attach to each other, creating what is known as a white-clot syndrome, but if secondary thrombin generation is created through antibody activation of the platelets, then a fibrin clot can be the result. In the absence of heparin, the heparin-PF4 antigen cannot form.

In the absence of an endothelial defect, the only responses to the antibody-antigen interaction are platelet consumption and thrombocytopenia. Atheroma rupture, endovascular interventions such as balloon angioplasty, vascular surgery, and other procedures that disrupt endothelium can provide a nidus for platelet adhesion and subsequent activation. PF4, released with platelet activation, binds to heparin locally, thus not only removing the inhibition of coagulation but also generating additional antigenic material (Fig. 27.5). Clumps of aggregated platelets thrombose vessels, resulting in organ and limb infarction. Amputation, death, or both often occur with established HITT. The presence of heparin-PF4 antibodies recently has been associated with other adverse effects. It appears that if a patient undergoes cardiac surgery with positive antibodies, the risk for mortality or MI, or both, may at least double.

Incidence and Diagnosis

Estimates of the true incidence of HIT are confounded by different diagnostic thresholds for platelet count, varying efforts to detect other causes, and incomplete reports. After 7 days of therapy with UFH, probably 1% of patients experience development of HIT; after 14 days of therapy, the prevalence rate is 3%. Using a platelet count of 100,000/mm^3, multiple reports comprising more than 1200 patients revealed an overall incidence rate of HIT of 5.5% with bovine heparin and 1.0% with porcine heparin. Other recent research has found the preoperative incidence rate of enzyme-linked immunosorbent assay (ELISA)–positive patients to be between 6.5% and 10%. This means that antibodies are present, and that may not mean that thrombocytopenia is occurring. Of great interest is that many more patients develop positive tests for

ELISA antibodies by days 7 to 30 after cardiac surgery. Somewhere between 25% and 50% of patients develop these antibodies.

Some particular lots of heparin may be more likely to cause HIT than others. HIT can occur not only during therapeutic heparin administration but with low prophylactic doses, although the incidence is dose-related. Even heparin flush solution or heparin-bonded intravascular catheters can incite HIT. Although HIT usually begins 3 to 15 days (median, 10 days) after heparin infusions commence, it can occur within hours in a patient previously exposed to heparin. Platelet count steadily decreases to a nadir between 20,000 and 150,000/mm³. Absolute thrombocytopenia is not necessary; only a significant decrease in platelet count matters, as witnessed by patients with thrombocytosis who experience development of thrombosis with normal platelet counts after prolonged exposure to heparin. Occasionally, thrombocytopenia resolves spontaneously despite continuation of heparin infusion.

Clinical diagnosis of HIT requires a new decrease in platelet count during heparin infusion. Laboratory confirmation is obtained from several available tests. In the serotonin release assay, patient plasma, donor platelets, and heparin are combined. The donor platelets contain radiolabeled serotonin, which is released when donor platelets are activated by the antigen-antibody complex. Measurement of serotonin release during platelet aggregation at both low and high heparin concentrations provides excellent sensitivity and specificity.

A second assay measures more traditional markers of platelet degranulation in a mixture of heparin, patient plasma, and donor platelets. The most specific test is an ELISA for antibodies to the heparin-PF4 complex.

Measurement of platelet-associated IgG is poorly specific for HIT because of numerous other causes of antiplatelet IgG. This test should not be used in the diagnosis of HIT.

Treatment and Prevention

In the absence of surgery, bleeding from thrombocytopenia with HIT is rare. In contrast with other drug-induced thrombocytopenia, in which severe thrombocytopenia commonly occurs, more moderate platelet count nadirs characterize HIT. Platelet transfusions are not indicated and may incite or worsen thrombosis. Heparin infusions must be discontinued, and an alternative anticoagulant should be instituted. LMWHs can be tested in the laboratory using serotonin release before patient administration. Although thrombosis may be treated with fibrinolytic therapy, surgery often is indicated. No heparin should be given for vascular surgery. Monitoring catheters should be purged of heparin flush, and heparin-bonded catheters should not be placed.

The patient presenting for cardiac surgery who has sustained HIT in the past presents a therapeutic dilemma. Antibodies may have regressed; if so, a negative serotonin release assay using the heparin planned for surgery will predict that transient exposure during surgery will be harmless. However, no heparin should be given at catheterization or in flush solutions after surgery.

Patients with HIT who require urgent surgery may receive heparin once platelet activation has been blocked with aspirin and ultrashort-acting platelet blocking agents, such as cangrelor, may help to create "platelet anesthesia."

Another alternative, delaying surgery to wait for antibodies to regress, may fail because of the variable offset of antibody presence and the unpredictable nature of platelet response to heparin rechallenge. Plasmapheresis may successfully eliminate antibodies and allow benign heparin administration. Finally, methods of instituting anticoagulation without heparin may be chosen.

Box 27.4 summarizes the therapeutic options available for urgent cardiac surgery in patients with HIT.

27

ALTERNATIVE MODES OF ANTICOAGULATION

The hemostatic goal during CPB is complete inhibition of the coagulation system. Unfortunately, even large doses of heparin do not provide this, as evidenced by formation of fibrinopeptides during surgery. Despite being far from the ideal anticoagulant, heparin still performs better than its alternatives. Current substitutes for heparin include ancrod, a proteinase obtained from snake venom that destroys fibrinogen; heparin fragments, which provide less thrombin inhibition than the parent, unfractionated molecule; direct factor Xa inhibitors; and direct thrombin inhibitors (Box 27.5).

Direct Thrombin Inhibitors

New direct thrombin inhibitors are now available (Fig. 27.6). These include argatroban and bivalirudin. Argatroban, a derivative of L-arginine, is a relatively small molecule and functions as a univalent direct thrombin inhibitor. It binds at the active cleavage site of thrombin and stops thrombin's action on serine proteases. It is completely

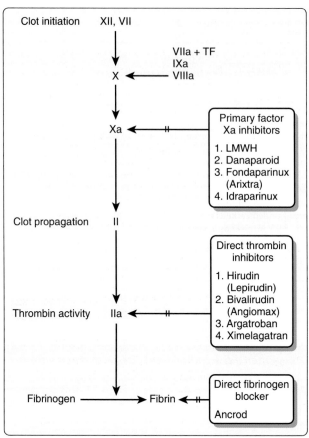

Fig. 27.6 Alternatives to heparin. New modes of anticoagulation are shown in the boxes on the right side of the figure where they inhibit either factor Xa, thrombin, or fibrinogen. *LMWH,* Low-molecular-weight heparin; *TF,* tissue factor.

hepatically cleared and has a reported half-life of 45 to 55 minutes with prolongation when liver function is depressed or liver blood flow is decreased. There is no reversal agent for argatroban, although factor VIIa has been given to increase thrombin generation. It has been approved by the US Food and Drug Administration (FDA) for anticoagulation in the face of HITT, but there has not been, to date, a large-scale, prospective, randomized trial for cardiac surgery or any type of comparison with heparin/protamine. Some case reports do exist of successful usage of argatroban in patients with HITT both on- and off-pump with acceptable amounts of postoperative bleeding.

Bivalirudin is a bivalent synthetic 20-amino acid peptide. Pharmacologists have taken the active amino acids at either end of the hirudin molecule and biosynthesized them. One active site competitively binds to the fibrinogen-binding site of thrombin; the other end of the molecule, the amino-terminal sequence, binds to the active serine cleavage site of thrombin. The two sequences of amino acids are connected together by a tetraglycine spacer. This fully manufactured molecule is highly specific for thrombin and has the unique property that it binds to both clot-bound and free thrombin. Heparin binds only to free plasma thrombin. Bivalirudin has a shorter half-life than argatroban; the $t_{1/2}$ is approximately 20 to 25 minutes (with normal renal function and not on CPB). One of the most unique features of bivalirudin is that its binding to thrombin is reversible and the molecule itself is cleaved by thrombin.

Bivalirudin also has no reversal agent analogous to protamine, so, when it is used, it must wear off. Bivalirudin undergoes destruction by the molecule to which it binds and deactivates, thrombin; it is destroyed by thrombin (proteolytic cleavage). The more thrombin activation that is present (ie, the less bivalirudin that is present), the shorter is the half-life. Only about 20% of the molecular activity is eliminated by renal clearance.

Several clinical trials of bivalirudin for cardiology procedures or cardiac surgery have been completed and published. Two pivotal trials aiming for FDA approval of bivalirudin for cardiac surgery with known/suspected HIT were conducted several years ago. In trials comparing bivalirudin with either heparin/protamine alone or heparin plus the use of a GP IIb/IIIa inhibitor for percutaneous interventions, bivalirudin was found to have at least equal or better safety and less bleeding than either of the other therapies. In a trial of 100 off-pump routine patients having CABG without suspected HIT, patients were randomized to receive either bivalirudin or heparin/protamine, and bleeding and outcome were equal between the groups. A phase I/II safety trial of bivalirudin in 30 on-pump patients having CABG has also shown good safety, but no comparison was conducted to look at advantages against heparin/protamine. When used, the doses for CPB have been a 0.50- to 0.75-mg/kg bolus followed by an infusion at 1.75 to 2.5 mg/kg/h titrated to the ACT (target, 2.5 times baseline). The CPB system also was primed with 50 mg, and no stasis can be allowed in the CPB circuit because of metabolism of bivalirudin during CPB. The infusion is stopped about 15 to 30 minutes before CPB is discontinued, and patients bleed for up to 4 to 6 hours. Off-pump coronary artery bypass (OPCAB) cases have used similar doses to ACT targets of 350 to 450 seconds. There certainly are some tricks to using bivalirudin for cardiac cases. The drug itself is broken down by thrombin, and thrombin is produced by CPB, as well as through tissue destruction. Any blood left alone without a continuous infusion of bivalirudin will, because of its generation of thrombin, overcome the anticoagulation of bivalirudin in time. Therefore it is expected that stagnant blood in the mediastinal or the chest cavities, or both, will clot. This is alarming to the first-time user of bivalirudin and completely different from what is seen in cases with heparin anticoagulation. Also, the use of mediastinal suction during bypass is not recommended because the mediastinum is a source of a great deal of thrombin activity. Suctioning that back into the CPB reservoir has led to clots being present in a hard-shell reservoir, wherein there is stasis or incomplete mixing of bivalirudin. Once the patient is separated from CPB, it is important to make a decision regarding whether the patient is likely to need to return to bypass. The bypass system, if left stagnant, will have ongoing production of thrombin. Over time, that thrombin will overcome the bivalirudin present in the plasma. Therefore within 10 minutes of separation from CPB, it is wise to decide to either drain the blood from the pump, process it through a cell-saver machine, or reestablish flow and have a slow infusion of bivalirudin into the pump. The reestablishment of flow can be easily accomplished by reattaching the ends of the venous and arterial cannulae. If it is necessary to reestablish CPB, the system should be maintained warm and either a bolus (25 to 50 mg) of bivalirudin should be put into the pump or the infusion that had been running to the patient should be switched to the pump. Furthermore, some surgeons have suggested that in areas of stasis, such as in an internal mammary artery, it is important to flush the artery every 10 to 15 minutes to allow for new bivalirudin to be perfused, or clot could build up in the "dead end" if it is clamped. The other option is not to completely clamp off the internal mammary artery until just before it is to be anastomosed.

27

There has been some confusion regarding how best to monitor anticoagulation with bivalirudin for cardiac surgery. The dose-responsiveness of bivalirudin is highly predictable. There is no secondary reaction necessary such as with AT III and UFH. Therefore, when bivalirudin is given, there is an absolute amount of AT available. The consensus is that ACT will work. The other reason for using an ACT is that, during CPB, if a drug pump malfunctions or the infusion is somehow disconnected, it is important to know that earlier rather than later. If the ACT begins to elevate to more than 500 seconds, then the team really does not know whether to back off on the bivalirudin infusion, stop it altogether, or attribute the effect to some other ACT-prolonging situation such as hemodilution or hypothermia. It is known that hypothermia retards the production of thrombin, but no studies have been done of bivalirudin half-lives in the face of mild-to-moderate hypothermia.

The two trials of bivalirudin in the face of known or suspected HIT antibodies did show effectiveness and safety. The CABG HIT On- and Off-Pump Safety and Efficacy (CHOOSE) study and the Evaluation of Patients During Coronary Artery Bypass Operation: Linking Utilization of Bivalirudin to Improved Outcomes and New Anticoagulant Strategies (EVOLUTION) trial were performed as parts of a program to get bivalirudin approved for patients undergoing cardiac surgery with known or suspected HIT. EVOLUTION (ON and OFF) trials randomized patients to receive either heparin-protamine or bivalirudin as the primary anticoagulant regimen for either on- or off-pump CABG surgery. There were no differences in death, MI, or need for repeat revascularization. However, there was a significant reduction in strokes seen with the use of bivalirudin. Bleeding was about the same with both groups. In the face of HITT syndrome, case reports continue to show effectiveness and utility of bivalirudin. This is an off-label use of the drug because it has not been FDA-approved.

New Oral Anticoagulants

The introduction of new oral anticoagulants (NOAC) that specifically target thrombin (factor IIa or FIIa) or factor Xa has increased the complexity of coagulation management in patients presenting for cardiac and noncardiac surgery. These NOACs or target-specific oral anticoagulants (TSOACs) include one FIIa inhibitor, dabigatran (Pradaxa), and three factor Xa inhibitors—rivaroxaban (Xarelto), apixaban (Eliquis), and edoxaban (Savaysa)—that are increasingly encountered in clinical practice. These drugs are prescribed in place of warfarin or LMWH for the prevention and treatment of thromboembolism in various clinical settings. Advantages for patients include shorter half-life, more favorable risk-benefit profile, and fixed daily dosing without the need for frequent laboratory tests because of more predictable pharmacokinetics (Table 27.3). Dabigatran has been found unsuitable for patients with artificial

Table 27.3 **New Oral Anticoagulants**				
	Dabigatran	Rivaroxaban	Apixaban	Edoxaban
Action	IIa Inhibitor	II Inhibitor	Xa Inhibitor	Xa Inhibitor
Administration	bid	daily	bid	daily
Peak plasma level	2 h	2–4 h	1–4 h	1–2 h
Half-life	12–14 h	11–13 h	8–15 h	9–11 h
Renal excretion	80%	35%	25%	50%
Protein binding	35%	90%	87%	—

valves in place, because it caused more bleeding and thromboembolic episodes than warfarin. Dabigatran has a half-life of 12 to 14 hours, whereas the factor Xa inhibitors' half-lives range from 5 to 15 hours. Dabigatran is 80% excreted by the kidneys, whereas the factor Xa inhibitors are protein-bound and metabolized by cytochrome P450s in the liver.

In the case of surgical bleeding, patients can be treated with the usual blood products. In addition, the prothrombin complex concentrates (PCCs) can be used, with or without FVIIa, to further improve coagulation in life-threatening situations. The four factor PCCs (eg, Kcentra) have been approved by the FDA for warfarin reversal and have had some positive results with the factor Xa inhibitors. The best ways to treat bleeding with dabigatran are to either prevent its absorption from the stomach with charcoal or to remove it from the blood with hemodialysis. Idarucizumab (Praxbind) is a fully humanized antibody fragment that has completely reversed dabigatran in clinical trials. It has been studied in more than 100 patients who are either bleeding or undergoing surgery in the RE-VERSE AD phase III trial. The thrombin time and coagulation time have been normalized very rapidly and sustained for 24 hours, whereas the plasma levels of dabigatran have been lowered significantly. Reversal agents are also being developed for the factor Xa inhibitors (eg, andexanet alfa, PER977), but these are at earlier stages of development.

PROTAMINE

Neutralization of heparin-induced anticoagulation remains the primary use of protamine. Formation of complexes with the sulfate groups of heparin forms the basis for this "antidote" effect. Protamine neutralizes the AT effect of heparin far better than its anti–factor Xa effect. This distinction may arise from the need for thrombin, but not factor Xa, to remain complexed to heparin for AT to exert its inhibitory effect. In the presence of circulating heparin, protamine forms large complexes with heparin. Excess protamine creates larger complexes. The reticuloendothelial system may then dispose of these particles by endocytosis. Macrophages in the lung may constitute the site for elimination of these complexes because intravenous administration of protamine permits formation of heparin-protamine complexes in the pulmonary circulation first.

The recommended dose of protamine to neutralize heparin varies widely. Box 27.6 lists factors accounting for this variability. The first factor is the proper ratio of protamine to heparin. Reports of the optimal ratio of milligrams of protamine to units of heparin cite values as low as zero (ie, they do not neutralize heparin) to as much as 4 mg/100 units. This variability has been accounted for by differences in

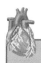

BOX 27.6   *Basis for Variability in Protamine Dose*

Ratio of protamine to heparin
Amount of heparin to neutralize
Heparin rebound
Protamine overdose

timing, temperature, and other environmental factors; choices for coagulation tests and outcome variables; and speculation and unproven assumptions. Second, the basis for calculating protamine dose, the total amount of heparin given or the amount remaining in the patient, must be determined. Protamine titration tests at the conclusion of CPB can determine the amount of heparin remaining in the patient. With automated versions of this test and simple assumptions regarding the volume of distribution of heparin, the amount needed to neutralize the heparin detected in the patient's vasculature can be calculated.

Adverse Reactions

The potential for a deleterious response to protamine administration raises serious questions and difficult choices in clinical care before, during, and after cardiac operations.

Slow administration of a neutralizing dose over 5 minutes or longer rarely will engender cardiovascular changes. Systemic hypotension from rapid injection in humans has been ascribed to pharmacologic displacement of histamine from mast cells by the highly alkaline protamine, similar to the mechanism by which curare, morphine, and alkaline antibiotics (eg, vancomycin and clindamycin) cause hypotension.

Some adverse responses to protamine are allergic reactions. The term *anaphylactoid reactions* includes not only severe immediate hypersensitivity allergy, termed *anaphylaxis*, but also other life-threatening idiosyncratic responses of nonimmunologic origin. The initial classification of protamine reactions split the anaphylactoid category (type II) into three subsets: anaphylaxis (IIA), nonimmunologic anaphylactoid reaction (IIB), and delayed noncardiogenic pulmonary edema (IIC).

■ BLEEDING PATIENT

After cardiac surgery, some patients bleed excessively (probably about 20%). Prompt diagnostic and therapeutic action will avoid impaired hemodynamics from hemorrhage, decreased oxygen-carrying capacity from anemia, and impaired hemostasis from depletion of endogenous hemostatic resources. Many factors govern whether a particular patient will experience excessive bleeding after cardiac surgery. Although many different criteria can define excessive bleeding, chest tube drainage of more than 10 mL/kg in the first hour after operation or a total of more than 20 mL/kg over the first 3 hours after operation for patients weighing more than 10 kg is considered significant. Also, any sudden increase of 300 mL/h or greater after minimal initial drainage in an adult usually indicates anatomic disruption warranting surgical intervention.

Insult of Cardiopulmonary Bypass

More so than patient factors, CPB itself acts to impair hemostasis. Bypass activates fibrinolysis, impairs platelets, and affects coagulation factors. Hypothermia, used in most centers during CPB, adversely affects hemostasis as well.

Synthetic Antifibrinolytics

Synthetic antifibrinolytics bind to plasminogen and plasmin, thus inhibiting binding of plasminogen at the lysine residues of fibrinogen. Antifibrinolytics may be administered intravenously and undergo renal concentration and excretion with a plasma half-life of about 80 minutes. Effective fibrinolysis inhibition requires an intravenous loading dose of 10 mg/kg for tranexamic acid (TA) followed by 1 mg/kg/h or 50 mg/kg of epsilon aminocaproic acid (EACA) followed by infusion of 25 mg/kg/h. Infusion rates require downward adjustment when serum creatinine concentration is increased.

Several investigations using prophylactic antifibrinolytics documented savings in blood loss, as well as in blood transfused in a general population of cardiac surgery patients. By commencing administration of TA before CPB, chest tube drainage in the first 12 hours after surgery decreased by 30%, and the likelihood of receiving banked blood within 5 days of operation decreased from 41% to 22%. Prophylactic antifibrinolytics may spare platelet function by inhibiting the deleterious effects of plasmin, but administration of very large doses of antifibrinolytics appears to offer no greater savings. Cardiac surgery patients undergoing repeat operation may benefit particularly from prophylactic antifibrinolytic administration.

Management of the Bleeding Patient

The initial approach to perioperative bleeding violates the medical paradigm of treatment based on diagnosis. The clinician must simultaneously initiate diagnostic tests, begin treating a presumed cause, and replace lost hemostatic resources.

Coagulation Products

The standard blood bank products available to the cardiovascular team include FFP, cryoprecipitate, and platelet concentrates (either pooled or apheresis single-donor platelets). These products should be used only if coagulation data from a laboratory point toward appropriate use or if a patient is bleeding severely enough that the team feels it necessary to attempt empiric therapy.

Platelet transfusions and FFP carry a higher risk of transfusion-related acute lung injury (TRALI) than do red blood cells from the blood bank. It is known that the causes of TRALI are manyfold and not limited to recipients receiving human leukocyte antigen (HLA) antibodies toward their pulmonary endothelium. Indeed, it has been shown that cytokines, red cell microparticles, and CD-40L (a platelet proinflammatory protein) all contribute to leaking pulmonary capillaries. The use of platelet concentrates makes a great deal of sense when a patient is bleeding and there is a proven or suspected platelet function or number deficit. Prophylactic platelet transfusions have never been shown to be of utility. Platelets are harvested by ultracentrifugation and stored in the blood bank at room temperature on a rocker that keeps them from aggregating. Platelet concentrates can be kept for only 5 days; therefore they are the blood product in shortest supply. Because they are kept at room temperature, they have the potential for growth of bacterial contamination. The risk of bacterial contamination is somewhere between 1/5000 and 20,000 units. Cryoprecipitate is a product that contains a very high concentration of fibrinogen and factor VIII. The product is manufactured from harvested plasma and represents the total available soluble fibrinogen in 1 unit of banked blood/plasma. That precipitate is packaged in approximately 15 mL of plasma. Unlike FFP, cryoprecipitate has a very low volume for the concentration of protein it delivers. Most often when used in cardiac surgery, a dose of cryo is from 10 donors representing the fibrinogen of 10 units of whole blood (roughly one circulating volume). Therefore if a patient is bleeding because of a low fibrinogen concentration or a dysfibrinogenemia, a single infusion of 10 units of cryo should restore the levels above 2 g/L. Cryo represents the exposure of 10 donors and still may carry viruses not tested for, such as Epstein-Barr virus and transfusion transmitted virus, both of which can cause hepatic failure in immuno-compromised hosts.

Table 27.4 lists a treatment plan for excessive bleeding after cardiac surgery. Interventions appear not in order of likelihood, but rather by priority of consideration.

Table 27.4   Treatment Plan for Excessive Bleeding After Cardiac Surgery

Action	Amount	Indication
Rule out surgical cause	—	No oozing at puncture sites; chest radiograph
More protamine	0.5–1 mg/kg	ACT >150 seconds or aPTT >1.5 times control
Warm the patient	—	"Core" temperature <35°C
Apply PEEP[a]	5–10 cm H_2O	—
Desmopressin	0.3 µg/kg IV	Prolonged bleeding time
Aminocaproic acid	50 mg/kg, then 25 mg/kg/h	Increased D-dimer or teardrop-shaped TEG tracing
Tranexamic acid	10 mg/kg, then 1 mg/kg/h	Increased D-dimer or teardrop-shaped TEG tracing
Platelet transfusion	1 U/10 kg	Platelet count <100,000/mm^3
Fresh-frozen plasma	15 mL/kg	PT or aPTT >1.5 times control
Cryoprecipitate	1 U/4 kg	Fibrinogen <1 g/L or 100 mg/dL
Fibrinogen	2 g	Fibrinogen <100 mg/dL

ACT, Activated coagulation time; *aPTT*, activated partial thromboplastin time; *IV*, intravenous; *TEG*, thromboelastograph.
[a]Positive end-expiratory pressure (PEEP) is contraindicated in hypovolemia.

Thus, surgical causes should be ruled out before seizing on the diagnosis of a consumptive coagulopathy. The priority will also vary among institutions, depending on the availability and cost of resources. This table provides a simple algorithm for treating postoperative bleeding.

REPLACEMENT THERAPY

Factor VIIa

Recombinant factor VIIa (rFVIIa, NovoSeven, Novo Nordisk, Bagsværd, Denmark) is approved for the treatment of bleeding in patients with hemophilia A or B with inhibitors against factors VIII and IX. Factor VII acts locally at the site of vessel injury by binding to tissue factor on subendothelial cells and facilitates transformation of factors IX and X to active forms, ultimately resulting in a thrombin burst and clot formation.

Off-label use of rFVIIa has been reported as a rescue therapy for patients with hemorrhage refractory to conventional therapy. However, the safety of rFVIIa in the cardiac surgical setting has not been clarified. Safety concerns are related to the risk for thrombosis, and reports of thrombotic events have tempered consideration for use in patients beyond rescue therapy, such as prophylactically in patients at high risk for bleeding to avoid blood transfusion.

Since the early 2000s, there have been numerous case reports and case series on the use of rFVIIa in cardiac surgery. Most suggest that rFVIIa is effective in reducing bleeding and decreasing red blood cell and component therapy requirements in the setting of refractory bleeding. Several, however, have reported increased complication rates associated with rFVIIa use.

Prevailing evidence suggests that rFVIIa is effective in refractory bleeding after cardiac surgery but that it does increase the risk of thromboembolic events. This has generated a dichotomy in approach. Although some think that its use should be limited to clinical studies, others maintain that it is appropriate to consider its use in the setting of life-threatening, refractory bleeding.

Fibrinogen Concentrates

Human fibrinogen concentrates have been used for substitution therapy in cases of hypofibrinogenemia, dysfibrinogenemia, and afibrinogenemia. Accumulating data suggest that fibrinogen, which is both the precursor of fibrin and a cofactor in platelet aggregation, plays a critical role in hemostasis, especially in bleeding patients with an acquired fibrinogen deficiency. Clinical use of fibrinogen concentrates is based on the supposition that plasma fibrinogen concentrations may become critically reduced somewhat early in a bleeding patient and that this may contribute to the coagulopathy associated with hemorrhage. A functional fibrinogen deficiency may develop with excessive hemodilution.

Normal plasma fibrinogen levels vary from 1.5 to 4.5 g/L and the minimum or critical fibrinogen level that is needed for proper clot formation in bleeding patients is unknown. The traditional critical level for fibrinogen replacement is 0.8 to 1.0 g/L, but several studies have found that clot formation and strength are impaired and that blood loss and transfusion rates are increased when fibrinogen levels are substantially higher than 1.0 g/L. Later guidelines recommend that the critical level should be increased to between 1.5 and 2.0 g/L.

Correction of fibrinogen deficits can be accomplished with administration of FFP, cryoprecipitate, and plasma-derived fibrinogen concentrates. Benefits of fibrinogen concentrates over FFP and cryoprecipitate include viral inactivation, rapid reconstitution, accurate dosing, and a lower volume of administration for equivalent fibrinogen supplementation.

Prothrombin Complex Concentrates

PCCs are virally inactivated, lyophilized products that are prepared from pooled plasma and primarily contain the vitamin K–dependent coagulation factors II, VII, IX, and X (Table 27.5). Other components include coagulation inhibitors proteins C and S, heparin, and AT. After reconstitution with small amounts of water, PCCs can be administered rapidly without the need for thawing or blood group matching.

Four-factor PCCs are approved for rapid reversal of oral vitamin K antagonists in patients requiring emergency surgery or invasive procedures. Recommended dosage is based on factor IX content, ranging from 25 to 50 IU of factor IX per 1 kg of body weight, depending on the patient's international normalized ratio (INR) (eg, 25 IU/kg for INR 2.0–3.9; 50 IU/kg for INR 4.0–5.9; 50 IU/kg for INR >5.9).

Three-factor PCCs contain low levels of factor VII, and activated PCCs such as FEIBA, a factor VIII inhibitor bypassing agent, contain trace amounts of activated factor VII and X. These products are primarily indicated for the prevention and treatment of hemophilia-related bleeding. There may be a role for PCCs in the management of surgical coagulopathy instead of FFP outside of vitamin K antagonist reversal; however, data on safety and efficacy are limited.

Table 27.5 Constituents of Commercially Available Prothrombin Complex Concentrates[a]

Product (Manufacturer), International Availability	Factor Content[b]								Antithrombotic Content				
	II		VII		IX		X		Protein C			ATIII	Heparin
	Label (U/mL)	Ratio (%)	Label (U/mL)	Ratio (%)	Label (U/mL)	Ratio (%)	Label (U/mL)	Ratio (%)	C Label (U/mL)	S Label (U/mL)	Z Label (U/mL)	Label (U/mL)	Label (U/mL)
Beriplex P/N (CSL Behring); major western European countries	20–48	133	10–25	69	20–31	100	22–60	161	15–45	13–26	Not in label	0.2–1.5	0.4–2.0
Octaplex (Octapharma); major western European countries	11–38	98	9–24	66	25	100	18–30	96	7–31	7–32	Not in label	Not in label	Not in label
Prothromplex Total/S-TIM 4 Immuno (Baxter); Sweden, Germany, Austria	30	100	25	83	30	100	30	100	20	Not in label	Not in label	0.75–1.5	15
Prothromplex TIM 3 (Baxter); Italy, Austria	25	100	Not in label	—	25	100	25	100	Not in label	Not in label	Not in label	Not in label	3.75
Cofact/PPSB SD (Sanquin/CAF); Netherlands, Belgium, Austria, Germany	15	75	5	25	20	100	15	75	Not in label	Not in label	Not in label	Present, not quantified	Not in label

V

Table 27.5 Constituents of Commercially Available Prothrombin Complex Concentrates—cont'd

Product (Manufacturer), International Availability	Factor Content[b]								Antithrombotic Content				
	II		VII		IX		X		Protein C			ATIII	Heparin
	Label (U/mL)	Ratio (%)	Label (U/mL)	Ratio (%)	Label (U/mL)	Ratio (%)	Label (U/mL)	Ratio (%)	C Label (U/mL)	S Label (U/mL)	Z Label (U/mL)	Label (U/mL)	Label (U/mL)
Kaskadil (LFB); France	40	160	25	100	25	100	40	160	Not in label	Not in label	Not in label	Not in label	Present, not quantified
Uman Complex D.I. (Kedrion); Italy	25	100	Not in label	0	25	100	20	80	Not in label	Not in label	Not in label	Present, not quantified	Present, not quantified
PPSB-human SD/Nano (Octapharma); Germany	25–55	130	7.5–20	45	24–37.5	100	25–55	130	20–50	5–25	Not in label	0.5–3	0.5–6
Profilnine (Grifols); United States	Present	150	Present	35	Present	100	Present	100	Not in label	Not in label	Not in label	Not in label	Not present
Bebulin (Baxter); United States	Present	—	Present (low)	—	Present	100	Present	—	Not in label	Not in label	Not in label	Not in label	0.15 U per U of factor IX
FEIBA (Baxter); USA	Present, not quantified (nonactivated)	Present, not quantified (activated)	500, 1000, or 2500 U per vial (nonactivated)	Present, not quantified (nonactivated)	—	Not in label	Not in label	Not in label	Not in label	Not present	—	—	—

[a]Information is based on product labeling. In Europe, ranges are usually given on the product label in accordance with the European Pharmacopoeia; single values usually are from older, national registrations.

[b]Factor content ratios are based on the content of factor IX.

AT/II, Antithrombin III.

From Levy JH, Tanaka KA, Dietrich W. Perioperative hemostatic management of patients treated with vitamin K antagonists. Anesthesiology. 2008;109:918–926.

SUGGESTED READINGS

Bhatt DL, Stone GW, Mahaffey KW, et al. Effect of platelet inhibition with cangrelor during percutaneous coronary interventions on ischemic events. *N Engl J Med*. 2013;368:1303.

Clifford L, Qing J, Subramanien A, et al. Characterizing the epidemiology of post operative transfusion-related acute lung injury. *Anesthesiology*. 2015;122:12–20.

Fassl J, Lurati Buse G, Filipovic M, et al. Perioperative administration of fibrinogen does not increase adverse cardiac and thromboembolic events after cardiac surgery. *Br J Anaesth*. 2015;114:225–234.

Greinacher A. Heparin-induced thrombocytopenia. *N Engl J Med*. 2015;373:252.

Hastings S, Myles P, McIlroy D. Aspirin and coronary artery surgery: a systematic review and meta-analysis. *Br J Anaesth*. 2015;115:376–385.

Karkouti K, Callum J, Crowther MA, et al. The relationship between fibrinogen levels after cardiopulmonary bypass and large volume red cell transfusion in cardiac surgery: an observational study. *Anesth Analg*. 2013;117:14–22.

Karkouti K, McCluskey SA, Callum J, et al. Evaluation of a novel transfusion algorithm employing point-of-care coagulation assays in cardiac surgery: a retrospective cohort study with interrupted time-series analysis. *Anesthesiology*. 2015;122:560–570.

Koster A, Spiess BD, Chew DP, et al. Effectiveness of bivalirudin as a replacement for heparin during cardiopulmonary bypass in patients undergoing coronary artery bypass grafting. *Am J Cardiol*. 2004;93:356.

Levy JH. Heparin resistance and antithrombin: should it still be called heparin resistance? *J Cardiothorac Vasc Anesth*. 2004;18:129.

Levy JH, Welsby I, Goodnough LT. Fibrinogen as a therapeutic target for bleeding: a review of critical levels and replacement therapy. *Transfusion*. 2014;54:1389–1405.

Mangano DT, Tudor JC, Dietzel C, et al; Multicenter Study of Perioperative Research Group of the Ischemic Research Foundation. The risk associated with aprotinin in cardiac surgery. *N Engl J Med*. 2006;254:353–365.

Meester ML, Vonk ABA, van der Weerdt EK, et al. Level of agreement between laboratory and point-of-care prothrombin time before and after cardiopulmonary bypass in cardiac surgery. *Thromb Res*. 2014;133:1141–1144.

Merry AF, Raudkivi P, White HD, et al. Anticoagulation with bivalirudin (a direct thrombin inhibitor) vs heparin. A randomized trial in OPCAB graft surgery. *Ann Thorac Surg*. 2004;77:925.

Murkin JM, Falter F, Granton J, et al. High dose tranexamic acid is associated with nonischemic clinical seizures in cardiac surgical patients. *Anesth Analg*. 2010;110:350–353.

Siegal DM. Managing target-specific oral anticoagulant-associated bleeding including an update on pharmacological reversal agents. *J Thromb Thrombolysis*. 2015;39:395–402.

Society of Thoracic Surgeons Guideline Task Force, Ferraris VA, Brown J, et al. 2011 update to the Society of Thoracic Surgeons and Society of Cardiovascular Anesthesiologists Blood Conservation Clinical Practice Guidelines. *Ann Thorac Surg*. 2011;91:944–982.

Tanaka KA, Mazzeffi M, Durila M. Role of prothrombin complex concentrate in perioperative coagulation therapy. *J Intensive Care*. 2014;2:60.

Welsby I, Newman M, Phillips-Bute B, et al. Hemodynamic changes after protamine administration. *Anesthesiology*. 2005;102:308.

Zatta A, Mcquilten Z, Kandane-Rathnayake R, et al. The Australian and New Zealand Haemostasis Registry: ten years of data on off-licence use of recombinant activated factor VII. *Blood Transfus*. 2015;13:86–99.

V

Chapter 28

Discontinuing Cardiopulmonary Bypass

Liem Nguyen, MD • David M. Roth, MD, PhD •
Jack S. Shanewise, MD • Joel A. Kaplan, MD, CPE, FACC

Key Points

1. The key to successful weaning from cardiopulmonary bypass (CPB) is proper preparation.
2. After rewarming the patient, correcting any abnormal blood gases, and inflating the lungs, make sure to turn on the ventilator.
3. To prepare the heart for discontinuing CPB, optimize the cardiac rate, rhythm, preload, myocardial contractility, and afterload.
4. The worse the heart's condition, the more gradually CPB should be weaned. If hemodynamic values are not adequate, immediately return to CPB. Assess the problem, and choose an appropriate pharmacologic, surgical, or mechanical intervention before trying to terminate CPB again.
5. Perioperative ventricular dysfunction usually is caused by myocardial stunning and is a temporary state of contractile dysfunction that should respond to positive inotropic drugs.
6. In addition to left ventricular dysfunction, right ventricular failure is a possible source of morbidity and mortality after cardiac surgical procedures.
7. The presence of diastolic dysfunction during the postbypass period may contribute to impaired chamber relaxation and poor compliance, resulting in reduced ventricular filling during separation.
8. Epinephrine is frequently chosen as an inotropic drug when terminating CPB because of its mixed α- and β-adrenergic stimulation.
9. Milrinone is an excellent inodilator drug that can be used alone or combined with other drugs such as epinephrine for discontinuing CPB in patients with poor ventricular function and diastolic dysfunction.
10. In patients with high preload and/or elevated systemic vascular resistance, vasodilators such as nitroglycerin, nicardipine, clevidipine, or nitroprusside may improve ventricular function.
11. Intraaortic balloon pump counterpulsation increases coronary blood flow during diastole and unloads the left ventricle during systole. These effects can help in weaning patients with poor left ventricular function and severe myocardial ischemia.

Cardiopulmonary bypass (CPB) has been used since the 1950s to facilitate surgical procedures of the heart and great vessels, and is a critical part of most cardiac operations. Managing patients undergoing CPB remains one of the defining characteristics of cardiac surgery and cardiac anesthesiology. Discontinuing CPB is a necessary part of every operation involving extracorporeal circulation. Through this process, the support of the circulation by the bypass pump and oxygenator is transferred back to the patient's heart and lungs. This chapter reviews important considerations for discontinuing CPB and presents an approach to managing this critical component of a cardiac operation, which may be routine and easy or extremely complex and difficult. The key to success in discontinuing CPB is proper preparation. The period during and immediately after weaning from CPB usually is busy for the anesthesiologist, and having to do tasks that could have been accomplished earlier in the operation is not helpful. The preparations for removing a patient from CPB may be organized into several parts: general preparations, preparing the lungs, preparing the heart, and final preparations.

GENERAL PREPARATIONS

Temperature

Because at least moderate hypothermia is used during CPB in most cardiac surgical cases, it is important that the patient is sufficiently rewarmed before attempts are made to wean the patient from CPB (Table 28.1). Initiation of rewarming is a good time to consider whether additional drugs must be given to keep the patient anesthetized and to prevent shivering. Monitoring the temperature of a highly perfused tissue such as the nasopharynx is useful to help prevent overheating of the brain during rewarming. Cerebral hyperthermia may lead to neurologic injury and postoperative cognitive dysfunction. The central nervous system receives a greater proportion of warm blood, thus resulting in a more rapid increase in temperature compared with other sites such as the bladder, rectum, or axilla. This situation may lead to inadequate rewarming and temperature dropoff after CPB as the heat continues to distribute throughout the body. Different institutions have various protocols for rewarming, but the important point is to warm gradually, avoiding hyperthermia of the central nervous system while providing enough heat to the patient to prevent significant dropoff after CPB. After CPB, the tendency is for the patient to lose heat, and measures to keep the patient warm (eg, fluid warmers, a circuit heater-humidifier, and forced-air warmers) should be set up and turned on before weaning from CPB is begun. The temperature of the operating room may need to be increased as well; this is probably an effective measure to keep a patient warm after CPB, but it may make the scrubbed and gowned personnel uncomfortable.

V

Table 28.1	General Preparations for Discontinuing Cardiopulmonary Bypass	
Temperature	**Laboratory Results**
Adequately rewarm before weaning from CPB	Correct metabolic acidosis
Avoid overheating the brain	Optimize hematocrit
Start measures to keep patient warm after CPB	Normalize potassium
Use fluid warmer, forced-air warmer	Consider giving magnesium or checking magnesium level
Warm operating room	Check calcium level and correct deficiencies

CPB, Cardiopulmonary bypass.

Laboratory Results

Arterial blood gases should be measured before the patient is weaned from CPB, and any abnormalities should be corrected. Severe metabolic acidosis depresses the myocardium and necessitates correction before separation from bypass. The optimal hematocrit for weaning from CPB is controversial and probably varies from patient to patient. It makes sense that sicker patients with lower cardiovascular reserve may benefit from a higher hematocrit (optimal is considered to be 30%), but the risks and adverse consequences of transfusion must be considered as well. The hematocrit should be measured and optimized before the patient is weaned from CPB. The serum potassium (K^+) level should be measured before weaning from CPB and may be high because of cardioplegia or low, especially in patients receiving loop diuretics. Hyperkalemia may make establishing an effective cardiac rhythm difficult and can be treated with sodium bicarbonate ($NaHCO_3$), calcium chloride ($CaCl_2$), or insulin, but the levels usually decrease quickly after cardioplegia has been stopped. Low serum K^+ levels should be corrected before CPB is discontinued, especially if arrhythmias are present. Administration of magnesium (Mg^{2+}) to patients on CPB decreases postoperative arrhythmias and may improve cardiac function, and many centers routinely give all CPB-treated patients magnesium sulfate. Theoretic disadvantages include aggravation of vasodilation and inhibition of platelet function. If Mg^{2+} is not given routinely, the level should be checked before weaning from CPB, and deficiencies should be corrected. The ionized calcium (Ca^{2+}) level should be measured, and significant deficiencies should be corrected before discontinuing CPB. Many centers give all patients a bolus of $CaCl_2$ just before coming off CPB because it transiently increases contractility and systemic vascular resistance (SVR). However, investigators have argued that this practice is to be avoided because Ca^{2+} may interfere with catecholamine action and aggravate reperfusion injury.

PREPARING THE LUNGS

As the patient is weaned from CPB and the heart starts to support the circulation, the lungs again become the site of gas exchange, by delivering oxygen and eliminating carbon dioxide. Before weaning from CPB, the patient's lung function must be restored (Box 28.1). The lungs are reinflated by hand gently and gradually, with sighs using up to 30 cm H_2O pressure, and then mechanically ventilated with 100% oxygen. Care should be taken not to allow the lungs to injure an in situ internal mammary artery

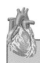

BOX 28.1 *Preparing the Lungs for Discontinuing Cardiopulmonary Bypass*

Suction trachea and endotracheal tube
Inflate lungs gently by hand
Ventilate with 100% oxygen
Treat bronchospasm with bronchodilators
Check for pneumothorax and pleural fluid
Consider the need for positive end-expiratory pressure, intensive care unit ventilator, and nitric oxide

graft as they are reinflated. The compliance of the lungs can be judged by their feel with hand ventilation; stiff lungs suggest more difficulty with oxygenation or ventilation after CPB. If visible, both lungs should be inspected for residual atelectasis, and they should be rising and falling with each breath. Ventilation alarms and monitors should be activated. If prolonged expiration or wheezing is detected, bronchodilators should be given. The surgeon should inspect both pleural spaces for pneumothorax, which should be treated by opening the pleural space. Examining the lung fields by trans-esophageal echocardiography (TEE) may assist in the detection of pleural effusions. Any fluid present in the pleural spaces should be removed before attempting to wean the patient from CPB.

The apneic period during CPB has been suggested to contribute to ventilator-associated pneumonia and postoperative pulmonary dysfunction through a variety of mechanisms. Continuing mechanical ventilation during CPB has been proposed as another option to attenuate the post-CPB impairment of lung function. Results of several small trials that used continued ventilation during CPB were mixed, with some trials showing benefit and others showing no outcome difference. At present, the evidence for intraoperative lung protection strategies such as continued ventilation is lacking and awaits larger randomized trials.

PREPARING THE HEART

Management of Intracardiac Air

During the bypass period, the heart is empty, cooled, and usually electrically silent to minimize consumption of adenosine triphosphate (ATP). Air is often introduced into the heart during the operation and can eventually cause deleterious effects during separation from CPB and in the postoperative period. TEE can be helpful in identifying and locating air in the heart and assisting in de-airing before CPB is discontinued. On TEE, air is often seen as echo-dense or bright foci floating to the highest point within the chamber.

The time to begin looking with TEE for intracardiac air on CPB is usually after all the chambers and the aorta are closed and the aortic cross-clamp is removed. It is essential to identify macroscopic accumulations of air within the left side of the heart to minimize systemic emboli. With the patient in the supine position, air often is visualized in the left atrium along the interatrial septum, left atrial (LA) appendage, and near the entry points of the pulmonary veins. In the left ventricle and aortic root, air often accumulates along the apical portion of the interventricular septum and right coronary sinus of Valsalva. As the heart ejects, close inspection of the left ventricular (LV) outflow tract (LVOT) and aortic root at this image plane may facilitate visualization of air emboli, mandating aggressive aspiration of the aortic root vent.

Although a correlation with the amount of intracardiac air seen with TEE and neurologic outcome has not been shown, one of the major concerns with systemic air emboli after CPB is the potential for cerebral injury. It is reasonable to proceed with the assumption that the less air pumped into the systemic circulation during and after CPB, the better. Another adverse consequence is the passage of air into the coronary circulation that leads to myocardial ischemia. In the supine patient, the right coronary artery takes off from the highest point of the aortic root, and intra-coronary air is most commonly manifested by dramatic inferior ST-segment elevation and acute right-sided heart dysfunction. Saphenous vein grafts typically are anastomosed to the anterior aspect of the ascending aorta and are susceptible to air emboli as well.

If this occurs while the patient is still on CPB or before decannulation, it is a simple matter to go back on CPB and wait a few minutes until the air clears from the coronary circulation, the ST segments normalize, and ventricular function improves before trying to wean the patient from CPB again. If, however, coronary air embolization occurs after decannulation, the hemodynamic status can quickly deteriorate to cardiac arrest. Smaller air emboli can be moved through the coronary vessels by acutely increasing the blood pressure with a vasopressor while dilating the coronary arteries with nitroglycerin (NTG). Perhaps the worst-case scenario is when a macroscopic air bubble in the left side of the heart is shaken loose while moving the patient from the operating table at the end of the case; acute right-sided heart failure (HF) and circulatory collapse may occur either then or while the patient is being transported to the intensive care unit.

Numerous maneuvers may be used to de-air the chambers. They may include shaking the vented heart on partial CPB to jar loose any pockets of air, elevating and aspirating LV air directly from the apex, applying positive pressure to the lungs to squeeze air out of the pulmonary veins, and tipping the table from side to side to help the passage of bubbles through the heart to the ascending aorta where they are released through a vent. Additional air may appear in the left side of the heart during weaning from CPB as increasing flow through the pulmonary veins flushes air out from the lungs into the left atrium. Passage of air from the left atrium to the left ventricle may be facilitated with the head and right-side-down position, as well as from the left ventricle to the ascending aorta with the head and right-side up. It may be impossible to evacuate every last trace of air from the left side of the heart before discontinuing CPB, especially tiny bubbles trapped in the trabeculae of the left ventricle; it therefore becomes a matter of judgment and experience to know when enough is enough. The persistence of a macroscopic air-fluid level in the left side of the heart visible with TEE, however, suggests that more de-airing probably is needed before closing the vent in the ascending aorta and weaning from CPB. After adequate de-airing, preparing the heart to resume its function of pumping blood involves optimizing the determinants of cardiac output (CO). The five hemodynamic parameters that can be controlled are rate, rhythm, preload, contractility, and afterload (Table 28.2).

Heart Rate

Establishing an effective heart rate (HR) is a critical prerequisite and major determinant of CO. In most situations for adult patients, the HR should be between 75 and 95 beats/minute for weaning from CPB. It may be prudent to establish electrical pacing early in the weaning process to ensure a means to control the HR precisely. Lower rates theoretically may be desirable for hearts with residual ischemia or incomplete revascularization. Higher HRs may be needed for hearts with limited stroke volume (SV) such as after ventricular aneurysmectomy. Slow HRs are best treated with electrical pacing, but β-agonist or vagolytic drugs also may be used to increase the HR. Tachycardia before weaning from CPB is more worrisome and difficult to manage, and treatable causes such as inadequate anesthesia, hypercarbia, and ischemia should be identified and corrected. The HR often decreases as the heart is filled in the weaning process, and electrical pacing always should be immediately available during cardiac operations to treat sudden bradycardias. Supraventricular tachycardias should be electrically cardioverted if possible, but drugs such as β-antagonists or Ca^{2+} channel antagonists may be needed to control the ventricular rate if these arrhythmias persist, most typically in patients with chronic atrial fibrillation. If drug therapy decreases the HR too much, pacing may be used.

28

Table 28.2 Preparing the Heart for Discontinuing Cardiopulmonary Bypass

Hemodynamic Parameters	Preparation
Heart rate	Rate should be between 75 and 95 beats/min in most cases
	Treat slow rates with electrical pacing
	Treat underlying causes of fast heart rates
	Heart rate may decrease as the heart fills
	Control fast supraventricular rates with drugs, and then pace as needed
	Always have pacing immediately available during heart operations
Rhythm	Normal sinus rhythm is ideal
	Defibrillate if necessary when temperature >30°C
	Consider antiarrhythmic drugs if ventricular fibrillation persists more than a few minutes
	Try synchronized cardioversion for atrial fibrillation or flutter
	Look at the heart to diagnose atrial rhythm
	Try atrial pacing if atrioventricular conduction exists
	Try atrioventricular pacing for heart block
Preload	End-diastolic volume is the best measure of preload and can be seen with TEE
	Filling pressures provide a less direct measure of preload
	Consider baseline filling pressures
	Assess RV volume with direct inspection
	Assess LV volume with TEE
	Cardiac distension may cause MR and TR
Contractility	Carefully examine heart for air and employ de-airing maneuvers
	Assess and quantify RV function with direct inspection and TEE
	Assess and quantify LV function with TEE
	Inspect for new regional wall motion abnormalities
	Inspect for new or worsening valvular abnormalities
	Quantify cardiac output by TEE or PAC
	Assess need for inotropic agent
Afterload	Systemic vascular resistance is a major component of afterload
	Keep MAP between 60 and 80 mm Hg at full CPB flow
	Consider a vasoconstrictor if the MAP is low and a vasodilator if the MAP is high

CPB, Cardiopulmonary bypass; *LV*, left ventricular; *MAP*, mean arterial pressure; *MR*, mitral regurgitation; *PAC*, pulmonary artery catheter; *RV*, right ventricular; *TEE*, transesophageal echocardiography; *TR*, tricuspid regurgitation.

Rhythm

The patient must have an organized, effective, and stable cardiac rhythm before attempts are made to wean the patient from CPB. This rhythm can occur spontaneously after removal of the aortic cross-clamp, but the heart may resume electrical activity with ventricular fibrillation. If the blood temperature is greater than 30°C, the heart may be defibrillated with internal paddles applied directly to the heart by using 10 to 20 J. Defibrillation at lower temperatures may be unsuccessful because extreme hypothermia can cause ventricular fibrillation. If ventricular fibrillation persists or recurs repeatedly, antiarrhythmic drugs such as lidocaine, amiodarone, or Mg^{2+} may be administered to help achieve a stable rhythm. It is not unusual for the rhythm to remain unstable for several minutes immediately after cross-clamp removal, but persistent or recurrent ventricular fibrillation should prompt concern about impaired coronary blood flow. Because it provides an atrial contribution to ventricular filling and a normal, synchronized contraction of the ventricles, normal sinus rhythm is the ideal cardiac rhythm for weaning from CPB. Atrial flutter or fibrillation, even if present before CPB, often can be converted to normal sinus rhythm with synchronized cardioversion, especially if antiarrhythmic drugs are administered. It often is helpful to look directly at the heart when any question exists about the cardiac rhythm. Atrial contraction, flutter, and fibrillation are easily seen on CPB when the heart is visible. Ventricular arrhythmias should be treated by correcting underlying causes such as K^+ or Mg^{2+} deficits and, if necessary, by administering antiarrhythmic drugs such as amiodarone. If asystole or complete heart block occurs after cross-clamp removal, electrical pacing with temporary epicardial pacing wires may be needed to achieve an effective rhythm before weaning from CPB. If atrioventricular conduction is present, atrial pacing should be attempted because, as with normal sinus rhythm, it provides atrial augmentation to filling and synchronized ventricular contraction. Atrioventricular sequential pacing is used in patients with heart block, which may be temporarily present for 30 to 60 minutes as the myocardium recovers after cardioplegia and cross-clamp removal. Ventricular pacing remains the only option if no organized atrial rhythm is present, but this sacrifices the atrial "kick" to ventricular filling and the more efficient synchronized ventricular contraction of the normal conduction system (see Table 28.2).

Preload

Once control of the rate and rhythm is established, priming the heart with volume or preload is the next step. Preload is the amount of stretch on the myocardial muscle fibers just before contraction. In the intact heart, the best measure of preload is end-diastolic volume. Less direct clinical measures of preload include LA pressure (LAP), pulmonary artery occlusion pressure, and pulmonary artery diastolic pressure, but the relationship between end-diastolic pressure and volume during cardiac surgical procedures may be poor. TEE is a useful tool for weaning from CPB because it provides direct visualization of the end-diastolic volume and contractility of the left ventricle. TEE may also provide a means to calculate serial CO measurements during volume loading of the heart. In addition, diastolic filling indices (transmitral and pulmonary venous inflow) may assist in assessing fluid responsiveness and elevations in LA and LV filling pressures. The process of weaning a patient from CPB involves increasing the preload (ie, filling the heart from its empty state on CPB) until an appropriate end-diastolic volume is achieved. When preparing to discontinue CPB, some thought should be given to the appropriate range of preload for the individual patient. The filling pressures before CPB may indicate what they need to be after CPB; a heart with high filling pressures before CPB may require high filling pressures after CPB to achieve an adequate preload.

Contractility

The contractile state of both the right and left sides of the heart should be considered individually before attempting to wean from CPB. The decision to institute inotropic support after CPB is complex, and intraoperative use of inotropes may be associated with higher mortality rates. Some of the factors associated with the low CO syndrome (LCOS) or the need for inotropic support after CPB include preexisting right ventricular (RV) or LV dysfunction, diastolic dysfunction, elevated LV end-diastolic pressure (LVEDP), advanced age, prolonged CPB time, and long aortic cross-clamp time (Table 28.3). Assessment of the right ventricle may be easily attainable because the

28

Table 28.3 Summary of Factors Associated With the Use of Inotropic Drug Support or Low Cardiac Output Syndrome

Variable	Odds Ratio
Age (>60 y)	4.3
Aortic cross-clamp time >90 min	2.32
Bypass time (min)	3.40
CABG + MVR	3.607
Cardiac index <2.5 L/m^2 per min	3.10
CHF (NYHA class >II)	1.85
CKD (stage 3–5; GFR <60 mL/1.73 m^2 per min	3.26
COPD	1.85
Diastolic dysfunction	4.31
Ejection fraction (%) <40	2.76
Emergency operation	9.15
Female sex	2.0
LVEDP >20 mm Hg	3.58
Myocardial infarction	2.01
Moderate-to-severe mitral regurgitation	2.277
Regional wall motion abnormality	4.21
Repeat operation	2.38

CABG, Coronary artery bypass graft; *CHF,* congestive heart failure; *CKD,* chronic kidney disease; *COPD,* chronic obstructive pulmonary disease; *GFR,* glomerular filtration rate; *LVEDP,* left ventricular end-diastolic pressure; *MVR,* mitral valve repair or replacement; *NYHA,* New York Heart Association.

right-sided chambers are directly visible to the anesthesiologist. Direct visualization of the left ventricle is difficult, and TEE may be the only modality by which to visualize left-sided heart function directly. Both right-sided and left-sided heart function and the corresponding atrioventricular valves should be systematically examined by TEE. The use of TEE during gradual weaning from the pump may provide essential information on chamber filling and the contractile state.

If evidence of poor contractility is visualized on TEE, initiation or titration of inotropic agents can begin at this time. As the pump flow is gradually reduced, the ability of the heart to fill and eject is continuously assessed, and drug therapy is titrated as needed. Once the heart has demonstrated the ability to maintain adequate hemodynamic status, separation from CPB is commenced. At this point, serial volume transfusions from the venous reservoir can be carefully titrated as needed, and the heart's response to volume can be monitored by TEE. After each volume bolus, assessments of biventricular function and the end-diastolic and end-systolic areas of the right and left ventricles are critical to prevent overdistension and unwanted wall tension. Reinstitution of CPB is warranted if the heart begins to distend or displays inadequate function.

Because the use of intraoperative and postoperative inotropic support may be associated with increased mortality rates, the decision to initiate pharmacologic therapy should be made with caution. A prudent approach, using a slow and gradual weaning process from the pump and assessing cardiac filling and biventricular contractility in a stepwise manner, may help reduce unnecessary use of inotropic agents. As the heart is allowed to fill gradually, if significant chamber distension or depression of contractility is evident on TEE or by direct visual inspection, the safest approach is to prevent cardiac distension by resuming CPB. At this point, the heart may benefit from a resting period of 10 to 20 minutes on CPB, and then the decision to start inotropes may be warranted before the patient is weaned from CPB.

Extreme depression of contractile function of the myocardium despite adequate pharmacologic therapy may require mechanical support with an intraaortic balloon pump (IABP), ventricular assist device, or extracorporeal membrane oxygenator.

Afterload

Afterload is the tension developed within the ventricular muscle during contraction. An important component of afterload in patients is the SVR. During CPB at full flow (usually $\approx$2.2 L/m^2 per min), mean arterial pressure (MAP) is directly related to SVR and indicates whether the SVR is appropriate, too high, or too low. Low SVR after CPB can cause inadequate systemic arterial perfusion pressure, and high SVR can significantly impair cardiac performance, especially in patients with poor ventricular function. SVR during CPB can be approximated by using the following equation:

$$SVR\,(dynes \cdot s \cdot cm^{-5}) = MAP \times 80 / pump\ flow$$

If the SVR is less than normal, infusion of a vasopressor may be needed to increase the SVR before attempting to wean the patient from CPB. If the MAP is high during CPB, vasodilator therapy may be needed.

▦ FINAL CONSIDERATIONS AND PREPARATIONS

The state of coagulation and the potential requirement for blood transfusion or component therapy must be considered before separation from CPB. Review of data from prebypass studies such as hemoglobin, platelet count, thromboelastography, and coagulation panels may help in recognizing preexisting coagulopathy and in predicting transfusion requirements in the presence of post-CPB bleeding after protamine administration. Risk factors that may be associated with higher rates of transfusion include emergency or urgent surgical procedures, reoperation, cardiogenic shock, older age, female sex, low body weight, and preoperative anemia. Preoperative use of antiplatelet agents, warfarin, and novel anticoagulants may also portend higher transfusion rates and warrant special attention. Assessing coagulation status and the need for transfusion is an important consideration before attempting to wean a patient from CPB.

The final preparations before discontinuing CPB include leveling the operating table, resetting the pressure transducers to zero, ensuring the proper function and location of all monitoring devices, confirming that the patient is receiving only intended drug infusions, ensuring the immediate availability of resuscitation drugs and appropriate fluid volume, and verifying that the lungs are being ventilated with 100% oxygen (Table 28.4).

The surgeon must confirm that he or she has completed the necessary preparations in the surgical field before CPB is discontinued. Macroscopic collections of air in the heart should be evacuated as described in detail earlier before starting to wean the patient from CPB. This is also an appropriate time to reassess the five major determinants of CO by using all available monitors and TEE. Major sites of bleeding should be controlled, cardiac vent suction should be off, all clamps on the heart and great vessels should be removed, coronary artery bypass grafts (CABGs) should be checked for kinks and bleeding, and tourniquets around the caval cannulas should be loosened or removed before starting to wean a patient from CPB.

28

Table 28.4	Final Preparations for Discontinuing Cardiopulmonary Bypass	
Anesthesiologist's Preparations	**Surgeon's Preparations**	
Level operating table	Remove macroscopic collections of air from the heart	
Reset transducers to zero	Control major sites of bleeding	
Activate monitors	Ensure CABG is lying nicely without kinks	
Check drug infusions	Turn off or remove cardiac vents	
Have resuscitation drugs and fluid volume at hand	Take clamps off the heart and great vessels	
Reestablish TEE or PAC monitoring	Loosen tourniquets around caval cannulas	

CABG, Coronary artery bypass graft; PAC, pulmonary artery catheter; TEE, transesophageal echocardiography.

ROUTINE WEANING FROM CARDIOPULMONARY BYPASS

The perfusionist, the surgeon, and the anesthesiologist should communicate closely and clearly while weaning a patient from CPB, and the surgeon or the anesthesiologist should be in charge of the process. The anesthesiologist should be positioned at the head of the table, able to see the CPB pump and perfusionist, the heart, the surgeon, and the anesthesia monitor display readily. The TEE display also should be easily in view. Weaning a patient from CPB is accomplished by diverting blood back into the patient's heart by occluding the venous drainage to the CPB pump. The arterial pump flow is decreased simultaneously as the pump reservoir volume empties into the patient, and the heart's contribution to systemic flow increases. This can be accomplished most abruptly by simply clamping the venous return cannula and transfusing blood from the pump until the heart fills and the preload appears to be adequate. Some patients tolerate this method of discontinuing CPB, but many do not, and a more gradual transfer from the pump to the heart usually is desirable. The worse the function of the heart is, the slower the transition from full CPB to off CPB needs to be.

Before beginning to wean the patient from CPB, the perfusionist should communicate to the physicians involved the following three important parameters: (1) the current flow rate of the pump; (2) the volume in the pump reservoir; and (3) the oxygen saturation of venous blood returning to the pump from the patient. The flow along with MAP can be used to gauge the SVR of the patient before weaning from CPB. The current flow rate of the pump indicates the stage of weaning as it is decreased. Weaning is just beginning at full flow, is well under way when down to 2 or 3 L/minute in adults, and is almost finished at less than 2 L/minute. The reservoir volume indicates how much blood is available for transfer to the patient to fill the heart and lungs as CPB is discontinued. If the volume is low (<400 to 500 mL in adults), more fluid may need to be added to the reservoir before weaning from CPB. The oxygen saturation of the venous return ($S\overline{v}O_2$) gives an indication of the adequacy of peripheral perfusion during CPB. If the $S\overline{v}O_2$ is greater than 60%, oxygen delivery during CPB is adequate; if it is less than 50%, oxygen delivery is inadequate, and measures to improve delivery (eg, increase pump flow or hematocrit) or decrease consumption (eg, give more anesthetic agents or neuromuscular blocking drugs) must be taken before CPB is discontinued. An $S\overline{v}O_2$ between 50% and 60% is marginal and must be followed closely. As the patient is weaned from CPB, an increasing $S\bar{v}O_2$ suggests that the net flow to the body is increasing and that the heart and lungs will support the circulation; a declining $S\bar{v}O_2$ indicates that tissue perfusion is decreasing and that further intervention to improve cardiac performance will be needed before CPB is discontinued.

The actual process of weaning from CPB begins with partially occluding the venous return cannula with a clamp. This may be done in the field by the surgeon or at the pump by the perfusionist. This maneuver causes blood to flow into the right ventricle. As the right ventricle fills and begins to pump blood through the lungs, the left heart begins to fill. When this occurs, the left ventricle begins to eject, and the arterial waveform becomes pulsatile. Next, the perfusionist gradually decreases the pump flow rate. As more of the venous return goes through the heart and less to the pump reservoir, it becomes necessary to decrease the pump flow gradually to avoid emptying the pump reservoir.

One approach to weaning from CPB is to bring the filling pressure being monitored (eg, central venous pressure, pulmonary artery pressure, LAP) to a specific, predetermined level somewhat lower than may be necessary and then assess the hemodynamic status. Volume (preload) of the heart also may be judged by direct observation of its size or with TEE. Further filling is done in small increments (50–100 mL) while closely monitoring the preload until the hemodynamic status appears satisfactory as judged by the arterial pressure, the appearance of the heart, the trend of the $S\bar{v}O_2$, and CO measurements by TEE or pulmonary artery catheter. It typically is easy to see the right-sided heart volume and function directly in the surgical field and the left side of the heart with TEE; combining the two observations is a useful approach for weaning from CPB. Overfilling and distension of the heart should be avoided because they may stretch the myofibrils beyond the most efficient length and dilate the annuli of the mitral and tricuspid valves, thus rendering them incompetent, which can be detected with TEE. If the patient has two venous cannulas, the smaller of the two may be removed when the pump flow is half of the full flow rate to improve movement of blood from the great veins into the right atrium. When the pump flow has been decreased to 1 L/minute or less in an adult and the hemodynamics findings are satisfactory, the venous cannula may be completely clamped and the pump flow turned off. At this point, the patient is "off bypass."

This is a critical juncture in the operation. The anesthesiologist should pause a moment to make a brief scan of the patient and monitors to confirm that the lungs are being ventilated with oxygen, the hemodynamic status is acceptable and stable, the electrocardiogram shows no new signs of ischemia, the heart does not appear to be distending, and the drug infusions are functioning as desired. Further fine-tuning of the preload is accomplished by transfusing 50- to 100-mL boluses from the pump reservoir through the arterial cannula and observing the effect on hemodynamics. If acute failure of the circulation occurs, as evidenced by an unstable rhythm, falling arterial and rising filling pressures, or visible distension of the heart, the patient is put back on CPB by unclamping the venous return cannula and turning on the arterial pump flow. Once CPB has resumed, an assessment of the cause of failure to wean is made, and appropriate interventions are undertaken before attempting to wean the patient from CPB again. Alternatively, if the hemodynamic status appears to be stable and adequate, the surgeon may remove the venous cannula from the heart.

The next step in discontinuing CPB is to transfuse as much of the blood remaining in the pump reservoir as possible into the patient before removal of the arterial cannula. This technique is usually easier and quicker than transfusing through the intravenous infusions after decannulation. The blood in the venous cannula and tubing (usually ≈500 mL) may be drained into the reservoir for transfusion. The patient's venous capacitance can be increased by raising the head of the bed (ie, reverse Trendelenburg position) and/or giving NTG; more caution is required with these maneuvers in patients with impaired cardiac function. Filling the vascular space with the patient's head up and while infusing NTG increases the ability to cope with volume loss after decannulation by allowing rapid augmentation of the central vascular volume by leveling the bed and decreasing the NTG infusion rate.

After discontinuing CPB, the anticoagulation by heparin is reversed with protamine. Depending on institutional preference, protamine may be administered before or after removal of the arterial cannula. Giving protamine before removal allows for continued transfusion from the pump and easier return to CPB if the patient has a severe protamine reaction. Giving protamine after removal of the arterial cannula may decrease the risk for thrombus formation and systemic embolization. After the infusion of protamine is started, pump suction return to the reservoir should be stopped to keep protamine out of the pump circuit in case subsequent return to CPB becomes necessary. Titrated dosing of protamine may be more effective in reducing postoperative bleeding compared with a standard protamine administration protocol. Titrated dosing involves adjusting the protamine concentration to reflect measured circulating heparin levels. Protamine should be given slowly through a peripheral intravenous catheter over 5 to 15 minutes while the clinician watches for systemic hypotension and pulmonary hypertension, which may indicate that an untoward (allergic) reaction to protamine is occurring. Technically flawed CABGs may thrombose after protamine administration, thus causing acute ischemia mimicking a protamine reaction.

When transfusion of the pump reservoir blood is completed, a thorough assessment of the patient's condition should be made before the arterial cannula is removed because, after this is done, returning to CPB becomes much more difficult. The cardiac rhythm should be stable. Cardiac function and hemodynamic status, as assessed by arterial and venous filling pressures, CO, and TEE, should be satisfactory and stable. A more detailed and comprehensive TEE examination can be performed as time permits. RV free wall motion to assess RV function qualitatively can be obtained in the midesophageal four-chamber view (0 degrees) and midesophageal RV inflow-outflow view (45–60 degrees). In the midesophageal four-four-chamber view, RV function can also be quantified by measuring tricuspid annular systolic plane excursion (TAPSE) and comparing it with prebypass assessments.

Findings of interatrial septal bowing into the left atrium may indicate volume or pressure overload of the right atrium. Interventricular septal motion after CPB should be interpreted with caution because abnormal septal movement may be caused by several factors, including epicardial pacing, stunned myocardium, volume or pressure overload, and ischemia. The midesophageal four-chamber view at 0 degrees and the RV inflow-outflow view at 45 to 60 degrees may be used to assess for new or worsening tricuspid regurgitation, thereby indicating the possibility of RV dysfunction. Advancing the probe to the transgastric level allows for further evaluation of RV function in the short-axis view. After examining the right-sided chambers, all segments of the left side of the heart should be reviewed. Special attention should be given to new regional wall motion abnormalities, systolic thickening, and excursion of all segments of the left ventricle, evidence of LVOT obstruction from systolic anterior motion of the mitral valve, new valvular abnormalities, and overall end-diastolic and systolic chamber dimensions. New regional wall motion abnormalities may signify a technically flawed CABG or intracoronary air. LVOT obstruction from systolic anterior motion may indicate the presence of inadequate chamber filling from hypovolemia and tachycardia or a hyperdynamic state of contractility. New valvular abnormalities may represent iatrogenic damage to the valvular apparatus, myocardial ischemia, volume overload, or ventricular dysfunction. It is also important to scan the aorta to rule out a new aortic dissection after aortic decannulation. As time permits, TEE can also be used to calculate SV and CO by Doppler interrogation of the LVOT and aortic outflow tract. Diastolic filling profiles of the left ventricle and left atrium may be obtained using transmitral and pulmonary venous inflow, respectively. Serial measurements of LA and LV inflow may allow for estimating filling pressures and chamber compliance.

Adequate oxygenation and ventilation should be confirmed by arterial blood gas or pulse oximetry and capnography. Bleeding from the heart should be at a manageable level before removal of the arterial cannula. Additionally, the perfusionist should not be transfusing significant amounts of blood through the arterial cannula before removing it because keeping up with the blood loss through intravenous infusions alone may be difficult. Bleeding sites behind the heart may have to be repaired on CPB if the patient cannot tolerate lifting of the heart to expose the problem area. At the time of arterial decannulation, the systolic pressure should be lowered to between 85 and 100 mm Hg to minimize the risk for dissection or tearing of the aorta. The head of the bed may be raised, or small boluses of a short-acting vasodilator may be given to lower the systemic blood pressure as necessary. Tight control of the arterial blood pressure may be needed for a few minutes until the cannulation site is secure. The routine process of discontinuing bypass is completed when removal of all cannulas is successful and full reversal of the anticoagulation is achieved.

PHARMACOLOGIC MANAGEMENT OF VENTRICULAR DYSFUNCTION

Perioperative ventricular dysfunction usually is a transient state of contractile impairment that may require temporary support with positive inotropic agents. In a subset of patients, contractility may be significantly depressed such that combination therapy with positive inotropes and vasodilator agents is needed to improve CO and tissue perfusion effectively. The use of mechanical assist devices is reserved for conditions of overt or evolving cardiogenic shock.

Severe ventricular dysfunction, specifically the LCOS, occurring after CPB and cardiac operations differs from chronic congestive HF (CHF) (Box 28.2). Patients emerging from CPB have hemodilution, moderate hypocalcemia, hypomagnesemia, and altered K^+ levels. Depending on temperature and depth of anesthesia, these patients may demonstrate low, normal, or high SVR. Increasing age, female sex, decreased LV ejection fraction (LVEF), diastolic dysfunction, prolonged aortic cross-clamp time,

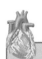

BOX 28.2   *Risk Factors for the Low Cardiac Output Syndrome After Cardiopulmonary Bypass*

Preoperative ventricular dysfunction
Myocardial ischemia
Poor myocardial preservation
Reperfusion injury
Inadequate cardiac surgical repair or revascularization

and increased duration of CPB are associated with a greater likelihood that inotropic support will be needed after CABG procedures (see Table 28.3).

Contractile dysfunction during or after cardiac operations can result from preexisting impairment in contractility or may be a new-onset condition. Abnormal contraction, especially in the setting of coronary artery disease (CAD), usually is caused by myocardial injury resulting in ischemia or infarction. The magnitude of contractile dysfunction corresponds to the extent and duration of injury. Brief periods of myocardial oxygen deprivation (<10 minutes) produce regional contractile dysfunction, which can be rapidly reversed by reperfusion. Extension of the ischemia to 15 to 20 minutes also is associated with restoration of cardiac function with reperfusion; however, this process is very slow and can take hours to days. This condition of postischemic reversible myocardial dysfunction in the presence of normal flow is referred to as *myocardial stunning*. Irreversible cell injury occurs with longer periods of ischemia and produces myocardial infarction characterized by release of intracellular enzymes, disruption of cell membranes, influx of Ca^{2+}, persistent contractile dysfunction, and eventual cellular swelling and necrosis.

In addition to the previously described factors, RV dysfunction and RV failure are potential sources of morbidity and death after cardiac operations. Numerous factors may predispose patients to the development of perioperative RV dysfunction, including CAD, RV hypertrophy, previous cardiac operation, and operative considerations such as inadequate revascularization or hypothermic protection. Technical and operative difficulties are associated with various cardiac surgical procedures (eg, right ventriculotomy), RV trauma, rhythm and conduction abnormalities, injury to the right ventricle during cessation of CPB, or protamine reaction.

The following discussion provides an overview of the pharmacologic approach to management of perioperative ventricular dysfunction in the setting of cardiac surgery. Management goals are described in Table 28.5. These are extensions of the routine preparations made for discontinuing CPB shown in Table 28.2.

Sympathomimetic Amines

Sympathomimetic drugs (ie, catecholamines) are pharmacologic agents capable of providing inotropic and vasoactive effects (Box 28.3). Catecholamines exert positive inotropic action by stimulation of the β_1- and β_2-receptors. The predominant hemodynamic effect of a specific catecholamine depends on the degree to which the various α, β, and dopaminergic receptors are stimulated (Tables 28.6 and 28.7).

The physiologic effect of an adrenergic agonist is determined by the sum of its actions on α, β, and dopaminergic receptors. The effectiveness of any adrenergic agent is influenced by the availability and responsiveness of adrenergic receptors. Chronically increased levels of plasma catecholamines (eg, chronic CHF and long

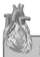

BOX 28.3   *Pharmacologic Approaches to Ventricular Dysfunction*

Inotropic drugs
Phosphodiesterase inhibitors
Calcium sensitizer
Vasodilators
Vasopressors
Metabolic supplements

Table 28.5 Goals and Management of Cardiac Dysfunction

Variable	Physiologic Management
Heart rate and rhythm	Maintain normal sinus rhythm, avoid tachycardia; for tachycardia or bradycardia, consider pacing or chronotropic agents (atropine, isoproterenol, epinephrine), correct acid-base, electrolytes, and review current medications
Contractility	Assess hemodynamics, perform TEE to assess cardiac function, inspect for RWMA, rule out ischemia or infarction, inspect for dynamic outflow obstruction, consider inotropes; consider combination therapy with inotropes and/or vasodilators, and evaluate need for assist devices (IABP/LVAD/RVAD)
Preload	Assess end-diastolic volumes and chamber dimensions on TEE, rule out ischemia, significant valvular lesions, tamponade, and intracardiac shunts; reduce increased preload with diuretics or venodilators (nitroglycerin); monitor CVP, PCWP, and SV; consider using inotropes, IABP, or both
Afterload	Avoid increased afterload (increased wall tension), use vasodilators; avoid hypotension; maintain coronary perfusion pressure; consider IABP, inotropes devoid of α_1-adrenergic effects (dobutamine or milrinone), or both IABP and inotropes
Oxygen delivery	Increase Fio_2 and CO; check ABGs and chest radiograph; confirm adequate ventilation and oxygenation; correct acid-base disturbances

ABG, Arterial blood gas; *CO,* cardiac output; *CVP,* central venous pressure; *Fio₂,* fraction of inspired oxygen concentration; *IABP,* intraaortic balloon pump; *LVAD,* left ventricular assist device; *PCWP,* pulmonary capillary wedge pressure; *RVAD,* right ventricular assist device; *RWMA,* regional wall motion abnormality; *SV,* stroke volume; *TEE,* transesophageal echocardiography.

Table 28.6 Sympathomimetic Agents

Drug	Dosage Intravenous Bolus	Dosage Infusion	Site of Action α	Site of Action β	Mechanism of Action
Dobutamine	—	2–20 µg/kg per min	+	++++	Direct
Dopamine	—	1–10 µg/kg per min	++	+++	Direct and indirect
Epinephrine	2–16 µg	2–10 µg/min Or 0.01–0.4 µg/kg per min	+++	+++	Direct
Ephedrine	5–25 mg	—	+	++	Direct and indirect
Isoproterenol	1–4 µg	0.5–10 µg/min Or 0.01–0.10 µg/kg per min		++++	Direct
Norepinephrine	—	2–16 µg/min Or 0.01–0.3 µg/kg per min	++++	+++	Direct

28

Table 28.7 Hemodynamic Effects of Inotropes

Drug	CO	dP/dt	HR	SVR	PVR	PCWP	Mv̇O$_2$
Dobutamine 2–20 µg/kg per min[a]	↑↑↑	↑	↑↑	↓	↓	↓ or ↔	↑
Dopamine 0–3 µg/kg per min	↑	↑	↑	↓	↓	↑	↑
3–10 µg/kg per min	↑↑	↑	↑	↓	↓	↑	↑
>10 µg/kg per min	↑↑	↑	↑↑	↑	(↑)	↑ or ↔	↑↑
Isoproterenol 0.5–10 µg/min	↑↑	↑↑	↑↑	↓↓	↓	↓	↑↑
Epinephrine 0.01–0.4 µg/kg per min	↑↑	↑	↑	↑ (↓)	(↑)	↑ or ↔	↑↑
Norepinephrine 0.01–0.3 µg/kg per min	↑	↑	↔ (↑↓)	↑↑	↔	↔	↑
Phosphodiesterase Inhibitors[b]	↑↑	↑	↑	↓↓	↓↓	↓↓	↓
Levosimendan[c]	↑↑↑	↑↑	↑	↓↓	↓↓	↓↓	↓ or ↔

[a]The indicated dosages represent the most common dosage ranges. For the individual patient, a deviation from these recommended doses may be indicated.

[b]Phosphodiesterase inhibitors are usually given as a loading dose followed by a continuous infusion: amrinone: 0.5 to 1.5 mg/kg loading dose, 5 to 10 µg/kg per minute continuous infusion; milrinone: 50 µg/kg loading dose, 0.375 to 0.75 µg/kg per minute continuous infusion.

[c]Levosimendan is usually administered as a loading dose followed by an infusion for 24 hours: 8 to 24 µg/kg loading dose, 0.1 to 0.2 µg/kg per minute.

CO, Cardiac output; dP/dt, myocardial contractility; HR, heart rate; Mv̇O$_2$, myocardial oxygen consumption; PCWP, pulmonary capillary wedge pressure; PVR, pulmonary vascular resistance; SVR, systemic vascular resistance; ↑, mild increase; ↑↑, moderate increase; ↑↑↑, major increase; ↔, no change; ↓, mild decrease; ↓↓, moderate decrease.

Modified from Lehmann A, Boldt J. New pharmacologic approaches for the perioperative treatment of ischemic cardiogenic shock. *J Cardiothorac Vasc Anesth.* 2005;19:97–108.

CPB time) cause downregulation of the number and sensitivity of β-receptors. Acute depression of β-adrenergic receptor signaling has been reported following CPB. Maintenance of normal acid-base status, normothermia, and electrolytes also improve the responsiveness to adrenergic-receptor stimulation.

The selection of a drug to treat ventricular dysfunction is influenced by pathophysiologic abnormalities, as well as by the physician's experience and preference. If LV performance is decreased primarily as a result of diminished contractility, the drug chosen should increase contractility. Although β-agonists improve contractility and tissue perfusion, their effects may increase myocardial oxygen consumption (Mv̇O$_2$) and reduce coronary perfusion pressure (CPP). However, if the factor most responsible for decreased cardiac function is hypotension with concomitantly reduced CPP, infusion of α-adrenergic agonists can increase blood pressure and improve diastolic coronary perfusion.

Catecholamines also are effective for treating primary RV contractile dysfunction, and all the β$_1$-adrenergic agonists augment RV contractility. Studies have documented the efficacy of epinephrine, norepinephrine, dobutamine, isoproterenol, dopamine, levosimendan, and phosphodiesterase fraction III (PDE III) inhibitors in managing RV contractile dysfunction. When decreased RV contractility is combined with increased afterload, agents that exert vasodilator and positive inotropic effects may be used, including epinephrine, isoproterenol, dobutamine, levosimendan, PDE III inhibitors, and inhaled nitric oxide or prostaglandins.

Epinephrine

Epinephrine is an endogenous catecholamine that stimulates both α- and β-adrenergic receptors in a dose-dependent fashion. The β-selective pharmacology of epinephrine is characterized by a higher binding affinity for the β-receptor at lower doses and a stronger preference for the α-receptor at higher doses. This provides the clinical basis for the biphasic response observed for epinephrine, in which at lower doses the hemodynamic effects are predominated by increased inotropy and chronotropy of the heart (β-effect), and at higher doses a vasopressor effect (α-effect) is primarily observed.

Epinephrine is often used to facilitate the separation from CPB (Box 28.4). In the earliest studies, epinephrine infusion at 0.03 µg/kg per minute following CPB resulted in an increase in cardiac index (CI), MAP, and HR by 30%, 27%, and 11%, respectively, compared with baseline.

Epinephrine infusion at dosages of 0.01, 0.02, and 0.04 µg/kg per minute was shown to increase SV by 2%, 12%, and 22%, respectively, corresponding to an increased CI of 0.1, 0.7, and 1.2 L/m^2 per minute. In the lower dose range (0.01–0.04 µg/kg per min), the effect on the HR was less pronounced, with a maximum increase of 10 beats/minute. Elevations in HR may be an effect observed at higher doses. Moreover, epinephrine is also used frequently after cardiac operations to support the function of the "stunned" reperfused heart following CPB. In summary, epinephrine (0.01–0.04 µg/kg per min) at certain doses effectively increases CO with minimal increases in HR following CPB (see Table 28.7).

Dobutamine

Dobutamine is a synthetic catecholamine that displays a strong affinity for the β-receptor and results in dose-dependent increases in CO and HR, as well as reductions in diastolic filling pressures. Administration of dobutamine in cardiac surgical patients produced a marked increase in CI and HR in several studies. In patients with the LCOS, dobutamine resulted in an increase in HR in excess of 25% and a significant concomitant decrease in SVR. The effects of epinephrine (0.03 µg/kg per min) were compared with those of dobutamine (5 µg/kg per min) in 52 patients recovering from CABG procedures. Both drugs significantly and similarly increased SV index (SVI), but epinephrine increased the HR by only 2 beats/minute, whereas dobutamine increased the HR by 16 beats/minute.

In addition to increasing contractility, dobutamine may have favorable metabolic effects on ischemic myocardium. Intravenous and intracoronary injections of dobutamine increased coronary blood flow in animal studies. In paced cardiac surgical

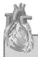

BOX 28.4 *Inotropic Drugs*

Epinephrine
Norepinephrine
Dopamine
Dobutamine
Isoproterenol

28

patients, dopamine increased oxygen demand without increasing oxygen supply, whereas dobutamine increased myocardial oxygen uptake and coronary blood flow. However, because increases in HR are a major determinant of $M\dot{v}O_2$, these favorable effects of dobutamine could be lost if dobutamine induces tachycardia. During dobutamine stress echocardiography, segmental wall motion abnormalities suggestive of myocardial ischemia can result from tachycardia and increases in $M\dot{v}O_2$.

Dopamine

Dopamine is an endogenous catecholamine and an immediate precursor of norepinephrine and epinephrine. Its actions are mediated by stimulation of adrenergic receptors and specific postjunctional dopaminergic receptors (D_1 receptors) in the renal, mesenteric, and coronary arterial beds. Dopamine is unique in comparison with other endogenous catecholamines because of its effects on the kidneys. It has been shown to increase renal artery blood flow by 20% to 40% by causing direct vasodilation of the afferent arteries and indirect vasoconstriction of the efferent arteries. This action results in increases in glomerular filtration rate and in oxygen delivery to the juxtamedullary nephrons. In low doses (0.5–3.0 µg/kg per minute), dopamine predominantly stimulates the dopaminergic receptors; at doses ranging from 3 to 10 µg/kg per minute, it activates most adrenergic receptors in a nonselective fashion; and at higher doses (>10 µg/kg per min), dopamine behaves as a vasoconstrictor. The dose-dependent effects of dopamine are not very specific and can be influenced by multiple factors, such as receptor regulation, concomitant drug use, and interindividual and intraindividual variability.

In patients undergoing cardiac surgical procedures, dopamine in the dose range of 2.5 and 5.0 µg/kg per minute was observed to produce significant increases in CI and HR. Doses greater than 5 µg/kg per minute may result in significant increases in MAP and pulmonary vascular resistance (PVR) without increasing CO. Dopamine caused more frequent and less predictable degrees of tachycardia than dobutamine or epinephrine at doses that produced comparable improvement in contractile function. The hemodynamic effects of dopamine at lower doses are predominantly characterized by marked elevations in HR and moderate increases in CI. At higher doses, increases in MAP and PVR predominate without an increase in CO. The propensity of dopamine to increase HR and induce tachyarrhythmias may limit its utility in the cardiac surgical patient emerging from CPB.

Norepinephrine

Norepinephrine is an endogenous catecholamine exhibiting potent α-adrenergic activity with a mild-to-modest effect on the β-adrenergic receptor. The higher affinity for norepinephrine for the α-adrenergic receptor provides the basis for its powerful vasoconstrictor effect and less potent inotropic and chronotropic properties. The overall hemodynamic effects of norepinephrine are characterized by an increase in systolic, diastolic, and pulse pressure, with minimal net impact on CO and HR. In this regard, norepinephrine is used primarily to manage low SVR secondary to vasodilation after CPB. Norepinephrine has been used in combination with milrinone, dobutamine, or levosimendan to counteract systemic vasodilation and hypotension in patients following CPB.

Isoproterenol

Isoproterenol is a potent, nonselective β-adrenergic agonist, devoid of α-adrenergic agonist activity. Isoproterenol dilates skeletal, renal, and mesenteric vascular beds and decreases diastolic blood pressure. The potent chronotropic action of isoproterenol, combined with its propensity to decrease CPP, limits its usefulness in patients with

CAD. Applications include treatment of bradycardia (especially after orthotopic heart transplantation), pulmonary hypertension, and HF after surgical treatment of congenital cardiac disease. Isoproterenol remains the inotrope of choice for stimulation of cardiac pacemaker cells in the management of acute bradyarrhythmias or atrioventricular heart block. Its use for this purpose during cardiac surgery is limited because artificial pacing is usually easily accomplished in this setting. The tachycardia seen with iso-proterenol is a result of direct effects of the drug on the sinoatrial and atrioventricular nodes and reflex effects caused by peripheral vasodilation.

Phosphodiesterase Inhibitors

The PDE III inhibitors milrinone and amrinone (inamrinone), increase cyclic adenosine monophosphate (cAMP), Ca^{2+} flux, and Ca^{2+} sensitivity of contractile proteins. PDE III inhibitors increase the level of cAMP by inhibiting its breakdown within the cell; this action leads to increased myocardial contractility. Their positive effects on inotropy are mediated primarily through an inhibition of the PDE enzyme and not through β-receptor stimulation. As a result, the effectiveness of the PDE III inhibitors is not altered by previous β-blockade, nor is it reduced in patients who may experience β-receptor downregulation. In addition to their positive inotropic effects, these agents produce systemic and pulmonary vasodilation and improve diastolic relaxation (lusitropy). For these reasons, the term *inodilator* has been used to describe this class of drugs (Box 28.5).

Milrinone has been shown to increase CO without increasing overall $M\dot{v}O_2$. Several studies also suggested that milrinone may improve myocardial diastolic relaxation and compliance (ie, positive "lusitropic" effect) while augmenting coronary perfusion. The proposed mechanism for this effect on diastolic performance is that, by decreasing LV wall tension, ventricular filling is enhanced, and myocardial blood flow and oxygen delivery are optimized (see Table 28.7). Amrinone represents the first-generation PDE III inhibitor used to wean from CPB. Compared with dobutamine, amrinone was found to be more effective for separation from CPB, with observed increases in SV and CO and decreases in SVR and PVR. Thrombocytopenia has been a potential clinical concern with the administration of PDE III inhibitors. Currently, amrinone has been implicated in causing dose-dependent thrombocytopenia, thus limiting its utility in cardiac surgical procedures. By contrast, the potential negative effects of PDE III inhibitors on platelets were not demonstrated with milrinone. In summary, the PDE III class of inodilators has a unique mechanism of action independent of the β-receptor. These agents combine increases in contractility with reductions in SVR and PVR. In addition, the properties that govern relaxation and compliance of

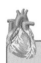

BOX 28.5 *Inodilator Drugs and Other Agents*

Inamrinone
Milrinone
Dobutamine
Epinephrine plus nitroprusside ("epipride")
Levosimendan
Nesiritide

the heart are enhanced with PDE III inhibitors and allow these drugs to improve diastolic filling. These unique properties render PDE III inhibitors particularly useful in patients with β-receptor downregulation, right-sided heart dysfunction, pulmonary hypertension, diastolic dysfunction, and the LCOS.

Calcium Sensitizers

Levosimendan is a positive inotropic drug belonging to the unique class of Ca^{2+} sensitizers. Levosimendan binds three distinct sites of action, and this property characterizes its unique tripartite mechanism of action and pharmacologic effects. In the myocardium, levosimendan selectively binds troponin C through a Ca^{2+}-dependent binding site stabilizing the cross-bridging mechanism and resulting in positive inotropy. Levosimendan also specifically binds to the ATP-dependent K^+ channel (K^+/ATP) in cardiac mitochondria, governing its protective effects against ischemia and reperfusion injury. By regulating Ca^{2+} influx in the mitochondria, opening of the K^+/ATP channel attenuates infarct size as a result of ischemia-reperfusion injury. The third site of action is at the level of the smooth muscle in the vasculature. At this site, levosimendan binds and opens K^+/ATP channels and thus leads to decreases in SVR and cardiac preload and afterload. The vasodilatory effect on the vasculature has been shown to increase coronary and renal blood flow. The salutary effects on the myocardium are achieved through an observed decrease in overall cardiac workload, cardioprotective effects, lusitropy, and a net increase in myocardial oxygen supply. Because the mechanism of action is independent of the β-receptor, concomitant administration of β-blocker therapy and levosimendan is not antagonistic. This property allows for earlier reinstitution of β-blocker therapy for prevention or management of postoperative tachyarrhythmias.

The effective perioperative use of levosimendan has been described in cardiac surgical patients with low LVEF. In summary, levosimendan improved myocardial performance with an observed increase in SVI and coronary blood flow, as well as a decrease in SVR while minimizing oxygen consumption. Currently, levosimendan is recommended by the European Society of Cardiology for treatment of acute worsening of HF and for acute HF after myocardial infarction. It also has been found to enhance contractile function of stunned myocardium in patients with acute coronary syndromes. It is available clinically in Europe and is now undergoing phase III trials in the United States. The use of levosimendan has been reported in cardiac surgical patients with high perioperative risk, compromised LV function, difficulties in weaning from CPB, and severe RV failure after mitral valve replacement. The drug has been used preoperatively, during emergence from CPB, and in the postoperative period for up to 28 days. The potential for levosimendan to produce increased contractility, decreased resistance, minimal metabolic cost, and minimal arrhythmias makes it a potentially useful addition to the treatments for patients with the LCOS or RV failure.

Vasodilators

The indications for using vasodilators such as NTG, sodium nitroprusside (SNP), nicardipine, and clevidipine in cardiac surgery include management of perioperative systemic or pulmonary hypertension, myocardial ischemia, and ventricular dysfunction complicated by excessive pressure or volume overload (Box 28.6). In most conditions, NTG, SNP, or clevidipine may be used because of their shared features, such as rapid onset, ultrashort half-lives, and easy titratability. Nevertheless, important pharmacologic differences exist among these vasodilators. In the setting of CAD or ischemia, NTG is preferred because it selectively vasodilates coronary arteries without producing

V

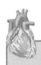

BOX 28.6 *Vasodilator Mechanisms Helpful in Discontinuing Cardiopulmonary Bypass*

Decreased right and left ventricular wall stress (afterload)
Decreased venous return (preload)
Improved lusitropy
Improved coronary blood flow

coronary "steal." Similarly, in the management of ventricular volume overload or RV pressure overload, NTG may offer some advantage over SNP. NTG has a predominant influence on the venous bed such that preload can be reduced without significantly compromising systemic arterial pressure. The benefits of NTG are improvement in SV, reduction in wall tension and $M\dot{v}O_2$, increased perfusion to the subendocardium as a result of a lower LVEDP, and maintenance of CPP. SNP is a more potent arterial vasodilator and may potentiate myocardial ischemia because of a coronary steal phenomenon or a reduction in CPP. Its greater potency, however, makes SNP a more rational choice for management of perioperative hypertensive disorders and for afterload reduction during or after operations for regurgitant valvular lesions.

Although NTG and SNP have been used for the management of hypertension during cardiac surgical procedures, they both have notable limitations. NTG use as a primary antihypertensive agent is limited by its weak effect on arterial vasodilation. SNP is a potent arterial dilator, but its use is associated with reflex tachycardia, tachyphylaxis, inhibition of hypoxic pulmonary vasoconstriction, increase in intracranial pressure, and reduced renal blood flow. The potential for cyanide toxicity is also an important consideration when administering SNP. This drug also may be difficult to titrate and often causes hypotension related to overshoot. In light of these limitations, the Ca^{2+} channel blocker class of antihypertensive agents, such as clevidipine and nicardipine, may prove to be valuable alternatives.

Clevidipine is an ultrafast-acting, dihydropyridine L-type Ca^{2+} channel blocker with a direct action on arteriolar resistance vessels and limited effects on venous capacitance vessels. The fast onset and offset of approximately 1 minute make clevidipine especially suited for intraoperative management of acute hypertension. Nicardipine is also a dihydropyridine Ca^{2+} channel blocker with a selective arterial vasodilator mode of action. Nicardipine has a beneficial hemodynamic profile in that the drug reduces systemic and coronary artery resistance while increasing coronary blood flow. However, its use may be limited to the postoperative setting because of its longer half-life and slower offset of action compared with clevidipine. Despite the benefits of vasodilator therapy in the management of CHF, these drugs can be difficult to use in treatment of perioperative ventricular dysfunction. This is most evident in cases of the LCOS when impaired pump function is complicated by inadequate perfusion pressure. In these situations, multidrug therapy with vasoactive and cardioactive agents is warranted (ie, NTG or SNP in combination with epinephrine or milrinone and norepinephrine). Combination therapy enables greater selectivity of effect. The unwanted side effects of one drug can be avoided while supplementing the desired effects with another agent. To maximize the desired effects of any particular combination of agents, frequent assessment of cardiac performance with a pulmonary artery catheter and TEE is needed. This approach allows the Starling curve and the pressure-volume loops to be visualized as they are shifted up and to the left with therapy.

28

Vasoplegic Syndrome and Cardiopulmonary Bypass

The concept of the vasoplegic syndrome, characterized by hypotension associated with profound vasodilation unresponsive to conventional catecholamines or vasopressors, was introduced in association with CPB in the late 1990s. It has been linked with preoperative use of vasodilators and shown to be a risk factor for increased morbidity and death after cardiac surgical procedures. Two pharmacologic agents have been reported to be used to treat vasoplegic syndrome after CPB: vasopressin and methylene blue (MB).

Vasopressin

Arginine vasopressin (antidiuretic hormone) is a peptide hormone normally produced in the posterior pituitary that plays a crucial role in water homeostasis by controlling water resorption in the renal collecting ducts. Administered as an intravenous infusion, vasopressin was initially used as a potent vasoconstrictor for vasodilatory shock associated with sepsis and ventricular assist device implantation. Because its vasopressor effect is mediated through a different mechanism (VP1 receptors) from that of the catecholamines, vasopressin can be infused at a constant rate as a strategy to decrease high doses of catecholamines such as norepinephrine and has been used in this way to treat vasodilation occurring after CPB. The vasoconstricting effects of vasopressin may spare the pulmonary vasculature, thus making it an attractive choice to treat hypotension associated with RV dysfunction, but this effect has not been clearly demonstrated in intact humans. Reported infusion doses vary widely from 0.01 to 0.6 IU/minute. Use of vasopressin has been associated with necrotic lesions of the skin, and this agent should be used with caution and in the lowest possible effective dose.

Methylene Blue

MB, a substance commonly used intravenously during surgical procedures for its ability to dye certain tissues, inhibits guanylate cyclase and hence the production of cyclic guanosine monophosphate, which is known to increase vascular smooth muscle relaxation. MB has been used as a rescue treatment for profound vasodilatory shock in several settings, including cardiac surgery. At a dose of 3 mg/kg given during CPB, MB was shown to increase SVR and MAP without adverse effects in a randomized trial of patients taking angiotensin-converting enzyme inhibitors, as well as decrease pressor requirements and serum lactate levels after CPB. MB causes transient discoloration of the urine and the skin and interferes with pulse oximetry measurements of arterial oxygen saturation. In a retrospective analysis of 57 patients with vasoplegia during cardiac surgical procedures and CPB, use of MB as treatment for vasoplegia was independently associated with poor outcomes. The use of MB has also been implicated in causing serotonin syndrome through its inhibition of monoamine oxidase-A enzyme. In another case report, MB was causally linked to the development of methemoglobinemia during CPB. These reports highlight the need for more studies on the safety and possible poor outcomes associated with MB. Although more studies are warranted, it may be prudent to reserve MB for rescue therapy, as opposed to using it as a preventive agent.

▦ INTRAAORTIC BALLOON PUMP COUNTERPULSATION

The IABP is a device that is designed to augment myocardial perfusion by increasing coronary blood flow during diastole and unloading the left ventricle during systole.

This is accomplished by mass displacement of a volume of blood (usually 30–50 mL) by alternately inflating and deflating a balloon positioned in the proximal segment of the descending aorta. The gas used for this purpose is carbon dioxide (because of its great solubility in blood) or helium (because of its inertial properties and rapid diffusion coefficients). Inflation and deflation are synchronized to the cardiac cycle by the electronics of the balloon console by producing counterpulsations. The results of effective use of the IABP are often quite dramatic. Improvements in CO, LVEF, coronary blood flow, and MAP frequently are seen, as well as decreases in aortic and ventricular systolic pressures, LVEDP, pulmonary capillary wedge pressure, LAP, HR, frequency of premature ventricular contractions, and suppression of atrial arrhythmias.

Indications and Contraindications

Since the introduction of the IABP, the indications for its use have grown (Table 28.8). The most common use of the IABP is for treatment of cardiogenic shock. This may occur after CPB or after cardiac operations in patients with preoperative shock, patients with acute postinfarction ventricular septal defects or mitral regurgitation, those who require preoperative stabilization or patients who decompensate hemodynamically during cardiac catheterization. Patients with myocardial ischemia refractory to coronary vasodilation and afterload reduction are stabilized with an IABP before cardiac catheterization, and some patients with severe CAD prophylactically have an IABP inserted before undergoing CABG or off-pump CABG procedures.

Contraindications to IABP use are relatively few. The presence of severe aortic regurgitation or aortic dissection is an absolute contraindication for the IABP, although successful reports of its use in patients with aortic insufficiency or acute trauma to the descending thoracic aorta have appeared. Other relative contraindications are listed; use of the IABP in these instances is at the discretion of the physician. Because the hemodynamic changes caused by an IABP theoretically would tend to worsen dynamic outflow tract obstruction caused by systolic anterior motion of the mitral valve, the device should be used with caution, if at all, in these patients.

Table 28.8   Intraaortic Balloon Pump Counterpulsation Indications and Contraindications

Indications	Contraindications

1. Cardiogenic shock
  a. Myocardial infarction
  b. Myocarditis
  c. Cardiomyopathy
2. Failure to separate from CPB
3. Stabilization of preoperative patient
  a. Ventricular septal defect
  b. Mitral regurgitation
4. Stabilization of noncardiac surgical patient
5. Procedural support during coronary angiography
6. Bridge to transplantation
	1. Aortic valvular insufficiency
	2. Aortic disease
	  a. Aortic dissection
	  b. Aortic aneurysm
	3. Severe peripheral vascular disease
	4. Severe noncardiac systemic disease
	5. Massive trauma
	6. Patients with "do not resuscitate" instructions
	7. Mitral SAM with dynamic outflow tract obstruction

CPB, Cardiopulmonary bypass; *SAM,* systolic anterior motion.

Timing and Weaning

IABP systems are commercially available from several different manufacturers. The basic console design includes electrocardiographic and arterial blood pressure waveform monitoring and printing, balloon volume monitoring, triggering selection switches, adjustments for inflation and deflation timing, battery backup power sources, and gas reservoir. Some of these systems have become quite sophisticated, with advanced computer microprocessor circuits allowing triggering based on pacemaker signals or detection of and compensation for aberrant rhythms such as atrial fibrillation. Portable models exist for transportation of patients by ground, helicopter, or air ambulances.

For optimal effect of the IABP, inflation and deflation must be correctly timed to the cardiac cycle. Although certain variables, including positioning of the balloon within the aorta, balloon volume, and the patient's cardiac rhythm, can affect the performance of the IABP, basic principles regarding the function of the balloon must be followed. Balloon inflation should be timed to coincide with aortic valve closure, or aortic insufficiency and LV strain will result. Similarly, late inflation results in a diminished perfusion pressure to the coronary arteries. Early deflation causes inappropriate loss of afterload reduction, and late deflation increases LV work by causing increased afterload, if only transiently. These errors and correct timing diagrams are shown in Fig. 28.1.

As the patient's cardiac performance improves, the IABP support must be removed in stages rather than abruptly. Judicious application and dosing of vasodilator and

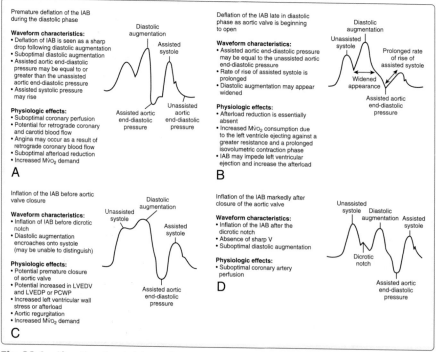

Fig. 28.1 Alterations in arterial waveform tracings caused by errors in timing of intraaortic balloon *(IAB)* pump. (A) The balloon was deflated too early. (B) The balloon was deflated too late. (C) The balloon was inflated too early. (D) The balloon was inflated too late. *LVEDP,* Left ventricular end-diastolic pressure; *LVEDV,* left ventricular end-diastolic volume; *MV̇O₂,* myocardial oxygen consumption; *PCWP,* pulmonary capillary wedge pressure. (Courtesy Datascope Corporation, Fairfield, NJ.)

Table 28.9	Intraaortic Balloon Pump Counterpulsation Complications		
Vascular	**Miscellaneous**	**Balloon**	
Arterial injury (perforation, dissection)	Hemolysis	Perforation (preinsertion)	
Aortic perforation	Thrombocytopenia	Tear (during insertion)	
Aortic dissection	Infection	Incorrect positioning	
Femoral artery thrombosis	Claudication (postremoval)	Gas embolization	
Peripheral embolization	Hemorrhage	Inadvertent removal	
Femoral vein cannulation	Paraplegia	—	
Pseudoaneurysm of femoral vessels	Entrapment	—	
Lower extremity ischemia	Spinal cord necrosis	—	
Compartment syndrome	Left internal mammary artery occlusion	—	
Visceral ischemia	Aggravation of dynamic outflow tract obstruction	—	

inotropic medications can assist this procedure. The balloon augmentation may be reduced in steps, from 1:1 counterpulsation to 1:2 and then to 1:4, with appropriate intervals at each stage to assess hemodynamic and neurologic stability, CO, and $S\overline{v}O_2$ changes. After appropriate observation at 1:4 or 1:8 counterpulsation, balloon assistance can be safely discontinued, and the device can be removed by one of the methods discussed. If percutaneous removal is chosen, an appropriate interval for reversal of anticoagulation (if used) before removal of the balloon should be allowed.

Complications

Several complications have been associated with IABP use (Table 28.9). The most frequently seen complications are vascular injuries, balloon malfunction, and infection.

SUGGESTED READINGS

Abraham WT, Fisher WG, Smith AL, et al. Cardiac resynchronization in chronic heart failure. *N Engl J Med.* 2002;346(24):1845–1853.

Apostolakis EE, Koletsis EN, Baikoussis NG, et al. Strategies to prevent intraoperative lung injury during cardiopulmonary bypass. *J Cardiothorac Surg.* 2010;5:1.

Aronson S, Dyke CM, Stierer KA, et al. The ECLIPSE trials: comparative studies of clevidipine to nitroglycerin, sodium nitroprusside, and nicardipine for acute hypertension treatment in cardiac surgery patients. *Anesth Analg.* 2008;107(4):1110–1121.

Bechtel A, Huffmyer J. Anesthetic management for cardiopulmonary bypass: update for 2014. *Semin Cardiothorac Vasc Anesth.* 2014;18:101–116.

De Hert SG, Lorsomradee S, Cromheecke S, et al. The effects of levosimendan in cardiac surgery patients with poor left ventricular function. *Anesth Analg.* 2007;104(4):766–773.

Felker GM, O'Connor CM. Inotropic therapy for heart failure: an evidence-based approach. *Am Heart J.* 2001;142(3):393–401.

George M, Rajaram M, Shanmugam E, et al. Novel drug targets in clinical development for heart failure. *Eur J Clin Pharmacol.* 2014;70(7):765–774.

Goldstein DJ, Oz MC. Mechanical support for postcardiotomy cardiogenic shock. *Semin Thorac Cardiovasc Surg.* 2000;12(3):220–228.

Greco T, Calabro MG, Covello RD, et al. Baysian Network meta-analysis on the effects of inodilatory agents on mortality. *Br J Anaesth.* 2015;114:746–756.

28

Haddad F, Couture P, Tousignant C, et al. The right ventricle in cardiac surgery, a perioperative perspective: II. Pathophysiology, clinical importance, and management. *Anesth Analg.* 2009;108(2):422–433.

Howell NJ, Ashrafian H, Drury NE, et al. Glucose-insulin-potassium reduces the incidence of low cardiac output episodes after aortic valve replacement for aortic stenosis in patients with left ventricular hypertrophy: results from the Hypertrophy, Insulin, Glucose, and Electrolytes (HINGE) trial. *Circulation.* 2011;123(2):170–177.

Kimmel SE, Sekeres M, Berlin JA, et al. Mortality and adverse events after protamine administration in patients undergoing cardiopulmonary bypass. *Anesth Analg.* 2002;94(6):1402–1408.

Levin R, Degrange M, Del Mazo C, et al. Preoperative levosimendan decreases mortality and the development of low cardiac output in high-risk patients with severe left ventricular dysfunction undergoing coronary artery bypass grafting with cardiopulmonary bypass. *Exp Clin Cardiol.* 2012;17(3):125–130.

Levy JH, Mancao MY, Gitter R, et al. Clevidipine effectively and rapidly controls blood pressure preoperatively in cardiac surgery patients: the results of the randomized, placebo-controlled efficacy study of clevidipine assessing its preoperative antihypertensive effect in cardiac surgery-1. *Anesth Analg.* 2007;105(4):918–925.

Moskowitz DM, Klein JJ, Shander A, et al. Predictors of transfusion requirements for cardiac surgical procedures at a blood conservation center. *Ann Thorac Surg.* 2004;77(2):626–634.

Nielsen DV, Algotsson L. Outcome of inotropic therapy: is less always more? *Curr Opin Anaesthesiol.* 2015;28(2):159–164.

Pathak A, Lebrin M, Vaccaro A, et al. Pharmacology of levosimendan: inotropic, vasodilatory and cardio-protective effects. *J Clin Pharm Ther.* 2013;38(5):341–349.

Porter TR, Shillcutt SK, Adams MS, et al. Guidelines for the use of echocardiography as a monitor for therapeutic intervention in adults: a report from the American Society of Echocardiography. *J Am Soc Echocardiogr.* 2015;28(1):40–56.

Treschan TA, Peters J. The vasopressin system: physiology and clinical strategies. *Anesthesiology.* 2006;105(3):599–612, quiz 639–640.

Weiner MM, Lin HM, Danforth D, et al. Methylene blue is associated with poor outcomes in vasoplegic shock. *J Cardiothorac Vasc Anesth.* 2013;27(6):1233–1238.

V

Postoperative Care

Chapter 29

Postoperative Respiratory Care

Daniel Bainbridge, MD • Davy C.H. Cheng, MD, MSC •
Thomas L. Higgins, MD, MBA • Daniel T. Engelman, MD

Key Points

1. Cardiac anesthesia has fundamentally shifted from a high-dose narcotic technique to a more balanced approach using moderate-dose narcotics, shorter-acting muscle relaxants, and volatile anesthetic agents.
2. This new paradigm has also led to renewed interest in perioperative pain management involving multimodal techniques that facilitate rapid tracheal extubation such as regional blocks, intrathecal morphine, and supplementary nonsteroidal antiinflammatory drugs.
3. This approach has prompted a change from the classical model of recovering patients in the traditional intensive care unit manner, with weaning protocols and intensive observation, to management more in keeping with the recovery room practice of early extubation and rapid discharge.
4. Fast-track cardiac anesthesia appears to be safe in comparison with conventional high-dose narcotic anesthesia, but if complications occur that would prevent early tracheal extubation, the management strategy should be modified accordingly.
5. The initial management in the postoperative care of fast-track cardiac surgical patients consists of ensuring an efficient transfer of care from operating room staff to cardiac recovery area staff, while at the same time maintaining stable patients' vital signs.
6. Pulmonary complications following cardiopulmonary bypass are relatively common, with up to 12% of patients experiencing some degree of acute lung injury and approximately 1% requiring tracheostomy for long-term ventilation.
7. Risk factors for respiratory insufficiency include advanced age, presence of diabetes or renal failure, smoking, chronic obstructive lung disease, peripheral vascular disease, previous cardiac operations, and emergency or unstable status.
8. Patients with preexisting chronic obstructive lung disease have higher rates of pulmonary complications, atrial fibrillation, and death.
9. Operating room events that increase risk include reoperation, blood transfusion, prolonged cardiopulmonary bypass time, and low–cardiac output states, particularly if a mechanical support device is required.
10. Hospital-acquired infections are important causes of postoperative morbidity. Strategies to reduce the incidence of ventilator-associated pneumonia include early removal of gastric and tracheal tubes, formal infection control programs, hand washing, semirecumbent positioning of the patient, use of disposable heat and moisture exchangers, and scheduled drainage of condensate from ventilator circuits.
11. Patients at risk for acute lung injury and those developing acute respiratory distress syndrome should be switched to a lung-protective ventilation strategy, which involves maintaining peak inspiratory pulmonary pressure less than 35 cm H_2O and restricting tidal volumes to 6 mL/kg of ideal body weight.
12. Permissive hypercapnia may be necessary to implement a lung-protective ventilation strategy. It should be used judiciously in patients with pulmonary hypertension because

13. Impediments to weaning from mechanical ventilation and extubation include delirium, unstable hemodynamic status, respiratory muscle dysfunction, renal failure with fluid overload, and sepsis.

14. Short-term weaning success can be achieved with any variety of ventilation modes. The patient receiving long-term ventilatory support requires an individualized approach that may encompass pressure-support ventilation, synchronized intermittent mandatory ventilation weaning, or T-piece trials. Noninvasive ventilation may assist in the transition from full support to liberation from mechanical ventilation.

15. A few patients are not able to be weaned from ventilation support. Characteristics of these patients include a persistent low-output state with multisystem organ failure. Long-term weaning may be best accomplished in a specialized unit rather than an acute cardiovascular recovery area.

Cardiac anesthesia itself has fundamentally shifted from a high-dose narcotic technique to a more balanced approach using moderate-dose narcotics, shorter-acting muscle relaxants, and volatile anesthetic agents. This change primarily has been driven by a realization that high-dose narcotics delay extubation and recovery after surgical procedures. This new paradigm also has led to renewed interest in perioperative pain management. In addition to changes in anesthetic practice, the type of patients presenting for cardiac operations is changing. Patients are now older and have more associated comorbidities (stroke, myocardial infarction [MI], renal failure). Change also has taken place in the recovery of patients undergoing cardiac procedures. Although cardiac surgical procedures often were associated with a high mortality rate and long intensive care unit (ICU) stays, the use of moderate doses of narcotics has allowed for rapid ventilator weaning and discharge from the ICU within 24 hours. This change has prompted a shift from the classical model of recovering patients in the traditional ICU manner, with weaning protocols and intensive observation, to management more in keeping with the recovery room practice of early extubation and rapid discharge.

29

◼ FAST-TRACK CARDIAC SURGICAL CARE

Anesthetic Techniques

Few trials have compared inhalation agents for fast-track cardiac anesthesia (FTCA). Several studies examined the effectiveness of propofol versus an inhalation agent; these studies demonstrated reductions in myocardial enzyme release (creatine kinase myocardium band [CK-MB], troponin I) and preservation of myocardial function in patients receiving inhalation agents.

The choice of muscle relaxant in FTCA is important to reduce the incidence of muscle weakness in the cardiac recovery area (CRA) that may delay tracheal extubation. Several randomized trials compared rocuronium (0.5–1 mg/kg) with pancuronium (0.1 mg/kg) and found significant differences in residual paralysis in the ICU, with delays in the time to extubation in the pancuronium-treated group.

Several trials examined the use of different short-acting narcotic agents during FTCA. In these trials, fentanyl, remifentanil, and sufentanil all were found to be efficacious for early tracheal extubation. The anesthetic drugs and their suggested dosages are listed in Box 29.1.

743

BOX 29.1 *Suggested Dosages for Fast-Track Cardiac Anesthesia*

Induction

Narcotic
    Fentanyl 5–10 µg/kg
    Sufentanil 1–3 µg/kg
    Remifentanil– infusions of 0.5–1.0 µg/kg per min
Muscle Relaxant
    Rocuronium 0.5–1 mg/kg
    Vecuronium 1–1.5 mg/kg
Hypnotic
    Midazolam 0.05–0.1 mg/kg
    Propofol 0.5–1.5 mg/kg

Maintenance

Narcotic
    Fentanyl 1–5 µg/kg
    Sufentanil 1–1.5 µg/kg
    Remifentanil infusions of 0.5–1.0 µg/kg per min
Hypnotic
    Inhalational 0.5–1 MAC
    Propofol 50–100 µg/kg per min

Transfer to Cardiac Recovery Area

Narcotic
    Morphine 0.1–0.2 mg/kg
Hypnotic
    Propofol 25–75 µg/kg per min

MAC, Minimum alveolar concentration.
Data from Mollhoff T, Herregods L, Moerman A, et al. Comparative efficacy and safety of remifentanil and fentanyl in 'fast track' coronary artery bypass graft surgery: a randomized, double-blind study. *Br J Anaesth.* 2001;87:718; Engoren M, Luther G, Fenn-Buderer N. A comparison of fentanyl, sufentanil, and remifentanil for fast-track cardiac anesthesia. *Anesth Analg.* 2001;93:859; and Cheng DC, Newman MF, Duke P, et al. The efficacy and resource utilization of remifentanil and fentanyl in fast-track coronary artery bypass graft surgery: a prospective randomized, double-blinded controlled, multi-center trial. *Anesth Analg.* 2001;92:1094.

Evidence Supporting Fast-Track Cardiac Recovery

Several randomized trials and one metaanalysis of randomized trials addressed the question of safety of FTCA. None of the trials was able to demonstrate differences in outcomes between the fast-track anesthesia group and the conventional anesthesia group. The metaanalysis of randomized trials demonstrated a reduction in the duration of intubation by 8 hours (Fig. 29.1) and in the ICU length of stay (LOS) by 5 hours in favor of the fast-track group. However, the hospital LOS was not statistically different.

FTCA appears safe in comparison with conventional high-dose narcotic anesthesia. It reduces the duration of ventilation and ICU LOS considerably without increasing the incidence of awareness or other adverse events. FTCA appears effective at reducing costs and resource use. As such, it is becoming the standard of care in many cardiac

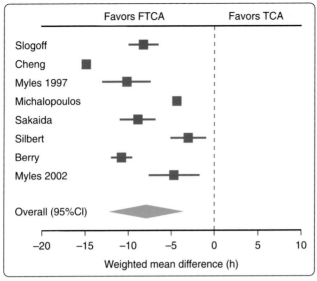

Fig. 29.1 Forrest plot showing the weighted mean difference in extubation times. The overall effect was an 8.1-hour reduction in extubation times. *CI,* Confidence interval; *FTCA,* fast-track cardiac anesthesia; *TCA,* traditional cardiac anesthesia. (Data from Myles PS, Daly DJ, Djaiani G, et al. A systematic review of the safety and effectiveness of fast-track cardiac anesthesia. *Anesthesiology.* 2003;99[4]:982–987.)

centers. The usual practice at many institutions is to treat all patients as candidates for FTCA with the goal of allowing early tracheal extubation for every patient. However, if complications occur that would prevent early tracheal extubation, the management strategy is modified accordingly. Investigators have demonstrated that the risk factors for delayed tracheal extubation (>10 hours) are increased age, female sex, postoperative use of intraaortic balloon pump (IABP), inotropes, bleeding, and atrial arrhythmia. The risk factors for prolonged ICU LOS (>48 hours) are those of delayed tracheal extubation in addition to preoperative MI and postoperative renal insufficiency. Care should be taken to avoid excessive bleeding (antifibrinolytic agents) and to treat arrhythmias either prophylactically or when they occur (β-blockers, amiodarone).

29

▨ INITIAL MANAGEMENT OF PATIENTS IN FAST-TRACK CARDIAC ANESTHESIA: THE FIRST 24 HOURS

On arrival in the CRA, initial management of cardiac patients consists of ensuring an efficient transfer of care from operating room (OR) staff to CRA staff while at the same time maintaining stable patient vital signs. The anesthesiologist should relay important clinical parameters to the CRA team. To accomplish this, many centers have devised handoff sheets to aid in the transfer of care. The patient's temperature should be recorded, and, if low, active rewarming measures should be initiated with the goal of rewarming the patient to 36.5°C. Shivering may be treated with low doses of meperidine (12.5–25 mg, intravenously). Hyperthermia, however, is common later within the first 24 hours after cardiac operations and may be associated with an increase in neurocognitive dysfunction, possibly a result of hyperthermia exacerbating cardiopulmonary bypass (CPB)–induced neurologic injury (Box 29.2).

BOX 29.2　*Initial Management of the Fast-Track Cardiac Anesthesia Patient*

Normothermia
Hemoglobin >7 g/dL
$Paco_2$ 35–45 mm Hg
Sao_2 >95%
Mean blood pressure >50–70 mm Hg
Potassium: 3.5–5.0 mEq/L
Blood glucose <10.0 mmol/L (<200 mg/dL)

$PaCO_2$, Partial pressure of arterial carbon dioxide; *SaO_2*, arterial oxygen saturation.

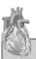

BOX 29.3　*Ventilation Management Goals During the Initial Trial of Weaning From Extubation*

Initial Ventilation Parameters

A/C at 10–12 beats/min
Tidal volume 8–10 mL/kg
PEEP 5 cm H_2O

Maintenance of Arterial Blood Gases

pH 7.35–7.45
$Paco_2$ 35–45 mm Hg
Pao_2 >90 mm Hg
Saturations >95%

Extubation Criteria

Arterial blood gases as above
Awake and alert
Hemodynamically stable
No active bleeding (<400 mL/2 h)
Temperature >36°C
Return of muscle strength (>5 s, head lift/strong hand grip)

A/C, Assist-controlled ventilation; *$PaCO_2$*, partial pressure of arterial carbon dioxide; *PaO_2*, partial pressure of arterial oxygen; *PEEP*, positive end-expiratory pressure.

Ventilation Management: Admission to Tracheal Extubation

Ventilatory requirements should be managed with the goal of early tracheal extubation in patients (Box 29.3). Arterial blood gases (ABGs) are initially drawn within one-half hour after admission and then repeated as needed. Patients should be awake and cooperative, hemodynamically stable, and have no active bleeding with coagulopathy. Respiratory strength should be assessed by hand grip or head lift to ensure complete reversal of neuromuscular blockade. The patient's temperature should be more than

36°C, preferably normothermic. When these conditions are met and ABG results are within the reference range, tracheal extubation may take place. ABGs should be drawn approximately 30 minutes after tracheal extubation to ensure adequate ventilation with maintenance of partial pressure of arterial oxygen (Pao_2) and partial pressure of arterial carbon dioxide ($Paco_2$). Inability to extubate patients as a result of respiratory failure, hemodynamic instability, or large amounts of mediastinal drainage necessitates more complex weaning strategies.

Some patients may arrive after extubation in the OR. Careful attention should be paid to these patients because they may subsequently develop respiratory failure. The patient's respiratory rate should be monitored every 5 minutes during the first several hours. ABGs should be drawn on admission and 30 minutes later to ensure that the patient is not retaining carbon dioxide. If the patient's respirations become compromised, ventilatory support should be provided. Simple measures such as reminders to breathe may be effective in the narcotized or anesthetized patient. Low doses of naloxone (0.04 mg, intravenously) also may be beneficial. Trials of continuous positive airway pressure (CPAP), bilevel positive airway pressure (BiPAP), or noninvasive ventilation (NIV) may provide enough support to allow adequate ventilation. Reintubation should be avoided because it may delay recovery; however, it may become necessary if the earlier mentioned measures fail, with resulting hypoxemia, hypercarbia, and a declining level of consciousness.

Management of Bleeding

Chest tube drainage should be checked every 15 minutes after ICU admission to assess a patient's coagulation status. Although blood loss is commonly divided into two types, surgical or medical, determining the cause of bleeding is often difficult. When bleeding exceeds 400 mL/hour during the first hour, 200 mL/hour for each of the first 2 hours, or 100 mL/hour over the first 4 hours, returning the patient to the OR for chest reexploration should be considered. The clinical situation must be individualized for each patient, however, and in patients with known coagulopathy, more liberal blood loss before chest reexploration may be acceptable (Box 29.4).

Electrolyte Management

Hypokalemia is common after cardiac surgical procedures, especially if diuretic agents were given intraoperatively. Hypokalemia contributes to increased automaticity and may lead to ventricular arrhythmias, ventricular tachycardia, or ventricular fibrillation.

BOX 29.4 *Management of the Bleeding Patient*

Review activated coagulation time, prothrombin time, international normalized ratio, and platelet count
Administer protamine if bleeding is caused by excess heparin (reinfusion of pump blood)
Treat the medical cause with platelets, fresh-frozen plasma, and cryoprecipitate if bleeding is secondary to decreased fibrinogen
Factor VIIa should be considered if bleeding continues despite a normal coagulation profile
Treat the surgical cause with reexploration

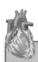

> **BOX 29.5**   *Common Electrolyte Abnormalities and Possible Treatment Options*
>
> **Hypokalemia (Potassium <3.5 mmol/L)**
>
> SSx: muscle weakness, ST-segment depression, "u" wave, T-wave flat, ventricular preexcitation
> Rx: IV KCl at 10–20 mEq/h by central catheter
>
> **Hyperkalemia (Potassium >5.2 mmol/L)**
>
> SSx: muscle weakness, peaked T wave, loss of P wave, prolonged PR/QRS
> Rx: $CaCl_2$ 1 g, insulin/glucose, HCO_3^-, diuretics, hyperventilation, dialysis
>
> **Hypocalcemia (Ionized Calcium <1.1 mmol/L)**
>
> SSx: hypotension, heart failure, prolonged QT interval
> Rx: $CaCl_2$ or calcium gluconate
>
> **Hypercalcemia (Ionized Calcium >1.3 mmol/L)**
>
> SSx: altered mental state, coma, ileus
> Rx: dialysis, diuretics, mithramycin, calcitonin
>
> **Hypermagnesemia (Magnesium >0.7 mmol/L)**
>
> SSx: weakness, absent reflexes
> Rx: stop magnesium infusion, diuresis
>
> **Hypomagnesemia (Magnesium <0.5 mmol/L)**
>
> SSx: arrhythmia, prolonged PR and QT intervals
> Rx: magnesium infusion 1 to 2 g
>
> *$CaCl_2$,* Calcium chloride; *HCO_3^-,* bicarbonate; *IV KCl,* intravenous potassium chloride; *Rx,* treatment; *SSx,* signs and symptoms.

Treatment consists of potassium infusions (20 mEq potassium in 50 mL of D_5W infused over 1 hour) until the potassium level exceeds 3.5 mEq/mL. In patients with frequent premature ventricular contractions caused by increased automaticity, a serum potassium level of 5.0 mEq/mL may be desirable. Hypomagnesemia contributes to ventricular preexcitation and may contribute to atrial fibrillation (AF). This disorder is common in malnourished and chronically ill patients, a frequent occurrence in the cardiac surgical setting. Management consists of intermittent boluses of magnesium: 1 to 2 g over 15 minutes. Hypocalcemia also is frequent during cardiac operations and may reduce cardiac contractility. Intermittent boluses of calcium chloride or calcium gluconate (1 g) may be required (Box 29.5).

Pain Control

Pain control after cardiac surgical procedures has become a concern as narcotic doses have been reduced to facilitate fast-track protocols. Intravenous morphine or hydromorphone is still the mainstay of treatment in patients after cardiac operations. The most common approach is patient-demanded, nurse-delivered intravenous morphine, and this treatment remains popular because of the 1:1 to 1:2 nursing typically

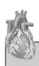

> ## BOX 29.6 *Pain Management Options After Cardiac Surgical Procedures*
>
> **Patient-Controlled Analgesia**
>
> Possible benefit in a step-down unit
> Reduced 24-hour morphine consumption in two of seven randomized trials
>
> **Intrathecal Morphine**
>
> Doses studied: 500 μg to 4 mg
> Possible benefit in reducing intravenous morphine use
> Possible benefit in reducing VAS pain scores
> Potential for respiratory depression
> Ideal dosing not ascertained; range, 250–400 μg
>
> **Thoracic Epidural Regimens**
>
> Common dosages from literature:
>   Ropivacaine 1% with 5 μg/mL fentanyl at 3–5 mL/h
>   Bupivacaine 0.5% with 25 μg/mL morphine at 3–10 mL/h
>   Bupivacaine 0.5–0.75% at 2–5 mL/h
> Reduced pain scores
> Shorter duration of intubation
> Risk for epidural hematoma difficult to quantify
>
> **Nonsteroidal Antiinflammatory Drugs**
>
> Common dosages from literature:
>   Indomethacin 50–100 mg PR bid
>   Diclofenac 50–75 mg PO/PR q8h
>   Ketorolac 10–30 mg IM/IV q8h
> Reduces narcotic utilization
> Many different drugs studied; difficult to determine superiority of a given agent
> Possible increase in serious adverse events (trial using cyclooxygenase-2–specific
>   inhibitors)
>
> *bid*, Twice daily; *IM*, intramuscularly; *IV*, intravenously; *PO*, orally; *PR*, rectally;
> *VAS*, visual analog scale.

29

provided during cardiac recovery. However, with a change to more flexible nurse coverage and therefore higher nurse-to-patient ratios, patient-controlled analgesia (PCA) morphine use has become increasingly popular. However, young patients, those who took opioids preoperatively, or patients transferred to a regular ward on the day of the operation may benefit from PCA for pain management (Box 29.6).

▓ MANAGEMENT OF POSTOPERATIVE COMPLICATIONS

Complications are frequent after cardiac surgical procedures. Although many are short-lived, some complications (eg, stroke) are long-term catastrophic events that seriously affect a patient's functional status. The incidence and predisposing risk factors are well studied for many of these complications. Many complications have specific management issues that may improve postoperative recovery (Box 29.7).

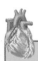

BOX 29.7 Treatment for Complications After Cardiac Surgical Procedures

Stroke

- Supportive treatment
- Avoidance of potential aggravating factors (eg, hyperglycemia, hyperthermia, severe anemia)

Delirium

- Usually self-limited
- Close observation required
- Sedatives (midazolam, lorazepam) possibly required

Atrial Fibrillation

- Rate control: calcium channel blockers, β-blockers, digoxin
- Rhythm control: amiodarone, sotalol, procainamide
- Thromboembolic prophylaxis: for atrial fibrillation >48 h

Left Ventricular Dysfunction

- Volume
- Inotropes: epinephrine, milrinone, norepinephrine
- Mechanical support: intraaortic balloon pump

Renal Failure

- Removal of the causative agent (nonsteroidal antiinflammatory drugs, antibiotics)
- Hemodynamic support if necessary
- Supportive care

🔲 RISK FACTORS FOR RESPIRATORY INSUFFICIENCY

Some cardiac surgical patients can be expected to have respiratory complications. Acute lung injury (ALI), sometimes progressing to acute respiratory distress syndrome (ARDS), can occur in up to 12% of postoperative cardiac patients. Approximately 6% of cardiovascular surgical patients require more than 72 hours on the ventilator, and approximately 1% of patients undergo tracheostomy to facilitate recovery and weaning from prolonged support with mechanical ventilation.

The lung is especially vulnerable because disturbances may affect it directly (atelectasis, effusions, pneumonia) or indirectly (from fluid overload in heart failure; as the result of mediator release from CPB, shock states, or infection; or from changes in respiratory pump function, as with phrenic nerve injury). Postoperative status is determined in part by the patient's preoperative pulmonary reserve, as well as by the level of stress imposed by the procedure. Thus a patient with reduced vital capacity as a result of restrictive lung disease who is undergoing a minimally invasive surgical procedure may have fewer postoperative pulmonary issues than a relatively healthy patient who is undergoing simultaneous coronary artery bypass grafting (CABG) and valve replacement with its longer accompanying operative, anesthetic, and CPB times. Respiratory muscle weakness contributes to postoperative pulmonary dysfunction, and prophylactic inspiratory muscle training has been shown to improve respiratory muscle function, pulmonary function test results, and gas exchange, as well as reducing the incidence of delayed extubation.

Assessing Risk Based on Preoperative Status

The Society of Thoracic Surgeons National Adult Cardiac Surgery Database is widely used in the United States, and it offers, in addition to a mortality prediction, a model customized to predict prolonged ventilation. The European System for Cardiac Operative Risk Evaluation (EuroSCORE) is commonly used in Europe. Factors common to outcome risk adjustment models include age, sex, body surface area, presence of diabetes or renal failure, chronic lung disease, peripheral vascular disease, cerebrovascular disease, previous cardiac operation, and emergency or unstable status. Patients with preexisting chronic obstructive pulmonary disease have higher rates of pulmonary complications (12%), atrial fibrillation (27%), and death (7%).

Operating Room Events

Identification of the patient who is difficult to intubate is important for planning extubation for a time when sufficient personnel and equipment are available to implement a potentially difficult reintubation. Patients undergoing reoperation are at risk partly because of longer CPB times with reoperation, increased use of blood transfusion, and the additional likelihood of bleeding in this population. Length of time on CPB is repeatedly identified as a risk factor, and a correlation between CPB time and inflammatory cytokine release has been demonstrated.

Postoperative Events

The expected ICU course, if the patient is not extubated "on the table," is a short period of ventilation support while the patient is warmed, allowed to awaken, and observed for bleeding or hemodynamic instability. In low-risk patients, short-stay (8-hour) protocols can deliver clinical results at lower cost comparable to a standard overnight ICU stay. Preoperative risks, issues with difficult intubation, and operating room events should be communicated from the operating room team to the ICU team at the time of ICU admission. Box 29.8 outlines criteria to be met before routine extubation.

Health care–acquired infections are important causes of postoperative morbidity and increased costs, and include pneumonia, sepsis, and *Clostridium difficile* colitis. Hospital-acquired pneumonia, and specifically ventilator-acquired pneumonia (VAP), may occur in any patient receiving continuous mechanical ventilation. Studies quote rates of hospital-acquired pneumonia of 3% to 8% for cardiac surgical patients, when assessed by criteria used by the Centers for Disease Control and Prevention (CDC), but these rates are lower when assessed by clinicians taking into account alternate explanations for new infiltrates, tachypnea, or hypoxemia. The historical risk of VAP in ICU patients was approximately 1%/day of ventilation when VAP was diagnosed using protected specimen brush and quantitative culture techniques. Strategies believed to be effective at reducing the incidence of VAP include early removal of nasogastric or endotracheal tubes, formal infection control programs, hand washing, semirecumbent positioning of the patient, daily sedation "vacations," avoidance of unnecessary reintubation, adequate nutritional support, avoidance of gastric overdistension, use of the oral rather than the nasal route for intubation, scheduled drainage of condensate from ventilator circuits, and maintenance of adequate endotracheal tube cuff pressure.

> **BOX 29.8** *Criteria to Be Met Before Early Postoperative Extubation*
>
> *Neurologic*: Awake, neuromuscular blockade fully dissipated (head lift ≥5 s); following instructions, able to cough and protect airway
> *Cardiac*: Stable without mechanical support; cardiac index ≥2.2 L/m² per min; MAP ≥70 mm Hg; no serious arrhythmias
> *Respiratory*: Acceptable CXR and ABGs (pH ≥7.35); minimal secretions, comfortable on CPAP or T-piece with spontaneous respiratory rate ≤20 breaths/min; MIP ≥25 cm H₂O; alternatively, a successful SBT defined as an RSBI <100 and a Pao_2/Fio_2 ≥200
> *Renal*: Undergoing diuresis well; urine output >0.8 mL/kg per h; not markedly fluid-overloaded from operative or CPB fluid administration or SIRS
> *Hematologic*: Chest tube drainage minimal
> *Temperature*: Fully rewarmed; not actively shivering
>
> *ABG*, Arterial blood gas; *CPAP*, continuous positive airway pressure; *CPB*, cardiopulmonary bypass; *CXR*, chest radiograph; *MAP*, mean arterial pressure; *MIP*, maximal inspiratory pressure; Pao_2/Fio_2, ratio of arterial partial pressure of oxygen to fraction of inspired oxygen; *RSBI*, rapid shallow breathing index; *SBT*, spontaneous breathing trial; *SIRS*, systemic immune response syndrome.

Diagnosis of Acute Lung Injury and Acute Respiratory Distress Syndrome

ARDS may develop as a sequela of blood transfusion or CPB, or, more commonly in the postoperative patient, it is associated with cardiogenic shock, sepsis, or multisystem organ failure. Components of ARDS include diffuse alveolar damage resulting from endothelial and type I epithelial cell necrosis and noncardiogenic pulmonary edema caused by breakdown of the endothelial barrier with subsequent vascular permeability. The exudative phase of ARDS occurs in the first 3 days after the precipitating event and is thought to be mediated by neutrophil activation and sequestration. Ultimately the alveolar spaces fill up with fluid as a result of increased endothelial permeability.

The clinical presentation is typically an acute onset of severe arterial hypoxemia refractory to oxygen therapy, with a ratio of arterial oxygen partial pressure to fraction of inspired oxygen (Pao_2/Fio_2 or P/F ratio) of less than 200 mm Hg. ARDS is classically diagnosed only in the absence of left ventricular failure, a factor that complicates the diagnosis in the postoperative cardiac patient, who may also be in heart failure. Other findings in ARDS include decreased lung compliance (<80 mL/cm H₂O) and bilateral infiltrates on chest radiographs.

The proliferative phase of ARDS occurs on days 3 to 7 as inflammatory cells accumulate in response to chemoattractants released by the neutrophils. At this stage, the normal repair process removes debris and begins repair, but a disordered repair process may result in exuberant fibrosis, stiff lungs, and inefficient gas exchange. Evidence suggests that careful fluid and ventilator management may affect this process. Current clinical practice in patients with known or suspected lung injury is to limit inflation pressures. The maximal "safe" inflation pressure is not known, but evidence favors keeping peak inspiratory pressures lower than 35 cm H₂O and restricting tidal volumes to less than 6 mL/kg of ideal body weight in patients at risk for ALI.

ADDITIONAL THERAPY IN PATIENTS WITH ACUTE LUNG INJURY OR ACUTE RESPIRATORY DISTRESS SYNDROME

Maintaining a lung-protective ventilatory strategy involves permissive hypercapnia if normal partial pressure of carbon dioxide (P_{CO_2}) levels cannot be achieved with low tidal volumes. The acid-base changes must be monitored carefully, especially in patients with reactive pulmonary vasculature. Lower tidal volumes with increasing amounts of positive end-expiratory pressure (PEEP) may promote alveolar recruitment and thus improve oxygenation. Taken to an extreme, patients with ALI may be ventilated with high-frequency oscillation, which is essentially high PEEP with tiny (smaller than dead space), frequently delivered tidal volumes. Other techniques for patients in whom conventional therapy is failing include extracorporeal CO_2 removal, extracorporeal membrane oxygenation (ECMO), inhaled nitric oxide, and inhaled prostacyclin. Inhaled nitric oxide has an established role in reducing right ventricular dysfunction when pulmonary hypertension compromises heart transplantation.

Healthy cardiac surgical patients generally do not require much PEEP. Higher levels of PEEP may decrease cardiac output, unless volume loading is used to stabilize preload by maintaining transmural filling pressures. The effects of PEEP are most marked in the presence of abnormal right ventricular function, particularly if the right coronary artery is compromised. PEEP neither protects against the development of ARDS nor reduces the amount of mediastinal bleeding after cardiac surgical procedures involving CPB. Most clinicians routinely use 5 cm H_2O of PEEP in ventilated patients. However, higher levels of PEEP (often 8–15+ cm H_2O) may be necessary to maintain adequate oxygenation with ALI or developing ARDS; application of PEEP in the postsurgical patient usually involves balancing cardiac and pulmonary goals.

IMPEDIMENTS TO WEANING AND EXTUBATION

Factors limiting the removal of mechanical ventilatory support include delirium, neurologic dysfunction, unstable hemodynamic status, respiratory muscle dysfunction, renal failure with fluid overload, and sepsis. Fig. 29.2 outlines one approach to identifying readiness to wean from ventilation and possible alternative approaches to weaning. Early mobilization, including formal exercise programs, can enhance recovery from the catabolic muscle loss with critical illness.

MODES OF VENTILATOR SUPPORT

Positive-pressure ventilators used outside the operating room have a non-rebreathing circuit, may be volume- or pressure-limited, and may be triggered by changes in flow or changes in pressure. All modern ventilators contain multiple modes of ventilation support that accommodate both mandatory and patient-triggered breaths. The most common modes of positive-pressure ventilation are assist-control (A/C), synchronized intermittent mandatory ventilation (SIMV), and pressure-support ventilation (PSV). With volume modes, the inspiratory flow rate, targeted volume, and inspiratory time are set by the clinician, and inspiratory peak pressure varies depending on the patient's lung compliance and synchrony with the ventilator. Volume cycling ensures consistent delivery of a set tidal volume, as long as the pressure limit is not exceeded. With nonhomogeneous lung disorders, however, delivered volume tends to flow to areas of low resistance; this may result in overdistension of healthy segments of lung and

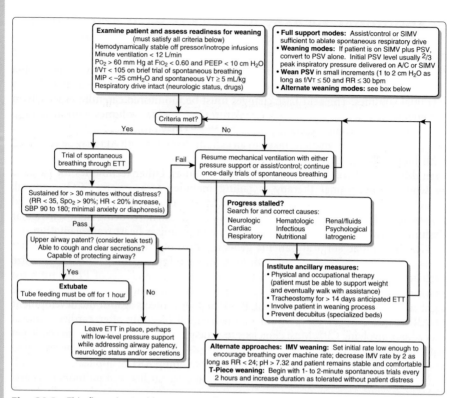

Fig. 29.2 This flow chart addresses care of patients receiving both short-term and long-term ventilatory support in the cardiothoracic intensive care unit. All patients require periodic assessment for readiness for weaning, and if they meet criteria they are eligible for spontaneous trials leading to extubation. Patients who do not meet the criteria should have mechanical ventilation maintained until criteria are met. Pressure-support ventilation *(PSV)* weaning may be possible; if not, alternative approaches include intermittent mandatory ventilation *(IMV)* weaning and T-piece weaning. Patients who stall in their weaning progress should have a comprehensive examination and an assessment of organ systems to search for correctable causes. *A/C,* Assist-control mode; *bpm,* breaths per minute; *ETT,* endotracheal tube; *FiO₂,* ratio of arterial partial pressure of oxygen to fraction of inspired oxygen; *f/VT,* frequency-to-tidal volume ratio; *HR,* heart rate; *MIP,* maximal inspiratory pressure; *PEEP,* positive end-expiratory pressure; *PO₂,* partial pressure of oxygen; *RR,* respiratory rate; *SBP,* systolic blood pressure; *SIMV,* synchronized intermittent mandatory ventilation; *SpO₂,* oxygen saturation measured with pulse oximetry.

underinflation of atelectatic segments with consequent ventilation/perfusion ($\dot{V}/\dot{Q}$) mismatching.

Intermittent mandatory ventilation (IMV) and later SIMV were developed to facilitate weaning from mechanical ventilatory support. With either IMV modality, a basal respiratory rate is set by the clinician that may be supplemented by patient-initiated breaths. In contrast to A/C ventilation, however, the tidal volume of the patient's spontaneous breaths is determined by the patient's own respiratory strength and lung compliance rather than delivered as a preset volume. SIMV mode is appropriate for patients with normal lungs who are recovering from opioid anesthesia. Weaning is accomplished by reducing the mandatory IMV rate and allowing the patient to assume more and more of the respiratory effort over time. SIMV mode has been used for weaning in patients with complex cases, but the weaning effort may stall at very low IMV rates if the patient cannot achieve spontaneous volumes sufficient to activate the pulmonary stretch receptors. Under these circumstances, the patient is likely to become tachypneic, and weaning attempts will fail.

Pressure-Support Ventilation

PSV, which is primarily a weaning tool, must be distinguished from pressure-control ventilation, which is generally used during the maintenance phase of ventilation. PSV may be used in conjunction with CPAP or SIMV modes. Pressure support augments the patient's spontaneous inspiratory effort with a clinician-selected level of pressure. Putative advantages include improved comfort for the patient, reduced ventilatory work, and faster weaning. The volume delivered with each PSV breath depends on the pressure set for inspiratory assist, as well as the patient's lung compliance. The utility of PSV in weaning from long-term ventilation support is that it allows the patient's ventilatory muscles to assume part of the workload while augmenting tidal volume, thus preventing atelectasis, sufficiently stretching lung receptors, and keeping the patient's spontaneous respiratory rate within a reasonable physiologic range.

■ LIBERATION FROM MECHANICAL SUPPORT (WEANING)

When terminating mechanical ventilation, two phases of decision making are involved. First, resolution of the initial process for which mechanical ventilation was begun should occur. The patient cannot have sepsis, be hemodynamically unstable, or be burdened with excessive respiratory secretions. If these general criteria are met, then specific weaning criteria can be examined. These include oxygenation (typically a PaO_2 >60 mm Hg on 35% inspired oxygen and low levels of PEEP), adequate oxygen transport (measurable by oxygen extraction ratio or assumed if the cardiac index is adequate and lactic acidosis is not present), adequate respiratory mechanics (tidal volume, maximal inspiratory pressure) and adequate respiratory reserve (minute ventilation at rest of <10 L/min), and a low frequency-to–tidal volume ratio (f/Vt <100; see next section) indicating adequate volume at a sustainable respiratory rate.

Weaning: the Process

The actual process of weaning from mechanical ventilatory support must be individualized. No "one size fits all" method exists. While gradually lowering the SIMV rate in increments of two breaths/minute generally works for short-term ventilatory support, patients receiving long-term ventilatory support often have difficulty making the transition from SIMV rates of two breaths/minute to CPAP. The time-honored method of weaning by maintaining a patient on full ventilatory support and alternating with increasingly longer periods of spontaneous ventilation on a T-piece is effective, but it is time consuming because it requires setting up additional equipment and also requires a nurse or respiratory therapist to be immediately available at the bedside during each weaning attempt. Diaphragmatic effort is significantly lower during a T-piece trial with a deflated tracheostomy tube cuff than with the cuff inflated. Weaning trials with the cuff deflated may thus be more physiologic when attempting weaning from the ventilator in a patient for whom this process is difficult. Breath-to-breath monitoring, display of tidal volumes, and ventilator alarms are not available during a T-piece trial. More commonly, pressure support is used as an adjunct to weaning either with IMV or CPAP while the patient is still connected to the ventilator and its alarm system.

29

Our preference is to conduct CPAP weaning with pressure support alone (ie, no additional IMV rate) because mechanical ventilation introduces one more variable into the evaluation of a patient's progress. Sufficient CPAP is applied to maintain open alveoli (generally 5–8 cm H_2O, but often higher when recovering from ALI or ARDS), and then the pressure-support level is titrated to provide the patient with sufficient tidal volume to achieve a respiratory rate lower than 24 breaths/minute. Rapid rates are detrimental to weaning, because diaphragmatic blood flow is limited during contraction. As the patient's exercise tolerance improves, the pressure-support level can be lowered in increments of 2 to 3 cm H_2O. It is usually necessary to address fluid overload, nutritional support, and other nonpulmonary factors to achieve the pressure-support reduction.

Specific Impediments to Weaning

Weaning from ventilator support affects cardiac output in response to changes in pulmonary vascular resistance. Increased pulmonary vascular resistance can lead to septal shifts and consequent changes in the efficiency of right ventricular and left ventricular function. Thus it makes little sense to attempt weaning in the hemodynamically unstable patient. Our approach has been to keep these patients on full ventilator support with sedation and neuromuscular blockade if necessary until the acute cardiac problem is resolved.

Tracheostomy

Prolonged endotracheal intubation results in damage to the respiratory epithelium and cilia and may lead to vocal cord damage and airway stenosis. If mechanical ventilation is anticipated for longer than 14 days, consideration should be given to early tracheostomy. Other indications for tracheostomy include copious or tenacious secretions in debilitated patients who are unable to clear secretions spontaneously. Tracheostomy is relatively contraindicated in patients with ongoing mediastinitis or local infection at the tracheostomy site because of the potential for mediastinal contamination with respiratory secretions.

Inability to Wean

A few patients are not able to be weaned from ventilator support despite all efforts. Predictive models, however, are rarely useful for deciding which patients will not benefit from further intensive care.

It is rarely a single problem, but rather the interactions among multiple morbidities that create a situation in which the patient may never be able to achieve the "escape velocity" needed to separate from the ventilator. At this point, a discussion with the patient (if he or she has decisional capacity) or the health care proxy can be helpful in defining the benefits and burdens of further therapy and the patient's desires. Consultation with the hospital's ethics team may be very helpful. A frank assessment of which problems can be "fixed" versus those that are irreversible will define care options. Patients who remain in low–cardiac output states cannot resolve their multiple organ failure, and thus their dependence on high-technology support continues, including ventilation and hemodialysis. Unless patients are candidates for long-term ventricular assist devices or heart transplantation, they are facing a slow, technology-assisted decline that will end in an untreatable infection. Conversely, malnutrition and deconditioning in the absence of ongoing sepsis and organ system failure sometimes respond to prolonged rehabilitation, which may be better handled by a long-term ventilation facility than an acute care hospital. The critical issue is the patient's reserve because, unless the patient has adequate cardiac and pulmonary reserve to tolerate stress once all remediable problems have been addressed, indefinite technologic support (ventilation, dialysis) will be required.

SUGGESTED READINGS

Badhwar V, Esper S, Brooks M, et al. Extubating in the operating room after adult cardiac surgery safely improves outcomes and lowers costs. *J Thorac Cardiovasc Surg.* 2014;148:3101–3109.

Baghban M, Paknejad O, Yousefshahi F, et al. Hospital-acquired pneumonia in patients undergoing coronary artery bypass graft: comparison of the center for disease control clinical criteria with physicians' judgment. *Anesth Pain Med.* 2014;17:e20733.

Bainbridge D, Martin JE, Cheng DC. Patient-controlled versus nurse-controlled analgesia after cardiac surgery: a meta-analysis. *Can J Anaesth.* 2006;53(5):492–499.

Branca P, McGaw P, Light R. Factors associated with prolonged mechanical ventilation following coronary artery bypass surgery. *Chest.* 2001;119:537–546.

Bucerius J, Gummert JF, Borger MA, et al. Predictors of delirium after cardiac surgery delirium: effect of beating-heart (off-pump) surgery. *J Thorac Cardiovasc Surg.* 2004;127(1):57–64.

Canver CC, Chanda J. Intraoperative and postoperative risk factors for respiratory failure after coronary bypass. *Ann Thorac Surg.* 2003;75:853–857.

Chacko B, Peter JV, Tharyan P, et al. Pressure-controlled versus volume-controlled ventilation for acute respiratory failure due to acute lung injury (ALI) or acute respiratory distress syndrome (ARDS). *Cochrane Database Syst Rev.* 2015;(1):CD008807.

Cheng DC, Newman MF, Duke P, et al. The efficacy and resource utilization of remifentanil and fentanyl in fast-track coronary artery bypass graft surgery: a prospective randomized, double-blinded controlled, multi-center trial. *Anesth Analg.* 2001;92(5):1094–1102.

Engelman D, Higgins TL, Talati R, et al. Maintaining situational awareness in a cardiac intensive care unit. *J Thorac Cardiovasc Surg.* 2014;147:1105–1106.

Gerstein NS, Gerstein WH, Carey MC, et al. The thrombotic and arrhythmogenic risks of perioperative NSAIDs. *J Cardiothorac Vasc Anesth.* 2014;28:369–374.

Gilstrap D, MacIntyre N. Patient-ventilator interactions: implications for clinical management. *Am J Respir Crit Care Med.* 2013;188:1058–1068.

Haddad F, Couture P, Tousignant C, et al. The right ventricle in cardiac surgery, a perioperative perspective: II. Pathophysiology, clinical importance, and management. *Anesth Analg.* 2009;108(2):422–433.

Kuiper AN, Trof RJ, Groeneveld AB. Mixed venous O_2 saturation and fluid responsiveness after cardiac or major vascular surgery. *J Cardiothorac Surg.* 2013;22(8):189.

Lopes CR, Brandao CM, Nozawa E, et al. Benefits of non-invasive ventilation after extubation in the postoperative period of heart surgery. *Rev Bras Cir Cardiovasc.* 2008;23:344–350.

Myles PS, Daly DJ, Djaiani G, et al. A systematic review of the safety and effectiveness of fast-track cardiac anesthesia. *Anesthesiology.* 2003;99(4):982–987.

Probst S, Cech C, Haentschel D, et al. A specialized post anaesthetic care unit improves fast-track management in cardiac surgery: a prospective randomized trial. *Crit Care.* 2014;18(4):468.

Pronovost P, Berenholtz S, Dorman T, et al. Improving communication in the ICU using daily goals. *J Crit Care.* 2003;18:71–75.

Raghunathan K, Murray PT, Beattie WS, et al. Choice of fluid in acute illness: what should be given? An international consensus. *Br J Anaesth.* 2014;113(5):772–783.

Schweickert WD, Gehlbach BK, Pohlman AS, et al. Daily interruption of sedative infusions and complications of critical illness in mechanically ventilated patients. *Crit Care Med.* 2004;32(6):1272–1276.

Zhu F, Gomersall CD, Ng SK, et al. A randomized controlled trial of adaptive support ventilation mode to wean patients after fast-track cardiac valvular surgery. *Anesthesiology.* 2015;122:832–840.

29

Chapter 30

Postoperative Cardiovascular Management

Jerrold H. Levy, MD, FAHA, FCCM •
Kamrouz Ghadimi, MD • James M. Bailey, MD •
James G. Ramsay, MD, PhD

Key Points

1. Maintaining oxygen transport and oxygen delivery appropriately to meet the tissue metabolic needs is the goal of postoperative circulatory control.
2. Cardiac function worsens after cardiac surgical procedures. Therapeutic approaches to reverse this dysfunction are important and often can be discontinued in the first few postoperative days.
3. Myocardial ischemia often occurs postoperatively, and it is associated with adverse cardiac outcomes. Multiple strategies have been studied to reduce this complication.
4. Postoperative biventricular dysfunction is common. It requires interventions to optimize the heart rate and rhythm, provide acceptable preload, and adjust afterload and contractility. In most patients, pharmacologic interventions can be rapidly weaned or stopped within the first 24 hours postoperatively.
5. Supraventricular tachyarrhythmias are common in the first postoperative days, with atrial fibrillation predominating. Preoperative and immediate postoperative pharmacotherapy can reduce the incidence and slow the ventricular response.
6. Postoperative hypertension has been a common complication of cardiac surgical procedures; newer vasodilator drugs are more arterial selective and allow greater circulatory stability than older, nonselective drugs.
7. Catecholamines, phosphodiesterase inhibitors, and the calcium sensitizer levosimendan have been studied for treating biventricular dysfunction.
8. Phosphodiesterase inhibitors and levosimendan are clinically effective inodilators that have important roles in patients with low cardiac output and biventricular dysfunction.
9. Long cardiopulmonary bypass times may cause a refractory vasodilated state ("vasoplegia") requiring combinations of pressors such as norepinephrine and vasopressin.
10. Positive-pressure ventilation has multiple effects on the cardiovascular system, with complex interactions that should be considered in patients after cardiac surgical procedures.
11. Critical care management of patients undergoing transcatheter aortic valve replacement who have experienced intraoperative complications includes understanding and managing the postoperative consequences of iatrogenic vascular injuries, stroke, significant paravalvular leaks, and/or cardiac conduction abnormalities.
12. Hemodynamic management after cardiothoracic operations may benefit from the use of transesophageal echocardiography to determine myocardial function and assess cardiovascular structures. Echocardiography is particularly helpful in the diagnosis of causes of obstructive shock, including pericardial effusions leading to tamponade physiology.

13. Echocardiography during the daily management of both venovenous and venoarterial extracorporeal membrane oxygenation (ECMO) may improve diagnosis of hemodynamic instability, troubleshoot common problems encountered during ECMO management, and aid in weaning the patient from mechanical support.

Postoperative cardiovascular dysfunction is becoming more common as older and increasingly critically ill patients undergo cardiac surgical procedures. Biventricular dysfunction and circulatory changes occur after cardiopulmonary bypass (CPB), but they can also occur in patients undergoing off-pump procedures. Pharmacologic therapy with suitable monitoring and mechanical support may be needed for patients in the postoperative period until ventricular or circulatory dysfunction improves.

OXYGEN TRANSPORT

Maintaining oxygen transport (ie, oxygen delivery [Do_2]) satisfactory to meet the tissue metabolic needs is the goal of postoperative circulatory control. Oxygen transport is the product of cardiac output (CO) times arterial content of oxygen (Cao_2) (ie, hemoglobin concentration $\times$ 1.34 mL of oxygen per 1 g of hemoglobin $\times$ oxygen saturation [Sao_2]), and it can be affected in many ways by the cardiovascular and respiratory systems, as shown in Fig. 30.1. Low CO, anemia from blood loss, and pulmonary disease can decrease Do_2. Before altering the determinants of CO, including the inotropic state of the ventricles, an acceptable hemoglobin concentration and adequate Sao_2 should be provided, thus enabling increases in CO to supply the maximum available Do_2.

Hypoxemia from any cause reduces Do_2, and acceptable arterial oxygenation (partial arterial pressure of oxygen [Pao_2]) may be achieved with the use of an elevated inspired oxygen fraction (Fio_2) or positive end-expiratory pressure (PEEP) in the ventilated patient. Use of PEEP or continuous positive airway pressure (CPAP) in the spontaneously breathing patient may improve Pao_2 by reducing intrapulmonary shunt; however, venous return may be reduced, causing a decrease in CO, with Do_2 decreased despite an increased Pao_2. It is important to measure CO as PEEP is applied. Intravascular volume expansion may be used to offset this damaging effect of PEEP.

Unexplained hypoxemia may be caused by right-to-left intracardiac shunting, most commonly by a patent foramen ovale. This situation is most likely to occur when right-sided pressures are abnormally increased; an example is the use of high

30

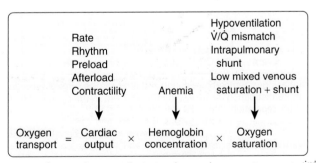

Fig. 30.1 Important factors that contribute to abnormal oxygen transport. $\dot{V}/\dot{Q}$, Ventilation/perfusion.

levels of PEEP. If this condition is suspected, echocardiography should be performed, and therapy to reduce right-sided pressures should be initiated.

Patients with pulmonary disease may experience dramatic worsening of oxygenation when vasodilator therapy is started because of release of hypoxic vasoconstriction in areas of diseased lung. Although CO may be increased, the worsening in CaO_2 results in a decrease in DO_2. Reduced doses of direct-acting vasodilators or trials of different agents may be indicated.

When DO_2 cannot be increased to an acceptable level as judged by decreased organ function or development of lactic acidemia, measures to decrease oxygen consumption ($\dot{V}O_2$) may be taken while awaiting improvement in cardiac or pulmonary function. For example, sedation and paralysis may buy time to allow reversible postoperative myocardial dysfunction to improve.

TEMPERATURE

Patients are often admitted to the intensive care unit (ICU) after cardiac operations with core temperatures lower than 35°C, especially after off-pump cardiac surgical procedures. The typical pattern of temperature change during and after cardiac operations and the hemodynamic outcomes are illustrated in Fig. 30.2. Decreases in temperature after CPB occur in part because of redistribution of heat within the body and in part because of heat loss. Monitoring of body sites other than the blood and brain (eg, urinary bladder, tympanic membrane temperatures) can help provide more complete rewarming, but the body temperature usually falls after CPB, especially when difficulties are encountered and the chest remains open for an extended period; in such cases, some degree of hypothermia is an almost unavoidable result. Intraoperative

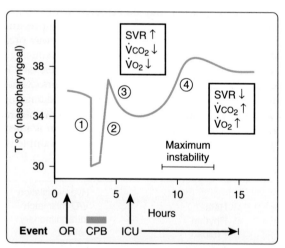

Fig. 30.2 Nasopharyngeal temperature during and after cardiac surgical procedures. *(1)* Core (ie, blood) cooling on cardiopulmonary bypass *(CPB)*. *(2)* Core warming on CPB. *(3)* Afterdrop in temperature *(T)* after separation from CPB. *(4)* Rewarming after admission to the intensive care unit *(ICU)*. Systemic vascular resistance *(SVR)* is increased, and carbon dioxide production *($\dot{V}CO_2$)* and oxygen consumption *($\dot{V}O_2$)* are decreased on admission to the ICU because of residual hypothermia. During rapid rewarming, SVR decreases and $\dot{V}CO_2$ and $\dot{V}O_2$ increase; these changes can cause marked cardiac and ventilatory instability. *OR,* Operating room. (From Sladen RN. Management of the adult cardiac patient in the intensive care unit. In: Ream AK, Fogdall RP, eds. *Acute cardiovascular management: anesthesia and intensive care.* Philadelphia: Lippincott; 1982:495.)

use of forced-air warming blankets or cutaneous gel pads can help reduce the temperature loss during and after surgical procedures.

The normal thermoregulatory and metabolic responses to hypothermia remain intact after cardiac operations and result in peripheral vasoconstriction that contributes to the hypertension commonly seen early in the ICU. As temperature decreases, CO is decreased because of bradycardia, whereas oxygen consumed per beat is actually increased. Another adverse consequence of postoperative hypothermia is a large increase in $\dot{V}O_2$ and carbon dioxide production during rewarming. When patients cannot increase CO (ie, DO_2), the effects of this large increase in $\dot{V}O_2$ include mixed venous desaturation and metabolic acidosis. Unless end-tidal carbon dioxide is monitored or arterial blood gases are analyzed often to show the increased carbon dioxide production and to guide increases in ventilation, hypercarbia will occur, causing catecholamine release, tachycardia, and pulmonary hypertension. The effects of rewarming are most intense when patients shiver. Shivering may be effectively treated with meperidine, which lowers the threshold for shivering. Muscle relaxation may provide more stable hemodynamic conditions than meperidine, but accompanying sedation must be administered to avoid having an awake and paralyzed patient.

As the temperature rises, usually to approximately 36°C, vasoconstriction and hypertension are replaced by vasodilation, tachycardia, and hypotension, even without hypercarbia. Often, over minutes, a patient who needs vasodilators for hypertension then requires vasopressors or large volumes of fluid for hypotension. Volume loading during the rewarming period can help reduce the rapid swings in blood pressure (BP) that may occur. It is important to recognize when these changes result from changes in body temperature, to avoid attributing them to other processes that may call for different therapy.

ASSESSMENT OF THE CIRCULATION

Surgical dressings, chest tubes attached to suction, fluid in the mediastinum and pleural spaces, peripheral edema, and temperature gradients can distort or mask information obtained by the classic techniques of inspection, palpation, and auscultation in the postoperative period. However, the physician should not be deterred from applying these basic techniques in view of their potential benefit. Physical examination may be of great value in diagnosing gross or acute disease, such as pneumothorax, hemothorax, or acute valvular insufficiency, but it is of limited value in diagnosing and managing ventricular failure. For example, in the critical care setting, experienced clinicians (eg, internists) using only physical findings often misjudge cardiac filling pressures by a large margin. Low CO in particular is not consistently recognized by clinical signs, and systemic BP does not correlate with CO after cardiac surgical procedures. Oliguria and metabolic acidosis, classic indicators of a low CO, are not always reliable because of the polyuria induced by hypothermia, oxygen debts induced during CPB that cause acidosis, and medications or fluids given during or immediately after bypass.

Although clinicians are taught that the adequacy of CO can be assessed by the quality of the pulses, capillary refill, and peripheral temperature, no relationship exists between these indicators of peripheral perfusion and CO or calculated systemic vascular resistance (SVR) in the postoperative period. Many patients arrive in the ICU in a hypothermic state, and residual anesthetic agents can decrease the threshold for peripheral vasoconstriction in response to this condition. A patient's extremities may therefore remain warm despite a hypothermic core or a decreasing CO. Even after temperature stabilization on the first postoperative day, the relationship between peripheral perfusion and CO is too crude to be used for hemodynamic management.

Despite the lack of a proven benefit with pulmonary artery catheter (PAC) use, many patients continue to have this monitor placed for cardiac surgical procedures. Cardiac anesthesiologists believe that the lack of evidence about the PAC may reflect the lack of a modern, well-designed randomized trial. That no such trials have been conducted in cardiac surgical patients probably attests to the reluctance of cardiac surgeons and anesthesiologists to manage their patients without what they consider to be important information. Postoperatively, many cardiac surgical centers do not have in-house physicians, and surgeons believe that the "objective" PAC data obtained over the telephone is valuable. As less invasive tools such as echocardiography or arterial waveform analysis devices become better known and more readily available, it seems likely that PAC use will diminish further in cardiac surgical patients.

Echocardiography is the technique of choice for acute assessment of cardiac function. Just as transesophageal echocardiography (TEE) has become essential for intraoperative management in various conditions, several studies document its utility in the post-operative period in the presence and absence of the PAC. It provides information that may lead to urgent surgery or prevent unnecessary surgery, gives important information about cardiac preload, and can detect acute structural and functional abnormalities. Although transthoracic echocardiography (TTE) can be performed more rapidly in this setting, satisfactory images can be obtained only in about 50% of patients in the ICU. A small lumen single plane disposable echocardiography device, Imacor, has been developed for use up to 72 hours for ICU management.

POSTOPERATIVE MYOCARDIAL DYSFUNCTION

Studies using hemodynamic, nuclear scanning, and metabolic techniques have documented worsening in cardiac function after coronary artery bypass grafting (CABG) procedures. All these studies showed significant declines in left ventricular (LV) or biventricular (when measured) function in the first postoperative hours, with a gradual return to preoperative values by 8 to 24 hours. Decreased ventricular performance at normal or elevated filling pressures occurs, suggesting decreased contractility. Similarly, "flattening" of the ventricular function curves is usually obvious; this finding suggests that preload expansion greater than 10 mm Hg for central venous pressure (CVP) or 12 mm Hg for pulmonary capillary wedge pressure (PCWP) is of little benefit.

Satisfactory myocardial protection is important to prevent postoperative dysfunction. In off-pump surgical procedures, the idea is to preserve coronary perfusion, but during mechanical manipulation, changes in CO and BP occur. For CABG with CPB, most surgeons use some combination of hypothermia and crystalloid or blood cardioplegia to arrest the heart and reduce its metabolism. Although little consensus exists that any one technique is preferable in all circumstances, cold intermittent crystalloid cardioplegia with systemic hypothermia is the most widely used technique clinically. Other proposed factors that contribute to postoperative ventricular dysfunction include myocardial ischemia, residual hypothermia, preoperative medications such as β-adrenergic antagonists, and ischemia-reperfusion injury (Box 30.1).

POSTOPERATIVE MYOCARDIAL ISCHEMIA

Although intraoperative myocardial ischemia has often been a focus, studies showed that ischemia frequently occurs postoperatively and is associated with adverse cardiac

> **BOX 30.1** *Risk Factors for Low Cardiac Output Syndrome After Cardiopulmonary Bypass*
>
> Preoperative left ventricular dysfunction
> Valvular heart disease requiring repair or replacement
> Long aortic cross-clamp time and total cardiopulmonary bypass time
> Inadequate cardiac surgical repair
> Myocardial ischemia and reperfusion
> Residual effects of cardioplegia solution
> Poor myocardial preservation
> Reperfusion injury and inflammatory changes

outcomes. Electrocardiographic (ECG) and segmental wall motion abnormality (SWMA) evidence of ischemia occur early postoperatively in up to 40% of patients undergoing CABG procedures. Postbypass SWMAs were significantly associated with adverse outcomes (eg, myocardial infarction [MI], death). Surprisingly, these abnormalities most often appeared in the regions of the heart that had been revascularized. Hemodynamic changes rarely preceded ischemia; however, postoperative heart rates (HRs) were significantly higher than intraoperative or preoperative values. Whether such changes occur because of operation and reperfusion or as a result of events after CPB is not known. These findings do suggest that monitoring for ischemia must continue after revascularization. It may be that early recognition and treatment of ischemia or prophylactic medication can help prevent or reduce myocardial ischemia and dysfunction after CABG procedures.

THERAPEUTIC INTERVENTIONS

Therapeutic interventions for postoperative biventricular dysfunction include the standard concerns of managing low-CO states by controlling the HR and rhythm, providing an acceptable preload, and adjusting afterload and contractility. In most patients, pharmacologic interventions can be rapidly weaned or stopped within the first 24 hours postoperatively.

Postoperative Arrhythmias

Patients with preoperative or newly acquired noncompliant ventricles need a correctly timed atrial contraction to provide satisfactory ventricular filling, especially when they are in sinus rhythm preoperatively. Although atrial contraction provides approximately 20% of ventricular filling, this may be more important in postoperative patients, when ventricular dysfunction and reduced compliance may be present. For example, in medical patients with acute MI, atrial systole contributed 35% of the stroke volume (SV). The SV is often relatively fixed in patients with ventricular dysfunction, and the HR is an important determinant of CO. Rate and rhythm disorders must be corrected when possible, using epicardial pacing wires. Approaches to postoperative rate and rhythm disturbances are shown in Table 30.1.

Later in the postoperative period (days 1 through 3), supraventricular tachyarrhythmias become a major problem, with atrial fibrillation (AF) predominating. The

30

Table 30.1	Postoperative Rate and Rhythm Disturbances	
Disturbance	Usual Causes	Treatments
Sinus bradycardia	Preoperative or intraoperative β-blockade	Atrial pacing, β-agonist, anticholinergic
Heart block (first, second, and third degree)	Ischemia Surgical trauma	Atrioventricular sequential pacing Catecholamines
Sinus tachycardia	Agitation or pain Hypovolemia Catecholamines	Sedation or analgesia Volume administration Change or discontinuance of drug
Atrial tachyarrhythmias	Catecholamines Chamber distension Electrolyte disorder (hypokalemia, hypomagnesemia)	Change or discontinuance of drug Treatment of underlying cause (eg, vasodilator, diuresis, potassium or magnesium administration) May require synchronized cardioversion or pharmacotherapy
Ventricular tachycardia or fibrillation	Ischemia Catecholamines	Cardioversion Treat ischemia, may require pharmacotherapy Change or discontinuance of drug

overall incidence is between 30% and 40%, but with increasing age and valvular surgical procedures, the incidence may be in excess of 60%. Many reasons are recognized for this development, including inadequate intraoperative atrial protection, electrolyte abnormalities, change in atrial size with fluid shifts, epicardial inflammation, stress, irritation, and genetic factors. When AF or other supraventricular arrhythmias develop, treatment is often urgently needed for symptomatic relief or hemodynamic benefit. The longer a patient remains in AF, the more difficult it may be to convert the rhythm, and the greater is the risk for thrombus formation and embolization. Treatable underlying conditions such as electrolyte disturbances or pain should be corrected while specific pharmacologic therapy is being instituted. Paroxysmal supraventricular tachycardia (uncommon in this setting) can be abolished or converted to sinus rhythm by intravenous adenosine, and atrial flutter can sometimes be converted by overdrive atrial pacing with temporary wires placed at the time of operation. Electrical cardioversion may be needed if hypotension is caused by the rapid HR; however, atrial arrhythmias tend to recur in this setting. Rate control for AF or atrial flutter can be achieved with various atrioventricular (AV) nodal blocking drugs, and conversion is facilitated by many of these drugs as well. Table 30.2 summarizes the various treatment modalities for supraventricular arrhythmias. If conversion to sinus rhythm does not occur, electrical cardioversion in the presence of antiarrhythmic drug therapy should be attempted, or anticoagulation should be started.

Preload

Assessment of preload is probably the single most important clinical skill for managing hemodynamic instability. Preload rapidly changes in the postoperative period because of bleeding, spontaneous diuresis, vasodilation during warming, the effects of positive-pressure ventilation and PEEP on venous return, capillary leak, and other causes.

Table 30.2 Treatment Modalities for Supraventricular Arrhythmias

Treatment	Specifics[a]	Indications
Overdrive pacing by atrial wires[b]	Requires rapid pacer ($\leq$800/min); start above arrhythmia rate and slowly decrease	PAT, atrial flutter
Adenosine	Bolus dose of 6–12 mg; may cause 10 s of complete heart block	AV nodal tachycardia, bypass-tract arrhythmia, atrial arrhythmia diagnosis
Amiodarone	150 mg IV over 10 min, followed by infusion	Rate control or conversion to NSR in atrial fibrillation or flutter
β-Blockade	Esmolol, up to 0.5 mg/kg load over 1 min, followed by infusion if tolerated	Rate control or conversion to NSR in atrial fibrillation or flutter
	Metoprolol, 0.5–5 mg, repeat effective dose q4–6h	Rate control or conversion to NSR in atrial fibrillation or/flutter
	Propranolol, 0.25–1 mg; repeat effective dose q4h[c]	
	Labetalol, 2.5–10 mg; repeat effective dose q4h[c]	Conversion of atrial fibrillation or flutter to NSR
	Sotalol, 40–80 mg PO q12h	Conversion of PAT to NSR
Ibutilide	1 mg over 10 min; may repeat after 10 min	Rate control or conversion to NSR in atrial fibrillation or flutter
Verapamil	2.5–5 mg IV, repeated PRN[c]	
Diltiazem	0.2 mg/kg over 2 min, followed by 10–15 mg/h[d]	Rate control or conversion to NSR in atrial fibrillation or flutter
Procainamide	50 mg/min up to 1 g, followed by 1–4 mg/min	Rate control or conversion to NSR in atrial fibrillation or flutter, prevention of recurrence of arrhythmias, treatment of wide-complex tachycardias[e]
Digoxin[f]	Load of 1 mg in divided doses over 4–24 h[g]; may give additional 0.125-mg doses 2 h apart (3–4 doses)	Rate control or conversion to NSR in atrial fibrillation or flutter
Synchronized cardioversion	50–300 J (external); most effective with anterior-posterior patches	Acute tachyarrhythmia with hemodynamic compromise (usually atrial fibrillation or flutter)

[a]See specific drug monographs for full descriptions of indications, contraindications, and dosages. Doses are for intravenous administration; use the lowest dose, and administer slowly in patients with hemodynamic compromise.

[b]Verify that the pacer is not capturing the ventricle.

[c]Infusion may provide better control. This drug is less useful than diltiazem because of myocardial depression.

[d]Limited experience; may cause less hypotension than verapamil.

[e]When diagnosis is unclear (ventricular versus supraventricular) and no acute hemodynamic compromise is present (ie, cardioversion not indicated).

[f]Less useful than other drugs because of its slow onset and modest effect.

[g]Rate of administration depends on the urgency of rate control.

AV, Atrioventricular; *IV,* intravenously; *NSR,* normal sinus rhythm; *PAT,* paroxysmal atrial tachycardia; *PO,* orally; *PRN,* as needed.

30

Direct assessment of preload is clinically feasible using echocardiography. A fair-to-good correlation exists between echocardiographic and radionuclide measures of end-diastolic volume and a good correlation between end-diastolic area measured by TEE and SV. Although the use of echocardiography to assess preload must always be tempered by the realization that the clinician is viewing a two-dimensional image of a three-dimensional object, this is the most direct technique clinically available. Greater awareness of the value of TEE in the ICU and increased availability of echocardiography in general have made this modality a first choice for the assessment of preload in the setting of acute unexplained or refractory hypotension. Without echocardiography, pressure measurements are used as surrogates for volume measurements. For example, in the absence of mitral valve disease, left atrial pressure (LAP) is almost equal to LV end-diastolic pressure (LVEDP), and pulmonary artery occlusion pressure (PAOP) is almost equivalent to these two pressures. In patients without LAP catheters, the PAOP or the pulmonary artery diastolic pressure is used.

When ventricular compliance is normal and the ventricle is not distended, small changes in end-diastolic volume are usually accompanied by small changes in end-diastolic pressure. In patients with noncompliant ventricles from preexisting congestive heart failure (HF), chronic hypertrophy resulting from hypertension or valvular disease, postoperative MI, or ventricular dysfunction, small increases in ventricular volume may produce rapid increases in end-diastolic pressure that require therapeutic intervention. Increased intraventricular pressure elevates myocardial oxygen demand ($M\dot{v}O_2$) and decreases subendocardial coronary artery blood flow. Myocardial ischemia may be the result. Elevations in LVEDP are transmitted to the pulmonary circulation, thus causing congestion and possibly hydrostatic pulmonary edema.

Contractility

Quantifying the contractility of the intact heart has been complicated by the difficulty of finding a variable to measure contractility that is also independent of preload and afterload. Therapy for decreased contractility should be directed toward correcting any reversible causes, such as myocardial depressants, metabolic abnormalities, or myocardial ischemia. If the cause of depressed myocardial contractility is irreversible, positive inotropic agents may be necessary to keep CO satisfactory to support organ function.

Afterload

Calculated SVR continues to be used in guiding therapy or drawing conclusions about the state of the circulation. This should be done only cautiously, if at all. SVR is not a complete indicator of afterload. Even if SVR were an accurate measure of impedance, the response to vasoactive agents depends on the coupling of ventricular-vascular function, not on impedance alone. Hemodynamic therapy should be guided based on the primary variables, BP and CO. If preload is appropriate, conditions of both low BP and low CO are treated with an inotropic drug. If BP is acceptable (and preload appropriate) but CO is low, a vasodilator alone or in combination with an inotropic drug is used. If the patient is hypertensive (with low CO), vasodilators are indicated; if the patient is vasodilated (low BP and high CO), vasoconstrictors are employed (Table 30.3).

▓ POSTOPERATIVE HYPERTENSION

Hypertension has been a common complication of cardiac surgical procedures, and it was reported to occur in 30% to 80% of patients. The current population of older,

Table 30.3 Hemodynamic Therapy Guidelines

Blood Pressure	Cardiac Output	Treatment
Low	Low	Inotrope
Normal	Low	Vasodilator with or without inotrope
High	Low	Vasodilator
Low	High	Vasopressor

Table 30.4 Novel Vasodilators

Drug	Mechanism of Action	Half-Life
Nicardipine	Calcium channel blocker	Intermediate
Clevidipine	Calcium channel blocker	Ultrashort
Fenoldopam	Dopamine₁-agonist	Ultrashort
Nesiritide	Brain natriuretic agonist	Short
Levosimendan	K$^+_{ATP}$ channel modulator	Intermediate

K^+_{ATP}, Adenosine triphosphate–sensitive potassium channel.

sicker patients appears to have fewer problems with hypertension than with low-output syndromes or vasodilation. Although hypertension most commonly occurs in patients with normal preoperative ventricular function, following aortic valve replacement or with a previous history of increased BP, any patient may develop hypertension. Multiple reasons contribute to postoperative hypertension, including preoperative hypertension, preexisting atherosclerotic vascular disease, awakening from general anesthesia, increases in endogenous catecholamines, activation of the plasma renin-angiotensin system, neural reflexes (eg, heart, coronary arteries, great vessels), and hypothermia. Arterial vasoconstriction with various degrees of intravascular hypovolemia is the hallmark of perioperative hypertension.

The hazards of untreated postoperative hypertension include depressed LV performance, increased M$\dot{V}O_2$, cerebrovascular accidents, suture line disruption, MI, rhythm disturbances, and increased bleeding. Historically, therapy for hypertension in cardiac surgery was sodium nitroprusside because of its rapid onset and short duration of action. With multiple vasodilators available in the current era, sodium nitroprusside is no longer the drug of choice. Many pharmaceutical alternatives to nitroprusside are available for treating hypertension after cardiac surgical procedures, including nitroglycerin, β-adrenergic blockers, and the mixed α- and β-adrenergic blocker labetalol. Direct-acting vasodilators, dihydropyridine calcium channel blockers (eg, nicardipine, isradipine, clevidipine), angiotensin-converting enzyme inhibitors, and fenoldopam (a dopamine₁ [D₁] receptor agonist) also have been used. Novel therapeutic approaches are listed in Table 30.4.

Dihydropyridine calcium channel blockers are particularly effective in cardiac surgical patients because these drugs relax arterial resistance vessels without negative inotropic actions or effects on AV nodal conduction and provide important therapeutic options. Dihydropyridines are arterial-specific vasodilators of peripheral resistance arteries that cause generalized vasodilation, including the renal, cerebral, intestinal, and coronary vascular beds. In doses that effectively reduce BP, the dihydropyridines have little or no direct negative effect on cardiac contractility or conduction. Nicardipine

30

is an important therapeutic agent to consider because of its lack of effects on vascular capacitance vessels and preload in patients after cardiac operations. The pharmacokinetic profile of nicardipine suggests that effective administration requires variable-rate infusions when trying to treat hypertension because of the half-life of 40 minutes. If even faster control of BP is essential, a dosing strategy consisting of a loading bolus or a rapid infusion dose with a constant-rate infusion may be more efficient. The effect of nicardipine may persist even though the infusion is stopped. Clevidipine, an ultrashort-acting dihydropyridine approved in 2008 in the United States for clinical use, has a half-life of only minutes; this drug represents an important alternative to nitroprusside.

POSTOPERATIVE VASODILATION

Vasodilation and a need for vasoconstrictor support are relatively frequent complications of cardiac surgical procedures, with and without CPB. Vasodilation alone should be associated with a hyperdynamic circulatory state manifesting as systemic hypotension in association with an increased CO (and a low calculated SVR). More commonly after cardiac operations, a combination of vasodilation and myocardial dysfunction occurs, requiring vasoconstrictor and inotropic therapy. *Vasoplegic syndrome* requires high doses of vasoconstrictors, and occurs after off-pump and on-pump surgical procedures.

While underlying causes are being sought and treated, the therapeutic approach to systemic vasodilation includes intravascular volume expansion, α-adrenergic agents, and vasopressin. Administration of vasoconstrictors for more than a brief period must be guided by measures of cardiac performance because restoration of BP may camouflage a low-output state.

CORONARY ARTERY SPASM

Coronary artery or internal mammary artery vasospasm can occur postoperatively. Mechanical manipulation and underlying atherosclerosis of the native coronary circulation and the internal mammary artery have the potential to produce transient endothelial dysfunction. The endothelium is responsible for releasing endothelium-derived relaxing factor (EDRF), which is nitric oxide (NO), a potent endogenous vasodilator substance that preserves normal endogenous vasodilation. Thromboxane can be liberated by heparin-protamine interactions, CPB, platelet activation, or anaphylactic reactions to produce coronary vasoconstriction. Calcium administration, increased α-adrenergic tone from vasoconstrictor administration (especially in bolus doses), platelet thromboxane liberation, and calcium channel blocker withdrawal represent added reasons that may put the cardiac surgical patient at risk for spasm of native coronary vessels and arterial grafts. The therapy of choice remains empiric. Nitroglycerin is a first-line drug, but nitrate tolerance can occur. Phosphodiesterase (PDE) inhibitors represent newer approaches to this problem and have been reported to be effective. Intravenous dihydropyridine calcium channel blockers are also important therapeutic considerations.

The radial artery is still used by some surgeons as a bypass conduit for revascularization. This conduit was abandoned by some groups because of its propensity to spasm. However, techniques developed in the use of the internal mammary artery have been applied to the radial artery, as well as prophylactic use of calcium channel blocker infusions. Which components of this approach are responsible for the reported success are not known, but use of a calcium channel blocking drug is recommended by many surgeons. The arterial selectivity of the dihydropyridine drugs (eg, nicardipine) should be an advantage in this setting.

DECREASED CONTRACTILITY

Drugs that increase contractility all augment calcium mobilization from intracellular sites to and from the contractile proteins or sensitize these proteins to calcium. Catecholamines, through β_1-receptor stimulation in the myocardium, increase intracellular cyclic adenosine monophosphate (cAMP). This second messenger increases intracellular calcium and thus improves myocardial contraction. Inhibition of the breakdown of cAMP by PDE inhibitors increases intracellular cAMP independent of the β-receptor. The "calcium sensitizers" constitute a newer class of inotropic agents. One drug in this class, levosimendan, is already available in certain countries and is currently being evaluated in the United States (Box 30.2).

Catecholamines

The catecholamines used postoperatively include dopamine, dobutamine, epinephrine, norepinephrine, and isoproterenol (Box 30.3). These drugs have various effects on α- and β-receptors and therefore various effects on HR, rhythm, and myocardial

BOX 30.2 *Pharmacologic Approaches for Perioperative Ventricular Dysfunction*

Inotropic Agents

- Catecholamines
- Phosphodiesterase inhibitors
- Levosimendan

Vasodilator Therapy

- Pulmonary vasodilators
- Phosphodiesterase inhibitors (milrinone, sildenafil)
- Inhaled nitric oxide
- Prostaglandins (PGI_2, PGE_1, iloprost, and derivatives)

30

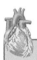

BOX 30.3 *Disadvantages of Catecholamines*

Increased myocardial oxygen consumption
Tachycardia
Arrhythmias
Excessive peripheral vasoconstriction
Coronary vasoconstriction
β-Receptor downregulation and decreased drug efficacy

Table 30.5 Catecholamines Used Postoperatively

Drug	Infusion Dose (µg/kg per min)
Dopamine[a,b]	2–10
Dobutamine[b]	2–10
Epinephrine[c]	0.03–0.20
Norepinephrine[c]	0.03–0.20
Isoproterenol[c]	0.02–0.10

[a]Less than 2 µg/kg per minute predominantly "dopaminergic" (renal and mesenteric artery dilatation).
[b]If 10 µg/kg per minute is ineffective, change to epinephrine or norepinephrine.
[c]Dose to effect; may require higher dose than indicated.

metabolism. Dosing recommendations for the catecholamines are provided in Table 30.5.

Isoproterenol

Isoproterenol is a potent β_1-agonist in the heart and a β_2-agonist in the periphery. Its positive inotropic effect is accompanied by an increase in HR and a propensity for arrhythmias. In patients with coronary artery disease, tachycardia and associated peripheral vasodilation increase M$\dot{v}o_2$ and decrease coronary perfusion pressure. In patients with bradycardias in whom pacing is not an immediate or practical option or in those in whom increased HR is desirable (eg, cardiac transplant recipients, patients with regurgitant valvular lesions), isoproterenol has long been used for this purpose, but increasingly dobutamine is used.

Epinephrine

Epinephrine is a potent adrenergic agonist with the desirable feature that, in low doses (<3 µg/min), β_1 and β_2 effects predominate. As the dose is increased, α effects (eg, vasoconstriction) and tachycardia occur. However, in the acutely failing heart postoperatively, only drugs such as epinephrine or norepinephrine provide positive inotropy and perfusion pressure. These features and its low cost make epinephrine a common first-line drug in the postoperative setting. Despite what is often stated in older literature, epinephrine causes less tachycardia than dopamine or dobutamine at equivalent inotropic doses. Because of the metabolic actions of α_2 stimulation, epinephrine infusion can cause hyperglycemia and increased serum lactate levels.

Norepinephrine

Norepinephrine, which has potent β_1- and α-receptor effects, preserves coronary perfusion pressure while not increasing HR, actions that are favorable to the ischemic, reperfused heart. When norepinephrine is used alone without a vasodilator or PDE inhibitor, the potent α_1 effects may have variable effects on CO. Ventricular filling pressures usually increase when this drug is given because of constriction of the capacitance vessels. Administration of a vasodilator, including the PDE inhibitors, with norepinephrine may partially oppose the vasoconstriction. End-organ ischemia would appear to be unlikely if CO can be preserved at normal levels when norepinephrine is given. PDE inhibitors in combination with norepinephrine attenuate the arterial vasoconstrictive effects.

Dopamine

A precursor of norepinephrine, dopamine probably achieves its therapeutic effects by releasing myocardial norepinephrine or preventing its reuptake, especially in high doses. This indirect action may result in reduced effectiveness when dopamine is given to patients with chronic HF or shock states because the myocardium becomes depleted of norepinephrine stores. In contrast to dobutamine, the α-agonist properties of dopamine cause increases in pulmonary artery pressure (PAP), pulmonary vascular resistance (PVR), and LV filling pressure. At doses higher than 10 μg/kg per minute, tachycardia and vasoconstriction become the predominant actions of this drug. Tachycardia is a consistent side effect, and in patients with cardiogenic shock, dopamine has been shown to increase mortality rates.

Dobutamine

In contrast to dopamine, dobutamine shows mainly β_1-agonist properties, with decreases in diastolic BP and sometimes systemic BP observed. Dobutamine is functionally similar to isoproterenol, with less tendency to induce tachycardia in the postoperative setting, although it is often infused at doses up to 40 μg/kg per minute to increase HR as part of a dobutamine stress echocardiographic evaluation. The favorable actions of dobutamine may be limited if tachycardia develops, and, as with dopamine, the inotropic potency of dobutamine is modest in comparison with that of epinephrine or norepinephrine.

Phosphodiesterase Inhibitors

The PDE inhibitors are nonglycosidic, nonsympathomimetic drugs that have positive inotropic effects independent of the β_1-adrenergic receptor and unique vasodilatory actions independent of endothelial function or nitrovasodilators. Patients with HF have downregulation of the β_1-receptor, with a decrease in receptor density and altered responses to catecholamine administration. Milrinone, amrinone, and enoximone bypass the β_1-receptor and increase intracellular cAMP by selective inhibition of PDE fraction III (ie, fraction IV), a cAMP-specific PDE enzyme. In vascular smooth muscle, these agents cause vasodilation in the arterial and capacitance beds. PDE inhibitors increase CO, decrease PAOP, and decrease SVR and PVR in patients with biventricular dysfunction, and they are important therapeutic agents in postoperative cardiac surgical patients. Sildenafil and other PDE 5 inhibitors are also increasingly used for pulmonary hypertension.

PDE III inhibitors have a clinical effect as inodilators; they produce dilation of arterial and venous beds and decrease the mean arterial pressure (MAP) and central filling pressures. Increases in CO are induced by multiple mechanisms, including afterload reduction and positive inotropy, but not by increasing HR. The net effect is a decrease in myocardial wall tension, representing an important contrast to most sympathomimetic agents. Catecholamine administration often needs the simultaneous administration of vasodilators to reduce ventricular wall tension. Milrinone and other PDE inhibitors also have unique mechanisms of vasodilation that may be favorable for coronary artery and internal mammary artery flow (Box 30.4).

Milrinone is a bipyridine derivative with inotropic activity that is almost 20 times more potent than that of amrinone and a shorter half-life. Milrinone is an effective inodilator for patients with decompensated HF and low CO after cardiac surgical procedures. Suggested administration of milrinone is a loading dose of 50 μg/kg over 10 minutes, followed by an infusion of 0.5 μg/kg per minute (0.375–0.75 μg/kg per min). By using slower loading doses, high peak concentrations can be prevented, and the vasodilation that is observed with rapid loading can be attenuated.

30

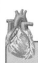

> **BOX 30.4   *Advantages of Preemptive Phosphodiesterase Inhibitor Administration***
>
> Increased myocardial contractility (left and right ventricles)
> Pulmonary vasodilation
> Resolution and prevention of ischemia
> Minimal drug side effects during cardiopulmonary bypass
> Dilation of internal mammary artery
> Avoidance of mechanical intervention
> Prevention of "failed weaning"

Levosimendan

Levosimendan is a calcium-sensitizing drug that exerts positive inotropic effects by sensitization of myofilaments to calcium and vasodilation through opening of ATP-dependent potassium channels on vascular smooth muscle. These effects occur without increasing intracellular cAMP or calcium and without an increase in $M\dot{V}O_2$ at therapeutic doses. As would be expected with an inodilator, the hemodynamic effects include a decrease in PAOP in association with an increase in CO. β-Blockade does not block the hemodynamic effects of this drug. Levosimendan itself has a short elimination half-life, but it has active metabolites with elimination half-lives up to 80 hours. A study in patients with decompensated HF found that hemodynamic improvements at 48 hours were similar whether patients received the drug for 24 hours or 48 hours. Increasing plasma levels of the active metabolite were found for 24 hours after the drug infusion was stopped. Levosimendan is approved in many European countries and is currently undergoing a cardiac surgical trial for use in the United States.

RIGHT-SIDED HEART FAILURE

HF after cardiac surgical procedures usually results from LV impairment. Although an isolated right-sided MI can occur perioperatively, most perioperative inferior MIs show variable involvement of the right ventricle. The myocardial preservation techniques that are best for the left ventricle may not offer ideal right ventricular (RV) protection because the right ventricle is thin-walled and more exposed to body and atmospheric temperature. Cardioplegic solution given through the coronary sinus (retrograde) may not reach parts of the right ventricle because of positioning of the cardioplegia cannula in relation to the venous outflow from this chamber and because the thebesian veins do not drain into the coronary sinus. Impairment of RV function postoperatively is more severe and persistent when preoperative right coronary artery stenosis is present. Although depression of the ejection fraction (EF) is compensated by preload augmentation, right ventricular ejection fraction (RVEF) cannot be preserved if coronary perfusion pressure is reduced or impedance to ejection is increased.

Certain aspects of the physiology of the right ventricle make it different from the left ventricle. Normally, the RV free wall receives its blood flow during systole and diastole; however, systemic hypotension or increased RV systolic and diastolic pressures may cause supply-dependent depression of contractility when $M\dot{V}O_2$ is increased while coronary perfusion pressure is decreased. The normal thin-walled right ventricle is at least twice as sensitive to increases in afterload as is the left ventricle. Relatively modest increases in outflow impedance from multiple causes in the postoperative period can exhaust preload reserve and cause a decrease in RVEF with ventricular dilation. RV pressure overload may be complicated by volume overload caused by functional tricuspid regurgitation. Decreases in RV SV reduce LV filling, and dilation of the right ventricle can cause a leftward shift of the interventricular septum that interferes with diastolic filling of the left ventricle (ie, ventricular interaction) (Fig. 30.3). A distended right ventricle limited by the pericardial cavity further decreases LV filling. RV failure has the potential to affect LV performance by decreasing pulmonary venous blood flow, decreasing diastolic distending pressure, and reducing LV diastolic compliance. The resulting decrease in LV output further impairs RV pump function. The mechanical outcomes of RV failure in postoperative cardiac surgical patients are depicted in Fig. 30.4. It can therefore be appreciated how, once established, RV failure is self-propagating, and aggressive treatment interventions may be needed to interrupt the vicious cycle.

Diagnosis

In the postoperative cardiac surgical patient, a low cardiac index with right atrial pressure (RAP) increased disproportionately compared with changes in left-sided filling pressures is highly suggestive of RV failure. The PAOP may also increase because of ventricular interaction, but the relationship of RAP with PAOP stays close to or higher than 1.0. The absence of a step-up in pressure in going from the right atrium

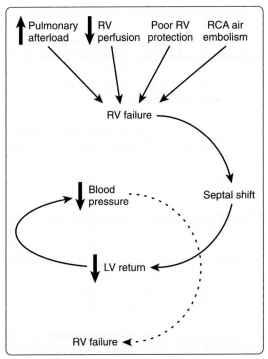

Fig. 30.3 Sequence inducing right ventricular failure and causing a downward spiral of events. *LV,* Left ventricular; *RCA,* right coronary artery; *RV,* right ventricular.

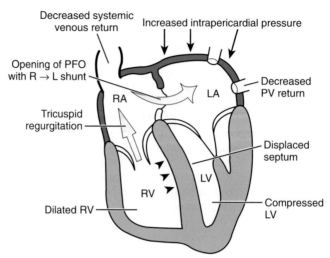

Fig. 30.4 Mechanical changes produced by acute right ventricular failure. *LA*, Left atrium; *LV*, left ventricle; *PFO*, patent foramen ovale; *PV*, pulmonary venous; *R → L*, right-to-left; *RA*, right atrium; *RV*, right ventricle.

to the pulmonary artery (mean), provided PVR is low, suggests that RV failure is severe and the right side of the heart is acting only as a conduit. This hemodynamic presentation is typical of cardiogenic shock associated with RV infarction. The venous waveforms are accentuated with a prominent Y descent similar to findings in constrictive pericarditis, thus suggesting reduced RV compliance. Large V waves may also be discernible and may relate to tricuspid regurgitation.

Echocardiography allows qualitative interpretation of RV size, contractility, and configuration of the interventricular septum, and it can enable the clinician to provide a definitive diagnosis of RV dysfunction or RV failure. Because of the crescent shape of the right ventricle, volume determination is not easy, but the qualitative examination and assessment for tricuspid regurgitation are very valuable. TEE is also useful to determine whether the increased RAP opens a patent foramen ovale, thus producing a right-to-left shunt. This is important because traditional methods to treat hypoxemia such as PEEP and larger tidal volumes in this setting will only increase the afterload of the right ventricle and potentially increase the shunt and hypoxemia.

Treatment

Treatment approaches in postoperative RV failure may differ from those used in LV failure, and they are affected by the presence of pulmonary hypertension (Box 30.5). In all cases, preload should be increased to the upper range of normal; however, the Frank-Starling relationship is flat in RV failure and, to avoid ventricular dilation, the CO response to an increasing CVP should be determined. Volume loading should be stopped when the CVP exceeds 10 mm Hg and the CO does not increase despite increases in this pressure. The CVP should not be permitted to exceed the PAOP because, if these pressures equalize, any increase obtained in pulmonary blood flow will be offset by decreased diastolic filling of the left ventricle by ventricular interdependence. The atrial contribution to RV filling is important when the ventricle is dilated and noncompliant. Maintenance of sinus rhythm and use of atrial pacing are important components of treating postoperative RV failure.

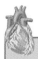

BOX 30.5 *Treatment Approaches in Postoperative Right-Sided Heart Failure*

Preload Augmentation

- Volume, vasopressors, or leg elevation (CVP/PCWP <1)
- Decrease juxtacardiac pressures (pericardium and/or chest open)
- Establishment of atrial kick and treatment of atrial arrhythmias (sinus rhythm, atrial pacing)

Afterload Reduction (Pulmonary Vasodilation)

- Nitroglycerin, isosorbide dinitrate nesiritide
- cAMP-specific phosphodiesterase inhibitors, α_2-adrenergic agonists
- Inhaled nitric oxide
- Nebulized PGI_2
- Intravenous PGE_1 (and left atrial norepinephrine)

Inotropic Support

- cAMP-specific phosphodiesterase inhibitors, isoproterenol, dobutamine
- Norepinephrine
- Levosimendan

Ventilatory Management

- Lower intrathoracic pressures (tidal volume <7 mL/kg, low PEEP)
- Attenuation of hypoxic vasoconstriction (high FIO_2)
- Avoidance of respiratory acidosis ($PaCO_2$ 30–35 mm Hg, metabolic control with meperidine or relaxants)

Mechanical Support

- Intraaortic counterpulsation
- Pulmonary artery counterpulsation
- Right ventricular assist devices

cAMP, Cyclic adenosine monophosphate; *CVP/PCWP,* central venous pressure/pulmonary capillary wedge pressure; *FIO₂,* fraction of inspired oxygen; *PaCO₂,* partial pressure of arterial carbon dioxide; *PEEP,* positive end-expiratory pressure; *PGI₂,* prostaglandin I₂; *PGE₁,* prostaglandin E₁.

30

Although vasodilators may lead to cardiovascular collapse in patients with RV infarction (as a result of decreases in RV filling and coronary perfusion), postoperative RV failure is often associated with increased PVR and pulmonary hypertension. In this context, attempts to decrease RV outflow impedance may be worthwhile. Intravenous vasodilators invariably reduce systemic BP and mandate the simultaneous administration of a vasoconstrictor. One way to reduce the pulmonary effects of the needed vasoconstrictor is to administer the vasoconstrictor through a left atrial (LA) catheter and treat RV dysfunction with intravenous prostaglandins and LA norepinephrine. The PDE inhibitors are commonly used for their effect on the pulmonary vasculature and RV function. Interest in and availability of aerosolized pulmonary vasodilators have increased. This route of administration reduces or even abolishes undesirable systemic vasodilation. Delivery of the drug directly to the alveoli improves pulmonary blood flow to these alveoli and potentially improves oxygenation by better matching blood flow to ventilation. Three drugs have been used: NO, PGI_2 (ie, epoprostenol or prostacyclin), and milrinone.

NO is an important signaling molecule throughout the body. In the lung, it rapidly diffuses across the alveolar-capillary membrane and activates soluble guanylate cyclase, thereby leading to smooth muscle relaxation by several mechanisms. Inhaled NO is given through a specialized delivery system in a concentration of 5 to 80 parts/million. It is commercially available in the United States, but it is costly. NO has been used successfully to treat RV dysfunction associated with pulmonary hypertension after heart operations, mitral valve replacement, cardiac transplantation, and placement of LV assist devices (LVADs). An intraaortic balloon pump may be of great benefit, even in patients with a right ventricle that is mainly responsible for circulatory decompensation. This beneficial effect is mediated by increased coronary perfusion. Right-sided heart assist devices have a place as temporizing measures in severe intractable right-sided HF. Pulmonary artery counterpulsation is experimental, and its clinical role is uncertain. In cases of severe RV failure it may be necessary to leave the sternum open or to reopen the chest if it has been closed. This approach decreases the tamponade-like compression of the left ventricle by the distended right ventricle, right atrium, and edematous mediastinal tissues.

Effects of Mechanical Ventilation in Heart Failure

HF at the time of a surgical procedure has been identified as a significant predictor of postoperative respiratory complications. Maintenance of gas exchange in these situations usually mandates prolonged ventilatory support. Besides improving Pao_2, mechanical ventilation can influence Do_2 through its effects on CO. Suppression of spontaneous respiratory efforts may substantially decrease the work of breathing and improve the oxygen supply-demand relationship. Traditionally, the influence of mechanical ventilation on hemodynamics has been viewed as negative. The unavoidable rise in intrathoracic pressure caused by positive-pressure ventilation or PEEP is associated with decreased CO. However, in the presence of HF or myocardial ischemia, raised intrathoracic pressure has the potential to affect the determinants of global cardiac performance favorably. Understanding these heart-lung interactions is essential for the integrated management of the ventilated patient with HF after cardiac operations. The effects of ventilation on RV and LV failure must receive independent consideration.

Raised intrathoracic pressure may significantly improve LV performance as a result of the reduced transmural pressure needed to give an acceptable systemic BP. This pressure can be viewed as afterload reduction, a favorable effect separate from the resistance to venous return that may also help such patients. Clinically significant improvements in cardiac function have been documented in patients ventilated for cardiogenic respiratory failure produced by myocardial ischemia and after CABG operations. High LV filling pressures may help identify a subgroup benefiting from reduced afterload with increased intrathoracic pressure.

The circulatory responses to changes in ventilation should always be assessed in patients with cardiac disease; the goal of improving or maintaining Do_2 must be kept in mind. This usually requires measurement of arterial oxygenation and CO. In RV and biventricular failure the increase in the airway pressure caused by ventilatory support should be kept at a minimum compatible with acceptable gas exchange. This means avoidance of high levels of PEEP and trials of decreased inspiratory times, flow rates, and tidal volumes. Breathing modes that emphasize spontaneous efforts such as intermittent mandatory ventilation, pressure support, or CPAP should be considered. Alternatively, if isolated LV failure is the reason for ventilatory therapy, improvements in cardiac performance may be achieved by positive-pressure ventilation with PEEP. In particular, patients with increased LV filling pressures, mitral regurgitation,

VI

and reversible ischemic dysfunction may improve from afterload reduction related to increased airway and intrathoracic pressures.

Effects of Ventilatory Weaning on Heart Failure

Traditional criteria for weaning of ventilatory support assess the adequacy of gas exchange and peak respiratory muscle strength. In the patient with HF, the response of global hemodynamics to spontaneous respirations must also be considered. The changes of the loading conditions of the heart brought about by resuming spontaneous ventilation can induce a vicious cycle resulting in hypoxemia and pulmonary edema.

Pulmonary congestion, often present in patients with LV dysfunction, decreases pulmonary compliance. Thus large decreases in inspiratory intrathoracic pressure are needed to cause satisfactory lung inflation. These negative swings of intrathoracic pressure increase venous return. Increased diaphragmatic movements may raise intraabdominal pressure and further increase the pressure gradient for venous return. Decreased intrathoracic pressure also raises the ventricular transmural pressures and the impedance to ventricular emptying. The increased afterload causes further increases in preload, and these changes jeopardize the myocardial oxygen balance. Accordingly, worsening of myocardial ischemia as shown by ST-segment deviations was demonstrated when ventilatory support was removed in patients ventilated after MI.

▧ CARDIAC TAMPONADE

Cardiac tamponade is an important cause of the low-CO state after cardiac operations and occurs when the heart is compressed by an external agent, most commonly blood accumulated in the mediastinum. Hemodynamic compromise, to some degree attributable to the constraining effect of blood accumulating within the chest, is often observed in the 3% to 6% of patients needing multiple blood transfusions for hemorrhage after cardiac surgical procedures. Postoperative cardiac tamponade usually manifests acutely during the first 24 hours postoperatively, but delayed tamponade may develop 10 to 14 days after the operation, and it has been associated with postpericardiotomy syndrome or postoperative anticoagulation.

The mechanism of hemodynamic deterioration during cardiac tamponade is the result of impaired filling of one or more of the cardiac chambers. As the external pressure on the heart increases, the distending or transmural pressure (external intracavitary pressure) is decreased. The intracavitary pressure increases in compensation lead to impaired venous return and elevation of the venous pressure. If the external pressure is high enough to exceed the ventricular pressure during diastole, diastolic ventricular collapse occurs. These changes have been documented in the right and the left sides of the heart after cardiac surgical procedures. As the end-diastolic volume and end-systolic volume decrease, a concomitant reduction in SV occurs. In the most severe form of cardiac tamponade, ventricular filling occurs only during atrial systole. Adrenergic and endocrine mechanisms are activated in an effort to maintain venous return and perfusion pressure. Intense sympathoadrenergic activation increases venous return by constricting venous capacitance vessels. Tachycardia helps maintain CO in the presence of reduced SV. Adrenergic mechanisms may explain decreased urinary output and sodium excretion, but these phenomena may also be caused by reduced CO or a reduction in atrial natriuretic factor from decreased distending pressure of the atria.

The diagnosis of cardiac tamponade depends on a high degree of suspicion. Tamponade after cardiac surgical procedures is a clinical entity distinct from the

30

tamponade typically seen in medical patients in whom the pericardium is intact and the heart is surrounded by a compressing fluid. In the setting of cardiac surgery, the pericardial space is often left open and in communication with one or both of the pleural spaces, and the compressing blood is at least in part in a clotted, nonfluid state and able to cause localized compression of the heart. Serious consideration should be given to the possibility of tamponade after cardiac surgical procedures in any patient with an inadequate or worsening hemodynamic status, as evidenced by hypotension, tachycardia, increased filling pressures, or low CO, especially when chest tube drainage has been excessive. A more subtle presentation of postoperative tamponade is characterized by gradually increasing needs for inotropic and pressor support. Many of the classic signs of cardiac tamponade may not be present in these patients, partly because the patients are usually sedated and ventilated, but also because the pericardium is usually left open, resulting in a more gradual increase in the restraining effects of blood accumulation. Patients may have localized accumulations that affect one chamber more than another. The classic findings of elevated CVP or equalization of CVP, pulmonary artery diastolic pressure, and PAOP may not occur. It may therefore be difficult in the presence of declining CO and elevated filling pressures to distinguish tamponade from biventricular failure. A useful clue may be the pronounced respiratory variation in BP with mechanical ventilation in association with high filling pressures and low CO because the additional external pressure applied to the heart by positive-pressure ventilation may further impair the already compromised ventricular filling in the presence of tamponade.

Echocardiography may provide strong evidence for the diagnosis of cardiac tamponade. Echolucent crescents between the RV wall and the pericardium or the posterior LV wall and the pericardium are visible with TTE or TEE. Echogenicity of grossly bloody pericardial effusions, especially when clots have been formed, may sometimes make delineation of the borders of the pericardium and the ventricular wall difficult, thus compromising the sensitivity of this technique. A classic echocardiographic sign of tamponade is diastolic collapse of the right atrium or right ventricle, with the duration of collapse bearing a relationship with the severity of the hemodynamic alteration, but such findings are often absent in patients after cardiac surgical procedures. Often, TTE is difficult because of mechanical ventilation, and TEE is required for satisfactory imaging.

The definitive treatment of cardiac tamponade is surgical exploration with evacuation of hematoma. The chest may have to be opened in the ICU if tamponade proceeds to hemodynamic collapse. For delayed tamponade, pericardiocentesis may be acceptable. Medical palliation in anticipation of reexploration consists of reinforcing the physiologic responses that are already occurring while preparing for definitive treatment. Venous return can be increased by volume administration and leg elevation. The lowest tidal volume and PEEP compatible with adequate gas exchange should be used. Epinephrine in high doses gives the needed chronotropic and inotropic boost to the ventricle and increases systemic venous pressures. Sedatives and opioids should be given cautiously because they may interfere with adrenergic discharge and precipitate abrupt hemodynamic collapse. Occasionally, patients develop significant cardiac tamponade without accumulation of blood in the chest. Edema of the heart, lungs, and other tissues in the chest after CPB may not allow chest closure at the first operation, and staged chest closure may be required after the edema has subsided. Similarly, some patients with an inadequate hemodynamic status after cardiac surgical procedures despite maximum support in the ICU improve with opening of the chest because this tamponade effect is relieved. Reclosure of the chest in the operating room is often possible after a few days of continued cardiovascular support and diuresis.

VI

Postoperative circulatory control in the heart transplant recipient differs in three major respects from that of the patient who has not received a heart transplant: (1) the transplanted heart is noncompliant, with a relatively fixed SV; (2) acute rejection must be considered when cardiac performance is poor or suddenly deteriorates; and (3) these patients are at risk for acute RV failure if pulmonary hypertension develops.

The fixed SV combined with denervation of the donor heart means that maintenance of CO often depends on therapy to maintain an elevated HR (110–120 beats/min). The drug most commonly used is isoproterenol because it is a potent inotropic agent and because it causes a dose-related increase in HR. Its vasodilating β_2-adrenergic effect on the pulmonary vasculature may be of benefit if PVR is greater than normal. Alternatively, atrial pacing may be used to maintain HR if contractility appears normal. Pacing is often used to allow the withdrawal of isoproterenol in the first postoperative days. Parasympatholytic drugs, such as atropine, do not have any effect on the transplanted heart.

Major concerns in monitoring and therapy for the transplant recipient are the potential for infection and rejection. Immunosuppressive therapy regimens include cyclosporine and usually steroids or azathioprine, or both. These drugs also suppress the patient's response to infection, and steroid therapy may induce elevations in the white blood cell count, thus further confusing the issue. Protocols for postoperative care stress strict aseptic technique and frequent careful clinical evaluations for infection.

Preoperative evaluation helps screen patients with fixed pulmonary hypertension because the normal donor right ventricle may acutely fail if it is presented with an elevated PAP in the recipient. However, patients may have progression of disease between the time of evaluation and operation, or the right ventricle may be inadequately protected during harvest or transport. When separation from CPB is attempted, acute RV dilation and failure occur, and such patients may emerge from the operating room receiving multiple drug therapy, including the inhaled agents NO and prostacyclin, as described earlier, to focus on treating RV dysfunction and/or pulmonary hypertension. Gradual withdrawal of these drugs occurs in the first postoperative days, with close monitoring of PAPs and oxygenation.

30

■ ADVANCES IN CARDIOVASCULAR SURGERY AND POSTOPERATIVE MANAGEMENT

Advances in cardiothoracic surgery include minimally invasive transcatheter aortic valve replacement (TAVR), the incorporation of echocardiography in the cardiothoracic ICU, and improved biotechnology and durability related to cardiopulmonary support by extracorporeal membrane oxygenation (ECMO). The following section explores these advances and highlights the major postoperative considerations for patients in the cardiothoracic ICU.

Postoperative Management of Complications After Transcatheter Aortic Valve Replacement

TAVR is increasingly used in clinical practice and is also described elsewhere. Although the benefits and indications for TAVR are well established, four major clinical challenges have emerged: vascular complications, stroke, paravalvular leak (PVL), and cardiac conduction abnormalities. The mechanisms of these intraoperative complications have immediate postoperative consequences and require appropriate management in the ICU.

Vascular Complications

Major vascular complications are independent predictors of major bleeding, transfusion, end-organ failure, and death. Atherosclerotic disease of the femoral arteries and operator experience are other notable predictors of clinical outcomes. Strategies to minimize vascular injury involve designing smaller and sleeker delivery systems. Major vascular complications are defined as thoracic aortic dissection, distal extremity or noncerebral vascular embolization requiring surgical intervention, and amputation. In addition, irreversible end-organ injury and iatrogenic access-related vascular injuries resulting in death, unplanned intervention, blood transfusion of 4 units or more, or permanent end-organ injury are considered major vascular complications related to TAVR. Access-related vascular injuries included dissection, stenosis, perforation, pseudoaneurysm formation, arteriovenous fistula, hematoma, compartment syndrome, and irreversible nerve injury.

Minor vascular complications include distal embolization not requiring surgical intervention or leading to irreversible end-organ damage. The incidence of major and minor vascular complications is 15.3% and 11.9%, respectively, within 30 days of TAVR. Furthermore, the most common major vascular complications were dissection, access-site hematoma, and arteriotomy of the posterior femoral arterial wall. Moreover, major vascular complications significantly increased the risks of major bleeding (and therefore blood transfusions), renal failure requiring continuous renal replacement therapy, and death at 30 days and again at 1 year. Postoperative cardiovascular management of the patient who has undergone TAVR complicated by intraoperative vascular injury includes assessment of the degree of vascular injury as well as continuous monitoring of peripheral arterial pulses (focus on access site), adequate perfusion, development and treatment of end-organ dysfunction, and hemodynamic and hemostatic resuscitation.

Stroke

Asymptomatic cerebral embolism is common during TAVR. Clinically silent cerebral embolism occurs in up to 70% of these patients. Major stroke, however, independently predicts prolonged recovery and increased mortality rates. Identified stroke predictors include history of previous stroke, functional disability, transapical approach, and AF. The long-term effects of asymptomatic cerebral embolism associated with TAVR are unknown. The predictors of stroke early after TAVR include previous stroke, severe arterial atheroma, and a smaller aortic valve area. Patients should be admitted to the ICU after undergoing TAVR and postoperatively monitored for immediate evidence of neurocognitive decline or focal neurologic deficit heralding a major stroke. Neurology consultation and activation of a stroke workup protocol native to the home institution should occur, and neuroimaging should be ordered to direct further clinical management. In the event of a stroke in the ICU, multidisciplinary decision making among physicians and patient care teams should be implemented regarding the initiation of permissive hypertension and procedural intervention.

Paravalvular Leak

PVL is common and significantly decreases survival. This undersizing is balanced against oversizing and aortic root trauma or rupture, which typically warrants emergency CPB and immediate repair. The formal grading of PVL severity in TAVR is based on its percentage of the circumferential extent of the aortic valve annulus. Further management strategies for PVL include a repositionable valve prosthesis and transcatheter plugging. The immediate postoperative importance of PVL after TAVR relates to the presence of aortic regurgitation in an otherwise noncompliant left ventricle with diastolic dysfunction, as commonly seen with severe aortic stenosis. The cardiothoracic ICU physician should be informed if a post-TAVR patient has moderate or higher degree of PVL because this finding may have consequences for clinical management.

Cardiac Conduction Abnormalities

Cardiac conduction disturbances after TAVR are common and important. New-onset AF is defined as an arrhythmia within the hospital stay that has the ECG characteristics of AF and lasts longer than 30 seconds. The types of heart block associated with TAVR may occur anywhere along the cardiac conduction pathway, including first-degree AV block, second-degree AV block (Mobitz I or Mobitz II), third-degree AV block, bundle branch block, and AV block requiring pacemaker insertion.

The native aortic valve lies in close proximity to the AV conduction system, a location that puts the ventricular septal conductive system at risk during aortic valve procedures. The basal attachments of the three aortic leaflets form an annulus that separates the aortic root from the LV outflow tract (LVOT). The noncoronary cusp lies adjacent to the membranous portion of the interventricular septum. The superior continuation of the membranous septum is an interleaflet triangle that separates the noncoronary from the right coronary cusp. Both structures, the membranous septum and the interleaflet triangle, are in fibrous continuity and overlie the bundle of His as it extends leftward from the AV node. The left bundle branch traverses below the membranous septum and penetrates superficially to traverse along the LV side of the interventricular septum. The circumferential forces of the bioprosthetic valve in TAVR on the adjacent, underlying cardiac conduction system are believed to be a cause of cardiac conduction disturbances after TAVR.

Prompt recognition and proper management of AV blockade remain essential in the management of patients undergoing TAVR because hemodynamically significant heart block after TAVR may be common in selected patients and require permanent pacemaker implantation (PPM). Certainly, in the postoperative ICU setting in the patient who does not have a preoperative pacemaker, new heart block and resulting hemodynamic instability may require swift intervention with transvenous pacing. This temporary measure may be implemented as a bridge to PPM.

30

Echocardiography in the Cardiothoracic Intensive Care Unit

Guidelines outlining basic TEE examinations have facilitated the adaptation of echocardiography in the ICU by intensivists without previous training in this modality. Outlining 11 TEE views that together comprise the full basic TEE perioperative examination: the midesophageal four-chamber view, the midesophageal two-chamber view, the midesophageal long-axis view, the midesophageal ascending aortic long-axis view, the midesophageal ascending aortic short-axis view, the midesophageal aortic valve short-axis view, the midesophageal RV inflow-outflow view, the midesophageal bicaval view, the transgastric midpapillary short-axis view, and the descending aortic long-axis and short-axis views. Additionally, TTE may be particularly useful in the ICU when determining the causes of hemodynamic instability after cardiothoracic operations. In the immediate postoperative period, TTE may yield poor visualization as a result of postoperative change and positioning of support devices. For this reason, TEE is advocated during this early point-of-care setting for definitive and accurate diagnoses of hemodynamic aberrancies.

Miniaturized Transesophageal Echocardiography Probe

The use of a miniaturized, monoplane TEE probe (ClariTEE; ImaCor, Uniondale, NY) may provide benefit in the assessment of hemodynamically unstable patients in the cardiothoracic ICU. This probe is capable of performing monoplane views of midesophageal four-chamber, midesophageal ascending aortic short-axis, and transgastric short-axis views. The probe is 5.5 mm in diameter and is approved by the Food and Drug Administration (FDA) to remain indwelling for up to 72 hours; it may connect to the portable ultrasound console. The probe may be disconnected when required from this portable ultrasound machine to facilitate evaluation of other patients with indwelling probes. The ultrasound machine (computer and monitor screen) is small and can be transported into patients' rooms. The ClariTEE probe uses a relatively high frequency (7 MHz) combined with specialized signal processing software to enhance penetration and contrast resolution. The inability to rotate the ultrasound scan sector, however, makes it difficult to obtain a complete diagnostic ultrasound scan of the cardiovascular structures.

Echocardiography During Postoperative Intensive Care Unit Management of Left Ventricular Assist Devices

Echocardiography is particularly useful for the postoperative management of patients after LVAD implantation. Assessment of RV function is central to the hemodynamic management of these patients in the immediate postoperative period, and echocardiography may help visualize interventricular septal position, RV systolic function, degree of the tricuspid valve regurgitation, and LV chamber size. TTE typically provides poor visualization of the cardiac chambers postoperatively as a result of inflammation, thoracostomy and mediastinal tubes, and echogenic dropout from the LVAD hardware.

RIGHT VENTRICULAR DYSFUNCTION AFTER LEFT VENTRICULAR ASSIST DEVICE PLACEMENT

Classically, the patient may present to the ICU with central venous access, a PAC, and invasive arterial monitoring. These hemodynamic data alert the ICU physician to aberrancies that may suggest RV dysfunction, venous hypertension, and inadequate LVAD filling and ejection. The use of echocardiography together with these hemodynamic variables allows the immediate titration of pharmacologic support and LVAD speed to optimize CO, right-sided filling pressures, mixed venous oxygenation, RV systolic function, and LV filling.

Akin to the TEE examination on separation from CPB in the operating room, the TEE examination in the ICU similarly focuses on the position of the interventricular septum. Equal filling and emptying of both the right ventricle and the left ventricle result in a midline position of the septum. When LVAD flows are relatively higher than the ability of the right ventricle to deliver CO to the left ventricle, the interventricular septum tends to bow toward the left ventricle, thus resulting in an LV "suckdown" effect, RV failure, and increased tricuspid regurgitation (Fig. 30.5A). Tricuspid regurgitation occurs as a result of tricuspid valve annular distortion (Fig. 30.5B). This effect may be somewhat offset by increasing SVR, increasing LV chamber size, and tempering the leftward interventricular septal shift. On occasion, titration of pharmacologic and mechanical support (LVAD settings) is ineffective, and a return to the operating room may be warranted for RV assist device (RVAD) placement.

ECHOCARDIOGRAPHY TO RULE OUT OBSTRUCTIVE SHOCK AFTER LEFT VENTRICULAR ASSIST DEVICE PLACEMENT

Increasing right-sided filling pressures, reduced cardiac index, and low mixed venous oxygenation saturation may alert the intensivist to problems with intrinsic RV function,

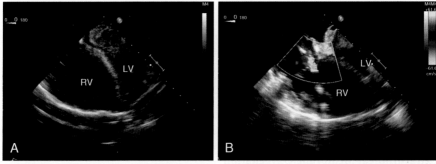

Fig. 30.5 Left ventricular assist device (LVAD) "suckdown" effect seen by transesophageal echocardiography (TEE) in the cardiothoracic intensive care unit. (A) Midesophageal four-chamber view using TEE to illustrate LVAD suckdown as a result of right ventricular failure and relatively increased and mismatched LVAD flows. (B) Midesophageal four-chamber view with color-flow Doppler illustrating severe tricuspid regurgitation during this suckdown event. *LV,* Left ventricle; *RV,* right ventricle. (Courtesy K. Ghadimi, MD.)

but causes of obstructive shock should be excluded. Invasive hemodynamic monitoring cannot always discern among different causes of poor RV function. However, TEE enables the clinician definitively to diagnose new pericardial effusions, large right-sided pleural effusions, or bleeding resulting in mass compression of the atria and/or ventricles. In the setting of cardiac tamponade physiology, immediate return to the operating room is warranted to relieve mass compression of the involved cardiac chambers.

Echocardiography in Patients Requiring Extracorporeal Membrane Oxygenation

ECMO is mechanical support of the lungs and/or heart for a period of days to weeks by a modified pulmonary or CPB machine; venovenous (VV) ECMO is primarily used for treating severe but potentially reversible respiratory failure, and venoarterial (VA) ECMO is primarily used for treating severe cardiac or cardiorespiratory failure.

With VV ECMO, deoxygenated blood is drained from the inflow cannula placed in a large central vein, typically the inferior vena cava (IVC), and oxygenated blood is returned through a cannula whose tip lies in or close to the right atrium. Ideally, all or most of the blood from the outflow cannula passes through the tricuspid valve into the pulmonary circulation. One single-cannula technique uses a double-lumen single cannula (Avalon Elite Bicaval Dual-Lumen Catheter and Vascular Access Kit, Maquet Cardiopulmonary, Rastatt, Germany), and it is designed for placement in the right internal jugular vein. The tip of the (larger) inflow lumen is situated within the IVC, thus taking care to avoid insertion into a hepatic vein. The inflow lumen has an end hole and side fenestrations at the tip, as well as side holes proximal to the exit site of the inflow lumen that allow drainage from the both the superior vena cava (SVC) and the IVC. The outflow lumen of the single cannula opens 10 cm above the inflow cannula tip and is designed to return blood to the right atrium. Once inserted, the outflow cannula lumen should be positioned inward and toward the tricuspid valve to direct flow through the valve. TEE may be used to illustrate flow within the inflow and outflow cannula lumina and to illustrate position of each limb within the IVC and the right atrium, respectively.

During VA ECMO, systemic venous blood drains into the circuit through a cannula placed in the right atrium through either the IVC (femoral approach) or SVC (internal

30

jugular vein approach). This may be visualized by TEE to establish flow through the cannula and correct positioning. If TEE is contraindicated, TTE may provide utility in selected patients who allow adequate echocardiographic visualization through the chest wall. Akin to VV ECMO, blood passes through the inflow cannula of the VA ECMO circuit into the pump and the oxygenator/heat exchanger before returning to the patient through a cannula placed within or grafted to a large artery (femoral, axillary, or aorta, commonly). Systemic arterial blood flow is the sum of the VA ECMO circuit flow and any ejection from the left ventricle. Systemic BP is determined by flow and vascular tone.

Using Echocardiography to Troubleshoot Common Complications of Venoarterial Extracorporeal Membrane Oxygenation

- **North-south syndrome:** This syndrome occurs in the specific circumstance of severely impaired lung function in conjunction with femoral placement of the VA ECMO outflow cannula. In this situation, the potential exists for upper body hypoxemia (coronary arteries, cerebral blood vessels, and upper limbs) because proximal branches of the aorta receive predominantly deoxygenated blood ejected from the left heart. This phenomenon of north-south syndrome may be seen on echocardiography as stagnant, "swirling" flow in the descending thoracic aorta as a result of the interface created by blood ejected from the left ventricle and blood returning to the patient from the outflow limb. Even in the presence of significant LV ejection, this situation does not arise if pulmonary function is good or the outflow cannula is transitioned to central placement (proximal aorta or axillary artery). For this reason, institutional practice may dictate transition from peripheral (through the femoral artery) to central (through the aortic or axillary artery) cannulation as soon as the patient is clinically stable enough to handle this transition. Alternatively, after recovery of LV function is confirmed by echocardiography, but lung function continues to suffer, transition to VV ECMO may be initiated.
- **Hemodynamic instability:** Hypotension during "full-flow" VA ECMO and complete circulatory support in the absence of native cardiac function suggests vasodilation or LV distension. LV distension may become particularly problematic in patients with aortic and mitral regurgitation. Clinically, the patient may present with pulmonary edema frothing from the endotracheal tube shortly after institution of VA ECMO and/or ventricular arrhythmia requiring defibrillation. The diagnosis may be confirmed by identifying a severely dilated left ventricle with TEE. Increasing pump flows reduce pulmonary blood flow and can ameliorate the issue. Failing this, the left side of the heart must be vented. Echocardiographic confirmation of LV vent placement is important to ensure that the left ventricle is decompressed and that the risk of developing LV thrombus has been significantly reduced.

Weaning and Discontinuing Venoarterial Extracorporeal Membrane Oxygenation

An early sign of recovery of myocardial function is the presence of pulsatility on the arterial waveform. Patients are usually weaned from VA ECMO onto moderate doses of inotropic support (eg, epinephrine 0.04–0.1 µg/kg per min). The planned inotropic regimen should be started several hours before weaning. Circuit flows are slowly reduced to 1 to 2 L/minute and cardiac function is assessed with TEE during hemodynamic monitoring. If the patient is hemodynamically stable and TEE imaging demonstrates preserved cardiac function on pharmacologic support, then decannulation and discontinuation of VA ECMO are planned.

In summary, understanding the process of initiation, management, weaning, and discontinuation from both VV and VA ECMO represents an important skill set for today's cardiothoracic intensivist. In particular, the utility of TEE in the care of these patients with complex conditions provides the intensive care physician with a tool that confirms the diagnosis of common complications or even routine management during VV and VA ECMO.

SUGGESTED READINGS

Aronson S, Dyke CM, Stierer KA, et al. The ECLIPSE Trials: comparative studies of clevidipine to nitroglycerin, sodium nitroprusside, and nicardipine for acute hypertension treatment in cardiac surgery patients. *Anesth Analg.* 2008;107(4):1110–1121.

Bellomo R, Chapman M, Finfer S, et al. Low-dose dopamine in patients with early renal dysfunction: a placebo-controlled randomized trial: Australian and New Zealand Intensive Care Society (ANZICS) Clinical Trials Group. *Lancet.* 2000;356:2139.

Esper SA, Levy JH, Waters JH, et al. Extracorporeal membrane oxygenation in the adult. *Anesth Analg.* 2014;118(4):731.

Feinman J, Weiss SJ. Hemodynamic transesophageal echocardiography in left ventricular assist device care: a complementary technology. *J Cardiothorac Vasc Anesth.* 2014;28:1181.

Fischer GW, Levin MA. Vasoplegia during cardiac surgery: current concepts and management. *Semin Thorac Cardiovasc Surg.* 2010;22:140.

Follath F, Cleland JG, Just H, et al. Efficacy and safety of intravenous levosimendan compared with dobutamine in severe low-output heart failure (the LIDO study): a randomized double-blind trial. *Lancet.* 2002;360:196.

Genereux P, Webb JG, Svensson LG, et al. Vascular complications after transcatheter aortic valve replacement: insights from the PARTNER (Placement of AoRTic TraNscathetER Valve) trial. *J Am Coll Cardiol.* 2012;60:1043–1052.

George I, Xydas S, Topkara VK, et al. Clinical indication for use and outcomes after inhaled nitric oxide therapy. *Ann Thorac Surg.* 2006;82(6):2161–2169.

Gomez WJ, Erlichman MR, Batista-Filho ML, et al. Vasoplegic syndrome after off-pump coronary artery bypass surgery. *Eur J Cardiothorac Surg.* 2003;23:165.

Hill LL, Kattapuram M, Hogue CW. Management of atrial fibrillation after cardiac surgery. Part 1. Pathophysiology and risks. *J Cardiothorac Vasc Anesth.* 2002;16:483.

Ichinose F, Roberts JD, Zapol WM. Inhaled nitric oxide: a selective pulmonary vasodilator; current uses and therapeutic potential. *Circulation.* 2004;109:3106.

Kodali SK, Williams MR, Smith CR, et al. Two-year outcomes after transcatheter or surgical aortic-valve replacement. *N Engl J Med.* 2012;366:1686–1695.

Lehmann A, Boldt J. New pharmacologic approaches for the perioperative treatment of ischemic cardiogenic shock. *J Cardiothorac Vasc Anesth.* 2005;19:97.

Levy JH. Treating shock: old drugs, new ideas. *N Engl J Med.* 2010;362:841.

Levy JH, Bailey JM, Deeb M. Intravenous milrinone in cardiac surgery. *Ann Thorac Surg.* 2002;73:325.

Lovich MA, Pezone MJ, Wakim MG, et al. Inhaled nitric oxide augments left ventricular assist device capacity by ameliorating secondary right ventricular failure. *ASAIO J.* 2015;61:379–385.

Nardi P, Pelligrino A, Scaferi A, et al. Long term outcome of CABG in patients with left ventricular dysfunction. *Ann Thorac Surg.* 2009;87:1401.

Puskas JD, Williams WH, Mahoney EM, et al. Off-pump versus conventional coronary artery bypass grafting: early and 1-year graft patency, cost, and quality of life outcomes. *JAMA.* 2004;291:1841.

Vincent JL, Rhodes A, Perel A, et al. Clinical review: update on hemodynamic monitoring: a consensus of 16. *Crit Care.* 2011;15:229.

Webb JG, Binder RK. Transcatheter aortic valve implantation: the evolution of prostheses, delivery systems and approaches. *Arch Cardiovasc Dis.* 2012;105:153–159.

Wiener RS, Welch HG. Trends in the use of pulmonary artery catheters in the United States, 1993–2004. *JAMA.* 2007;298:423.

30

Chapter 31

Central Nervous System Dysfunction After Cardiopulmonary Bypass

Suzanne Flier, MD, MSc • John M. Murkin, MD, FRCPC

Key Points

1. Despite a progressive decrease in cardiac surgical mortality, the incidence of postoperative neurologic complications has remained relatively unchanged over the decades.
2. The risk for stroke in patients undergoing coronary artery surgery increases progressively with increasing age, ranging from 0.5% for patients younger than 55 years to 2.3% for those older than 75 years.
3. Neurologic events in cardiac surgical patients are associated with increased postoperative mortality, prolonged intensive care unit stay, longer hospital stay, decreased quality of life, and decreased long-term survival.
4. Mechanisms for neurologic injury in cardiac surgery include some combination of cerebral embolism, hypoperfusion, and inflammation, associated vascular disease, and altered cerebral autoregulation, rendering the brain more susceptible to injury.
5. While occlusive carotid disease is associated with increased risk of perioperative stroke, such stroke is not infrequently contralateral, and concomitant perioperative carotid endarterectomy may increase risk of stroke and other major adverse events.
6. Perioperative risk factors for neurologic complications include renal dysfunction, diabetes mellitus, hypertension, prior cerebrovascular disease, aortic atheromatosis, manipulation of ascending aorta, complex surgical procedures, bypass time longer than 2 hours, hypothermic circulatory arrest, hemodynamic instability during and after bypass, new-onset atrial fibrillation, hyperglycemia, hyperthermia, and hypoxemia.
7. Routine epiaortic scanning before instrumentation of the ascending aorta is a sensitive and specific technique used to detect nonpalpable aortic atheromatosis.
8. In patients with significant ascending aorta atheromatosis, avoidance of aortic manipulation ("no-touch technique") is associated with decreased perioperative stroke.
9. Strategies to decrease the impact of cardiopulmonary bypass (CPB) on embolization, inflammation, and coagulation will decrease neurologic complications.
10. Cerebrovascular disease renders patients who experience wide hemodynamic perturbations during CPB at greater risk for perioperative stroke.
11. Cerebral near-infrared spectroscopy (cerebral oximetry) can detect cerebral ischemia and is associated with decreased incidence of stroke and improved outcomes after cardiac surgery.
12. There is a greater incidence of early postoperative cognitive dysfunction in patients exposed to conventional CPB compared with off-pump and noncardiac surgical patients.

13. The incidence of late cognitive dysfunction and stroke appears to be similar between groups undergoing conventional CPB, percutaneous coronary intervention, or medical management, implying progression of underlying disease and atrial arrhythmias as primary mechanisms of late stroke.

From 2001 to 2011, coronary artery bypass graft (CABG) procedures decreased by nearly 50% to 213,700 procedures, whereas percutaneous coronary intervention (PCI) decreased by more than 25% to 560,500 procedures in 2011. Although these trends may reflect a variety of environmental, lifestyle, and therapeutic factors, overt and subclinical perioperative cerebral injury remains a compelling problem and continues to influence the debate over optimal strategy for coronary revascularization. Accordingly, the risk factors, causes, and potential for mitigation of perioperative stroke and neurobehavioral outcomes associated with cardiac surgery and cardiopulmonary bypass (CPB) are the topic of this chapter.

CATEGORIZATION OF CENTRAL NERVOUS SYSTEM INJURY

In a seminal study, central nervous system (CNS) injury was classified into two broad categories: type I (focal injury, stupor, or coma at discharge) and type II (deterioration in intellectual function, memory deficit, or seizures). Cerebral injury can also be broadly classified as stroke, delirium (encephalopathy), or postoperative cognitive dysfunction. *Stroke* is defined clinically as any new focalized sensorimotor deficit persisting longer than 24 hours, identified either on clinical grounds only or, ideally, as confirmed by magnetic resonance imaging (MRI), computed tomography, or other form of brain imaging.

Transient ischemic attack (TIA) is defined as brief neurologic dysfunction persisting for less than 24 hours. Neurologic dysfunction lasting longer than 24 hours but less than 72 hours is termed a *reversible ischemic neurologic deficit.*

Delirium is described as a transient global impairment of cognitive function, reduced level of consciousness, profound changes in sleep pattern, and attention abnormalities.

Cognitive dysfunction is defined as a decrease in score falling below some predetermined threshold, such as a decrease in postoperative score of magnitude 1 standard deviation or more derived from the preoperative performance.

Seizure is categorized as either convulsive or nonconvulsive and may be related to overt CNS injury or, alternatively, may reflect transient biochemical or pharmacologically mediated neuroexcitation.

The incidence of stroke or type I injury after closed-chamber cardiac procedures is generally considered to be approximately 1%. For isolated single valve surgical repair or replacement, a stroke rate of 1.6% is reported and this increases to 2.9% for combined CABG and valve surgery. The incidence of cognitive dysfunction (type II) is reported as ranging in rate from 30% to 80% in the early postoperative period. The difference in the incidence of cerebral injury after cardiac surgery is related to the type and complexity of the procedure, whether it is off-pump coronary artery bypass (OPCAB), CABG, open chamber, combined CABG and valvular surgery, or aortic arch and related procedures. The increasing usage of minimally invasive valvular

31

and coronary revascularization techniques, as well as the expanding role for catheter-based valve replacement, has independently impacted the risk of CNS injury. Overall, the increased length of stay and increased mortality rates associated with any form of cerebral complication in cardiac surgical patients are striking. Predictors of both types of cerebral complications included advanced age of older than 70 years and a history or the presence of significant hypertension. Predictors of type I deficits include the presence of proximal aortic atherosclerosis, a history of prior neurologic disease, use of the intraaortic balloon pump, diabetes, a history of hypertension, a history of unstable angina, and increasing age. Perioperative hypotension and the use of ventricular venting were also weakly associated with this type of outcome.

Early, Delayed, and Late Stroke

In considering the incidence of perioperative stroke it is apparent that distinguishing stroke as early (ie, neurologic deficit apparent on emergence from anesthesia), delayed (ie, neurologic deficit developing more than 24 hours postoperatively), or late (ie, stroke developing more than 30 days postoperatively) is important to better discriminate causative factors and potential risk reduction strategies. Such an analysis facilitates identification of potentially causal intraoperative events (eg, hypotension, atherosclerotic aorta) from perioperative occurrences (eg, atrial fibrillation) and later progression of underlying disease (eg, cerebrovascular atherosclerosis).

Studies strongly indicate that patient comorbidities, particularly aortic atherosclerosis, in concert with intraoperative factors, whether associated with CABG, OPCAB, or PCI, fundamentally impact the incidence of early stroke and are thus potentially modifiable, whereas late stroke reflects progression of comorbid disease and atrial arrhythmias.

Age-Associated Risk for Central Nervous System Injury

In a review of 67,764 cardiac surgical patients, of whom 4743 were octogenarians, and who underwent cardiac surgery at 22 centers in the National Cardiovascular Network, the incidence of type I cerebral injury was 10.2% in patients older than 80 years versus 4.2% in patients younger than 80. Although global mortality for cardiac surgery in octogenarians was greater than in younger patients, the researchers reported that, when octogenarians without significant comorbidities were considered, their mortality rates were similar to those of younger patients.

In addition to the age-related factor, reports from Europe and North America consistently describe previous cerebrovascular disease, diabetes mellitus, hypertension, peripheral vascular disease (including carotid disease), aortic atherosclerosis, renal dysfunction, infarction or unstable angina within 24 hours before surgery, and intraoperative and postoperative complications as being additional factors increasing the incidence of cerebral injury in cardiac surgical patients (Box 31.1). Determining the impact of age-associated cerebral injury in cardiac surgery is becoming more relevant because of the progressive increase in the average age of the general population and, in particular, of the cardiac surgical population. The presence of preoperative comorbidities is increasingly recognized as the primary determinant of the age-associated risk for CNS complications. As overall survival and quality of life after cardiac surgery continue to improve in older patients, advanced age alone is no longer considered a deterrent when evaluating a patient for cardiac surgery. The presence and extent of comorbidities should be considered as being of equal or greater importance than age itself as a risk factor for cerebral injury in cardiac surgical patients.

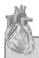

BOX 31.1 *Factors Related to Cerebral Injury in Cardiac Surgery*

Age
Aorta atheromatosis
Carotid disease
Diabetes mellitus
Hypertension
Peripheral vascular disease
Renal dysfunction
Stroke or cerebrovascular disease
Recent unstable angina or acute myocardial infarction
Preoperative low output/low ejection fraction
Combined/complex procedures
Redo surgery
Prolonged cardiopulmonary bypass time
Intraoperative hemodynamic instability
Postoperative atrial fibrillation

Risk factors consistently reported for perioperative cerebral injury in cardiac surgery patients; see discussion in the text.

Retrospective Versus Prospective Neurologic Assessment

The detection of CNS injury depends critically on the methodology used, and retrospective studies have been demonstrated as insensitive in various studies. A retrospective chart review is inadequate as an assessment of the overall incidence of postoperative neurologic dysfunction. The reasons for the inability of retrospective chart audit to detect the majority of patients with neurologic dysfunction are readily apparent and include incompleteness of records, a reluctance to document apparently minor complications, and, most important, an insensitivity to subtle neurologic dysfunction. The timing, thoroughness, and reproducibility (single examiner) of the neurologic examinations, as well as the incorporation of a preoperative assessment for comparison, all determine the sensitivity and accuracy with which postoperative CNS injury can be detected. Many of the types of neurologic impairment now being documented are subclinical and not readily detectable by a standard "foot-of-the-bed" assessment and have currently unknown implications for longer-term patient outcomes.

■ NEUROPSYCHOLOGIC DYSFUNCTION

Compared with stroke, cognitive dysfunction (neurocognitive dysfunction) is a considerably more frequent sequela of cardiac surgery and has been demonstrated in up to 80% of patients early after surgery. The pathogenesis of cognitive dysfunction after cardiac surgery is still uncertain. Variables that have been postulated to explain the development of postoperative neurocognitive decline include advanced age, concomitant cerebrovascular disease, and severity of cardiovascular disease, as well as progression of underlying disease. Various intraoperative factors, such as cerebral emboli, hypoperfusion or hypoxia, activation of inflammatory processes, aortic cross-clamp or CPB time, low mean arterial pressure (MAP), and cerebral venous

31

hypertension, have all been implicated. In many instances, subtle signs of neuropsychological dysfunction are detectable only with sophisticated cognitive testing strategies, although depression and personality changes may be noted by family members. It should be recognized that formalized cognitive testing is reproducible and quantifiable and represents an objective outcome measure; as such, it can act as a benchmark to assess various therapeutic interventions (eg, the efficacy of putative cerebroprotectants, equipment modifications, pH management strategies). In addition, a number of studies have made correlations between early postoperative cognitive dysfunction and intraoperative cerebral oxygen desaturation, as well as new ischemic lesions on MRI. Assessment of early cognitive dysfunction can be used to discriminate between various intraoperative treatment modalities (eg, pH management, use of cell saver, epiaortic scanning [EAS]). However, whether early postoperative cognitive dysfunction represents permanent neurologic damage remains controversial.

Several more recent studies have demonstrated similar incidences of later cognitive dysfunction whether patients underwent CABG, off-pump surgery, PCIs, or were managed medically. These results strongly imply that underlying comorbidities and progression of cerebrovascular disease are the most relevant factors in late postoperative cognitive dysfunction rather than cardiac surgery per se.

MECHANISMS OF BRAIN INJURY

Determining which factor or, more likely, which combination of factors is responsible for postoperative neurologic or behavioral dysfunction in patients undergoing cardiac surgery using CPB is problematic (Box 31.2). From the few studies in which a surgical control group has been used, it appears that elements inherent to CPB are causative, particularly in dysfunction occurring in the immediate postoperative period. How much of this dysfunction is as a direct result of exposure to CABG and CPB or occurs as a result of underlying comorbid disease is an area of active ongoing investigation. Based on postmortem studies, as well as correlative analyses of intraoperative events with neurologic outcomes, two primary mechanisms appear to be responsible for brain injury in otherwise uncomplicated cardiac operations: cerebral hypoperfusion and cerebral emboli.

Intraoperative cerebral embolization of particulate and microgaseous elements has a significant role in the genesis of cerebral events in postoperative cardiac surgical

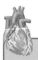

BOX 31.2   *Risk Factors for Neurologic Complications in Cardiac Surgery*

Hemodynamic instability
Diabetes mellitus
Advanced age
Combined/complex procedures
Prolonged cardiopulmonary bypass time
Prior stroke/cerebrovascular disease
Aortic atheromatosis
Renal dysfunction
Peripheral vascular disease

VI

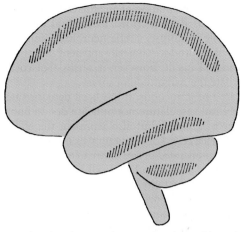

Fig. 31.1 Hatched areas showing the most frequent locations of boundary area, or watershed zone infarcts in the brain, situated between the territories of major cerebral or cerebellar arteries. (From Torvik A. The pathogenesis of watershed infarcts in the brain. *Stroke.* 1984;2:221–223.)

patients. Increasing attention is also being paid to the role of perioperative hypoperfusion, particularly in patients with intracranial and extracranial atherosclerosis, and to the effect of inflammatory processes triggered during exposure to surgery and CPB.

More recent evidence is also focusing on new-onset postoperative atrial fibrillation (POAF) as being associated with increased long-term mortality and stroke. Formerly, POAF was thought to be relatively benign and self-limited, whereas a recent meta-analysis identified new-onset POAF following CABG as associated with significantly higher risk of mortality in short- and long-term follow-up and higher rates of stroke and other complications.

Watershed Infarctions

Watershed, or boundary zone, infarcts are ischemic lesions that are situated along border zones between the territories of two major cerebral arteries (eg, the middle and posterior, or the anterior and middle cerebral arteries) where terminal arteriolar anastomoses exist (Fig. 31.1).

By the same rationale, however, these areas are also highly susceptible to ischemia because of end-artery embolization, and it is also recognized that, although severe hypotension is the most common cause, showers of microemboli may lodge preferentially in these areas and cause infarcts in the underlying brain. As such, although they commonly arise from profoundly hypotensive episodes, watershed lesions are not pathognomonic of a hypotensive episode and may be the result of cerebral emboli. Embolization and hypoperfusion acting together play a synergistic role and either cause or magnify the brain damage of cardiac surgical patients.

Cerebral Emboli and Outcome

Cerebral emboli during CPB can be arbitrarily differentiated into macroemboli (eg, calcific or atherosclerotic debris) and microemboli (eg, microgaseous bubbles, microparticulate matter). Overt and focal neurologic damage likely reflects the occurrence of cerebral macroemboli (eg, calcific and atheromatous debris generated during valve tissue removal or instrumentation of an atheromatous aorta), whereas less focal neurologic dysfunction has been ascribed to cerebral microemboli. Microemboli appear to have some role in diffuse, subtle neurologic and cognitive disturbances, whereas macroemboli likely produce clinically apparent catastrophic strokes. Whatever the nature of the cerebral insult, however, it seems that coexistent inflammatory processes can exacerbate the magnitude of injury.

Gaseous emboli are not innocuous. It has been demonstrated that the effects of air emboli on the cerebral vasculature not only are due to bubble entrapment with direct blockage of cerebral vessels but also represent the effects that such bubbles have on vascular endothelial cells. Ultrastructural examinations of pial vessels exposed to cerebral air emboli demonstrated severe injury to endothelial plasmalemma, leading to loss of cellular integrity and endothelial cell swelling. Such endothelial damage produces disruptions of vasoreactivity. Air embolism also produces changes in blood elements leading to formation of a proteinaceous capsule around the bubbles, marked dilation of pial vessels, platelet sequestration, and damage to endothelial cells. Air-induced mechanical trauma to the endothelium causes basement membrane disruption, thrombin production, release of P-selectin from intracellular vesicles, synthesis of platelet-activating factor, and a reperfusion-like injury with perturbations in inflammation and thrombotic processes. These phenomena likely impair nitric oxide production, causing alterations in cerebral microvascular regulation. Whether heparin anticoagulation during CPB mitigates the impact of cerebral gas embolization as demonstrated during cerebral angiography remains speculative.

Cerebral Perfusion Pressure

Intraoperative hypotension during cardiac surgery has been related to postoperative neurologic dysfunction. Electroencephalographic (EEG) patterns consistent with ischemia—increased slow wave activity, diffuse slowing of EEG activity—have been reported to occur during CPB episodes thought to be associated with cerebral hypoperfusion. Episodes of flow reduction during normothermia frequently produced ischemic changes, whereas similar decreases during stable hypothermia were not associated with EEG changes. Indeed, ischemic EEG changes are frequently seen in association with reductions in perfusion flow rate during the initiation of CPB.

During the transition to CPB, the brain is particularly vulnerable to ischemia, inasmuch as cerebral metabolic rate for oxygen ($CMRO_2$) is apparently unchanged, yet the brain is initially perfused with an asanguineous prime, and even after equilibration during established CPB, hematocrit is generally maintained at a range between 20% and 30%. As a result, any further decreases in cerebral perfusion, in the absence of concomitant decreases in $CMRO_2$, are poorly tolerated. During hypothermic conditions, there is a profound decrease in $CMRO_2$, exceeding 50% for a 10°C reduction in temperature. It is clear that under anesthesia, and particularly during hypothermic CPB, cerebral blood flow (CBF) is maintained at very low levels of cerebral perfusion pressure. Using radioisotope techniques for measurement of CBF, and incorporating a jugular venous catheter for calculation of $CMRO_2$, it was determined that there is a profound reduction in $CMRO_2$ during hypothermic CPB and that CBF is decreased proportionately and will autoregulate down to a cerebral perfusion pressure of 20 mm Hg, in the presence of alpha-stat pH management. Low arterial pressure during the hypothermic phase of CPB is thus unlikely to result in cerebral ischemia in the absence of cerebrovascular disease. As the average age and extent of disease in patients presenting for CABG continue to increase, the number of patients with concomitant cerebrovascular disease, and thus potentially deranged cerebral autoregulation, presents an increasingly important group.

Cerebral Venous Obstruction

It should also be appreciated that, during CPB, cerebral venous hypertension can result from partial obstruction of the superior vena cava, particularly in the presence of a single two-stage venous cannula, and may cause cerebral edema and produce a disproportionate decline in cerebral perfusion pressure relative to arterial pressure. Cerebral venous hypertension, as can occur during CPB with myocardial dislocation and impaired drainage of superior vena cava, may result in cerebral ischemia if unrecognized and untreated. It is feasible that such unrecognized cerebral venous hypertension has resulted in some of the postoperative neurologic syndromes that have been reported.

Although the association between arterial hypotension during CPB and cerebral dysfunction remains contentious, there is some evidence that certain subsets of patients may be at particular risk. MAP and rewarming are not primary determinants of cognitive decline, but hypotension and rapid rewarming contribute significantly to cognitive dysfunction in older patients. Again, because older patients comprise an increasing segment of the population undergoing cardiac surgical procedures, these aspects are becoming increasingly important clinical management issues.

Hemodynamic Instability During Cardiopulmonary Bypass

Hemodynamic complications, either before, during, or after surgery, have been found to increase cerebral injury in cardiac surgical patients. Studies indicate an increased susceptibility of the brain in cardiac surgical patients to apparently "benign" hemodynamic alterations that either produce or enhance cerebral injury, probably through hypoperfusion of the brain tissue. This is of particular importance since it has been estimated that more than 50% of patients undergoing CABG have coexisting cerebrovascular disease. The interaction of emboli, perfusion pressure, and the particular conditions of the regional cerebral circulation (eg, preexisting cerebral intravascular lesions) determine the final expression of brain damage in the cardiac surgical patient. Patients with cerebrovascular disease who undergo CPB procedures with large fluctuations in hemodynamic parameters are at particularly increased risk for the development of postoperative neurologic complications.

31

Aortic Atherosclerosis

Atheroembolism from an atheromatous ascending aorta and aortic arch is recognized as a major risk factor in the patient undergoing cardiac surgical procedures and is a widespread problem. The prevalence rate of aortic arch atheroma increases with age, such that severe atheroma is seen in more than 20% of patients older than 74 years—a primary factor in the age-associated increase in risk of perioperative stroke.

Atheroembolism in cardiac surgery has a broad spectrum of clinical presentations, including devastating injuries and death, yet its true incidence is probably underestimated. Thoracic aorta atheromatosis is associated with coronary artery disease and stroke in the general population. Investigators have concluded that the risk for stroke is four times greater in patients with severe arch atheroma. Yahia and colleagues prospectively studied patients with diagnoses of TIA or stroke using transesophageal echocardiography (TEE) to assess aortic atheromatosis. Thoracic aortic atheromas were present in 141 of 237 patients (59%); mild plaque (<2 mm) was present in 5%, moderate plaque (2–4 mm) in 21%, severe plaque (≥4 mm) in 33%, and complex plaque in 27%. Plaques were more frequently present in the descending aorta and the arch of the aorta than in the ascending aorta. Significant atherosclerosis of the ascending aorta is present in 20% to 40% of cardiac surgical patients, the percentage increases with age, and it is an independent risk factor for stroke (type I cerebral injury).

Diabetes Mellitus and Hyperglycemia

The presence of diabetes is recognized as a factor related to increased morbidity and mortality in cardiac surgical patients. The incidence of diabetes mellitus increases with age, and its presence is known to accelerate the damage caused by atherosclerosis; thus, an increasingly greater percentage of patients presenting for CABG have concomitant diabetes, currently estimated as a comorbidity in approximately 30% to 40% of patients having CABG. Investigators have linked diabetes to increased incidences of stroke and mortality. Part of the risk may involve cerebral hypoperfusion because increased extent and duration of cerebral oxygen desaturation during CPB has been documented in diabetic patients, with patients with insulin-dependent diabetes demonstrating the lowest values (as measured via jugular oximetry) and the poorest response to increases in MAP.

Studies identify normoglycemia as a desirable perioperative goal in cardiac surgical patients regardless of whether they are diabetic. Experimental and clinical evidence shows that hyperglycemia is associated with exacerbation of neurologic injury. Approaches to maintain serum glucose values less than 150 mg/dL have shown favorable results. The ideal value of serum glucose in cardiac surgical patients remains unknown, but the evidence available suggests that maintenance of euglycemia is related to a better prognosis.

In accordance with these data, Society of Thoracic Surgeons' (STS) guidelines for glucose control in patients undergoing cardiac surgery recommend that, in both diabetic and nondiabetic patients, blood glucose levels should be maintained at less than or equal to 180 mg/dL with intravenous insulin as required. However, there are concerns regarding potential adverse effects associated with hypoglycemia, including increased risk for mortality associated with even a single episode of severe hypoglycemia as seen in medical/surgical intensive care patients. Furthermore, in a randomized, prospective study of 400 cardiac surgical patients managed either with tight glucose control (intravenous insulin to maintain intraoperative glucose between 80 and 100 mg/dL) or conventional management (glucose level <200 mg/dL), a significantly greater incidence of stroke was found in the treatment group. Hence, avoidance of hypoglycemia should be paramount. Accordingly, an important caveat recommending preservation of lower limit of glucose level greater than 100 mg/dL should be appended to the guidelines. Overall, it would appear that maintenance of perioperative serum glucose between 100 and 180 mg/dL in both diabetic and nondiabetic patients is desirable.

CEREBRAL BLOOD FLOW

pH Management and Cerebral Blood Flow

Relatively little new information regarding the cerebral circulation in human beings during CPB appeared until 1983, when Henriksen and colleagues reported evidence of cerebral hyperemia occurring during CPB. This report was followed in 1984 by a seminal paper from Govier and coworkers, who incited controversy with their observations of ischemic threshold levels of CBF during CPB, in direct contrast with the hyperperfusion reported by Henriksen. It was hypothesized that differences in pH management accounted for the divergent values previously reported for CBF during hypothermic CPB. Accordingly, patients were managed with either alpha-stat or pH-stat pH management during hypothermic CPB. A similar and pronounced reduction in $CMRo_2$ was observed in both groups during hypothermia and, in the alpha-stat group, global cerebral flow/metabolism coupling was preserved in comparison with the group managed with pH-stat. Alpha-stat management preserved autoregulation and the relation between CBF and metabolism and has become the standard of care for adult patients undergoing CPB with mild and moderate hypothermia.

Cerebral Hyperthermia

Cerebral hyperthermia during the rewarming phase of CPB can exacerbate a preexisting injury before rewarming and may be detrimental itself. Hyperthermia can have a strong impact on cerebral oxygen transfer and neurologic outcome. Glutamate levels can increase during cerebral hyperthermia, leading to eventual cell death. Rapid rewarming decreases jugular venous hemoglobin saturation, creating a mismatch between cerebral oxygen consumption and delivery. Slower rewarming rate with lower peak temperatures during CPB may be an important factor in the prevention of neurocognitive decline after hypothermic CPB, and interventions to avoid postoperative hyperthermia may be warranted to improve cerebral outcome after cardiac surgery.

▣ CARDIOPULMONARY BYPASS EQUIPMENT

Early studies demonstrated increased microemboli in patients undergoing CPB using bubble oxygenators, with a reduction in cerebral embolization with the use of membrane oxygenators and arterial line filtration (Box 31.3).

BOX 31.3 *Clinical Strategies That May Decrease Neurologic Complications in Cardiac Surgery*

Early and aggressive control of hemodynamic instability
Perioperative euglycemia between 100 and 180 mg/dL
Routine epiaortic scanning before manipulation of ascending aorta
Avoidance of manipulation of ascending aorta in severe atheromatosis
Maintenance of adequate cerebral perfusion pressure (neuromonitoring/cerebral oximetry)
Monitoring of cerebral venous pressure via a proximal central venous pressure catheter or the introducer port of a pulmonary artery catheter
Alpha-stat pH management during moderate hypothermic cardiopulmonary bypass (CPB)
Avoidance of arterial inflow temperature greater than 37°C
Use of CPB circuitry incorporating membrane oxygenator and 40-µm arterial line filter
Use of surface-modified and reduced-area CPB circuitry
Use of cerebral oximetry

31

Modification of the inflammatory response to the CPB using modified surface CPB circuits and leukocyte-depleting filters has also been explored.

In addition, various intraoperative manipulations, particularly instrumentation of the atherosclerotic aorta, are independent risks for the generation of cerebral emboli and likely produce particulate and microparticulate emboli rather than oxygenator-generated microgaseous and microaggregate emboli. Avoidance of manipulation of a diseased aorta seems to decrease embolization and cerebral injury. An alternative approach, emboli reduction by capture using an intraaortic filter inserted through a side chamber of a modified aortic cannula, has also been assessed.

Minimally Invasive Extracorporeal Circulation

A recent development in the drive for more physiologic CPB has been the advent of minimally invasive extracorporeal circulation (MiECC). This system consists of a modular biocompatible closed circuit of minimal priming volume, incorporating a centrifugal pump and membrane oxygenator, and has been shown to result in significantly decreased inflammatory markers. MiECC was also associated with reduced systemic inflammatory response as measured by polymorphonuclear elastase, hemodilution as calculated by hematocrit drop after procedure, need for red blood cell transfusion, reduced levels of peak troponin release, incidence of low cardiac output syndrome, need for inotropic support, peak creatinine level, occurrence of POAF, duration of mechanical ventilation, and ICU stay.

Because the technique of modular MiECC has been employed for combined CABG and valve surgery, as well as in high-risk patients, and shown to result in less cerebral microembolization and improved cerebral tissue oxygenation, as well as improved neurocognitive outcomes, there is significant potential that such an approach to CPB may well become the standard of care in the near future.

CEREBROPROTECTIVE STRATEGIES

Risk Assessment

Major perioperative neurologic event key predictors are age, history of neurologic disease, diabetes, previous CABG, unstable angina, and history of pulmonary disease. The Stroke Risk Index allows neurologic risk to be estimated for each patient, thus enabling the most appropriate perioperative therapy to be used, whether this be surgical modification, change in perfusion management, applied neuromonitoring, or administration of putative pharmacologic cerebroprotectants. It is also useful as a scale to compare risk indices and thus the efficacy of different interventions across clinical outcome studies.

Carotid Endarterectomy

In the current cardiac surgical population, 17% to 22% of patients have a moderate carotid artery stenosis of 50% or more, and 6% to 12% have a severe stenosis of 80% or more. The risk for postoperative stroke is 10% in patients with moderate and 11% to 19% in patients with severe stenosis, whereas it remains 2% or less in patients with a stenosis of less than 50%. Although in patients presenting for cardiac surgery severe bilateral carotid artery disease is rare, the risk for perioperative stroke is as high as 20%. However, it is not clear that carotid endarterectomy decreases this rate, because in a meta-analysis, pooled data for stroke or death did not support carotid endarter-ectomy for risk reduction from asymptomatic carotid stenosis during CABG (relative risk, 0.9; $P = .5$). In a review, it was estimated that only about 40% of perioperative strokes (at most) could be directly attributable to ipsilateral carotid artery disease. Accordingly, in a patient with asymptomatic carotid stenosis, combined surgery should not be undertaken unless the surgical team is very experienced in combined carotid endarterectomy/CABG procedures. Concomitant carotid endarterectomy is unlikely to decrease a patient's stroke risk. Rather, carotid stenosis should be regarded as indicating a high likelihood of aortic and/or concomitant intracerebral disease, and that use of EAS with appropriate modification of surgical approach and applied neuromonitoring can be of particular benefit in this high-risk group.

Transesophageal Echocardiography Versus Epiaortic Scanning

The detection of ascending aorta atheromatosis is a cornerstone of strategies to decrease the incidence of stroke during and after cardiac surgical procedures. Manual palpation of the aorta, despite its widespread utilization, has a very low sensitivity for this purpose. The association between severe thoracic aortic plaques (defined as 5-mm-thick focal hyperechogenic zones of the aortic intima and/or lumen irregularities with mobile structures or ulcerations) and coronary artery disease is well established. Identifying severe aortic disease has important clinical implications because surgical technique, including surgical procedure and siting of cannulation and anastomotic sites for proximal grafts, can be altered to avoid producing emboli and stroke.

Multiple studies have documented that most of the significant atherosclerotic lesions in the ascending aorta are missed by intraoperative palpation by the surgeon, and intraoperative echocardiographic studies of the aorta have been recommended (Fig. 31.2). However, the ability of TEE to detect ascending aorta and aortic arch lesions reliably is limited. The high acoustic reflectance attributable to the air-tissue interface resulting from overlying right main bronchus and trachea limits TEE

31

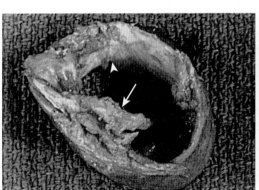
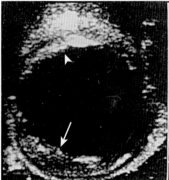

Fig. 31.2 Transverse ultrasonic image of the ascending aorta and the corresponding segment of aorta in a patient with severe atherosclerosis. Note the calcification *(arrowhead)* and the projection of atheroma *(arrow)* into the lumen. (From Wareing TH, Davila-Roman VG, Barzilai B, et al. Management of the severely atherosclerotic ascending aorta during cardiac operations. A strategy for detection and treatment. *J Thorac Cardiovasc Surg.* 1992;103:453–462.)

assessment of the upper ascending aorta, where cannulation is generally undertaken. If the complete biplane TEE examination is negative for plaque, it is highly unlikely that there is significant plaque in the ascending aorta. If the TEE examination is positive for plaque, there is a 34% chance that there is significant disease of the ascending aorta, and EAS should be considered. TEE is a sensitive but only mildly specific method of determining whether ascending aortic atherosclerosis is present.

The standard for aortic assessment before instrumentation continues to be visual inspection and palpation by the surgeon, despite the fact that this has been shown to identify atheromatous disease in only 25% to 50% of patients and, even when identified, to underestimate its severity significantly. Management strategies for the diseased ascending aorta range from minimally invasive aortic "no-touch" techniques (NTTs) to maximally invasive procedures, including ascending aorta replacement or extensive aortic debridement under deep hypothermic circulatory arrest (HCA). Operative modifications in CABG include avoidance of aortic cross-clamping, alternative sites of aortic cross-clamping, and avoidance of proximal anastomoses by usage of all arterial conduit or Y-grafts.

"No-Touch" Technique

Avoidance of instrumentation of the ascending aorta in patients with severe aortic atheromatosis has been advocated.

In these patients, revascularization is performed with single or bilateral internal thoracic arteries and by connecting additional coronary grafts (saphenous vein, radial artery) in a T or Y configuration.

Powerful evidence implicating aortic instrumentation comes from a 12,079-patient study of isolated coronary artery bypass surgery in which aortic manipulation was completely avoided by using in situ internal thoracic arteries for inflow in 1552 patients (no-touch), a clampless facilitating device for proximal anastomoses in 1548 patients, and aortic clamping in 8979 patients. The study demonstrated an overall incidence of postoperative stroke of 1.4% ($n = 165$), with an unadjusted incidence of 0.6% ($n = 10$) in the no-touch group, 1.2% ($n = 18$) in the clampless facilitating device group, and 1.5% ($n = 137$) in the clamp group ($P < .01$ for no-touch vs clamp). The ratio of observed to expected stroke rate increased as the degree of aortic manipulation increased from 0.48 in the no-touch group to 0.61 in the clampless facilitating device group, and to 0.95 in the clamp group, demonstrating that aortic clamping was independently associated with an increase in postoperative stroke compared with a no-touch technique. Even after correcting for use of CPB, aortic clamping was an independent risk factor for postoperative stroke, since both the OPCAB partial clamp and the on-pump cross-clamp techniques increased the risk of postoperative stroke compared to no-touch.

Carbon Dioxide Insufflation During Open-Chamber Procedures

A primary determinant of the number and duration of microgaseous emboli during open-chamber procedures relates to methodologies for removal of intracavitary air. Although needle aspiration and/or aortic root venting are standard techniques for air removal, use of CO_2 insufflation, either continuously or immediately before closure of ventriculotomy, has been shown to significantly increase the efficacy of de-airing, resulting in decreased systemic gaseous emboli. However, although there has been a general expectation of improvements in neurologic and cognitive outcomes resulting from such CO_2 insufflation, it has been surprisingly difficult to demonstrate.

VI

Temperature and Coronary Artery Bypass Grafting

It is known that the vulnerability of the normothermic brain to focal ischemic insult demonstrates a surprising variability in the presence of small gradations in temperature. Small increases in brain temperature, such as to 39°C, as may occur during CABG, have been shown to profoundly enhance the susceptibility of the brain to focal ischemic insult and result in ischemic lesions of much greater extent in comparison with controls at 37°C.

Applied Neuromonitoring

Intraoperative neurophysiologic monitoring may be of benefit to decrease CNS injury. Intraoperative transcranial Doppler (TCD) has been demonstrated to detect embolic events in real time and allows modification of perfusion and surgical techniques. Alternatively, brain oximetry studies using noninvasive near-infrared spectroscopy (NIRS) have shown promising results. Combined electroencephalography and cerebral oximetry identified episodes of cerebral ischemia in 15% of a series of 550 beating-heart patients; all were treated successfully by a combination of pharmacologically improved cardiac output, increased perfusion pressure, and cardiac repositioning.

A physiologically derived treatment algorithm for management of perioperative cerebral oxygen desaturation has been proposed and is shown in Fig. 31.3.

Some of the concerns associated with cerebral oximetry, including extracerebral signal contamination, and change in arterial/venous partitioning, have been addressed in a new generation device. The incorporation of a Doppler ultrasound to focus NIRS photons has permitted the direct measurement of changes in microcirculatory CBF using ultrasound-tagged photons, and a series of preliminary studies has demonstrated the utility of this approach to assess the integrity and the lower limit of cerebral autoregulation.

Neuromonitoring During Deep Hypothermic Circulatory Arrest

Moderate (25–30°C) and deep (<25°C) hypothermia remain a mainstay for cerebral and systemic protection during complex aortic arch repair because surgical access may require interruption of systemic perfusion for relatively protracted periods. As there is relatively little ability to monitor cerebral well-being during such times because electroencephalography becomes progressively attenuated at less than 25°C, cerebral NIRS has been advocated as a means of monitoring and detecting onset of cerebral ischemia during deep HCA. Although some groups monitor jugular venous oxygen saturation (SjO_2) using retrograde cannulation of the internal jugular vein as an index of cerebral metabolic suppression during cooling, correlation has not been demonstrated between SjO_2 and cerebral NIRS during deep HCA. A possible explanation could be that NIRS is a highly regional measure of cerebral cortical oxygen tissue saturation, whereas SjO_2 is a measure of cerebral mixed venous oxygen saturation and thus reflective of global changes in venous oxygenation and, as such, potentially less sensitive to regional perfusion inhomogeneities.

In addition to deep HCA, some centers use retrograde cerebral perfusion (RCP) via the superior vena cava or, increasingly, selective anterograde cerebral perfusion (SACP) via the innominate or subclavian artery. There have been a variety of case reports of the ability of cerebral NIRS to detect onset of cerebral ischemia during aortic arch surgeries, and there is growing interest in the role of cerebral NIRS as a measure of adequacy of perfusion in this setting. It is increasingly recognized that RCP does not provide sufficient nutritive flow to sustain cerebral integrity for an

31

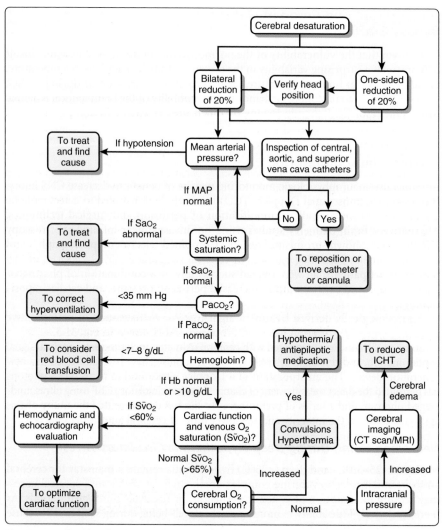

Fig. 31.3 Algorithm for the use of brain oximetry. *CT,* Computed tomography; *Hb,* hemoglobin; *ICHT,* intracranial hypertension; *MAP,* mean arterial pressure; *MRI,* magnetic resonance imaging; *Paco₂,* arterial partial pressure of carbon dioxide; *Sao₂,* arterial oxygen saturation; *Sv̄o₂,* mixed venous oxygen saturation. (Reprinted from Denault A, Deschamps A, Murkin JM. A proposed algorithm for the intraoperative use of cerebral near-infrared spectroscopy. *Semin Cardiothorac Vasc Anesth.* 2007;11:274–281.)

extended interval, as has been reflected in lower regional hemoglobin oxygen saturation (rSo₂) values seen during NIRS monitoring in RCP versus SACP.

In adult patients, cerebral malperfusion can occur either as a consequence of ascending aortic dissection with occlusion of carotid lumen, kinking or obstruction of perfusion cannula during selective cerebral perfusion for circulatory arrest procedures, or migration of aortic endoclamp cannula during minimal-access cardiac surgery with potential compromise of cerebral perfusion. Reports are increasing that bilateral rSo₂ monitoring can detect contralateral desaturation during unilateral selective cerebral perfusion. This can result from an incomplete circle of Willis, which, in some

VI

series, has a prevalence rate of up to 50% and has been estimated to be a factor in cerebral malperfusion in approximately 15% of patients.

Pharmacologic Cerebral Protection

Whereas multiple advances toward understanding the basic mechanisms of brain injury have led to the development of multiple pharmacologic strategies for neuroprotection, in general, pharmacologic protection from cerebral ischemia remains an elusive goal. Based on sound experimental evidence, including data from animal studies, a number of putative neuroprotective agents have been examined in cardiac surgical patients, but the results have been mostly negative. Agents tested have included those that reduce brain oxygen consumption to increase tolerance to ischemia (thiopental and propofol) and those that target established neuroprotective pathways, including the N-methyl-D-aspartate (NMDA) receptor, calcium channels, oxidant stress, the gamma-aminobutyric acid (GABA) receptor, and others. Post hoc analyses of several trials have suggested encouraging neuroprotective effects from remacemide and complement-inhibiting agents. However, for the most part, there are no widely accepted pharmacologic agents with proven efficacy to reduce the extent of brain injury associated with cardiac surgery.

As a broad-spectrum antiinflammatory agent, the serine protease inhibitor aprotinin has been shown to positively impact coagulation and inflammatory alterations triggered by CPB and has also been associated with decreased incidences of stroke and major CNS injury in cardiac surgical patients. However, because the clinical usage of aprotinin has been suspended indefinitely because of several reports of increased mortality and adverse events associated with aprotinin therapy in cardiac surgical patients, the future of this drug remains controversial.

There are some other interesting associations between certain drug therapies having antiinflammatory and antiplatelet properties and lowered incidences of stroke and adverse CNS events. Findings are strongly supportive of perioperative aspirin therapy and suggest that platelets have a fundamental role in orchestrating the ischemic response to reperfusion injury of multiple organ systems in patients undergoing cardiac surgery.

Another promising line of investigation for cerebral protection is the role for 3-hydroxy-3-methyl-glutaryl coenzyme–A (HMG CoA) reductase inhibitors (eg, statins). With evidence accruing that statins not only have a lowering effect on low-density lipoprotein cholesterol but also present pleiotropic and neuroprotective effects, evidence for stroke reduction is accumulating. Currently statins are thought to possess antiatherosclerotic properties, increase plaque stability, and exert favorable effects on inflammation, vasomotor function, local fibrinolysis, and platelet activity. Another plausible mechanism for statin-induced neuroprotection could be the prevention of POAF, possibly inflammation-induced, leading to less postoperative stroke. However, blunt systemic inhibition of inflammation (eg, dexamethasone) does not seem to provide protection of the brain in cardiac surgery.

Theoretically, volatile anesthetics and nonvolatile xenon possess neuroprotective effects as well. There is experimental evidence for increased perfusion of ischemic areas, decreased cerebral metabolism, inhibition of glutamate receptor activity and neurotransmitter activity, inhibition of ion channels thereby preventing pathologic calcium or sodium influx, reduction of injurious oxidative stress, maintenance of mitochondrial function, and inhibition of apoptosis. However, apart from an abundance of animal data, clinical evidence is still scarce. Although there is as yet no pharmacologic magic bullet that can be used to reduce neurologic injury in patients undergoing cardiac surgery, a combination of technical and pharmacologic measures is currently available that might positively affect the CNS outcomes of these patients. In patients identified as being at risk for

31

perioperative cerebral injury, preventive measures should be instituted with organ-targeted management to guide the whole intraoperative and postoperative period.

These neuroprotective strategies include:

- the use of alpha-stat pH management during moderate hypothermic CPB,
- avoidance of cerebral hyperthermia by limiting arterial line temperature to 37°C,
- avoidance of direct reinfusion of unprocessed cardiotomy suction blood by use of blood cell processing and secondary filtration,
- intraoperative TEE or epiaortic ultrasonographic EAS in all patients,
- use of arterial line filters to minimize embolic load,
- maintenance of euglycemia,
- reduction of CPB circuit and use of biocompatible surface-modified circuits, and
- reduced hemodilution to avoid subsequent allogeneic blood transfusion.

Further recommendations would include monitoring cerebral venous outflow pressure via proximal jugular venous pressure, avoidance of hypotension, and the use of tepid rather than normothermic perfusion during CPB. As the age and incidence of comorbid disease in the cardiac surgical population continue to increase, the importance of these issues becomes ever more acute. In summary, primary prevention continues to be the only effective measure to decrease the incidence of cerebral injury in patients undergoing cardiac surgical procedures.

SUGGESTED READINGS

Alexander KP, Anstrom KJ, Muhlbaier LH, et al. Outcomes of cardiac surgery in patients > or = 80 years: results from the National Cardiovascular Network. *J Am Coll Cardiol.* 2000;35(3):731–738.

Anastasiadis K, Bauer A, Antonitsis P, et al. Minimal invasive extra-corporeal circulation (MiECC): a revolutionary evolution in perfusion. *Interact Cardiovasc Thorac Surg.* 2014;19(4):541–542.

Doty JR, Wilentz RE, Salazar JD, et al. Atheroembolism in cardiac surgery. *Ann Thorac Surg.* 2003;75(4):1221–1226.

Ebert AD, Walzer TA, Huth C, et al. Early neurobehavioral disorders after cardiac surgery: a comparative analysis of coronary artery bypass graft surgery and valve replacement. *J Cardiothorac Vasc Anesth.* 2001;15(1):15–19.

Eckmann DM, Armstead SC, Mardini F. Surfactants reduce platelet-bubble and platelet-platelet binding induced by in vitro air embolism. *Anesthesiology.* 2005;103(6):1204–1210.

Gandhi GY, Nuttall GA, Abel MD, et al. Intensive intraoperative insulin therapy versus conventional glucose management during cardiac surgery: a randomized trial. *Ann Intern Med.* 2007;146(4):233–243.

Grigore AM, Grocott HP, Mathew JP, et al. The rewarming rate and increased peak temperature alter neurocognitive outcome after cardiac surgery. *Anesth Analg.* 2002;94(1):4–10, table.

Hillis LD, Smith PK, Anderson JL, et al. 2011 ACCF/AHA Guideline for Coronary Artery Bypass Graft Surgery: a report of the American College of Cardiology Foundation/American Heart Association Task Force on Practice Guidelines. *Circulation.* 2011;124(23):e652–e735.

Knipp SC, Matatko N, Wilhelm H, et al. Evaluation of brain injury after coronary artery bypass grafting. A prospective study using neuropsychological assessment and diffusion-weighted magnetic resonance imaging. *Eur J Cardiothorac Surg.* 2004;25(5):791–800.

Koster S, Hensens AG, van der Palen J. The long-term cognitive and functional outcomes of postoperative delirium after cardiac surgery. *Ann Thorac Surg.* 2009;87(5):1469–1474.

Lazar HL, McDonnell M, Chipkin SR, et al. The Society of Thoracic Surgeons practice guideline series: blood glucose management during adult cardiac surgery. *Ann Thorac Surg.* 2009;87(2):663–669.

Maruff P, Silbert B, Evered L. Cognitive decline following cardiac surgery. *Br J Anaesth.* 2001;87(3):518–519.

Millar K, Asbury AJ, Murray GD. Pre-existing cognitive impairment as a factor influencing outcome after cardiac surgery. *Br J Anaesth.* 2001;86(1):63–67.

Murkin JM. Perioperative multimodality neuromonitoring: an overview. *Semin Cardiothorac Vasc Anesth.* 2004;8(2):167–171.

Murkin JM, Falter F, Granton J, et al. High-dose tranexamic acid is associated with nonischemic clinical seizures in cardiac surgical patients. *Anesth Analg.* 2010;110(2):350–353.

Okita Y, Minatoya K, Tagusari O, et al. Prospective comparative study of brain protection in total aortic arch replacement: deep hypothermic circulatory arrest with retrograde cerebral perfusion or selective antegrade cerebral perfusion. *Ann Thorac Surg.* 2001;72(1):72–79.

Palerme LP, Hill AB, Obrand D, et al. Is Canadian cardiac surgeons' management of asymptomatic carotid artery stenosis at coronary artery bypass supported by the literature? A survey and a critical appraisal of the literature. *Can J Surg.* 2000;43(2):93–103.

Selnes OA, Gottesman RF. Neuropsychological outcomes after coronary artery bypass grafting. *J Int Neuropsychol Soc.* 2010;16(2):221–226.

Slater JP, Guarino T, Stack J, et al. Cerebral oxygen desaturation predicts cognitive decline and longer hospital stay after cardiac surgery. *Ann Thorac Surg.* 2009;87(1):36–44.

Wang D, Wu X, Li J, et al. The effect of lidocaine on early postoperative cognitive dysfunction after coronary artery bypass surgery. *Anesth Analg.* 2002;95(5):1134–1141, table.

Yahia AM, Kirmani JF, Xavier AR, et al. Characteristics and predictors of aortic plaques in patients with transient ischemic attacks and strokes. *J Neuroimaging.* 2004;14(1):16–22.

Chapter 32

Long-Term Complications and Management

Martin Birch, MD • Monica I. Lupei, MD •
Michael Wall, MD, FCCM • Julia Weinkauf, MD

Key Points

1. Cardiac surgical patients are at significant risk from preventable adverse events. These events occur through human error, by either faulty decision making (diagnosis, decision for treatment) or faulty actions (failure to implement the plan correctly).
2. Human error is ubiquitous and cannot be prevented or eliminated by trying harder or by eliminating the one who errs. Reduction in human error requires system changes that prevent errors from occurring (forcing functions) or prevent errors from reaching the patient.
3. Sleep deprivation and fatigue can render a person more likely to make an error. Although residents' hours are limited, those of other physicians in the United States are not, unlike in other countries.
4. Nontechnical skills such as leadership, communication, cooperation, and situational awareness are critical to patient safety, but they are rarely taught. Distractions, disruptions, noise, and alarms contribute to technical errors and increase mortality rates in cardiac surgery.
5. Communication is the leading root cause of sentinel events, whether through missing information or through misunderstanding. Use of structured communication protocols reduces errors. Handoffs performed without a protocol involve significant numbers of omitted items.
6. Team training reduces surgical mortality rates, but it must be done with careful preparation and with regular retraining.
7. Surgical briefings that use a checklist significantly reduce surgical mortality rates ("World Health Organization Safe Surgery Saves Lives"). Debriefings allow teams to identify hazards and formulate improvements.
8. Simulation is an effective means to teach both technical and nontechnical skills and to allow teams to train for rare but dangerous events.
9. Cognitive aids should be available in every operating room to provide direction during rare crisis events (eg, malignant hyperthermia, pulseless electrical activity).
10. Medication errors occur approximately in 1 in every 150 to 200 anesthetic cases. The Anesthesia Patient Safety Foundation published a set of recommendations to reduce medication errors, including standardization, use of technology such as bar codes and smart infusion pumps, having pharmacy involvement in every step of the medication process, and building a culture of safety.
11. Awareness during anesthesia occurs approximately 1 to 2 times per 1000 anesthetic cases, and it occurs more often in cardiac surgical procedures. Use of a processed electroencephalogram or achieving an end-tidal concentration of 0.7 minimum alveolar concentration is effective in reducing the incidence of awareness.

12. The culture of an organization or a unit contributes significantly to patient safety or danger. Strict hierarchical cultures typically harbor a culture of blame and shame, which inhibits identification and correction of hazards. A "Just Culture" acknowledges that human error occurs and seeks to redesign the system to prevent future errors, but also holds individual persons accountable for willful violations.

This chapter focuses on the long-term complications and management of patients after cardiac surgery in the intensive care unit (ICU) and includes a discussion of specific infections observed in patients after surgery, the management of acute renal failure, and the role of nutritional support in the critically ill. The chapter also covers complications after newer surgical procedures such as transcatheter aortic valve replacement (TAVR), other minimally, invasive hybrid procedures, and long-term complications of ventricular assist devices (VADs) and extracorporeal membrane oxygenation (ECMO). Finally, this chapter concludes with an overview of the numerous ethical dilemmas that this technology has created for patients, families, and clinicians.

INFECTIONS AFTER CARDIAC SURGERY

Device-Related Infections

Cardiac-Implanted Electronic Devices

As the number of cardiac-implanted electronic devices (CIEDs; eg, pacemakers, cardioverter-defibrillators, cardiac resynchronization therapy) is gradually increasing, their complications, such as infections, are also increasing. CIED-related infections can be difficult to diagnose since echocardiography is less accurate and blood cultures are less sensitive than in endocarditis. Most of the patients exhibit nonspecific symptoms, and fewer than 10% of the patients develop septic shock. The incidence of CIED-related infections varies among studies from between 0.5% and 2.2%, with a twofold to fivefold increase in incidence after a revision. The most common pathogens identified across different studies were staphylococci and other gram-positive bacteria. All-cause mortality associated with CIED-related infection varied between 0% and 35%.

The management of suspected CIED-related infections, including the number and sequence of blood cultures and antibiotic therapy, should be guided by the clinical severity. The treatment recommendations for definite CIED-related infections include early removal of the entire system (ie, all leads and generator) along with appropriate antibiotic therapy.

Ventricular Assist Devices

Left ventricular assist device (LVAD) driveline-related infections occur with an incidence up to 20% and commonly develop more than 30 days after implantation. Infections in patients with LVADs are associated with increased hospitalization, frequent need for reoperation, increased risk of stroke, and delay in heart transplantation. Some authors report a trend toward decreased survival in patients with an LVAD who develop infections.

Patients with LVAD infections tend to have a larger body mass index and frequently have a history of diabetes mellitus. *Staphylococcus aureus* was the most common organism identified in patients with an LVAD and with sepsis complications. The management of LVAD driveline-related infections potentially requires driveline

32

repositioning or LVAD exchange with antibiotic bead implantation and systemic antibiotic treatment.

Intravascular Devices

Intravascular devices such as arterial, central venous, or pulmonary artery catheters are universally used in patients after cardiac surgery. Patients who have intravascular catheters often acquire bloodstream infections (BSIs), which are associated with prolonged hospitalization and increased risk of mortality. Central line–associated BSI (CLABSI) is defined by the Centers for Disease Control and Prevention (CDC) as bacteremia not related to an infection at another site or two or more positive blood cultures with a common skin contaminant associated with signs and symptoms of infection. CLABSIs are prevalent worldwide, and the rate is almost fourfold higher internationally (7.6 per 1000 central-line days) than the national rate in the United States (2 per 1000 central-line days). The CDC reported a significant reduction of CLABSI incidence in ICUs in the United States in recent years: a 58% reduction from 2001 to 2009. The risk of a BSI for arterial catheters is lower than the risk associated with noncoated, uncuffed, nontunneled short-term central vascular catheters (1.7 vs 2.7 per 1000 catheter days). If arterial catheters are inserted using maximum barrier precautions, then a very low risk of BSIs (0.41 per 1000 catheter days) can be achieved.

The recognized risk factors for the development of CLABSIs were prolonged hospitalization before catheter insertion, femoral and internal jugular catheterization, longer catheterization duration, neutropenia, use of total parenteral nutrition, extensive catheter manipulation, and reduced nurse-to-patient ratio. The majority of CLABSI cases are caused by gram-positive organisms (60%), including coagulase-negative staphylococci (34%), the *Enterococcus* species (16%), and *Staphylococcus aureus* (10%); approximately 18% of the reported CLABSI cases were attributable to gram-negative organisms (18%) and to the *Candida* species (12%).

The prominent reduction of the CLABSI rate with the implementation of various prevention initiatives has prompted the development of many quality improvement initiatives with the goal to achieve a minimum-to-none CLABSI incidence. The CDC published guidelines for the prevention of catheter-related infections (CRIs) in 2011. The summary of the guidelines is presented in Box 32.1.

Sternal Wound Infections

The CDC classifies this surgical site infection as superficial or deep. Based on the CDC definition of a deep sternal wound infection (DSWI), this surgical site infection occurs within 30 to 90 days after a surgical procedure. The incision is dehiscent or deliberately opened, an association exists with fever or localized pain and tenderness, or an abscess has formed. The DSWI is an uncommon but serious complication after cardiac surgery that is associated with unfavorable morbidity and increased mortality.

Old age, diabetes, previous stroke and transient ischemic attacks, congestive heart failure (CHF), and bilateral internal mammary artery grafts for the coronary artery bypass graft (CABG) procedure are risk factors for DSWI after cardiac surgery. Mechanical ventilation duration and ICU and hospital lengths of stay were longer in patients diagnosed with DSWI as compared with patients without DSWI. *Staphylococcus aureus* and gram-positive bacteria were the most common pathogens. The recommended treatment for DSWI is adequate systemic antibiotic therapy, along with either surgical débridement with antibiotic irrigation and primary closure or sternotomy with flap reconstruction.

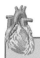

> **BOX 32.1** *Prevention of Intravascular Catheter–Related Infections*
>
> **Central Venous Catheter Infection Prevention**
>
> - Use the subclavian site if possible, and avoid using the femoral site
> - Use ultrasound, if available, to reduce the number of imaging attempts
> - Use the catheter with the minimum number of lumens necessary
> - Use strict hand hygiene, skin preparation with an antiseptic, and full barrier precaution for insertion
> - Maintain aseptic technique through the insertion and care of the catheter
> - Regularly monitor the catheter insertion site for signs of infection
> - Use 2% chlorhexidine for daily skin cleansing
> - Do not routinely replace the catheter to prevent infection
> - Do not use guidewire to exchange the catheter in case of suspected infection
> - Remove the catheter when it is no longer necessary
>
> **Arterial Catheter Infection Prevention**
>
> - In adults, radial, brachial, and dorsalis pedis are preferred over axillary and femoral sites
> - Use a minimum of cap, mask, sterile gloves for arterial catheter insertion, and full barrier precautions for the femoral site
> - Replace the arterial catheter only when clinically indicated
> - Remove the arterial catheter when no longer necessary
>
> Adapted from O'Grady NP, Alexander M, Burns LA, et al. Guidelines for the prevention of intravascular catheter-related infections. *Am J Infect Control.* 2011;39(4 Suppl 1):S1–S34.

Prosthetic Valve Endocarditis

The diagnosis of endocarditis requires a high level of clinical suspicion, considering that the clinical presentation is frequently nonspecific with fever, chills, fatigue, or weight loss. The modified Duke criteria are the gold standard for infective endocarditis (IE) diagnosis: two major, one major and three minor, or five minor clinical criteria are required (Table 32.1). Prosthetic valve IE can occur early (less than 1 year after valve replacement) or late (more than 1 year after surgery). The risk of IE was found to be 1% to 4% early after surgery, and 0.5% to 1% per patient year of prosthetic valve later after surgery. The prosthetic valve and CIED-associated IE incidence has increased in recent years. The reported risk was similar for mitral or aortic valve replacement (AVR), regardless of the type of prosthesis; however, it was higher if more than one valve was replaced. *Staphylococcus aureus* was reported to be the most common pathogen in prosthetic valve IE (34%), followed by the *Streptococcus* species (23%), the *Enterococcus* species (19%), and coagulase-negative *Staphylococcus* (18%).

Despite the low level of evidence regarding the benefit of antibiotic prophylaxis in the prevention of IE, the current recommendation remains that all patients with prosthetic valves receive antibiotic prophylaxis before dental or surgical procedures. Evidence also suggests that antibiotic treatment decreases the risk of stroke after IE. Based on current guidelines of the American College of Cardiology and the American Heart Association (ACC/AHA), surgery is indicated in prosthetic valve–related IE, resulting in hemodynamic instability, heart failure, or valvular complications such as

32

Table 32.1	Modified Duke Criteria for Diagnosing Infective Endocarditis
Major Criteria	**Minor Criteria**
1. Two positive blood cultures with typical microorganisms collected at least 12 hours apart (or one positive blood culture for *Coxiella burnetii*) 2. Evidence of endocardial involvement (new murmur, echocardiographic evidence of a cardiac mass, abscess, valve dehiscence)	1. Fever >38°C 2. Vascular phenomena (systemic emboli, Janeway lesions) 3. Immunologic phenomena (Osler nodes, Roth spots) 4. Predisposition to infective endocarditis (previous infective endocarditis or intravenous drug abuse) 5. Microbiologic evidence that does not meet major criteria

Adapted from Thanavaro KL, Nixon JV. Endocarditis 2014: an update. *Heart Lung.* 2014;43(4):334–337.

dysfunction or dehiscence, obstruction or regurgitation, and abscess or fistula formation, but it is not indicated in uncomplicated cases.

Systemic Inflammatory Response Syndrome and Sepsis

Systemic inflammatory response syndrome (SIRS) and sepsis are clinical entities that result from an infection with an inflammatory response. Box 32.2 summarizes the diagnostic criteria for sepsis. The number of sepsis cases reported in the United States exceeds 750,000 per year, of which 50% were treated in ICUs. Fifteen million to 19 million new sepsis cases per year are estimated to develop worldwide each year. Most studies have reported that sepsis mortality remained high over time, and septic shock accounted for the highest mortality, approaching 50%.

Some authors report that infections are the most common noncardiac complication after cardiac surgery. Hospital costs, lengths of stay, and readmissions were significantly associated with hospital-acquired infections after cardiac surgery. Another large prospective study revealed that nearly 5% of the patients were diagnosed with major infections (eg, DSWI, mediastinitis, infectious myocarditis or pericarditis, endocarditis, cardiac device infection, pneumonia, empyema, *Clostridium difficile* colitis, BSI) after cardiac surgery. The risk factors associated with increased infections were chronic lung disease, heart failure, long surgery, emergent surgery, prolonged mechanical ventilation, and postoperative antibiotic administration for longer than 48 hours. Major infections significantly increased the mortality rate after cardiac surgery.

Considering the high mortality and morbidity risk of sepsis, a group of experts representing numerous international organizations launched the Surviving Sepsis Campaign (SSC) and published guidelines in 2003, which were updated in 2012. The SSC guidelines are outlined in Box 32.3.

Pneumonia

Pneumonia is a difficult diagnosis to make in patients after cardiac surgery because the typical radiographic signs might be confused with postsurgical changes. Pneumonia

BOX 32.2 *Diagnostic Criteria for Sepsis*

Infection Documented or Suspected With Some of the Following Criteria

General Variables

- Fever
- Hypothermia
- Tachycardia
- Tachypnea
- Altered mental status
- Positive fluid balance
- Hyperglycemia in the absence of diabetes

Inflammatory Variables

- Leukocytosis
- Leucopenia
- Greater than 10% immature leukocytes
- Increased plasma C-reactive protein
- Increase plasma procalcitonin

Hemodynamic Variables

- Arterial hypotension

Organ Dysfunction Variables

- Hypoxemia
- Oliguria
- Creatinine increase
- Coagulation abnormalities
- Ileus
- Hyperbilirubinemia

Tissue Perfusion Variables

- Increased lactic acid
- Decreased capillary refill

Adapted from Dellinger RP, Levy MM, Rhodes A, et al. Surviving Sepsis Campaign Guidelines Committee including the Pediatric Subgroup. *Crit Care Med.* 2013;41(2):580–637

is an important complication after cardiac surgery. A multicenter study revealed that pneumonia represented 48% of hospital-acquired infections in patients who underwent cardiac surgery. A history of chronic obstructive lung disease is significantly associated with respiratory infection after cardiac surgery.

Approximately 5.5% of patients require prolonged mechanical ventilation after cardiac surgery. Considering the increased mortality and health care costs related to ventilator-assisted pneumonia (VAP), the Institute for Healthcare Improvement (IHI) recommends the use of a five-component ventilator bundle, which has been associated with a lower incidence of VAP: (1) head of the bed elevation; (2) daily sedation interruption and spontaneous breathing trials; (3) peptic ulcer disease prophylaxis; (4) deep vein thrombosis (DVT) prophylaxis; and (5) daily oral care with chlorhexidine.

> **BOX 32.3** *Summary of the Surviving Sepsis Campaign Guidelines*
>
> Routine screening of patients who are potentially infected and seriously ill is recommended for severe sepsis.
>
> Protocolized resuscitation of patients with hypoperfusion should be initiated during the first 6 hours of recognizing septic shock.
>
> Effective intravenous antimicrobials should be administrated within the first hour of recognizing severe sepsis or septic shock, ideally after culture collection.
>
> Crystalloids should be the initial fluid of choice in the resuscitation of severe sepsis and septic shock. Albumin may be added when substantial amounts of crystalloids are needed.
>
> Norepinephrine should be the first vasopressor of choice. Epinephrine may be added when an additional agent is needed.
>
> Hydrocortisone is not indicated if fluid therapy and vasopressor restores hemodynamic stability. If hemodynamic stability is not achievable, then 200 mg daily hydrocortisone might be beneficial.
>
> Empiric antibiotic combination therapy should not be administered for more than 3 to 5 days. De-escalation to the appropriate single therapy should be performed when available.
>
> The typical antibiotic therapy duration should be 7 to 10 days.
>
> Glucose management in the intensive care unit to maintain glycemia <180 mg/dL is indicated.
>
> Transfusion is indicated only for hemoglobin levels <7 g/dL (with a goal range of 7–9 g/dL) unless severe hypoxemia, myocardial ischemia, coronary artery disease, or acute hemorrhage is present.
>
> Adapted from Dellinger RP, Levy MM, Rhodes A, et al. Surviving Sepsis Campaign Guidelines Committee including the Pediatric Subgroup. *Crit Care Med.* 2013;41(2):580–637

Urinary Tract Infection

Urinary tract infection (UTI) is one of the most common hospital-acquired infections and accounts for 4.4% of infections after cardiac surgery. Diabetes mellitus and advanced age are associated with increased incidences of UTI in patients after cardiac surgery. Bacteriuria rapidly develops in patients with a urinary catheter, with an average of 3% to 10% per day of catheterization. Bacteriuria is frequently asymptomatic (approximately 90% of cases), and therefore the diagnosis of UTI is primarily clinical. Traditional diagnostic criteria for UTI include the presence of pyuria and great than 10^5 colony-forming units (CFU)/mL urine. UTI treatment is not indicated unless laboratory data are associated with clinical signs and symptoms of infection (eg, temperature >38°C, urgency, frequency, dysuria, suprapubic tenderness). Because 80% of UTIs are attributable to the presence of an indwelling catheter, the removal of unnecessary catheters is recommended.

▓ ACUTE KIDNEY INJURY

Acute kidney injury (AKI) is a frequent and potentially devastating complication after cardiac surgery. When severe, dialysis may be necessary. Risk factors are multiple, and the etiology and pathogenesis is complex and only incompletely understood. Multiple preventative strategies have been tried. Unfortunately, the benefit is unclear, especially pharmacologic prevention. After the onset of AKI, multiple therapeutic interventions also have been tried, and these, too, have been mostly unsuccessful. The consequences of cardiac–associated AKI (CSA-AKI) are severe. Mortality after routine CABG surgery can increase from less than 1% to 20% when moderate AKI develops. If dialysis is required, then mortality can exceed 50%. Additionally, costs dramatically increase. The incidence of CSA-AKI can vary from approximately 9% to 40%, depending on the definition used and the procedure performed. Patient risk factors are well studied. They include advanced age, female gender, chronic obstructive pulmonary disease (COPD), diabetes, peripheral vascular disease, CHF, baseline renal insufficiency, cardiogenic shock, need for emergent surgery, and left main coronary artery disease. Procedural risk factors include cardiopulmonary bypass (CPB) time, aortic cross-clamp time, transfusion requirements, valvular surgery, combined procedures, and on-pump versus off-pump procedures.

Multiple perioperative insults lead to the development of CSA-AKI, and it is unlikely that one particular insult is the primary causative factor. Preoperative hemodynamic instability coupled with the administration of nephrotoxins, such as intravenous contrast dye, is an early insult. During CPB, blood loss and transfusion, atheroembolism, and further hemodynamic instability add further injury. After CPB, hemodynamic instability is not uncommon, and insults can continue if complications such as infections and sepsis occur. The renal medulla is exceptionally prone to hypoxemia and, even under normal conditions, has a very low tissue oxygen tension. The oxygen tension becomes virtually undetectable during CPB.

Unfortunately, many of the risk factors for and injuries that cause CSA-AKI are not modifiable. Although some are, they are generally surgical in nature. Careful and timely surgery, with shorter CPB and cross-clamp times, will lead to lower rates of renal injury. Less bleeding with fewer transfusions will also be renoprotective. The ACC/AHA Guidelines recommend potentially delaying surgery in patients with preexisting renal dysfunction until the effects of contrast can be assessed.

Treatment

Unfortunately, there is no treatment for CSA-AKI once it occurs. The best practice is to optimize hemodynamics, avoid nephrotoxins, and hope that renal function recovers. If renal function does not recover or if it worsens, then the patient may require dialysis. Standard indications for dialysis initiation are presented in Box 32.4.

32

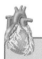

BOX 32.4   *Indications for Renal Replacement Therapy*

Uremia
Hyperkalemia that cannot be medically managed
Significant volume overload unresponsive to diuretics
Severe metabolic acidosis
Removal of dialyzable toxins

Adapted from Liu Y, Davari-Farid S, Arora P, et al. Early versus late initiation of renal replacement therapy in critically ill patients with acute kidney injury after cardiac surgery: a systematic review and meta-analysis. *J Cardiothorac Vasc Anesth.* 2014;28(3):557–563

Determining when renal replacement should be initiated is not always clear. Although this remains an area of great controversy and ongoing research, it appears that initiating renal replacement therapy (RRT) *early* in the course of oliguric AKI not responsive to diuretic medications improves outcomes.

RRT can be prescribed in two basic ways, continuous or intermittent. Each has its own advantages and disadvantages. Continuous therapy provides greater hemodynamic stability and the ability for more controlled and well-tolerated fluid removal, whereas intermittent treatment has the ability to clear blood of harmful electrolytes or toxins more quickly. No data are available that clearly demonstrate the superiority of one technique over the other. Continuous RRT can usually be changed to intermittent therapy after a period of relative hemodynamic stability and when the ability to manage volume status improves.

No evidence-based criteria exist for the cessation of RRT. Cessation depends on multiple criteria, such as the return of renal function and increased urine output, the ability to manage volume status without RRT, the risk outweighs the benefit, or potential medical futility in the moribund patient.

COMPLICATIONS OF TRANSCATHETER AORTIC VALVE REPLACEMENT

TAVR has been used in many high-risk patients and, to some extent, in intermediate-risk patients with severe aortic stenosis (AS) since its introduction in Europe in 2001. This procedure was developed to offer an alternative treatment for patients with severe AS classified as at too high risk for open surgical aortic valve replacement (SAVR). In 2011, the Food and Drug Administration (FDA) granted the approval of this procedure for the replacement of severely stenosed aortic valves.

The first large, multicenter, prospectively randomized trial, the Placement of Aortic Transcatheter Valve (PARTNER) Trial, was conducted in 25 centers in the United States and comprised two cohorts: PARTNER A compared the outcomes of the high-risk patients treated with TAVR versus SAVR, and PARTNER B compared the outcomes of the inoperable patients treated with TAVR versus standard therapy. Cohort A enrolled 699 high-risk patients and revealed that the 30-day mortality rate was 3.4% for TAVR and 6.5% for SAVR, the 1-year mortality rate was 24.2% and 26.8%, respectively, and the 2-year mortality rate remained similar between TAVR and SAVR. In Cohort B, 358 inoperable patients were enrolled. The 30-day mortality rate was 5% for transfemoral (TF)-TAVR and 2.8% for standard therapy; the 1-year mortality rate was 30.7% and 50.7%, respectively; and the 2-year mortality rate was 43.3% and 68%, respectively.

At 30 days, the incidence of stroke in the PARTNER trial cohort A was significantly higher after TAVR (4.6%) versus SAVR (2.4%), and stroke increased the hazard of death. This stroke hazard peaked early after TAVR and remained constant thereafter in relation to SAVR. The overall rate of stroke was significantly higher after TAVR (13.8%), as compared with medical treatment (5.5%) in inoperable patients.

A paravalvular leak post-TAVR could be the result of incomplete prosthesis apposition to the annulus, annular eccentricity, undersized prosthetic valve, or malposition of the implanted device. Moderate-to-severe paravalvular aortic regurgitation (AR) was more frequent after TAVR at 1 and 2 years (7% and 6.9%), as compared with SAVR (1.9% and 0.9%) in the PARTNER trial cohort A and was associated with increased late mortality.

Major vascular complications were more frequent 1 year after TAVR (11.3%), as compared with SAVR (3.8%), whereas major bleeding was less frequent 1 year after

TAVR (15.7%) than after SAVR (26.7%) in the PARTNER trial cohort A, and the differences were maintained at 2 years. The common major bleeding complications after TAVR were gastrointestinal (40.8%), neurologic (15.5%), trauma or fall (7.8%), and genitourinary (6.3%). The occurrence of a major late bleeding complication was a strong independent predictor of mortality, and it was associated with a fourfold increase in late mortality.

COMPLICATIONS OF MECHANICAL ASSIST DEVICES

Long-Term Complications of Ventricular Assist Device Implantation

The landmark Randomized Evaluation of Mechanical Assistance for the Treatment of Congestive Heart Failure (REMATCH) trial of 2001 demonstrated that implanting LVAD improved survival and the quality of life for patients with heart failure over medical management. This trial paved the way for a new paradigm in heart failure management, during which VADs are not only solely used in patients who are failing medical management as a bridge-to-transplant but are also used as destination therapy (DT) for patients in end-stage heart failure who are not candidates for heart transplantation. Furthermore, as devices have improved, survival rates in patients who have a nonemergent VAD implant have started to approach that of heart transplant patients, with a 2-year survival for heart transplantation unchanged at approximately 80% over the last 10 years. Thus VADs are increasingly chosen as DT in lieu of transplantation, even in patients who are transplant-eligible. This development could lead to a future in which a heart for transplant may not be quite in such short supply when compared with the demand.

The adverse event burden that patients with an implanted VAD experience is key to the long-term success of their implant and is increasingly critical in this new era of DT VADs. The original pulsatile-flow VADs (eg, HeartMate XVE) have been replaced by continuous-flow devices (eg, HeartMate II, HeartWare HVAD, DuraHeart II) for DT, as they generally show improved outcomes. Many long-term complications of VAD use still remain, however, which are discussed in the following text.

32

Device Infection

Recently reported rates of all infections in patients with a VAD range up to 49%, with a range of serious infections, such as interior pump infections, occurring in less than 1%, to less serious infections such as percutaneous site infections ranging from 12% to 32%. Overall sepsis rates are relatively high at 11% to 36%. The only independent characteristic predictive of infection was increased duration of support. *Staphylococcus* and *Pseudomonas* species were the most commonly cultured organisms, likely attributable to these organisms' ability to create a biofilm.

Although most VAD-related infections are superficial and can be treated with antibiotics and local débridement, serious infectious complications lead to 11% of device failures. More aggressive treatment strategies that have been reported include vacuum-assisted wound closure and antibiotic-impregnated beads. Curbing an infection as soon as possible is particularly important to prevent the need for device exchange, which carries significantly lower survival rates with each exchange.

Device Thrombosis

Mechanical propulsion of blood within the VAD has several consequences, including stasis and contact with the nonbiologic material, which can lead to thrombosis. Hematologic effects differ, depending on the type of device. Continuous axial flow pumps, such as the HeartMate II, spin at higher revolutions per minute and have more surface-area contact with blood, whereas centrifugal flow pumps such as the HeartWare have fewer and slower moving parts that contact the blood, resulting in less shear stress, less hemostasis, and less blood component activation. Because of this, axial flow pumps have higher rates of hemolysis than centrifugal flow models. Centrifugal flow pumps may ultimately prove to have fewer hemocompatibility issues such as thrombosis as well.

Device-related thrombosis is a feared complication of long-term VAD use; it requires device exchange or transplant. Furthermore, device-related thrombosis is the most common cause of device failure, at 50%. Rates of device-related thrombosis in the HeartMate II original studies were 2% to 4% of patients. Thrombosis is diagnosed by elevated lactate dehydrogenase levels, reflecting associated hemolysis attributable to increased turbulence near the thrombus, echocardiographic findings, computed tomographic (CT) angiography, and increasing pump power use. Conservative treatment strategies that have been reported with success include glycoprotein IIb/IIIa inhibitors and thrombolytic therapy. If these fail or if hemodynamic compromise occurs, then the device must be exchanged.

Gastrointestinal Bleeding

Many factors predispose the patient with a VAD to bleeding events. First, patients require chronic anticoagulation therapy to avoid thrombotic complications. Typical regimens include full-dose aspirin and warfarin with an international normalized ratio (INR) of 2 to 2.5. Another factor predisposing patients to bleeding events is a consequence of the mechanical propulsion of blood, which causes shear stress on the blood components. This leads to acquired von Willebrand (vWB) disease attributable to cleavage of the vWB factor multimers, leading to increased rates of bleeding events.

Gastrointestinal bleeding (GIB) is the most frequently experienced bleeding event in patients with a VAD, with reported rates ranging from 10% to 40%. Patients with continuous-flow VADS tend to form arteriovenous malformations (AVMs) in the intestines, which are thought to be the result of the low pulse-pressure state, and further increase the risk for GIB. Management of the patient with a VAD and GIB is similar to a patient without a VAD, primarily consisting of transfusion, anticoagulation cessation, and endoscopic evaluation. Bleeding of a large number of AVMs in the small intestine may result in more capsule endoscopic studies. Aspirin should be restarted after the cessation of the bleeding and warfarin after individual patient consideration.

Neurovascular Events

Between 2% and 14% of patients with a VAD will experience a stroke, and 4% to 11% will have a stroke leading to disability or death. Disabling stroke is a dreaded event with possibly the greatest impact on the quality of life and the potential to complicate the course of a patient with an otherwise perfectly functioning VAD. Rates of neurologic events are less in continuous-flow devices, as compared with pulsatile-flow devices. The rates of neurologic events have also declined over time in continuous-flow devices, but the explanation remains unclear.

An important patient factor in stroke is anticoagulation status. Multiple studies have found that patients with laboratory values favoring coagulation (high platelet count, low INR and prothrombin time [PT]) correlate with ischemic stroke, and patients with values reflecting anticoagulation (high INR and PT) correlate with hemorrhagic stroke. Careful monitoring of chronic anticoagulation therapy is, no doubt, critical to balance the risk of thrombotic events with hemorrhage.

Device Failure

One-year survival after nonemergent implant of a continuous-flow device is now 80%; 1-year survival drops to 65% after a second implant and 50% after a third. Whether this decrease is due to underlying conditions that may have predisposed to a problem with the pump or to the device exchange itself remains unclear, but exchange is still avoided until deemed absolutely necessary. Device failure occurs at rates of approximately 4%, with a median duration of support of around 500 days. Pump thrombosis was the most common cause of failure at 50%. Lead or cable damage was the next cause at 22%, followed by mechanical failure at 12%, and infection at 11%.

Long-Term Complications of Extracorporeal Membrane Oxygenation

Extracorporeal life support (ECLS) has been used in thousands of patients with respiratory or cardiovascular failure who have not responded to medical management. However, indications and guidelines for the use of ECLS/ECMO remain controversial. The mortality rate in patients undergoing ECMO remains high. Mortality rates range from 21% to 50% in patients undergoing ECMO for respiratory failure, whereas in patients with heart failure, the mortality rate is in the 40% range.

Complications are extremely common in patients undergoing ECMO; approximately 57% of all patients undergoing ECMO for cardiac failure had at least one major complication. Complications are divided into two general categories: device-related and patient-related. The ECMO circuit, itself, is complex, and failures from each component (eg, cannula, tubing, pump, oxygenator, heat exchanger, tubing and return cannula [arterial or venous]) have been reported. Fortunately, with modern cannulas, centrifugal pumps, heparin-coated circuits, and hollow-filter oxygenators, the incidence of circuit-related failures seems to be decreasing. Problems with venous drainage cannulas may include partial obstruction that will increase venous pressure in the patient (an increase in venous pressure may also decrease organ perfusion pressure) and decrease flow rates that will affect oxygenation, ventilation, and blood pressure if using venoarterial (VA) ECMO. Venous drainage may also be decreased if the pump flows are too high, which results in "suck down" where the cannula is occluded because the vein collapses around it, preventing venous drainage. When vein collapse happens, the circuit tubing often "shakes" or "chatters." The collapse can usually be treated by transiently decreasing flows, a fluid bolus, or both. Echocardiography is useful to confirm cannula position. Another cannula problem with venovenous (VV) ECMO can occur when the venous drainage cannula is too close to the venous return cannula from the oxygenator and the oxygenated blood is drained back into the ECMO circuit, which results in inadequate tissue oxygenation. This problem is usually treated by adjusting the position of the cannulas.

A newer bicaval Avalon Elite dual lumen cannula (Avalon Laboratories, Rancho Dominguez, CA) is now being used for VV-ECMO that drains blood from both the superior vena cava and the inferior vena cava and returns it to the right atrium. When

815

32

properly positioned by echocardiography or fluoroscopy, femoral cannulation is avoided. However, a high rate (up to 80%) of upper extremity DVT is associated with the use of this cannula. Hemolysis is also a common complication that has been reported and can lead to anemia, hyperbilirubinemia, AKI, and neurologic complications. Risk factors for hemolysis include the type of oxygenator used, mean venous inlet pressure, and mean pump speed. Hemolysis can be limited by using the largest cannula and the lowest pump speeds possible.

Thrombosis of the pump and/or oxygenator is another dreaded complication of ECMO that must be balanced against over-anticoagulation and bleeding. Unfortunately, no standardized, universally accepted guidelines are available for anticoagulation or for the monitoring of adequate anticoagulation in patients on ECMO.

ECMO is also incredibly expensive, costing $65,519 more in the patients randomized to the conventional ventilation or ECMO for Severe Adult Respiratory failure (CESAR) trial. In this study, ECMO showed a favorable lifetime predicted cost utility of $131,000 per life year.

Finally, ECMO has created numerous ethical problems for patients, families, and clinicians. The most stressful for everyone is the so-called "bridge to nowhere" in which patients on ECMO have no long-term alternative for life support. In conclusion, ECMO is an expensive intervention that has a mortality rate of 20% to 50% and a morbidity rate of approximately 50%. Further studies are underway to continue to define the indications and management of ECMO to improve outcomes.

PATIENT AND FAMILY SUPPORT, PALLIATIVE CARE, AND END-OF-LIFE ISSUES

Twenty percent of Americans who die each year do so during or shortly after a stay in the ICU. This fact places ICU providers in a key position of helping families and patients begin to navigate a difficult process that has the potential to end in an unforeseen and undesirable way. Certainly, helping patients live with a good quality of life for as long as possible is preferable, but when the end inevitably comes, helping patients and their families experience a "good death" can also be invaluable.

Patient care in the cardiothoracic ICU is extremely technology heavy and is becoming more so with time. Supporting organ vital functions is almost indefinitely possible, moving the interventions and care from what used to be "can we" questions to "should we" questions, which result in far more difficult decisions for practitioners, patients, and families.

One complexity particular to surgical ICUs is that the ongoing goals of care may differ among practitioners. A covenant of care often exists between surgeons and their patients. This covenant is described by medical anthropologist Joan Cassell, in which the surgeon's commitment to the patient is characterized as not "giving up" and defeating death at all costs. This commitment can lead to conflicts with intensivists, who more often emphasize the quality of life, and this can create confusion for the patient and their families, who may be hearing mixed messages.

Patients in the cardiac surgical ICU tend to be older and have chronic medical conditions. These patients have often been prompted to create an advanced directive or living will. Patients and families can feel forearmed when this has already been discussed and is in place. Unfortunately, when unforeseen circumstances and questions of whether to continue curative treatment arise, the wording is often unhelpful when it comes to making practical decisions in the ICU. Typical standardized documents say something to the effect that the patient would not want to continue to receive medical intervention or "heroic procedures" if no "realistic" hope of recovery exists.

Unfortunately, having no hope or no chance is extremely rare, and physicians do not know how to predict whether or when a patient will die.

Prognosticating

Patients coming through the ICU are having major surgery and have underlying medical comorbidities; their chance of a poor outcome is not insignificant. A patient having CABG surgery has an overall 3.2% chance of death by 30 days. If a patient has a left ventricle ejection fraction of less than 20%, then that risk increases to 8% by 30 days. In patients 80 years of age and older, the 30-day mortality rate for an AVR is 6.6%. Often, these patients are also approaching the end of their lives, with a 2-year mortality rate of 35%. At the extreme end of the morbidity spectrum is the patient who receives VA-ECMO for a cardiac arrest, severe cardiogenic shock, or failure to wean from CPB; hospital survival is a mere 35% to 43%. This scenario is not infrequently encountered in the cardiac surgical ICU.

Scoring systems can be helpful in getting a sense of a patient's likelihood of doing poorly. Several scoring systems for patients undergoing cardiac surgery have been validated. Another system that predicts morbidity and mortality is the cardiac anesthesia risk evaluation (CARE) score (Box 32.5). The CARE model incorporates severity of cardiac disease, comorbidities, nature of the surgery, and urgency into a scale of 1 to 5 with an E that designates emergency. For example, a 4E patient would be a patient with an uncontrolled medical problem having a complex surgery that is also an emergency; the risk of hospital mortality is 17% (Table 32.2).

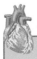

> **BOX 32.5   *Cardiac Anesthesia Risk Evaluation Score***
>
> 1. Patient with stable cardiac disease and no other medical problem: a noncomplex surgery is undertaken.
> 2. Patient with stable cardiac disease and one or more controlled medical problems[a]: a noncomplex surgery is undertaken.
> 3. Patient with any uncontrolled medical problem[b] *or* patient in whom a complex surgery is undertaken.[c]
> 4. Patient with any uncontrolled medical problem *and* in whom a complex surgery is undertaken.
> 5. Patient with chronic or advanced cardiac disease for whom cardiac surgery is undertaken as a last hope to save or improve life.
> 6. Emergency: surgery is performed as soon as the diagnosis is made and the surgical unit is available.
>
> [a]Examples: Controlled hypertension, diabetes mellitus, peripheral vascular disease, chronic obstructive pulmonary disease, controlled systemic diseases, and others as judged by clinicians.
> [b]Examples: Unstable angina treated with intravenous heparin or nitroglycerin, preoperative intraaortic balloon pump, heart failure with pulmonary or peripheral edema, uncontrolled hypertension, renal insufficiency (creatinine level >140 μmol/L), debilitating systemic diseases, and others as judged by clinicians.
> [c]Examples: Reoperation, combined valve and coronary artery surgery, multiple valve surgery, left ventricular aneurysmectomy, repair of ventricular septal defect after myocardial infarction, coronary artery bypass of diffuse or heavily calcified vessels, and other as judged by clinicians.
> Adapted from Dupuis JY, Wang F, Nathan H, et al. The cardiac anesthesia risk evaluation score: a clinically useful predictor of mortality and morbidity after cardiac surgery. *Anesthesiology.* 2001; 94(2):194–204.

32

Table 32.2 **Probabilities of Mortality, Morbidity, and Prolonged Postoperative Length of Stay in Hospital, as Predicted by the CARE Score**

CARE Score	Mortality (%)	Morbidity (%)	Prolonged LOS (days)
1	0.5 (0.3–0.9)	5.4 (4.3–6.8)	2.9 (2.2–3.9)
2	1.1 (0.7–1.7)	10.3 (8.9–12.1)	5.1 (4.2–6.3)
3	2.2 (1.6–3.1)	19.0 (17.2–20.9)	8.8 (7.6–10.2)
3E	4.5 (3.5–5.7)	32.1 (29.3–35.0)	14.7 (12.8–16.8)
4	8.8 (6.9–11.3)	48.8 (44.1–53.6)	23.5 (20.1–27.3)
4E	16.7 (12.4–22.1)	65.8 (59.5–71.6)	35.4 (29.3–42.0)
5	29.3 (20.8–39.6)	79.6 (73.2–84.7)	49.4 (40.4–58.5)
5E	46.2 (32.4–60.5)	88.7 (83.5–92.5)	63.6 (52.5–73.4)

Values obtained from the logistic regression analysis performed in the reference population (n=2000). Numbers in parentheses are 95% confidence intervals.
CARE, Cardiac anesthesia risk evaluation; LOS, length of stay.
Adapted from Dupuis JY, Wang F, Nathan H, et al. The cardiac anesthesia risk evaluation score: a clinically useful predictor of mortality and morbidity after cardiac surgery. Anesthesiology. 2001;94(2):194–204.

Palliative Care

Recognizing that palliative care does not exclude curative treatment is important. Palliative care is a concept that incorporates symptom management into medical and surgical disease therapy. It recognizes that the patient has a chronic disease that must be managed and is designed to relieve suffering and to improve the quality of life, which can enhance disease-specific therapies but need not replace them. Almost without exception, the cardiac surgery patient has a chronic disease that must be indefinitely managed. Thus palliative care, with the goals of managing symptoms and improving the quality of life, is often appropriate to incorporate into the care plan, even if stopping therapy is not expected in the near future.

Palliative care consults have been shown to increase life span, decrease costs, and improve patient satisfaction. Thus early integration of a palliative care approach to a patient's care plan has no apparent drawbacks. If disease-specific therapies become ineffective or exhausted or if the goals of care change to sole palliation, then palliative therapies can be ramped up accordingly.

Recommendations for Patient and Family Support

Some ICUs have instituted a set schedule for family meetings starting from admission, or a set time for "family rounds" when families can be at the bedside and expect care providers to visit. This practice has many potential benefits. It allows family members and patients to become familiar with the care providers before a potential complication or urgent situation arises, and it can improve patient and family satisfaction, in that they believe they are more regularly informed. Family meetings also provide opportunities to discuss a patient's goals of care in a nonurgent manner, while eliminating some of the anxiety that can be provoked by a hastily scheduled meeting should the patient's status unexpectedly decline.

Facilitating a family meeting is a skill that requires practice. Meetings should include members of all disciplines as appropriate, and introductions of all participants should be made. The family's understanding of the patient's condition should be assessed. A clear, coherent message should be delivered to the family about the patient's condition, including clear prognosticating as much as possible.

If decisions need to be made about further treatment, then the goal is to discover what the patient's goals of care would be in this situation. It is the surrogates' role to help interpret those wishes, based on their knowledge of the patient, not to express their own wishes for care plans. It can then be appropriate for providers to make recommendations to the decision maker about further care, taking into consideration the patient's perceived wishes and the clinical situation. Thus decisions to limit or change the goals of care are a joint decision between practitioners and family members, based on the patient's perceived wishes within the clinical context.

Withdrawal of Life-Sustaining Treatments and Palliative Sedation

If the decision is made that curative treatment has been exhausted and that the goals of care are changed to palliative only, then disease-specific treatment and life-sustaining therapies can be stopped or not escalated, according to the surrogates' and providers' judgment. Excellent resources exist that can guide the mechanics of this process.

SUGGESTED READINGS

Athappan G, Gajulapalli RD, Sengodan P, et al. Influence of transcatheter aortic valve replacement strategy and valve design on stroke after transcatheter aortic valve replacement: a meta-analysis and systematic review of literature. *J Am Coll Cardiol.* 2014;63(20):2101–2110.

Cheng R, Hachamovitch R, Kittleson M, et al. Complications of extracorporeal membrane oxygenation for treatment of cardiogenic shock and cardiac arrest: a meta-analysis of 1,866 adult patients. *Ann Thorac Surg.* 2014;97(2):610–616.

Dellinger RP, Levy MM, Rhodes A, et al. Surviving Sepsis Campaign Guidelines Committee including the Pediatric, S. Surviving sepsis campaign: international guidelines for management of severe sepsis and septic shock: 2012. *Crit Care Med.* 2013;41(2):580–637.

Gaffney AM, Sladen RN. Acute kidney injury in cardiac surgery. *Curr Opin Anaesthesiol.* 2015;28(1):50–59.

Genereux P, Head SJ, Hahn R, et al. Paravalvular leak after transcatheter aortic valve replacement: the new Achilles' heel? A comprehensive review of the literature. *J Am Coll Cardiol.* 2013;61(11):1125–1136.

Greco G, Shi W, Michler RE, et al. Costs associated with health care-associated infections in cardiac surgery. *J Am Coll Cardiol.* 2015;65(1):15–23.

Klein AA, Skubas NJ, Ender J. Controversies and complications in the perioperative management of transcatheter aortic valve replacement. *Anesth Analg.* 2014;119(4):784–798.

Lund LH, Edwards LB, Kucheryavaya AY, et al. The registry of the International Society for Heart and Lung Transplantation: thirty-first official adult heart transplant report–2014; focus theme: retransplantation. *J Heart Lung Transplant.* 2014;33(10):996–1008.

Maki DG, Kluger DM, Crnich CJ. The risk of bloodstream infection in adults with different intravascular devices: a systematic review of 200 published prospective studies. *Mayo Clin Proc.* 2006;81(9):1159–1171.

Mandal K, Alwair H, Nifong WL, et al. Robotically assisted minimally invasive mitral valve surgery. *J Thorac Dis.* 2013;5(suppl 6):S694–S703.

Nicolle LE. The prevention of hospital-acquired urinary tract infection. *Clin Infect Dis.* 2008;46(2):251–253.

Rose EA, Gelijns AC, Moskowitz AJ, et al. Randomized evaluation of mechanical assistance for the treatment of congestive heart failure study, G. Long-term use of a left ventricular assist device for end-stage heart failure. *N Engl J Med.* 2001;345(20):1435–1443.

Salehi Omran A, Karimi A, Ahmadi SH, et al. Superficial and deep sternal wound infection after more than 9000 coronary artery bypass grafts (CABG): incidence, risk factors and mortality. *BMC Infect Dis.* 2007;7:112.

Sandoe JA, Barlow G, Chambers JB, et al. Guidelines for the diagnosis, prevention and management of implantable cardiac electronic device infection. Report of a joint Working Party project on behalf of the British Society for Antimicrobial Chemotherapy (BSAC, host organization), British Heart Rhythm

32

Society (BHRS), British Cardiovascular Society (BCS), British Heart Valve Society (BHVS) and British Society for Echocardiography (BSE). *J Antimicrob Chemother*. 2015;70(2):325–359.

Slaughter MS, Rogers JG, Milano CA, et al. Advanced heart failure treated with continuous-flow left ventricular assist device. *N Engl J Med*. 2009;361(23):2241–2251.

Strueber M, Larbalestier R, Jansz P, et al. Results of the post-market Registry to Evaluate the HeartWare Left Ventricular Assist System (ReVOLVE). *J Heart Lung Transplant*. 2014;33(5):486–491.

Thuny F, Grisoli D, Cautela J, et al. Infective endocarditis: prevention, diagnosis, and management. *Can J Cardiol*. 2014;30(9):1046–1057.

Topkara VK, Kondareddy S, Malik F, et al. Infectious complications in patients with left ventricular assist device: etiology and outcomes in the continuous-flow era. *Ann Thorac Surg*. 2010;90(4):1270–1277.

Turner KR, Fisher EC, Hade EM, et al. The role of perioperative sodium bicarbonate infusion affecting renal function after cardiothoracic surgery. *Front Pharmacol*. 2014;5:127.

Ventetuolo CE, Muratore CS. Extracorporeal life support in critically ill adults. *Am J Respir Crit Care Med*. 2014;190(5):497–508.

Chapter 33

Postoperative Pain Management for the Cardiac Patient

Mark A. Chaney, MD

Key Points

1. Inadequate postoperative analgesia and/or an uninhibited perioperative surgical stress response has the potential to initiate pathophysiologic changes in all major organ systems, which may lead to substantial postoperative morbidity. Adequate postoperative analgesia prevents unnecessary patient discomfort, may decrease morbidity, hospital lengths of stay, and thus may decrease costs.

2. Pain after cardiac surgery may be intense and originates from many sources, including the incision (sternotomy or thoracotomy), intraoperative tissue retraction and dissection, vascular cannulation sites, vein-harvesting sites, and chest tubes. Achieving optimal pain relief after cardiac surgery is often difficult, yet it may be attained through a wide variety of techniques, including local anesthetic infiltration, nerve blocks, intravenous agents, intrathecal techniques, and epidural techniques.

3. Traditionally, analgesia after cardiac surgery has been obtained with intravenous opioids (specifically morphine). However, intravenous opioid use is associated with definite detrimental side effects and longer-acting opioids such as morphine may delay tracheal extubation during the immediate postoperative period via excessive sedation and/or respiratory depression. Thus in the current era of early extubation (eg, fast-tracking), cardiac anesthesiologists are exploring unique options for the control of postoperative pain in patients after cardiac surgery.

4. Although patient-controlled analgesia is a well-established technique and offers potential unique benefits, whether it truly offers significant clinical advantages (compared with traditional nurse-administered analgesic techniques) to patients immediately after cardiac surgery remains to be determined.

5. Administration of intrathecal morphine to patients initiates reliable postoperative analgesia after cardiac surgery. Intrathecal opioids or local anesthetics cannot reliably attenuate the perioperative stress response associated with cardiac surgery that persists during the immediate postoperative period. Although intrathecal local anesthetics (not opioids) may induce perioperative thoracic cardiac sympathectomy, the hemodynamic changes associated with total spinal anesthesia make the technique unpalatable in patients with cardiac disease.

6. Administration of thoracic epidural opioids or local anesthetics to patients initiates reliable postoperative analgesia after cardiac surgery. The quality of analgesia obtained with thoracic epidural anesthetic techniques is sufficient to allow cardiac surgery to be performed in "awake" patients.

7. Use of intrathecal and epidural techniques in patients undergoing cardiac surgery remains extremely controversial. Concerns regard the risk of hematoma formations.

8. The last decade has seen a resurgence of nerve blocks (including catheter-based techniques) in patients undergoing cardiac surgery. Recent clinical studies using intercostal, intrapleural, and paravertebral blocks indicate that these techniques may have unique clinical advantages, even when compared with traditional intrathecal and epidural techniques. The emergence of liposomal bupivacaine, which has the potential to provide clinical analgesia for 96 hours after a single injection, may revolutionize the use of single-shot nerve blocks for patients undergoing cardiac surgery.

9. As a general rule, avoiding intense, single-modality therapy for the treatment of acute postoperative pain is best. The administration of two analgesic agents that act by different mechanisms (multimodal or balanced analgesia) provides superior analgesic efficacy with equivalent or reduced adverse effects.

Adequate postoperative analgesia prevents unnecessary patient discomfort, may decrease morbidity, may decrease postoperative hospital lengths of stay, and thus may decrease costs. Because postoperative pain management has been deemed important, the American Society of Anesthesiologists has published practice guidelines regarding this topic. Furthermore, in recognition of the need for improved pain management, the Joint Commission has developed standards for the assessment and management of pain in accredited hospitals and other health care settings. Patient satisfaction (no doubt linked to adequacy of postoperative analgesia) has become an essential element that influences clinical activity of not only anesthesiologists but all health care professionals.

Achieving optimal pain relief after cardiac surgery is often difficult. Pain may be associated with many interventions, including sternotomy, thoracotomy, leg vein harvesting, pericardiotomy, and/or chest tube insertion, among other interventions. Inadequate analgesia and/or an uninhibited stress response during the postoperative period may increase morbidity by causing adverse hemodynamic, metabolic, immunologic, and hemostatic alterations. Aggressive control of postoperative pain, associated with an attenuated stress response, may decrease morbidity and mortality in high-risk patients after noncardiac surgery and may also decrease morbidity and mortality in patients after cardiac surgery. Adequate postoperative analgesia may be attained via a wide variety of techniques (Box 33.1). Traditionally, analgesia after cardiac surgery has been obtained with intravenous opioids (specifically morphine). However, intravenous opioid use is associated with definite detrimental side effects (eg, nausea and vomiting, pruritus, urinary retention, respiratory depression), and longer-acting opioids such as morphine may delay tracheal extubation during the immediate

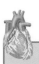

BOX 33.1   *Techniques Available for Postoperative Analgesia*

Local anesthetic infiltration
Nerve blocks
Opioids
Nonsteroidal antiinflammatory agents
α-Adrenergic agents
Intrathecal techniques
Epidural techniques
Multimodal analgesia

VI

postoperative period via excessive sedation and/or respiratory depression. Thus in the current era of early extubation (fast-tracking), cardiac anesthesiologists are exploring unique options other than traditional intravenous opioids for the control of postoperative pain in patients after cardiac surgery. The last decade has witnessed increased use of smaller incisions by cardiac surgeons, prompting clinical investigations into the use of intercostal, intrapleural, and paravertebral blocks (with and without catheters), and the emergence of long-acting liposomal bupivacaine may revolutionize the use of these techniques. No single technique is clearly superior; each possesses distinct advantages and disadvantages. It is becoming increasingly clear that a multimodal approach and/or a combined analgesic regimen (using a variety of techniques) is the best way to approach postoperative pain in all patients after surgery to maximize analgesia and minimize side effects. When addressing postoperative analgesia in cardiac surgical patients, the choice of technique (or techniques) should be made only after a thorough analysis of the risk-benefit ratio of each technique in the specific patient in whom analgesia is desired.

▦ PAIN AND CARDIAC SURGERY

Surgical or traumatic injury initiates changes in the peripheral and central nervous systems that must be addressed therapeutically to promote postoperative analgesia and, it is hoped, positively influence clinical outcomes (Box 33.2). The physical processes of incision, traction, and cutting of tissues stimulate free nerve endings and a wide variety of specific nociceptors. Receptor activation and activity are further modified by the local release of chemical mediators of inflammation and sympathetic amines released via the perioperative surgical stress response. The perioperative surgical stress response peaks during the immediate postoperative period and exerts major effects on many physiologic processes. The potential clinical benefits of attenuating the perioperative surgical stress response (above and beyond simply attaining adequate clinical analgesia) have received significant attention during the 2000s and remain fairly controversial. However, inadequate postoperative analgesia and/or an uninhibited perioperative surgical stress response clearly has the potential to initiate pathophysiologic changes in all major organ systems, including the cardiovascular, pulmonary, gastrointestinal, renal, endocrine, immunologic, and/or central nervous systems, all of which may lead to substantial postoperative morbidity.

Pain after cardiac surgery may be intense, and it originates from many sources, including the incision (eg, sternotomy, thoracotomy), intraoperative tissue retraction and dissection, vascular cannulation sites, vein-harvesting sites, and chest tubes, among other sources. Patients in whom an internal mammary artery is surgically exposed and used as a bypass graft may have substantially more postoperative pain.

33

BOX 33.2   *Pain and Cardiac Surgery*

Originates from many sources
Most commonly originates from the chest wall
Preoperative expectations influence postoperative satisfaction
Quality of postoperative analgesia may influence morbidity

Persistent pain after cardiac surgery, although rare, can be problematic. The cause of persistent pain after sternotomy is multifactorial, yet tissue destruction, intercostal nerve trauma, scar formation, rib fractures, sternal infection, stainless-steel wire sutures, and/or costochondral separation may all play roles. Such chronic pain is often localized to the arms, shoulders, or legs. Postoperative brachial plexus neuropathies also may occur and have been attributed to rib fracture fragments, internal mammary artery dissection, suboptimal positioning of the patient during surgery, and/or central venous catheter placement. Postoperative neuralgia of the saphenous nerve has also been reported after harvesting of saphenous veins for coronary artery bypass grafting (CABG). Younger patients appear to be at greater risk for the development of chronic, long-lasting pain. The correlation of severity of acute postoperative pain and the development of chronic pain syndromes has been suggested (patients requiring more postoperative analgesics may be more likely to develop chronic pain), yet this link is still vague.

Patient satisfaction with quality of postoperative analgesia is as much related to the comparison between anticipated and experienced pain as it is to the actual level of pain experienced. Satisfaction is related to a situation that is better than predicted, dissatisfaction to one that is worse than expected. Patients undergoing cardiac surgery remain concerned regarding the adequacy of postoperative pain relief and preoperatively tend to expect a greater amount of postoperative pain than that which is actually experienced. Because of these unique preoperative expectations, patients after cardiac surgery who postoperatively receive only moderate analgesia will likely still be satisfied with their pain control. Thus patients may experience pain of moderate intensity after cardiac surgery yet still express very high satisfaction levels.

POTENTIAL CLINICAL BENEFITS OF ADEQUATE POSTOPERATIVE ANALGESIA

Inadequate analgesia (coupled with an uninhibited stress response) during the postoperative period may lead to many adverse hemodynamic (tachycardia, hypertension, vasoconstriction), metabolic (increased catabolism), immunologic (impaired immune response), and hemostatic (platelet activation) alterations. In patients undergoing cardiac surgery, perioperative myocardial ischemia is most commonly observed during the immediate postoperative period and appears to be related to outcome. Intraoperatively, initiation of cardiopulmonary bypass (CPB) causes substantial increases in stress response hormones (eg, norepinephrine, epinephrine) that persist into the immediate postoperative period and may contribute to myocardial ischemia observed during this time. Furthermore, postoperative myocardial ischemia may be aggravated by cardiac sympathetic nerve activation, which disrupts the balance between coronary blood flow and myocardial oxygen demand. Thus during the pivotal immediate postoperative period after cardiac surgery, adequate analgesia coupled with stress-response attenuation may potentially decrease morbidity and enhance health-related quality of life.

LOCAL ANESTHETIC INFILTRATION

Pain after cardiac surgery is often related to median sternotomy, peaking during the first 2 postoperative days. Because of problems associated with traditional intravenous opioid analgesia and with the nonsteroidal antiinflammatory drugs (NSAIDs) and cyclooxygenase (COX) inhibitors, alternative methods of achieving postoperative analgesia in cardiac surgical patients have been sought. One such alternative method that may hold promise is the continuous infusion of a local anesthetic.

Clinical investigations have revealed the potential benefits of using a continuous infusion of a local anesthetic in patients after cardiac surgery. Patients undergoing elective CABG via median sternotomy were randomized to either ropivacaine or placebo groups. At the end of the surgery but before wound closure, bilateral intercostal nerve injections from T1 to T12 were performed using 20 mL of either 0.2% ropivacaine or normal saline. After sternal reapproximation with wires, two catheters with multiple side openings were placed anterior to the sternum (Fig. 33.1). These catheters were connected to a pressurized elastomeric pump containing a flow regulator, which allowed for the delivery of 0.2% ropivacaine or normal saline at approximately 4 mL/h. The postoperative pain management was via intravenous patient-controlled anesthesia (PCA) morphine (for 72 hours). The sternal catheters were removed after 48 hours. Total mean PCA morphine consumption during the immediate postoperative period (72 hours) was significantly decreased in the ropivacaine group (47.3 vs 78.7 mg, respectively; $P = .038$). Mean overall pain scores (scale ranging from 0 for no pain to 10 for maximum pain imaginable) were also significantly decreased in the ropivacaine group (1.6 vs 2.6, respectively; $P = .005$). Most interestingly, patients receiving ropivacaine had a mean hospital length of stay of 5.2 ± 1.3 days compared with 8.2 ± 7.9 days for patients receiving normal saline, a difference that was statistically significant ($P = .001$). No difference was observed in wound infections or wound healing between

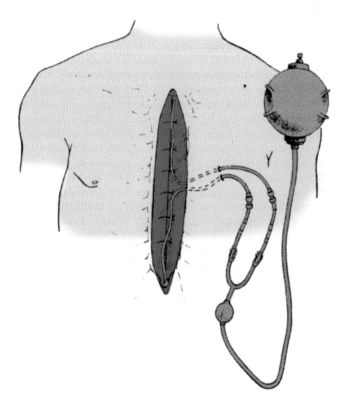

Fig. 33.1 Intraoperative placement of the pressurized elastomeric pump and catheters. (From Dowling R, Thielmeier K, Ghaly A, et al. Improved pain control after cardiac surgery: results of a randomized, double-blind, clinical trial. *J Thorac Cardiovasc Surg*. 2003;126:1271–1278.)

the two groups during hospitalization or after hospital discharge. No complications related to placement of the sternal wound catheters or performance of the intercostal nerve blocks were encountered. The authors concluded that their analgesic technique significantly improves postoperative pain control while decreasing the amount of opioid analgesia required in patients subjected to standard median sternotomy.

NERVE BLOCKS

With the increasing popularity of minimally invasive cardiac surgery, which uses nonsternotomy incisions (minithoracotomy), the use of nerve blocks for the management of postoperative pain has increased. Thoracotomy incisions (transverse anterolateral minithoracotomy, vertical anterolateral minithoracotomy), because of costal cartilage tissue trauma to ribs, muscles, or peripheral nerves, may induce more intense postoperative pain than that resulting from median sternotomy. Adequate analgesia after thoracotomy incisions is important because pain is a key component in the alteration of lung function after this type of incision. Uncontrolled pain causes a reduction in respiratory mechanics, reduced mobility, and increases in hormonal and metabolic activity. Perioperative deterioration in respiratory mechanics may lead to pulmonary complications and hypoxemia, which may in turn lead to myocardial ischemia or infarction, cerebrovascular accidents, thromboembolism, delayed wound healing, increased morbidity, and prolonged hospital stay. Various analgesic techniques have been developed to treat postoperative thoracotomy pain. The most commonly used techniques include intercostal nerve block, intrapleural administration of a local anesthetic, and thoracic paravertebral block. Intrathecal techniques and epidural techniques are also effective in controlling postthoracotomy pain.

Intercostal nerve block has been extensively used for analgesia after thoracic surgery and can be performed either intraoperatively or postoperatively. It usually provides sufficient analgesia lasting approximately 6 to 12 hours (depending on the amount and type of local anesthetic used) and may need to be repeated if additional analgesia is required. Local anesthetics may be administered as a single injection under direct vision before chest closure, as a single preoperative percutaneous injection, as multiple percutaneous serial injections, or via an indwelling intercostal catheter. Blockade of intercostal nerves interrupts C-fiber afferent transmission of impulses to the spinal cord. A continuous intercostal catheter allows frequent dosing or infusions of local anesthetic agents and avoids multiple needle injections. Various clinical studies have confirmed the analgesic efficacy of this technique, and the technique compares favorably with thoracic epidural analgesic techniques. A major concern associated with intercostal nerve block is the potentially high amount of local anesthetic systemic absorption. However, multiple clinical studies involving patients undergoing thoracic surgery have documented safe blood levels with standard techniques. Clinical investigations involving patients undergoing thoracic surgery indicate that intercostal nerve blockade by intermittent or continuous infusion of bupivacaine (0.25% to 0.5%) or ropivacaine (0.5% to 0.75%) through indwelling intercostal catheters is an effective method for supplementing systemic intravenous opioid analgesia for postthoracotomy pain. Intrapleural administration of local anesthetics initiates analgesia via mechanisms that remain incompletely understood. However, the mechanism of action of extrapleural analgesia seems to depend primarily on diffusion of the local anesthetic into the paravertebral region. Local anesthetics then affect not only the ventral nerve root but also afferent fibers of the posterior primary ramus. Posterior ligaments of the posterior primary ramus innervate posterior spinal muscles and skin and are traumatized during posterolateral thoracotomy. Intrapleural administration of a local anesthetic

826

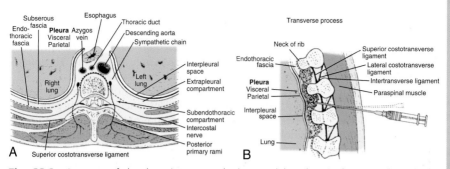

Fig. 33.2 Anatomy of the thoracic paravertebral space (A) and sagittal section through the thoracic paravertebral space showing a needle that has been advanced above the transverse process (B). (From Karmakar MK. Thoracic paravertebral block. *Anesthesiology.* 2001;95:771–780.)

to this region through a catheter inserted in the extrapleural space creates an analgesic region in the skin. The depth and width of this region depend on the diffusion of the local anesthetic in the extrapleural space. Thoracic paravertebral block involves the injection of a local anesthetic adjacent to the thoracic vertebrae close to where the spinal nerves emerge from the intervertebral foramina (Fig. 33.2). Thoracic paravertebral block, compared with thoracic epidural analgesic techniques, appears to provide equivalent analgesia, is technically easier, and may harbor less risk. Several different techniques exist for successful thoracic paravertebral block. The classic technique, most commonly used, involves eliciting loss of resistance. Injection of a local anesthetic results in ipsilateral somatic and sympathetic nerve blockade in multiple contiguous thoracic dermatomes above and below the site of injection, together with the possible suppression of the neuroendocrine stress response to surgery. These blocks may be effective in alleviating acute and chronic pain of unilateral origin from the chest. Continuous thoracic paravertebral infusion of a local anesthetic via a catheter placed under direct vision at thoracotomy is also a safe, simple, and an effective method of providing analgesia after thoracotomy. It is usually used in conjunction with adjunct intravenous opioid or other analgesics to provide optimal relief after thoracotomy. For a wide variety of reasons, including the increased use of small thoracic incisions by cardiac surgeons, the last decade has seen a resurgence of nerve blocks (usually catheter-based techniques) in patients undergoing cardiac surgery. Specifically, recent clinical studies using intercostal catheters, intrapleural catheters, and paravertebral blockade indicate that these techniques may have unique advantages, even when compared with traditional intrathecal and epidural techniques. Lastly, the emergence of liposomal bupivacaine, which has the potential to provide clinical analgesia for 96 hours after a single injection, may revolutionize the use of single-shot nerve blocks for thoracic and cardiac surgeries.

OPIOIDS

The classic pharmacologic effect of opioids is analgesia, and these drugs have traditionally been the initial choice when a potent postoperative analgesic is required. Two anatomically distinct sites exist for opioid receptor–mediated analgesia: supraspinal and spinal. Systemically administered opioids produce analgesia at both sites. Supraspinally, the μ_1 receptor is primarily involved in analgesia, whereas the μ_2 receptor is the receptor predominantly involved in the spinal modulation of nociceptive processing. κ Receptors are important in mediating spinal and supraspinal analgesia as well.

δ Ligands may have a modulatory rather than a primary analgesic role. All three types of opioid receptors (μ, κ, and δ) have been demonstrated in peripheral terminals of sensory nerves. Activation of these receptors seems to require an inflammatory reaction because locally applied opioids do not produce analgesia in healthy tissue. The inflammatory process also may activate previously inactive opioid receptors.

Morphine is the prototype opioid agonist with which all opioids are compared and is perhaps the most popular analgesic used in patients after cardiac surgery. Many semisynthetic derivatives are made by simple modifications of the morphine molecule. Morphine is poorly lipid-soluble and binds approximately 35% to plasma proteins, particularly albumin. Morphine is primarily metabolized in the liver, principally by conjugation to water-soluble glucuronides. The liver is the predominant site for morphine biotransformation, although extrahepatic metabolism also occurs in the kidney, brain, and possibly the gut. Extrahepatic clearance accounts for approximately 30% of the total body clearance. The terminal elimination half-life of morphine is 2 to 3 hours. In patients with liver cirrhosis, morphine pharmacokinetic actions are variable, probably reflecting the variability of liver disease in patients. Morphine's terminal elimination half-life in patients with renal disease is comparable with that of patients without renal disease. Although morphine is perhaps the most popular intravenous analgesic used in patients after cardiac surgery, other synthetically derived opioids have been developed and may be used as well. These include fentanyl, alfentanil, sufentanil, and remifentanil.

Transdermal delivery of fentanyl has also been investigated extensively. This modality is simple, noninvasive, and allows continuous release of fentanyl into the systemic circulation. However, the steady release of fentanyl in such a manner does not allow flexibility in dose adjustment, which may result in inadequate treatment of postoperative pain during rapidly changing intensity. Thus intravenous opioids are often necessary to supplement analgesia when transdermal fentanyl is used to manage acute postoperative pain.

Alfentanil is approximately 5 to 10 times less potent than fentanyl. The drug acts rapidly; its peak effect is reached within minutes after intravenous administration. Its duration of action after bolus administration is also shorter than fentanyl. Alfentanil is highly lipid-soluble (approximately 100 times more lipid-soluble than morphine) and rapidly crosses the blood-brain barrier. Alfentanil pharmacokinetics is minimally affected by renal disease, and hepatic extraction is more a function of intrinsic hepatic enzyme capacity and protein binding than liver blood flow.

The performance of a patient-demand, target-controlled alfentanil infusion system has compared favorably with traditional morphine PCA in patients after cardiac surgery. Morphine PCA versus alfentanil PCA for postoperative analgesia after undergoing elective cardiac surgery was evaluated in a nonblinded fashion. All patients received a similar standardized intraoperative anesthetic technique and were extubated during the immediate postoperative period. Overall median visual analogue pain scores were significantly lower in patients receiving alfentanil, yet both alfentanil and morphine delivered high-quality postoperative analgesia (Fig. 33.3). Although the clinical impression of these investigators was that alfentanil patients were less sedated in the immediate postoperative period, this clinical observation was not substantiated after statistical analysis of sedation scores. The two groups did not differ with respect to overall sedation scores, frequency of nausea and vomiting, hemodynamic instability, myocardial ischemia, or hypoxemia during the immediate postoperative period.

Sufentanil is approximately 10 times more potent than fentanyl. The drug is extremely lipid-soluble and is highly bound to plasma proteins. Because of its high potency, conventional clinical doses of sufentanil result in plasma concentrations that rapidly decline to less than the sensitivity of most assayed methods, making it difficult to

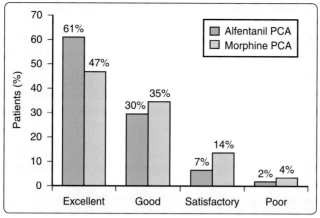

Fig. 33.3 Overall patient satisfaction with postoperative analgesia. Ninety-one percent of patients using alfentanil rated their postoperative analgesia as excellent or good, whereas 82% of patients using morphine rated their postoperative analgesia similarly (differences not statistically significant). *PCA*, Patient-controlled analgesia. (From Checketts MR, Gilhooly CJ, Kenny GN. Patient-maintained analgesia with target-controlled alfentanil infusion after cardiac surgery: a comparison with morphine PCA. *Br J Anaesth*. 1998;80:748–751.)

determine accurate pharmacokinetic parameters. However, sufentanil pharmacokinetic actions appear not to be altered in patients with renal disease. Because hepatic sufentanil clearance approaches liver blood flow, the drug's pharmacokinetic properties are expected to change with hepatic disease yet the clinical relevance remains undetermined. Sufentanil undergoes substantial (approximately 60%) first-pass uptake in the lungs.

Remifentanil has a very fast onset and an ultrashort duration of action; it is unique in that it is readily susceptible to rapid hydrolysis by nonspecific esterases in the blood and tissues. The drug is moderately lipophilic and is half as potent as fentanyl when blood concentrations causing equivalent analgesia are compared. Remifentanil has an elimination half-life of 10 to 20 minutes, and the time required for a 50% reduction in blood concentration after discontinuation of an infusion that has attained a steady state is approximately 3 minutes and does not increase with the duration of infusion. Available evidence suggests that neither the pharmacokinetics nor the pharmacodynamics of remifentanil are significantly altered in patients with severe hepatic or renal disease. These properties should confer ease of titration to changing analgesic conditions. However, the quick offset of action, although desirable, may result in inadequate postoperative analgesia. Because of the rapid offset of analgesic effect of remifentanil, the continued requirement for postoperative analgesia needs to be considered before the remifentanil are discontinued. A transition must be made from remifentanil to some other longer-acting analgesic agent for the initiation of substantial postoperative analgesia. Although the transition to postoperative pain management can be made using a remifentanil infusion alone, this appears to be associated with a high incidence of adverse respiratory effects.

The use of a remifentanil infusion to provide postoperative analgesia was evaluated during recovery from total intravenous anesthesia with remifentanil and propofol from a wide variety of noncardiac surgeries (eg, abdominal, spine, joint replacement, thoracic). This multiinstitutional study had a detailed protocol that specified doses and method of administration of all anesthetic drugs. Total intraoperative intravenous anesthesia consisted of midazolam (premedication only), remifentanil, propofol, and vecuronium. Propofol was stopped immediately before intraoperative extubation,

33

and the remifentanil infusion was continued for postoperative analgesia. During the immediate postoperative period, intravenous morphine was administered during tapering of remifentanil infusion. Adverse respiratory events that included oxygen saturation via pulse oximetry less than 90%, respiratory rate less than 12 per minute, and apnea, affected 45 patients (29%; two required naloxone). Apnea occurred in 11 patients (7% treated with mask ventilation and downward titration of remifentanil infusion; one required naloxone). The administration of a bolus of remifentanil preceded the onset of adverse respiratory events in 19 of 45 cases and in 9 of 11 cases of apnea.

These data suggest that remifentanil boluses plus an infusion are particularly likely to produce clinically significant adverse respiratory events. This open, dose-ranging study concluded that, although remifentanil certainly initiates analgesia, its use in the immediate postoperative period may pose dangers. Additional studies are needed to investigate the transition from remifentanil to longer-lasting analgesics and to refine strategies that minimize respiratory depression while optimizing pain control. The administration of a potent, rapid-acting opioid such as remifentanil by continuous infusion for postoperative analgesia must be performed with meticulous attention to detail and constant vigilance. Extreme caution should be exercised in the postoperative administration of bolus doses of remifentanil because substantial respiratory depression (including apnea) may develop. Furthermore, the remifentanil infusion should be inserted into the intravenous line as close as possible to the patient to minimize dead space, and the rate of the main intravenous infusion should be controlled at a rate that is high enough to flush remifentanil from the tubing continuously. A more dilute remifentanil solution that runs at greater rates (on a volume-per-time basis) helps minimize the effect of variations in flow rate of the main intravenous tubing on delivery of remifentanil to the patient. Remifentanil also may possess detrimental cardiovascular effects via bradycardia and decreases in systemic vascular resistance, leading to decreased cardiac output and hypotension. Such changes may occur during clinically used doses for cardiac surgery (0.1 to 1.0 μg/kg/min), inducing significant cardiovascular disturbances that are potentially deleterious to patients with cardiac disease.

PATIENT-CONTROLLED ANALGESIA

When intravenous opioids are used for controlling postoperative pain, PCA technology is generally used. Essentials in the successful use of PCA technology include loading the patient with intravenous opioids to the point of patient comfort before initiating PCA, ensuring that the patient wants to control analgesic treatment, using an appropriate PCA dose and lockout interval, and considering the use of a basal rate infusion. Focused guidance of PCA dosing by a dedicated acute pain service, compared with surgeon-directed PCA, may result in more effective analgesia with fewer adverse effects.

NONSTEROIDAL ANTIINFLAMMATORY AGENTS

NSAIDs, in contrast with the opioids' central nervous system mechanism of action, primarily exert their analgesic, antipyretic, and antiinflammatory effects peripherally by interfering with prostaglandin synthesis after tissue injury. NSAIDs inhibit COX, the enzyme responsible for the conversion of arachidonic acid to prostaglandin. Combining NSAIDs with traditional intravenous opioids may allow a patient to

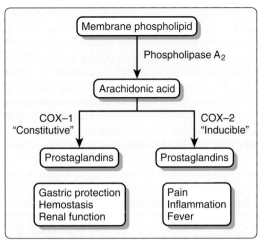

Fig. 33.4 Cyclooxygenase *(COX)* Pathways. Molecular studies distinguishing between COX-1 and COX-2 enzymes have led to the exciting hypothesis that the therapeutic and adverse effects of the nonspecific inhibitors (nonsteroidal antiinflammatory drugs) could be uncoupled. (From Gajraj NM. Cyclooxygenase-2 inhibitors. *Anesth Analg.* 2003;96:1720–1738.)

achieve an adequate level of analgesia with fewer side effects than if a similar level of analgesia was obtained with intravenous opioids alone. Unlike opioids, which preferentially reduce spontaneous postoperative pain, NSAIDs have comparable efficacy for both spontaneous and movement-evoked pain, the latter of which may be more important in causing postoperative physiologic impairment. Concerns regarding NSAID side effects, including alterations in the gastric mucosal barrier, renal tubular function, and inhibition of platelet aggregation, have likely made clinicians reluctant to use NSAIDs in patients undergoing cardiac surgery.

NSAIDs are not a homogenous group and vary considerably in analgesic efficacy as a result of differences in pharmacodynamic and pharmacokinetic parameters. NSAIDs are nonspecific inhibitors of COX, which is the rate-limiting enzyme involved in the synthesis of prostaglandins. COX-1 is ubiquitously and constitutively expressed and has a homeostatic role in platelet aggregation, gastrointestinal mucosal integrity, and renal function, whereas COX-2 is inducible and primarily expressed at the sites of injury (and in the kidney and brain) and mediates pain and inflammation. NSAIDs are nonspecific inhibitors of both forms of COX yet vary in their ratio of COX-1 to COX-2 inhibition. Molecular studies distinguishing between constitutive COX-1 and inflammation-inducible COX-2 enzymes have led to the exciting hypothesis that the therapeutic and adverse effects of NSAIDs could be uncoupled (Fig. 33.4). Subsequently, clinicians have witnessed the growing use of COX-2 inhibitors in the perioperative period after noncardiac surgery. The primary advantage of COX-2 inhibitors, compared with NSAIDs, is their lack of effect on platelet function and bleeding.

ALPHA₂-ADRENERGIC AGONISTS

The α_2-adrenergic agonists provide analgesia, sedation, and sympatholysis.

The potential perioperative analgesic benefits of α_2 agonists when administered to patients undergoing cardiac surgery were demonstrated 30 years ago. Most of the clinical investigations regarding perioperative use of this class of drugs remain focused on exploiting the sedative effects and beneficial cardiovascular effects (decreasing

33

hypertension and tachycardia) associated with their use. α_2-Adrenergic agonists have been used perioperatively in patients undergoing cardiac surgery. However, the focus of such clinical investigations has been on the intraoperative period and the potential for enhanced postoperative hemodynamic stability, potentially leading to reduced postoperative myocardial ischemia (but not specifically to enhance postoperative analgesia). Taken together, these clinical investigations indicate that perioperative administration of α_2-adrenergic agonists to patients undergoing cardiac surgery decreases intraoperative anesthetic requirements, may enhance perioperative hemodynamic stability, and may decrease perioperative myocardial ischemia. The potential ability of this class of drugs to initiate reliable postoperative analgesia awaits definitive investigation.

INTRATHECAL AND EPIDURAL TECHNIQUES

Numerous clinical investigations clearly indicate that intrathecal and/or epidural techniques (using opioids and/or local anesthetics) initiate reliable postoperative analgesia in patients after cardiac surgery (Boxes 33.3 and 33.4). Additional potential advantages of using intrathecal and/or epidural techniques in patients undergoing cardiac surgery include stress-response attenuation and thoracic cardiac sympathectomy.

BOX 33.3 *Intrathecal Techniques*

Advantages
- Simple, reliable analgesia
- Stress-response attenuation
- Less hematoma risk than epidural techniques

Disadvantages
- No cardiac sympathectomy
- Hematoma risk increased
- Side effects of intrathecal opioids

BOX 33.4 *Epidural Techniques*

Advantages
- Reliable analgesia
- Stress-response attenuation
- Cardiac sympathectomy

Disadvantages
- Labor-intensive
- Hematoma formation risk increased
- Side effects of epidural opioids

Intrathecal Techniques

Most clinical investigators have used intrathecal morphine in hopes of providing prolonged postoperative analgesia. Some clinical investigators have used intrathecal fentanyl, sufentanil, and/or local anesthetics for intraoperative anesthesia and analgesia (with stress-response attenuation) and/or thoracic cardiac sympathectomy. An anonymous survey of members of the Society of Cardiovascular Anesthesiologists published in 2001 indicated that almost 8% of practicing anesthesiologists incorporate intrathecal techniques into their anesthetic management of adults undergoing cardiac surgery. Of these anesthesiologists, 75% practice in the United States, 72% perform the intrathecal injection before the induction of anesthesia, 97% use morphine, 13% use fentanyl, 2% use sufentanil, 10% use lidocaine, and 3% use tetracaine.

The mid-1990s saw the emergence of fast-track cardiac surgery, with the goal being tracheal extubation in the immediate postoperative period. Some clinical investigators have revealed that certain combinations of intraoperative anesthetic techniques coupled with appropriate doses of intrathecal morphine will allow tracheal extubation after cardiac surgery within the immediate postoperative period to coexist with enhanced analgesia. Many clinical investigations involving the use of intrathecal analgesic techniques in patients undergoing cardiac surgery indicate that the administration of intrathecal morphine to patients before CPB initiates reliable postoperative analgesia after cardiac surgery. Intrathecal opioids or local anesthetics cannot reliably attenuate the perioperative stress response associated with CPB that persists during the immediate postoperative period. A recently published metaanalysis of randomized, controlled trials (25 randomized trials, 1106 patients) concluded that spinal analgesia does not improve clinically relevant outcomes in patients undergoing cardiac surgery.

Epidural Techniques

Since this initial impressive display of potential benefits (eg, reliable postoperative analgesia, stress-response attenuation, facilitation of early tracheal extubation), other clinical investigators have subsequently applied thoracic epidural anesthesia (TEA) to patients undergoing cardiac surgery. Most clinical investigators have used thoracic epidural local anesthetics in hopes of providing perioperative stress-response attenuation and/or perioperative thoracic cardiac sympathectomy. Some clinical investigators have used thoracic epidural opioids to provide intraoperative and/or postoperative analgesia. An anonymous survey of members of the Society of Cardiovascular Anesthesiologists published in 2001 indicated that 7% of practicing anesthesiologists incorporate thoracic epidural techniques into their anesthetic management of adults undergoing cardiac surgery. Of these anesthesiologists, 58% practice in the United States.

Many clinical investigations have proved that TEA with local anesthetics significantly attenuates the perioperative stress response in patients undergoing cardiac surgery. Patients randomized to receive intermittent boluses of thoracic epidural bupivacaine intraoperatively, followed by continuous infusion postoperatively, exhibited significantly decreased blood levels of norepinephrine and epinephrine perioperatively when compared with patients similarly managed without thoracic epidural catheters. The February 2011 issue of *Anesthesiology* highlights the controversial nature of this topic as two clinical studies with opposite conclusions were published. These authors concluded, "Given the potentially devastating complications of epidural hematoma after insertion of an epidural catheter, it is questionable whether this procedure should be applied routinely in cardiac surgical patients who require full heparinization." These two clinical studies were accompanied by an editorial that stated that "we continue to try and show that regional anesthesia and analgesia can substantially alter surgical outcomes without success … perhaps it is time to move away from trying to prove that anesthetic interventions will reduce morbidity or mortality and to focus on tangible benefits to patients or their families." Despite enhanced postoperative analgesia offered via TEA techniques, such analgesia does not appear to decrease the incidence of persistent pain after cardiac surgery. Persistent pain, defined as pain still present 2 or more months after surgery, was similar in the two cohorts (reported in almost 30% of patients).

The quality of analgesia obtained with TEA techniques is sufficient to allow cardiac surgery to be performed in awake patients without general endotracheal anesthesia. The initial report of awake cardiac surgery was published in the *Annals of Thoracic Surgery* in 2000. Since these initial small clinical reports appeared, larger series of patients have been published, demonstrating that awake cardiac surgery is feasible and safe. In 2003, the first case report of awake cardiac surgery requiring CPB was published. In this astonishing case report from Austria, a 70-year-old man with aortic stenosis underwent aortic valve replacement with the assistance of normothermic CPB (total time: 123 minutes; cross-clamp time: 82 minutes) solely via TEA. Verbal communication with the patient was possible on demand throughout the CPB surgery. The patient did well and experienced an unremarkable postoperative course.

Risk for Hematoma Formation

Intrathecal or epidural instrumentation entails risk, the most feared complication being epidural hematoma formation. The estimated incidence of hematoma formation is approximately 1:220,000 after intrathecal instrumentation. Hematoma formation is more common (approximately 1:150,000) after epidural instrumentation because larger needles are used, catheters are inserted, and the venous plexus in the epidural space is prominent. Furthermore, hematoma formation does not exclusively occur during epidural catheter insertion; almost one half of all cases develop after catheter removal.

Risk is increased when intrathecal or epidural instrumentation is performed before systemic heparinization, and hematoma formation has occurred in patients when diagnostic or therapeutic lumbar puncture has been followed by systemic heparinization. When lumbar puncture is followed by systemic heparinization, concurrent use of aspirin, difficult or traumatic instrumentation, and the administration of intravenous heparin within 1 hour of instrumentation increase the risk for hematoma formation. However, by observing certain precautions, intrathecal or epidural instrumentation can be safely performed in patients who will subsequently receive intravenous heparin. By delaying surgery 24 hours in the event of a traumatic tap, by delaying heparinization 60 minutes after catheter insertion, and by maintaining tight perioperative control of anticoagulation, more than 4000 intrathecal or epidural catheterizations were safely performed in patients undergoing peripheral vascular surgery who received intravenous heparin after catheter insertion. However, the magnitude of anticoagulation in these two studies (activated partial thromboplastin time of approximately 100 seconds and activated coagulation time approximately twice the baseline value) involving patients undergoing peripheral vascular surgery was substantially less than the degree of anticoagulation required in patients subjected to CPB.

Most clinical studies investigating the use of intrathecal or epidural anesthesia and analgesia techniques in patients undergoing cardiac surgery include precautions to decrease the risk for hematoma formation. Some used the technique only after the demonstration of laboratory evidence of normal coagulation parameters, delayed surgery 24 hours in the event of traumatic tap, or required that the time from instrumentation to systemic heparinization exceed 60 minutes. Although most clinicians investigating the use of epidural anesthesia and analgesia techniques in patients undergoing cardiac surgery insert the catheters the day before scheduled surgery, investigators have performed instrumentation on the same day of surgery. Institutional practice (same-day admit surgery) may eliminate the option of epidural catheter insertion on the day before scheduled surgery. An alternative is to perform epidural instrumentation postoperatively (before or after tracheal extubation) after laboratory evidence demonstrates normal coagulation parameters.

The use of regional anesthetic techniques in patients undergoing cardiac surgery remains extremely controversial, prompting numerous editorials by recognized experts in the field of cardiac anesthesia. One of the primary reasons such controversy exists (and likely will continue for some time) is that the numerous clinical investigations regarding this topic are suboptimally designed and use a wide array of disparate techniques, preventing clinically useful conclusions on which all can agree.

MULTIMODAL ANALGESIA

The possibility of synergism among analgesic drugs is a concept that is nearly a century old. Although subsequent research has demonstrated the difference between additivity and synergy, the fundamental strategy behind such combinations (multimodal or balanced analgesia) remains unchanged—enhanced analgesia with the minimization of adverse physiologic effects. The use of analgesic combinations during the postoperative period, specifically the combination of traditional intravenous opioids with other analgesics (eg, NSAIDs, COX-2 inhibitors, ketamine), has been proven clinically effective in noncardiac patients for decades.

SUGGESTED READINGS

Allen MS, Halgren L, Nichols FC, et al. A randomized controlled trial of bupivacaine through intercostal catheters for pain management after thoracotomy. *Ann Thorac Surg.* 2009;88:903.

American Society of Anesthesiologists Task Force on Acute Pain Management. Practice guidelines for acute pain management in the perioperative setting: an updated report by the American Society of Anesthesiologists Task Force on Acute Pain Management. *Anesthesiology.* 2012;116:248.

Bettex DA, Schmidlin D, Chassot PG, et al. Intrathecal sufentanil-morphine shortens the duration of intubation and improves analgesia in fast-track cardiac surgery. *Can J Anaesth.* 2002;49:711.

Bignami E, Landoni G, Biondi-Zoccai GGL, et al. Epidural analgesia improves outcome in cardiac surgery: a meta-analysis of randomized controlled trials. *J Cardiothorac Vasc Anesth.* 2010;24:586.

Blaudszun G, Lysakowski C, Elia N, et al. Effect of perioperative systemic α2 agonists on postoperative morphine consumption and pain intensity; systematic review and meta-analysis of randomized controlled trials. *Anesthesiology.* 2012;116:1312.

Goldstein S, Dean D, Kim SJ, et al. A survey of spinal and epidural techniques in adult cardiac surgery. *J Cardiothorac Vasc Anesth.* 2001;15:158.

Hansdottir V, Philip J, Olsen MF, et al. Thoracic epidural versus intravenous patient-controlled analgesia after cardiac surgery. *Anesthesiology.* 2006;104:142.

Lena P, Balarac N, Lena D, et al. Fast-track anesthesia with remifentanil and spinal analgesia for cardiac surgery: the effect on pain control and quality of recovery. *J Cardiothorac Vasc Anesth.* 2008;22:536.

Lynch JJ, Mauermann WJ, Pulido JN, et al. Use of paravertebral blockade to facilitate early extubation after minimally invasive cardiac surgery. *Semin Cardiothorac Vasc Anesth.* 2010;14:47.

Mazzeffi M, Khelemsky Y. Poststernotomy pain: a clinical review. *J Cardiothorac Vasc Anesth.* 2011;25:1163.

Metz S, Schwann N, Hassanein W, et al. Intrathecal morphine for off-pump coronary artery bypass grafting. *J Cardiothorac Vasc Anesth.* 2004;18:451.

Monaco F, Biselli C, Landoni G, et al. Thoracic epidural anesthesia improves early outcome in patients undergoing cardiac surgery for mitral regurgitation: a propensity-matched study. *J Cardiothorac Vasc Anesth.* 2013;27:1301.

33

Myles PS, Bain C. Underutilization of paravertebral block in thoracic surgery. *J Cardiothorac Vasc Anesth.* 2006;20:635.

Ried M, Schilling C, Potzger T, et al. Prospective, comparative study of the On-Q painbuster postoperative pain relief system and thoracic epidural analgesia after thoracic surgery. *J Cardiothorac Vasc Anesth.* 2014;28:973.

Royse C. Epidurals for cardiac surgery; can we substantially reduce surgical morbidity or should we focus on quality of recovery? *Anesthesiology.* 2011;114:232.

Royse C, Royse A, Soeding P, et al. Prospective randomized trial of high thoracic epidural analgesia for coronary artery bypass surgery. *Ann Thorac Surg.* 2003;75:93.

Viscusi ER, Candiotti KA, Onel E, et al. The pharmacokinetics and pharmacodynamics of liposome bupivacaine administered via a single epidural injection to healthy volunteers. *Reg Anesth Pain Med.* 2012;37:616.

White PF, Rawal S, Latham P, et al. Use of a continuous local anesthetic infusion for pain management after median sternotomy. *Anesthesiology.* 2003;99:918.

Zangrillo A, Bignami E, Biondi-Zuccai GGL, et al. Spinal analgesia in cardiac surgery: a meta-analysis of randomized controlled trials. *J Cardiothorac Vasc Anesth.* 2009;23:813.

VI

Index

Page numbers followed by *t* indicate table, by *f* figure,
and by *b* box.

Extracorporeal membrane oxygenation (ECMO)
    (Continued)
  in lung transplantation, 496
  physiology of, 678–679
  standard circuit, 678f
  venoarterial, 679–680
    implementation of, 680b
    initiation of, 679–680, 679b
    weaning from, 680
  venovenous, 681–683
    care of patients on, 682
    complications of, 683, 683b
    initial, 682
    weaning of, 682–683
Extrinsic fibrinolysis, 695
Extrinsic system, in protein coagulation activation,
    688–689
Extubation, postoperative, 752b
  impediments to, 753

F

Factor VIIa, 457, 710–711
Failing Fontan, 396–397
Fast-track cardiac anesthesia (FTCA), 743
  extubation times for, 745f
  initial management of, 745–749, 746b
    bleeding, 747, 747b
    electrolyte, 747–748, 748b
    pain control, 748–749, 749b
    tracheal extubation, admission to, 746–747, 746b
  safety of, 744
  suggested dosages for, 744b
Femoral artery, arterial pressure monitoring and,
    205–206
Fenoldopam, 628
Fenoldopam mesylate, 142t
Fentanyl, 828
  for coronary artery bypass grafting, 335
  dilated cardiomyopathy and, 443
Fetal heart rate, of gravid patient, 656
Fiberoptic bronchoscope, in lung transplantation, 492
Fiberoptic bronchoscope, in lung transplantation, 492
Fibrinogen concentrates, 711
Fibrinogen level, 307
Fibrinolysis, 695–696
  clinical applications of, 696, 696f
  exogenous activators of, 695–696
  extrinsic, 695
  intrinsic, 695
Fibrinopeptides, 689
Fibroelastic deficiency, 451
Fibroma, incidence of, 427t
Flecainide, 97
Flexible bronchoscopy, for pulmonary hemorrhage, 457
Fluoroscopy
  for cerebral blood flow monitoring, 662t
  in hybrid operating room, 535–536
  intraoperative, transcatheter aortic valve replacement
    and, 544
Fontan operation, modern, 395–396, 396f
Fontan physiology, 395–398, 395f
  modern operation in, 395–396, 396f
  preoperative assessment in, 396–397
  ventilatory management of, 397–398, 397b
Foramen ovale, 455–456
Forward stroke volume (FSV), 25–26
Fourier spectra, 282–283
Frequency-domain analysis, 282–285, 283f, 284b, 284t,
    286b
FSV. *see* Forward stroke volume
Funny current inhibitors, 152
Furosemide, 628

G

G-protein-coupled receptors (GPCRs), 99, 99b, 100f
GABA-specific agonist, on sensory- and motor-evoked
    responses, 289t
Gas embolism, in cardiopulmonary bypass, massive
    arterial, 653–654
Gastrointestinal bleeding, 814
Gastrointestinal complications, 634–636
  causative factors in, 634–635
  gastrointestinal tract protection, during cardiac
    surgery, 635–636, 635b
  incidence of, 634
  pathophysiology of, 634–635
  risk factors for, 634
  significance of, 634
Gender, central nervous system injury and, 612
Gene therapy, 105–106
Genes, cognitive dysfunction and, 615b, 615t
Genetic cardiovascular medicine, 102–106, 103b, 104f
Global cerebral hypoperfusion
  cognitive dysfunction and, 615b, 615t
  during CPB, 615–616
Glucocorticoids, for heart-lung transplantation, 502
Glucose
  control of, 794
  management of, during cardiopulmonary bypass, 620
Glycemia, control of, during CPB, 627
Glycoprotein IIB/IIIA receptor inhibitors, platelet
    function and, 695
Gorlin formula, 370
Gott shunt, 414
GPCRs. *see* G-protein-coupled receptors
Graft dysfunction, in lung transplantation, 499
Graft harvest
  for heart transplantation, 475–476
  for lung transplantation, 485–486
Gravid patient, cardiopulmonary bypass for, 655–658
  blood flow of, 657
  blood pressure of, 657–658
  conducting procedure, 656–658
  extracorporeal circulation in, 657t
  maternal and fetal monitor information, 655–656
  premedication and patient positioning, 655
  temperature, 658
Great arteries, transposition of (D-transposition),
    399–400

H

Halothane, 113
Handoffs, 599
HCM. *see* Hypertrophic cardiomyopathy
HDR. *see* Heparin dose-response
Heart, 62
  blood supply to, 63–64
  catheterization
    left-sided, 22, 23b
    right-sided, 22, 23b
  conduction in, 64–65, 64t
  hemodynamic monitoring of, 203–204, 204b
  monitoring of, 203–225
  myocyte of, 65–66
  physiology of, 62–79
  preparation of, in discontinuing cardiopulmonary
    bypass, 718–723, 720t
    afterload in, 723
    contractility in, 721–723, 722t
    heart rate in, 719
    intracardiac air, management of, 718–719
    preload in, 721
    rhythm in, 720–721
  right, evaluation of, 13

849

Platelets
  abnormalities, drug-induced, 693–695
  activation of, 692–693, 699
  count of, 308–309, 309b
  endothelial inhibition of, 82–83, 83b, 84f
  function
    hemostasis and, 692–695, 694t
    monitoring of, 308–309, 309b
    testing of, 309–316, 318b
Pleural effusions, after cardiac surgery, 637
PMC. see Percutaneous mitral commissurotomy
Pneumonia, 808–809
  after cardiac surgery, 637
  hospital-acquired, 751
  ventilator-acquired, 751
Pneumothorax
  electrocardiogram for, 195, 195f
  in lung transplantation, 498
Point-of-care tests, of platelet, 299, 310t, 316
  Platelet Function Analyzer for, 310t, 316, 318b
  VerifyNow for, 310t, 316
Port-access bypass circuit, 659–661, 660f
Port-access cardiac surgery, outcome data of, 661, 662t
Positive end-expiratory pressure (PEEP), increasing
    amounts of, 753
Post-pulmonary thromboendarterectomy hemodynamic
    management, 524–525
Postanesthesia pacemaker evaluation, 57
Postcapillary patterns, in pulmonary hypertension, 505
Posterior descending artery (PDA), 324
Postinfarct septal rupture, 6t
Postoperative analgesia, 822b
  adequate, 822
    potential clinical benefits and, 824
    overall patient satisfaction with, 829f
Postoperative arrhythmias, 763–764, 764t–765t
Postoperative atrial fibrillation (POAF), 791
Postoperative biventricular dysfunction, therapeutic
    interventions for, 763
Postoperative cardiovascular management, 758–785
  advances in, 779–785
  circulation during, 761–762
  oxygen transport and, 759–760, 759f
  temperature during, 760–761, 760f
Postoperative hypothermia, 760–761
Postoperative myocardial dysfunction, 762, 763b
Postoperative myocardial ischemia, 762–763
Postoperative pain management, for cardiac patient,
    821–836
  α_2-adrenergic agonists, 831–832
  intrathecal and epidural techniques, 832–835
  local anesthetic infiltration, 824–826, 825f
  multimodal analgesia, 835
  nerve blocks, 826–827
  NSAIDs, 830–831
  opioids, 827–830
  patient-controlled analgesia, 830
  potential clinical benefits of adequate postoperative
      analgesia, 824
Postoperative thrombosis prophylaxis, in pulmonary
    thromboendarterectomy, 526
Postoperative vasodilation, 768
Potassium, 165
  cardiopulmonary bypass and, 650
  in discontinuing cardiopulmonary bypass,
      717
  disturbance in, electrocardiogram for, 192
Potassium channel blockers, 160t–161t, 162–163
Potts shunt, 389–390, 389f, 390t
Power M-mode Doppler (PMD), 290–292, 291f
Prasugrel (Effient), 693–695

Preanesthetic pulse generator (pacemaker, implantable
    cardioverter-defibrillator) evaluation, 53b
Precapillary patterns, in pulmonary hypertension, 505
Pregnancy
  cardiac surgery during, 463–464
    anesthetic considerations for, 464
  during CPB, 655
Prekallikrein, 687–688
Preload
  assessment of, 764–766
  in cardiac dysfunction, 729t
  as determinant of pump performance, 70–71,
      71f
  in discontinuing cardiopulmonary bypass, 720t, 721
Preload augmentation, right-sided heart failure, 775b
Pressure gradient, 354
Pressure-overload hypertrophy, 357t
Pressure-support ventilation (PSV), 755
Pressure-volume loop
  in aortic regurgitation, 365, 365f
  in aortic stenosis, 355, 355f
  in mitral stenosis, 370, 371f
Primary benign tumors, cardiac, 428–430
  myxoma and, 428–429, 429f
  papillary fibroelastoma and, 430, 430f
Primary cardiomyopathies, 435, 435f
Primary malignant tumors, cardiac, 430–431
Probe passage, technique of, 231–232
Procainamide, 159, 160t–161t
  for supraventricular arrhythmias, 765t
Propafenone, 159–160
Prophylaxis, 55t
Propofol, 124, 622
  cardiovascular effects of, 120t, 124
  for coronary artery bypass grafting, 335
  dilated cardiomyopathy and, 443
  for myocardial contractility, 116
  for sedation, 341
  uses of, 124
Propranolol
  for cardiac arrhythmias, 161–162, 161t
  for ischemia, 136, 137t
Prostacyclin (PGI$_2$), 81
  aerosolized inhaled, in lung transplantation, 491
Prostaglandin E$_1$ (PGE$_1$), for mitral regurgitation,
    377–378
Prostaglandins, 693
Prosthetic valve endocarditis, 807–808
Protamine, 707–708, 707b
  in discontinuing cardiopulmonary bypass, 726
  effects, on coagulation monitoring, of heparin,
      304
  in heart transplantation, 482
Protamine-response test (PRT), 304
Protein C, 690
Protein coagulation activation, of hemostasis, 687–690,
    688f
Protein S, 690
Proteins, of contractile apparatus, 66
Prothrombin complex concentrates (PCCs), 582, 707,
    711
Prothrombin time (PT), 21, 306–307
Prothrombinase complex, 689
Pseudo-MVP, in chronic thromboembolic pulmonary
    hypertension, 531
PT. see Prothrombin time
PTCA. see Percutaneous transluminal coronary
    angioplasty
PTT. see Partial thromboplastin time
Pulmonary allograft, endothelial damage in, lung
    transplantation and, 490–491